D1708231

EIGHTH **edition**

Clinical Chemistry

Principles, Techniques, and Correlatons

EIGHTH edition

Clinical Chemistry
Principles, Techniques, and Correlations

Michael L. Bishop, MS, MLS(ASCP)^CM

Campus Department Chair
Medical Laboratory Science
Keiser University
Orlando, Florida

Edward P. Fody, MD

Clinical Professor
Department of Pathology, Microbiology and Immunology
Vanderbilt University School of Medicine
Nashville, Tennessee
Medical Director
Department of Pathology
Holland Hospital
Holland, Michigan

Larry E. Schoeff, MS, MT(ASCP)

Professor (Retired), Medical Laboratory Science Program
Department of Pathology
University of Utah School of Medicine
Salt Lake City, Utah

 Wolters Kluwer

Philadelphia • Baltimore • New York • London
Buenos Aires • Hong Kong • Sydney • Tokyo

Acquisitions Editor: Jonathan Joyce
Product Development Editor: John Larkin
Marketing Manager: Leah Thomson
Production Project Manager: Kim Cox
Design Coordinator: Joan Wendt
Manufacturing Coordinator: Margie Orzech
Prepress Vendor: SPi Global

Eighth edition

Copyright © 2018 Wolters Kluwer

Copyright © 2013, 2010, 2005, 2000, 1996, 1992, 1985 Wolters Kluwer Health/Lippincott Williams & Wilkins. All rights reserved. This book is protected by copyright. No part of this book may be reproduced or transmitted in any form or by any means, including as photocopies or scanned-in or other electronic copies, or utilized by any information storage and retrieval system without written permission from the copyright owner, except for brief quotations embodied in critical articles and reviews. Materials appearing in this book prepared by individuals as part of their official duties as U.S. government employees are not covered by the above-mentioned copyright. To request permission, please contact Wolters Kluwer at Two Commerce Square, 2001 Market Street, Philadelphia, PA 19103, via email at permissions@lww.com, or via our website at lww.com (products and services).

9 8 7 6 5 4 3

Printed in China

Library of Congress Cataloging-in-Publication Data
Names: Bishop, Michael L., editor. | Fody, Edward P., editor. | Schoeff, Larry E., editor.
Title: Clinical chemistry : principles, techniques, and correlations / [edited by] Michael L. Bishop, Edward P. Fody, Larry E. Schoeff.
Other titles: Clinical chemistry (Bishop)
Description: Eighth edition. | Philadelphia : Wolters Kluwer, [2018] | Includes bibliographical references and index.
Identifiers: LCCN 2016031591 | ISBN 9781496335586
Subjects: | MESH: Clinical Chemistry Tests | Chemistry, Clinical—methods
Classification: LCC RB40 | NLM QY 90 | DDC 616.07/56—dc23 LC record available at https://lccn.loc.gov/2016031591

This work is provided "as is," and the publisher disclaims any and all warranties, express or implied, including any warranties as to accuracy, comprehensiveness, or currency of the content of this work.

This work is no substitute for individual patient assessment based upon healthcare professionals' examination of each patient and consideration of, among other things, age, weight, gender, current or prior medical conditions, medication history, laboratory data and other factors unique to the patient. The publisher does not provide medical advice or guidance and this work is merely a reference tool. Healthcare professionals, and not the publisher, are solely responsible for the use of this work including all medical judgments and for any resulting diagnosis and treatments.

Given continuous, rapid advances in medical science and health information, independent professional verification of medical diagnoses, indications, appropriate pharmaceutical selections and dosages, and treatment options should be made and healthcare professionals should consult a variety of sources. When prescribing medication, healthcare professionals are advised to consult the product information sheet (the manufacturer's package insert) accompanying each drug to verify, among other things, conditions of use, warnings and side effects and identify any changes in dosage schedule or contraindications, particularly if the medication to be administered is new, infrequently used or has a narrow therapeutic range. To the maximum extent permitted under applicable law, no responsibility is assumed by the publisher for any injury and/or damage to persons or property, as a matter of products liability, negligence law or otherwise, or from any reference to or use by any person of this work.

LWW.com

In memory of my mother, Betty Beck Bishop, for her constant support, guidance, and encouragement.

MLB

To Nancy, my wife, for continuing support and dedication.

EPF

To my wife, Anita, for continuing support.

LES

Dev Abraham, MD
Professor of Medicine
Division of Endocrinology
University of Utah
Salt Lake City, Utah

Josephine Abraham, MD, MPH
Professor of Medicine
Division of Nephrology
University of Utah
Salt Lake City, Utah

Michael J. Bennett, PhD, FRCPath, FACB, DABCC
Professor of Pathology and Laboratory Medicine
University of Pennsylvania
Director, Metabolic Disease Laboratory
Children's Hospital of Philadelphia
Abramson Pediatric Research Center
Philadelphia, Pennsylvania

Takara L. Blamires, M.S., MLS(ASCP)^{CM}
Medical Laboratory Science Program
Department of Pathology
University of Utah School of Medicine
Salt Lake City, Utah

Maria G. Boosalis, PhD, MPH, RD, LD
Professor, College of Health and Wellness
Northwestern Health Sciences University
Bloomington, Minnesota

Raffick A. R. Bowen, PhD, MHA, MT(CSMLS), DClChem, FCACB, DABCC, FACB
Clinical Associate Professor of Pathology
Associate Director of Clinical Chemistry and Immunology
    Laboratory
Department of Pathology
Stanford Health Care
Stanford, California

Janelle M. Chiasera, PhD
Department Chair, Clinical and Diagnostic Sciences
University of Alabama – Birmingham
Birmingham, Alabama

Heather Corn, MD
Internal Medicine – Clinical Instructor
Endocrinology and Diabetes Center
University of Utah
Salt Lake City, Utah

Heather Crookston, PhD
Point of Care Coordinator
Nemours Children's Hospital
Orlando, Florida

Julia C. Drees, PhD, DABCC
Clinical Research and Development Scientist
Kaiser Permanente Regional Laboratory
Berkeley, California

Kathryn Dugan, MEd, MT(ASCP)
Instructor Medical and Clinical Laboratory Sciences
Auburn University at Montgomery
Montgomery, Alabama

Michael Durando, MD, PhD
Research Track Resident, Internal Medicine and
    Hematology/Oncology
Emory University
Atlanta, Georgia

Edward P. Fody, MD
Clinical Professor
Department of Pathology, Microbiology and
    Immunology
Vanderbilt University School of Medicine
Nashville, Tennessee
Medical Director
Department of Pathology
Holland Hospital
Holland, Michigan

Elizabeth L. Frank, PhD
Associate Professor, Department of Pathology
University of Utah School of Medicine
Medical Director, Analytic Biochemistry and Calculi
ARUP Laboratories, Inc.
Salt Lake City, Utah

Vicki S. Freeman, PhD, MLS(ASCP)^{CM} SC, FACB
Department Chair and Associate Professor, Clinical
    Laboratory Sciences
University of Texas Medical Branch
Galveston, Texas

Linda S. Gorman, PhD
Retired Associate Professor
Medical Laboratory Science
University of Kentucky
Lexington, Kentucky

Ryan W. Greer, MS, I&C(ASCP)
Assistant Vice President, Group Manager Chemistry
    Group III, Technical Operations
ARUP Laboratories, Inc.
Salt Lake City, Utah

Marissa Grotzke, MD
Assistant Professor
Endocrinology and Metabolism
Internal Medicine
University of Utah
Salt Lake City, Utah

Mahima Gulati, MD
Endocrinologist
Middlesex Hospital
Danbury, Connecticut

Carrie J. Haglock-Adler, MSFS, C(ASCP)
Research Scientist
ARUP Institute for Clinical and Experimental
    Pathology
Salt Lake City, Utah

Matthew P. A. Henderson, PhD, FCACB
Clinical Biochemist and Laboratory Director for the
    Children's Hospital of Eastern Ontario
Ottawa Hospital
Assistant Professor
Department of Pathology and Laboratory Medicine at the
    University of Ottawa
University of Ottawa
Ottawa, Ontario, Canada

Ronald R. Henriquez, PhD, NRCC
Fellow, Clinical Chemistry
University of North Carolina at Chapel Hill, Pathology and
    Laboratory Medicine
University of North Carolina
Chapel Hill, North Carolina
Clinical Chemist, Department of Pathology
Walter Reed National Military Medical Center, United
    States Army
Bethesda, Maryland

Laura M. Hickes, PhD
Chemistry and Applications Support Manager
Roche Diagnostics
Greensboro, North Carolina

Brian C. Jensen, MD
Assistant Professor of Medicine and Pharmacology
UNC Division of Cardiology
UNC McAllister Heart Institute
University of North Carolina
Chapel Hill, North Carolina

Kamisha L. Johnson-Davis, PhD, DABCC (CC, TC), FACB
Assistant Professor (Clinical)
Department of Pathology
University of Utah
Medical Director, Clinical Toxicology
ARUP Laboratories
Salt Lake City, Utah

Robert E. Jones, MD
Professor of Medicine
Endocrinology and Diabetes Center
Division of Endocrinology
University of Utah
Salt Lake City, Utah

Yachana Kataria, Phd
Clinical Chemistry Fellow
Department of Laboratory Medicine
Boston Children's Hospital
Research Fellow
Harvard Medical School
Boston, Massachusetts

Mark D. Kellogg, PhD, MT(ASCP), DABCC, FACB
Director of Quality Programs
Associate Director of Chemistry
Department of Laboratory Medicine
Boston Children's Hospital
Assistant Professor of Pathology
Harvard Medical School
Boston, Massachusetts

Cindi Bullock Letsos, MT(ASCP)
Lean Six Sigma Black Belt Consultant
Retired from University of North Carolina Health Care
Chapel Hill, North Carolina

Kara L. Lynch, PhD
Associate Division Chief, Chemistry and Toxicology
    Laboratory
San Francisco General Hospital
San Francisco, California

J. Marvin McBride, MD, MBA
Assistant Clinical Professor
Division of Geriatric Medicine
UNC School of Medicine
Chapel Hill, North Carolina

Christoper R. McCudden, PhD
Clinical Biochemist, Pathology and Laboratory Medicine
The Ottawa Hospital
Assistant Professor
Department of Pathology and Laboratory Medicine at the
    University of Ottawa
University of Ottawa
Ottawa, Ontario, Canada

Shashi Mehta, PhD
Associate Professor
Department of Clinical Laboratory Sciences
School of Health Related Professions
University of Medicine and Dentistry of New Jersey
Newark, New Jersey

James March Mistler, MS, MLS
Lecturer
Department of Medical Laboratory Science
University of Massachusetts Dartmouth
North Dartmouth, Massachusetts

Matthew S. Petrie, PhD
Clinical Chemistry Fellow, Department of Laboratory
    Medicine
University of California San Francisco
San Francisco, California

Tracey G. Polsky, MD, PhD
Assistant Professor of Clinical Pathology and Laboratory
    Medicine
University of Pennsylvania Perelman School of
    Medicine
Assistant Director of the Clinical Chemistry
    Laboratory
Children's Hospital of Philadelphia
Philadelphia, Pennsylvania

Deepika S. Reddy, MD
Assistant Professor (Clinical)
Internal Medicine
Endocrinology and Diabetes Center
University of Utah
Salt Lake City, Utah

Alan T. Remaley, MD, PhD
Senior Staff, Department of Laboratory Medicine
National Institutes of Health
Bethesda, Maryland

Kyle B. Riding, PhD, MLS(ASCP)
Instructor, Medical Laboratory Science
Teaching and Learning Center Coordinator
Keiser University – Orlando Campus
Orlando, Florida

Michael W. Rogers, MT(ASCP), MBA
Clinical Laboratory Quality Management Consultant
Retired from University of North Carolina Health Care
Chapel Hill, North Carolina

Amar A. Sethi, PhD
Chief Scientific Officer, Research and Development
Pacific Biomarkers
Seattle, Washington

Joely A. Straseski, PhD
Assistant Professor, Pathology
University of Utah
Salt Lake City, Utah

Frederick G. Strathmann, PhD, DABCC (CC, TC)
Assistant Professor
Department of Pathology
University of Utah
Medical Director of Toxicology
ARUP Laboratories
Salt Lake City, Utah

Vishnu Sundaresh, MD, CCD
Assistant Professor (Clinical)
Internal Medicine
Endocrinology and Diabetes Center
University of Utah
Salt Lake City, Utah

Sara A. Taylor, PhD, MLS(ASCP), MB
Associate Professor and Graduate Advisor
Department of Medical Laboratory Science
Tarleton State University
Fort Worth, Texas

Tolmie E. Wachter, MBA/HCM, SLS(ASCP)
Assistant Vice President
Director of Corporate Safety/RSO
ARUP Laboratories
Salt Lake City, Utah

G. Russell Warnick, MS, MBA
Chief Scientific Officer
Health Diagnostic Laboratory
Richmond, Virginia

Elizabeth Warning, MS, MLS(ASCP)CM
Adjunct Faculty
MLS Program
University of Cincinnati
Cincinnati, Ohio

Monte S. Willis, MD, PhD, FCAP, FASCP, FAHA
Associate Professor, Vice Chair of Academic Affairs
    Department of Pathology & Laboratory Medicine,
    Director, Campus Health Services Laboratory
University of North Carolina at Chapel Hill, Pathology &
    Laboratory Medicine
Director, Sweat Chloride Testing
Assistant Director Clinical Core (Chemistry)
    Laboratory Services
University of North Carolina Healthcare
University of North Carolina
Chapel Hill, North Carolina

Alan H. B. Wu, PhD, DABCC
Director, Clinical Chemistry Laboratory, San Francisco
  General Hospital
Professor, Laboratory Medicine, University of California,
  San Francisco
San Francisco, California

Xin Xu, MD, PhD, MLS(ASCP)
Division of Pulmonary, Allergy, and Critical Care
  Medicine
Department of Medicine
University of Alabama at Birmingham
Birmingham, AL

For many years, the health care and medical laboratory communities have been preparing for an impending workforce shortage that could threaten to compromise patient care and safety. It is vital that the medical laboratory community continue to educate and prepare credentialed professionals who can work efficiently, have essential analytical and critical thinking skills, and can communicate test results and test needs to health care providers. While the shortage of qualified laboratory practitioners has been in the forefront of our collective thoughts, a more insidious shortage has also arisen among the ranks of faculty within medical laboratory education programs.

As a profession, we have long been blessed with dedicated faculty who strive to impart their knowledge and experience onto countless students. We know, however, that many of these dedicated faculty members have and will continue to step aside to pursue other passions through retirement. As new dedicated faculty step up to take over, we must support these new educators in their roles as program directors and content specialists. Furthermore, we must provide tools for these educators about techniques and theories that are appropriate as they continue to develop their curricula.

One potential tool to assist educators is the American Society for Clinical Laboratory Science (ASCLS) Entry Level Curriculum. At the 2016 ASCLS Annual Meeting, the House of Delegates adopted a newly formatted version of the entry level curriculum for MLT and MLS programs. This document had not been updated since 2002, and a subcommittee of the ASCLS Education Scientific Assembly was charged with editing the document to better represent the field's expectations of new graduates. Subcommittee members solicited feedback from educators and professionals in all subdisciplines and reviewed the content for currency. New material was added to reflect techniques and theories that have emerged since the last edition while material was removed if it was no longer deemed relevant. After this extensive process, the final document is reflective of what the industry demands of a new professional.

Similarly, the material presented throughout *Clinical Chemistry: Principles, Techniques, and Correlations* has always kept current with changes in the laboratory industry. This exceptional ability of authors and editors to keep pace with the needs of an ever-changing profession has not diminished through its, now, eight editions. The content inherent to the discipline of clinical chemistry is foundational to all other areas of laboratory medicine. The eighth edition of this textbook is ideal for students learning the principles of clinical chemistry while helping them build connections to other areas of the laboratory. The chapters have a perfect blend of basic theory and practical information that allows the student to comprehend each area of clinical chemistry. The text is well organized to help MLT and MLS educators distinguish what each unique student population needs to be successful in the marketplace. The online materials, powerpoints, and exam questions, for educators, are an invaluable resource for those creating a new course or revising a current course.

As we face this transition of laboratory practitioners who perform testing and faculty who train and educate our students, products that stay current with the times and help facilitate better understanding of the unique levels of practice within our field are the most essential element to success. The eighth edition of *Clinical Chemistry: Principles, Techniques, and Correlations* accomplishes this and serves as an invaluable tool for any new educator looking for guidance, or seasoned educator looking to refresh their teachings.

As educators we are thrilled that students continue to find the field of medical laboratory science an avenue to build a professional career. We wish all students and educators who use this book the best to carry on a tradition of excellence!

Joan Polancic, MSEd, MLS(ASCP)^CM
Director, School of Medical Laboratory Science
Denver Health Medical Center
Denver, Colorado

Kyle B. Riding, PhD, MLS(ASCP)
Instructor, Medical Laboratory Science
Teaching and Learning Center Coordinator
Keiser University – Orlando Campus
Orlando, Florida

You should not be surprised to learn that the delivery of health care has been undergoing major transformation for several decades. The clinical laboratory has been transformed in innumerable ways as well. At one time, the laboratory students' greatest asset was motor ability. That is not the case any longer. Now the need is for a laboratory professional who is well educated, an analytical thinker, and problem solver, and one who can add value to the information generated in the laboratory regarding a specific patient.

This change impacts the laboratory professional in a very positive manner. Today the students' greatest asset is their mental skill and their ability to acquire and apply knowledge. The laboratory professional is now considered a knowledge worker, and a student's ability to successfully become this knowledge worker depends on their instruction and exposure to quality education. Herein lies the need for the seventh edition of *Clinical Chemistry: Principles, Techniques, and Correlations*. It contributes to the indispensable solid science foundation in medical laboratory sciences and the application of its principles in improving patient outcomes needed by the laboratory professional of today. This edition provides not only a comprehensive understanding of clinical chemistry but also the foundation upon which all the other major laboratory science disciplines can be further understood and integrated. It does so by providing a strong discussion of organ function and a solid emphasis on pathophysiology, clinical correlations, and differential diagnosis. This information offers a springboard to better understand the many concepts related to the effectiveness of a particular test for a particular patient.

Reduction of health care costs, while ensuring quality patient care, remains the goal of health care reform efforts. Laboratory information is a critical element of such care. It is estimated that $65 billion is spent each year to perform more than 4.3 billion laboratory tests. This impressive figure has also focused a bright light on laboratory medicine, and appropriate laboratory test utilization is now under major scrutiny. The main emphasis is on reducing costly overutilization and unnecessary diagnostic testing; however, the issue of under- and misutilization of laboratory tests must be a cause for concern as well. The role of laboratorians in providing guidance to clinicians regarding appropriate test utilization is becoming not only accepted but also welcomed as clinicians try to maneuver their way through an increasingly complex and expensive test menu. These new roles lie in the pre- and postanalytic functions of laboratorians. The authors of this text have successfully described the importance of these phases as well as the more traditional analytic phase. It does not matter how precise or accurate a test is during the analytic phase if the sample has been compromised or if an inappropriate test has been ordered on the patient. In addition, the validation of results with respect to a patient's condition is an important step in the postanalytic phase. Participation with other health care providers in the proper interpretation of test results and appropriate follow-up will be important abilities of future graduates as the profession moves into providing greater consultative services for a patient-centered medical delivery system. Understanding these principles is a necessary requirement of the knowledge worker in the clinical laboratory. This significant professional role provides effective laboratory services that will improve medical decision making and thus patient safety while reducing medical errors. This edition of *Clinical Chemistry: Principles, Techniques, and Correlations* is a crucial element in graduating such professionals.

Diana Mass, MA, MT(ASCP)
Clinical Professor and Director (Retired)
Clinical Laboratory Sciences Program
Arizona State University
Tempe, Arizona
President
Associated Laboratory Consultants
Valley Center, California

Make no mistake: There are few specialties in medicine that have a wider impact on today's health care than laboratory medicine. For example, in the emergency room, a troponin result can not only tell an ER physician if a patient with chest pain has had a heart attack but also assess the likelihood of that patient suffering an acute myocardial infarction in 30 days. In the operating room during a parathyroidectomy, a parathyroid hormone assay can tell a surgeon that it is appropriate to close the procedure because he has successfully removed all of the affected glands or go back and look for more glands to excise. In labor and delivery, testing for pulmonary surfactants from amniotic fluid can tell an obstetrician if a child can be safely delivered or if the infant is likely to develop life-threatening respiratory distress syndrome. In the neonatal intensive care unit, measurement of bilirubin in a premature infant is used to determine when the ultraviolet lights can be turned off. These are just a handful of the thousands of medical decisions that are made each day based on results from clinical laboratory testing.

Despite our current success, there is still much more to learn and do. For example, there are no good laboratory tests for the diagnosis of stroke or traumatic brain injury.

The work on Alzheimer's and Parkinson's disease prediction and treatment is in the early stages. And when it comes to cancer, while our laboratory tests are good for monitoring therapy, they fail in the detection of early cancer, essential for improving treatment and prolonging survival. Finally, personalized medicine including pharmacogenomics will play an increasingly important role in the future. Pharmacogenomic testing will be used to select the right drug at the best dose for a particular patient in order to maximize efficacy and minimize side effects.

If you are reading this book, you are probably studying to be a part of the field. As a clinical chemist for over 30 years, I welcome you to our profession.

Alan H. B. Wu, PhD, DABCC
Director, Clinical Chemistry Laboratory, San Francisco
General Hospital
Professor, Laboratory Medicine, University of California,
San Francisco
San Francisco, California

Clinical chemistry continues to be one of the most rapidly advancing areas of laboratory medicine. Since the initial idea for this textbook was discussed in a meeting of the Biochemistry/Urinalysis section of ASMT (now ASCLS) in the late 1970s, the only constant has been changed. New technologies and analytical techniques have been introduced, with a dramatic impact on the practice of clinical chemistry and laboratory medicine. In addition, the health care system is rapidly changing. There is ever increasing emphasis on improving the quality of patient care, individual patient outcomes, financial responsibility, and total quality management. Now, more than ever, clinical laboratorians need to be concerned with disease correlations, interpretations, problem solving, quality assurance, and cost-effectiveness; they need to know not only the *how* of tests but more importantly the *what, why, and when*. The editors of *Clinical Chemistry: Principles, Techniques, and Correlations* have designed the eighth edition to be an even more valuable resource to both students and practitioners.

Now almost 40 years since the initiation of this effort, the editors have had the privilege of completing the eighth edition with another diverse team of dedicated clinical laboratory professionals. In this era of focusing on metrics, the editors would like to share the following information. The 330 contributors in the 8 editions represent 70 clinical laboratory science programs, 83 clinical laboratories, 13 medical device companies, 4 government agencies, and 3 professional societies. One hundred and thirty contributors were clinical laboratory scientists with advanced degrees. With today's global focus, the previous editions of the text have been translated into at least six languages. By definition, a profession is a calling requiring specialized knowledge and intensive academic preparation to define its scope of work and produce its own literature. The profession of Clinical Laboratory Science has evolved significantly over the past four decades.

The eighth edition of *Clinical Chemistry: Principles, Techniques, and Correlations* is comprehensive, up-to-date, and easy to understand for students at all levels. It is also intended to be a practically organized resource for both instructors and practitioners. The editors have tried to maintain the book's readability and further improve its content. Because clinical laboratorians use their interpretive and analytic skills in the daily practice of clinical chemistry, an effort has been made to maintain an appropriate balance between analytic principles, techniques, and the correlation of results with disease states.

In this edition, the editors have maintained features in response to requests from our readers, students, instructors, and practitioners. Ancillary materials have been updated and expanded. Chapters now include current, more frequently encountered case studies and practice questions or exercises. To provide a thorough, up-to-date study of clinical chemistry, all chapters have been updated and reviewed by professionals who practice clinical chemistry and laboratory medicine on a daily basis. The basic principles of the analytic procedures discussed in the chapters reflect the most recent or commonly performed techniques in the clinical chemistry laboratory. Detailed procedures have been omitted because of the variety of equipment and commercial kits used in today's clinical laboratories. Instrument manuals and kit package inserts are the most reliable reference for detailed instructions on current analytic procedures. All chapter material has been updated, improved, and rearranged for better continuity and readability. thePoint*, a Web site with additional case studies, review questions, teaching resources, teaching tips, additional references, and teaching aids for instructors and students, is available from the publisher to assist in the use of this textbook.

Michael L. Bishop
Edward P. Fody
Larry E. Schoeff

acknowledgments

A project as large as this requires the assistance and support of many clinical laboratorians. The editors wish to express their appreciation to the contributors of all the editions of *Clinical Chemistry: Principles, Techniques, and Correlations*—the dedicated laboratory professionals and educators whom the editors have had the privilege of knowing and exchanging ideas with over the years. These individuals were selected because of their expertise in particular areas and their commitment to the education of clinical laboratorians. Many have spent their professional careers in the clinical laboratory, at the bench, teaching students, or consulting with clinicians. In these frontline positions, they have developed a perspective of what is important for the next generation of clinical laboratorians.

We extend appreciation to our students, colleagues, teachers, and mentors in the profession who have helped shape our ideas about clinical chemistry practice and education. Also, we want to thank the many companies and professional organizations that provided product information and photographs or granted permission to reproduce diagrams and tables from their publications. Many Clinical and Laboratory Standards Institute (CLSI) documents have also been important sources of information. These documents are directly referenced in the appropriate chapters.

The editors would like to acknowledge the contribution and effort of all individuals to previous editions. Their efforts provided the framework for many of the current chapters. Finally, we gratefully acknowledge the cooperation and assistance of the staff at Wolters Kluwer for their advice and support.

The editors are continually striving to improve future editions of this book. We again request and welcome our readers' comments, criticisms, and ideas for improvement.

contents

PART one

Basic Principles and Practice of Clinical Chemistry

Basic Principles and Practices

KATHRYN DUGAN and ELIZABETH WARNING

chapter outline

key terms

Analyte
Anhydrous
Arterial blood
Beer's law
Buffer
Centrifugation
Cerebrospinal fluid (CSF)
Colligative property
Conductivity
Deionized water
Deliquescent substance
Delta absorbance
Density
Desiccant
Desiccator
Dilution
Dilution factor
Distilled water
Equivalent weight
Erlenmeyer flasks
Filtration
Graduated cylinder
Griffin Beaker
Hemolysis
Henderson-Hasselbalch equation
Hydrate
Hygroscopic
Icterus
International unit
Ionic strength
Lipemia
Molality
Molarity
Normality
One-point calibration
Osmotic pressure
Oxidized
Oxidizing agent
Percent solution
pH
Pipette
Primary standard

chapter objectives

Upon completion of this chapter, the clinical laboratorian should be able to do the following:

- Convert results from one unit format to another using the SI and traditional systems.
- Describe the classifications used for reagent grade water.
- Identify the varying chemical grades used in reagent preparation and indicate their correct use.
- Define primary standard and standard reference materials.
- Describe the following terms that are associated with solutions and, when appropriate, provide the respective units: percent, molarity, normality, molality, saturation, colligative properties, redox potential, and conductivity.
- Define a buffer and give the formula for pH and pK calculations.
- Use the Henderson-Hasselbalch equation to determine the missing variable when given either the pK and pH or the pK and concentration of the weak acid and its conjugate base.
- List and describe the types of thermometers used in the clinical laboratory.

(continues on page 4)

For additional student resources, please visit thePoint® at http://thepoint.lww.com

chapter objectives (continued)

- Classify the type of pipette when given an actual pipette or its description.
- Demonstrate the proper use of a measuring and volumetric pipette.
- Describe two ways to calibrate a pipetting device.
- Define a desiccant and discuss how it is used in the clinical laboratory.
- Describe how to properly care for and balance a centrifuge.
- Correctly perform the laboratory mathematical calculations provided in this chapter.
- Identify and describe the types of samples used in clinical chemistry.
- Outline the general steps for processing blood samples.
- Apply Beer's law to determine the concentration of a sample when the absorbance or change in absorbance is provided.
- Identify the preanalytic variables that can adversely affect laboratory results as presented in this chapter.

key terms (continued)

Ratio
Reagent grade water
Redox potential
Reduced
Reducing agent
Reverse osmosis
Serial dilution
Serum
Significant figures
Solute
Solution
Solvent
Specific gravity
Standard
Standard reference materials (SRMs)
Système International d'Unités (SI)
Thermistor
Ultrafiltration
Valence
Whole blood

The primary purpose of a clinical chemistry laboratory is to perform analytic procedures that yield accurate and precise information, aiding in patient diagnosis and treatment. The achievement of reliable results requires that the clinical laboratory scientist be able to correctly use basic supplies and equipment and possess an understanding of fundamental concepts critical to any analytic procedure. The topics in this chapter include units of measure, basic laboratory supplies, and introductory laboratory mathematics, plus a brief discussion of specimen collection, processing, and reporting.

UNITS OF MEASURE

Any meaningful *quantitative* laboratory result consists of two components: the first component represents the number related to the actual test value and the second is a label identifying the units. The unit defines the physical quantity or dimension, such as mass, length, time, or volume.[1] Not all laboratory tests have well-defined units, but whenever possible, the units used should be reported.

Although several systems of units have traditionally been utilized by various scientific divisions, the **Système International d'Unités (SI)**, adopted internationally in 1960, is preferred in scientific literature and clinical laboratories and is the only system employed in many countries. This system was devised to provide the global scientific community with a uniform method of describing physical quantities. The SI system units (referred to as *SI units*) are based on the metric system. Several subclassifications exist within the SI system, one of which is the *basic unit*. There are seven basic units (Table 1.1), with length (meter), mass (kilogram), and quantity of a substance (mole) being the units most frequently encountered. Another set of

SI-recognized units is termed *derived units*. A derived unit, as the name implies, is a derivative or a mathematical function describing one of the basic units. An example of an SI-derived unit is meters per second (m/s), used to express velocity. Some non-SI units are so widely used that they have become acceptable for use within the SI system (Table 1.1). These include long-standing units such as hour, minute, day, gram, liter, and plane angles expressed as degrees. The SI uses **standard** *prefixes* that, when added to a given basic unit, can indicate decimal fractions or multiples of that unit (Table 1.2). For example, 0.001 liter can be expressed using the prefix *milli*, or 10^{-3}, and since it requires moving the decimal point three places to the right, it can then be written as 1 milliliter, or abbreviated as 1 mL. It may also be written in scientific notation as 1×10^{-3} L. Likewise, 1,000 liters would use the prefix of kilo (10^3) and could be written as 1 kiloliter or expressed in scientific notation as 1×10^3 L.

It is important to understand the relationship these prefixes have to the basic unit. The highlighted upper portion of Table 1.2 indicates prefixes that are smaller than the basic unit and are frequently used in clinical laboratories. When converting between prefixes, simply note the relationship between the two prefixes based on whether you are changing to a smaller or larger prefix. For example, if converting from one liter (1.0×10^0 or 1.0) to milliliters (1.0×10^{-3} or 0.001), the starting unit (L) is larger than the desired unit by a factor of 1,000 or 10^3. This means that the decimal place would be moved to the *right* three places, so 1.0 liter (L) equals 1,000 milliliters (mL). When changing 1,000 milliliters (mL) to 1.0 liter (L), the process is reversed and the decimal point would be moved three places to the left to become 1.0 L. Note that the SI term for mass is *kilogram*; it is the only basic unit that contains a prefix as part of its name. Generally, the standard prefixes for mass use the term *gram* rather than *kilogram*.

TABLE 1.1 SI Units

Base Quantity	Name	Symbol
Length	Meter	m
Mass	Kilogram	kg
Time	Second	s
Electric current	Ampere	A
Thermodynamic temperature	Kelvin	K
Amount of substance	Mole	mol
Luminous intensity	Candela	cd
Selected Derived		
Frequency	Hertz	Hz
Force	Newton	N
Celsius temperature	Degree Celsius	°C
Catalytic activity	Katal	kat
Selected Accepted Non-Si		
Minute (time)	(60 s)	min
Hour	(3,600 s)	h
Day	(86,400 s)	d
Liter (volume)	($1\ dm^3 = 10^{-3}\ m^3$)	L
Angstrom	($0.1\ nm = 10^{-10}\ m$)	Å

TABLE 1.2 Prefixes Used with SI Units

Factor	Prefix	Symbol	Select Decimals
10^{-18}	atto	a	—
10^{-15}	femto	f	—
10^{-12}	pico	p	—
10^{-9}	nano	n	—
10^{-6}	micro	μ	0.000001
10^{-3}	milli	m	0.001
10^{-2}	centi	c	0.01
10^{-1}	deci	d	0.1
10^{0}	Liter, meter, gram	Basic unit	1.0
10^{1}	deka	da	10.0
10^{2}	hecto	h	100.0
10^{3}	kilo	k	1,000.0
10^{4}	mega	M	—
10^{9}	giga	G	—
10^{12}	tera	T	—
10^{15}	peta	P	—
10^{18}	exa	E	—

Prefixes are used to indicate a subunit or multiple of a basic SI unit.

Example 1: Convert 1.0 L to μL

$1.0\ L\ (1 \times 10^0) = ?\ \mu L$ (micro = 10^{-6}); move the decimal place six places to the right and it becomes 1,000,000 μL; reverse the process to determine the expression in L (move the decimal six places to the left of 1,000,000 μL to get 1.0 L).

SI CONVERSIONS

To convert between SI units, move the decimal by the difference between the exponents represented by the prefix either to the right (from a larger to a smaller unit) or to the left (from a smaller to a larger one) of the number given:

decimal point
←000 #.000→
smaller to larger unit larger to smaller unit
Convert to larger unit: smaller to larger unit—move to the left
Convert to a smaller unit: larger to smaller—move to the right
= the numeric value given

Example 2: Convert 5 mL to μL

5 mL (milli = 10^{-3}, larger) = ? μL (micro = 10^{-6}, smaller); move the decimal by three places to the right and it becomes 5,000 μL.

Example 3: Convert 5.3 mL to dL

5.3 mL (milli = 10^{-3}, smaller) = ? dL (deci = 10^{-1}, larger); move the decimal place by two places to the left and it becomes 0.053 dL.

Reporting of laboratory results is often expressed in terms of substance concentration (e.g., moles) or the mass of a substance (e.g., mg/dL, g/dL, g/L, mmol/L, and IU) rather than in SI units. These familiar and traditional units can cause confusion during interpretation. Appendix D (on thePoint), *Conversion of Traditional Units to SI Units for Common Clinical Chemistry Analytes*, lists both reference and SI units together with the conversion factor from traditional to SI units for common analytes. As with other areas of industry, the laboratory and the rest of medicine are moving toward adopting universal standards promoted by the International Organization for Standardization, often referred to as ISO. This group develops standards of practice, definitions, and guidelines that can be adopted by everyone in a given field, providing for more uniform terminology and less confusion. Many national initiatives have recommended common units for laboratory test results, but none have been widely adopted.[2] As with any transition, clinical laboratory scientists should be familiar with all the terms currently used in their field.

REAGENTS

In today's highly automated laboratory, there seems to be little need for reagent preparation by the clinical laboratory scientist. Most instrument manufacturers make the reagents in a ready-to-use form or "kit" where all necessary reagents and respective storage containers are prepackaged as a unit requiring only the addition of water or buffer to the prepackaged components for reconstitution. A heightened awareness of the hazards of certain chemicals and the numerous regulatory agency requirements has caused clinical chemistry laboratories to readily eliminate massive stocks of chemicals and opt instead for the ease of using prepared reagents. Periodically, especially in hospital laboratories involved in research and development, biotechnology applications, specialized analyses, or method validation, the laboratorian may still face preparing various reagents or solutions.

Chemicals

Analytic chemicals exist in varying grades of purity: analytic reagent (AR); ultrapure, chemically pure (CP); United States Pharmacopeia (USP); National Formulary (NF); and technical or commercial grade.[3] A committee of the American Chemical Society (ACS) established specifications for AR grade chemicals, and chemical manufacturers will either meet or exceed these requirements. Labels on reagents state the actual impurities for each chemical lot or list the maximum allowable impurities. The labels should be clearly printed with the percentage of impurities present and either the initials *AR* or *ACS* or the term *For laboratory use* or *ACS Standard-Grade Reference Materials*. Chemicals of this category are suitable for use in most analytic laboratory procedures. Ultrapure chemicals have been put through additional purification steps for use in specific procedures such as chromatography, atomic absorption, immunoassays, molecular diagnostics, standardization, or other techniques that require extremely pure chemicals. These reagents may carry designations of HPLC (high-performance liquid chromatography) or chromatographic on their labels.

Because USP and NF grade chemicals are used to manufacture drugs, the limitations established for this group of chemicals are based only on the criterion of not being injurious to individuals. Chemicals in this group may be pure enough for use in most chemical procedures; however, it should be recognized that the purity standards are not based on the needs of the laboratory and, therefore, may or may not meet all assay requirements.

Reagent designations of CP or pure grade indicate that the impurity limitations are not stated and that preparation of these chemicals is not uniform. It is not recommended that clinical laboratories use these chemicals for reagent preparation unless further purification or a reagent blank is included. Technical or commercial grade reagents are used primarily in manufacturing and should never be used in the clinical laboratory.

Organic reagents also have varying grades of purity that differ from those used to classify inorganic reagents. These grades include a practical grade with some impurities; CP, which approaches the purity level of reagent grade chemicals; spectroscopic (spectrally pure) and chromatographic grade organic reagents, with purity levels attained by their respective procedures; and reagent grade (ACS), which is certified to contain impurities below certain levels established by the ACS. As in any analytic method, the desired organic reagent purity is dictated by the particular application.

Other than the purity aspects of the chemicals, laws related to the Occupational Safety and Health Administration (OSHA)[4] require manufacturers to indicate any physical or biologic health hazards and precautions needed for the safe use, storage, and disposal of any chemical. A manufacturer is required to provide technical data sheets for each chemical manufactured on a document called a Safety Data Sheet (SDS).

Reference Materials

Unlike other areas of chemistry, clinical chemistry is involved in the analysis of biochemical by-products found in *biological* fluids, such as serum, plasma, or urine, making purification and a known *exact* composition of the material almost impossible. For this reason, traditionally defined standards used in analytical chemistry do not readily apply in clinical chemistry.

A **primary standard** is a highly purified chemical that can be measured directly to produce a substance of *exact* known concentration and purity. The ACS has purity tolerances for primary standards, because most biologic constituents are unavailable within these tolerance limitations; the National Institute of Standards and Technology (NIST)-certified **standard reference materials (SRMs)** are used instead of ACS primary standard materials.[5–7]

The NIST developed certified reference materials/SRMs for use in clinical chemistry laboratories. They are assigned a value after careful analysis, using state-of-the-art methods and equipment. The chemical composition of these substances is then certified; however, they may not possess the purity equivalent of a primary standard. Because each substance has been characterized for certain chemical or physical properties, it can be used in place of an ACS primary standard in clinical work and is often used to verify calibration or accuracy/bias assessments. Many manufacturers use an NIST SRM when producing calibrator and standard materials, and in this way, these materials are considered "traceable to NIST" and may meet certain accreditation requirements. There are SRMs for a number of routine analytes, hormones, drugs, and blood gases, with others being added.[5]

Water Specifications[8]

Water is the most frequently used reagent in the laboratory. Because tap water is unsuitable for laboratory applications, most procedures, including reagent and standard preparation, use water that has been substantially purified. There are various methods for water purification including distillation, ion exchange, reverse osmosis, ultrafiltration, ultraviolet light, sterilization, and ozone treatment. Laboratory requirements generally call for **reagent grade water** that, according to the Clinical and Laboratory Standards Institute (CLSI), is classified into one of six categories based on the specifications needed for its use rather than the method of purification or preparation.[9,10] These categories include clinical laboratory reagent water (CLRW), special reagent water (SRW), instrument feed water, water supplied by method manufacturer, autoclave and wash water, and commercially bottled purified water. Laboratories need to assess whether the water meets the specifications needed for its application.

Most water-monitoring parameters include at least microbiological count, pH, resistivity (measure of resistance in ohms and influenced by the number of ions present), silicate, particulate matter, and organics. Each category has a specific acceptable limit. A long-held convention for categorizing water purity was based on three types, I through III, with type I water having the most stringent requirements and generally suitable for routine laboratory use.

Prefiltration can remove particulate matter from municipal water supplies before any additional treatments. Filtration cartridges are composed of glass; cotton; activated charcoal, which removes organic materials and chlorine; and submicron filters ($\leq$0.2 mm), which remove any substances larger than the filter's pores, including bacteria. The use of these filters depends on the quality of the municipal water and the other purification methods used. For example, hard water (containing calcium, iron, and other dissolved elements) may require prefiltration with a glass or cotton filter rather than activated charcoal or submicron filters, which quickly become clogged and are expensive to use. The submicron filter may be better suited after distillation, deionization, or reverse osmosis treatment.

Distilled water has been purified to remove almost all organic materials, using a technique of distillation much like that found in organic chemistry laboratory distillation experiments in which water is boiled and vaporized. Many impurities do not rise in the water vapor and will remain in the boiling apparatus so that the water collected after condensation has less contamination. Water may be distilled more than once, with each distillation cycle removing additional impurities. **Ultrafiltration** and nanofiltration, like distillation, are excellent in removing particulate matter, microorganisms, and any pyrogens or endotoxins.

Deionized water has some or all ions removed, although organic material may still be present, so it is neither pure nor sterile. Generally, deionized water is purified from previously treated water, such as prefiltered or distilled water. Deionized water is produced using either an anion or a cation exchange resin, followed by replacement of the removed ions with hydroxyl or hydrogen ions. The ions that are anticipated to be removed from the water will dictate the type of ion exchange resin to be used. One column cannot service all ions present in water. A combination of several resins will produce different grades of deionized water. A two-bed system uses an anion resin followed by a cation resin. The different resins may be in separate columns or in the same column. This process is excellent in removing dissolved ionized solids and dissolved gases.

Reverse osmosis is a process that uses pressure to force water through a semipermeable membrane, producing water that reflects a filtered product of the original water. It does not remove dissolved gases. Reverse osmosis may be used for the pretreatment of water.

Ultraviolet oxidation, which removes some trace organic material or sterilization processes at specific wavelengths, when used in combination with ozone treatment, can destroy bacteria but may leave behind residual products.

These techniques are often used after other purification processes have been completed.

Production of reagent grade water largely depends on the condition of the feed water. Generally, reagent grade water can be obtained by initially filtering it to remove particulate matter, followed by reverse osmosis, deionization, and a 0.2-mm filter or more restrictive filtration process. Type III/autoclave wash water is acceptable for glassware washing but not for analysis or reagent preparation. Traditionally, type II water was acceptable for most analytic requirements, including reagent, quality control, and standard preparation, while type I water was used for test methods requiring minimum interference, such as trace metal, iron, and enzyme analyses. Use with HPLC may require less than a 0.2-mm final **filtration** step and falls into the SRW category. Some molecular diagnostic or mass spectrophotometric techniques may require special reagent grade water; some reagent grade water should be used immediately, so storage is discouraged because the resistivity changes. Depending on the application, CLRW should be stored in a manner that reduces any chemical or bacterial contamination and for short periods.

Testing procedures to determine the quality of reagent grade water include measurements of resistance, pH, colony counts on selective and nonselective media for the detection of bacterial contamination, chlorine, ammonia, nitrate or nitrite, iron, hardness, phosphate, sodium, silica, carbon dioxide, chemical oxygen demand, and metal detection. Some accreditation agencies[11] recommend that laboratories document culture growth, pH, and specific resistance on water used in reagent preparation. Resistance is measured because pure water, devoid of ions, is a poor conductor of electricity and has increased resistance. The relationship of water purity to resistance is linear. Generally, as purity increases, so does resistance. This one measurement does not suffice for determination of true water purity because a nonionic contaminant may be present that has little effect on resistance. Note that reagent water meeting specifications from other organizations, such as the ASTM, may not be equivalent to those established by the CLSI, and care should be taken to meet the assay procedural requirements for water type requirements.

Solution Properties

In clinical chemistry, substances found in biologic fluids including serum, plasma, urine, and spinal fluid are quantified. A substance that is dissolved in a liquid is called a **solute**; in laboratory science, these biologic solutes are also known as *analytes*. The liquid in which the solute is dissolved—in this instance, a biologic fluid—is the **solvent**. Together they represent a **solution**. Any chemical or biologic solution is described by its basic properties, including concentration, saturation, colligative properties, redox potential, conductivity, density, pH, and ionic strength.

Concentration

Analyte concentration in solution can be expressed in many ways. Routinely, concentration is expressed as percent solution, molarity, molality, or normality, Note that these are non-SI units, and the SI expression for the amount of a substance is the mole.

Percent solution is expressed as the amount of solute per 100 total units of solution. Three expressions of percent solutions are weight per weight (w/w), volume per volume (v/v), and weight per volume (w/v). Weight per weight (% w/w) refers to the number of grams of solute per 100 g of solution. Volume per volume (% v/v) is used for liquid solutes and gives the milliliters of solute in 100 mL of solution. For v/v solutions, it is recommended that grams per deciliter (g/dL) be used instead of % v/v. Weight per volume (% w/v) is the most commonly used percent solution in the clinical laboratory and is defined as the number of grams of solute in 100 mL of solution. This is not the same as molarity and care must be taken to not confuse the two.

Molarity (M) is expressed as the number of moles per 1 L of solution. One mole of a substance equals its gram molecular weight (gmw), so the customary units of molarity (M) are moles/liter. The SI representation for the traditional molar concentration is moles of solute per volume of solution, with the volume of the solution given in liters. The SI expression for concentration should be represented as moles per liter (mol/L), millimoles per liter (mmol/L), micromoles per liter (μmol/L), and nanomoles per liter (nmol/L). The familiar concentration term *molarity* has not been adopted by the SI as an expression of concentration. It should also be noted that molarity depends on volume, and any significant physical changes that influence volume, such as changes in temperature and pressure, will also influence molarity.

Molality (m) represents the amount of solute per 1 kg of solvent. Molality is sometimes confused with molarity; however, it can be easily distinguished from molarity because molality is always expressed in terms of moles per kilogram (weight per weight) and describes moles per 1,000 g (1 kg) of solvent. Note that the common abbreviation (m) for molality is a lowercase "m," while the uppercase (M) refers to molarity. The preferred expression for molality is moles per kilogram (mol/kg) to avoid any confusion. Unlike molarity, molality is not influenced by temperature or pressure because it is based on mass rather than volume.

Normality is the least likely of the four concentration expressions to be encountered in clinical laboratories, but it is often used in chemical titrations and chemical reagent classification. It is defined as the number of gram equivalent weights per 1 L of solution. An **equivalent weight** is equal to the gmw of a substance divided by its valence. The **valence** is the number of units that can combine with or replace 1 mole of hydrogen ions for acids and hydroxyl ions for bases and the number of electrons exchanged in oxidation–reduction reactions. Normality is always equal to or greater than the molarity of the compound. Normality was previously used for reporting electrolyte values, such as sodium [Na^+], potassium [K^+], and chloride [Cl^-], expressed as milliequivalents per liter (mEq/L); however, this convention has been replaced with the more familiar units of millimoles per liter (mmol/L).

Solution saturation gives little specific information about the concentration of solutes in a solution. A solution is considered saturated when no more solvent can be dissolved in the solution. Temperature, as well as the presence of other ions, can influence the solubility constant for a solute in a given solution and thus affect the saturation. Routine terms in the clinical laboratory that describe the extent of saturation are *dilute, concentrated, saturated,* and *supersaturated*. A *dilute solution* is one in which there is relatively little solute or one that has a lower solute concentration per volume of solvent than the original, such as when making a dilution. In contrast, a *concentrated solution* has a large quantity of solute in solution. A solution in which there is an excess of undissolved solute particles can be referred to as a *saturated solution*. As the name implies, a *supersaturated solution* has an even greater concentration of undissolved solute particles than a saturated solution of the same substance. Because of the greater concentration of solute particles, a supersaturated solution is thermodynamically unstable. The addition of a crystal of solute or mechanical agitation disturbs the supersaturated solution, resulting in crystallization of any excess material out of solution. An example is seen when measuring serum osmolality by freezing point depression.

Colligative Properties

Colligative properties are those properties related to the number of solute particles per solvent molecules, not on the type of particles present. The behavior of particles or solutes in solution demonstrates four repeatable properties, osmotic pressure, vapor pressure, freezing point, and boiling point, these are called **colligative properties**. *Vapor pressure* is the pressure exerted by the vapor when the liquid solvent is in equilibrium with the vapor. *Freezing point* is the temperature at which the first crystal (solid) of solvent forms in equilibrium with the solution. *Boiling point* is the temperature at which the vapor pressure of the solvent reaches atmospheric pressure (usually one atmosphere).

Osmotic pressure is the pressure that opposes osmosis when a solvent flows through a semipermeable membrane to establish equilibrium between compartments of differing concentration. The osmotic pressure of a dilute solution is directly proportional to the concentration of the molecules in solution. The expression for concentration is the osmole. One osmole of a substance equals the molarity or molality multiplied by the number of particles, not the kind of particle, at dissociation. If molarity is used, the resulting expression would be termed osmolarity; if molality is used, the expression changes to osmolality. Osmolality is preferred since it depends on the weight rather than volume and is not readily influenced by temperature and pressure changes. When a solute is dissolved in a solvent, the colligative properties change in a predictable manner for each osmole of substance present. In the clinical setting, freezing point and vapor pressure depression can be measured as a function of osmolality. Freezing point is preferred since vapor pressure measurements can give inaccurate readings when some substances, such as alcohols, are present in the samples.

Redox Potential

Redox potential, or *oxidation–reduction potential*, is a measure of the ability of a solution to accept or donate electrons. Substances that donate electrons are called **reducing agents**; those that accept electrons are considered **oxidizing agents**. The pneumonic—LEO (lose electrons **oxidized**) the lion says GER (gain electrons **reduced**)—may prove useful when trying to recall the relationship between reducing/oxidizing agents and redox potential.

Conductivity

Conductivity is a measure of how well electricity passes through a solution. A solution's conductivity quality depends principally on the number of respective charges of the ions present. *Resistivity*, the reciprocal of conductivity, is a measure of a substance's resistance to the passage of electrical current. The primary application of resistivity in the clinical laboratory is for assessing the purity of water. Resistivity or resistance is expressed as ohms and conductivity is expressed as ohms^{-1}.

pH and Buffers

Buffers are weak acids or bases and their related salts that, as a result of their dissociation characteristics, minimize changes in the hydrogen ion concentration. Hydrogen ion concentration is often expressed as pH. A lowercase *p* in front of certain letters or abbreviations operationally means the "negative logarithm of" or "inverse log of" that substance. In keeping with this convention, the term **pH** represents the negative or inverse log of the hydrogen ion concentration. Mathematically, pH is expressed as

$$pH = \log\left(\frac{1}{[H^+]}\right)$$
$$pH = -\log[H^+] \qquad \text{(Eq. 1-1)}$$

where [H$^+$] equals the concentration of hydrogen ions in moles per liter (M).

The pH scale ranges from 0 to 14 and is a convenient way to express hydrogen ion concentration.

Unlike a strong acid or base, which dissociates almost completely, the dissociation constant for a weak acid or base solution (like a buffer) tends to be very small, meaning little dissociation occurs.

The dissociation of acetic acid (CH$_3$COOH), a weak acid, can be illustrated as follows:

$$[HA] \leftrightarrow [A^-] + [H^+]$$
$$[CH_3COOH] \leftrightarrow [CH_3COO^-] + [H^+] \qquad \text{(Eq. 1-2)}$$

HA = weak acid, A$^-$ = conjugate base, H$^+$ = hydrogen ions, [] = concentration of anything in the bracket.
Sometimes, the conjugate base (A$^-$) will be referred to as a "salt" since, physiologically, it will be associated with some type of cation such as sodium (Na$^+$).

Note that the dissociation constant, K_a, for a weak acid may be calculated using the following equation:

$$K_a = \frac{[A^-][H^+]}{[HA]} \qquad \text{(Eq. 1-3)}$$

Rearrangement of this equation reveals

$$[H^+] = K_a \times \frac{[HA]}{[A^+]} \qquad \text{(Eq. 1-4)}$$

Taking the log of each quantity and then multiplying by minus 1 (−1), the equation can be rewritten as

$$-\log[H^+] = -\log K_a \times -\log\frac{[HA]}{[A^-]} \qquad \text{(Eq. 1-5)}$$

By convention, lowercase *p* means "negative log of"; therefore, −log[H$^+$] may be written as pH, and −K_a may be written as pK_a. The equation now becomes

$$pH = pK_a - \log\frac{[HA]}{[A^-]} \qquad \text{(Eq. 1-6)}$$

Eliminating the minus sign in front of the log of the quantity $\frac{[HA]}{[A^-]}$ results in an equation known as the **Henderson-Hasselbalch equation**, which mathematically describes the dissociation characteristics of weak acids (pK_a) and bases (pK_b) and the effect on pH:

$$pH = pK_a + \log\frac{[A^-]}{[HA]} \qquad \text{(Eq. 1-7)}$$

When the **ratio** of [A$^-$] to [HA] is 1, the pH equals the pK and the buffer has its greatest buffering capacity. The dissociation constant K_a, and therefore the pK_a, remains the same for a given substance. Any changes in pH are solely due to the ratio of conjugate base [A$^-$] concentration to weak acid [HA] concentration.

Ionic strength is another important aspect of buffers, particularly in separation techniques. **Ionic strength** is the concentration or activity of ions in a solution or buffer. Increasing ionic strength increases the ionic cloud surrounding a compound and decreases the rate of particle migration. It can also promote compound dissociation into ions effectively increasing the solubility of some salts, along with changes in current, which can also affect electrophoretic separation.

CLINICAL LABORATORY SUPPLIES

In today's clinical chemistry laboratory, many different types of equipment are in use. Most of the manual techniques have been replaced by automation, but it is still necessary for the laboratory scientist to be knowledgeable in the operation and use of certain equipment. The following

TABLE 1.3	Common Temperature Conversions
Celsius (Centigrade) to Fahrenheit	°C (9/5) + 32 (multiply Celsius temperature by 9; divide the answer by 5, then add 32)
Fahrenheit to Celsius (Centigrade)	(°F − 32)5/9 (subtract 32 and divide the answer by 9; then multiply that answer by 5)

is a brief discussion of the composition and general use of common equipment found in a clinical chemistry laboratory, including thermometers, pipettes, flasks, beakers, and dessicators.

Thermometers/Temperature

The predominant practice for temperature measurement uses the Celsius (°C) scale; however, Fahrenheit (°F) and Kelvin (°K) scales are also used.[12] The SI designation for temperature is the Kelvin scale. Table 1.3 gives the conversion formulas between Fahrenheit and Celsius scales and Appendix C (thePoint) lists the various conversion formulas.

All analytic reactions occur at an optimal temperature. Some laboratory procedures, such as enzyme determinations, require precise temperature control, whereas others work well over a wide range of temperatures. Reactions that are temperature dependent use some type of heating/cooling cell, heating/cooling block, or water/ice bath to provide the correct temperature environment. Laboratory refrigerator temperatures are often critical and need periodic verification. Thermometers either are an integral part of an instrument or need to be placed in the device for temperature maintenance. The two types of thermometers discussed include liquid-in-glass and electronic thermometer or **thermistor** probe; however, several other types of temperature-indicating devices are in use. Regardless of which is being used, all temperature-reading devices must be calibrated to ascertain accuracy. Liquid-in-glass thermometers use a colored liquid (red or other colored material), encased in plastic or glass material. They usually measure temperatures between 20°C and 400°C. Visual inspection of the liquid-in-glass thermometer should reveal a continuous line of liquid, free from separation or bubbles. The accuracy range for a thermometer used in clinical laboratories is determined by the specific application.

Liquid-in-glass thermometers should be calibrated against an NIST-certified or NIST-traceable thermometer for critical laboratory applications.[13] NIST has an SRM thermometer with various calibration points (0°C, 25°C, 30°C, and 37°C) for use with liquid-in-glass thermometers. Gallium, another SRM, has a known melting point and can also be used for thermometer verification.

As automation advances and miniaturizes, the need for an accurate, fast-reading electronic thermometer (thermistor) has increased and is now routinely incorporated in many devices. The advantages of a thermistor over the more traditional liquid-in-glass thermometers are size and millisecond response time. Similar to the liquid-in-glass thermometers, the thermistor can be calibrated against an SRM thermometer.

Glassware and Plasticware

Until recently, laboratory supplies (e.g., pipettes, flasks, beakers, and burettes) consisted of some type of glass and could be correctly termed *glassware*. As plastic material was refined and made available to manufacturers, plastic has been increasingly used to make laboratory equipment. Before discussing general laboratory supplies, a brief summary of the types and uses of glass and plastic commonly seen today in laboratories is given (see Appendices G, H, and I on thePoint). Regardless of design, most laboratory supplies must satisfy certain tolerances of accuracy and fall into two classes of precision tolerance, either Class A or Class B as given by the American Society for Testing and Materials (ASTM).[14,15] Those that satisfy Class A ASTM precision criteria are stamped with the letter "A" on the glassware and are preferred for laboratory applications. Class B glassware generally have twice the tolerance limits of Class A, even if they appear identical, and are often found in student laboratories where durability is needed. Vessels holding or transferring liquid are designed either to contain (TC) or to deliver (TD) a specified volume. As the names imply, the major difference is that TC devices do not deliver that same volume when the liquid is transferred into a container, whereas the TD designation means that the labware will deliver that amount.

Glassware used in the clinical laboratory usually fall into one of the following categories: Kimax/Pyrex (borosilicate), Corex (aluminosilicate), high silica, Vycor (acid and alkali resistant), low actinic (amber colored), or flint (soda lime) glass used for disposable material.[16] Whenever possible, routinely used clinical chemistry glassware should consist of high thermal borosilicate or aluminosilicate glass and meet the Class A tolerances recommended by the NIST/ASTM/ISO 9000. The manufacturer is the best source of information about specific uses, limitations, and accuracy specifications for glassware.

Plasticware is beginning to replace glassware in the laboratory setting. The unique high resistance to corrosion and breakage, as well as varying flexibility, has made plasticware appealing. Relatively inexpensive, it allows most items to be completely disposable after each use. The major types of resins frequently used in the clinical chemistry laboratory are polystyrene, polyethylene, polypropylene, Tygon, Teflon, polycarbonate, and polyvinyl chloride. Again, the individual manufacturer is the best source of information concerning the proper use and limitations of any plastic material.

In most laboratories, glass or plastic that is in direct contact with biohazardous material is usually disposable. If not, it must be decontaminated according to appropriate protocols. Should the need arise, however, cleaning of glass or plastic may require special techniques. Immediately rinsing glass or plastic supplies after use, followed by washing with a powder or liquid detergent designed for cleaning laboratory supplies and several distilled water rinses, may be sufficient. Presoaking glassware in soapy water is highly recommended whenever immediate cleaning is impractical. Many laboratories use automatic dishwashers and dryers for cleaning. Detergents and temperature levels should be compatible with the material and the manufacturer's recommendations. To ensure that all detergent has been removed from the labware, multiple rinses with appropriate grade water is recommended. Check the pH of the final rinse water and compare it with the initial pH of the pre-rinse water. Detergent-contaminated water will have a more alkaline pH as compared with the pH of the appropriate grade water. Visual inspection should reveal spotless vessel walls. Any biologically contaminated labware should be disposed of according to the precautions followed by that laboratory.

Some determinations, such as those used in assessing heavy metals or assays associated with molecular testing, require scrupulously clean or disposable glassware. Some applications may require plastic rather than glass because glass can absorb metal ions. Successful cleaning solutions are acid dichromate and nitric acid. It is suggested that disposable glass and plastic be used whenever possible.

Dirty reusable pipettes should be placed immediately in a container of soapy water with the pipette tips up. The container should be long enough to allow the pipette tips to be covered with solution. A specially designed pipette-soaking jar and washing/drying apparatus are recommended. For each final water rinse, fresh reagent grade water should be provided. If possible, designate a pipette container for final rinses only. Cleaning brushes are available to fit almost any size glassware and are recommended for any articles that are washed routinely.

Although plastic material is often easier to clean because of its nonwettable surface, it may not be appropriate for some applications involving organic solvents or autoclaving. Brushes or harsh abrasive cleaners should not be used on plasticware. Acid rinses or washes are not required. The initial cleaning procedure described in Appendix J (thePoint) can be adapted for plasticware as well. Ultrasonic cleaners can help remove debris coating the surfaces of glass or plasticware. Properly cleaned laboratory ware should be completely dried before using.

Laboratory Vessels

Flasks, beakers, and graduated cylinders are used to hold solutions. Volumetric and Erlenmeyer flasks are two types of containers in general use in the clinical laboratory.

A *volumetric flask* is calibrated to hold one exact volume of liquid (TC). The flask has a round, lower portion with a flat bottom and a long, thin neck with an etched calibration line. Volumetric flasks are used to bring a given reagent to its final volume with the prescribed diluent. When bringing

the bottom of the meniscus to the calibration mark, a pipette should be used when adding the final drops of diluent to ensure maximum control is maintained and the calibration line is not missed.

Erlenmeyer flasks and **Griffin beakers** are designed to hold different volumes rather than one exact amount. Because Erlenmeyer flasks and Griffin beakers are often used in reagent preparation, flask size, chemical inertness, and thermal stability should be considered. The Erlenmeyer flask has a wide bottom that gradually evolves into a smaller, short neck. The Griffin beaker has a flat bottom, straight sides, and an opening as wide as the flat base, with a small spout in the lip.

Graduated cylinders are long, cylindrical tubes usually held upright by an octagonal or circular base. The cylinder has calibration marks along its length and is used to measure volumes of liquids. Graduated cylinders do not have the accuracy of volumetric labware. The sizes routinely used are 10, 25, 50, 100, 500, 1,000, and 2,000 mL.

All laboratory utensils used in critical measurement should be Class A whenever possible to maximize accuracy and precision and thus decrease calibration time (Fig. 1.1 illustrates representative laboratory glassware).

Pipettes

Pipettes are glass or plastic equipment used to transfer liquids; they may be reusable or disposable. Although pipettes may transfer any volume, they are usually used for volumes of 20 mL or less; larger volumes are usually transferred or dispensed using automated pipetting devices. Table 1.4 outlines the classification applied here.

Similar to other laboratory equipment, pipettes are designed to contain (TC) or to deliver (TD) a particular volume of liquid. The major difference is the amount of liquid needed to wet the interior surface of the pipette and the amount of any residual liquid left in the pipette tip. Most manufacturers stamp *TC* or *TD* near the top of the pipette to alert the user as to the type of pipette. Like other TC-designated labware, a TC pipette holds or contains a particular volume but does not dispense that exact volume, whereas a TD

FIGURE 1.1 Laboratory glassware.

TABLE 1.4   Pipette Classification

I. Design
   A. To contain (TC)
   B. To deliver (TD)
II. Drainage characteristics
   A. Blowout
   B. Self-draining
III. Type
   A. Measuring or graduated
      1. Serologic
      2. Mohr
      3. Bacteriologic
      4. Ball, Kolmer, or Kahn
      5. Micropipette
   B. Transfer
      1. Volumetric
      2. Ostwald-Folin
      3. Pasteur pipettes
      4. Automatic macropipettes or micropipettes

FIGURE 1.3 Pipetting technique. **(A)** Meniscus is brought above the desired graduation line. **(B)** Liquid is allowed to drain until the bottom of the meniscus touches the desired calibration mark.

a slight suction is applied to the opposite end until the liquid enters the pipette and the meniscus is brought above the desired graduation line (Fig. 1.3A), and suction is then stopped. While the meniscus level is held in place, the pipette tip is raised slightly out of the solution and wiped with a laboratory tissue of any adhering liquid. The liquid is allowed to drain until the bottom of the meniscus touches the desired calibration mark (Fig. 1.3B). With the pipette held in a vertical position and the tip against the side of the receiving vessel, the pipette contents are allowed to drain into the vessel (e.g., test tube, cuvette, or flask). A *blowout pipette* has a continuous etched ring or two small, close, continuous rings located near the top of the pipette. This means that the last drop of liquid should be expelled into the receiving vessel. Without these markings, a pipette is *self-draining*, and the user allows the contents of the pipette to drain by gravity. The tip of the pipette should not be in contact with the accumulating fluid in the receiving vessel during drainage. With the exception of the Mohr pipette, the tip should remain in contact with the side of the vessel for several seconds after the liquid has drained. The pipette is then removed (Fig. 1.2).

Measuring or graduated pipettes are capable of dispensing several different volumes. Measuring pipettes are used to transfer reagents and to make dilutions and can be used to repeatedly transfer a particular solution. Because the graduation lines located on the pipette may vary, they should be indicated on the top of each pipette. For example, a 5-mL pipette can be used to measure 5, 4, 3, 2, or 1 mL of liquid, with further graduations between each milliliter. The pipette is designated as 5 in 1/10 increments

pipette will dispense the volume indicated. When using either pipette, the tip must be immersed in the intended transfer liquid to a level that will allow the tip to remain in solution after the volume of liquid has entered the pipette—without touching the vessel walls. The pipette is held upright, not at an angle (Fig. 1.2). Using a pipette bulb or similar device,

Serologic/Mohr

Correct

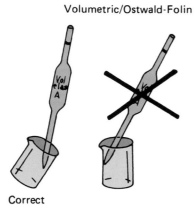

Volumetric/Ostwald-Folin

Correct

FIGURE 1.2 Correct and incorrect pipette positions.

FIGURE 1.4 Disposable transfer pipettes.

FIGURE 1.5 Volume indication of a pipette.

(Fig. 1.5) and could deliver any volume in tenths of a milliliter, up to 5 mL. Another pipette, such as a 1-mL pipette, may be designed to dispense 1 mL and have subdivisions of hundredths of a milliliter. The markings at the top of a measuring or graduated pipette indicate the volume(s) it is designed to dispense. The subgroups of measuring or graduated pipettes are Mohr, serologic, and micropipettes. A *Mohr pipette* does not have graduations to the tip. It is a self-draining pipette, but the tip should not be allowed to touch the vessel while the pipette is draining. A *serologic pipette* has graduation marks to the tip and is generally a blowout pipette. A *micropipette* is a pipette with a total holding volume of less than 1 mL; it may be designed as either a Mohr or a serologic pipette.

The next major category is the *transfer pipettes*. These pipettes are designed to dispense one volume without further subdivisions. Ostwald-Folin pipettes are used with biologic fluids having a viscosity greater than that of water. They are blowout pipettes, indicated by two etched continuous rings at the top. The volumetric pipette is designed to dispense or transfer aqueous solutions and is always self-draining. *The bulb-like enlargement in the pipette stem easily identifies the volumetric pipette.* This type of pipette usually has the greatest degree of accuracy and precision and should be used when diluting standards, calibrators, or quality control material. They should only be used once prior to cleaning. *Disposable transfer pipettes may or may* not have calibration marks and are used to transfer solutions or biologic fluids without consideration of a specific volume. These pipettes should not be used in any quantitative analytic techniques (Fig. 1.4).

The *automatic pipette* is the most routinely used pipette in today's clinical chemistry laboratory. Automatic pipettes come in a variety of types including fixed volume, variable volume, and multichannel. The term *automatic*, as used here, implies that the mechanism that draws up and dispenses the liquid is an integral part of the pipette. It may be a fully automated/self-operating, semiautomatic, or completely manually operated device. Automatic and semiautomatic pipettes have many advantages, including safety, stability, ease of use, increased precision, the ability to save time, and less cleaning required as a result of the contaminated portions of the pipette (e.g., the tips) often being disposable. Figure 1.6 illustrates many common

FIGURE 1.6 **(A)** Adjustable volume pipette. **(B)** Fixed volume pipette with disposable tips. **(C)** Multichannel pipette. **(D)** Multichannel pipette in use.

automatic pipettes. A pipette associated with only one volume is termed a *fixed* volume, and models able to select different volumes are termed *variable*; however, only one volume may be used at a time. The available range of volumes is 1 μL to 5,000 mL. The widest volume range usually seen in a single pipette is 0.5 μL to 1,000 μL. A pipette with a pipetting capability of less than 1 mL is considered a *micropipette*, and a pipette that dispenses greater than 1 mL is called an *automatic macropipette*. Multichannel pipettes are able to attach multiple pipette tips to a single handle and can then be used to dispense a fixed volume of fluid to multiple wells, such as in delivery to a multiwell microtiter plate. In addition to classification by volume delivery amounts, automatic pipettes can also be categorized according to their mechanism: air-displacement, positive-displacement, and dispenser pipettes. An *air-displacement pipette* relies on a piston for creating suction to draw the sample into a disposable tip that must be changed after each use. The piston does not come in contact with the liquid. A *positive-displacement pipette* operates by moving the piston in the pipette tip or barrel, much like a hypodermic syringe. It does not require a different tip for each use. Because of carryover concerns, rinsing and blotting between samples may be required. *Dispensers* and *dilutor/dispensers* are automatic pipettes that obtain the liquid from a common reservoir and dispense it repeatedly. The dispensing pipettes may be bottle-top, motorized, handheld, or attached to a dilutor. The dilutor often combines sampling and dispensing functions. Many automated pipettes use a wash between samples to eliminate carryover problems. However, to minimize carryover contamination with manual or semiautomatic pipettes, careful wiping of the tip may remove any liquid that adhered to the outside of the tip before dispensing any liquid. Care should be taken to ensure that the orifice of the pipette tip is not blotted, drawing sample from the tip. Another precaution in using manually operated semiautomatic pipettes is to move the plunger in a continuous and steady manner. These pipettes should be used according to the individual manufacturer's directions.

Disposable one-use pipette tips are designed for use with air-displacement pipettes. The laboratory scientist should ensure that the pipette tip is seated snugly onto the end of the pipette and free from any deformity. Plastic tips used on air-displacement pipettes can vary. Different brands can be used for one particular pipette but they do not necessarily perform in an identical manner. Tips for positive-displacement pipettes are made of straight columns of glass or plastic. These tips must fit snugly to avoid carryover and can be used repeatedly without being changed after each use. As previously mentioned, these devices may need to be rinsed and dried between samples to minimize carryover.

Class A pipettes, like all other Class A labware, do not need to be recalibrated by the laboratory. Automatic pipetting devices, as well as non–Class A materials, do need recalibration.[17,18] Calibration of pipettes is done to verify accuracy and precision of the device and may be required by the laboratory's accrediting agency. A gravimetric method (see Box 1-1) can accomplish this task by delivering and weighing a solution of known specific gravity, such as water. A currently calibrated analytic balance and at least Class 2 weights should be used. A pipette should be used only if it is within ±1.0% of the expected value following calibration.

Although gravimetric validation is the most desirable method, pipette calibration may also be accomplished by using photometric methods, particularly for automatic pipetting devices. When a spectrophotometer is used, the molar absorptivity of a compound, such as potassium dichromate, is obtained. After an aliquot of diluent is pipetted, the change in concentration will reflect the volume of the pipette. Another photometric technique used to assess pipette accuracy compares the absorbances of dilutions of potassium dichromate, or another colored liquid with appropriate absorbance spectra, using Class A volumetric labware versus equivalent dilutions made with the pipetting device.

These calibration techniques are time consuming and, therefore, impractical for use in daily checks. It is recommended that pipettes be checked initially and subsequently three or four times per year, or as dictated by the laboratory's accrediting agency. Many companies offer calibration services; the one chosen should also satisfy any accreditation requirements. A quick, daily check for many larger volume automatic pipetting devices involves the use of volumetric flasks. For example, a bottle-top dispenser that routinely delivers 2.5 mL of reagent may be checked by dispensing four aliquots of the reagent into a 10-mL Class A volumetric flask. The bottom of the meniscus should meet with the calibration line on the volumetric flask.

Syringes

Syringes are sometimes used for transfer of small volumes (< 500 μL) in blood gas analysis or in separation techniques such as chromatography or electrophoresis (Fig. 1.7). The syringes are glass and have fine barrels. The plunger is often made of a fine piece of wire. Tips are not used when syringes are used for injection of sample into a gas chromatographic or high-pressure liquid chromatographic system. In electrophoresis work, however, disposable Teflon tips may be used.

Desiccators and Desiccants

Many compounds combine with water molecules to form loose chemical crystals. The compound and the associated water are called a **hydrate**. When the water of crystallization is removed from the compound, it is said to be **anhydrous**. Substances that take up water on exposure to atmospheric conditions are called **hygroscopic**. Materials that are very hygroscopic can remove moisture from the air as well as from other materials. These materials make excellent drying substances and are sometimes used as **desiccants** (drying agents) to keep other chemicals from becoming hydrated. If these compounds absorb enough

BOX 1-1 Gravimetric Pipette Calibration

Materials

Pipette
10 to 20 pipette tips, if needed
Balance capable of accuracy and resolution to ±0.1% of
    dispensed volumetric weight
Weighing vessel large enough to hold volume of liquid
Type I/CLRW
Thermometer and barometer

Procedure

1. Record the weight of the vessel. Record the temperature of the water. It is recommended that all materials be at room temperature. Obtain the barometric pressure.
2. Place a small volume (0.5 mL) of the water into the container. To prevent effects from evaporation, it is desirable to loosely cover each container with a substance such as Parafilm. Avoid handling of the containers.
3. Weigh each container plus water to the nearest 0.1 mg *or* set the balance to zero.
4. Using the pipette to be tested, draw up the specified amount. Carefully wipe the outside of the tip. Care should be taken not to touch the end of the tip; this will cause liquid to be wicked out of the tip, introducing an inaccuracy as a result of technique.
5. Dispense the water into the weighed vessel. Touch the tip to the side.
6. Record the weight of the vessel.
7. Subtract the weight obtained in step 3 from that obtained in step 6. Record the result.
8. If plastic tips are used, change the tip between each dispensing. Repeat steps 1 to 6 for a minimum of nine additional times.

9. Obtain the average or mean of the weight of the water. Multiply the mean weight by the corresponding density of water at the given temperature and pressure. At 20°C, the density of water is 0.9982.
10. Determine the accuracy or the ability of the pipette to dispense the expected (selected or stated) volume according to the following formula:

$$\frac{\textbf{Mean volume}}{\textbf{Expected volume}} \times \textbf{100\%} \qquad \textbf{(Eq. 1-8)}$$

The manufacturer usually gives acceptable limitations for a particular pipette, but they should not be used if the value differs by more than 1.0% from the expected value.

Precision can be indicated as the percent coefficient of variation (%CV) or standard deviation (SD) for a series of repetitive pipetting steps. A discussion of %CV and SD can be found in Chapter 3. The equations to calculate the SD and %CV are as follows:

$$SD = \sqrt{\frac{\Sigma\,(x-x)^2}{n-1}} \qquad \textbf{(Eq. 1-9)}$$

$$\%CV = \frac{SD}{x} \times 100$$

Required imprecision is usually ±1 SD. The %CV will vary with the expected volume of the pipette, but the smaller the %CV value, the greater the precision. When *n* is large, the data are more statistically valid.[19,23]

---

water from the atmosphere to cause dissolution, they are known as **deliquescent substances.** Closed and sealed containers that contain desiccant material are referred to as desiccators and may be used to store more hygroscopic substances. Many sealed packets or shipping containers, often those that require refrigeration, include some type of small packet of desiccant material to prolong storage.

Balances

A properly operating balance is essential in producing high-quality reagents and standards. However, because many laboratories discontinued in-house reagent preparation, balances may no longer be as widely used. Balances are classified according to their design, number of pans (single or double), and whether they are mechanical or electronic or classified by operating ranges.

Analytic and electronic balances are currently the most popular in the clinical laboratory. Analytic balances (Fig. 1.8) are required for the preparation of any primary standard. It has a single pan enclosed by sliding transparent doors, which minimize environmental influences on pan movement, a tared weighing vessel, on the sample pan. An optical scale allows the operator to visualize the mass of the substance. The weight range for certain analytic balances is from 0.01 mg to 160 g.

FIGURE 1.7 Microliter glass syringe.

FIGURE 1.8 Analytic balance.

Electronic balances (Fig. 1.9) are single-pan balances that use an electromagnetic force to counterbalance the weighed sample's mass. Their measurements equal the accuracy and precision of any available mechanical balance, with the advantage of a fast response time (< 10 seconds).

Test weights used for calibrating balances should be selected from the appropriate ANSI/ASTM Classes 1 through 4.[20] The frequency of calibration is dictated by the accreditation/licensing guidelines for a specific laboratory. Balances should be kept scrupulously clean and be located

FIGURE 1.9 Electronic top-loading balance.

in an area away from heavy traffic, large pieces of electrical equipment, and open windows. The level checkpoint should always be corrected before weighing occurs.

CENTRIFUGATION

Centrifugation is a process in which centrifugal force is used to separate solid matter from a liquid suspension. It is used to prepare samples, blood and body fluids, in clinical chemistry for analysis and also to concentrate urine sediment in urinalysis for microscopic viewing. When samples are not properly centrifuged, small fibrin clots and cells can cause erroneous results during analysis. The centrifuge separates the mixture based on mass and density of the component parts. It consists of a head or rotor, carriers, or shields that are attached to the vertical shaft of a motor or air compressor and enclosed in a metal covering. The centrifuge always has a lid; new models will have a locking lid for safety and an on/off switch; however, many models include a brake or a built-in tachometer, which indicates speed, and some centrifuges are refrigerated. Centrifugal force depends on three variables: mass, speed, and radius. The speed is expressed in revolutions per minute (rpm), and the centrifugal force generated is expressed in terms of relative centrifugal force (RCF) or gravities (g). The speed of the centrifuge is related to the RCF by the following equation:

$$RCF = 1.118 \times 10^{-5} \times r \times (rpm)^2 \qquad (Eq. 1-10)$$

where 1.118×10^{-5} is a constant, determined from the angular velocity, and r is the radius in centimeters, measured from the center of the centrifuge axis to the bottom of the test tube shield or bucket. The RCF value may also be obtained from a nomogram similar to that found in Appendix F on thePoint. Centrifuge classification is based on several criteria, including benchtop (Fig. 1.10A) or floor model; refrigeration, rotor head (e.g., fixed, hematocrit, cytocentrifuge, swinging bucket [Fig. 1.10B], or angled Fig. 1.10); or maximum speed attainable (i.e., ultracentrifuge). Centrifuges are generally used to separate serum or plasma from the blood cells as the blood samples are being processed; to separate a supernatant from a precipitate during an analytic reaction; to separate two immiscible liquids, such as a lipid-laden sample; or to expel air.

Centrifuge care includes daily cleaning of any spills or debris, such as blood or glass, and ensuring that the centrifuge is properly balanced and free from any excessive vibrations. Balancing the centrifuge load is critical (Fig. 1.11). Many newer centrifuges will automatically decrease their speed if the load is not evenly distributed, but more often, the centrifuge will shake and vibrate or make more noise than expected. A centrifuge needs to be balanced based on equalizing both the volume and weight distribution across the centrifuge head. Many laboratories will make up "balance" tubes that approximate routinely used volumes and

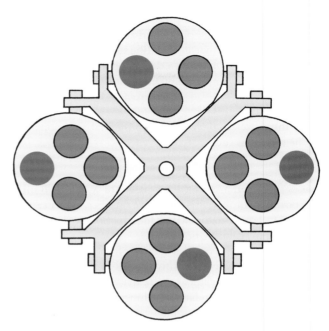

FIGURE 1.11 Properly balanced centrifuge. *Colored circles* represent counterbalanced positions for sample tubes.

FIGURE 1.10 **(A)** Benchtop centrifuge. **(B)** Swinging-bucket rotor.

LABORATORY MATHEMATICS AND CALCULATIONS

Significant Figures

Significant figures are the minimum number of digits needed to express a particular value in scientific notation without loss of accuracy. There are several rules in regard to identifying significant figures:

1. All nonzero numbers are significant (1, 2, 3, 4, 5, 6, 7, 8, 9).
2. All zeros between nonzero numbers are significant.
3. All zeros to the right of the decimal are not significant when followed by a nonzero number.
4. All zeros to the left of the decimal are not significant.

The number 814.2 has four significant figures, because in scientific notation, it is written as 8.142×10^2. The number 0.000641 has three significant figures, because the scientific notation expression for this value is 6.41×10^{-4}. The zeros

tube sizes, including the stopper on phlebotomy tubes, which can be used to match those needed from patient samples. A good rule of thumb is one of even placement and one of "opposition" (Fig. 1.12). Exact positioning of tubes depends on the design of the centrifuge holders.

The centrifuge cover should remain closed until the centrifuge has come to a complete stop to avoid any aerosol contamination. It is recommended that the timer, brushes (if present), and speed be periodically checked. The brushes, which are graphite bars attached to a retainer spring, create an electrical contact in the motor. The specific manufacturer's service manual should be consulted for details on how to change brushes and on lubrication requirements. The speed of a centrifuge is easily checked using a tachometer or strobe light. The hole located in the lid of many centrifuges is designed for speed verification using these devices but may also represent an aerosol biohazard if the hole is uncovered. Accreditation agencies require periodic verification of centrifuge speeds.

FIGURE 1.12 Properly loaded centrifuge.

to the right of the decimal preceding the nonzero digits are merely holding decimal places and are not needed to properly express the number in scientific notation. However, by convention, zeros following a decimal point are considered significant. For example, 10.00 has four significant figures.

Logarithms

Logarithms are the inverse of exponential functions and can be related as such:

$$x = A^B \text{ or } B = \log_A(x)$$

This is then read as B is the log base a of X, where B must be a positive number, A is a positive number, and A cannot be equal to 1. Calculators with a log function do not require conversion to scientific notation.

To determine the original number from a log value, the process is done in reverse. This process is termed the *antilogarithm*. Most calculators require that you enter this value, use an inverse or secondary/shift function, and enter log. If given a log of 3.1525, the resulting value should be 1.424×10^3. Consult the specific manufacturer's directions of the calculator to become acquainted with the proper use of these functions.

pH (Negative Logarithms)

In certain circumstances, the laboratory scientist must deal with negative logs. Such is the case with pH or pK_a. As previously stated, the pH of a solution is defined as the negative log of the hydrogen ion concentration. The following is a convenient formula to determine the negative logarithm when working with pH or pK_a:

$$\frac{pH}{pK_a} = x - \log N \quad \text{(Eq. 1-11)}$$

where x is negative exponent base 10 expressed and N is the decimal portion of the scientific notation expression.

For example, if the hydrogen ion concentration of a solution is 5.4×10^{-6}, then $x = 6$ and $N = 5.4$. Substitute this information into Equation 1-11, and it becomes

$$pH = 6 - \log 5.4 \quad \text{(Eq. 1-12)}$$

The logarithm of N (5.4) is equal to 0.7324, or 0.73. The pH becomes

$$pH = 6 - 0.73 = 5.27 \quad \text{(Eq. 1-13)}$$

The same formula can be applied to obtain the hydrogen ion concentration of a solution when only the pH is given. Using a pH of 5.27, the equation becomes

$$5.27 = x - \log N \quad \text{(Eq. 1-14)}$$

In this instance, the x term is always the next largest whole number. For this example, the next largest whole number is 6. Substituting for x, the equation becomes

$$5.27 = 6 - \log N \quad \text{(Eq. 1-15)}$$

A shortcut is to simply subtract the pH from x ($6 - 5.27 = 0.73$) and take the antilog of that answer 5.73. The final answer is 5.73×10^{-6}. Note that rounding, while allowed, can alter the answer. A more algebraically correct approach follows in Equations 1-16 through 1-18. Multiply all the variables by -1:

$$(-1)(5.27) = (-1)(6) - (-1)(\log N)$$
$$-5.27 = -6 + \log N \quad \text{(Eq. 1-16)}$$

Solve the equation for the unknown quantity by adding a positive 6 to both sides of the equal sign and the equation becomes

$$6 - 5.27 = \log N$$
$$0.73 = \log N \quad \text{(Eq. 1-17)}$$

The result is 0.73, which is the antilogarithm value of N, which is 5.37, or 5.4:

$$\text{Antilog } 0.73 = N; \ N = 5.37 = 5.4 \quad \text{(Eq. 1-18)}$$

The hydrogen ion concentration for a solution with a pH of 5.27 is 5.4×10^{-6}. Many scientific calculators have an inverse function that allows for more direct calculation of negative logarithms.

Concentration

A detailed description of each concentration term (e.g., molarity and normality) may be found at the beginning of this chapter. The following discussion focuses on the basic mathematical expressions needed to prepare reagents of a stated concentration.

Percent Solution

A percent solution is determined in the same manner regardless of whether weight/weight, volume/volume, or weight/volume units are used. *Percent* implies "parts per 100," which is represented as percent (%) and is independent of the molecular weight of a substance.

Example 1.1 Weight/Weight (w/w)

To make up 250 g of a 5% aqueous solution of hydrochloric acid (using 12 M HCl), multiply the total amount by the percent expressed as a decimal. The 5% aqueous solution can be expressed as

$$5\% = \frac{5}{100} = 0.050 \quad \text{(Eq. 1-19)}$$

Therefore, the calculation becomes

$$0.050 \times 250 \text{ g} = 12.5 \text{ g of 12M HCl} \quad \text{(Eq. 1-20)}$$

Another way of arriving at the answer is to set up a ratio so that

Desired solution concentration = Final product of 12 M HCl

$$\frac{5}{100} = \frac{x}{250}$$
$$x = 12.5 \quad \text{(Eq. 1-21)}$$

Example 1.2 Weight/Volume (w/v)

The most frequently used term for a percent solution is weight per volume, which is often expressed as grams per 100 mL of the diluent. To make up 1,000 mL of a 10% (w/v) solution of NaOH, use the preceding approach. Restate the w/v as a fraction:

$$10\% = \frac{10\,g}{100\,mL} = 0.10$$

Then, the calculation becomes $0.10 \times 1{,}000\,mL = 100\,g$ or setting up a ratio so that

$$\frac{10\,g}{100\,mL} = \frac{x}{1{,}000\,mL} \qquad \text{(Eq. 1-22)}$$
$$x = 100\,g$$

Therefore, add 100 g of 10% NaOH to a 1,000-mL volumetric Class A flask and dilute to the calibration mark with reagent grade water.

Example 1.3 Volume/Volume (v/v)

Make up 50 mL of a 2% (v/v) concentrated hydrochloric acid solution.

$$\text{Restate 2\% as a fraction } \frac{2\,mL}{100\,mL} = 0.02$$

Then, the calculation becomes

$$0.02 \times 50\,mL = 1\,mL$$

or using a ratio

$$\frac{2\,mL}{100} = \frac{x}{50\,mL} \qquad \text{(Eq. 1-23)}$$
$$x = 1\,mL$$

Therefore, add 40 mL of reagent grade water to a 50-mL Class A volumetric flask, add 1 mL of concentrated HCl, mix, and dilute up to the calibration mark with reagent grade water. Remember, always add acid to water!

Molarity

Molarity (M) is routinely expressed in units of moles per liter (mol/L) or sometimes millimoles per milliliter (mmol/mL). Remember that 1 mol of a substance is equal to the gmw (gram molecular weight) of that substance. When trying to determine the amount of substance needed to yield a particular concentration, initially decide what final concentration units are needed. For molarity, the final units will be moles per liter (mol/L) or millimoles per milliliter (mmol/mL). The second step is to consider the existing units and the relationship they have to the final desired units. Essentially, try to put as many units as possible into like terms and arrange so that the same units cancel each other out, leaving only those needed in the final answer. To accomplish this, it is important to remember what units are used to define each concentration term. It is key to understand the relationship between molarity (moles/liter),

moles, and gmw. While molarity is given in these examples, the approach for molality is the same except that one molal is expressed as one mole of solute per kilogram of solvent. For water, one kilogram is proportional to one liter, so molarity and molality are equivalent.

Example 1.4

How many *grams* are needed to make 1 L of a 2 M solution of HCl?
Step 1: Which *units* are needed in the final answer? *Answer:* Grams per liter (g/L).
Step 2: Assess other mass/volume terms used in the problem. In this case, moles are also needed for the calculation: How many grams are equal to 1 mole? The gmw of HCl, which can be determined from the periodic table, will be equal to 1 mole. For HCl, the gmw is 36.5, so the equation may be written as

$$\frac{36.5\,g\,HCl}{mol} \times \frac{2\,mol}{L} = \frac{73\,g\,HCl}{L} \quad \text{(Eq. 1-24)}$$

Cancel out like units, and the final units should be grams per liter. In this example, 73 g HCl per liter is needed to make up a 2 M solution of HCl.

Example 1.5

A solution of NaOH is contained within a Class A 1-L volumetric flask filled to the calibration mark. The content label reads 24 g of NaOH. Determine the molarity.
Step 1: What *units* are ultimately needed? *Answer:* Moles per liter (mol/L).
Step 2: The units that exist are grams and L. NaOH may be expressed as moles and grams. The gmw of NaOH is calculated to equal 40 g/mol. Rearrange the equation so that grams can be canceled and the remaining units reflect those needed in the answer, which are mole/L.
Step 3: The equation becomes

$$\frac{24\,g\,NaOH}{L} \times \frac{1\,mol}{40\,g\,NaOH} = 0.6\,\frac{mol}{L} \quad \text{(Eq. 1-25)}$$

By canceling out like units and performing the appropriate calculations, the final answer of 0.6 M or 0.6 mol/L is derived.

Example 1.6

Make up 250 mL of a 4.8 M solution of HCl.
Step 1: *Units* needed? *Answer:* Grams (g).
Step 2: Determine the gmw of HCl (36.5 g), which is needed to calculate the molarity.
Step 3: Set up the equation, cancel out like units, and perform the appropriate calculations:

$$\frac{36.5\,g\,HCl}{mol} \times \frac{4.8\,mol\,HCl}{L} \times \frac{250\,mL \times L}{1{,}000\,mL} \quad \text{(Eq. 1-26)}$$
$$= 43.8\,g\,HCl$$

In a 250-mL Class A volumetric flask, add 200 mL of reagent grade water. Add 43.8 g of HCl and mix. Dilute up to the calibration mark with reagent grade water.

Although there are various methods to calculate laboratory mathematical problems, this technique of canceling like units can be used in most clinical chemistry situations, regardless of whether the problem requests molarity and normality or exchanging one concentration term for another. However, it is necessary to recall the interrelationship between all the units in the expression.

Normality

Normality (N) is expressed as the number of equivalent weights per liter (Eq/L) or milliequivalents per milliliter (mmol/mL). Equivalent weight is equal to gmw divided by the valence (V). Normality has often been used in acid–base calculations because an equivalent weight of a substance is also equal to its combining weight. Another advantage in using equivalent weight is that an equivalent weight of one substance is equal to the equivalent weight of any other chemical.

Example 1.7

Give the equivalent weight, in grams, for each substance listed below.
1. NaCl (gmw = 58 g/mol, valence = 1)

$$\frac{58\,g}{L} = 58\,g \text{ per equivalent weight} \quad (Eq.\,1\text{-}27)$$

2. H_2SO_4 (gmw = 98 g/mol, valence = 2)

$$\frac{98\,g}{2} = 49\,g \text{ per equivalent weight} \quad (Eq.\,1\text{-}28)$$

Example 1.8

What is the normality of a 500 mL solution that contains 7 g of H_2SO_4? The approach used to calculate molarity could be used to solve this problem as well.
Step 1: Units needed? *Answer:* Normality expressed as equivalents per liter (Eq/L).
Step 2: Units you have? *Answer:* Milliliters and grams. Now, determine how they are related to equivalents per liter. (There are 49 g per equivalent—see Equation 1-28 above.)
Step 3: Rearrange the equation so that like terms cancel out, leaving Eq/L. This equation is

$$\frac{7\,g\,H_2SO_4}{500\,mL} \times \frac{1\,Eq}{49\,g\,H_2SO_4} \times \frac{1,000\,mL}{1\,L} \quad (Eq.\,1\text{-}29)$$
$$= 0.285\,Eq/L = 0.285\,N$$

Because 500 mL is equal to 0.5 L, the final equation could be written by substituting 0.5 L for 500 mL, eliminating the need to include the 1,000-mL/L conversion factor in the equation.

Example 1.9

What is the normality of a 0.5 M solution of H_2SO_4? Continuing with the previous approach, the final equation is

$$\frac{0.5\,mol\,H_2SO_4}{L} \times \frac{98\,g\,H_2SO_4}{mol\,H_2SO_4} \times \frac{1\,Eq\,H_2SO_4}{49\,g\,H_2SO_4} \quad (Eq.\,1\text{-}30)$$
$$= 1\,Eq/L = 1N$$

When changing molarity into normality or vice versa, the following conversion formula may be applied:

$$M \times V = N \quad (Eq.\,1\text{-}31)$$

where V is the valence of the compound. Using this formula, Example 1.9 becomes

$$0.5\,M \times 2 = 1N \quad (Eq.\,1\text{-}32)$$

Example 1.10

What is the molarity of a 2.5 N solution of HCl? This problem may be solved in several ways. One way is to use the stepwise approach in which existing units are exchanged for units needed. The equation is

$$\frac{2.5\,Eq\,HCl}{L} \times \frac{36.5\,g\,HCl}{1\,Eq} \times \frac{1\,mol\,HCl}{36.5\,g\,HCl} \quad (Eq.\,1\text{-}33)$$
$$= 2.5\,mol/L\,HCl$$

The second approach is to use the normality-to-molarity conversion formula. The equation now becomes

$$M \times V = 2.5\,N$$
$$V = 1 \quad (Eq.\,1\text{-}34)$$
$$M = \frac{2.5\,N}{1} = 2.5\,N$$

When the valence of a substance is 1, the molarity will equal the normality. As previously mentioned, normality either equals or is greater than the molarity.

Specific Gravity

Density is expressed as mass per unit volume of a substance. The specific gravity is the ratio of the density of a material when compared with the density of pure water at a given temperature and allows the laboratory scientist a means of expressing density in terms of volume. The units for density are grams per milliliter. Specific gravity is often used with very concentrated materials, such as commercial acids (e.g., sulfuric and hydrochloric acids).

The density of a concentrated acid can also be expressed in terms of an assay or percent purity. The actual concentration is equal to the **specific gravity** multiplied by the *assay* or *percent purity value* (expressed as a decimal) stated on the label of the container.

Example 1.11

What is the actual weight of a supply of concentrated HCl whose label reads specific gravity 1.19 with an assay value of 37%?

$$1.19 \, g/mL \times 0.37 = 0.44 \, g/mL \text{ of } HCl \quad \text{(Eq. 1-35)}$$

Example 1.12

What is the molarity of this stock solution? The final units desired are moles per liter (mol/L). The molarity of the solution is

$$\frac{0.44 \, g \, HCl}{mL} \times \frac{1 \, mol \, HCl}{36.5 \, g \, HCl} \times \frac{1,000 \, mL}{L} \quad \text{(Eq. 1-36)}$$

$$= 12.05 \, mol/L \text{ or } 12 M$$

Conversions

To convert one unit into another, the same approach of canceling out like units can be applied. In some instances, a chemistry laboratory may report a given analyte using two different concentration units—for example, calcium. The recommended SI unit for calcium is millimoles per liter. The better known and more traditional units are milligrams per deciliter (mg/dL). Again, it is important to understand the relationship between the units given and those needed in the final answer.

Example 1.13

Convert 8.2 mg/dL calcium to millimoles per liter (mmol/L). The gmw of calcium is 40 g. So, if there are 40 g per mol, then it follows that there are 40 mg per mmol. The final units wanted are mmol/L. The equation becomes

$$\frac{8.2 \, mg}{dL} \times \frac{1 \, dL}{100 \, mL} \times \frac{1,000 \, mL}{L} \times \frac{1 \, mmol}{40 \, mg} \quad \text{(Eq. 1-37)}$$

$$= \frac{2.05 \, mmol}{L}$$

Once again, the systematic stepwise approach of deleting similar units can be used for this conversion problem.

A frequently encountered conversion problem or, more precisely, a dilution problem occurs when a weaker concentration or different volume is needed than the stock substance available, but the concentration *terms* are the same. The following formula is used where V_1 is the volume of the first substance, C_1 is the concentration of the first substance, V_2 is the volume of the second substance, and C_2 is the concentration of the second substance:

$$V_1 \times C_1 = V_2 \times C_2 \quad \text{(Eq. 1-38)}$$

This formula is useful only if the concentration and volume units between the substances are the *same* and if three of four variables are known.

Example 1.14

What volume is needed to make 500 mL of a 0.1 M solution of Tris buffer from a solution of 2 M Tris buffer?

Identify the known values:
Concentration of initial substance (C_1) = 2 M
Volume of the product (V_2) = 500 mL
Concentration of the product (C_2) = 0.1 M

And the equation becomes:

$$V_1 \times 2 M = 0.1 M \times 500 \, mL$$

$$(V_1)(2 M) = (0.1 M)(500 \, mL); (V_1)(2 M) = 50 \, mL$$

$$\text{Therefore, } V_1 = \frac{50 \, mL}{2} = 25 \, mL \quad \text{(Eq. 1-39)}$$

It requires 25 mL of the 2 M solution to make up 500 mL of a 0.1 M solution.

This problem differs from the other conversions in that it is actually a dilution of a stock solution. While this approach will provide how much stock is needed when making the solution, the laboratory scientist must subtract that volume from the final volume to determine the amount of diluent needed, in this case 475 mL. A more involved discussion of dilution problems follows.

Dilutions

A **dilution** represents the ratio of concentrated or stock material to the total final volume of a solution and consists of the volume or weight of the concentrate plus the volume of the diluent, with the concentration units remaining the same. This ratio of concentrated or stock solution to the total solution volume equals the **dilution factor**. Because a dilution is made by adding a more concentrated substance to a diluent, the dilution is always less concentrated than the original substance. The relationship of the dilution factor to concentration is an inverse one; thus, the *dilution factor* increases as the *concentration decreases*. To determine the dilution factor, simply take the concentration needed and divide by the stock concentration, leaving it in a reduced fraction form.

Example 1.15

What is the dilution factor needed to make a 100 mmol/L sodium solution from a 3,000 mmol/L stock solution? The dilution factor becomes

$$\frac{100 \, mmol}{L} \times \frac{L}{3,000 \, mmol} = \frac{1}{30} \quad \text{(Eq. 1-40)}$$

The dilution factor indicates that the ratio of stock material is 1 part stock made to a *total volume* of 30 mL. To actually make this dilution, 1 mL of stock is added to 29 mL of diluent to achieve a total final volume of 30 mL. Note that the dilution factor indicates the parts per total amount; however, in *making* the dilution, the sum of the amount of the stock material plus the amount of the diluent must equal the *total volume* or dilution fraction denominator. The dilution factor may be correctly written as either a fraction or a ratio.

Confusion arises when distinction is not made between a ratio and a dilution, which by its very nature is a ratio of stock to diluent. A ratio is always expressed using a colon; a dilution can be expressed as either a fraction or a ratio.[21] Many directions in the laboratory are given orally. For example, making a "1-**in**-4" dilution means adding one part stock to a *total* of four parts. That is, one part of stock would be added to three parts of diluent. The dilution factor would be 1/4. Analyses performed on the diluted material would need to be multiplied by 4, the dilution factor, to get the final concentration. The dilution factor is the reciprocal of the dilution. Stating the dilution factor is ¼ is very different from saying make a "1-**to**-4" dilution! In this instance, the dilution factor would be 1/5! It is important during procedures that you fully understand the meaning of these expressions. Patient sample or stock dilutions should be made using reagent grade water, saline, or method-specific diluent using Class A glassware. The sample and diluent should be thoroughly mixed before use. It is not recommended that sample dilutions be made in smaller volume sample cups or holders. Any total volume can be used as long as the fraction reduces to give the dilution factor.

Example 1.16

If in the preceding example 150 mL of the 100 mmol/L sodium solution was required, the dilution ratio of stock to total volume must be maintained. Set up a ratio between the desired total volume and the dilution factor to determine the amount of stock needed. The equation becomes

$$\frac{1\,\text{part}}{30\,\text{parts}} = \frac{x\,\text{mL}}{150\,\text{mL}}$$

$$x = 5\,\text{mL}$$

(Eq. 1-41)

Note that 5/150 reduces to the dilution factor of 1/30. To make up this solution, 5 mL of stock is added to 145 mL of the appropriate diluent, making the ratio of *stock volume* to *diluent volume* equal to 5/145. Recall that the dilution factor includes the total volume of *both* stock plus diluent in the denominator and differs from the amount of diluent to stock that is needed.

Example 1.17

Many laboratory scientists like using $(V_1)(C_1) = (V_2)(C_2)$ for simple dilution calculations. This is acceptable, as long as you recall that you will need to subtract the stock volume from the total final volume for the correct *diluent* volume.

$$(V_1)(C_1) = (V_2)(C_2)(x)(3{,}000\,\text{mmol/L})$$
$$= (150\,\text{mL})(100\,\text{mmol/L})$$

$$x = 5;\ 150 - 5 = 145\,\text{mL of diluent}$$
$$\textbf{should be added to 5 mL of stock}$$

(Eq. 1-42)

Simple Dilutions

When making a *simple dilution*, the laboratory scientist must decide on the total volume desired and the amount of stock to be used.

Example 1.18

A 1:10 (1/10) dilution of serum can be achieved by using any of the following approaches. A ratio of 1:9—one part serum and nine parts diluent (saline):

- 100 µL of serum added to 900 µL of saline
- 20 µL of serum added to 180 µL of saline
- 1 mL of serum added to 9 mL of saline
- 2 mL of serum added to 18 mL of saline

Note that the sum of the ratio of serum to diluent (1:9) needed to make up each dilution satisfies the dilution factor (1:10 or 1/10) of stock material to total volume. When thinking about the stock to diluent volume, subtract the parts of stock needed from the total volume or parts to get the number of diluent "parts" needed. Once the volume of each part, usually stock, is known, multiply the diluent parts needed to obtain the correct volume.

Example 1.19

You have a 10 g/dL stock of protein standard. You need a 2 g/dL standard. You only have 0.200 mL of 10 g/dL stock to use. The procedure requires 0.100 mL.

Solution:

$$\frac{2\,\text{g/dL}}{10\,\text{g/dL}} = \frac{1}{5} = \textbf{Dilution factor}$$

(Eq. 1-43)

You will need 1 part or volume of stock of a total of 5 parts or volumes. Subtracting 1 from 5 yields that 4 parts or volumes of diluent is needed (Fig. 1.13). In this instance, you need at least 0.100 mL for the procedure. You have 0.200 mL of stock. You can make the dilution in various ways, as seen in Example 1.20.

FIGURE 1.13 Simple dilution. Consider this diagram depicting a substance having a 1/5 dilution factor. The dilution factor represents that 1 part of stock is needed from a total of 5 parts. To *make* this dilution, you would determine the volume of 1 "part," usually the stock or patient sample. The remainder of the "parts" or total would constitute the amount of diluent needed or four times the volume used for the stock.

Example 1.20

There are several ways to make a 1/5 dilution having only 0.200 mL of stock and needing a total minimum volume of 0.100 mL.

- Add 0.050 mL stock (1 part) to 0.200 mL of diluent (4 parts × 0.050 mL).
- Add 0.100 mL of stock (1 part) to 0.400 mL of diluent (4 parts × 0.100 mL).
- Add 0.200 mL of stock (1 part) to 0.800 mL of diluent (4 parts × 0.200 mL).

The dilution factor is also used to determine the final concentration of a dilution by multiplying the original concentration by the inverse of the dilution factor or the dilution factor denominator when it is expressed as a fraction.

Example 1.21

Determine the concentration of a 200 µmol/mL human chorionic gonadotropin (hCG) standard that was diluted 1/50. This value is obtained by multiplying the original concentration, 200 µmol/mL hCG, by the dilution factor, 1/50. The result is 4 µmol/mL hCG. Quite often, the concentration of the original material is needed.

Example 1.22

A 1:2 dilution of serum with saline had a creatinine result of 8.6 mg/dL. Calculate the actual serum creatinine concentration.

Dilution factor: 1/2
Dilution result = 8.6 mg/dL

Because this result represents 1/2 of the concentration, the inverse of the dilution is used, and the actual serum creatinine value is

$$2 \times 8.6 \, \text{mg/dL} = 17.2 \, \text{mg/dL} \qquad \text{(Eq. 1-44)}$$

Serial Dilutions

A **serial dilution** may be defined as multiple progressive dilutions ranging from more concentrated solutions to less concentrated solutions. Serial dilutions are extremely useful when the volume of concentrate or diluent is in short supply and needs to be minimized or a number of dilutions are required, such as in determining a titer. The volume of patient sample available to the laboratory may be small (e.g., pediatric samples), and a serial dilution may be needed to ensure that sufficient sample is available. The serial dilution is initially made in the same manner as a simple dilution. Subsequent dilutions will then be made from each preceding dilution. When a serial dilution is made, certain criteria may need to be satisfied. The criteria vary with each situation but usually include such considerations as the total volume desired, the amount of diluent or concentrate available, the dilution factor, the final concentration needed, and the support materials required.

Example 1.23

A three tube, twofold serial dilution is to be made on a sample. To start, the tubes must be labeled. It is arbitrarily decided that the total volume for each dilution is to be 1 mL. Into the first tube, 0.5 mL of diluent is added and then 0.5 mL of patient sample. This satisfies the "twofold" or 1:2 dilution for tube 1. In the next tube, 0.5 mL of diluent is again added, along with 0.5 mL of well-mixed liquid from tube 1. This satisfies the 1:2 dilution in tube 2, bringing the total tube dilution to 1:4. For the third tube, 0.5 mL of diluent is added, along with 0.5 mL of well-mixed liquid from tube 2. This satisfies the 1:2 dilution within the tube but brings the total tube dilution to 1:8. The calculation for these values is

$$\text{Dilution Tube 1} \frac{1}{2} \times \text{Dilution Tube 2} \frac{1}{2}$$
$$= \frac{1}{4} \text{ total tube dilution Tube 2} \qquad \text{(Eq. 1-45)}$$

Making a 1:2 dilution of the 1:4 dilution will result in the next dilution (1:8) in Tube 3. To establish the dilution factor needed for subsequent dilutions, it is helpful to solve the following equation for (x):

$$\text{Stock/preceding concentration} \times (x)$$
$$= (\text{final dilution factor}) \qquad \text{(Eq. 1-46)}$$

Refer to Figure 1.14 for an illustration of this serial dilution.

Example 1.24

Another type of dilution combines several dilution factors that are not multiples of one another. In our previous example, 1:2, 1:4, and 1:8 dilutions are all related to one another by a factor of 2. Consider the situation when 1:10, 1:20, 1:100, and 1:200 dilution factors are required. There are several approaches to solving this type of dilution problem. One method is to treat the 1:10 and 1:20 dilutions as one serial dilution problem, the 1:20 and 1:100 dilutions as a second serial dilution, and the 1:100 and 1:200 dilutions as the last serial dilution. Another approach is to consider what dilution factor of the concentrate is needed to yield the final dilution. In this example, the initial dilution is 1:10, with subsequent dilutions of 1:20, 1:100, and 1:200. The first dilution

FIGURE 1.14 Serial dilution.

may be accomplished by adding 1 mL of stock to 9 mL of diluent. The total volume of solution is 10 mL. Our initial dilution factor has been satisfied. In making the remaining dilutions, 2 mL of diluent is added to each test tube.

$$\text{Initial/preceding dilution} \times (x) = \text{dilution needed}$$

Solve for (x).

Using the dilution factors listed above and solving for (x), the equations become

$$1:10 \times (x) = 1:20$$
$$\text{where } (x) = 2 \text{ (or 1 part stock to 1 part diluent)}$$
$$1:20 \times (x) = 1:100$$
$$\text{where } (x) = 5 \text{ (or 1 part stock to 4 parts diluent)}$$
$$1:100 \times (x) = 1:200$$
$$\text{where } (x) = 2 \text{ (or 1 part stock to 1 part diluent)}$$

(Eq. 1-47)

In practice, the 1:10 dilution must be diluted by a factor of 2 to obtain a subsequent 1:20 dilution. Because the second tube already contains 2 mL of diluent, 2 mL of the 1:10 dilution should be added (1 part stock to 1 part diluent). In preparing the 1:100 dilution from this, a 1:5 dilution factor of the 1:20 mixture is required (1 part stock to 4 parts diluent). Because this tube already contains 2 mL, the volume of diluent in the tube is divided by its parts, which is 4; thus, 500 µL, or 0.500 mL, of stock should be added. The 1:200 dilution is prepared in the same manner using a 1:2 dilution factor (1 part stock to 1 part diluent) and adding 2 mL of the 1:100 to the 2 mL of diluent already in the tube.

Water of Hydration

Some compounds are available in a hydrated form. To obtain a correct gmw for these chemicals, the attached water molecule(s) must be included.

Example 1.25

How much $CuSO_4 \cdot 5H_2O$ must be weighed to prepare 1 L of 0.5 M $CuSO_4$? When calculating the gmw of this substance, the water weight must be considered so that the gmw is 250 g rather than gmw of $CuSO_4$ alone (160 g). Therefore,

$$\frac{250 \text{ g } CuSO_4 \cdot 5H_2O}{\text{mol}} \times \frac{0.5 \text{ mol}}{1 \text{ g}} = 125 \text{ g/L} \quad \text{(Eq. 1-48)}$$

Cancel out like terms to obtain the result of 125 g/L. A reagent protocol often designates the use of an anhydrous form of a chemical; frequently, however, all that is available is a hydrated form.

Example 1.26

A procedure requires 0.9 g of $CuSO_4$. All that is available is $CuSO_4 \cdot 5H_2O$. What weight of $CuSO_4 \cdot 5H_2O$ is needed?

Calculate the percentage of $CuSO_4$ present in $CuSO_4 \cdot 5H_2O$. The percentage is

$$\frac{160}{250} = 0.64, \text{ or } 64\% \quad \text{(Eq. 1-49)}$$

Therefore, 1 g of $CuSO_4 \cdot 5H_2O$ contains 0.64 g of $CuSO_4$, so the equation becomes

$$\frac{0.9 \text{ g } CuSO_4 \text{ needed}}{0.64 \text{ } CuSO_4 \text{ in } CuSO_4 \cdot 5H_2O} \quad \text{(Eq. 1-50)}$$
$$= 1.41 \text{ g } CuSO_4 \cdot 5H_2O \text{ required}$$

Graphing and Beer's Law

The Beer-Lambert law (Beer's law) mathematically establishes the relationship between concentration and absorbance in many photometric determinations. Beer's law is expressed as

$$A = abc \quad \text{(Eq. 1-51)}$$

where A is absorbance; a is the absorptivity constant for a particular compound at a given wavelength under specified conditions of temperature, pH, and so on; b is the length of the light path; and c is the concentration.

If a method follows Beer's law, then absorbance is proportional to concentration as long as the length of the light path and the absorptivity of the absorbing species remain unaltered during the analysis. In practice, however, there are limits to the predictability of a linear response. In automated systems, adherence to Beer's law is often determined by checking the linearity of the test method over a wide concentration range. The *limits of linearity* often represent the reportable range of an assay. This term should not be confused with the reference ranges associated with clinical significance of a test. Assays measuring absorbance generally obtain the concentration results by using a graph of Beer's law, known as a standard graph or curve. This graph is made by plotting absorbance versus the concentration of known standards (Fig. 1.15). Because most photometric assays set the initial absorbance to zero (0) using a reagent blank, the initial data points are 0,0. Graphs should be labeled properly and the concentration units must be given. The horizontal axis is referred to as the x-axis, whereas the

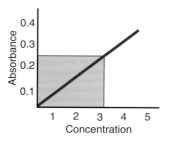

Unknown absorbance = 0.250
Concentration from graph = 3.2

FIGURE 1.15 Standard curve.

vertical line is the *y*-axis. By convention in the clinical laboratory, concentration is usually plotted on the *x*-axis. On a standard graph, only the standard and their associated absorbances are plotted.

Once a standard graph has been established, it is permissible to run just one standard, or calibrator, as long as the system remains the same. One-point calculation or calibration refers to the calculation of the comparison of the known standard/calibrator concentration and its corresponding absorbance to the absorbance of the unknown value according to the following ratio:

$$\frac{\text{Concentration of standard }(C_s)}{\text{Absorbance of standard }(A_s)} = \frac{\text{Concentration of unknown }(C_u)}{\text{Absorbance of unknown }(A_u)} \quad \text{(Eq. 1-52)}$$

Solving for the concentration of the unknown, the equation becomes

$$C_u = \frac{(A_u)(C_s)}{A_s} \quad \text{(Eq. 1-53)}$$

Example 1.27

The biuret protein assay is very stable and follows Beer's law. Rather than make up a completely new standard graph, one standard (6 g/dL) was assayed. The absorbance of the standard was 0.400, and the absorbance of the unknown was 0.350. Determine the value of the unknown in g/dL.

$$C_u = \frac{(0.350)(6\,\text{g/dL})}{(0.400)} = 5.25\,\text{g/dL} \quad \text{(Eq. 1-54)}$$

This method of calculation is acceptable as long as everything in the system, including the instrument and lot of reagents, remains the same. If anything in the system changes, a new standard graph should be done. Verification of linearity and/or calibration is required whenever a system changes or becomes unstable. Regulatory agencies often prescribe the condition of verification as well as how often the linearity needs to be checked.

Enzyme Calculations

Another application of Beer's law is the calculation of enzyme assay results. When calculating enzyme results, the *rate of change in absorbance* is often monitored continuously during the reaction to give the difference in absorbance, known as the **delta absorbance**, or ΔA. Instead of using a standard graph or a one-point calculation, the molar absorptivity of the product is used. If the absorptivity constant and absorbance, in this case ΔA, are given, Beer's law can be used to calculate the enzyme concentration directly without initially needing a standard graph, as follows:

$$A = abC$$
$$C = \frac{A}{ab} \quad \text{(Eq. 1-55)}$$

When the absorptivity constant (*a*) is given in units of grams per liter (moles) through a 1-centimeter (cm) light path, the term *molar absorptivity* (ε) is used. Substitution of ε for *a* and ΔA for *A* produces the following Beer's law formula:

$$C = \frac{\Delta A}{\varepsilon} \quad \text{(Eq. 1-56)}$$

For reporting enzyme activity, the IU, or **international unit**, is defined as the amount of enzyme that will catalyze 1 μmol of substrate per minute per liter. These units were often expressed as units per liter (U/L). The designations IU, U, and IU/L were adopted by many clinical laboratories to represent the IU. Although the reporting unit is the same, unless the analysis conditions are identical, use of the IU does not standardize the actual enzyme activity, and therefore, results between different methods of the same enzyme do not result in equivalent activity of the enzyme. For example, an alkaline phosphatase performed at 37°C will catalyze more substrate than if it is run at lower temperature, such as 25°C, even though the unit of expression, U/L, will be the same. The SI recommended unit is the *katal*, which is expressed as moles per liter per second. Whichever unit is used, calculation of the activity using Beer's law requires inclusion of the dilution and, depending on the reporting unit, possible conversion to the appropriate term (e.g., μmol to mol, mL to L, minute to second, and temperature factors). Beer's law for the IU now becomes

$$C = \frac{(\Delta A)10^{-6}(\text{TV})}{(\varepsilon)(b)(\text{SV})} \quad \text{(Eq. 1-57)}$$

where TV is the total volume of sample plus reagents in mL and SV is the sample volume used in mL. The 10^{-6} converts moles to μmol for the IU. If another unit of activity is used, such as the katal, conversion into liters and seconds would be needed, but the conversions to and from micromoles are excluded.

Example 1.28

The ΔA per minute for an enzyme reaction is 0.250. The product measured has a molar absorptivity of 12.2×10^3 at 425 nm at 30°C. The incubation and reaction temperature are also kept at 30°C. The assay calls for 1 mL of reagent and 0.050 mL of sample. Give the enzyme activity results in international units.

Applying Beer's law and the necessary conversion information, the equation becomes

$$C = \frac{(0.250)(10^{-6})(1.050\,\text{mL})}{(12.2\times10^3)(1)(0.050\,\text{mL})} = 430\,\text{U} \quad \text{(Eq. 1-58)}$$

Note: *b* is usually given as 1 cm; because it is a constant, it may not be considered in the calculation.

SPECIMEN CONSIDERATIONS

The process of specimen collection, handling, and processing remains one of the primary areas of *preanalytic* error. Careful attention to each phase is necessary to ensure proper subsequent testing and reporting of meaningful results. All accreditation agencies require laboratories to clearly define and delineate the procedures used for proper collection, transport, and processing of patient samples and the steps used to minimize and detect any errors, along with the documentation of the resolution of any errors. The Clinical Laboratory Improvement Amendments Act of 1988 (CLIA 88)[22] specifies that procedures for specimen submission and proper handling, including the disposition of any specimen that does not meet the laboratories' criteria of acceptability, be documented.

Types of Samples

Phlebotomy, or *venipuncture*, is the act of obtaining a blood sample from a vein using a needle attached to a collection device or a stoppered *evacuated tube*. These tubes come in different volume sizes: from pediatric sizes (≈150 μL) to larger 5 mL tubes. The most frequent site for venipuncture is the medial antecubital vein of the arm. A tourniquet made of pliable nonlatex rubber flat band or tubing is wrapped around the arm, causing cessation of blood flow and dilation of the veins, making for easier detection. The gauge of the needle is inversely related to the size of the needle; the larger the number, the smaller the needle bore and length. Routine venipuncture uses a 23- or 21-gauge needle. An intravenous (IV) infusion set, sometimes referred to as a butterfly because of the appearance of the setup, may be used whenever the veins are fragile, small, or hard to reach or find. The butterfly is attached to a piece of tubing, which is then attached to a hub or barrel. Because of potential needlesticks and cost of the product, this practice may be discouraged. Sites adjacent to IV therapy should be avoided; however, if both arms are involved in IV therapy and the IV cannot be discontinued for a short time, a site *below* the IV site should be sought. The initial sample drawn (5 mL) should be discarded because it is most likely contaminated with IV fluid and only subsequent sample tubes should be used for analytic purposes.

In addition to venipuncture, blood samples can be collected using a skin puncture technique that customarily involves the outer area of the bottom of the foot (a heel stick) for infants or the fleshy part of the middle of the last phalanx of the third or fourth (ring) finger (finger stick). A sharp lancet device is used to pierce the skin and an appropriate capillary or microtainer tubes are used for sample collection.[23]

Analytic testing of blood involves the use of whole blood, serum, or plasma. **Whole blood**, as the name implies, uses both the liquid portion of the blood called *plasma* and the cellular components (red blood cells, white blood cells, and platelets). This requires blood collection into a vacuum tube containing an anticoagulant. Complete mixing of the blood immediately following venipuncture is necessary to ensure the anticoagulant can adequately inhibit the blood's clotting factors. As whole blood sits or is centrifuged, the cells fall toward the bottom, leaving a clear yellow supernate on top called *plasma*. If a tube does *not* contain an anticoagulant, the blood's clotting factors are active in forming a clot incorporating the cells. The clot is encapsulated by the large protein fibrinogen. The remaining liquid is called **serum** rather than plasma (Fig. 1.16). Most testing in the clinical chemistry laboratory is performed on either plasma or serum. The major difference between plasma and serum is that serum does not contain fibrinogen (i.e., there is less protein in serum than plasma) and some potassium is released from platelets (serum potassium is slightly higher in serum than in plasma). It is important that serum samples be allowed to completely clot (≈20 minutes) before being centrifuged. Plasma samples also require centrifugation but do not need to allow for clotting time and their use can decrease turnaround time for reporting results.

Centrifugation of the sample accelerates the process of separating the plasma and cells. Specimens should be centrifuged for approximately 10 minutes at an RCF of 1,000 to 2,000 *g* but should avoid mechanical destruction of red cells that can result in hemoglobin release, called **hemolysis**.

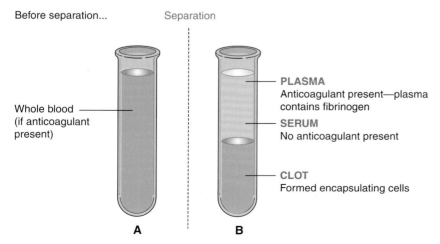

Before separation...   Separation

Whole blood (if anticoagulant present)

PLASMA
Anticoagulant present—plasma contains fibrinogen

SERUM
No anticoagulant present

CLOT
Formed encapsulating cells

A   B

FIGURE 1.16 Blood sample. **(A)** Whole blood. **(B)** Whole blood after separation.

Arterial blood samples measure blood gases (partial pressures of oxygen and carbon dioxide) and pH. Syringes containing heparin anticoagulant are used instead of evacuated tubes because of the pressure in an arterial blood vessel. The radial, brachial, and femoral arteries are the primary arterial sites. Arterial punctures are more difficult to perform because of inherent arterial pressure, difficulty in stopping bleeding afterward, and the undesirable development of a hematoma, which cuts off the blood supply to the surrounding tissue.[24]

Continued metabolism may occur if the serum or plasma remains in contact with the cells for any period. Evacuated tubes may incorporate plastic, gel-like material that serves as a barrier between the cells and the plasma or serum and seals these compartments from one another during centrifugation. Some gels can interfere with certain analytes, notably trace metals and drugs such as the tricyclic antidepressants.

Proper patient identification is the first step in sample collection. The importance of using the proper collection tube, avoiding prolonged tourniquet application, drawing tubes in the proper order, and proper labeling of tubes cannot be stressed strongly enough. Prolonged tourniquet application causes a stasis of blood flow and an increase in hemoconcentration and anything bound to proteins or the cells. Having patients open and close their fist during phlebotomy is of no value and may cause an increase in potassium and, therefore, should be avoided. IV contamination should be considered if a large increase occurs in the substances being infused, such as glucose, potassium, sodium, and chloride, with a decrease of other analytes such as urea and creatinine. In addition, the proper antiseptic must be used. Isopropyl alcohol wipes, for example, are used for cleaning and disinfecting the collection site; however, this is not the proper antiseptic for disinfecting the site when drawing blood alcohol levels (which is then soap and water only as the disinfectant).

Blood is not the only sample analyzed in the clinical chemistry laboratory. Urine is the next most common fluid for determination. Most quantitative analyses of urine require a timed sample (usually 24 hours); a complete sample (all urine must be collected in the specified time) can be difficult because many timed samples are collected by the patient in an outpatient situation. Creatinine analysis is often used to assess the completeness of a 24-hour urine sample because creatinine output is relatively free from interference and is stable, with little change in output within individuals. The average adult excretes 1 to 2 g of creatinine per 24 hours. Urine volume differs widely among individuals; however, a 4-L container is adequate (average output is ≈2 L). It should be noted that this analysis differs from the creatinine clearance test used to assess glomerular filtration rate, which compares urine creatinine output with that in the serum or plasma in a specified time interval and urine volume (often correcting for the surface area).

Other body fluids analyzed by the clinical chemistry laboratory include **cerebrospinal fluid (CSF)**, *paracentesis* fluids (pleural, pericardial, and peritoneal), and amniotic fluids. The color and characteristics of the fluid *before* centrifugation should be noted for these samples. *Before* centrifugation, a laboratorian should also verify that the sample is designated for clinical chemistry analysis *only* because a single fluid sample may be shared among several departments (i.e., hematology or microbiology) and centrifugation could invalidate certain tests in those areas.

CSF is an ultrafiltrate of the plasma and will, ordinarily, reflect the values seen in the plasma. For glucose and protein analysis (total and specific proteins), it is recommended that a blood sample be analyzed concurrently with the analysis of those analytes in the CSF. This will assist in determining the clinical utility of the values obtained on the CSF sample. This is also true for lactate dehydrogenase and protein assays requested on paracentesis fluids. All fluid samples should be handled immediately without delay between sample procurement, transport, and analysis.

Amniotic fluid is used to assess fetal lung maturity, congenital diseases, hemolytic diseases, genetic defects, and gestational age. The laboratory scientist should verify the specific handling of this fluid with the manufacturer of the testing procedure(s).

Sample Processing

When samples arrive in the laboratory, they are first processed. In the clinical chemistry laboratory, this means correctly matching the blood collection tube(s) with the appropriate test requisition and patient identification labels. This is a particularly sensitive area of preanalytic error. Bar code labels on primary sample tubes are vital in detecting errors and to minimizing clerical errors at this point of the processing. The laboratory scientist must also ascertain if the sample is acceptable for further processing. The criteria used depend on the test involved but usually include volume considerations (i.e., is there sufficient volume for testing needs?), use of proper anticoagulants or preservatives (i.e., was it collected in the correct evacuated tube), whether timing is clearly indicated and appropriate for timed testing, and whether the specimen is intact and has been properly transported (e.g., cooled or on ice, within a reasonable period, protected from light). Unless a whole blood analysis is being performed, the sample is then centrifuged as previously described and the serum or plasma should be separated from the cells if not analyzed immediately.

Once processed, the laboratory scientist should note the presence of any serum or plasma characteristics such as *hemolysis* and **icterus** (increased bilirubin pigment) or the presence of turbidity often associated with **lipemia** (increased lipids). Samples should be analyzed within 4 hours; to minimize the effects of evaporation, samples should be properly capped and kept away from areas of rapid airflow, light, and heat. If testing is to occur after that time, samples should be appropriately stored. For most, this means refrigeration at 4°C for 8 hours. Many analytes are stable at this temperature, with the exception of alkaline phosphatase (increases) and lactate dehydrogenase (decreases as a result of temperature labile fractions). Samples may be frozen at −20°C and stored for longer periods without deleterious effects on the results. Repeated cycles of freezing and thawing, like those that occur in so-called frost-free freezers, should be avoided.

Sample Variables

Sample variables include physiologic considerations, proper patient preparation, and problems in collection, transportation, processing, and storage. Although laboratorians must include mechanisms to minimize the effect of these variables on testing and must document each preanalytic incident, it is often frustrating to try to control the variables that largely depend on individuals outside of the laboratory. The best course of action is to critically assess or predict the weak areas, identify potential problems, and put an action plan in place that contains policies, procedures, or checkpoints throughout the sample's journey to the laboratory scientist who is actually performing the test. Good communication with all personnel involved helps ensure that whatever plans are in place meet the needs of the laboratory and, ultimately, the patient and physician. Most accreditation agencies require that laboratories consider all aspects of preanalytic variation as part of their quality assurance plans, including effective problem solving and documentation.

Physiologic variation refers to changes that occur within the body, such as cyclic changes (diurnal or circadian variation) or those resulting from exercise, diet, stress, gender, age, underlying medical conditions (e.g., fever, asthma, and obesity), drugs, or posture (Table 1.5). Samples may be drawn on patients who are fasting (usually overnight for at least 8 hours). When fasting, many patients may avoid drinking water and they may become dehydrated, which can be reflected in higher than expected results. Patient preparation for timed samples or those requiring specific diets or other instructions must be well written and verbally explained to patients. Elderly patients often misunderstand or are overwhelmed by the directions given to them by physician office personnel. Drugs can affect various analytes.[25] It is important to ascertain what, if any, medications the patient is taking that may interfere with the test. Unfortunately, many laboratorians do not have access to this information and the interest in this type of interference only arises when the physician questions a result. Some frequently encountered influences are smoking, which causes an increase in glucose as a result of the action of nicotine, growth hormone, cortisol, cholesterol, triglycerides, and urea. High amounts or chronic consumption of alcohol causes hypoglycemia, increased triglycerides, and an increase in the enzyme gamma-glutamyltransferase and other liver function tests. Intramuscular injections increase the enzyme

TABLE 1.5 Variables Affecting Select Chemistry Analytes

Factor	Examples of Analytes Affected
Age	Creatinine clearance, hormone levels (↓ with age)
Gender	(↑ males): albumin, ALP, creatine, Ca^{2+}, uric acid, CK, AST, phosphate (PO_4), blood urea nitrogen, Mg^{2+}, bilirubin, cholesterol
	(↑ females): Fe, cholesterol, γ-globulins, α-lipoproteins
Diurnal variation	↑ in AM: ACTH, cortisol, Fe, aldosterone
	↑ in PM: ACP, growth hormone, PTH, TSH
Day-to-day variation	≥20% for ALT, bilirubin, Fe, TSH, triglycerides
Recent food ingestion	↑ glucose, insulin, triglycerides, gastrin, ionized Ca^{2+}
	↓ chloride, phosphorus, potassium, amylase, ALP
Posture	↑ when standing: albumin, cholesterol, aldosterone, Ca^{2+}
Activity	↑ in ambulatory patients: CK
	↑ with exercise: lactic acid, creatine, protein, CK, AST, LD, K+, glucose
	↓ with exercise: cholesterol, triglycerides, pH
Stress	↑ ACTH, cortisol, catecholamines, TSH
Race	TP ↑ (black), albumin ↓ (black); IgG 40% ↑, and IgA 20%↑ (black male vs. white male); CK/LD ↑ black males; ↑ cholesterol and triglycerides > white >40 years old (glucose incidence diabetes in Asian, Black, Native American, Hispanic)
Require fasting	Fasting blood sugar, glucose tolerance test, triglycerides, lipid panel, gastrin, insulin, aldosterone/renin
Anaerobic and require ICE slurry (immediate cooling)	Lactic acid, ammonia, blood gas (if not analyzed within 30 min = ↓ pH, and pO_2), iCa^{+2} (heparinized whole blood if not analyzed within 30 min)
Hemolysis	↑ K+, ammonia, PO_4, Fe, Mg^{2+}, ALT, AST, LD, ALP, ACP, catecholamines, CK (marked hemolysis)

ALP, alkaline phosphatase; CK, creatine kinase; AST, aspartate aminotransferase; ACTH, adrenocorticotropic hormone; ACP, acid phosphatase; PTH, parathyroid hormone; TSH, thyroid-stimulating hormone; ALT, alanine aminotransferase; LD, lactate dehydrogenase; TP, total protein; K+, potassium.

creatine kinase and the skeletal muscle fraction of lactate dehydrogenase. Opiates, such as morphine or meperidine, cause increases in liver and pancreatic enzymes, and oral contraceptives may affect many analytic results. Many drugs affect liver function tests. Diuretics can cause decreased potassium and hyponatremia. Thiazide-type medications can cause hyperglycemia and prerenal azotemia secondary to the decrease in blood volume. Postcollection variations are related to those factors discussed under specimen processing. Clerical errors are the most frequently encountered, followed by inadequate separation of cells from serum, improper storage, and collection.

Chain of Custody

When laboratory tests are likely linked to a crime or accident, they become forensic in nature. In these cases, documented specimen identification is required at each phase of the process. Each facility has its own forms and protocols; however, the patient, and usually a witness, must identify the sample. It should be collected and then sealed with a tamper-proof seal. Any individual in contact with the sample must document receipt of the sample, the condition of the sample at the time of receipt, and the date and time it was received. In some instances, one witness verifies the entire process and cosigns as the sample moves along. Any analytic test could be used as part of legal testimony; therefore, the laboratory scientist should give each sample—even without the documentation—the same attention given to a forensic sample.

Electronic and Paper Reporting of Results

Electronic transmission of laboratory data and the more routine use of an electronic medical record, coding, billing, and other data management systems have caused much debate regarding appropriate standards needed in terms of both reporting guidelines and safeguards to ensure privacy of the data and records. Complicating matters is that there are many different data management systems in use by health care agencies that all use laboratory information. For example, the Logical Observation Identifiers Names and Codes (LOINC) system, International Federation of Clinical Chemistry/International Union of Pure and Applied Chemistry (IFCC/IUPAC), ASTM, Health Level 7 (HL7), and Systematized Nomenclature of Medicine, Reference Technology (SNOMED RT) are databases that use their own coding systems for laboratory observations. There are also additional proprietary systems in use, adding to the confusion. In an attempt to standardize these processes and to protect the confidentiality of patient information as required by the Health Insurance Portability and Accountability Act (HIPAA), the Healthcare Common Procedure Coding System (HCPCS) test and services coding system was developed to be recognized by all insurers for reimbursement purposes. The International Classification of Diseases (ICD) developed by the World Health Organization (WHO) uses codes identifying patient diseases and conditions. In the United States, ICD-10 is currently in place. The clinical modifications are maintained by the National Center for Health Statistics. Incorporated into the HCPCS system is the Current Procedural Terminology (CPT) codes, developed by the American Medical Association, which identify almost all laboratory tests and procedures. The CPT codes are divided into different subcategories, with tests or services assigned five-digit numbers followed by the name of the test or service. Together, these standard coding systems help patient data and tracking of disease transmission between all stakeholders such as physicians, patients, epidemiologists, and insurers.

Clinical laboratory procedures are found in CPT Category I with coding numbers falling between 80,000 and 89,000. There can be several codes for a given test based on the reason and type of testing and there are codes given for common profiles or array of tests that represent each test's separate codes. For example, blood glucose testing includes the codes 82947 (quantitative except for strip reading), 82948 (strip reading), and 82962 (self-monitoring by FDA-cleared device) and the comprehensive metabolic panel (80053) includes albumin, alkaline phosphatase, total bilirubin, blood urea nitrogen, total calcium, carbon dioxide, chloride, creatinine, glucose, potassium, total protein, sodium, and alanine and aspartate transaminases and their associated codes. At a minimum, any system must include a unique patient identifier, test name, and code that relates back to the HCPCS and ICD databases. For reporting purposes, whether paper or electronic, the report should include the unique patient identifier and test name including any appropriate abbreviations, the test value with the unit of measure, date and time of collection, sample information, reference ranges, plus any other pertinent information for proper test interpretation. Results that are subject to autoverification should be indicated in the report. Table 1.6 lists the information that is often required by accreditation agencies.[26]

TABLE 1.6 Minimum Elements of Paper or Electronic Patient Reports

Name and address of laboratory performing the analysis including any reference laboratories used

Patient name and identification number or unique identifier

Name of physician or person ordering the test

Date and time of specimen collection

Date and time of release of results (or available if needed)

Specimen source or type

Test results and units of measure if applicable

Reference ranges, when available

Comments relating to any sample or testing interferences that may alter interpretation

For additional student resources, please visit thePoint® at http://thepoint.lww.com

questions

1. What is the *molarity* for a solution containing 100 g of NaCl made up to 500 mL with distilled water? Assume a gram molecular weight (from periodic table) of approximately 58 grams.
   a. 3.45 M
   b. 1.72 M
   c. 290 M
   d. 5.27 M

2. What is the *normality* for a solution containing 100 g of NaCl made up to 500 mL with distilled water? Assume a gram molecular weight (from periodic table) of approximately 58 g.
   a. 3.45
   b. 0.86
   c. 1.72
   d. 6.9

3. What is the *percent* (*w/v*) for a solution containing 100 g of NaCl made up to 500 mL with distilled water?
   a. 20%
   b. 5%
   c. 29%
   d. 58%

4. What is the *dilution factor* for a solution containing 100 g of NaCl made up to 500 mL with distilled water?
   a. 1:5 or 1/5
   b. 5
   c. 50 or 1/50
   d. 10

5. What is the value in mg/dL for a solution containing 10 mg of $CaCl_2$ made with 100 mL of distilled water?
   a. 10
   b. 100
   c. 50
   d. Cannot determine without additional information

6. What is the molarity of a solution containing 10 mg of $CaCl_2$ made with 100 mL of distilled water? Assume a gram molecular weight from the periodic table of approximately 111 g.
   a. 9×10^{-4}
   b. 1.1×10^{-3}
   c. 11.1
   d. 90

7. You must make 1 L of 0.2 M acetic acid (CH_3COOH). All you have available is concentrated glacial acetic acid (assay value, 98%; specific gravity, 1.05 g/mL). It will take _____ milliliters of acetic acid to make this solution. Assume a gram molecular weight of 60.05 grams.
   a. 11.7
   b. 1.029
   c. 3.42
   d. 12.01

8. What is the hydrogen ion concentration of an acetate buffer having a pH of 3.85?
   a. 1.41×10^{-4}
   b. 3.90×10^{-1}
   c. 0.048
   d. 0.15×10^{-6}

9. Using the Henderson-Hasselbalch equation, give the ratio of salt to weak acid for a Veronal buffer with a pH of 8.6 and a pK_a of 7.43.
   a. 14.7/1
   b. 1/8.6
   c. 1.17/1
   d. 1/4.3

10. The pK_a for acetic acid is 4.76. If the concentration of salt is 2 mmol/L and that of acetic acid is 6 mmol/L, what is the expected pH?
    a. 4.43
    b. 6.19
    c. 104
    d. 56

11. The hydrogen ion concentration of a solution is 0.000439. What is the pH?
    a. 3.36
    b. 4.39×10^{-5}
    c. 4.39
    d. 8.03

12. Perform the following conversions:
    a. 4×10^4 mg = _____ g
    b. 1.3×10^2 mL = _____ dL
    c. 0.02 mL = _____ μL
    d. 5×10^{-3} mL = _____ μL
    e. 5×10^{-2} L = _____ mL
    f. 4 cm = _____ mm

review questions (continued)

13. What volume of 14 N H_2SO_4 is needed to make 250 mL of 3.2 M H_2SO_4 solution? Assume a gram molecular weight of 98.08 g.
- **a.** 114 mL
- **b.** 1.82 mL
- **c.** 1.75 mL
- **d.** 7 mL

14. A 24-hour urine has a total volume of 1,200 mL. A 1:200 dilution of the urine specimen gives a creatinine result of 0.8 mg/dL. The serum value is 1.2 mg/dL. What is the final value of creatinine in mg/dL in the undiluted urine sample?
- **a.** 160
- **b.** 0.8
- **c.** 960
- **d.** 860

15. A 24-hour urine has a total volume of 1,200 mL. A 1:200 dilution of the urine specimen gives a creatinine result of 0.8 mg/dL. The serum value is 1.2 mg/dL. What is the result in terms of grams per 24 hours?
- **a.** 1.92
- **b.** 0.08
- **c.** 80
- **d.** 19

16. A new medical technologist was selecting analyte standards to develop a standard curve for a high-performance liquid chromatography (HPLC) procedure. This analyte must have a 100% purity level and must be suitable for HPLC. Which of the following labels would be most appropriate for this procedure?
- **a.** ACS with no impurities listed
- **b.** USP
- **c.** NF
- **d.** CP
- **e.** ACS with impurities listed

17. When selecting quality control reagents for measuring an analyte in urine, the medical technologist should select:
- **a.** A quality control reagent prepared in a urine matrix.
- **b.** A quality control reagent prepared in a serum matrix.
- **c.** A quality control reagent prepared in deionized water.
- **d.** The matrix does not matter; any quality control reagent as long as the analyte of measure is chemically pure.

18. A patient's serum sample was placed on the chemistry analyzer and the output indicated "out of range" for the measurement of creatine kinase (CK) enzyme. A dilution of the patient serum was required. Which of the following should be used to prepare a dilution of patient serum?
- **a.** Deionized water
- **b.** Tap water
- **c.** Another patient's serum with confirmed, low levels of CK
- **d.** Type III water
- **e.** Type I water

19. True or False? Laboratory liquid-in-glass thermometers should be calibrated against an NIST-certified thermometer.

20. Which of the following containers is calibrated to hold only one exact volume of liquid?
- **a.** Volumetric flask
- **b.** Erlenmeyer flask
- **c.** Griffin beaker
- **d.** Graduated cylinder

21. Which of the following does NOT require calibration in the clinical laboratory?
- **a.** Electronic balance
- **b.** Liquid-in-glass thermometer
- **c.** Centrifuge
- **d.** Volumetric flask
- **e.** Air-displacement pipette

22. Which of the following errors is NOT considered a preanalytical error?
- **a.** During a phlebotomy procedure, the patient is opening and clenching his fist multiple times.
- **b.** The blood was not permitted to clot and spun in a centrifuge after 6 minutes of collection.
- **c.** The patient was improperly identified leading to a mislabeled blood sample.
- **d.** The serum sample was diluted with tap water.
- **e.** During phlebotomy, the EDTA tube was collected prior to the red clot tube.

references

1. National Institute of Standards and Technology (NIST). *Reference on Constants, Units, and Uncertainty.* Washington, DC: U.S. Department of Commerce; 1991/1993. http://physics.nist. gov/cuu/Units/introduction.html. Accessed December 2, 2015 [Adapted from Special Publications (SP) Nos. 811 and 330].
2. Miller WG, Tate JR, Barth J, et al. Harmonization: the sample, the measurement, and the report. *Annals of Laboratory Medicine.* 2014;34(3):187–197, doi: 10.33431/alm.2014.34.3.
3. American Chemical Society (ACS). *Reagent Chemicals.* 9th ed. Washington, DC: ACS Press; 2000.
4. Department of Labor and Occupational Safety and Health Administration (OSHA). *Occupational Exposure to Hazardous Chemicals in Laboratories.* Washington, DC: OSHA; 2011. (Federal Register, 29 CFR, Part 1910.1450.)
5. National Institute of Standards and Technology (NIST). *Standard Reference Materials Program.* Washington, DC: U.S. Department of Commerce; 2008. www.nist.gov/srm/ definitons.cfm. Accessed December 10, 2015.
6. IUPAC. *Compendium of Chemical Terminology.* 2nd ed. (the "Gold Book"). Compiled by A.D. McNaught and A. Wilkinson. Oxford: Blackwell Scientific Publications; 1997. XML on-line corrected version: http://goldbook.iupac.org (2006-) created by M. Nic, J. Jirat, Kosata; updates compiled by A. Jenkins, ISBN 0-9678550-9-8. Doi: 10.1351/goldbook. Last update 2014-02-24; version 2.3.3
7. International Organization for Standardization, European Committee for Standardization (ISO). *In Vitro Diagnostic Medical Devices—Measurement of Quantities in Samples of Biological Origin—Metrological Traceability of Values Assigned to Calibrators and Control Material.* Geneva, Switzerland: ISO; 2003. (Publication No. ISO/TC 212/WG2 N65/EN 17511.)
8. Carreiro-Lewandowski E. Basic principles and practice of clinical chemistry. In: Bishop M, Schoeff L, Fody P, eds. *Clinical Chemistry, Principles, Procedures, and Correlations.* 7th ed. Baltimore, MD: Lippincott Williams & Wilkins; 2010:3–32.
9. Clinical Laboratory Standards Institute/National Committee for Clinical Laboratory Standards. *Preparation and Testing of Reagent Water in the Clinical Laboratory; Approved Guideline.* 4th ed. Wayne, PA: CLSI; 2006. (Publication No. C3-A4.) Amended June, 2012.
10. National Institutes of Health. *Laboratory Water: Its Importance and Applications.* NIH. http://orf.od.nih.gov/ Policies and Guidelines/Documents. Published March, 2013. Accessed December 11, 2015.
11. College of American Pathologists (CAP). *Laboratory General Checklist: Quality of Water and Glassware Washing.* Northfield, IL: September, 25, 2012.
12. National Institute of Standards and Technology (NIST). *Calibration Uncertainties of Liquid-in-Glass Thermometers Over the Range from −20°C to 400°C.* Gaithersburg, MD: U.S. Department of Commerce; 2003.
13. NIH, National Institute of Allergy and Infectious Diseases. *DAIDS Guidelines for Good Clinical Laboratory Practice Standards.* https://www.niaid.nih.gov/LabsAndResources/ resources/DAIDSClinRsrch/Documents/gclp.pdf. Published July, 2013. Accessed December 8, 2015.
14. American Society for Testing and Materials (ASTM), E969-02 (2012). *Standards Specification for Volumetric (Transfer) Pipets.* West Conshohocken, PA: ASTM International; 2012. doi: 10.1520/E0969-02R12
15. American Society for Testing and Materials (ASTM), E288-10. *Standard Specification for Glass, Volumetric flasks.* West Conshohocken, PA: ASTM International; 2010. doi: 10.1520/ E0288-10
16. American Society for Testing and Materials (ASTM), E438-92 (2011). *Standard Specification for Glasses in Laboratory Apparatus.* West Conshohocken, PA: ASTM International; 2011. doi: 10.1520/E0438-92R11.
17. Eppendorf. *Standard Operating Procedure for Pipettes.* AESOP13640-08 05213_en_online. Hamburg: Eppendorf AG; 2013. Accessed October 2015.
18. Gilson. *Verification Procedure for Accuracy and Precision.* Middleton, WI. Procedure LT 8022921C; 2003. http://www. sipoch.cz/download/overeni_pipety.pdf. Accessed December 15, 2015.
19. McCall RE, Tankersley CM. *Phlebotomy Essentials.* 6th ed. Philadelphia, PA: LWW; 2016.
20. American Society for Testing and Materials (ASTM) E617-13. *Standard Specification for Laboratory Weights and Precision Mass Standards.* West Conshohocken, PA: ASTM; 2013. www. astm.org. doi: 10.1520/E0617
21. Doucette, Lorraine J. *Mathematics for the Clinical Laboratory.* 2nd ed. Philadelphia, PA: Saunders; 2010.
22. Clinical Laboratory Standards Institute (CLSI). *Procedures for the Handling and Processing of Blood Specimens.* 4th ed. Wayne, PA: CLSI; 2010. (Publication No. H18-A4, Vol. 30.)
23. Centers for Disease Control and Prevention, Division of Laboratory Systems. *Clinical Laboratory Improvement Amendments.* CFR Part 493, Laboratory requirements. http://wwwn.cdc.gov/clia/default.aspx. Accessed November 2015.
24. Clinical Laboratory Standards Institute (CLSI). *Procedures and Devices for the Collection of Diagnostic Blood Specimens by Skin Puncture.* 6th ed. Wayne, PA: CLSI; 2010. (Publication No. H3-A6, Vol. 27)
25. Young DS. *Effects of Drugs on Clinical Laboratory Tests.* 5th ed. Washington, DC: AACC Press; 2000.
26. College of American Pathology; Commission on Laboratory Accreditation; Laboratory Accreditation Program Laboratory General Checklist Website. http://www.cap.org/apps/docs/ laboratory_accreditation/checklists/laboratory. Accessed November 2015.

2

Laboratory Safety and Regulations

TOLMIE E. WACHTER

chapter outline

key terms

Airborne pathogens
Biohazard
Bloodborne pathogens
Carcinogens
Chemical hygiene plan
Corrosive chemicals
Cryogenic material
Fire tetrahedron
Hazard Communication Standard
Hazardous materials
High-efficiency particulate air (HEPA) filters
Laboratory standard
Mechanical hazards
Medical waste
National Fire Protection Association (NFPA)
Occupational Safety and Health Act (OSHA)
Radioactive materials
Reactive chemicals
Safety Data Sheets (SDSs)
Teratogens
Universal precautions

chapter objectives

Upon completion of this chapter, the clinical laboratorian should be able to do the following:

- Discuss safety awareness for clinical laboratory personnel.
- List the responsibilities of employer and employee in providing a safe workplace.
- Identify hazards related to handling chemicals, biologic specimens, and radiologic materials.
- Choose appropriate personal protective equipment when working in the clinical laboratory.
- Identify the classes of fires and the types of fire extinguishers to use for each.

(continues on page 34)

For additional student resources, please visit thePoint®
at http://thepoint.lww.com

chapter objectives (continued)

- Describe steps used as precautionary measures when working with electrical equipment, cryogenic materials, and compressed gases and avoiding mechanical hazards associated with laboratory equipment.
- Select the correct means for disposal of waste generated in the clinical laboratory.
- Outline the steps required in documentation of an accident in the workplace.

LABORATORY SAFETY AND REGULATIONS

Clinical laboratory personnel, by the nature of the work they perform, are exposed daily to a variety of real or potential hazards: electric shock, toxic vapors, compressed gases, flammable liquids, radioactive material, corrosive substances, mechanical trauma, poisons, and the inherent risks of handling biologic materials, to name a few. Each clinician should develop an understanding of the risks associated with these hazards and must be "safety conscious" at all times.

Laboratory safety necessitates the effective control of all hazards that exist in the clinical laboratory at any given time. Safety begins with the recognition of hazards and is achieved through the application of common sense, a safety-focused attitude, good personal behavior, good housekeeping in all laboratory work and storage areas, and, above all, the continual practice of good laboratory technique. In most cases, accidents can be traced directly to two primary causes: unsafe acts (not always recognized by personnel) and unsafe environmental conditions. This chapter discusses laboratory safety as it applies to the clinical laboratory.

Occupational Safety and Health Act

Public Law 91-596, better known as the **Occupational Safety and Health Act (OSHA)**, was enacted by the U.S. Congress in 1970. The goal of this federal regulation was to provide all employees (clinical laboratory personnel included) with a safe work environment. Under this legislation, the Occupational Safety and Health Administration (also known as OSHA) is authorized to conduct on-site inspections to determine whether an employer is complying with the mandatory standards. Safety is no longer only a moral obligation but also a federal law. In about half of the states, this law is administered by individual state agencies rather than by the federal OSHA. These states still fall within delineated OSHA regions, but otherwise they bear all administrative, consultation, and enforcement responsibilities. The state regulations must be at least as stringent as the federal ones, and many states incorporate large sections of the federal regulations verbatim.

OSHA standards that regulate safety in the laboratory include the Bloodborne Pathogen Standard, Formaldehyde Standard, Laboratory Standard, Hazard Communication Standard, Respiratory Protection Standard, Air Contaminants Standard, and Personal Protective Equipment Standard. Because laws, codes, and ordinances are updated frequently,

current reference materials should be reviewed. Assistance can be obtained from local libraries, the Internet, and federal, state, and local regulatory agencies. The primary standards applicable to clinical laboratory safety are summarized next.

Bloodborne Pathogens [29 CFR 1910.1030]

This standard applies to all exposure to blood or other potentially infectious materials in any occupational setting. It defines terminology relevant to such exposures and mandates the development of an *exposure control plan*. This plan must cover specific preventative measures including exposure evaluation, engineering controls, work practice controls, and administrative oversight of the program. Universal precautions and personal protective equipment (PPE) are foremost among these infection control measures. The *universal precautions* concept is basically an approach to infection control in which all human blood, tissue, and most fluids are handled as if known to be infectious for the human immunodeficiency virus (HIV), hepatitis B virus (HBV), and other bloodborne pathogens. The standard also provides fairly detailed directions for decontamination and the safe handling of potentially infectious laboratory supplies and equipment, including practices for managing laundry and infectious wastes. Employee information and training are covered regarding recognition of hazards and risk of infection. There is also a requirement for HBV vaccination or formal declination within 10 days of assuming duties that present exposure. In the event of an actual exposure, the standard outlines the procedure for postexposure medical evaluation, counseling, and recommended testing or postexposure prophylaxis.

Hazard Communication [29 CFR 1910.1200]

This subpart to OSHA's Toxic and Hazardous Substances regulations is intended to ensure that the hazards of all chemicals used in the workplace have been evaluated and that this hazard information is successfully transmitted to employers and their employees who use the substances. Informally referred to as the OSHA "HazCom Standard," it defines *hazardous substances* and provides guidance for evaluating and communicating identified hazards. The primary means of communication are through proper labeling, the development and use of **safety data sheets (SDSs)**, and employee education.

Occupational Exposure to Hazardous Chemicals in Laboratories [29 CFR 1910.1450]

This second subpart to OSHA's Toxic and Hazardous Substances regulations is also known as the "OSHA Lab

Standard." It was intended to address the shortcomings of the Hazard Communication Standard regarding its application peculiar to the handling of hazardous chemicals in laboratories, whose multiple small-scale manipulations differ from the industrial volumes and processes targeted by the original HazCom Standard. The Lab Standard requires the appointment of a *chemical hygiene officer* and the development of a *chemical hygiene plan* to reduce or eliminate occupational exposure to hazardous chemicals. This plan is required to describe the laboratory's methods of identifying and controlling physical and health hazards presented by chemical manipulations, containment, and storage. The chemical hygiene plan must detail engineering controls, PPE, safe work practices, and administrative controls, including provisions for medical surveillance and consultation, when necessary.

Other Regulations and Guidelines

There are other federal regulations relating to laboratory safety, such as the Clean Water Act, the Resource Conservation and Recovery Act (RCRA), and the Toxic Substances Control Act. In addition, clinical laboratories are required to comply with applicable local and state laws, such as fire and building codes. The Clinical and Laboratory Standards Institute (CLSI, formerly National Committee for Clinical Laboratory Standards [NCCLS]) provides excellent general laboratory safety and infection control guidelines in their documents GP17-A3 (*Clinical Laboratory Safety; Approved Guideline*, Second Edition) and M29-A4 (*Protection of Laboratory Workers from Occupationally Acquired Infections; Approved Guideline*, Third Edition).

Safety is also an important part of the requirements for initial and continued accreditation of health care institutions and laboratories by voluntary accrediting bodies such as The Joint Commission (TJC; formerly the Joint Commission on Accreditation of Health Care Organizations [JCAHO]) and the Commission on Laboratory Accreditation of the College of American Pathologists (CAP). TJC publishes a yearly accreditation manual for hospitals and the *Accreditation Manual for Pathology and Clinical Laboratory Services*, which includes a detailed section on safety requirements. CAP publishes an extensive inspection checklist (*Laboratory General Checklist*) as part of their *Laboratory Accreditation Program*, which includes a section dedicated to laboratory safety.

Over the past decade, several new laws and directives have been emplaced regarding enhanced security measures for particular hazardous substances with potential for nefarious use in terrorist activities. These initiatives are typically promulgated by the Department of Homeland Security in cooperation with the respective agency regulating chemical, nuclear, or biological agents of concern. Although most laboratories do not store or use the large volumes of chemicals required to trigger chemical security requirements, many laboratories do surpass the thresholds for radiological and biological agents. Management and employees must be cognizant of security requirements for substances in quantities qualifying them for regulation under enhanced security measures for chemical (Chemical Facilities Anti-Terrorism Standards, 6 CFR 27), radiological (Nuclear Regulatory Commission [NRC] *Security Orders* and *Increased Controls* for licensees holding sources above *Quantities of Concern*), and biological (Select Agents and Toxins, 42 CFR 73) agents. Most security measures involve restriction of access to only approved or authorized individuals, assessment of security vulnerabilities, secure physical containment of the agents, and inventory monitoring and tracking.

SAFETY AWARENESS FOR CLINICAL LABORATORY PERSONNEL

Safety Responsibility

The employer and the employee share safety responsibility. While the individual employee has an obligation to follow safe work practices and be attentive to potential hazards, the employer has the ultimate responsibility for safety and delegates authority for safe operations to laboratory managers and supervisors. In order to ensure clarity and consistency, safety management in the laboratory should start with a written safety policy. Laboratory supervisors, who reflect the attitudes of management toward safety, are essential members of the safety program.

Employer's Responsibilities
- Establish laboratory work methods and safety policies.
- Provide supervision and guidance to employees.
- Provide safety information, training, PPE, and medical surveillance to employees.
- Provide and maintain equipment and laboratory facilities that are free of recognized hazards and adequate for the tasks required.

The employee also has a responsibility for his or her own safety and the safety of coworkers. Employee conduct in the laboratory is a vital factor in the achievement of a workplace without accidents or injuries.

Employee's Responsibilities
- Know and comply with the established laboratory safe work practices.
- Have a positive attitude toward supervisors, coworkers, facilities, and safety training.
- Be alert and give prompt notification of unsafe conditions or practices to the immediate supervisor and ensure that unsafe conditions and practices are corrected.
- Engage in the conduct of safe work practices and use of PPE.

Signage and Labeling

Appropriate signs to identify hazards are critical, not only to alert laboratory personnel to potential hazards but also to identify specific hazards that may arise because of emergencies such as fire or explosion. The **National Fire Protection Association (NFPA)** developed a standard hazard identification system (diamond-shaped, color-coded symbol), which has been adopted by many clinical laboratories. At a glance, emergency personnel can assess health hazards (blue quadrant), flammable hazards (red quadrant), reactivity/stability hazards (yellow quadrant), and other special information (white quadrant). In addition, each quadrant shows the magnitude of severity, graded from a low of 0 to a high of 4, of the hazards within the posted area. (Note the NFPA hazard code symbol in Fig. 2.1.)

Manufacturers of laboratory chemicals also provide precautionary labeling information for users. Information indicated on the product label includes statement of the hazard, precautionary measures, specific hazard class, first aid instructions for internal/external contact, the storage code, the safety code, and personal protective gear and equipment needed. This information is in addition to specifications on the actual lot analysis of the chemical constituents and other product notes (Fig. 2.1). Over the last two decades, there has been an effort to standardize hazard terminology and classification under an internationally recognized guideline, titled the *Globally Harmonized System of Classification and Labeling of Hazardous Chemicals* (GHS). This system incorporates universal definitions and symbols to clearly communicate specific hazards in a single concise label format (Fig. 2.2).

Although not yet law, or codified as a regulatory standard, OSHA is presently working to align the existing Hazard Communication Standard with provisions of the GHS and encourages employers to begin adopting the program.

All in-house prepared reagents and solutions should be labeled in a standard manner and include the chemical identity, concentration, hazard warning, special handling, storage conditions, date prepared, expiration date (if applicable), and preparer's initials.

SAFETY EQUIPMENT

Safety equipment has been developed specifically for use in the clinical laboratory. The employer is required by law to have designated safety equipment available, but it is also the responsibility of the employee to comply with all safety rules and to use safety equipment.

All laboratories are required to have safety showers, eyewash stations, and fire extinguishers and to periodically test and inspect the equipment for proper operation. It is recommended that safety showers deliver 30 to 50 gallons of water per minute at 20 to 50 pounds per square in. (psi) and be located in areas where corrosive liquids are stored or used. Eyewash stations must be accessible (i.e., within 100 ft

FIGURE 2.1 Sample chemical label: **(1)** statement of hazard, **(2)** hazard class, **(3)** safety precautions, **(4)** NFPA hazard code, **(5)** fire extinguisher type, **(6)** safety instructions, **(7)** formula weight, and **(8)** lot number. Color of the diamond in the NFPA label indicates hazard: Red = flammable. Store in an area segregated for flammable reagents. Blue = health hazard. Toxic if inhaled, ingested, or absorbed through the skin. Store in a secure area. Yellow = reactive and oxidizing reagents. May react violently with air, water, or other substances. Store away from flammable and combustible materials. White = corrosive. May harm skin, eyes, or mucous membranes. Store away from red-, blue-, and yellow-coded reagents. Gray = presents no more than moderate hazard in any of the categories. For general chemical storage. Exception = reagent incompatible with other reagents of same color bar. Store separately. Hazard code **(4)**—Following the NFPA use, each diamond shows a red segment (flammability), a blue segment (health; i.e., toxicity), and a yellow segment (reactivity). Printed over each color-coded segment is a black number showing the degree of hazard involved. The fourth segment, as stipulated by the NFPA, is left blank. It is reserved for special warnings, such as radioactivity. The numeric ratings indicate degree of hazard: 4 = extreme, 3 = severe, 2 = moderate, 1 = slight, and 0 = none according to present data. (Courtesy of Baxter International Inc.)

ToxiFlam (Contains: XYZ)

Danger! Toxic If Swallowed, Flammable Liquid and Vapor

Do not eat, drink or use tobacco when using this product. Wash hands
thoroughly after handling. Keep container tightly closed. Keep away
from heat/sparks/open flame. - No smoking. Wear protective gloves
and eye/face protection. Ground container and receiving equipment.
Use explosion-proof electrical equipment. Take precautionary measures against static discharge.
Use only non-sparking tools. Store in cool/well-ventilated place.

IF SWALLOWED: Immediately call a POISON CONTROL CENTER or doctor/physician. Rinse mouth.

In case of fire, use water fog, dry chemical, CO_2, or "alcohol" foam.

See Safety Data Sheet for further details regarding safe use of this product.

MyCompany, MyStreet, MyTown NJ 00000, Tel: 111 222 3333

FIGURE 2.2 Example of a GHS inner container label (e.g., bottle inside a shipping box).

or 10 s travel) in laboratory areas presenting chemical or biological exposure hazards. Other items that must be available for personnel include fire blankets, spill kits, and first aid supplies.

Mechanical pipetting devices must be used for manipulating all types of liquids in the laboratory, including water. Mouth pipetting is strictly prohibited.

Chemical Fume Hoods and Biosafety Cabinets

Fume Hoods

Fume hoods are required to contain and expel noxious and hazardous fumes from chemical reagents. Fume hoods should be visually inspected for blockages. A piece of tissue paper placed at the hood opening will indicate airflow direction. The hood should never be operated with the sash fully opened, and a maximum operating sash height should be established and conspicuously marked. Containers and equipment positioned within hoods should not block airflow. Periodically, ventilation should be evaluated by measuring the face velocity with a calibrated velocity meter. The velocity at the face of the hood (with the sash in normal operating position) should be 100 to 120 ft per minute and fairly uniform across the entire opening. Smoke testing is also recommended to locate no flow or turbulent areas in the working space. As an added precaution, personal air monitoring should be conducted in accordance with the chemical hygiene plan of the facility.

Biosafety Cabinets

Biological safety cabinets (BSCs) remove particles that may be harmful to the employee who is working with potentially infectious biologic specimens. The Centers for Disease Control and Prevention (CDC) and the National Institutes of Health have described four levels of biosafety, which consist of combinations of laboratory practices and techniques, safety equipment, and laboratory facilities. The biosafety level of a laboratory is based on the operations performed, the routes of transmission of the infectious agents, and the laboratory function or activity. Accordingly, biosafety cabinets are designed to offer various levels of protection, depending on the biosafety level of the specific laboratory (Table 2.1). BSCs should be periodically recertified to ensure continued optimal performance as filter occlusion or rupture can compromise their effectiveness.

Chemical Storage Equipment

Safety equipment is available for the storage and handling of hazardous chemicals and compressed gases. Safety carriers should always be used to transport glass bottles of acids, alkalis, or organic solvents in volumes larger than 500 mL, and approved safety cans should be used for storing, dispensing, or disposing of flammables in volumes greater than 1 quart. Steel safety cabinets with self-closing doors are required for the storage of flammable liquids, and only specially designed, explosion-proof refrigerators may be used to store flammable materials. Only the amount of chemical needed for that day should be available at the bench. Gas cylinder supports or clamps must be used at all times, and larger cylinders should be transported with valve caps on, using handcarts.

PPE and Hygiene

The parts of the body most frequently subject to injury in the clinical laboratory are the eyes, skin, and respiratory and digestive tracts. Hence, the use of PPE and proper hygiene is very important. Safety glasses, goggles, visors, or work shields protect the eyes and face from splashes and impact. Contact lenses do not offer eye protection; it is strongly recommended that they not be worn in the clinical chemistry laboratory, unless additional protective eyewear is also utilized. If any solution is accidentally splashed into the eye(s), thorough irrigation is required.

Gloves and rubberized sleeves protect the hands and arms when using caustic chemicals. Gloves are required for routine laboratory use; however, polyvinyl or other nonlatex gloves are an acceptable alternative for people with latex

TABLE 2.1   Comparison of Biosafety Cabinet Characteristics

BSC Class	Face Velocity	Airflow Pattern	Applications	
			Nonvolatile Toxic Chemicals and Radionuclides	Volatile Toxic Chemicals and Radionuclides
I	75	In at front through HEPA to the outside or into the room through HEPA	Yes	When exhausted outdoors
II, A1	75	70% recirculated to the cabinet work area through HEPA; 30% balance can be exhausted through HEPA back into the room or to outside through a canopy unit	Yes (minute amounts)	No
II, B1	100	30% recirculated, 70% exhausted. Exhaust cabinet air must pass through a dedicated duct to the outside through a HEPA filter	Yes	Yes (minute amounts)
I, B2	100	No recirculation; total exhaust to the outside through a HEPA filter	Yes	Yes (small amounts)
II, A2	100	Similar to II, A1, but has 100 lfm intake air velocity and plenums are under negative pressure to room; exhaust air can be ducted to the outside through a canopy unit	Yes	When exhausted outdoors (*formally* "B3") (minute amounts)

BSC, biological safety cabinet; HEPA, high-efficiency particulate air; lfm, linear feet per minute.
Adapted from Centers for Disease Control and Prevention, National Institutes of Health. *Biosafety in Microbiological and Biomedical Laboratories*. 5th ed. Washington, DC: U.S. Government Printing Office; 2009.

allergies. Certain glove materials offer better protection against particular reagent formulations. Nitrile gloves, for example, offer a wider range of compatibility with organic solvents than do latex gloves. Laboratory coats, preferably with knit-cuffed sleeves, should be full length and buttoned and made of liquid-resistant material. When performing manipulations prone to splash hazards, the laboratory coat should be supplemented with an impermeable apron and/or sleeve garters, constructed of suitable material to guard against the substances. Proper footwear is required; shoes constructed of porous materials, open-toed shoes, and sandals are considered ineffective against spilled hazardous liquids.

Respirators may be required for various procedures in the clinical laboratory. Whether used for biologic or chemical hazards, the correct type of respirator must be used for the specific hazard. Respirators with **high-efficiency particulate air (HEPA) filters** must be worn when engineering controls are not feasible, such as when working directly with patients with tuberculosis (TB) or when performing procedures that may aerosolize specimens of patients with a suspected or confirmed case of TB. Training, maintenance, and written protocol for use of respirators are required according to the respiratory protection standard.

Each employer must provide (at no charge) laboratory coats, gloves, or other protective equipment to all employees who may be exposed to biologic or chemical hazards. It is the employer's responsibility to clean and maintain any PPE used by more than one person. All contaminated

PPE must be removed and properly cleaned or disposed off before leaving the laboratory.

Hand washing is a crucial component of both infection control and chemical hygiene. After removing gloves, hands should be washed thoroughly with soap and warm water, even if glove breakthrough or contamination is not suspected. The use of antimicrobial soap is not as important as the physical action of washing the hands with water and any mild soap. After any work with highly toxic or carcinogenic chemicals, the face should also be washed.

BIOLOGIC SAFETY

General Considerations

All blood samples and other body fluids should be collected, transported, handled, and processed using **universal precautions** (i.e., presumed to be infectious). Gloves, gowns, and face protection must be used during manipulations or transfers when splashing or splattering is most likely to occur. Consistent and thorough hand washing is an essential component of infection control. Antiseptic gels and foams may be used at waterless stations between washes, but they should not take the place of an actual hand wash.

Centrifugation of biologic specimens produces finely dispersed aerosols that are a high-risk source of infection. Ideally, specimens should remain capped during centrifugation, or several minutes should be allowed to elapse after centrifugation is complete before opening the lid. As a preferred option, the use of a sealed-cup centrifuge is recommended. These sealed vessels can then be brought to a biosafety cabinet to be opened.

Spills

Any blood, body fluid, or other potentially infectious material spill must be promptly cleaned up, and the area or equipment must be disinfected immediately. Safe cleanup includes the following recommendations:

- Alert others in area of the spill.
- Wear appropriate protective equipment.
- Use mechanical devices to pick up broken glass or other sharp objects.
- Absorb the spill with paper towels, gauze pads, or tissue.
- Clean the spill site using a common aqueous detergent.
- Disinfect the spill site using approved disinfectant or 10% bleach, using appropriate contact time.
- Rinse the spill site with water.
- Dispose off all materials in appropriate biohazard containers.

Bloodborne Pathogens

In December 1991, OSHA issued the final rule for occupational exposure to **bloodborne pathogens**. To minimize employee exposure, each employer must have a written *exposure control plan*. The plan must be available to all employees whose duties may result in reasonably anticipated occupational exposure to blood or other potentially infectious materials. The exposure control plan must be discussed with all employees and be available to them while they are working. The employee must be provided with adequate training in all techniques described in the exposure control plan at initial work assignment and annually thereafter. All necessary safety equipment and supplies must be readily available and inspected on a regular basis.

Clinical laboratory personnel are knowingly or unknowingly in frequent contact with potentially biohazardous materials. In recent years, new and serious occupational hazards to personnel have arisen, and this problem has been complicated because of the general lack of understanding of the epidemiology, mechanisms of transmission of the disease, or inactivation of the causative agent. Special precautions must be taken when handling all specimens because of the continual increase in the proportion of infectious samples received in the laboratory. Therefore, in practice, specimens from patients with confirmed or suspected hepatitis, acquired immunodeficiency syndrome (AIDS), or other potentially infectious diseases should be handled no differently than other routine specimens. Adopting a universal precautions policy, which considers blood and other body fluids from all patients as potentially infective, is required.

Airborne Pathogens

Because of a global resurgence of TB, OSHA issued a statement in 1993 that the agency would enforce CDC Guidelines for Preventing the Transmission of Tuberculosis in Health Care Facilities. The purpose of the guidelines is to encourage early detection, isolation, and treatment of active cases. A TB exposure control program must be established, and risks to laboratory workers must be assessed. In 1997, a proposed standard (29 CFR 1910.1035, Tuberculosis) was issued by OSHA only to be withdrawn again when it was determined that existing CDC guidelines could be enforced by OSHA through its "general duty" clause and Respiratory Protection Standard. The CDC guidelines require the development of a *tuberculosis infection control program* by any facility involved in the diagnosis or treatment of cases of confirmed infectious TB. TB isolation areas with specific ventilation controls must be established in health care facilities. Those workers in high-risk areas may be required to wear a respirator for protection. All health care workers considered to be at risk must be screened for TB infection.

Other specific pathogens, including viruses, bacteria, and fungi, may be considered airborne transmission risks. Protective measures in the clinical laboratory generally involve work practice and engineering controls focused on prevention of aerosolization, containment/isolation, and respiratory protection of N-95 (filtration of 95% of particles >0.3 μm) or better.

Shipping

Clinical laboratories routinely ship regulated material. The U.S. Department of Transportation (DOT) and the International Air Transport Association (IATA) have specific requirements for carrying regulated materials. There are two types of specimen classifications. Known or suspect infectious specimens are labeled *infectious substances* if the pathogen can be readily transmitted to humans or animals. *Diagnostic specimens* are those tested as routine screening or for initial diagnosis. Each type of specimen has rules and packaging requirements. The DOT guidelines are found in the *Code of Federal Regulations, Title 49, Subchapter C*; IATA publishes its own manual, *Dangerous Goods Regulations*.

CHEMICAL SAFETY

Hazard Communication

In the August 1987 issue of the *Federal Register*, OSHA published the new **Hazard Communication Standard** (Right to Know Law, 29 CFR 1910.1200). The Right to Know Law was developed for employees who may be exposed to hazardous chemicals in the workplace. Employees must be informed of the health risks associated with those chemicals. The intent of the law is to ensure that health hazards are evaluated for all chemicals that are produced and that this information is relayed to employees.

To comply with the regulation, clinical laboratories must

- Plan and implement a written hazard communication program.
- Obtain *SDSs* for each hazardous compound present in the workplace and have the SDSs readily accessible to employees.

- Educate all employees annually on how to interpret chemical labels, SDSs, and health hazards of the chemicals and how to work safely with the chemicals.
- Maintain hazard warning labels on containers received or filled on-site.

In 2012, OSHA adopted significant changes to the Hazard Communication Standard to facilitate a standardization of international hazard communication programs. This new initiative was titled the Globally Harmonized System of Classification and Labelling of Chemicals, or GHS. The primary improvements to the program involved more specific criteria for classification of chemicals; a uniform system of chemical labeling, including intuitive pictographs; and, replacing the existing Material Safety Data Sheet (MSDS) program with the new SDS format. These changes were phased in over a 3-year period, with the final requirements effective in June of 2016.

Safety Data Sheet

The SDS is a major source of safety information for employees who may use **hazardous materials** in their occupations. Employers are responsible for obtaining the SDS from the chemical manufacturer or developing an SDS for each hazardous agent used in the workplace. The information contained in the SDS must follow a specific format, addressing each of the following 16 items:

- Section 1: Identification
- Section 2: Hazard identification
- Section 3: Ingredients information
- Section 4: First aid procedures
- Section 5: Fire-fighting procedures
- Section 6: Accidental-release measures
- Section 7: Handling and storage
- Section 8: Exposure controls and personal protection
- Section 9: Physical and chemical properties
- Section 10: Stability and reactivity
- Section 11: Toxicological information
- Section 12: Ecological information
- Section 13: Disposal considerations
- Section 14: Transport information
- Section 15: Regulatory information
- Section 16: Other information, including date of preparation or last revision

The SDS must provide the specific compound identity, together with all common names. All information sections must be completed, and the date that the SDS was printed must be indicated. Copies of the SDS must be readily accessible to employees during all shifts.

OSHA Laboratory Standard

Occupational Exposure to Hazardous Chemicals in Laboratories (29 CFR 1910.1450), also known as the **laboratory standard**, was enacted in May 1990 to provide laboratories with specific guidelines for handling hazardous

chemicals. This OSHA standard requires each laboratory that uses hazardous chemicals to have a written **chemical hygiene plan**. This plan provides procedures and work practices for regulating and reducing exposure of laboratory personnel to hazardous chemicals. *Hazardous chemicals* are those that pose a physical or health hazard from acute or chronic exposure. Procedures describing how to protect employees against **teratogens** (substances that affect cellular development in a fetus or embryo), carcinogens, and other toxic chemicals must be described in the plan. Training in the use of hazardous chemicals must be provided to all employees and must include recognition of signs and symptoms of exposure, location of SDS, the chemical hygiene plan, and how to protect themselves against hazardous chemicals. A chemical hygiene officer must be designated for any laboratory using hazardous chemicals. The protocol must be reviewed annually and updated when regulations are modified or chemical inventory changes. Remember that practicing consistent and thorough hand washing is an essential component of preventative chemical hygiene.

Toxic Effects from Hazardous Substances

Toxic substances have the potential of producing deleterious effects (local or systemic) by direct chemical action or interference with the function of body systems. They can cause acute or chronic effects related to the duration of exposure (i.e., short-term, or single contact, versus long-term, or prolonged, repeated contact). Almost any substance, even the most benign seeming, can pose risk of damage to a worker's lungs, skin, eyes, or mucous membranes following long- or short-term exposure and can be toxic in excess. Moreover, some chemicals are toxic at very low concentrations. Exposure to toxic agents can be through direct contact (absorption), inhalation, ingestion, or inoculation/injection.

In the clinical chemistry laboratory, personnel should be particularly aware of toxic vapors from chemical solvents, such as acetone, chloroform, methanol, or carbon tetrachloride, that do not give explicit sensory irritation warnings, as do bromide, ammonia, and formaldehyde. Air sampling or routine monitoring may be necessary to quantify dangerous levels. Mercury is another frequently disregarded source of poisonous vapors. It is highly volatile and toxic and is rapidly absorbed through the skin and respiratory tract. Mercury spill kits should be available in areas where mercury thermometers are used. Most laboratories are phasing out the use of mercury and mercury-containing compounds. Laboratories should have a policy on mercury reduction or elimination and a method for legally disposing off mercury. Several compounds, including formaldehyde and methylene chloride, have substance-specific OSHA standards, which require periodic monitoring of air concentrations. Laboratory engineering controls, PPE, and procedural controls must be adequate to protect employees from these substances.

Storage and Handling of Chemicals

To avoid accidents when handling chemicals, it is important to develop respect for all chemicals and to have a complete knowledge of their properties. This is particularly important when transporting, dispensing, or using chemicals that, when in contact with certain other chemicals, could result in the formation of substances that are toxic, flammable, or explosive. For example, acetic acid is incompatible with other acids such as chromic and nitric acid, carbon tetrachloride is incompatible with sodium, and flammable liquids are incompatible with hydrogen peroxide and nitric acid.

Arrangements for the storage of chemicals will depend on the quantities of chemicals needed and the nature or type of chemicals. Proper storage is essential to prevent and control laboratory fires and accidents. Ideally, the storeroom should be organized so that each class of chemicals is isolated in an area that is not used for routine work. An up-to-date inventory should be kept that indicates location of chemicals, minimum/maximum quantities required, and shelf life. Some chemicals deteriorate over time and become hazardous (e.g., many ethers and tetrahydrofuran form explosive peroxides). Storage should not be based solely on alphabetical order because incompatible chemicals may be stored next to each other and react chemically. They must be separated for storage, as shown in Table 2.2.

Flammable/Combustible Chemicals

Flammable and combustible liquids, which are used in numerous routine procedures, are among the most hazardous materials in the clinical chemistry laboratory because of possible fire or explosion. They are classified according to flash point, which is the temperature at which sufficient vapor is given off to form an ignitable mixture with air. A flammable liquid has a flash point below 37.8°C (100°F), and combustible liquids, by definition, have a flash point at or above 37.8°C (100°F). Some commonly used flammable and combustible solvents are acetone, benzene, ethanol, heptane, isopropanol, methanol, toluene, and xylene. It is important to remember that flammable or combustible chemicals also include certain gases, such as hydrogen, and solids, such as paraffin.

Corrosive Chemicals

Corrosive chemicals are injurious to the skin or eyes by direct contact or to the tissue of the respiratory and gastrointestinal tracts if inhaled or ingested. Typical examples include acids (acetic, sulfuric, nitric, and hydrochloric) and bases (ammonium hydroxide, potassium hydroxide, and sodium hydroxide). External exposures to concentrated corrosives can cause severe burns and require immediate flushing with copious amounts of clean water.

Reactive Chemicals

Reactive chemicals are substances that, under certain conditions, can spontaneously explode or ignite or that evolve heat or flammable or explosive gases. Some strong acids or bases react with water to generate heat (exothermic reactions). Hydrogen is liberated if alkali metals (sodium or potassium) are mixed with water or acids, and spontaneous combustion also may occur. The mixture of oxidizing agents, such as peroxides, and reducing agents, such as hydrogen, generates heat and may be explosive.

Carcinogenic Chemicals

Carcinogens are substances that have been determined to be cancer-causing agents. OSHA has issued lists of confirmed and suspected carcinogens and detailed standards for the handling of these substances. Benzidine is a common example of a known carcinogen. If possible, a substitute chemical or different procedure should be used to avoid exposure to carcinogenic agents. For regulatory (OSHA) and institutional safety requirements, the laboratory must maintain an accurate inventory of carcinogens.

Chemical Spills

Strict attention to good laboratory technique can help prevent chemical spills. However, emergency procedures should be established to handle any accidents. If a spill occurs, the first step should be to assist/evacuate personnel, and then confinement and cleanup of the spill can begin. There are several commercial spill kits available for neutralizing and absorbing spilled chemical solutions (Fig. 2.3). However, no single kit is suitable for all types of spills. Emergency procedures for spills should also include a reporting system.

RADIATION SAFETY

Environmental Protection

A radiation safety policy should include environmental and personnel protection. All areas where **radioactive materials** are used or stored must be posted with caution signs, and traffic in these areas should be restricted to essential personnel only. Regular and systematic monitoring must be emphasized, and decontamination of laboratory equipment, glassware, and work areas should be scheduled as part of routine procedures. Records must be maintained as to the quantity of radioactive material on hand as well as the quantity that is disposed. A NRC or agreement state license

TABLE 2.2	Storage Requirements
Substance	**Stored Separately**
Flammable liquids	Flammable solids
Mineral acids	Organic acids
Caustics	Oxidizers
Perchloric acid	Water-reactive substances
Air-reactive substances	Others
Heat-reactive substances requiring refrigeration	
Unstable substances (shock-sensitive explosives)	

FIGURE 2.3 Spill cleanup kit.

is required if the amount of radioactive material exceeds a certain level. The laboratory safety officer must consult with the institutional safety officer about these requirements.

Personal Protection

It is essential that only properly trained personnel work with radioisotopes. Good work practices must consistently be employed to ensure that contamination and inadvertent internalization are avoided. Users should be monitored to ensure that the maximal permissible dose of radiation is not exceeded. Radiation monitors must be evaluated regularly to detect degree of exposure for the laboratory employee. Records must be maintained for the length of employment plus 30 years.

Nonionizing Radiation

Nonionizing forms of radiation are also a concern in the clinical laboratory. Equipment often emits a variety of wavelengths of electromagnetic radiation that must be protected against through engineered shielding or use of PPE (Table 2.3). These energies have varying biologic effects, depending on wavelength, power intensity, and duration of exposure. Laboratorians must be knowledgeable regarding the hazards presented by their equipment to protect themselves and ancillary personnel.

FIRE SAFETY

The Chemistry of Fire

Fire is basically a chemical reaction that involves the rapid oxidation of a combustible material or fuel, with the subsequent liberation of heat and light. In the clinical chemistry laboratory, all the elements essential for fire to begin are present—fuel, heat or ignition source, and oxygen (air). However, recent research suggests that a fourth factor is present. This factor has been classified as a reaction chain in which burning continues and even accelerates. It is caused by the breakdown and recombination of the molecules from the material burning with the oxygen in the atmosphere.

The fire triangle has been modified into a three-dimensional pyramid known as the **fire tetrahedron** (Fig. 2.4). This modification does not contradict established procedures in dealing with a fire but does provide additional means by which fires may be prevented or extinguished. A fire will extinguish if any of the three basic elements (heat, air, or fuel) are removed.

Classification of Fires

Fires have been divided into four classes based on the nature of the combustible material and requirements for extinguishment:

Class A: ordinary combustible solid materials, such as paper, wood, plastic, and fabric
Class B: flammable liquids/gases and combustible petroleum products

TABLE 2.3	Examples of Nonionizing Radiation in Clinical Laboratories		
Type	**Approximate Wavelength**	**Source Equipment Example**	**Protective Measures**
Low frequency	>1 cm	Radiofrequency coil in inductively coupled plasma–mass spectrometer	Engineered shielding and posted pacemaker warning
Microwaves	3 m–3 mm	Energy beam microwave used to accelerate tissue staining in histology prep processes	Engineered shielding
Infrared	750 nm–0.3 cm	Heat lamps, lasers	Containment and appropriate warning labels
Visible spectrum	400–750 nm	General illumination and glare	Filters, diffusers, and nonreflective surfaces
Ultraviolet	4–400 nm	Germicidal lamps used in biologic safety cabinets	Eye and skin protection; UV warning labels

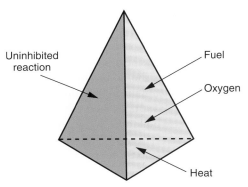

FIGURE 2.4 Fire tetrahedron.

Class C: energized electrical equipment
Class D: combustible/reactive metals, such as magnesium, sodium, and potassium

Types and Applications of Fire Extinguishers

Just as fires have been divided into classes, fire extinguishers are divided into classes that correspond to the type of fire to be extinguished. Be certain to choose the right type—using the wrong type of extinguisher may be dangerous. For example, do not use water on burning liquids or electrical equipment.

Pressurized water extinguishers, as well as foam and multipurpose dry chemical types, are used for Class A fires. Multipurpose dry-chemical and carbon dioxide extinguishers are used for Class B and C fires. Halogenated hydrocarbon

extinguishers are particularly recommended for use with computer equipment. Class D fires present special problems, and extinguishment is left to trained firefighters using special dry chemical extinguishers (Fig. 2.5). Generally, all that can be done for a Class D fire in the laboratory is to try and isolate the burning metal from combustible surfaces with sand or ceramic barrier material. Personnel should know the location and type of portable fire extinguisher near their work area and know how to use an extinguisher before a fire occurs. In the event of a fire, first evacuate all personnel, patients, and visitors who are in immediate danger and then activate the fire alarm, report the fire, and, if possible, attempt to extinguish the fire. Personnel should work as a team to carry out emergency procedures. Fire drills must be conducted regularly and with appropriate documentation. Fire extinguishers must be inspected monthly to ensure that they are mounted, visible, accessible, and charged.

CONTROL OF OTHER HAZARDS
Electrical Hazards

Most individuals are aware of the potential hazards associated with the use of electrical appliances and equipment. Direct hazards of electrical energy can result in death, shock, or burns. Indirect hazards can result in fire or explosion. Therefore, there are many precautionary procedures to follow when operating or working around electrical equipment:

• Use only explosion-rated (intrinsically wired) equipment in hazardous atmospheres.

FIGURE 2.5 Proper use of fire extinguishers. (Adapted from the Clinical and Laboratory Safety Department, The University of Texas Health Science Center at Houston.)

- Be particularly careful when operating high-voltage equipment, such as electrophoresis apparatus.
- Use only properly grounded equipment (three-prong plug).
- Check for frayed electrical cords.
- Promptly report any malfunctions or equipment producing a "tingle" for repair.
- Do not work on "live" electrical equipment.
- Never operate electrical equipment with wet hands.
- Know the exact location of the electrical control panel for the electricity to your work area.
- Use only approved extension cords in temporary applications and do not overload circuits. (Some local regulations prohibit the use of any extension cord.)
- Have ground, polarity, and leakage checks and other periodic preventive maintenance performed on outlets and equipment.

Compressed Gas Hazards

Compressed gases, which serve a number of functions in the laboratory, present a unique combination of hazards in the clinical laboratory: danger of fire, explosion, asphyxiation, or mechanical injuries. There are several general requirements for safely handling compressed gases:

- Know the gas that you will use.
- Store tanks in a vertical position.
- Keep cylinders secured at all times.
- Never store flammable liquids and compressed gases in the same area.
- Use the proper regulator, tubing, and fittings for the type of gas in use.
- Do not attempt to control or shut off gas flow with the pressure relief regulator.
- Keep removable protection caps in place until the cylinder is in use.
- Make certain that acetylene tanks are properly piped (the gas is incompatible with copper tubing).
- Do not force a "frozen" or stuck cylinder valve.
- Use a hand truck to transport large cylinders.
- Always check cylinders on receipt and then periodically for any problems such as leaks.
- Make certain that the cylinder is properly labeled to identify the contents.
- Empty tanks should be marked "empty."

Cryogenic Materials Hazards

Liquid nitrogen is probably one of the most widely used cryogenic fluids (liquefied gases) in the laboratory. There are, however, several hazards associated with the use of any **cryogenic material**: fire or explosion, asphyxiation, pressure buildup, embrittlement of materials, and tissue damage similar to that of thermal burns.

Only containers constructed of materials designed to withstand ultralow temperatures should be used for cryogenic work. In addition to the use of eye/face protection, hand protection to guard against the hazards of touching supercooled surfaces is recommended. The gloves, of impermeable material, should fit loosely so that they can be taken off quickly if liquid spills on or into them. Also, to minimize violent boiling/frothing and splashing, specimens to be frozen should always be inserted into the coolant very slowly. Cryogenic fluids should be stored in well-insulated but loosely stoppered containers that minimize loss of fluid resulting from evaporation by boil-off and that prevent plugging and pressure buildup.

Mechanical Hazards

In addition to physical hazards such as fire and electric shock, laboratory personnel should be aware of the **mechanical hazards** of equipment such as centrifuges, autoclaves, and homogenizers.

Centrifuges, for example, must be balanced to distribute the load equally. The operator should never open the lid until the rotor has come to a complete stop. Safety interlocks on equipment should never be rendered inoperable.

Laboratory glassware itself is another potential hazard. Agents, such as glass beads or boiling chips, should be added to help eliminate bumping/boilover when liquids are heated. Tongs or insulated gloves should be used to remove hot glassware from ovens, hot plates, or water baths. Glass pipettes should be handled with extra care, as should sharp instruments such as cork borers, needles, scalpel blades, and other tools. A glassware inspection program should be in place to detect signs of wear or fatigue that could contribute to breakage or injury. All infectious *sharps* must be disposed in OSHA-approved containers to reduce the risk of injury and infection.

Ergonomic Hazards

Although increased mechanization and automation have made many tedious and repetitive manual tasks obsolete, laboratory processes often require repeated manipulation of instruments, containers, and equipment. These physical actions can, over time, contribute to repetitive strain disorders such as tenosynovitis, bursitis, and ganglion cysts. The primary contributing factors associated with repetitive strain disorders are position/posture, applied force, and frequency of repetition. Remember to consider the design of hand tools (e.g., ergonomic pipettes), adherence to ergonomically correct technique, and equipment positioning when engaging in any repetitive task. Chronic symptoms of pain, numbness, or tingling in extremities may indicate the onset of repetitive strain disorders. Other hazards include acute musculoskeletal injury. Remember to lift heavy objects properly, keeping the load close to the body and using the muscles of the legs rather than the back. Gradually increase force when pushing or pulling, and avoid pounding actions with the extremities.

DISPOSAL OF HAZARDOUS MATERIALS

The safe handling and disposal of chemicals and other materials require a thorough knowledge of their properties and hazards. Generators of hazardous wastes have a moral and legal responsibility, as defined in applicable local, state, and federal regulations, to protect both the individual and the environment when disposing off waste. There are four basic waste disposal techniques: flushing down the drain to the sewer system, incineration, landfill burial, and recycling.

Chemical Waste

In some cases, it is permissible to flush water-soluble substances down the drain with copious quantities of water. However, strong acids or bases should be neutralized before disposal. The laboratory must adhere to institutional, local, and state regulations regarding the disposal of strong acids and bases. Foul-smelling chemicals should never be disposed off down the drain. Possible reaction of chemicals in the drain and potential toxicity must be considered when deciding if a particular chemical can be dissolved or diluted and then flushed down the drain. For example, sodium azide, which is used as a preservative, forms explosive salts with metals, such as the copper, in pipes. Many institutions ban the use of sodium azide due to this hazard. In all cases, check with the local water reclamation district or publicly owned treatment works for specific limitations before utilizing sewer disposal.

Other liquid wastes, including flammable solvents, must be collected in approved containers and segregated into compatible classes. If practical, solvents such as xylene and acetone may be filtered or redistilled for reuse. If recycling is not feasible, disposal arrangements should be made by specifically trained personnel. Flammable material can also be burned in specially designed incinerators with afterburners and scrubbers to remove toxic products of combustion.

Also, before disposal, hazardous substances that are explosive (e.g., peroxides) and carcinogens should be transformed to less hazardous forms whenever feasible. Solid chemical wastes that are unsuitable for incineration may be amenable to other treatments or buried in an approved, permitted landfill. Note that certain chemical wastes are subject to strict "cradle to grave" tracking under the RCRA, and severe penalties are associated with improper storage, transportation, and disposal.

Radioactive Waste

The manner of use and disposal of isotopes is strictly regulated by the NRC or NRC agreement states and depends on the type of waste (soluble or nonsoluble), its level of radioactivity, and the radiotoxicity and half-life of the isotopes involved. The radiation safety officer should always be consulted about policies dealing with radioactive waste disposal. Many clinical laboratories transfer radioactive materials to a licensed receiver for disposal.

Biohazardous Waste

On November 2, 1988, President Reagan signed into law The Medical Waste Tracking Act of 1988. Its purpose was to (1) charge the Environmental Protection Agency with the responsibility to establish a program to track medical waste from generation to disposal, (2) define medical waste, (3) establish acceptable techniques for treatment and disposal, and (4) establish a department with jurisdiction to enforce the new laws. Several states have implemented the federal guidelines and incorporated additional requirements. Some entities covered by the rules are any health care–related facility including, but not limited to, ambulatory surgical centers; blood banks and blood drawing centers; clinics, including medical, dental, and veterinary; clinical, diagnostic, pathologic, or biomedical research laboratories; emergency medical services; hospitals; long-term care facilities; minor emergency centers; occupational health clinics and clinical laboratories; and professional offices of physicians and dentists.

Medical waste is defined as *special waste from health care facilities* and is further defined as solid waste that, if improperly treated or handled, "may transmit infectious diseases." (For additional information, see the TJC Web site: http://www.jointcommission.org/). It comprises animal waste, bulk blood and blood products, microbiologic waste, pathologic waste, and sharps. The approved methods for treatment and disposition of medical waste are incineration, steam sterilization, burial, thermal inactivation, chemical disinfection, or encapsulation in a solid matrix.

Generators of medical waste must implement the following procedures:

- Employers of health care workers must establish and implement an infectious waste program.
- All biomedical waste should be placed in a bag marked with the biohazard symbol and then placed into a leak-proof container that is puncture resistant and equipped with a solid, tight-fitting lid. All containers must be clearly marked with the word **biohazard** or its symbol.
- All sharp instruments, such as needles, blades, and glass objects, should be placed into special puncture-resistant containers before placing them inside the bag and container.
- Needles should not be transported, recapped, bent, or broken by hand.
- All biomedical waste must then be disposed off according to one of the recommended procedures.
- Highly pathogenic waste should undergo preliminary treatment on-site.
- Potentially biohazardous material, such as blood or blood products and contaminated laboratory waste, cannot be directly discarded. Contaminated combustible waste can be incinerated. Contaminated noncombustible waste, such as glassware, should be autoclaved before being discarded. Special attention should be given to the discarding of syringes, needles, and broken glass that could also inflict accidental cuts or punctures. Appropriate containers should be used for discarding these sharp objects.

ACCIDENT DOCUMENTATION AND INVESTIGATION

Any accidents involving personal injuries, even minor ones, should be reported immediately to a supervisor. Manifestation of occupational illnesses and exposures to hazardous substances should also be reported. Serious injuries and illnesses, including those resulting in hospitalization, disability, or death, must be reported to OSHA or the state-administered program within 8 hours. Under OSHA regulations, employers are required to maintain records of occupational injuries and illnesses for the length of employment plus 30 years. The record-keeping requirements include a first report of injury, an accident investigation report, and an annual summary that is recorded on an OSHA injury and illness log (Form 300).

The first report of injury is used to notify the insurance company and the human resources or safety department that a workplace injury has occurred. The employee and the supervisor usually complete the report, which contains information on the employer and injured person, as well as the time and place, cause, and nature of the injury. The report is signed and dated; then, it is forwarded to the institution's risk manager or insurance representative.

The investigation report should include information on the injured person, a description of what happened, the cause of the accident (environmental or personal), other contributing factors, witnesses, the nature of the injury, and actions to be taken to prevent a recurrence. This report should be signed and dated by the person who conducted the investigation.

Annually, a log and summary of occupational injuries and illnesses should be completed and forwarded to the U.S. Department of Labor, Bureau of Labor Statistics'

OSHA injury and illness log (Form 300). The standardized form requests depersonalized information similar to the first report of injury and the accident investigation report. Information about every occupational death, nonfatal occupational illness, biologic or chemical exposure, and nonfatal occupational injury that involved loss of consciousness, restriction of work or motion, transfer to another job, or medical treatment (other than first aid) must be reported.

Because it is important to determine why and how an accident occurred, an accident investigation should be conducted. Most accidents can be traced to one of two underlying causes: environmental (unsafe conditions) or personal (unsafe acts). Environmental factors include inadequate safeguards, use of improper or defective equipment, hazards associated with the location, or poor housekeeping. Personal factors include improper laboratory attire, lack of skills or knowledge, specific physical or mental conditions, and attitude. The employee's positive motivation is important in all aspects of safety promotion and accident prevention.

It is particularly important that the appropriate authority be notified immediately if any individual sustains a contaminated needle puncture during blood collection or a cut during subsequent specimen processing or handling. For a summary of recommendations for the protection of laboratory workers, refer to *Protection of Laboratory Workers from Occupationally Acquired Infections; Approved Guideline*, Third Edition, M29-A3 (CLSI).

For additional student resources, please visit **the**Point® at http://thepoint.lww.com

---

questions

1. Which of the following standards requires that SDSs are accessible to all employees who come in contact with a hazardous compound?
   a. Hazard Communication Standard
   b. Bloodborne Pathogen Standard
   c. CDC Regulations
   d. Personal Protection Equipment Standard

2. Chemicals should be stored
   a. According to their chemical properties and classification
   b. Alphabetically, for easy accessibility
   c. Inside a safety cabinet with proper ventilation
   d. Inside a fume hood, if toxic vapors can be released when opened

3. Proper PPE in the chemistry laboratory for routine testing includes
   a. Impermeable lab coat with eye/face protection and appropriate disposable gloves

   b. Respirators with HEPA filter
   c. Gloves with rubberized sleeves
   d. Safety glasses for individuals not wearing contact lenses

4. A fire caused by a flammable liquid should be extinguished using which type of extinguisher?
   a. Class B
   b. Halogen
   c. Pressurized water
   d. Class C

5. Which of the following is the proper means of disposal for the type of waste?
   a. Microbiologic waste by steam sterilization
   b. Xylene into the sewer system
   c. Mercury by burial
   d. Radioactive waste by incineration

review questions (continued)

6. What are the major contributing factors to repetitive strain injuries?
   a. Position/posture, applied force, and frequency of repetition
   b. Inattention on the part of the laboratorian
   c. Temperature and vibration
   d. Fatigue, clumsiness, and lack of coordination

7. Which of the following are examples of nonionizing radiation?
   a. Ultraviolet light and microwaves
   b. Gamma rays and x-rays
   c. Alpha and beta radiation
   d. Neutron radiation

8. One liter of 4 N sodium hydroxide (strong base) in a glass 1 L beaker accidentally fell and spilled on the laboratory floor. The first step is to:
   a. Call 911
   b. Alert and evacuate those in the immediate area out of harm's way

   c. Throw some kitty litter on the spill
   d. Squirt water on the spill to dilute the chemical
   e. Neutralize with absorbing materials in a nearby spill kit

9. Of the following, which is NOT reportable to the Department of Labor?
   a. A laboratorian with a persistent cough that is only triggered at work
   b. A laboratorian that experienced a chemical burn
   c. A laboratorian that tripped in the lab and hit her head on the lab bench rendering her unconscious
   d. A laboratorian that was stuck by a contaminated needle after performing phlebotomy on a patient
   e. A laboratorian that forgot to wear his lab coat and gloves while diluting patient serum

bibliography and suggested reading

Allocca JA, Levenson HE. *Electrical and Electronic Safety*. Reston, VA: Reston Publishing Company; 1985.

American Chemical Society, Committee on Chemical Safety. Smith GW, ed. *Safety in Academic Chemistry Laboratories*. Washington, DC: American Chemical Society; 1985.

Boyle MP. Hazardous chemical waste disposal management. *Clin Lab Sci*. 1992;5:6.

Brown JW. Tuberculosis alert: an old killer returns. *MLO Med Lab Obs*. 1993;25:5.

Bryan RA. Recommendations for handling specimens from patients with confirmed or suspected Creutzfeldt-Jakob disease. *Lab Med*. 1984;15:50.

Centers for Disease Control and Prevention, National Institutes of Health. *Biosafety in Microbiological and Biomedical Laboratories*. 5th ed. Washington, DC: U.S. Government Printing Office; 2009.

Chervinski D. Environmental awareness: it's time to close the loop on waste reduction in the health care industry. *Adv Admin Lab*. 1994;3:4.

Clinical Laboratory Standards Institute (CLSI). *Clinical Laboratory Waste Management (Approved Guideline, GP05-A3)*. Wayne, PA: CLSI; 2011.

Clinical Laboratory Standards Institute (CLSI). *Clinical Laboratory Safety (Approved Guideline, GP17-A3)*. Wayne, PA: CLSI; 2012.

Clinical Laboratory Standards Institute (CLSI). *Protection of Laboratory Workers from Occupationally Acquired Infection (Approved Guideline, M29-A4)*. Wayne, PA: CLSI; 2014.

Committee on Hazardous Substances in the Laboratory, Assembly of Mathematical and Physical Sciences, National Research Council. *Prudent Practices for Handling Hazardous Chemicals in Laboratories*. Washington, DC: National Academies Press; 1981.

Furr AK. *Handbook of Laboratory Safety*. 5th ed. Boca Raton, FL: CRC Press; 2000.

Gile TJ. Hazard-communication program for clinical laboratories. *Clin Lab*. 1988;1:2.

Gile TJ. An update on lab safety regulations. *MLO Med Lab Obs*. 1995;27:3.

Gile TJ. *Complete Guide to Laboratory Safety*. Marblehead, MA: HCPro, Inc.; 2004.

Hayes DD. Safety considerations in the physician office laboratory. *Lab Med*. 1994;25:3.

Hazard communication. *Federal Register*. 1994;59:27.

Karcher RE. Is your chemical hygiene plan OSHA proof? *MLO Med Lab Obs*. 1993;25:7.

Le Sueur CL. A three-pronged attack against AIDS infection in the lab. *MLO Med Lab Obs*. 1989;21:37.

Miller SM. Clinical safety: dangers and risk control. *Clin Lab Sci*. 1992;5:6.

National Institute for Occupational Safety and Health (NIOSH). *NIOSH Pocket Guide to Chemical Hazards*. Atlanta, GA: Center for Disease Control; 2007.

National Institutes of Health, Radiation Safety Branch. *Radiation: The National Institutes of Health Safety Guide*. Washington, DC: U.S. Government Printing Office; 1979.

National Regulatory Committee, Committee on Hazardous Substances in the Laboratory. *Prudent Practices for the Handling of Hazardous Chemicals in Laboratories*. Washington, DC: National Academies Press; 1981.

National Regulatory Committee, Committee on Hazardous Substances in the Laboratory. *Prudent Practices for Disposal of Chemicals from Laboratories*. Washington, DC: National Academies Press; 1983.

National Regulatory Committee, Committee on the Hazardous Biological Substances in the Laboratory. *Biosafety in the Laboratory: Prudent Practices for the Handling and Disposal of Infectious Materials*. Washington, DC: National Academies Press; 1989.

National Safety Council (NSC). *Fundamentals of Industrial Hygiene*. 5th ed. Chicago, IL: NSC; 2002.

Occupational exposure to bloodborne pathogens; final rule. *Federal Register*. 1991;56:235.

Occupational Safety and Health Administration. Subpart Z 29CFR 1910.1000-1450.

Otto CH. Safety in health care: prevention of bloodborne diseases. *Clin Lab Sci*. 1992;5:6.

Pipitone DA. *Safe Storage of Laboratory Chemicals*. New York, NY: Wiley; 1984.

Rose SL. *Clinical Laboratory Safety*. Philadelphia, PA: JB Lippincott; 1984.

Rudmann SV, Jarus C, Ward KM, et al. Safety in the student laboratory: a national survey of university-based programs. *Lab Med*. 1993;24:5.

Stern A, Ries H, Flynn D, et al. Fire safety in the laboratory: part I. *Lab Med*. 1993;24:5.

Stern A, Ries H, Flynn D, et al. Fire safety in the laboratory: part II. *Lab Med*. 1993;24:6.

United Nations. *Globally Harmonized System of Classification and Labelling of Chemicals*. New York, NY; Geneva: United Nations; 2003.

Wald PH, Stave GM. *Physical and Biological Hazards of the Workplace*. New York, NY: Van Nostrand Reinhold; 1994.

3

Method Evaluation and Quality Control

MICHAEL W. ROGERS, CINDI BULLOCK LETSOS, MATTHEW P. A. HENDERSON, MONTE S. WILLIS, and CHRISTOPER R. McCUDDEN

chapter outline

(continues on page 50)

key terms

Accuracy
AMR
Bias
CLIA
Constant error
CRR
Descriptive statistics
Dispersion
Histograms
Levey-Jennings control chart
Limit of detection
Linear regression
Precision
Predictive values
Proficiency testing
Proportional error
Quality control
Random error
Reference interval
Reference method
SDI
Sensitivity
Shifts
Specificity
Systematic error
Trends

For additional student resources, please visit thePoint® at http://thepoint.lww.com

49

chapter objectives

Upon completion of this chapter, the clinical laboratorian should be able to do the following:

- Define the following terms: quality control, accuracy, precision, descriptive statistics, reference interval, random error, sensitivity, specificity, systematic error, and confidence intervals.
- Calculate the following: sensitivity, specificity, efficiency, predictive value, mean, median, range, variance, and standard deviation.
- Understand why statistics are needed for effective quality management.
- Read a descriptive statistics equation without fear.
- Understand the types, uses, and requirements for reference intervals.
- Understand the basic protocols used to verify or establish a reference interval.
- Appreciate how the test cutoff affects diagnostic performance.
- Evaluate laboratory data using multirules for quality control.
- Graph laboratory data and determine significant constant or proportional errors.
- Determine if there is a trend or a shift, given laboratory data.
- Discuss the processes involved in method selection and evaluation.
- Discuss proficiency testing programs in the clinical laboratory.
- Describe how a process can be systematically improved.

It is widely accepted that the majority of medical decisions are supported using laboratory data. It is therefore critical that results generated by the laboratory are accurate and provide the appropriate laboratory diagnostic information to assist the health care provider in treating patients. Determining and maintaining **accuracy** requires considerable effort and cost, entailing the use of a series of approaches depending on the complexity of the test. To begin, one must appreciate what *quality* is and how quality is measured and managed. To this end, it is vital to understand basic statistical concepts that enable the laboratorian to measure quality. Before implementing a new test, it is important to determine if the test is capable of performing acceptably by meeting or exceeding defined quality criteria; *method evaluation* is used to verify the acceptability of new methods prior to reporting patient results. Once a method has been implemented, it is essential that the laboratory ensures it remains valid over time; this is achieved by a process known as **quality control** (QC) and Quality Improvement/Assurance (see Chapter 4). This chapter describes basic statistical concepts and provides an overview of the procedures necessary to implement a new method and ensure its continued accuracy.

BASIC CONCEPTS

Each day, high-volume clinical laboratories generate thousands of results. This wealth of clinical laboratory data must be summarized and critically be reviewed to monitor test performance. The foundation for monitoring performance (known as QC) is **descriptive statistics**.

Descriptive Statistics: Measures of Center, Spread, and Shape

When examined closely, a collection of seemingly similar things always has at least slight differences for any given characteristic (e.g., smoothness, size, color, weight, volume, and potency). Similarly, laboratory data will have at least slight measurement differences. For example, if glucose on a given specimen is measured 100 times in a row, there would be a range of values obtained. Such differences in laboratory values can be a result of a variety of sources. Although measurements will differ, their values form patterns that can be visualized and analyzed collectively. Laboratorians view and describe these patterns using graphical representations and descriptive statistics (Fig. 3.1).

When comparing and analyzing collections or sets of laboratory data, patterns can be described by their center, spread, and shape. Although comparing the center of data is most common, comparing the spread can be even more powerful. Assessment of data **dispersion**, or spread, allows laboratorians to assess the predictability (and the lack of) in a laboratory test or measurement.

Measures of Center

The three most commonly used descriptions of the center of a data set (Fig. 3.2) are the mean, the median, and the mode. The *mean* is most commonly used and often called the *average*. The *median* is the "middle" point and is often used with skewed data so its calculation is not significantly affected by outliers. The *mode* is rarely used as a measure of the data's center but is more often used to describe data that seem to have two centers (i.e., bimodal). The mean is calculated by summing the observations and dividing by the number of the critically evaluated observations (Box 3.1).

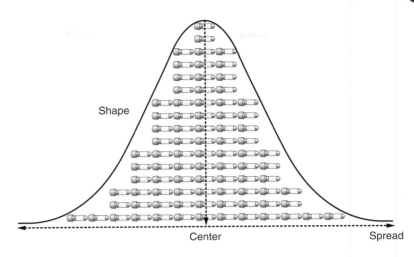

FIGURE 3.1 Basic measures of data include the center, spread, and shape.

Mean Equation:

$\sum$ — Add up ...

$\sum_{i=1}^{n} x_i$ — the data points (the x's) and ...

$\sum_{i=1}^{n} x_i / n$ — divide by the total number of data points (n)   (Eq. 3-1)

$\bar{x} \sum_{i=1}^{n} x_i / n$ — to find the mean ("$x$bar")

The summation sign, Σ, is an abbreviation for $(x_1 + x_2 + x_3 + \cdots + x_n)$ and is used in many statistical formulas. Often, the mean of a specific data set is called $\bar{x}$, or "x bar."

The median is the middle of the data after the data have been rank ordered. It is the value that divides the data in half. To determine the median, values are rank ordered from least to greatest and the middle value is selected. For example, given a sample of 5, 4, 6, 5, 3, 7, 5, the rank order of the points is 3, 4, 5, 5, 5, 6, 7. Because there are an odd number of values in the sample, the middle value (median) is 5; the value 5 divides the data in half. Given another sample with an even number of values 5, 4, 6, 8, 9, 7, the rank order

of the points is 4, 5, 6, 7, 8, 9. The two "middle" values are 6 and 7. Adding them yields 13 (6 + 7 = 13); division by 2 provides the median (13/2 = 6.5). The median value of 6.5 divides the data in half.

The mode is the most frequently occurring value in a data set. Although it is seldom used to describe data, it is referred to when in reference to the shape of data, a bimodal distribution, for example. In the sample 3, 4, 5, 5, 5, 6, 7, the value that occurs most often is 5. The mode of this set is then 5. The data set 3, 4, 5, 5, 5, 6, 7, 8, 9, 9, 9 has two modes, 5 and 9.

After describing the center of the data set, it is very useful to indicate how the data are distributed (spread). The spread represents the relationship of all the data points to the mean (Fig. 3.3). There are four commonly used descriptions of spread: (1) range, (2) standard deviation (SD), (3) coefficient of variation (CV), and (4) standard deviation index (SDI). The easiest measure of spread to understand is the range. The range is simply the largest value in the data minus the smallest value, which represents the extremes of data one might encounter. Standard deviation (also called "s," SD, or σ) is the most frequently used measure of variation. Although calculating SD can seem somewhat intimidating, the concept is straightforward; in fact, all of the descriptive statistics and even the inferential statistics have a combination of mathematical operations that are by themselves no more complex than a square root. The SD and, more specifically, the variance represent the "average" distance from the center of the data (the mean) and every value in the data set. The CV

FIGURE 3.2 The center can be defined by the mean (x-bar character), median, or mode.

BOX 3.1 Sources of Analytic Variability

Operator technique	Environmental conditions (e.g., temperature, humidity)
Instrument differences	Reagents
Test accessories	Power surges
Contamination	Matrix effects (hemolysis, lipemia, serum proteins)

FIGURE 3.3 Spread is defined by the standard deviation and coefficient of variation.

Spread

allows a laboratorian to compare SDs with different units and reflects the SDs in percentages. The **SDI** is a calculation to show the number of SDs a value is from the target mean. Similar to CV, it is a way to reflect ranges in a relative manner regardless of how low or high the values are.

Range is one description of the spread of data. It is simply the difference between the highest and lowest data points: range = high − low. For the sample 5, 4, 6, 5, 3, 7, 5, the range is 7 − 3 = 4. The range is often a good measure of dispersion for small samples of data. It does have a serious drawback; the range is susceptible to extreme values or outliers (i.e., wrong quality control material or wrong data entry).

To calculate the SD of a data set, it is easiest to first determine the variance (s^2). Variance is similar to the mean in that it is an average. Variance is the average of the squared distances of all values from the mean:

$$s^2 = \sum_{i=1}^{n}(x_i - \bar{x})/n - 1 \qquad \text{(Eq. 3-2)}$$

As a measure of dispersion, variance represents the difference between each value and the average of the data. Given the values 5, 4, 6, 5, 3, 7, 5, variance can be calculated as shown below:

$\bar{x}$	$(5+4+6+5+3+7+5)/7 = 5$
$(x_i - \bar{x})$	$(5-5)+(4-5)+(6-5)$
	$+(5-5)+(3-5)$
	$+(7-5)+(5-5)$
$(x_i - \bar{x})^2$	$(0)2+(-1)2+(1)2+(0)^2$
	$+(-2)2+(2)2+(0)^2$ (Eq. 3-3)
$\sum_{i=1}^{n}(x_i - \bar{x})^2$	$0+1+1+0+4+4$
	$+0 = 10$
$\sum_{i=1}^{n}(x_i - \bar{x})^2/n - 1$	$10/(7-1) = 10/6$
$s^2 \sum_{i=1}^{n}(x_i - \bar{x})^2/n - 1$	1.67

To calculate the SD (or "s"), simply take the square root of the variance:

$$s(\sigma) = \sqrt{s^2} = \sqrt{\sum_{i=1}^{n}(x_i - \bar{x})^2/n - 1} \qquad \text{(Eq. 3-4)}$$

Although it is important to understand how these measures are calculated, most analyzer/instruments, laboratory information systems, and laboratory statistical software packages determine these automatically. SD describes the distribution of all data points around the mean.

Another way of expressing SD is in terms of the CV. The CV is calculated by dividing the SD by the mean and multiplying by 100 to express it as a percentage:

$$CV(\%) = \frac{100s}{x} \qquad \text{(Eq. 3-5)}$$

The CV simplifies comparison of SDs of test results expressed in different units and concentrations. As shown in Table 3.1, analytes measured at different concentrations can have a drastically different SD but a comparable CV. The CV is used extensively to summarize QC data. The CV of highly precise analyzers can be lower than 1%. For values at the low end of the analytical measurement, the acceptable CV can range as high as 50% as allowed by CLIA.

Another way of expressing SD is in terms of the SDI, where the SDI is calculated by dividing the difference of the (measured laboratory value or mean − target or group mean)/assigned or group SD. The SDI can be a negative or positive value.

$$SDI = \frac{(\text{laboratory mean} - \text{group mean})}{\text{Group SD}} \qquad \text{(Eq. 3-6)}$$

Measures of Shape

Although there are hundreds of different "shapes"—distributions—that data sets can exhibit, the most commonly discussed is the Gaussian distribution (also called normal distribution; Fig. 3.4). The Gaussian distribution describes many continuous laboratory variables and shares several unique characteristics: the mean, median, and mode are identical; the distribution is symmetric—meaning half

FSH Concentration	SD	CV	βhCG Concentration	SD	CV
1	0.09	9.0	10	0.8	8.0
5	0.25	5.0	100	5.5	5.5
10	0.40	4.0	1,000	52.0	5.2
25	1.20	4.8	10,000	500.00	5.0
100	3.80	3.8	100,000	4,897.0	4.9

TABLE 3.1   Comparison of SD and CV for Two Different Analytes

SD, standard deviation; CV, coefficient of variation; FSH, follicle-stimulating hormone; βhCG, β-human chorionic gonadotropin.

the values fall to the left of the mean and the other half fall to the right with the peak of the curve representing the average of the data. This symmetrical shape is often called a "bell curve."

The total area under the Gaussian curve is 1.0, or 100%. Much of the area—68.3%—under the "normal" curve is between ±1 SD ($\mu \pm 1\sigma$) (Fig. 3.5A). Most of the area—95.4%—under the "normal" curve is between ±2 SDs ($\mu \pm 2\sigma$; Fig. 3.5B). And almost all of the area—99.7%—under the "normal" curve is between ±3 SDs ($\mu \pm 3\sigma$) (Fig. 3.5C). (Note that μ represents the average of the total population, whereas the mean of a specific data set is $\bar{x}$, or "x bar.")

The "68–95–99 Rule" summarizes the above relationships between the area under a Gaussian distribution and the SD. In other words, given any Gaussian distributed data, ≈68% of the data fall between ±1 SD from the mean; ≈95% of the data fall between ±2 SDs from the mean; and ≈99% fall between ±3 SDs from the mean. Likewise, if you selected a value in a data set that is Gaussian distributed, there is a 0.68 chance of it lying between ±1 SD from the mean; there is a 0.95 likelihood of it lying between ±2 SDs; and there is a 0.99 probability of it lying between ±3 SDs. (Note: the terms "chance," "likelihood," and "probability" are synonymous in this example.)

As will be discussed in the **reference interval** section, most patient data are not normally distributed. These data may be skewed or exhibit multiple centers (bimodal, trimodal, etc.) as shown in Figure 3.6. Plotting data in **histograms** as shown in the figure is a useful and an

easy way to visualize distribution. However, there are also mathematical analyses (e.g., normality tests) that can confirm if data fit a given distribution. The importance of recognizing whether data are or are not normally distributed is related to the way it can be statistically analyzed.

Descriptive Statistics of Groups of Paired Observations

While the use of basic descriptive statistics is satisfactory for examining a single method, laboratorians frequently need to compare two different methods. This is most commonly encountered in comparison of methods (COM) experiments. A COM experiment involves measuring patient specimens by both an existing (reference) method and a new (test) method (described in the Reference Interval and Method Evaluation sections later). The data obtained from these comparisons consist of two measurements for each patient specimen. It is easiest to visualize and summarize the paired-method comparison data graphically (Fig. 3.7). By convention, the values obtained by the **reference method** are plotted on the x-axis, and the values obtained by the test method are plotted on the y-axis.

In Figure 3.7, the agreement between the two methods is estimated from the straight line that best fits the points. Whereas visual estimation may be used to draw the line, a statistical technique known as **linear regression** analysis provides objective an objective measure of the line of best fit for the data. Three factors are generated in a linear regression—the slope, the y-intercept, and the

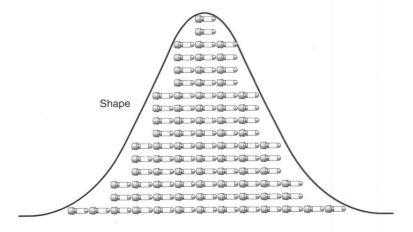

FIGURE 3.4 Shape is defined by how the distribution of data relates the center. This is an example of data that have "normal" or Gaussian distribution.

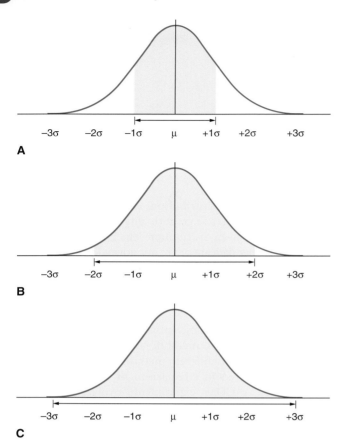

FIGURE 3.5 A normal distribution contains **(A)** ≈68% of the results within ±1 SD (1s or 1σ), **(B)** 95% of the results within ±2s (2σ), and **(C)** ≈99% of the results within ±3σ.

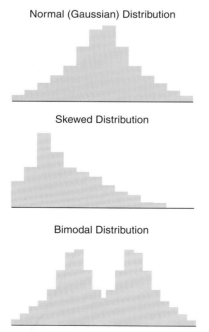

FIGURE 3.6 Examples of normal (Gaussian), skewed, and bimodal distributions. The type of statistical analysis that is performed to analyze the data depends on the distribution (shape).

FIGURE 3.7 A generic example of a linear regression. A linear regression compares two tests and yields important information about systematic and random error. Systematic error is indicated by changes in the y-intercept (constant error) and the slope (proportional error). Random error is indicated by the standard error of the estimate ($S_{y/x}$); $S_{y/x}$ basically represents the distance of each point from the regression line. The correlation coefficient indicates the strength of the relationship between the tests.

correlation coefficient (r). In Figure 3.7, there is a linear relationship between the two methods over the entire range of values. The linear regression is defined by the equation $y = mx + b$. The slope of the line is described by m, and the value of the y-intercept (b) is determined by plugging $x = 0$ into the equation and solving for y. The correlation coefficient (r) is a measure of the strength of the relationship between the two methods. The correlation coefficient can have values from −1 to 1, with the sign indicating the direction of relationship between the two variables. A positive r indicates that both variables increase and decrease together, whereas a negative r indicates that as one variable increases, the other decreases. An r value of 0 indicates no relationship, whereas $r = 1.0$ indicates a perfect relationship. Although many equate high positive values of r (0.95 or higher) with excellent agreement between the test and comparative methods, most clinical chemistry comparisons should have correlation coefficients greater than 0.98. When r is less than 0.99, the regression formula can underestimate the slope and overestimate the y-intercept. The absolute value of the correlation coefficient can be increased by widening the concentration range of samples being compared. However, if the correlation coefficient remains less than 0.99, then alternate regression statistics or modified COM value sets should be used to derive more realistic estimates of the regression, slope, and y-intercept.[1,2] Visual inspection of data is essential prior to drawing conclusions from

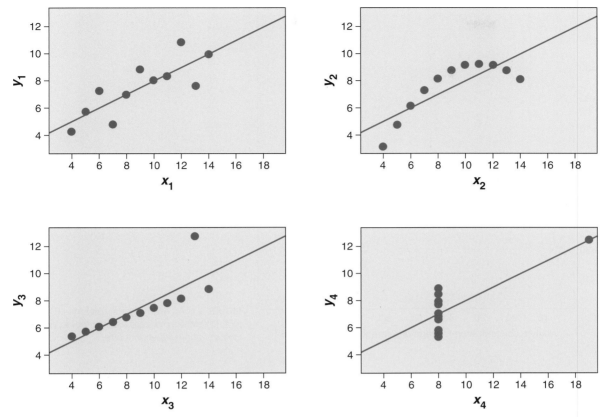

FIGURE 3.8 Anscombe's quartet demonstrates the need to visually inspect data. In each panel, $y = 0.5\,x + 3$, $r^2 = 0.816$, $S_{y/x} = 4.1$.

the summary statistics as demonstrated by the famous Anscombe quartet (Fig. 3.8). In this data set, the slope, y-intercept, and correlation coefficients are all identical, yet visual inspection reveals that the underlying data are completely different.

An alternate approach to visualizing paired data is the difference plot, which is also known as the Bland-Altman plot (Fig. 3.9). A difference plot indicates either the percent or absolute **bias** (difference) between the reference and test method values over the average range of values. This approach permits simple comparison of the differences to previously established maximum limits. As is evident in Figure 3.9, it is easier to visualize any concentration-dependent differences than by linear regression analysis. In this example, the percent difference is clearly greatest at lower concentrations, which may not be obvious from a regression plot.

The difference between test and reference method results is called *error*. There are two kinds of error measured in COM experiments: random and systematic. **Random error** is present in all measurements and can be either positive or negative, typically a combination of both positive and negative errors on both sides of the assigned target value. Random error can be a result of many factors including instrument, operator, reagent, and environmental variation. Random error is calculated as the SD of the points about the regression line ($S_{y/x}$). $S_{y/x}$ essentially refers to average

distance of the data from the regression line (Fig. 3.7). The higher the $S_{y/x}$, the wider is the scatter and the higher is the amount of random error. In Figure 3.7, the $S_{y/x}$ is 5.0. If the points were perfectly in line with the linear regression, the $S_{y/x}$ would equal 0.0, indicating there would not be any random error. $S_{y/x}$ is also known as the standard error of the estimate S_E (Box 3.2).

Systematic error influences observations consistently in one direction (higher or lower). The measures of slope and y-intercept provide estimates of the systematic error. Systematic error can be further broken down into **constant error** and **proportional error**. Constant systematic error exists when there is a continual difference between the test method and the comparative method values, regardless of the concentration. In Figure 3.7, there is a constant difference of 6.0 between the test method values and the comparative method values. This constant difference, reflected in the y-intercept, is called *constant systematic error*. Proportional error exists when the differences between the test method and the comparative method values are proportional to the analyte concentration. Proportional error is present when the slope is 1. In the example, the slope of 0.89 represents the proportional error, where samples will be underestimated in a concentration-dependent fashion by the test method compared with the reference method; the error is proportional, because it will increase with the analyte concentration.

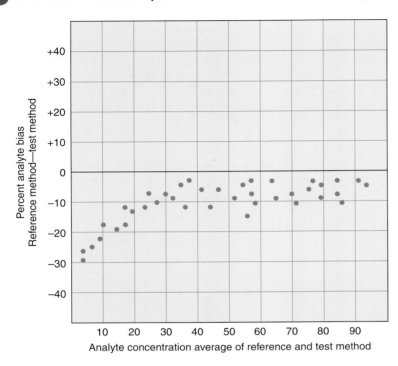

FIGURE 3.9 An example of a difference (Bland-Altman) plot. Difference plots are a useful tool to visualize concentration-dependent error.

Inferential Statistics

The next level of complexity beyond paired descriptive statistics is inferential statistics. Inferential statistics are used to draw conclusions (inferences) regarding the means or SDs of two sets of data. Inferential statistical analyses are most commonly encountered in research studies, but can also be used in COM studies.

An important consideration for inferential statistics is the distribution of the data (shape). The distribution of the data determines what kind of inferential statistics can be used to analyze the data. Normally distributed (Gaussian) data are typically analyzed using what are known as "parametric" tests, which include a Student's *t*-test or analysis of variance (ANOVA). Data that are not normally distributed require a "nonparametric" analysis. Nonparametric tests are encountered in reference interval studies, where population data are often skewed. For reference interval studies, nonparametric methods typically rely on ranking or ordering the values in order to determine upper and lower percentiles. While many software packages are capable of performing either parametric or nonparametric analyses, it is important for the user to understand that the type of data (shape) dictates which statistical test is

appropriate for the analysis. An inappropriate analysis of sound data can yield the wrong conclusion and lead to erroneous provider decisions and patient care/impact consequences.

METHOD EVALUATION

The value of clinical laboratory service is based on its ability to provide reliable, accurate test results and optimal test information for patient management. At the heart of providing these services is the performance of a testing method. To maximize the usefulness of a test, laboratorians undergo a process in which a method is selected and evaluated for its usefulness to those who will be using the test. This process is carefully undertaken to produce results within medically acceptable error limits to help providers maximally manage/treat their patients.

Currently, clinical laboratories more often select and evaluate methods that were commercially developed instead of developing their own. Most commercially developed tests have U.S. Food and Drug Administration (FDA) approval, only requiring a laboratory to provide a limited but regulatory mandated evaluation of a method to verify the manufacturer's performance claims and to see how well the method works specifically in the laboratory and patient population served.

Regulatory Aspects of Method Evaluation (Alphabet Soup)

The Centers for Medicare and Medicaid Services (CMS) and the Federal Drug Agency (FDA) are the primary government agencies that influence laboratory testing methods in the United States. The FDA regulates laboratory instruments and reagents, and the CMS regulates the

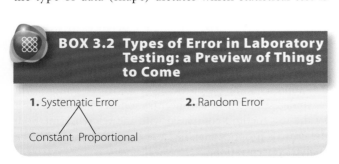

BOX 3.2 Types of Error in Laboratory Testing: a Preview of Things to Come

1. Systematic Error   2. Random Error

Constant   Proportional

Clinical Laboratory Improvement Amendments (**CLIA**).[3] Most large laboratories in the United States are accredited by the College of American Pathologists (CAP) and The Joint Commission (TJC; formerly the Joint Commission on Accreditation of Healthcare Organizations [JCAHO]), which impacts how method evaluations need to be performed. Professional organizations such as the National Academy of Clinical Biochemistry (NACB) and the American Association for Clinical Chemistry (AACC) also contribute important guidelines and method evaluations that influence how method evaluations are performed. Future trends are seeing additional regulatory services being used by both larger laboratories and smaller laboratories (i.e., Physician clinics and public health departments), Commission of Office Laboratory Accreditation (COLA) is an example of additional regulatory services available to clinical laboratories regardless of their size, test menu, and test volume. Regardless of which regulatory agency is used the acceptable and mandatory standards of compliance guidelines are set by CLIA, FDA, and TJC.

The FDA "Office of In Vitro Diagnostic Device Evaluation and Safety" (OIVD) regulates diagnostic tests. Tests are categorized into one of three groups: (1) waived, (2) moderate complexity, and (3) high complexity. Waived tests are cleared by the FDA to be so simple that they are most likely accurate and most importantly would pose negligible risk of harm to the patient if not performed correctly. A few examples of waived testing include dipstick tests, qualitative pregnancy testing, rapid strep, rapid HIV, rapid HCV, and glucose monitors. For waived testing, personnel requirements are not as stringent as moderately complex testing or high-complexity testing, but there are still training, competency, and quality control mandatory requirements. Most automated methods are rated as moderate complexity, while manual methods and methods requiring more interpretation are rated as high complexity. The patient management/treatment impact is also a factor in determining whether a test is waived, moderate complexity or high complexity. The CLIA final rule requires that waived tests simply follow the manufacturer's instructions. Both moderate- and high-complexity tests require in-laboratory validation. However, FDA-approved nonwaived tests may undergo a more basic validation process (Table 3.2), whereas a more extensive validation is required for tests developed by laboratories (Table 3.2). While the major requirements for testing validation are driven by the CLIA, TJC and CAP essentially require the same types of experiments to be performed, with a few additions. It is these rules that guide the way tests in the clinical chemistry laboratory are selected and validated.

DEFINITIONS BOX

AACC American Association for Clinical Chemistry

CAP College of American Pathologists

CLIA Clinical Laboratory Improvement Amendments

CLSI Clinical Laboratory and Standards Institute (formerly NCCLS)

CMS Centers for Medicare and Medicaid Services

COLA Commission of Office Laboratory Accreditation

FDA Food and Drug Administration

NACB National Academy of Clinical Biochemistry

OIVD Office of In Vitro Diagnostic Device Evaluation and Safety

TJC The Joint Commission

 TABLE 3.2 **General CLIA Regulations of Method Validation**

Nonwaived FDA–Approved Tests	1. Demonstrate test performance comparable to that established by the manufacturer.
	   a. Accuracy
	   b. Precision
	   c. Reportable range
	2. Verify reference (normal) values appropriate for patient population

Nonwaived FDA–Approved Tests Modified or Developed by Laboratory	1. Determine
	   a. Accuracy
	   b. Precision
	   c. Analytic sensitivity
	   d. Analytic specificity (including interfering substances)
	   e. Reportable range of test results
	   f. Reference/normal ranges
	   g. Other performance characteristics
	   h. Calibration and control procedures

From Clinical Laboratory Improvement Amendments of 1988; final rule. *Fed Regist.* 7164 [42 CFR 493 1253]: Department of Health and Human Services, Centers for Medicare and Medicaid Services; 1992.

FIGURE 3.10 A flowchart on the process of method selection, evaluation, and monitoring. (Adapted from Westgard JO, Quam E, Barry T. *Basic QC Practices: Training in Statistical Quality Control for Healthcare Laboratories*. Madison, WI: Westgard Quality Corp.; 1998.)

Method Selection

Evaluating a method is a labor-intensive costly process—so why select a new method? There are many reasons, including enhanced provider utilization in effectively treating/managing patients, reducing costs, staffing needs, improving the overall quality of results, increasing provider satisfaction, and improving overall efficiency. Selecting a test method starts with the collection of technical information about a particular test from colleagues, scientific presentations, the scientific literature, and manufacturer claims. Practical considerations should also be addressed at this point, such as the type and volume of specimen to be tested, the required throughput and turnaround time, your testing needs, testing volumes, cost, break-even financial analysis, calibration, Quality Control Plan, space needs, disposal needs, personnel requirements, safety considerations, alternative strategies to supply testing (i.e., referral testing laboratories), etc. Most importantly, the test should be able to meet the clinical task by having specific analytic performance standards that will accurately assist in the management and ultimately the treatment of patients. Specific information that should be discovered about a test you might bring into the laboratory includes analytic sensitivity, analytic specificity, linear range, interfering substances, estimates of precision and accuracy, and test-specific regulatory requirements. The process of method selection is the beginning of a process to bring in a new test for routine use (Fig. 3.10).

Method Evaluation

A short, initial evaluation should be carried out before the complete method evaluation. This preliminary evaluation should include the analysis of a series of *standards* to verify the linear range and the replicate analysis (at least eight measurements) of two controls to obtain estimates of short-term precision. If any results fall short of the specifications published in the method's product information sheet (package insert), the method's manufacturer should be consulted. Without a successful initial evaluation, including precision and linear range minimal studies, there is no opportunity

to proceed with the method evaluation until the initial issues have been resolved. Also, without improvement in the method, more extensive evaluations are pointless.[4]

First Things First: Determine Imprecision and Inaccuracy

The first determinations (estimates) to be made in a method evaluation are the *precision* and *accuracy*, which should be compared with the maximum allowable error budgets based on medical criteria and regulatory guidelines. If the precision or accuracy exceeds the maximum allowable error budgets, it is unacceptable and must be modified and reevaluated or rejected. Precision is the dispersion of repeated measurements around a mean (true level), as shown in Figure 3.11A with the mean represented as the bull's-eye. Random analytic error is the cause of lack of precision or the imprecision in a test. Precision is estimated from studies in which multiple aliquots of the same specimen (with a constant concentration) are analyzed repetitively.

Accuracy, or the difference between a measured value and its actual value, is due to the presence of a systematic error, as represented in Figure 3.11B. Systematic error can be due to constant or proportional error and is estimated from three types of study: (1) recovery, (2) interference, and (3) a COM study.

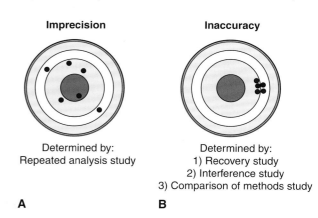

FIGURE 3.11 Graphic representation of **(A)** imprecision and **(B)** inaccuracy on a dartboard configuration with bull's-eye in the center.

DEFINITIONS BOX

Analytic sensitivity Ability of a method to detect small quantities or small changes in concentration of an analyte.

Analytic specificity Ability of a method to detect only the analyte it is designed to determine, also known as cross-reactivity.

AMR (analytic measurement range) Also known as linear or dynamic range. Range of analyte concentrations that can be directly measured without dilution, concentration, or other pretreatment.

CRR (clinically reportable range) Range of analyte that a method can quantitatively report, allowing for dilution, concentration, or other pretreatment used to extend AMR.

LoD (limit of detection) Lowest amount of analyte accurately detected by a method.

LoQ (limit of quantitation) Lowest amount of analyte that can be reported while achieving a precision target (e.g., lowest concentration at which a CV of 10% may be achieved).

SDI (standard deviation index) Refers to the difference between the measured value and the mean expressed as a number of SDs. An SDI = 0 indicates the value is accurate or in 100% agreement; an SDI = 3 is 3 SDs away from the target (mean) and indicates inaccuracy. SDI may be positive or negative.

DEFINITIONS BOX

Precision Dispersion of repeated measurements about the mean due to analytic error.

Accuracy How close the measured value is to the true value due to systematic error, which can be either constant or proportional.

Bias Difference between the true value and the measured value.

Systematic error Error always in one direction (may be constant or proportional).

Constant error Type of systematic error in the sample direction and magnitude; the magnitude of change is constant and not dependent on the amount of analyte.

Proportional error Type of systematic error where the magnitude changes as a percent of the analyte present, error dependent on analyte concentration.

Random error Error varies from sample to sample. Causes include instrument instability, temperature variations, reagent variation, handling techniques, and operator variables.

Total error Random error plus systematic error.

SDI Standard deviation index. ((Test method value) – (Reference method value))/(Reference method SD), analogous to **Z-score**.

Measurement of Imprecision

Method evaluation begins with a **precision** study. This estimates the random error associated with the test method and detects any problems affecting its reproducibility. It is recommended that this study be performed over a 10- to 20-day period, incorporating one or two analytic runs (runs with patient samples or QC materials) per day, preferred is an AM run and a PM run.[5,6] A common precision study is a $2 \times 2 \times 10$ study, where two controls are run twice a day (AM and PM) for 10 days. The rationale for performing the evaluation of precision over many days is logical. Running multiple samples on the same day does a good job of estimating precision within a single day (simple precision) but underestimates long-term changes and testing variables that occur over time. By running multiple samples on different days, a better estimation of the random error over time is given. It is important that more than one concentration be tested in these studies, with materials ideally spanning the clinically appropriate and analytical measurement range of concentrations. For glucose, this might include samples in the hyperglycemic range (150 mg/dL) and the hypoglycemic range (50 mg/dL). After these data are collected, the mean, SD, CV, and SDI are calculated. An example of a precision study from our laboratory is shown in Figure 3.12.

The random error or imprecision associated with the test procedure is indicated by the SD and the CV. The within-run imprecision is indicated by the SD of the controls analyzed within one run. The total imprecision may be obtained from the SD of control data with one or two data points accumulated per day. The total imprecision is the most accurate assessment of performance that would affect the values a provider might see and reflects differences in operators, pipettes, and variations in environmental changes such as temperature, reagent stability, etc. In practice, however, within-run imprecision is used more commonly than total imprecision. An inferential statistical technique, ANOVA, is then used to analyze the available precision data to provide estimates of the within-run, between-run, and total imprecision.[7]

Acceptable Performance Criteria: Precision Studies

During an evaluation of vitamin B_{12} in the laboratory, a precision study was performed for a new test method (Fig. 3.12). Several concentrations of vitamin B_{12} were run twice daily (in duplicate) for 10 days, as shown in Figure 3.12 (for simplicity, only one concentration is shown). The data are represented in the precision plot in Figure 3.12 ($\approx$76 pg/mL). The amount of variability between runs is represented by different colors, over 10 days (x-axis). The CV was then calculated for within-run, between-run, and between-days. The total SD, estimated at 2.3, is then compared with medical decision levels or medically required standards based on the analyte (Table 3.3). The acceptability of analytic error is based on how the test is to be used to make clinical interpretations.[8,9] In this case, the medically required SD limit is 4.8, based on mandated CLIA error budgets. The determination

FIGURE 3.12 An example of a precision study for vitamin B_{12}. The data represent analysis of a control sample run in duplicate twice a day (*red* and *black circles*) for 10 days (*x*-axis). Data are presented as standard deviation index (SDI). SDI refers to the difference between the measured value and the mean expressed as a number of SDs. An imprecision study is designed to detect random error.

Precision estimate
User's Concentration: 76.78

	Within Run	Between Run	Between Day	Total	Medically Required	Verification Value (95%)	Pass/Fail
Std. Dev	1.06	0.45	1.37	**1.79**	**4.80**	6.2	Pass
% CV	1.4	0.6	1.8	**2.3**	6.3		
df	18	–	–	**15**			

of whether long-term precision is adequate is based on the total imprecision being less than one-third of the total allowable error (total imprecision, in this case, 1.6; selection of one-third total allowable error for imprecision is based on Westgard[10]). In the case that the value is greater than the total allowable error (1.79 in our example), the test can pass as long as the difference between one-third total allowable error and the determined allowable error is not statistically significant. In our case, the 1.79 was not statistically different from 1.6 (1/3 × 4.8), and the test passed our imprecision studies (Fig. 3.12). The one-third of total error is a run of thumb; some laboratories may choose one-fourth of the total error for analytes that are very precise and accurate. It is not recommended to use all of the allowable error for imprecision (random error) as it leaves no room for systematic error (bias or inaccuracy).

DEFINITIONS BOX

Recovery Ability of an analytic test to measure a known amount of analyte; a known amount of analyte is added to real sample matrices.

Interference Effect of (a) compound(s) on the accuracy of detection of a particular analyte.

Interferents Substances that cause interference.

Matrix Body component (e.g., fluid and urine) in which the analyte is to be measured.

TABLE 3.3 **Performance Standards for Common Clinical Chemistry Analytes as Defined by the CLIA**

Calcium, total	Target ±1.0 mg/dL
Chloride	Target ±5%
Cholesterol, total	Target ±10%
Cholesterol, HDL	Target ±30%
Glucose	Greater of target ±6 mg/dL or ±10%
Potassium	Target ±0.5 mmol/L
Sodium	Target ±4 mmol/L
Total protein	Target ±10%
Triglycerides	Target ±25%
Urea nitrogen	Greater of target ±2 mg/dL or ±9%
Uric acid	Target ±17%

Reprinted from Centers for Disease Control and Prevention (CDC), Centers for Medicare and Medicaid Services (CMS), Health and Human Services. Medicare, Medicaid, and CLIA programs; laboratory requirements relating to quality systems and certain personnel qualifications. *Final rule. Fed Regist.* 2003;68:3639–3714, with permission.

Estimation of Inaccuracy

Once method imprecision is estimated and deemed acceptable, the determination of accuracy can begin.[6] Accuracy is estimated using three different types of studies: (1) recovery, (2) interference, and (3) patient sample comparison.

Recovery Studies

Recovery studies will show whether a method is able to accurately measure an analyte. In a recovery experiment, a small aliquot of concentrated analyte is added (spiked) into a patient sample (matrix) and then measured by the method being evaluated. The amount recovered is the

	Ca²⁺ Measured in Matrix	Ca²⁺ Added	Ca²⁺ Recovered	% Recovery
Baseline	7.5 mg/dL	NA	NA	NA
Sample 1	8.35 mg/dL	0.95 mg/dL	0.85 mg/dL	89%
Sample 2	9.79 mg/dL	2.38 mg/dL	2.29 mg/dL	96%

Calculation of % recovery

$$\% \text{ Recovered} = \frac{(\text{Measured in spike sample}) - (\text{Measured in baseline})}{\text{Concentration added}} \times 100$$

e.g., Calculation for Sample 1

$$\% \text{ Recovered} = \frac{(8.35 \text{ mg/dL}) - (7.5 \text{ mg/dL})}{0.95 \text{ mg/dL}} \times 100$$

% Recovered = 89%

FIGURE 3.13 An example of a sample recovery study for total calcium. A sample is spiked with known amounts of calcium in a standard matrix, and recovery is determined as shown. Recovery studies are designed to detect proportional error in an assay.

difference between the spiked sample and the patient sample (unmodified). The purpose of this type of study is to determine how much of the analyte can be detected (recovered) in the presence of all the other compounds in the matrix. The original patient samples (matrix) should not be diluted more than 10% so that the physiological (biological and protein components) matrix solution is minimally affected. An actual example of a recovery study for total calcium is illustrated in Figure 3.13; the results are expressed as percentage recovered. The performance standard for calcium, defined by CLIA, is the target value ±1.0 mg/dL (see Table 3.3). Recovery of calcium in this example exceeds this standard at the two calcium levels tested and therefore acceptable (Fig. 3.13).

Interference Studies

Interference studies are designed to determine if specific compounds affect the accuracy of laboratory tests. Common interferences encountered in the laboratory include hemolysis (broken red blood cells and their contents), icterus (high bilirubin), and turbidity (particulate matter or lipids), which can affect the measurement of many analytes. Interferents often affect tests by absorbing or scattering light, but they can also react with the reagents or affect reaction rates used to measure a given analyte.

Interference experiments are typically performed by adding the potential interferent to patient samples.[11] If an effect is observed, the concentration of the interferent is lowered sequentially to determine the concentration at which test results are not clinically affected (or minimally affected). It is common practice to flag results with unacceptably high levels of an interferent. Results may be reported with cautionary comments or not reported at all. An example of an interference study performed in one laboratory is shown in Figure 3.14. When designing a method validation study, potential interferents should be selected from literature reviews and specific references. Other excellent resources include Young[12] and Siest and Galteau.[13] Common interferences, such as hemolysis,

lipemia, bilirubin, anticoagulant, and preservatives, are tested by the manufacturer. Glick and Ryder[14,15] published "interferographs" for clinical chemistry instruments, which relate analyte concentration measure to interferent concentration. They have also demonstrated that considerable expense can be saved by the acquisition of instruments that minimize hemoglobin, triglyceride, and bilirubin interference.[16] It is good laboratory practice and a regulatory requirement to consider interferences as part of any method validation. In the clinical laboratory, interference studies "in vitro" are often difficult, and standardized experiments are often suspect as to reflecting the actual actions "in vivo." Proper instrumentation and critical literature reviews are often the best options for determining interference acceptability guidelines.

Pooled TnI Concentration = 0.0295 ng/mL			
Sample #	Hemolysate (Hg) g/dL	TnI (ng/mL)	% Bias
1	<0.15	0.0295	
2	0.14	0.0255	−13.6
3	0.25	0.0220	−25.4
4	0.36	0.0205	−30.5
5	0.48	0.0200	−32.0
6	0.60	0.0180	−39.0

Calculation of Interference

$$\text{Interference} = \frac{\text{Concentration with interference added}}{\text{Concentration without interference}}$$

Bias = Interference − concentration without interference
Bias % = Bias × 100

FIGURE 3.14 An example of an interference study for troponin I (TnI). Increasing amounts of hemolysate (lysed red blood cells, a common interference) were added to a sample with elevated TnI of 0.295 ng/mL. Bias is calculated based on the difference between the baseline and hemolyzed samples. The data are corrected for the dilution with hemolysate.

COM Studies

A method comparison experiment examines patient samples by the method being evaluated (test method) with a reference method. It is used primarily to estimate systematic error in actual patient samples, and it may offer the type of systematic error (proportional vs. constant). Ideally, the test method is compared with a standardized reference method (gold standard), a method with acceptable accuracy in comparison with its imprecision. Many times, reference methods are laborious and time consuming, as is the case with the ultracentrifugation methods of determining cholesterol. Because most laboratories are understaffed or do not have the technical expertise required to perform reference methods, most test methods are compared with those routinely used. These routine tests have their own particular inaccuracies, so it is important to determine what inaccuracies they might have that are documented in the literature. If the new test method is to replace the routine method, differences between the two should be well characterized. Also extensive documented communications with all providers and staff must be performed before implementation.

To compare a test method with a comparative method, it is recommended by Westgard et al.[6] and CLIA[17] that 40 to 100 specimens be run by each method on the same day over 8 to 20 days (preferably within 4 hours), with specimens spanning the clinical range and representing a diversity of pathologic conditions. Samples should cover the full analytical measurement range, and it is recommended that 25% be lower than the reference range, 50% should be in the reference range, and 25% should be higher than the reference range. Additional samples at the medical decision points should be a priority during the COM. As an extra measure of QC, specimens should be analyzed in duplicate. Otherwise, experimental results must be critically reviewed by the laboratory director and evaluation staff comparing test and comparative method results immediately after analysis. Samples with large differences should be repeated to rule out technical errors as the source of variation. Daily analysis of two to five patient specimens should be followed for at least 8 days if 40 specimens are compared and for 20 days if 100 specimens are compared in replication studies.[17]

A plot of the test method data (y-axis) versus the comparative method (x-axis) helps to visualize the data generated in a COM test (Fig. 3.15A).[18] As described earlier, if the two methods correlate perfectly, the data pairs plotted as concentration values from the reference method (x) versus the evaluation method (y) will produce a straight line ($y = mx + b$), with a slope of 1.0, a y-intercept of 0, and a correlation coefficient (r) of 1. Data should be plotted daily and inspected for outliers so that original samples can be reanalyzed as needed. While linearity can be confirmed visually in most cases, it may be necessary to evaluate linearity more quantitatively.[19]

DEFINITIONS BOX

Deming regression Linear regression analysis (orthogonal least squares) used to compare two methodologies using the best fit line through the data points (see Figs. 3.24 and 3.25).

Passing-Bablok regression A nonparametric regression method for comparison studies. It is a robust method that is resistant to outliers.

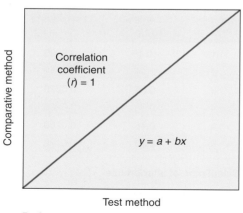

A

Perfect correlation (Hypothetical)
Slope (b) = 1
y-intercept (a) = 0
Correlation coefficient (r) = 1

B

FIGURE 3.15 A comparison of methods experiment. **(A)** A model of a perfect method comparison. **(B)** An actual method comparison of beta-human chorionic gonadotropin (βhCG) between the Elecsys 2010 (Roche, Nutley, NJ) and the IMx (Abbott Laboratories, Abbott Park, IL). (Adapted from Shahzad K, Kim DH, Kang MJ. Analytic evaluation of the beta-human chorionic gonadotropin assay on the Abbott IMx and Elecsys2010 for its use in doping control. *Clin Biochem.* 2007;40:1259–1265.)

Statistical Analysis of COM Studies

While a visual inspection of method comparisons is essential, statistical analysis can be used to make objective decisions about the performance of a method. The first and most fundamental statistical analysis for COM studies is the linear regression. Linear regression analysis yields the slope (b), the y-intercept (a), the SD of the points about the regression line ($S_{y/x}$), and the correlation coefficient (r); regression also yields the coefficient of determination (r^2) (see DEFINITIONS BOX). An example of these calculations can be found in Figure 3.15, where a comparison of β-human chorionic gonadotropin (βhCG) concentrations on an existing immunoassay system (Reference Method) and to a new system (Test Method). Statistics are calculated to determine the types and amounts of error that a method has, which is the basis for deciding if the test is still valid to make clinical decisions. Several types of errors can be seen looking at a plot of test method versus comparative method (Fig. 3.16). When random errors occur (Fig. 3.16A), points are randomly distributed around the regression line. Increases in the $S_{y/x}$ statistic reflect random error. Constant error (Fig. 3.16B) is seen visually as a shift in the y-intercept; a t-test can be used to determine if two sets of data are significantly different from each other. Proportional error (Fig. 3.16C) is reflected in alterations in line slope and can also be analyzed with a t-test (see Fig. 3.1).

DEFINITIONS BOX

Correlation Coefficient (r) Defines the strength of relationship between two variables. Ranges from −1 (perfect inverse correlation) to +1 (perfect positive correlation). A value of 0 indicates no correlation or a random relationship between variables.

Coefficient of Determination (r^2 or R^2) Indicates the proportion of variation explained by one variable to predict another. Ranges from 0 to 1. Where $r^2 = 0.95$, one variable explains 95% of the variation of the other. In the case of regression, it indicates how well the line represents the data.

Note that a statistical difference does not necessarily indicate that the method is not clinically usable, just that it is different. The size and nature (systematic and random error) of the differences determines if a method is clinical useable.[20] For this reason, linear regression analysis is more useful than the t-test for evaluating COM studies,[20] as the constant systematic error can be determined by the y-intercept and the proportional systematic error can be determined by the slope. Random error can also be determined by the standard error of the estimate ($S_{y/x}$). Importantly, if a nonlinear relationship occurs between the test and comparative methods, linear regression analysis can be used

FIGURE 3.16 Examples of **(A)** random, **(B)** constant, and **(C)** proportional error using linear regression analysis. (Adapted from Westgard JO. *Basic Method Evaluation*. 2nd ed. Madison, WI: Westgard Quality Corp.; 2003.)

only over the values in the linear range. To make accurate conclusions about the relationship between two tests, it is important to confirm that outliers are true outliers and not the result of technical errors.[21–23]

So far, we have described how we estimate error test methods in terms of imprecision and inaccuracy. However, tests are performed to answer clinical questions, so to assess how this error might affect clinical judgments, it is assessed in terms of *allowable (analytical) error* (E_a).[24] Allowable error is determined for each test based on the amount of error that will not negatively affect clinical decisions. If the combined random and systematic error (total error) is less than E_a, then the performance of the test is considered acceptable. However, if the error is larger than E_a, corrections (calibration, new reagents, or hardware improvements) must be made to reduce the error or the method rejected. This process ensures that the laboratory provides accurate, clinically usable information to physicians to manage their patients effectively. To emphasize this point, laboratorians should consider that physicians are rarely aware of the imprecision, bias, and performance of a given test that they rely on to make decisions. It is the responsibility of the laboratory to ensure quality.

Allowable Analytical Error

An important aspect of method evaluation is to determine if the random and systematic errors (total error) are less than the total allowable analytical error (E_a). In the past, there have been several methodologies that have been used to establish E_a, including physiologic variation, multiples of the reference interval, and pathologist judgment.[25–28] The Clinical Laboratory Improvement Amendments of 1988 (CLIA 88) published allowable error (Ea) for an array of clinical tests.[29] The E_a limits published by the CLIA specify the maximum error allowable by federally mandated **proficiency testing** (see examples in Table 3.3). These performance standards are now being used to determine the acceptability of clinical chemistry analyzer performance.[30,31] The E_a is specifically calculated based on the types of studies described in the previous section (Table 3.4). An example of calculations made for the single-value criteria is shown in Table 3.4. Here, estimates of random and systematic errors are calculated and then compared with the published allowable error at critical concentrations of the analyte. If the test

does not meet the allowable error criteria, it must be modified to reduce error or be rejected.

Comprehensive COM studies are demanding on personnel, time, and budgets. This has led to the description of abbreviated experiments that could be undertaken to estimate imprecision and inaccuracy.[32] CLIA has published guidelines for such an abbreviated application, which can be used by a laboratory to confirm that the precision and accuracy performance is consistent with the manufacturer's reported claims. These studies can be completed in 5 working days, making it likely laboratories will use these guidelines to set up new methodologies. The Clinical Laboratory Standards Institute (CLSI) also has several documents that describe best practices for method evaluation with worked examples.

Method Evaluation Acceptance Criteria

Collectively, the data gathered in precision, linearity, interference, recovery, and method comparison studies are used to guide test implementation decisions. That is, the data do not define if a test method is acceptable by itself. Clinical judgment is required to determine if the analytical performance is acceptable for clinical use with consideration for the nature and application of the analyte. For example, imprecision for a pregnancy test around the cutoff value of 5 or 10 mIU/mL is more of a concern than it would be at 15,000 mIU/mL. Likewise, proportional bias for troponin at a high concentration is of less concern than it is near the clinical decision point. Thus, method evaluation studies and statistical analysis are necessary, but not sufficient to determine if a test is valid. The validation and statistics serve as the basis on which to make the decision.

QUALITY CONTROL

QC in the laboratory involves the systematic monitoring of analytic processes to detect analytic errors that occur during analysis and to ultimately prevent the reporting of incorrect patient test results. In the context of what we have discussed so far, QC is part of the performance monitoring that occurs after a test has been established (see Fig. 3.10). In general, monitoring of analytic methods is performed by assaying stable control materials and comparing their determined values with their expected values. The expected values are represented by intervals of acceptable values with

TABLE 3.4 Single-Value Criteria of Westgard et al.

Type of Error	Test Used to Determine	Criteria
Random error	Replication experiment	$2.58\,s < E_a$
Proportional error	Recovery experiment	$\lvert (\text{Recovery} - 100) \times X_C/100 \rvert < E_a$
Constant error	Interference experiment	$\lvert \text{Bias} \rvert < E_a$
Systematic error	Comparison of methods	$X0 \rvert < E_a \lvert (y_0 + mX_C)$
Total error	Replication and comparison	$2.58\,s + \lvert (y_0 + mX_C) - X_C \rvert < E_a$

Based on National Committee for Clinical Laboratory Standards (NCCLS). *Approved Guideline for Handling and Processing of Blood Specimens.* 3rd ed. Villanova, PA: NCCLS; 2004 (Document no. H18-A3).
Medically acceptable error (E_a) based on performance standards set by CLIA, as shown in Table 3.12.

upper and lower limits, known as control limits. When the expected values are within the control limits, the operator can be reasonably assured that the analytic method is properly reporting values as approved during the method validation. However, when observed values fall outside the control limits, the operator must be aware of possible problems and the need for further investigation before reporting potentially erroneously patient results. The principles of visualizing QC data were initially applied to the clinical laboratory in the 1950s by Levey and Jennings.[33] Many important modifications have been made to these systems since that time, and they are discussed in general in this section.

DEFINITIONS BOX

Control limits Threshold at which the value is statistically unlikely.

Control material Material analyzed only for QC purposes.

Levey-Jennings control chart Graphical representation of observed values of a control material over time in the context of the upper and lower control limits.

Multirule procedure Decision criteria to determine if an analytic run is in control; used to detect random and systematic errors over time (e.g., 1-3S, 2-2S, R4-S in combination).

Specimens analyzed for QC purposes are known as *QC materials.* These materials must be available in sufficient quantity to last for extended periods of time determined by QC material stability and vendor determined expiration dates. QC materials should be the same matrix as the specimens actually to be tested. For example, a glucose assay performed on serum should have QC materials that are prepared in serum. Variation between vials should be minimal so that differences seen over time can be attributed to the analytic method itself and not variation in the QC material. Control material concentrations should span the clinically important range of the analyte at appropriate decision levels. For example, sodium QC materials might be tested at 130 and 150 mmol/L, representing cutoff values for hyponatremia and hypernatremia, respectively. QC for general chemistry assays generally uses two levels of control, while immunoassays commonly use three. Today, laboratories more often purchase manufactured control materials for QC, instead of preparing the materials themselves. These materials are often lyophilized (dehydrated to powder) for stability and can be reconstituted in specific diluents or matrices representing urine, blood, or cerebrospinal fluid (CSF). Control materials can be purchased with or without previously assayed ranges. Assayed materials give expected target ranges, often including the mean and SD using common analytic methods. While these products are more expensive because of the additional characterization, they allow another external check of method accuracy. Some laboratories will prepare internal quality control materials

using human serum (i.e., serum pools) as an attempt to address concerns about artificial matrixes and analyte values used in commercial materials.

Because most commercially prepared control materials are lyophilized and require reconstitution before use, the diluent should be carefully added and mixed. Incomplete mixing yields a partition of supernatant liquid and underlying sediment and will result in incorrect control values. Frequently, the reconstituted material will be more turbid (cloudy) than the actual patient specimen. Stabilized frozen controls do not require reconstitution but may behave differently from patient specimens in some analytic systems. It is important to carefully evaluate these stabilized controls with any new instrument system. Improper preparation and handling of QC materials is the main reason for QC failures in the laboratory and requires staff education and material management to minimize. For example, if one user mixes the QC material thoroughly after warming it for several hours, while another user runs it cold with minimal mixing, it may be expected that the QC results will vary while the process itself may be perfectly stable. More manufactured liquid QC is becoming available; however, it is usually more expensive, but it does remove any variation due to the preparation of the QC materials.

QC Charts

A common method to assess the determination of control materials over time is by the use of a **Levey-Jennings control chart** (Fig. 3.17). Control charts graphically

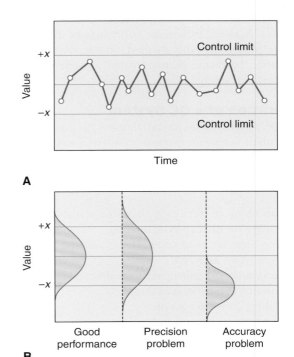

FIGURE 3.17 Levey-Jennings control chart. Data are plotted over time to identify quality control failures. (Adapted from Westgard JO, Klee GG. Quality management. In: Tietz NW, Burtis CA, Ashwood ER, Bruns DE, eds. *Tietz Textbook of Clinical Chemistry and Molecular Diagnostics.* 4th ed. St. Louis, MO: Elsevier Saunders; 2006:485–529.)

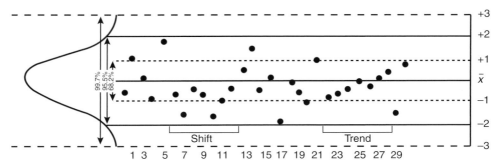

FIGURE 3.18 Control chart showing the relationship of control limits to the Gaussian distribution. Daily control values are graphed, and they show examples of a shift, an abrupt change in the analytic process, and a trend, a gradual change in the analytic process.

represent the observed values of a control material over time in the context of the upper and lower control limits in relation to the target value. When the observed value falls with the control limits, it can be interpreted that the method is performed adequately. Points falling outside the control limits suggest that problems may be developing. Control limits are expressed as the mean ± SD using formulas previously described in this chapter. Control charts can detect errors in accuracy and imprecision over time (Fig. 3.17A). Analytic errors that can occur can be separated into random and systematic errors. The underlying rationale for running repeated assays is to detect random errors that affect precision (Fig. 3.17B, *middle*). Random errors may be caused by variations in technique. Systematic errors arise from factors that contribute to constant differences between measurements; these errors may be either positive or negative (Fig. 3.17B, *right*). Systematic errors may be due to several factors, including poorly made standards, reagents, instrumentation problems, poorly written procedures, or inadequate staff training.

Operation of a QC System

The QC system in the clinical laboratory is used to monitor the analytic variations that can occur (refer to Chapter 4 for Quality Control Plan additional information)

The QC program can be thought of as a three-stage process:

1. Establishing or verifying allowable statistical limits of variation for each analytic method
2. Using these limits as criteria for evaluating the QC data generated for each test
3. Taking action to remedy errors real time when indicated
   a. Finding the cause(s) of error
   b. Taking corrective action
   c. Reanalyzing control and patient data

Establishing Statistical Quality Control Limits

With a new instrument or with new lots of control material, the different levels of control material must be analyzed for 20 days. Exceptions include assays that are highly precise (CV < 1%), such as blood gases, where 5 days is adequate. Also, if the QC materials is a new lot with similar ranges for an existing analyte to be implemented, a modified precision

study can be done with as few as 10 values and monitoring post implementation. Repeat analysis of the control materials allows the determination of the mean and SD of control materials. Initial estimates of the mean and control limits may be somewhat inaccurate because of the low number of data points. In order to produce more reliable data, estimates of the mean and SDs should be reviewed and updated to include cumulative data. When changing to a new lot of similar material, laboratorians use the newly obtained mean (or manufacturer mean and SD) as the target mean but retain the previous SD. As more data are obtained, all data should be averaged to derive the best estimates of the mean and SD.[34]

The distribution of error is assumed to be symmetrical and bell shaped (Gaussian) as shown in Figure 3.18. Control limits are set to include most observed values (95% to 99.7%), corresponding to the mean ±2 or 3 SDs. Observation of values in the distribution tails should therefore be rare (1/20 for 2 SDs; 3/1,000 for 3 SDs). Observations outside the control limits suggest changes in the analytic methods. If the process is in control, no more than 0.3% of the points will be outside the 3 SDs (3s) limits. Analytic methods are considered in control if a symmetrical distribution of control values about the mean is seen, and few values outside the 2 SDs (2s) control limits are observed. Some laboratories define a method out of control if a control value exceeds the 2s limits. Other laboratories use the 2s limit as a warning limit and the 3s limit as an error limit. In this particular case, a control point between 2s and 3s would alert the technologist to a potential problem, while a point greater than 3s would require a corrective action. The selection of control rules and numbers should be related to the goals set by the laboratory.[35]

It is essential to recognize the distinction between QC limits and QC goals or specifications (Figure 3.19 control_v_specification.png). *QC specifications are the criteria used to decide that a given method meets the clinical requirements.* QC specifications may be derived from the total allowable error, biological variation, or other medical decision criteria. *QC limits are defined by the process itself based on its natural variation.* A good description of the difference is that QC specifications are the "voice of the customer," while QC limits are the "voice of the process." Thus,

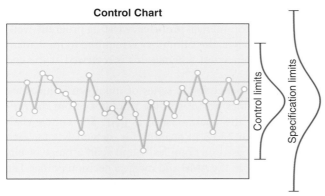

Control Chart

FIGURE 3.19 QC specifications limits are the criteria used to decide that a given method meets the clinical requirements based on the needs of the health care provider. QC control limits are defined by the process itself based on its natural variation.

QC specifications are "the performance the health care provider needs," whereas QC limits are the "natural variation of a given test"; more simply, QC specifications are what you want and QC limits are what you have. A process tells the user its limits and the user decides if those limits meet their specification.

From a practical perspective, QC limits define if a process is in control on a daily basis, and QC specifications define if the overall performance of the process meets the quality goals. Consider that a process may be out of control (e.g., have a 1-3S flag), but still meet the QC specification limits. Conversely, a poorly performing method might have natural variation QC limits, which exceed the QC specification. QC limits must be within QC specifications or the lab will not be able to consistently report accurate results. Importantly, QC specifications do not have any effect on or causal relationship with QC limits; setting QC specifications to a CV of 0.1% will not make a method more precise any more than widening specifications to a CV of 100% would make the method become imprecise. However, the relationship between QC limits and QC specifications *can* be used to establish which multirules to use.

Multirules RULE!

The use of the statistical process control chart (Levey-Jennings) was pioneered by Shewhart in the 1920s.

Multirules were formalized by the Western Electric Company and later applied to the clinical laboratory by Westgard and Groth.[36] Multirules establish a criterion for judging whether an analytic process is out of control. To simplify the various control rules, abbreviations are used to refer to the various control rules (Table 3.14). Control rules indicate the number of control observations per analytic run, followed by the control amount in subscript.[37] For example, the 1_{3s} rule indicates that a data point cannot exceed 3 SDs (3s). If the 1_{3s} rule is not triggered, the analytic run will be accepted (i.e., results will be reported). If the QC results are more than 3 SDs (the 1_{3s} rule is violated), the run may be rejected and there will be additional investigation. The type of rule violated indicates what type of error exists. For example, a 1_{3s} rule violation may indicate a loss of precision or "random error" (Table 3.5).

Analogous to overlapping diseased and healthy patient results, it is important to consider that not every rule violation indicates that a process is out of control. The 1_{2s} rule, for example, will be outside the 2s limit in 5% of the runs with normal analytic variation (Fig. 3.19A). The 8_X rule is violated if 8 consecutive control observations fall on one side or the other of the mean (Fig. 3.19B). The more levels of QC material analyzed, the higher the probability of a rule violation even in the absence of true error. When two controls are used, there is an approximately 10% chance that at least one control will be outside the 2s limits; when four controls are used, there is a 17% chance. For this reason, many laboratories use 2s limits either as a warning or not at all when used with other QC rules rather than criteria for run rejection. QC rules should be selected based on the performance of the test relative to the QC specifications. If a test is very precise and well within the QC specification, fewer QC rules are needed. For example, if there are 6 standard deviations between the natural process variation and the QC specification limits, a simple 1-3S rule will easily detect that a process is out of control long before it exceeds the specification limits. Conversely, a test that just meets the QC specification would need multiple rules to ensure that error is detected before exceeding the specification. By judiciously selecting QC rules based on method performance and specifications, error detection can be maximized while minimized false rejections.

 TABLE 3.5 | Multirule Procedures

- 1_{2s} One control observation exceeding the mean ±2s. A warning rule that initiates testing of control data by other rules.
- 1_{3s} One control observation exceeding the mean ±3s. Allows high sensitivity to random error.
- 2_{2s} Two control observations consecutively exceeding the same +2s or –2s. Allows high sensitivity to systematic error.
- R_{4s} One control exceeding the +2s and another exceeding the –2s. Allows detection of random error.
- 4_{1s} Four consecutive control observations exceeding +1s or –1s. This allows the detection of systematic error.
- 10_X Ten consecutive control observations falling on one side or the other of the mean (no requirement for SD size). This allows the detection of systematic error.

SD, standard deviation.

A final practical concept related to QC materials is repeats. It is common practice is to repeat a control when a QC rule is violated. In the context of imprecision, this practice does not make much sense. A repeat sample is likely to regress to the mean and therefore falls within the limits, even if the process is out of control. If ever, QC repeats only make sense in the context of a shift or bias, where the bias would persist between samples. Collectively, operators should review the Levey-Jennings chart and think about their process and what a given QC violation means before acting. The operators' job is not get QC to pass, but to report accurate results.

Proficiency Testing

In addition to daily QC practices, laboratories are required to participate in external proficiency testing programs. Acceptable performance in proficiency testing programs is required by the CAP, the CLIA, and TJC to maintain laboratory accreditation. Even more important, proficiency testing is another tool in the ongoing process of monitoring test performance.

Indicators of Analytic Performance

Proficiency testing

Internal quality control

Laboratory inspections (accreditation)

Quality assurance monitoring (see Chapter 4)

Clinical utilization

DEFINITIONS BOX

Proficiency test Method used to validate a particular measurement process. The results are compared with other external laboratories to give an objective indication of test accuracy.

Proficiency samples Specimens that have known concentrations of an analyte for the test of interest. The testing laboratory does not know the targeted concentration when tested.

The majority of clinical laboratories subscribe to the proficiency program provided by the CAP. The CAP program has been in existence for 50 years, and it is the gold standard for clinical laboratory proficiency testing. In our laboratory, the majority of analytes are monitored with the CAP proficiency surveys. Other proficiency testing programs are often used when analytes of interest are not tested through CAP (e.g., esoteric tests) or as a means to supplement CAP proficiency testing programs. Additional proficiency programs used in our laboratory include the International Sirolimus Proficiency Testing Scheme (IST), the Binding Site, the American Proficiency Institute (API),

and the Centers for Disease Control and Prevention (CDC). If there is no commercial proficiency testing program available for an analyte, the laboratory is required to implement a non–proficiency test scheme; this is reviewed at the end of this section.

For a proficiency test, a series of unknown samples are sent several times per year to the laboratory from the program offering this analysis, such as CAP. The sample challenges are from 2 to 5 in quantity for each analyte for each testing event based on complexity and span a range of target values within the **AMR** and medical decision points. The samples are analyzed in the same manner as patient specimens as much as possible, and the results are reported to the proficiency program. The program then compiles the results from all of the laboratories participating in the survey and sends a performance report back to each participating laboratory. Each analyte has a defined performance criteria (e.g., ±3 SDs to peer mean), where laboratories using the same method are graded by comparing them with the group. Some proficiency tests are not quantitative and are qualitatively or semiquantitatively (i.e., rapid pregnancy test, RPR titers) compared with other laboratories. Areas of pathology other than clinical chemistry are also subjected to mandatory proficiency qualitative/interpretive testing, including anatomic pathology, clinical microbiology, and clinical microscopy.

Example of Proficiency Test Results for βhCG

βhCG-08: CAP value = 75.58; SD = 4.80; CV = 6.4%; n = 47 peer laboratories

Evaluation criteria: Peer group ±3 SDs; acceptable range 65.7–85.2 mIU/mL

Testing laboratory value = 71.54; SDI = –0.84 acceptable

An example of a hypothetical survey is shown in the text box above. The βhCG survey was the eighth sample sent in that year (βhCG-08). The mean of all the laboratories using the same method was 75.58 mIU/mL. The SD and CV are indicated, as is the number of laboratories that participate in that survey ($n = 47$). The acceptance criteria for this test is established as within ±3 SDs (i.e., between 65.7 and 85.2 mIU/mL). The laboratory's result was 71.54 mIU/mL, which is –0.84 SD from the mean and is within the acceptable limits.

When a laboratory performs proficiency testing, there are strict requirements as follows:

1. The laboratory must incorporate proficiency testing into its routine workflow as much as possible.
2. The test values/samples must not be shared with other laboratories until after the deadline of submission of results to the proficiency provider. Referral of proficiency samples to another lab is prohibited as well as acceptance of proficiency samples from another lab is prohibited.

3. Proficiency samples are tested by bench technical staff who normally conduct patient testing; there can be no unnecessary repeats or actions outside of how a patient sample would be tested and reported.
4. Testing should be completed within the usual time it would take for routine patient testing.
5. Proficiency samples are to be performed and submitted on the primary analyzer when there are multiple analyzers in the laboratory following CLIA guidelines (D2006 493.801). In addition, at least twice per year, other analyzers within the laboratory are to be compared to the primary analyzer.
6. All proficiency failures and significant shifts and trends must be reviewed, investigated, and resolved with 30 days of final receipt of proficiency results. Emphasis must be placed on investigating potential patient impact during the time of proficiency testing.
7. Proficiency testing program must demonstrate a dynamic and real-time review time of all proficiency results by the laboratory director and delegated management personnel.

The bottom line is that the sample should be treated like a patient sample to yield a true indication of test accuracy. Proficiency samples are not to be analyzed more than once unless this is the standard policy for patient testing at your laboratory.

The acceptability criteria for proficiency testing are provided by the proficiency program. For regulated analytes, these criteria are often the CLIA limits (see Table 3.3). For nonregulated analytes, acceptable criteria are often determined by the scientific community at large. For example, the acceptability criterion for lactate dehydrogenase is ±20% or 3 SDs (whichever is greater) based on peer group data.

Proficiency testing allows each laboratory to compare its test results with those of peer laboratories that use the same or similar instruments and methods. Proficiency testing provides performance data for a given analyte at a specific point in time. Comparison of performance to a robust, statistically valid peer group is essential to identify areas for improvement. Areas of improvement that may be identified in a single proficiency testing event or over multiple events include variation from peer group results, imprecision, and/or results that trend above or below the mean consistently or at specific analyte concentrations. Use of these data allows laboratories to continuously monitor and improve their test performance. The proficiency testing samples also can serve as valuable troubleshooting aids when investigating problem analytes. In our hospital, proficiency samples are also included in the technologist competency or new employee training program. Proficiency tests can also be beneficial in validating the laboratory's measurement method, technical training, and total allowable error limits for new tests.

Proficiency testing programs require thorough investigation of discrepant results for any analyte (i.e., failure). Laboratories may be asked to submit information that could include current and historical proficiency testing reports, QC and equipment monitoring, analysis and corrective action of the problem that caused the failure, and the steps taken to ensure the reliability of patient test results (patient impact). If the laboratory cannot resolve analyte testing discrepancies over several testing events, the testing facility may be at risk of losing the authority to perform patient testing for the analyte(s) in question. Also if the laboratory violates any of the mandatory proficiency requirements referenced earlier, it may be at risk of losing its accreditation and authority to perform patient testing for all tests.

To develop and manage a successful proficiency testing program for the clinical laboratory, it is important to understand the documented requirements from the two main accreditation bodies. A large proficiency testing program often requires considerable personnel resources and costs for the laboratory and is an essential factor of several in providing a quality management system. As an example of the scale and volume of proficiency tests, our laboratory (for a 800-bed hospital with outreach clinics) performed ≈10,000 proficiency tests in a year for ≈500 individual analytes. Even a smaller laboratory with a limited test menu and 3 analyzers and waived testing performs several hundred proficiencies per year. Besides meeting required accreditation standards, proficiency testing allows the laboratory to objectively ensure patient results are accurate.

REFERENCE INTERVAL STUDIES

Laboratory test data is used to make medical diagnoses, assess physiologic function, and manage therapy. When interpreting laboratory data, clinicians compare the measured test result from a patient with a reference interval.

Reference intervals include all the data points that define the range of observations (e.g., if the interval is 5 to 10, a patient result of 5 would be considered within the interval). The upper and lower reference limits are set to define a specified percentage (usually 95%) of the values for a population; this means that a percentage (usually 5%) of patients will fall outside the reference interval in the absence of any condition or disease. Reference intervals are sometimes erroneously called "normal ranges." While all normal ranges are in fact reference intervals, not all reference intervals are normal ranges. This is exemplified by the reference interval for therapeutic drug levels. In this case, a "normal" individual would not have any drug in their system, whereas a patient on therapy has a defined target range. Reference intervals are also sometimes called reference ranges; the preferred term is reference interval because range implies the absolute maximum and minimum values.

DEFINITIONS BOX

Reference interval A pair of medical decision points that span the limits of results expected for a defined healthy population.

The theory for the development of reference intervals was the work of two main expert committees.[38–41] These committees established the importance of standardizing collection procedures, the use of statistical methods for analysis of reference values and estimation of reference intervals, and the selection of reference populations. Reference intervals are usually established by the scientific community or the manufacturers of reagents and new methodologies. Developing reference intervals often has a financial impact on vendors and marketing of the laboratory products. Laboratorians must be aware of these scientific and economic forces when reviewing vendor data and determining the need for reference interval studies. The two main types of reference interval studies that are reviewed in this section are (1) establishing a reference interval and (2) transferring and verifying a reference interval.

The clinical laboratory is required by good laboratory practice and accreditation agencies (i.e., the CAP checklist) to either verify or establish reference intervals for any new tests or significant changes in methodology (Box 3.3).

DEFINITIONS BOX

Establishing a reference interval A new reference interval is established when there is no existing analyte or methodology in the clinical or reference laboratory with which to conduct comparative studies. It is a costly and labor-intensive study that will involve laboratory resources at all levels and may require from 120 to as many as ≈700 study individuals.

Transference and validation of a reference interval In many cases, a reference interval will be transferred from a similar instrument or laboratory. The reference interval is then validated using the method comparison and patient population and/or using a smaller sample of healthy individuals. These are the most common reference interval studies performed in the clinical laboratory and often include as few as 40 study individuals.

The core protocols for both establishing and verifying reference ranges are reviewed in this section. Other terms are used for values or ranges that help the clinician determine the relationship of patients' test results to statistically determined values or ranges for the clinical condition under treatment.

DEFINITIONS BOX

Medical decision level Value for an analyte that represents the boundary between different therapeutic approaches.

Normal range Range of results between two medical decision points that correspond to the central 95% of results from a healthy patient population. Note: Of the results, 2.5% will be above the upper limit, and 2.5% will be below the lower limit of the normal range.

Therapeutic range Reference interval applied to a therapeutic drug. Reference intervals are needed for all tests in the clinical laboratory, and the provision of reliable reference intervals is an important task for clinical laboratories and test manufacturers. The review of existing reference intervals by the health care team (scientific community, manufacturers, and clinical laboratory) is crucial to meeting the challenges of providing optimal laboratory data for patient care.

The application of reference intervals can be grouped into three main categories: diagnosis of a disease or condition (Table 3.6), monitoring of a physiologic condition (Table 3.7), or monitoring therapeutic drugs (Table 3.8). These different applications require different approaches for determination of a reference interval. Specifically, therapeutic drug targets are not derived from a healthy population and unique physiologically conditions require the appropriate reference population.

 BOX 3.3 Examples of CAP Checklist Questions Regarding Reference Intervals for Laboratory Inspection

The Laboratory Establishes or Verifies Its Reference Intervals (Normal Values)

NOTE: Reference intervals are important to allow a clinician to assess patient results against an appropriate population. The reference range must be established or verified for each analyte and specimen source (e.g., blood, urine, and CSF), when appropriate. For many analytes (e.g., therapeutic drugs and CSF total protein), literature references or a manufacturer's package insert information may be appropriate.

Evidence of Compliance

Record of reference range study or records of verification of manufacturer's stated range when reference range study is not practical (e.g., unavailable normal population) or other methods approved by the laboratory director.[47–49]

The Laboratory Evaluates the Appropriateness of Its Reference Intervals and Takes Corrective Action if Necessary

Criteria for evaluation of reference intervals include the following:

1. Introduction of a new analyte to the test repertoire
2. Change of analytic methodology
3. Change in patient population

If it is determined that the range is no longer appropriate for the patient population, corrective action must be taken.[42–44]

Evidence of Compliance

Records of evaluation and corrective action, if indicated

Adapted from Sarewitz SJ, ed. *Laboratory Accreditation Program Inspection Checklists.* Northfield, IL: College of American Pathologists; 2009, with permission.

TABLE 3.6	Thyroid-Stimulating Hormone (TSH) Thyroid Disease	
Patients	**Age**	**TSH Reference Ranges (µIU/ML)**
Pediatric	0–3 d	1.00–20.00
	3–30 d	0.50–6.50
	31 d–5 m	0.50–6.00
	6 m–18 y	0.50–4.50
Adults, ambulatory, healthy	>18 y	0.60–3.30

Based on Dugaw KA, Jack RM, Rutledge J. Pediatric reference ranges for TSH, free T4, total T4 total T3 and T3 uptake on the vitros ECi analyzer. *Clin Chem.* 2001;47:A108.

Tables 3.6 to 3.8 also demonstrate the complexity of reference intervals when multiple levels (partitions) of reference intervals are required by the clinician. The framework for verifying or establishing reference intervals is one that can be overwhelming and not feasible for many valid reasons for large and small clinical laboratories. The costs, personnel, and resource requirements mandate that the reference interval experiment be feasible, well defined, and structured in such a manner to provide accurate and timely reference intervals for optimal clinical use. Where possible, the clinical laboratory director may determine that a review of literature references or manufacturer's package inserts is appropriate in assigning reference intervals for an analyte or this additional information may allow for the shorter reference interval verification study (i.e., 20 study individuals).

Establishing Reference Intervals

The Clinical and Laboratory Standards Institute (CLSI, formerly National Committee for Clinical Laboratory Standards [NCCLS]) has published a preferred guideline/

TABLE 3.7	hCG at Defined Gestational Age

Approximate βhCG Levels at Defined Gestational Age Units MIU/ML (U/L)

Weeks of Pregnancy	Mean	Range	N
4	1,110	40–4,480	42
5	8,050	270–28,700	52
6	29,700	3,700–84,900	67
7	58,800	9,700–120,000	62
8	79,500	31,000–184,000	37
9	91,500	61,200–152,000	25
10	71,000	22,000–143,000	12
14	33,100	14,300–75,800	219
15	27,500	12,300–60,300	355
16	21,900	8,800–54,500	163
17	18,000	8,100–51,300	68
18	18,400	3,900–49,400	30
19	20,900	3,600–56,600	14

TABLE 3.8	Therapeutic Management Targets for Digoxin	
Normal	0.8–1.8 ng/mL (collected 6 h after dose)	
Critical	>2.0 ng/mL	

resource for establishing or verification of reference intervals (Box 3.4).[45]

Selection of Reference Interval Study Individuals

The selection of individuals who can be included in a reference interval study requires defining detailed inclusion/exclusion criteria. Inclusion criteria define what factors (e.g., age and gender) are required to be used for the study, while exclusion criteria list factors that render individuals inappropriate for the study (Table 3.9). It is essential to select the appropriate individuals to obtain the optimal set of specimens with an acceptable level of confidence. Determination of the necessary inclusion and exclusion criteria for donor selection may require extensive literature searches and review with laboratory directors and clinicians. Initially, it must be exactly defined what is a "healthy"/"normal" donor for associated reference values. For example, for a βhCG reference interval study, one would exclude pregnant women or those who may be pregnant, as well as individuals with βhCG-producing tumors. An important note to make is that laboratories are often challenged to locate donors outside the laboratory working

BOX 3.4 To Establish a Reference Range Study

1. Define an appropriate list of biological variations and analytic interferences from medical literature.
2. Choose selection and partition (e.g., age or gender) criteria.
3. Complete a written consent form and questionnaire to capture selection criteria.
4. Categorize the potential reference individuals based on the questionnaire findings.
5. Exclude individuals from the reference sample group based on exclusion criteria.
6. Define the number of reference individuals in consideration of desired confidence limits and statistical accuracy.
7. Standardize collection and analysis of reference specimens for the measurement of a given analyte consistent with the routine practice of patients.
8. Inspect the reference value data and prepare a histogram to evaluate the distribution of data.
9. Identify possible data errors and/or outliers and then analyze the reference values.
10. Document all of the previously mentioned steps and procedures.

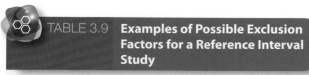

TABLE 3.9 Examples of Possible Exclusion Factors for a Reference Interval Study

Fasting or nonfasting	Pregnancy
Genetic factors	Illness, recent
Drugs: prescription or over the counter	Exercise pattern

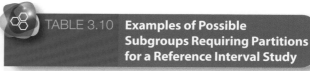

TABLE 3.10 Examples of Possible Subgroups Requiring Partitions for a Reference Interval Study

Age (adult and childhood)	Stage of pregnancy
Fasting or nonfasting	Sex
Diet	Tobacco use

environment, who may be largely females under 40 years of age. The use of donors who may not represent the population of interest has the potential to skew the evaluation data used to establish the reference interval. Inpatient samples generally cannot be used for reference interval studies that are designed to reflect a healthy population. Often, donors are recruited from unlikely sources out of necessity, that is, medical or university students and public health patients. Practical considerations must be built into the study to include adequate sample procurement areas, staffing, legal disclaimers, and patient financial incentives (Box 3.5).

Capturing the appropriate information for the inclusion and exclusion criteria, such as donor health status, often requires a well-written confidential questionnaire and consent form. Another consideration when selecting individuals for a reference interval study is additional factors that may require partitioning individuals into subgroups (Table 3.10). These subgroups may require separate reference interval studies. Fortunately, a large number of laboratory tests do not require partitioning and can be used with only one reference interval that is not dependent on a variety of factors (Table 3.11). These examples are testimony to the complexity and variability of conducting reference interval studies. The initial selection of individual donors is crucial to the successful evaluation of reference intervals.

Preanalytic and Analytic Considerations

Once individuals are selected for a reference interval study, it is important to consider both preanalytic and analytic variables that can affect specific laboratory tests (Table 3.12). Preanalytic and analytic variables must be controlled and standardized to generate a valid reference interval. To illustrate these points, consider establishing a reference

interval for fasting glucose. An obvious preanalytic variable that should be addressed for this test is that individuals should not eat for at least 8 hours prior to sample collection. In terms of analytic factors, it is important to define acceptable levels of common interferences, such as hemolysis or lipemia. For fasting glucose, the laboratorian must define whether samples with excess hemolysis or lipemia will be included in the study; this depends, in part, on whether the interferences affect the methods (in this case, glucose). If specific interferences do affect the accuracy of the test, it is essential that interferences can be flagged, to appropriately deal with the results and interpretation. Hemolysis and lipemia can be detected automatically by large chemistry analyzers. It is also worth considering that some methods are more sensitive to interferences. It is also necessary to consider what specific reagents are used in an assay. Changing to a new reagent lot in the middle of a reference study could widen the reference interval or change the data distribution (e.g., change from normal to bimodal). Thus, an effective reference interval study requires extensive knowledge of the analyte, analytic parameters, methodology, and instrumentation and management of all study variables.

Determining Whether to Establish or Transfer and Verify Reference Intervals

Whether to transfer and verify a reference interval or establish an entirely new reference interval for a new method/analyte depends on several factors, such as the presence of an existing reference interval for assay and on the results of a statistical analysis comparing the test method with the reference method. The most basic method comparison involves plotting a reference method against a test method and fitting a linear regression (described in Fig. 3.7). If the correlation coefficient is 1.0, slope is 1, and intercept is 0, the two methods agree and may not require new reference ranges. In this case, a simple reference interval verification study is all that may be required. Conversely, if the two methods differ considerably, then a new reference interval needs to be established or external resources reviewed.

BOX 3.5 Example Questionnaire

Creatinine Clearance Example

Time Urine Instructions Creatinine
Donor Number: _____
Sex: _____
Height: _____
Weight: _____
Exercise routine: _____
Pregnancy: Yes/No
Medications: _____

TABLE 3.11 Example of a Simple Reference Interval

Plasma potassium	3.5–5.0 mmol/L

TABLE 3.12	**Preanalytic and Analytic Considerations for Reference Interval Studies**

Preanalytic Factors

Subject preparation	Sample storage
Prescription medications	Stress
Collection time	Food/beverage ingestion

Analytic Factors

Precision	Linearity
Accuracy	Interference
Lot-to-lot reagents	Recovery

Analysis of Reference Values

DEFINITIONS BOX

Nonparametric method Statistical test that makes no specific assumption about the distribution of data. Nonparametric methods rank the reference data in order of increasing size. Because the majority of analytes are not normally (Gaussian) distributed (see Fig. 3.6), nonparametric tests are the recommended analysis for most reference range intervals.

Parametric method Statistical test that assumes the observed values, or some mathematical transformation of those values, follow a (normal) Gaussian distribution (see Fig. 3.6).

Confidence interval Range of values that include a specified probability, usually 90% or 95%. For example, consider a 95% confidence interval for slope = 0.972–0.988 from a method comparison experiment. If this same experiment were conducted 100 times, then the slope would fall between 0.972 and 0.988 in 95 of the 100 times. Confidence intervals serve to convey the variability of estimates and quantify the variability.

Data Analysis to Establish a Reference Interval

To establish a reference interval, it is recommended that the study includes at least 120 individuals. This can be challenging and costly, but it may be necessary for esoteric and laboratory-developed tests. Once the acceptable raw data have been generated, the next step is to actually define the reference interval. The reference interval is calculated statistically using methods that depend on the distribution of the data. In the most basic sense, data may be either normally distributed (Gaussian) or skewed (non-Gaussian) (see Fig. 3.6). If reference data are normally distributed, the reference interval can be determined using a parametric method. A parametric method defines the interval by the mean ±1.96 SDs; by centering on the mean, this formula will include the central 95% of values as given in the example in Figure 3.20A.

Most analytes do not display a normal (Gaussian) distribution. For example, the distribution of βhCG in pregnant individuals over a range of gestational ages is skewed (Fig. 3.20B); although the selection of a wide range of gestational ages makes this a poor population for a reference interval study, it was selected as an example to emphasize the need for nonparametric intervals. Data that are not normally distributed (i.e., non-Gaussian) must be analyzed using nonparametric analyses. Nonparametric determination of the reference interval is analyzed using percentiles, which do not depend on the distribution. The reference interval is determined by using the central 95% of values; the reference range is therefore defined by the 2.5th to the 97.5th percentiles, as demonstrated in Figure 3.20B. To calculate the interval, values are ranked from lowest to highest and the 2.5th and 97.5th percentiles are then calculated as follows:

$$n = \text{number of reference specimens}$$
$$2.5\text{th percentile} = 0.025(n+1) \qquad \text{(Eq. 3-7)}$$
$$97.5\text{th percentile} = 0.975(n+1)$$

Most reference interval analyses are determined using nonparametric analysis. This is because nonparametric analysis can be used on Gaussian distributed data and it is the CLSI-recommended method (Fig. 3.20B).[45]

With the development of statistical software packages such as Analyse-it, EP Evaluator, GraphPad Prism, JMP, MedCalc, Minitab, R, and SAS, reference intervals are rarely determined manually, although basic reference range verification can be done with in a spreadsheet with minimal effort just reviewing patient results (>90% or $n \geq 36$ out of $n = 40$ total) that fall within the proposed reference range. However they are determined, it is important to understand how basic statistical concepts are used to establish reference intervals. For more information on these software programs, the interested reader can access the references and online resources listed at the end of the chapter.

Data Analysis to Transfer and Verify a Reference Interval

When possible, clinical laboratories rely on assay manufacturers or on published primary literature as a source of reference intervals. This avoids the expensive and lengthy process of establishing a reference range interval on a minimum of 120 healthy people. The CLSI allows less vigorous studies to verify a reference interval with as few as 40 subject specimens.[45] Method verification studies can be used if the test method and study subjects are similar to the vendor's reference data and package insert information. The main assumption in using transference studies is that the reference method is of high quality and the subject populations are similar. The manufacturer's reported 95% reference limits may be considered valid if no more than 10% of the tested subjects fall outside the original reported limits. Figure 3.21 shows an example from our laboratory where we verify the manufacturer's reference range for free thyroxine (fT_4). In this example, fewer than 10% are outside the manufacturer's limits, enabling the reference interval to be adopted by the laboratory. If more than 10% of the

A

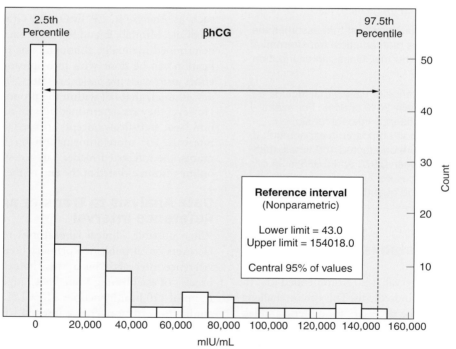

B

FIGURE 3.20 **(A)** Histogram of total thyroxine (TT$_4$) levels in a real population illustrating a shape indicative of a Gaussian distribution, which is analyzed by parametric statistics. The reference interval is determined from the mean ±1.96 SDs. **(B)** Histogram of beta-human chorionic gonadotropin (βhCG) levels in a population of pregnant women demonstrating non-Gaussian data and nonparametric determination of the reference interval. The reference interval is determined from percentiles to include the central 95% of values. Although the selection of a wide range of gestational ages makes this a poor population for a reference interval study, it does demonstrate the application of nonparametric intervals.

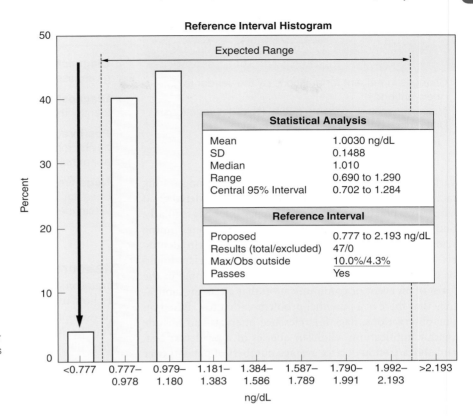

FIGURE 3.21 Reference verification test for free thyroxine (fT₄). Only 4.3% of the values are outside the expected range (*arrow*). The test passes because this is less than the allowable number of outlying samples (10%) (underlined in *red*).

values fall outside the proposed interval, an additional 20 or more specimens should be analyzed. If the second attempt at verification fails, the laboratorian should reexamine the analytic procedure and identify any differences between the laboratory's population and the population used by the manufacturer for their analysis. If no differences are identified, the laboratory may need to establish the reference interval using at least 120 individuals. Figure 3.22 demonstrates a simple algorithm to verify reference intervals.

Once a reference interval is completed, determined, and approved by the laboratory director, it needs to be effectively communicated and documented to the physicians and providers interpreting test results at the time the test results are reported. This is important given the slight

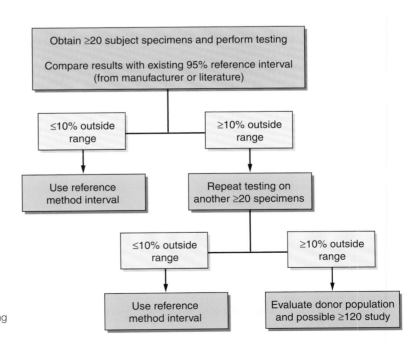

FIGURE 3.22 Algorithm to test whether a reference interval can be verified. A published reference interval (from a manufacturer or scientific literature) can be adopted if only a few samples fall outside the range. When possible, laboratory reference intervals are verified because of the time and expense of establishing a new interval.

TABLE 3.13	Common Problems Encountered when Monitoring Reference Intervals
Changes in reagent formulations by the vendor (e.g., new antibody)	
Minor changes in reagents due to lot-to-lot variations	
Differences between reference interval and test populations—selection bias	

DEFINITIONS BOX

Diagnostic sensitivity Ability of a test to detect a given disease or condition.

Diagnostic specificity Ability of a test to correctly identify the absence of a given disease or condition.

Positive predictive value Chance of an individual having a given disease or condition if the test is abnormal.

Negative predictive value Chance an individual does not have a given disease or condition if the test is within the reference interval.

variations in reference intervals seen even among testing facilities using similar methodologies. It is considered good laboratory practice to monitor reference intervals regularly. Some common problems that occur when determining reference intervals are given in Table 3.13. To help identify reference interval problems, the clinical laboratorian should be aware of common flags. These flags often come in the form of an event or communication that alerts the laboratory that there is a potential problem with a test. Based on our observations, flags for reference intervals can include vendor notifications, clinician queries of a particular test, and **shifts/trends** in large average numbers of patients over time. Review of a large number of patient results over time requires a laboratory information system capable of retrieving patient result data. In addition, all studies need to be evaluated as to patient population sampled and does it represent the desired donor population. Any of these or other related factors may warrant a review of existing reference intervals.

Not all analytes use population/gender/age-based reference intervals. For example, therapeutic drugs are not found in healthy individuals, such that the target values are based either on toxicity limits or on minimum effective concentrations. The target limits are derived from clinical or pharmacological studies rather than the healthy population studies described above. In these situations, the need for analytical accuracy is essential. One cannot apply a clinical cut point for a test if the results do not agree with the method used to determine the cut point. Cholesterol and HbA1c are also used in the context of clinical outcomes rather than reflecting values in a healthy population. The quintessential example of this is vitamin D testing in extreme latitudes or smog-ridden large cities, where a healthy population will be deficient.

DIAGNOSTIC EFFICIENCY

Ideally, healthy patients would have completely distinct laboratory values from patients with disease (Fig. 3.23A). However, the reality is that laboratory values usually overlap significantly between these populations (Fig. 3.23B). To determine how good a given test is at detecting and predicting the presence of disease (or a physiologic condition), there are a number of different parameters that are used. These parameters are broadly defined as *diagnostic efficiency*, which can be broken down into **sensitivity**, specificity, and **predictive values**.

Measures of Diagnostic Efficiency

Parameters of diagnostic efficiency are intended to quantify how useful a test is for a given disease or condition.[46] For example, βhCG is used as a test to diagnose pregnancy. While βhCG is excellent for this purpose, there are instances where βhCG may be increased because of other causes, such as cancer (trophoblastic tumors), or below the cutoff, as is the case very early in pregnancy.

It is important to recognize that there is both diagnostic and clinical sensitivity. Analytic sensitivity refers to the lower **limit of detection** for a given analyte, whereas clinical sensitivity refers to the proportion of individuals with that disease who test positively with the test. *Sensitivity* can be calculated from simple ratios (Fig. 3.24A). Patients with a condition who are correctly classified by a test to have the condition are called true positives (TPs). Patients with the condition who are classified by the test as not having the condition are called false negatives (FNs). Using the βhCG test as an example, sensitivity can be calculated as follows:

$$\text{Diagnostic sensitivity (\%)} = \frac{(\text{No. of pregnant with positive test})}{(\text{No. of pregnant individuals tested})}$$
$$= (\text{TP})/(\text{TP} + \text{FN})$$

(Eq. 3-8)

Another measure of clinical performance is diagnostic **specificity**. *Diagnostic specificity* is defined as the proportion of individuals without a condition who have a negative test for that condition (Fig. 3.24B). Note that there is also an analytic specificity (described in the Method Evaluation section), which refers to cross-reactivity with other substances. Continuing with βhCG as an example, diagnostic specificity refers to the percentage of nonpregnant individuals that have a negative test compared with the number of nonpregnant individuals tested. Patients who are not pregnant and have a negative βhCG test are called true negatives (TNs), whereas those who are incorrectly classified as pregnant by the test are called false positives (FPs). Clinical specificity can be calculated as follows:

FIGURE 3.23 Comparison of an ideal and true laboratory values for healthy and abnormal populations. **(A)** In the ideal case, the healthy population is completely distinct from those with the condition. **(B)** In reality, values show significant overlap that affects the diagnostic efficiency of the test.

FIGURE 3.24 The sensitivity and specificity of beta-human chorionic gonadotropin (βhCG) for pregnancy. **(A)** Sensitivity refers to the ability to detect pregnancy. **(B)** Specificity refers to the ability of the test to correctly classify nonpregnant women. FN, false negative; FP, false positive; TN, true negative; TP, true positive.

$$\text{Specificity (\%)} = \frac{(\text{No. of nonpregnant with negative test})}{(\text{No. of nonpregnant individuals tested})}$$
$$(\text{TN})/(\text{TN}+\text{FP})$$

(Eq. 3-9)

For example, a sensitivity of 100% plus a specificity of 100% means that the test detects every patient with disease and that the test is negative for every patient without the disease. Because of the overlap in laboratory values between people with and without disease, this is, of course, almost never the case (see Fig. 3.23B).

There are other measures of diagnostic efficiency such as predictive values. There are predictive values for both positive and negative test results. The predictive value of a positive (PPV) test refers to the probability of an individual having the disease if the result is abnormal ("positive" for the condition). Conversely, the predictive value of a negative (NPV) test refers to the probability that a patient does not have a disease if a result is within the reference range (test is negative for the disease) (Fig. 3.25). Predictive values are also calculated using ratios of TPs, TNs, FPs, and FNs as follows:

$$\text{PPV} = \frac{(\text{No. of pregnant with positive test})}{(\text{No. with positive test})}$$ (Eq. 3-10)
$$(\text{TP})/(\text{TP}+\text{FP})$$

$$\text{NPV} = \frac{(\text{No. of nonpregnant with negative test})}{(\text{No. with negative test})}$$ (Eq. 3-11)
$$(\text{TN})/(\text{TN}+\text{FN})$$

Using the data from Figure 3.25, if the βhCG test is "positive," there is a 72% chance the patient is pregnant; if the test is negative, then there is a 78% chance the patient is not pregnant. It is important to understand that unlike sensitivity and specificity, predictive values depend on the prevalence of the condition in the population studied. Prevalence refers to the proportion of individuals within a given population who have a particular condition. If one were testing for βhCG, the prevalence of pregnancy would be quite different between female Olympic athletes and young women shopping for baby clothes (Table 3.14). Accordingly, the predictive values would change drastically, while the sensitivity and specificity of the test would remain unchanged.

Measures of diagnostic efficiency depend entirely on the distribution of test results for a population with and without the condition and the cutoff used to define abnormal levels. The laboratory does not have control of the overlap between populations but does have control of the test cutoff. Thus, we will consider what happens when the cutoff is adjusted. The test cutoff (also known as a "medical decision limit") is the analyte concentration that separates a "positive" test from a "negative" one. For qualitative tests, such as a urine βhCG, the cutoff is defined by the manufacturer and can be visualized directly (Fig. 3.26). For quantitative tests, the cutoff is a concentration; in the case of pregnancy, a serum βhCG concentration greater than 5 mIU/mL could be considered "positive." By changing the cutoff, from 8 mIU/mL (Fig. 3.27A) to 5 mIU/mL (Fig. 3.27B) or 2 mIU/mL (Fig. 3.27C), it becomes apparent that the diagnostic efficiency changes. As the cutoff is lowered, the sensitivity of the test for pregnancy improves from 40% (Fig. 3.27A) to 90% (Fig. 3.27C). However, this

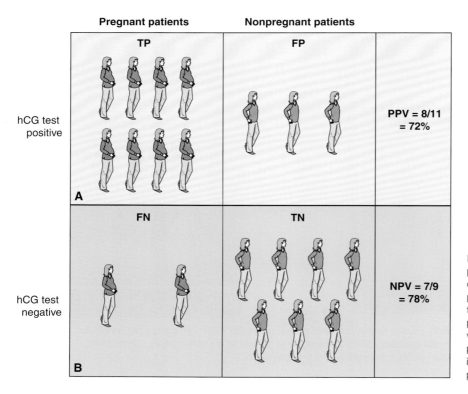

Pregnant patients   **Nonpregnant patients**

TP   FP

hCG test positive

PPV = 8/11 = 72%

FN   TN

hCG test negative

NPV = 7/9 = 78%

A

B

FIGURE 3.25 Positive and negative predictive values using beta-human chorionic gonadotropin (βhCG) as a test for pregnancy. **(A)** Predictive value of a positive test (PPV) indicates the probability of being pregnant if the test is positive. **(B)** Predictive value of a negative test (NPV) refers to the probability of being nonpregnant if the test is negative. FN, false negative; FP, false positive; TN, true negative; TP, true positive.

TABLE 3.14 Dependence of Predictive Value on Condition Prevalence[a]

Population[b]	Prevalence of Pregnancy	+PPV (%)	NPV (%)
Olympic athletes	1/10,000	0.03	99.99
Ob/gyn clinic patients aged 18–35 y	1/50	5.16	99.42
Babies "R" Us shoppers	3/10	53.33	89.09

[a]Based on a constant sensitivity of 80% and specificity of 70%.
[b]Hypothetical.
PPV, positive predictive value; NPV, negative predictive value.

occurs at the expense of specificity, which decreases from 80% (Fig. 3.27A) to 40% (Fig. 3.27C) at the same cutoff. The best test with the wrong cutoff would be clinically useless. Accordingly, it is imperative to use an appropriate cutoff for the testing purpose. In the most rudimentary sense, a high sensitivity is desirable for a screening test, whereas a high specificity is appropriate for confirmation testing.

To define an appropriate cutoff, laboratorians often use a graphical tool called the receiver operator characteristic (ROC).[47] ROC curves are generated by plotting the true-positive rate against the false-positive rate (sensitivity vs. 1 − specificity; Fig. 3.28). Each point on the curve represents an actual cutoff concentration. ROC curves can be used to determine the most efficient cutoff for a test and are an excellent tool for comparing two different tests. The area under the curve represents the efficiency of the test, that is, how often the test correctly classifies individuals as having a condition or not. The higher the area under the ROC curve, the greater the efficiency. Figure 3.28 shows a hypothetical comparison of two tests used to diagnose pregnancy. The βhCG test has a larger area under the curve and has an overall higher performance than test B. Based on these ROC curves, βhCG represents a superior test compared with hypothetical test B, for diagnosing pregnancy.

ROC curves can also be used to determine the optimal cutoff point for a test. The optimal cutoff maximizes the number of correct tests (i.e., fewest FPs and FNs). A perfect test would have an area under the curve of 1.0 and reach the top-left corner of the graph (where sensitivity and specificity equal 100%). Clinical evaluations of diagnostic tests frequently use ROC curves to establish optimal cutoffs and compare different tests.[47] As with the other statistical measures described, there are many software applications that can be used to generate ROC curves.

In addition to sensitivity, specificity, and predictive values, there are a number of other measures of diagnostic efficiency. These include odds ratios, likelihood ratios, and multivariate analysis.[48,49] While these have increasingly higher degrees of complexity, they all represent efforts to make clinical sense of data postanalytically. It is worth remembering the bigger picture, which is that laboratory values are not used in isolation. Laboratory tests are interpreted in the context of a patient's physical exam, symptoms, and clinical history to achieve a diagnosis.

SUMMARY

Collectively, method validation is the first step toward establishing quality for a new method. Once a method has an established acceptable performance, quality control, proficiency testing, and reference interval review are employed to ensure that quality is maintained. Underpinning all decisions about quality are allowable error limits and the clinical requirements of a given test. Given a set of clinical requirements, visual inspection and basic statistics are used to help decide if a method meets the clinical need. Beyond the analytical performance of a test is the diagnostic efficiency, the measure of how well a test can differentiate a diseased state from a healthy one. Diligent method evaluation and ongoing quality monitoring ensure that a test consistently meets analytical and clinical requirements to maximize diagnostic utility.

FIGURE 3.26 An example of a point-of-care device for beta-human chorionic gonadotropin. This is an example of a qualitative test, where the test line (T) represents whether the patient has a positive test, and the control (C) line is used to indicate that the test was successful.

Positive control (C) line

Test result (T) line

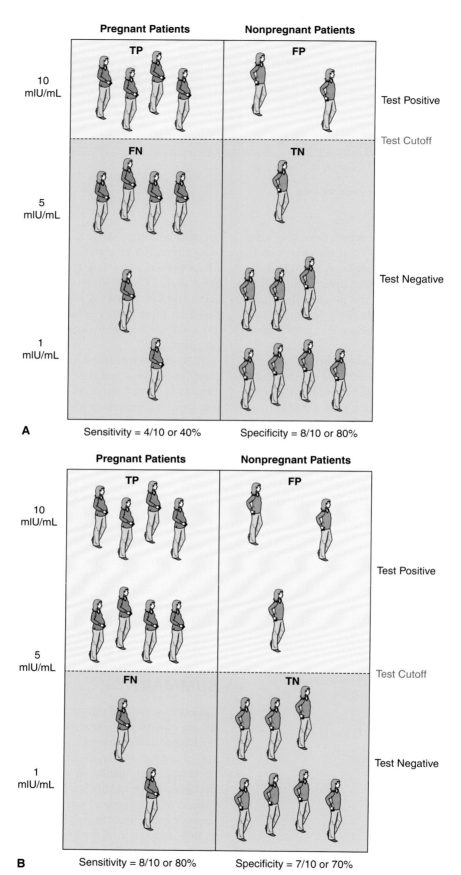

FIGURE 3.27 The effect of adjusting the beta-human chorionic gonadotropin test cutoff on sensitivity and specificity for pregnancy. **(A)** Using a high cutoff, sensitivity is low and specificity is high. **(B, C)** As the cutoff is lowered, the sensitivity improves at the expense of specificity. The predictive values also change as the cutoff is adjusted. TP, true positive; FP, false positive; FN, false negative; TN, true negative.

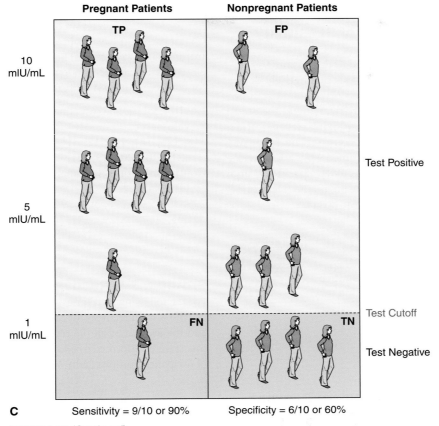

C

Sensitivity = 9/10 or 90%   Specificity = 6/10 or 60%

FIGURE 3.27 (*Continued*)

FIGURE 3.28 A receiver operator characteristic curve for beta-human chorionic gonadotropin (βhCG) and a hypothetical "test B." The area under the βhCG curve is greater than "test B" at all points, indicating that it is a superior test for pregnancy. The *thin dotted line* represents a test of no value (equal to diagnosis by a coin toss). The maximum (optimal) efficiency is indicated by the *arrow* and corresponds to the βhCG cutoff concentration with the fewest incorrect patient classifications.

Total area under the curve (AUC)

	βhCG	Test B	Difference
AUC	0.993	0.813	0.180

PRACTICE PROBLEMS

Problem 3-1. Calculation of Sensitivity and Specificity

Urine hCG tests are commonly used to determine if someone is pregnant. Urine pregnancy tests qualitatively detect the presence of hCG in the urine. While manufacturers often state 99.99% accuracy, they are referring to the accuracy of a test in a patient who has a highly elevated urine hCG, effectively testing a positive control. The following data are based on population of women only a few weeks into pregnancy. Calculate the sensitivity, specificity, and efficiency of urine hCG for detecting pregnancy. Determine the predictive value of a positive urine hCG test.

Number of Pregnancies/Interpretation of hCG Findings			
Pregnant?	Positive Urine hCG	Negative Urine hCG	Total
Yes	32	8	40
No	5	143	148
Total	37	151	188

Problem 3-2. A Quality Control Decision

Glucose Control Values		
Day	Low	High
1	86	215
2	82	212
3	83	218
4	87	214
5	85	220
6	81	217
7	88	223
8	83	224
9	82	217
10	85	222

1. Calculate the mean and standard deviation for the above data set.
2. Plot these control data by day (one graph for each level, x-axis = day, y-axis = concentration). Indicate the mean and the upper and lower control limits (mean ±2 standard deviations) with horizontal lines (see Fig. 3.28).
3. You are working in the night shift at a community hospital and are the only person in the laboratory. You are running glucose quality control and obtain the following:

   Low control value = 90; High control value = 230
   Plot these controls on the process control chart (Levey-Jennings) you created above.

4. Are these values within the control limits?
5. What do you observe about these control data?
6. What might be a potential problem?
7. What is an appropriate next step?

Problem 3-3. Precision (Replication)

For the following precision data, calculate the mean, SD, and CV for each of the two control solutions A and B. These control solutions were chosen because their concentrations were close to medical decision levels (X_C) for glucose: 120 mg/dL for control solution A and 300 mg/dL for control solution B.

Control solution A was analyzed daily, and the following values were obtained:
118, 120, 121, 119, 125, 118, 122, 116, 124, 123, 117, 117, 121, 120, 120, 119, 121, 123, 120, and 122 mg/dL.
Control solution B was analyzed daily and gave the following results:
295, 308, 296, 298, 304, 294, 308, 310, 296, 300, 295, 303, 305, 300, 308, 297, 297, 305, 292, and 300 mg/dL.
Does the precision exceed the total allowable error defined by the CLIA?

Problem 3-4. Recovery

For the following tacrolimus immunosuppressant data, calculate the percent recovery for each of the individual experiments and the average of all the recovery experiments. The experiments were performed by adding two levels of standard to each of five patient samples (A through E) with the following results:

Sample	0.9 mL Blood + 0.1 mL Water	0.9 mL Blood + 0.1 mL 50 µg/L STD	0.9 mL Blood + 0.1 mL 100 µg/L STD
A	6.0	11.0	15.6
B	6.3	11.2	16.0
C	8.6	13.6	18.5
D	13.0	17.8	23.1
E	22.5	27.0	32.0

What do the results of this study indicate?

Problem 3-5. Interference

For the interference data that follow for glucose, calculate the concentration of bilirubin added, the interference for each individual sample, and the average interference for the group of patient samples. The experiments were performed by adding 0.1 mL of a 150 mg/dL ascorbic acid standard to 0.9 mL of five different patient samples (A through E). A similar dilution was prepared for each patient sample using water as the diluent. The results follow:

Sample	Glucose (mg/dL) 0.9 mL Serum + 0.1 mL Water	Glucose (mg/dL) 0.9 mL Serum + 0.1 mL 150 mg/dL Bilirubin STD
A	54	40
B	99	80
C	122	101
D	162	133
E	297	256

What do the results of this study indicate?

Problem 3-6. Sample Labeling

You receive an urine specimen in the laboratory with a request for a complete urinalysis. The cup is labeled and you begin your testing. You finish the testing and report the results to the ward. Several minutes later, you receive a telephone call from the ward informing you that the urine was reported on the wrong patient. You are told that the cup was labeled incorrectly before it was brought to the laboratory.

1. What is the problem in this case, and where did it occur?
2. Would your laboratory's QC system be able to detect or prevent this type of problem?

Problem 3-7. QC Program for POCT Testing

Your laboratory is in charge of overseeing the QC program for the glucometers (POCT) in use at your hospital. You notice that the ward staff is not following proper procedure for running QC. For example, in this case, the glucometer QC was rerun three times in a row in an effort to have the results in control. The first two runs were both 3 SD high. The last run did return to less than 2 SDs. Explain the correct follow-up procedure for dealing with the out-of-control results.

Problem 3-8. QC Rule Interpretation

Explain the R_{4s} rule, including what type of error it detects.

Problem 3-9. Reference Interval Study Design

You are asked to design a reference interval study for a new test. The results are known to be different in men and women and is affected by the consumption of aspirin, age, and time of day. Create a questionnaire to collect the appropriate information needed to perform a reference interval study. How would you account for these variables in the data collection?

For additional student resources, please visit thePoint® at http://thepoint.lww.com

questions

1. A Gaussian distribution is usually
   a. Bell shaped
   b. Rectangular
   c. Uniform
   d. Skewed

2. The following chloride (mmol/L) results were obtained using a new analyzer:

106	111	104	106	112	110
115	127	83	110	108	109
83	119	105	106	108	114
120	100	107	110	109	102

   What is the mean?
   a. 108
   b. 105
   c. 109
   d. 107

3. The following chloride (mmol/L) results were obtained using a new analyzer:

106	111	104	106	112	110
115	127	83	110	108	109
83	119	105	106	108	114
120	100	107	110	109	102

   What is the median?
   a. 108.5
   b. 105
   c. 112
   d. 107

4. For a data value set that is Gaussian distributed, what is the likelihood (%) that a data point will be within ±1 SD from the mean?
   a. 68%
   b. 99%
   c. 95%
   d. 100%

5. The correlation coefficient
   a. Indicates the strength of relationship in a linear regression
   b. Determines the regression type used to derive the slope and y-intercept
   c. Is always expressed as "b"
   d. Expresses method imprecision

6. If two methods agree perfectly in a method comparison study, the slope equals _____ and the y-intercept equals _____.
   a. 1.0, 0.0
   b. 0.0, 1.0
   c. 1.0, 1.0
   d. 0.0, 0.0
   e. 0.5, 0.5

7. Systematic error can best be described as consisting of
   a. Constant and proportional error
   b. Constant error
   c. Proportional error
   d. Random error
   e. Syntax error

(continues on page 84)

review questions (continued)

8. Examples of typical reference interval data distribution plots include all of the following except
   a. ROC
   b. Nonparametric
   c. Parametric
   d. Bimodal

9. A reference range can be verified by
   a. Testing as few as 20 normal donor specimens
   b. Literature and vendor material review
   c. Using samples from previously tested hospital patients
   d. Using pharmacy-provided Plasmanate spiked with target analyte concentrations

10. Reference interval transference studies
   a. Are used to verify a reference interval
   b. Are used to establish a reference interval
   c. Require as many as 120 normal donors
   d. Use a 68% reference limit for acceptability

11. Diagnostic specificity is the
   a. Ability of a test to correctly identify the absence of a given disease or condition
   b. Chance an individual does not have a given disease or condition if the test is within the reference interval
   c. Chance of an individual having a given disease or condition if the test is abnormal
   d. Ability of a test to detect a given disease or condition

12. To evaluate a moderately complex laboratory test, all of the following must be done except:
   a. Analytical sensitivity and specificity
   b. Verification of the reference interval
   c. Accuracy and precision
   d. Reportable range

13. An ROC includes all of the following except:
   a. Perfect test = an area under the curve <1.0
   b. Equals receiver operator characteristic
   c. Plots sensitivity and 1 – specificity
   d. Can be used to compare two different tests

14. For method development studies, which analytical performance test should be done first?
   a. Imprecision studies
   b. Comparison of methods (COM)
   c. Recovery
   d. Interference studies
   e. Does not matter, they all need to be done

15. For the following series of laboratory values, the vendor has indicated that a true value is 6.0. Series = 5, 4, 5, 6, 7, 5, 3, 8, 5, 9, 5, 4, 5, 6. The SDI (standard deviation index) is:
   a. −0.3
   b. +0.3
   c. +1.0
   d. −0.7

16. Comparison of method studies:
   a. Estimate systematic error.
   b. Use primary QC material and standards that span the reportable range.
   c. Are usually completed within 4 working days.
   d. Are not required for nonwaived tests.

17. Interference studies typically use _____ as an interferent.
   a. All of these
   b. Hemolyzed red cells
   c. Highly icteric samples
   d. Highly lipemic samples

18. Allowable analytical error is
   a. A combination of random and systematic error
   b. Best if it is greater than the total error
   c. Used only for research and initial evaluation studies

online resources

AACC	http://aacc.org	JMP	http://www.jmp.com
Centers for Disease Control and Prevention	http://www.cdc.gov	Labs Online	http://www.labtestsonline.org
CLIA	http://www.cms.hhs.gov/clia	McLendon Clinical Laboratories	http://labs.unchealthcare.org
CLSI	http://www.clsi.org	OIVD	http://www.fda.gov/CDRH/oivd
College of American Pathologists	http://CAP.org	R	http://www.r-project.org/
EP Evaluator	http://www.dgrhoads.com	SAS	http://www.sas.com
FDA	http://www.FDA.gov	Westgard Laboratory pages	http://www.westgard.com
GraphPAD	http://www.graphpad.com		http://www.fda.gov/MedicalDevices

references

1. Westgard JO, de Vos DJ, Hunt MR, et al. Concepts and practices in the evaluation of clinical chemistry methods. V. Applications. *Am J Med Technol.* 1978;44:803–813.
2. Wakkers PJ, Hellendoorn HB, Op de Weegh GJ, et al. Applications of statistics in clinical chemistry. A critical evaluation of regression lines. *Clin Chim Acta.* 1975;64:173–184.
3. Centers for Disease Control and Prevention (CDC), Centers for Medicare and Medicaid Services (CMS), Health and Human Services. Medicare, Medicaid, and CLIA programs; laboratory requirements relating to quality systems and certain personnel qualifications. Final rule. *Fed Regist.* 2003;68:3639–3714.
4. Westgard JO, de Vos DJ, Hunt MR, et al. Concepts and practices in the evaluation of clinical chemistry methods. I. Background and approach. *Am J Med Technol.* 1978;44:290–300.
5. National Committee for Clinical Laboratory Standards (NCCLS). *Approved Guideline for Precision Performance of Clinical Chemistry Devices.* Villanova, PA: NCCLS; 1999 (Document no. EP05-A).
6. Westgard JO, de Vos DJ, Hunt MR, et al. Concepts and practices in the evaluation of clinical chemistry methods. II. Experimental procedures. *Am J Med Technol.* 1978;44:420–430.
7. Krouwer JS, Rabinowitz R. How to improve estimates of imprecision. *Clin Chem.* 1984;30:290–292.
8. Westgard JO, Burnett RW. Precision requirements for cost-effective operation of analytic processes. *Clin Chem.* 1990;36:1629–1632.
9. Westgard JO, Carey RN, Wold S. Criteria for judging precision and accuracy in method development and evaluation. *Clin Chem.* 1974;20:825–833.
10. Westgard JO. *Basic Method Evaluation.* 2nd ed. Madison, WI: Westgard Quality Corp; 2003.
11. National Committee for Clinical Laboratory Standards (NCCLS). *Proposed Guideline for Interference Testing in Clinical Chemistry.* Villanova, PA: NCCLS; 1986 (Document no. EP07-A).
12. Young DS. *Effects of Drugs on Clinical Laboratory Tests.* 4th ed. Washington, DC: American Association of Clinical Chemistry; 2000.
13. Siest G, Galteau MM. *Drug Effects on Laboratory Tests.* Littleton, MA: PSG Publishing; 1988.
14. Glick MR, Ryder KW. Analytical systems ranked by freedom from interferences. *Clin Chem.* 1987;33:1453–1458.
15. Glick MR, Ryder KW, Jackson SA. Graphical comparisons of interferences in clinical chemistry instrumentation. *Clin Chem.* 1986;32:470–475.
16. Ryder KW, Glick MR. Erroneous laboratory results from hemolyzed, icteric, and lipemic specimens. *Clin Chem.* 1993;39:175–176.
17. National Committee for Clinical Laboratory Standards (NCCLS). *Approved Guideline for Method Comparison and Bias Estimation Using Patient Samples.* Villanova, PA: NCCLS; 2002 (Document no. EP09-A2).
18. Shahzad K, Kim DH, Kang MJ. Analytic evaluation of the beta-human chorionic gonadotropin assay on the Abbott IMx and Elecsys2010 for its use in doping control. *Clin Biochem.* 2007;40:1259–1265.
19. National Committee for Clinical Laboratory Standards (NCCLS). *Proposed Guideline for Evaluation of Linearity of Quantitative Analytical Methods.* Villanova, PA: NCCLS; 2001 (Document no. EP6-P2).
20. Westgard JO, Hunt MR. Use and interpretation of common statistical tests in method-comparison studies. *Clin Chem.* 1973;19:49–57.
21. Westgard JO. Precision and accuracy: concepts and assessment by method evaluation testing. *Crit Rev Clin Lab Sci.* 1981;13:283–330.
22. Cornbleet PJ, Gochman N. Incorrect least-squares regression coefficients in method-comparison analysis. *Clin Chem.* 1979;25:432–438.
23. Feldmann U, Schneider B, Klinkers H, et al. A multivariate approach for the biometric comparison of analytical methods in clinical chemistry. *J Clin Chem Clin Biochem.* 1981;19:121–137.
24. Westgard JO, de Vos DJ, Hunt MR, et al. Concepts and practices in the evaluation of clinical chemistry methods: IV. Decisions of acceptability. *Am J Med Technol.* 1978;44:727–742.
25. Barnett RN. Medical significance of laboratory results. *Am J Clin Pathol.* 1968;50:671–676.
26. Fraser CG. Data on biological variation: essential prerequisites for introducing new procedures? *Clin Chem.* 1994;40:1671–1673.
27. Fraser CG. *Biological Variation: From Principles to Practice.* Washington, DC: AACC Press; 2001.
28. Tonks DB. A study of the accuracy and precision of clinical chemistry determinations in 170 Canadian laboratories. *Clin Chem.* 1963;9:217–233.
29. Medicare, Medicaid and CLIA programs; regulations implementing the Clinical Laboratory Improvement Amendments of 1988 (CLIA)—HCFA. Final rule with comment period. *Fed Regist.* 1992;57:7002–7186.
30. Ehrmeyer SS, Laessig RH, Leinweber JE, et al. 1990 Medicare/CLIA final rules for proficiency testing: minimum intralaboratory performance characteristics (CV and bias) needed to pass. *Clin Chem.* 1990;36:1736–1740.
31. Westgard JO, Seehafer JJ, Barry PL. European specifications for imprecision and inaccuracy compared with operating specifications that assure the quality required by US CLIA proficiency-testing criteria. *Clin Chem.* 1994;40(7 pt 1):1228–1232.
32. Bland JM, Altman DG. Statistical methods for assessing agreement between two methods of clinical measurement. *Lancet.* 1986;1:307–310.
33. Levey S, Jennings ER. The use of control charts in the clinical laboratory. *Am J Clin Pathol.* 1950;20:1059–1066.
34. Westgard JO, Barry PL, Hunt MR, et al. A multi-rule Shewhart chart for quality control in clinical chemistry. *Clin Chem.* 1981;27:493–501.
35. Clinical and Laboratory Standards Institute (CLSI). *Statistical Quality Control for Quantitative Measurements: Principles and Definitions.* Wayne, PA: CLSI; 2006.
36. Westgard JO, Groth T. Power functions for statistical control rules. *Clin Chem.* 1979;25:863–869.
37. Westgard JO, Groth T, Aronsson T, et al. Performance characteristics of rules for internal quality control: probabilities for false rejection and error detection. *Clin Chem.* 1977;23:1857–1867.
38. Solberg HE. The IFCC recommendation on estimation of reference intervals. The RefVal program. *Clin Chem Lab Med.* 2004;42:710–714.
39. Solberg HE. International Federation of Clinical Chemistry. Scientific Committee, Clinical Section. Expert Panel on Theory of Reference Values and International Committee for Standardization in Haematology Standing Committee on Reference Values. Approved recommendation (1986) on the

theory of reference values. Part 1. The concept of reference values. *Clin Chim Acta.* 1987;165:111–118.

40. Solberg HE. International Federation of Clinical Chemistry (IFCC), Scientific Committee, Clinical Section, Expert Panel on Theory of Reference Values, and International Committee for Standardization in Haematology (ICSH), Standing Committee on Reference Values. Approved Recommendation (1986) on the theory of reference values. Part 1. The concept of reference values. *J Clin Chem Clin Biochem.* 1987;25:337–342.

41. International Committee for Standardization in Haematology (ICSH). Standardization of blood specimen collection procedure for reference values. *Clin Lab Haematol.* 1982;4:83–86.

42. Clinical Laboratory Improvement Amendments of 1988; final rule. *Fed Regist.* 7164 [42 CFR 493.1213]: Department of Health and Human Services, Centers for Medicare and Medicaid Services; 1992.

43. van der Meulen EA, Boogaard PJ, van Sittert NJ. Use of small-sample-based reference limits on a group basis. *Clin Chem.* 1994;40:1698–1702.

44. National Committee for Clinical Laboratory Standards (NCCLS). *How to Define and Determine Reference Intervals in the Clinical Laboratory; Approved Guideline C28-A2.* Wayne, PA: NCCLS; 2000.

45. Clinical and Laboratory Standards Institute (CLSI). C28-A2: *How to Define and Determine Reference Intervals in the Clinical Laboratory; Approved Guideline.* 2nd ed. Villanova, PA: CLSI; 2008.

46. Galen RS, Gambino SR. *Beyond Normality: The Predictive Value and Efficiency of Medical Diagnoses.* New York, NY: Wiley; 1975.

47. Zweig MH, Campbell G. Receiver-operating characteristic (ROC) plots: a fundamental evaluation tool in clinical medicine [published erratum appears in *Clin Chem.* 1993;39:1589]. *Clin Chem.* 1993;39:561–577.

48. van der Helm HJ, Hische EA, Bolhuis PA. Bayes' theorem and the estimation of the likelihood ratio. *Clin Chem.* 1982;28:1250–1251.

49. Reibnegger G, Fuchs D, Hausen A, et al. Generalized likelihood ratio concept and logistic regression analysis for multiple diagnostic categories. *Clin Chem.* 1989;35:990–994.

4

Lean Six Sigma Methodology Basics and Quality Improvement in the Clinical Chemistry Laboratory

CINDI BULLOCK LETSOS, MICHAEL W. ROGERS, CHRISTOPER R. McCUDDEN, and MONTE S. WILLIS

chapter outline

key terms

chapter objectives

Upon completion of this chapter, the clinical laboratorian should be able to do the following:

- Discuss the basic concepts of Lean Six Sigma process improvement.
- Apply the DMAIC methodology in laboratory process improvement projects.
- Explain the role of Six Sigma Metrics in laboratory quality control.
- Discuss new concepts in Clinical Laboratory Quality Management, including Individual Quality Control Program (IQCP) and ISO 151189.

For additional student resources, please visit thePoint at http://thepoint.lww.com

LEAN SIX SIGMA METHODOLOGY

In the previous chapter, we discussed how laboratory tests are established by method evaluation and how **quality control (QC)** continuously monitors their processes. In this chapter, we expand on these ideas to discuss the concept of quality improvement (QI) and **quality assurance (QA)** (Fig. 4.1). Quality improvement and quality assurance (QI/QA) goes beyond monitoring, detecting, and preventing errors and eliminates potential negative patient impact events. QI/QA achieves new levels of performance, not otherwise realized through QC, and addresses chronic problems. **Lean Six Sigma** is the combination of Six Sigma methodology and Lean principles. The Six Sigma business management strategy developed by Motorola, Inc. in the 1980s seeks to improve the performance of a process by identifying and eliminating causes of defects and errors, resulting in eliminating variation in the process. Lean principles work to eliminate the waste, such as streamlining a process to reduce wait times or modifying a process to reduce cost. Lean manufacturing strategy, pioneered by Toyota Motor Company Management, provides tangible metrics for QI. In its simplest form, Six Sigma asks the question, "How can this process be improved?" Lean manufacturing asks the question, "Does this process (or step) need to exist?" Together as Lean Six Sigma, sometimes abbreviated as LSS, they are being increasingly used to reduce error (Six Sigma) and waste (Lean) within the health care system. These tools are increasingly being used in health care, including laboratory services, to reduce error and waste.

FIGURE 4.1 QI for a given process. QI seeks to eliminate inefficiencies in a process through reduction of variation and waste. The current process exhibits high variation and waste, and QC measures do not adequately manage the process. After a period of QI, the desired process shows much smaller variation and waste and tighter control of the process using the new QC measures. Lean Six Sigma methodology seeks to identify, measure, and eliminate the large gaps of inefficiency in a process. Examples from the laboratory include data accuracy, turnaround times, and reagent inventory.

ADOPTION AND IMPLEMENTATION OF LEAN SIX SIGMA

Effective adoption of Lean Six Sigma for process improvement requires an organization-wide dedication and support for a continuous process improvement culture. A pioneer in this field, Dr. J. M. Juran taught that continuous improvement does not make an organization distinctive or "excellent." Instead, it is the rate of improvement that distinguishes an organization.[1] Effecting change will not occur without support from senior members within the organization. These leaders select and assign QI projects to teams within the organization.

The most common team roles are the project coaches/leaders (black belts), project team members (green belts and yellow belts), and project sponsors or champions that may or may not have much experience with LSS but are critical to the success of implementing change within an organization. The colored belt designations are given to different levels and types of training in either Lean or Six Sigma, with some overlap (e.g., the highest levels are Black Belts in both Lean and Six Sigma). Their application to health care and mixing of the complementary methodologies has led to the use of varied designations, which we here discuss in general terms only. Black belt–trained coaches dedicate as much as 100% of their time to QI projects, proactively addressing process and quality opportunities for improvement. Black belt training includes training at all levels (e.g., yellow, green) in addition to significant additional training in statistical analysis, coaching, and facilitation. Black belt certification additionally involves the successful completion of multiple projects and written test. Green belt training focuses on understanding and applying the five phases of the Six Sigma process, including completion of a project for certification. Green Belt trainees contribute approximately 20% of their time to improvement projects while delivering their normal job functions. Yellow belt training includes a full day basic Lean Six Sigma training, including interactive and didactic training program, as a perquisite for all participation in projects. Sponsors or Champions attend a 1-day training class and are usually mid- to senior-level leaders who review the project, remove organizational barriers, and encourage the team members. In the laboratory, a team may consist of technologists with subject matter expertise (and trained as yellow or green belts in our organization), supervisors, directors, and a black belt or an expert consultant who will coach the team (Boxes 4.1 to 4.4).

PROCESS IMPROVEMENT

All work is a dynamic process, and every process has variation, overlap, and waste. Variation results in unpredictable and undesirable outcomes. Waste results in increased cost and delays and thereby limiting efficiency. Lean Six Sigma uses a problem–cause–solution methodology to improve any process through waste elimination and variation reduction. The **DMAIC** (Define, Measure, Analyze, Improve,

BOX 4.1

Each phase of a Six Sigma project is data driven. Examples of projects included in our laboratory organization have included (1) Reducing Billing Errors in the Laboratory, which provided a significant monetary savings to the organization and (2) Reducing Blood Wastage in the Blood Bank, which modified

processes to ensure there were continued sufficient blood product supply for our patients and also provided monetary savings to the organization. These usually target quality or time-related problems expressed as numbers, percentages, or dollars with unknown causes. Remember these are very data driven.

BOX 4.2

Lean improvement projects are typically headed by black belts using staff trained in Lean principles. This is usually a 3- to 5-day project to reduce waste, such as turnaround times, wait times, flow or cycle times, and causes that can be seen by observation. The team actually does a "Gemba Walk" by going to the area and personally observing the "thing" going through the process. A Lean project is fast and is done in conjunction with the staff. It is very helpful to share some of the Lean basics so that all staff are knowledgeable and included in the process prior to the actual event. Planning is intense for several weeks prior to the event; however, the actual event is a 3- to 5-day project called a Kaizen event. Laboratories lend themselves well to Lean projects to create better workflow and reduce walking

or motion time and to produce a more value-added system and reduce waste. Some of the common Lean tools used include process mapping, value stream analysis, spaghetti charts, visual management, 6S (5S plus safety), impact effort grids, Kanban cards, and the identification of the eight Wastes of Lean or Muda (transportation, inventory, movement, waiting, overproduction, overprocessing, defects, underutilization of resources). Other Lean opportunities include shifting from push to pull, single piece flow, work leveling, and the focus of "doing it right, the first time." Lean allows for rapid improvement projects. Staff are dedicated to the project for the entire Kaizen event. Effective planning makes the Kaizen more productive and more fun for the team and develops ownership.

BOX 4.3

Most of our Lean improvement projects start with organizing the areas using 5S (Set, Sort, Shine, Standardize, Sustain, and Safety has been added to make it 6S). One project involving 6S ultimately resulted in enough workbench space cleared in conjunction with some renovations that another workstation was able to be added. This was a significant improvement as we needed another workstation to keep up with the workload due to the opening of our new cancer center. Also with the changes, we were to ensure that each product had a dedicated space, which improved patient safety for the processing of these products. Other projects in addition to 6S have improved ergonomics for staff, a significant reduction in motion and transportation, added recycling of plastics collecting 96 gallons

per week that have tripled since implementation, and Kanban systems to help with supply ordering have been implemented to prevent laboratories from "running out" of supplies and reagents as well as prevent overstocking. Other changes that have occurred due to our Kaizens are one-piece flow, development of a "cell" workflow, visual aids using color designations that have helped staff, use of value stream mapping to determine the most efficient workflow to redesign an area, and time savings on locating supplies by reorganizing and use of visual aids. To document our Kaizen events, we utilize A3 worksheets that consist of nine boxes (Reason for Action, Current State, Target State, Gap analysis, Solution approach, Experiments, Completion plan, Confirmed State and Insights).

BOX 4.4

Two other project types are Express Workouts and Process Design. If there is a well-understood focused problem for which the cause is known, then an Express Workout concept is utilized by working with a team over 6 weeks to improve the process and ultimately addressing process control. We utilized this technique in our lab for Serum Protein Electrophoresis testing and Interpretation. We knew there were duplication and overlapping of efforts by the technologists and the attending physicians. By mapping

out each part of the process by groups and then bringing all participants back together, we were able to streamline the total process by eliminating 16 steps and a time saving of 1.5 to 2 hours per day. Note that savings are not used to eliminate staff but allows for other responsibilities to be performed. Process design is utilized in the planning for a new facility or laboratory. A team of black belts and senior level executives work together over a 6- to 12-month period.

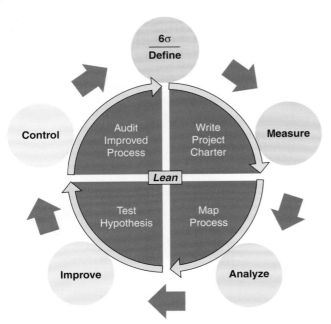

FIGURE 4.2 Integration of Six Sigma and Lean principles. The methodologies of Six Sigma manufacturing and Lean process optimization are combined to an iterative cycle of QI. Applications of Lean Six Sigma are now being applied to all aspects of the laboratory and the health care system as a whole.

the importance of the project, the scope of the project and the measures, and the project schedule and resources. This should be modified by the team as the project progresses. In the Measure phase, the team collects data to measure the process and establish a baseline. The Analyze phase verifies the root causes. In the Improve phase, the team pilots process changes and evaluates and fine-tunes the new process. The Control phase maintains process gains. See Table 4.1 for the detailed listing of the general steps of process improvement. At the end of each phase, a tollgate review is set up with the entire team and their sponsor. All information in that phase is then shared, and questions and discussion follow, including testing staff as well as the team involved in the process assessment. If the work has been performed as indicated in the project plan and the objectives achieved, the team is allowed by the sponsor to proceed to the next phase.

Let's apply the DMAIC methodology. The following generic example will not include all of the Six Sigma tools; however, it will provide a representation of a real Green Belt project and how the tools were used.

The project begins in the Define phase by setting a goal to reduce variation. The project charter states the overall purpose and potential impact, the scope of the project (what is included and what is not), resources (e.g., who is on the team and what resources are available to implement changes), and expectations—what will be delivered and the total project timetable. A high-level map is also created, called a **SIPOC (Supply–Input–Process–Output–Customer)**. This encourages system thinking by focusing the team to see the process through the customer's eyes. Team members listen and gather the **voice of the customer (VOC)** to identify key drivers of customer satisfaction and expand this further into a Critical to Quality (CTQ) tree to provide clarity around the aspects of the VOC and establish a specific "measurable" characteristic. The charter is a modifiable document intended to keep everyone involved and focused on the defined problem and improve the outcomes throughout the project. By the end of the Define phase, both the project team and the management team have validated the "project charter."

Control) methodology is the QI team's project management road map (Fig. 4.2). The five phases allow for the identification of the root cause for error and waste through establishment of the following:

1. A universally accepted framework for QI
2. Common language throughout the organization
3. A checklist to guide the process
4. Control measures to sustain improvements and offer long-term monitoring

The Define phase validates the problem(s) and explicitly describes the QI issues starting with a project charter. In constructing the charter, establish a problem statement,

TABLE 4.1 General Steps Within Each Phase of Process Improvement: DMAIC

Define	Measure	Analyze	Improve	Control
Create charter	Map and analyze current process	Brainstorm potential root causes	Develop potential solutions	Document process changes
Create SIPOC-hi level map	Develop data collection plan	Select potential root causes	Prioritize select solutions	Develop SOPs, training
Create VOC	Collect baseline data	Cause and effect data	Develop plans and pilots	Implement solutions and ongoing process measurements
			Implement pilots	
Use VOC present in CTQ tree	Calculate process sigma	Verify root causes	Develop full-scale implementation plans	Initiate dashboard
				Summarize lessons learned
Plan project including communication plan	Focus on charter and problem statement		Evaluate results	Transition to process owner

The Measure phase maps, measures, and assesses the current process. This would include mapping the entire process, collecting data, and graphing, which could include histograms, box plots, dot plots, run charts (time series charts), control charts (p, np, u, or c charts depending on the type of data), and frequency charts (Pareto charts) as well as descriptive statistics. Black Belts "crunch" the data and share with the Green Belts. The collection and plotting of real data will lead the team to review the current situation in detail. Then the Process Sigma is calculated. The higher the process sigma, the less variation in the process and the better the outcome. The Process Sigma metric focuses on defects and customer expectation. The goal is to achieve Six Sigma; however, in health care, it is often in the 3 to 4 sigma range leaving many opportunities for improvement.

In the Analyze phase, the team drills down to identify the root causes of the problem using some of the following techniques: (1) brainstorming, which can be used to consider a range of root causes; (2) applying a process called the 5 Whys (to continue to drill down what the root causes of identified problems are); (3) creating Fishbone Diagrams to facilitate brainstorming and recognizing relationships; (4) creating and applying Affinity Diagrams to finding commonalities in processes; and (5) using a Failure Mode and Effect Analysis (FMEA) tool to analyze risk and highlight aspects of a process that should be targeted for improvement. Using all of the data collected, a hypothesis is created and tested and statistically analyzed. This is used by the Black Belts and Green Belts to determine if there is a difference or relationship in the data.

The team next develops strategies that address each of these specific problems and pilots the changes in the Improve phase. The team brainstorms to develop possible solutions and then prioritizes them. They develop plans and implement pilots of the possible solutions. These are then fine-tuned as needed and developed into full-scale plans. Data are collected to compare the before and after of the pilot(s) to ensure that the process has indeed improved.

The Control phase ensures that the gains made by implemented improvements are maintained by QA mechanisms. Any changes in the process are documented in procedures, and training of staff and competencies are put in place to ensure the gains are sustained. Dashboards are initiated to share the improvements, and visuals are posted to help maintain those gains. The group summarizes Lessons Learned, which can be shared with other teams to provide insight to improve future projects. Often there are subsequent projects that spin off from completed ones. Additional items arise during the project that may need solutions but are not within the scope of this project. These are noted and are called "parking lot" items, so that these items are not forgotten. These need to be reviewed to see if future projects are needed to address these or shared with the appropriate staff as needed. The DMAIC methodology (Fig. 4.2) applies to problems in the laboratory of unknown causes and allows the team to quantitatively measure the error of the process, identify the root cause(s) of the problem, develop improvement strategies, and monitor the changes in a defined manner.

MEASUREMENTS OF SUCCESS USING LEAN AND SIX SIGMA

Originally, Lean and Six Sigma were separate ideas designed to improve two related metrics: time and error. Lean was designed to eliminate non–value-adding steps or waste, and Six Sigma, which is data driven, aims to reduce variation. The metrics for measuring QI with Lean Six Sigma still reflects those original principles. The combination of these two ideas provides a positive synergistic impact on process and QI.

The Lean approach seeks to streamline the process by eliminating duplication, excess, and barriers for a more optimized flow. The major measurement for Lean is generally time, but it can also include things such as cost, inventory, distance, time, and distribution. A common method of Lean improvement is the concept of a Kaizen event. The Kaizen event is 3 to 5 days of QI by a cross-functional team that analyzes the current steps associated with a particular process and makes real-time changes to improve its efficiency. With detailed study, most teams find unnecessary complexity in their work process. This complexity often contributes to errors as well as delays. Teams typically find that only 5% of the activities in any process add value; this means that a vast majority of activities do not contribute to the process. Graphically, this might look like the redundant and nonlinear process shown in Figure 4.3. Note that for laboratories, certain steps that do not appear to add value will need to be maintained to satisfy accreditation standards. Lean Six Sigma measures the amount of non–value-adding steps in a process as part of its core metrics, by including Six Sigma methodology and Lean principles. The implemented solutions (based on charter goals) are represented by the final process in Figure 4.3 where inefficiency has been removed to illustrate a more streamlined, efficient process.

Six Sigma metrics seek to quantitatively measure the amount of error or variation that occurs within a system. A **process sigma** represents the capability of a process to meet (or exceed) its defined criteria for acceptability. In the laboratory, this could refer to staffing assignments, assay performance, turnaround times, number of rejected samples, specimen transport, or relay of critical values. The process sigma is usually represented as the number of defects (errors) per million opportunities (DPMO). The sigma (σ) value refers to the number of standard deviations (SDs) away from the mean a process can move before it is outside the acceptable limits (Fig. 4.4). For example, if a sodium test has Six Sigma performance, then the mean could shift by 6 SDs (6σ) and still meet the laboratory requirements for precision and accuracy for sodium measurement. If a test achieves Six Sigma (6σ), it has a narrow process SD (i.e., it is very precise) and produces only three errors for every million tests performed. A test that performs at a three sigma

FIGURE 4.3 Application of Six Sigma and Lean methodologies toward process improvement. Steps in a process can have duplication, failure, and waste, all of which contribute to delay, increased cost, inefficiency, and longer turnaround times.

(3σ) has a much wider process SD and produces about 26,674 errors per million tests (Fig. 4.4).

To calculate the sigma, defects must be clearly defined. In the laboratory, any test that does not meet its requirements (i.e., correctly quantified or delivered on time) is considered a defect. The most straightforward method uses the process yield—the percentage of times that a process is defect free. Another method to calculate the process sigma is to calculate the DPMO. For example, in the laboratory, this might be measured by the number of errors that occurs for every 1 million tests. The process sigma can be estimated from a Process Sigma table (Table 4.2) using either the process yield or the DPMO.

As stated earlier, eliminating non–value-adding steps and reducing variation have a synergistic positive impact on process performance (Table 4.3). Several examples illustrate this concept. Assume that there are four steps involved in testing a specimen and each step is performed at a 3σ level (each step is 93.3% accurate and timely). With this performance, approximately three out of four test results will be accurate and delivered on time (75.8%)! Now imagine

that a team improves the quality of the process so that each step is performed correctly and timely at a 4σ level (99.38% accurate and timely). The new level of performance produces 97.5% of the results accurately and delivered on time. Alternatively, if a test has 10 steps, each of which operates at a 3σ level (93.3% accurate and timely) the increase in the number of slightly inaccurate steps, 50% of the tests will be inaccurate and late. Simply by eliminating unnecessary steps and maintaining a high level of performance, the team can drastically reduce the number of total errors. If the improvement team can both eliminate six steps and increase the quality of each step to a 4σ level, the process will improve so that 97.5% of the tests are accurate and on time (Table 4.3). These improvement strategies are designed to be continuous. Once changes have been realized, the improvement process should start again to make the system even better with each cycle. Eliminating non–value-added steps in any process reduces the possibility of error defects.

LEAN SIX SIGMA APPLICATIONS IN THE LABORATORY AND THE GREATER HEALTH CARE SYSTEM

The popularity of the combination of Lean and Six Sigma principles as an approach to quality management in health care has grown in the last 12 years. In 2004, there were two articles published describing specifically the application

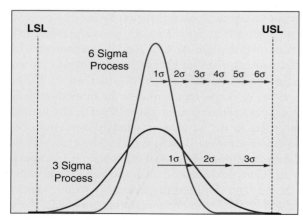

FIGURE 4.4 Comparison of Sigma performance for results distributed between the lower satisfactory limit (LSL) and the upper satisfactory limit (USL).

TABLE 4.2	**Process Sigma Table**	
Yield	**Errors/Million Results**	**Process Sigma**
99.9999%	1	6.27
99.9997%	3	6.04
99.999%	10	5.77
99.99%	100	5.22
99.9%	1,000	4.59

Definition of "Sigma" for a process with a given error rate.

TABLE 4.3 Example of Yield at Given Performance (R): % of Data Reported Correctly

No. of Steps	™3σ	™4σ	™5σ	™6σ
1	93.3%	99.38%	99.977%	99.9999%
3	82.7%	98.16%	99.931%	99.9953%
4	77.4%	97.56%	99.908%	99.9930%
7	61.6%	95.73%	99.839%	99.9976%
10	50.1%	93.96%	99.768%	99.9966%
20	25.1%	88.29%	99.536%	99.9932%
40	6.3%	77.94%	99.074%	99.9864%
80	1.6%	68.81%	98.614%	99.9796%
100	0.4%	60.75%	98.156%	99.9728%

of Lean Six Sigma, according to a PubMed search utilizing the phrase "Lean Six Sigma." This number has significantly risen since introduction of Lean and Six Sigma. Since 1997, there have been more than 300 publications on Six Sigma QI strategies alone in the health care field. Application of Lean and Six Sigma methodology at the Virginia Mason Medical Center showed numerous improvements to patient care.[2] Table 4.4 highlights the major improvements achieved in Lean Six Sigma Quality Management. Prior to the adoption of Lean Six Sigma strategies, no laboratory result was reported (the time the result was available until mailing) within less than 3 days, and every physician had an average of 1,800 results waiting to be reported. After application of Lean methodology, 89% of the test results were reported in less than 3 days. Patient waiting time was significantly reduced for chemotherapy infusion time, clinic waiting time decreased by 50%, and discharge time decreased from 2.5 to 1.5 hours. All of these aspects for organizational improvement represent tangible metrics that can be measured and quantified by Lean Six Sigma tools. The results of the improvement process provide superior patient care, improve customer service, and positively impact patient satisfaction, which all contribute toward enhanced customer retention by the individual health care organization.

A similar application of Lean Six Sigma Methodology was used to develop a new phlebotomy staffing model that better matched demand at Brigham and Women's Hospital in Boston.[3] The project was initiated in response to excessive safety reports filed for missed inpatient collections, thereby delaying laboratory results. Discrepancies between estimated and actual collection demand identified periods of understaffing for the phlebotomy service during peak demand times. After application of the Lean Six Sigma Methodology, new, staggered shifts were implemented to better handle the high-volume times between 5 and 9 AM and 7 and 9 PM (Fig. 4.5). Four new shifts were created that increased available personnel during peak hours and decreased available personnel during periods of low collections. The number of full-time equivalents remained the same between the old and new staffing model. The new staffing model improved collection by 17 minutes, accelerated results for basic chemistry such as potassium by 15 minutes, and reduced by 80% the number of filed safety reports from delayed or missed collections.[3]

These Lean Six Sigma Methodologies were applied to our own clinical laboratory at the University of North Carolina Hospitals. In an effort to decrease health care costs, we applied **DMAIC methodology** to review the laboratory billing processes, to better capture revenue that had been earned but not received.[4] In the Define and Measure Phase, we were able to narrow the scope of the project by determining that 27% of the tests not billed originated from outreach services. Applying the tools to determine the root cause analysis identified two clinics that were responsible for 20% of the total charges not billed. In the Analyze Phase, our group identified that insufficient medical necessity was a potential root cause, accounting for 67% of tests performed but not billed. In the Improve Phase, solutions were ranked based on their greatest impact with the least effort. The top three areas of focus were (1) revising requisitions to match medical necessity to the appropriate laboratory tests, (2) educating physicians and clinic managers to link the correct medical necessity with the laboratory tests ordered, and (3) providing feedback to the clinic managers on their performance. Before the pilot, the one physician with the highest amount of ordered tests not billed was averaging $10,430 per month and after the intervention $3,465 per month, a significant improvement. In the Control Phase, these gains were sustained; however, this justified the need for a long-term electronic solution to provide correct medical necessity needed to properly bill a laboratory test at the time it is ordered.

TABLE 4.4 Major Improvements Achieved from Lean Six Sigma Quality Management

	Before Lean Six Sigma	After Lean Six Sigma
Results report mailed	100% >3 d	89% <3 d
Patient waiting time	[Data not published]	Decreased by 50%
Discharge time	2.5 h	1.5 h
Chemotherapy time	[Data not published]	Decreased by 50%

Source: Bush RW. Reducing waste in US health care systems. *JAMA*. 2007;297(8):871–874.

FIGURE 4.5 The revised staffing model that better matches the collection pattern (*black line*) modified through Six Sigma QI strategies. Blocked colors represent different staff shifts. (Reprinted with permission from Morrison AP, Tanasijevic MJ, Torrence-Hill JN, et al. A strategy for optimizing staffing to improve the timeliness of inpatient phlebotomy collections. *Arch Pathol Lab Med.* 2011;135(12):1576–1580.)

PRACTICAL APPLICATION OF SIX SIGMA METRICS

Detecting Laboratory Errors

Recent studies have highlighted that medical errors occur with greater frequency than previously thought.[5–9] As part of the health care system, the laboratory is a potential source of error. Error rates in laboratory tests have been estimated to occur between 1:164 and 1:8,300 results (Table 4.5).[10–17] Converting these error rates to the standard Six Sigma metric DPMO, laboratory error rates would be expected to occur at a rate of between 120 and 6,098 DPMO; this corresponds to a 4σ to 5σ rating. A 6σ quality level would require less than 3.4 DPMO (Table 4.2).

While an estimated 12.5% of laboratory errors impact patient health, only 37.5 of every 100,000 (0.0375%) errors place patients at risk due to analytical testing mistakes.[9,16,18] Previously, laboratory QI focused on errors that occur in the analytic phase of testing. But currently, analytical testing errors constitute only 4% to 32% of all errors in the laboratory.[19] Most laboratory errors are now attributed to processes

TABLE 4.5	**Rate of Laboratory Error Detection**
Estimated Laboratory Error Rate	**Errors/Million (DPMO)**
1:164	6,098
1:214	4,672
1:283	3,534
1:8,300	20
Risk of dying in a plane crash 1:7,000,000 passengers	0.14

Table adapted from Bonini P, Plebani M, Ceriotti F, Rubboli F. Errors in laboratory medicine. *Clin Chem.* 2002;48(5):691–698, with permission.

occurring either before (preanalytic) or immediately after (postanalytic) the test. Preanalytic errors are estimated at between 32% and 75%, and postanalytic errors account for 9% to 55%. As outlined in Figure 4.6, the preanalytic phase involves steps such as the actual ordering of the tests by physicians, as well as sample collection. Because many of the preanalytic errors are outside the physical laboratory (i.e., phlebotomy), it is imperative that the process as a whole be considered when reorganizing laboratory processes to improve quality. This often requires collaboration between other departments within the system. With the current emphasis on QI in the health care setting,[2,20–22] clinical laboratories have been early adopters of Lean Six Sigma methodology to improve the quality of laboratory testing by identifying and reducing pre- and postanalytical sources of error.[3,23–27]

Defining the Sigma Performance of an Assay

From a quality management perspective, Six Sigma metrics can determine how well an analytic process performs and assist in choosing appropriate QC rules based on test performance. For example, if a given test has excellent performance (very precise and accurate over time), then fewer errors will occur. It would take a large shift in the mean for the test to fail the quality requirements. Accordingly, fewer QC rules would be needed to identify errors. These rules are designed to maximize the chance of detecting a problem, while simultaneously minimizing the risk of rejecting a result when it is actually correct (false rejection).

FIGURE 4.6 Schematic representation of the process components involved in clinical laboratory testing.

Six Sigma metrics can be plotted graphically using an operational process specification "OPSpecs" chart. This chart incorporates many of the measures described in the Method Evaluation chapter into one graph, including (1) total allowable error, (2) systematic error (inaccuracy), and (3) random error (imprecision) (Fig. 4.7). From the QC section, total allowable error is defined by CLIA (Clinical Laboratory Improvement Amendments) regulations (see Table 3.12 from Chapter 3). Systematic and random errors are derived from method comparison experiments, described in Chapter 3 (see Fig. 3.16). Consider the following hypothetical example for total calcium.

The performance of the assay is defined by the following linear regression equation:

$$y = 0.91x + 0.2$$
The total allowable error for calcium is 1 mg/dL
The assay has an impression of 2%
What is the systemic error for the assay at 10 mg/dL?
$$y = (0.91 \times 10) + 0.2$$
$$y = 9.3 \, mg/dL$$
$$10 \, mg/dL - 9.3 \, mg/dL = 0.7 \, mg/dL$$
0.7 mg/dL represents 70% of the total allowable error for calcium (1 mg/dL)
What is the random error of the assay at 10 mg/dL
$$Impression = 10 \, mg/dL \times 0.02$$
$$Impression = 0.2 \, mg/dL$$
0.2 mg/dL represents 20% of the total allowable error for calcium (1 mg/dL)   (Eq. 4-1)

Plotting the random error of 20% on the x-axis and the systemic error of 70% on the y-axis using the OPSpecs chart (Fig. 4.7) reveals that the assay has a 2σ performance; this is considered poor performance and would require extensive QC measurements to detect the high number of errors. Many rules are needed because only a small shift in the mean would result in a failure (this principle is evident in Fig. 4.4). If the systemic error (bias) could be eliminated (as demonstrated with point 2, Fig. 4.7), the performance would fall into the 5σ range, which is considered to be very good; only a few QC measurements would be necessary with a minimal use of control rules to detect the low number of errors.

Choosing the Appropriate Westgard Rules

Recently, a straightforward methodology has been published detailing how Six Sigma metrics can be used to choose appropriate Westgard QC rules for any assay (as initially introduced in Chapter 3).[28] A sigma value for every Westgard rule or set of rules can be deduced from the slope of the line it generates in an OPSpecs chart (Fig. 4.7). In short, the slope of the line is equal to the—(negative) sigma value.

Furthermore, the sigma value for an assay can be calculated by the following equation:

$$Sigma = \frac{(total \; allowable \; error - bias)}{coefficient \; of \; variation}$$ (Eq. 4-2)

Total allowable error represents the error budget based on the biological variation of the specific analyte. Bias refers to the systematic error of the assay, and the coefficient of variation (CV) is the analytical SD of the assay. If the calculated sigma for an assay is greater than the sigma of the Westgard rule, that rule is suitable for monitoring the error of the test. Values for total allowable error for specific analytes have been published and are readily available (Table 3.12) so the laboratory must simply calculate bias and for the assay in question. Consider the following hypothetical example using potassium:

The total allowable error for potassium = 5.8%
The bias for your laboratory's assay for potassium = 0.7%
The CV for your laboratory's assay for potassium = 1%
$$Sigma_{potassium} = \frac{(5.8 - 0.7)}{1}$$
$$Sigma_{potassium} = 5.1$$

Using Table 4.6, the Westgard rule with the sigma value closest, but below 5.1 is the 1 2.5 s rule. Therefore, a QC rule of 1 2.5 s would provide the optimum control to detect error in the laboratory's potassium assay while minimizing false rejection of accurate results.

PRESENT AND EVOLVING APPROACHES TO QUALITY IMPROVEMENT AND QUALITY ASSURANCE IN THE CLINICAL LABORATORY: FROM QCP TO IQCP AND ISO5189

Today's Standard: Quality Control Plan

A **quality control plan** (QCP) is a written document describing the practices and procedures performed by

FIGURE 4.7 OPSpecs chart used to determine process performance. The allowable imprecision is plotted against the allowable inaccuracy as percentage of the total allowable error. Assay performance changing from point 1 to point 2 by reducing inaccuracy improves the performance from a 2σ process to a 5σ process.

TABLE 4.6 Hypothetical Sigma Values for Westgard Rules (When Using Two Controls)

Westgard Rule	Sigma Value
1 3.5s	6
1 3s	5.6
1 2.5s	5.0
1 3s/2 2s/R 4s/4 1s	4.0

Source: Schoenmakers CHH, Naus AJM, Vermeer HJ, et al. Practical application of Sigma Metrics QC procedures in clinical chemistry. *Clin Chem Lab Med.* 2011;49(11):1837–1843.

BOX 4.5 What Is Included in a QCP?

At a minimum, the QCP must include the number, type, and frequency of testing quality control materials, as well as criteria for acceptable quality control. If indicated by the risk assessment, the QCP may also incorporate the use of:

- Electronic controls
- Equipment maintenance
- Internal controls
- Personnel training and competency assessment
- Equipment calibration
- Other specified quality control activities

your laboratory to reduce the chance of possible failures and errors in test processes. The QCP must ensure that the accuracy and reliability of test results, for a specific process, are appropriate for patient care. Practices, procedures, and resources that are incorporated in your QCP may include, but are not limited to, an instrument's (1) electronic controls, (2) internal controls, (3) proficiency testing (PT) performance of unknown samples, (4) calibration, (5) maintenance, and (6) training and competency assessment of the users.

A QCP describes practices, procedures, and resources needed by the laboratory to ensure the quality of a testing process. The QCP includes measures to assure the accuracy and reliability of test results and that the quality of testing is adequate for patient care. The QCP must provide for immediate detection of errors that occur due to test system failure, adverse environmental conditions, and operator performance. It must also monitor, over time, the accuracy and precision of test performance that may be influenced by changes in the specimen, test system, reagent, environment, or variance in operator performance. A plan includes activities to reduce the likelihood of failures and errors identified from **risk assessment** (Table 4.7).

Below, we describe four programs in use for monitoring quality in the laboratory, including QCP, QA, **Individual Quality Control Program (IQCP)**, ISO 15189. All of these programs require a highly qualified, skilled, and motivated staff, trained in implementing, monitoring, resolving, and controlling programs.

Regulatory compliance and laboratory accreditation are also driving forces in these processes, in addition to the primary goal of assuring the accuracy and reliability of test results, and that the quality of testing is adequate for patient care (Box 4.5).

QUALITY CONTROL PLAN BASED ON RISK MANAGEMENT: CLSI EP23-A DOCUMENT

Under Clinical Laboratory Improvement Amendments (CLIA) quality control (QC) policies, the Centers for Medicare and Medicaid Services (CMS) created a policy for regulating QC in moderately complex tests (42CFR493.1250). In 2011, the Clinical & Laboratory Standards Institute (CLSI) Guidelines built upon these guidelines to create a system of Quality Control in the context of the patient, specifically with the potential patient care impact. The CLSI "Quality Control Based on Risk Management" guidelines (EP23-A)[29] provided for more than just determining an individual test's quality control specifications, it also took into account the intended medical application of the test and the risk to the patient. The purpose of developing a QCP is to prevent laboratory test errors and ensures that the correct results are reported and appropriately followed up upon with the clinical staff. Development of a QCP requires understanding of the preanalytical, analytical, and postanalytical processes so that potential failures in the entire process can be

TABLE 4.7 Risk Acceptability Table: Occurrence versus Severity

Probability of Harm	Severity of Harm				
	Negligible	Minor	Serious	Critical	Catastrophic
Frequent	Unacceptable	Unacceptable	Unacceptable	Unacceptable	Unacceptable
Probable	Acceptable	Unacceptable	Unacceptable	Unacceptable	Unacceptable
Occasional	Acceptable	Acceptable	Acceptable	Unacceptable	Unacceptable
Remote	Acceptable	Acceptable	Acceptable	Unacceptable	Unacceptable
Improbable	Acceptable	Acceptable	Acceptable	Acceptable	Acceptable

Adapted from CLSI EP23A Laboratory Quality Control Based on Risk Assessment, Oct 2011.

determined, resolved, and controlled (see Fig. 4.7). These actions taken throughout the organization increase the efficiency of the processes to add benefits to the patient.

QUALITY ASSESSMENT

Quality assessment (QA) is the continuous process of monitoring the effectiveness of the QCP. Practices, processes, and resources to consider for monitoring effectiveness of a QCP may include but are not limited to (1) routine reviews of Quality Control Performance, (2) proficiency performance reviews, (3) patient chart reviews, (4) specimen rejection logs, (5) turnaround time reports, (6) complaint reports, (7) variance reports, and (8) safety reports. The process of QA involves ongoing monitoring and assessing of performance in a defined way. The laboratory must establish and follow written policies and procedures to monitor and assess, and when indicated, correct problems identified. The monitoring should include, but is not limited to, the following risk assessment components: specimen, test system, reagents, environment, and testing personnel. The QA must also include a review of the effectiveness of corrective actions taken to resolve and monitor problems identified. The laboratory must update the risk assessment and modify the QCP, as necessary based on the information obtained from the QA. A common confusion when first being introduced to the concepts of QA is understanding how it is different from the quality control assessments that are done in parallel and are closely related. An example of a QC activity may be recording the room temperature on a log sheet; the parallel QA activity may then be reviewing the room temperature log for problems and evidence of corrective actions. Similarly, A QC activity may be documenting personnel training, and a parallel QA activity would be reviewing personnel training records for completion of required training and competency assessments. QA is an integral part of the QCP, receiving input from the QCP and being used to assess risk, as outlined in Figure 4.8.

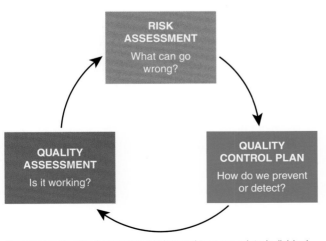

FIGURE 4.8 Quality Assessment is integral to a complete Individual Quality Control Program (IQCP).

INDIVIDUAL QUALITY CONTROL PROGRAM: AN OPTION TO STREAMLINE QCP

Under CLIA, the CMS has implemented IQCP as an acceptable QC option. The new requirements for IQCP provide laboratories with the framework to implement IQCP, when appropriate, and offer flexibility to design a QC plan that meets the needs of the laboratory. These changes will ensure that accredited laboratories remain in compliance with the CLIA and CMS regulations. As one of the leading accrediting organization, the College of American Pathologists (CAP) revised its checklists in the 2015 edition to address the IQCP changes. These adjustments ensure that CAP-accredited laboratories will remain CLIA and CMS compliant. For more information, the Centers for Medicare and Medicaid Services has downloadable information regarding implementation. Like the QCP, the IQCP integrates QCP with QA and risk assessment, customized to individual laboratories.

ISO5189—QUALITY MANAGEMENT IN MEDICAL LABORATORIES: ADDING RISK ASSESSMENT TO THE FORMULA INTERNATIONALLY (GLOBAL INITIATIVE)

The International Organization for Standards (ISO) assigned technical committee 212 (ISO/TC 212) the task of creating global standards for quality and competence in medical laboratories. The ISO/TC 212 published these standards in a technical document, called **ISO 15189** in 2003. This was later revised in 2007 and updated to its current form in 2012 and represents an important contribution to laboratory science, given the diversity of laboratory settings in the world. The standard has developed initiatives to promote competence and responsibility in medical laboratory processes, equipment, and outcomes. Implemented in over 200 countries, the process involves testing of the effectiveness of laboratory equipment and the impact those particular equipment has on the processes in the labs and their outcomes. The approach takes into account a lot of perspectives, including the interpretation of test results, the method patient samples are actually collected, as well as the time required for the tests to be carried out.

The basic requirements for ISO 15189 certification include a well-documented procedure analysis by the laboratories and a training manual provided by the laboratories. ISO 15189 requires an effective detailed analysis of medical laboratory procedures in a bid to make sure that all weaknesses have been identified. A detailed evaluation report of the existing quality management system as well as other monitoring and evaluation reports is required in addition to a detail audit of management reviews.

The ISO 15189 certification has a set of very unique benefits, and the main objective of certification is QA. An

ISO 15189 certification promotes development of an international reputable image for your organization through Quality Assurance and Management Systems. It also promotes a strong degree of consistency in compliance to medical laboratory laws and legislation both from an international and national perspective. ISO 15189 certification program has been very critical in promoting modern laboratory practices that include professionalism and expertise in conduction of medical activities in the labs. By promoting laboratory efficiency and responsibility for better results and service delivery, it has ultimately promoted the growth of customer satisfaction in organizations involved in medical laboratory testing across the world.

CONCLUSIONS

Lean Six Sigma Methodology has emerged as a powerful technique to effectively improve the quality and efficiency of the clinical laboratory. It provides a framework to define, measure, and reduce waste and variation associated with the total testing process. Furthermore, it supplies mathematically sound metrics to assess laboratory processes and assay performance, define QC rules, and develop QI and QA strategies. Lean Six Sigma's role in clinical chemistry will continue to grow in importance and scope as the need for improved quality and reduced cost becomes paramount in the health care system. Knowledge of Lean Six Sigma methodology will be critical for laboratorians going forward to achieve the mission of delivering quality health care to patients. Major hospitals have made institutional-wide commitments to QI using Lean Six Sigma. Yellow belt training is currently offered at certain institutions to all laboratory personnel with the goal of having the entire laboratory staff trained. Supervisors and directors are trained at the sponsor level. Lead technologists are trained at the Lean level. Black belt training is for a few with commitment to Lean and Six Sigma who plan to participate in QI and QA projects across departments within the institution. For all laboratory professionals, this training provides an unprecedented opportunity to be an agent for change in the health care system and allows the laboratorian to take greater ownership in enhancing customer service and ultimately improving patient care.

ACKNOWLEDGMENTS

The authors wish to acknowledge Glen Spivak, Vice President of Business Development and Operational Efficiency, and more broadly the University of North Carolina Hospitals for its support and training in Lean Six Sigma Methodologies utilized in writing this chapter and used in our clinical laboratories.

For additional student resources, please visit thePoint® at http://thepoint.lww.com

questions

1. The methodology for a Lean Six Sigma QI team will include consideration of all of the following factors EXCEPT:
   a. Define
   b. Measure
   c. Analyze
   d. Improve
   e. Communicate

2. It is reported that the greatest percentage of laboratory errors occur during the _____ phase.
   a. Preanalytical
   b. Analytical
   c. Postanalytical
   d. Proficiency
   e. Phlebotomy

3. Calculate the Sigma value for sodium given that the total allowable error is 8%, the bias is 0.9%, and the CV is 2%.
   a. 3.6
   b. 2.7

   c. 7.1
   d. 4.5
   e. 6.7

4. Process Sigma is usually represented by:
   a. SIPOC
   b. DPMO
   c. DMAIC
   d. OPSpec
   e. CLIA

5. Which team member is the coach in a Lean Six Sigma project?
   a. Yellow Belts
   b. Green Belts
   c. Black Belts
   d. Blue Belts
   e. Sponsors or Champions

review questions (continued)

6. Lean addresses which of the following?
   a. Variation
   b. Eliminating waste
   c. Data-driven errors
   d. 7 to 9 month project
   e. DMAIC Phases

7. Which one of these is a best fit for a Kaizen project (Lean)?
   a. Design of a new laboratory
   b. Improving the flow of a laboratory
   c. Improving the turnaround times for the laboratory
   d. Reducing laboratory billing errors
   e. Both b and c

8. Which one of these is best for a Six Sigma project?
   a. Design of a new lab
   b. Reducing defects of the billing process
   c. Reducing defects of blood wastage
   d. Both b and c
   e. Selecting QC rules for a lab test

9. What is not a major component of the IQCP?
   a. Quality Assurance
   b. Risk Assessment
   c. SDS
   d. Quality Control Plan

10. An IQCP replaces what quality control program?
   a. CMS
   b. CAP
   c. Six Sigma
   d. ECP

11. What are key components of Risk Assessment in IQCP
   a. Testing personnel
   b. Environment
   c. Reagents
   d. Test system
   e. Specimens
   f. All of the above

references

1. Juran JM. *Juran on Leadership for Quality*. 1st ed. New York, NY: Free Press; 1989.
2. Bush RW. Reducing waste in US health care systems. *JAMA*. 2007;297(8):871–874.
3. Morrison AP, Tanasijevic MJ, Torrence-Hill JN, et al. A strategy for optimizing staffing to improve the timeliness of inpatient phlebotomy collections. *Arch Pathol Lab Med*. 2011;135(12):1576–1580.
4. Levtzow CB, Willis MS. Reducing laboratory billing defects using Six Sigma principles. *Lab Med*. 2013;44(4):358–371.
5. Institute of Medicine (U.S.). Committee on Crossing the Quality Chasm: Adaptation to Mental Health and Addictive Disorders. *Improving the Quality of Health Care for Mental and Substance-Use Conditions*. Washington, DC: National Academies Press; 2006.
6. Committee on Quality of Health Care in America, Institute of Medicine. *Crossing the Quality Chasm: A New Health System for the 21st Century*. 1st ed. Washington, DC: National Academies Press; 2001.
7. Institute of Medicine. IOM report: patient safety—achieving a new standard for care. *Acad Emerg Med*. 2005;12(10):1011–1012.
8. Committee on Quality of Health Care in America. Institute of Medicine. *To Err Is Human: Building a Safer Health System*. 1st ed. Washington, DC: National Academies Press; 2000.
9. Committee on Identifying Priority Areas for Quality Improvement. *Priority Areas for National Action: Transforming Health Care Quality*. 1st ed. Washington, DC: National Academies Press; 2003.
10. Siebers R. Laboratory blunders revisited. *Ann Clin Biochem*. 1994;31(pt 4):390–391.
11. Chambers AM, Johnston J, O'Reilly DS. Laboratory blunders revisited. *Ann Clin Biochem*. 1994;31(pt 4):390; author reply 391.
12. Lapworth R, Teal TK. Laboratory blunders revisited. *Ann Clin Biochem*. 1994;31(pt 1):78–84.
13. Stankovic AK. The laboratory is a key partner in assuring patient safety. *Clin Lab Med*. 2004;24(4):1023–1035.
14. Kalra J. Medical errors: impact on clinical laboratories and other critical areas. *Clin Biochem*. 2004;37(12):1052–1062.
15. Hollensead SC, Lockwood WB, Elin RJ. Errors in pathology and laboratory medicine: consequences and prevention. *J Surg Oncol*. 2004;88(3):161–181.
16. Plebani M. Errors in clinical laboratories or errors in laboratory medicine? *Clin Chem Lab Med*. 2006;44(6):750–759.
17. Singla P, Parkash AA, Bhattacharjee J. Preanalytical error occurrence rate in clinical chemistry laboratory of a public hospital in India. *Clin Lab*. 2011;57(9–10):749–752.
18. Plebani M. Exploring the iceberg of errors in laboratory medicine. *Clin Chim Acta*. 2009;404(1):16–23.
19. Bonini P, Plebani M, Ceriotti F, et al. Errors in laboratory medicine. *Clin Chem*. 2002;48(5):691–698.
20. Nicolay CR, Purkayastha S, Greenhalgh A, et al. Systematic review of the application of quality improvement methodologies from the manufacturing industry to surgical healthcare. *Br J Surg*. 2012;99(3):324–335. Retrieved from http://www.ncbi.nlm.nih.gov/pubmed/22101509
21. Sciacovelli L, Sonntag O, Padoan A, et al. Monitoring quality indicators in laboratory medicine does not automatically result in quality improvement. *Clin Chem Lab Med*. 2011;50(3):463–469. Retrieved from http://www.ncbi.nlm.nih.gov/pubmed/22149744

22. Signori C, Ceriotti F, Sanna A, et al. Process and risk analysis to reduce errors in clinical laboratories. *Clin Chem Lab Med.* 2007;45(6):742–748.

23. DelliFraine JL, Langabeer JR II, Nembhard IM. Assessing the evidence of Six Sigma and Lean in the health care industry. *Qual Manag Health Care.* 2010;19(3):211–225.

24. Gras JM, Philippe M. Application of the Six Sigma concept in clinical laboratories: a review. *Clin Chem Lab Med.* 2007;45(6):789–796.

25. Kuo AM-H, Borycki E, Kushniruk A, et al. A healthcare Lean Six Sigma System for postanesthesia care unit workflow improvement. *Qual Manag Health Care.* 2011;20(1):4–14.

26. Pocha C. Lean Six Sigma in health care and the challenge of implementation of Six Sigma methodologies at a Veterans Affairs Medical Center. *Qual Manag Health Care.* 2010;19(4):312–318.

27. Vanker N, van Wyk J, Zemlin AE, et al. A Six Sigma approach to the rate and clinical effect of registration errors in a laboratory. *J Clin Pathol.* 2010;63(5):434–437.

28. Schoenmakers CHH, Naus AJM, Vermeer HJ, et al. Practical application of Sigma Metrics QC procedures in clinical chemistry. *Clin Chem Lab Med.* 2011;49(11):1837–1843.

29. CLSI Document, EP23A Laboratory Quality Control Based on Risk Management, Approved guideline, October 2011.

resources for further information on:

CMS.Gov Individual Quality Control Plan—http://www.cms.gov/Regulations-and-Guidance/Legislation/CLIA/Individualized_Quality_Control_Plan_IQCP.html

CMS Workbook for IQCP—http://www.cms.gov/Regulations-and-Guidance/Legislation/CLIA/Downloads/IQCP-Workbook.pdf

Individualized Quality Control Plan (IQCP)—https://www.cms.gov/regulations-and-guidance/legislation/CLIA/Individualized_Quality_Control_Plan_IQCP.html

ISO 15189:2012(en), Medical laboratories—Requirements for quality and competence—https://www.iso.org/obp/ui/#iso:std:iso:15189:ed-3:v2:en

CAP 15189 Program—http://www.cap.org/apps/docs/laboratory_accreditation/15189/15189_accreditation_faq.pdf

5

Analytic Techniques

JULIA C. DREES, MATTHEW S. PETRIE, and ALAN H. B. WU

chapter outline

key terms

Atomic absorption
Chemiluminescence
Electrochemistry
Electrophoresis
Fluorometry
Ion-selective electrodes
Spectrophotometry

chapter objectives

Upon completion of this chapter, the clinical laboratorian should be able to do the following:

- Explain the general principles of each analytic method.
- Discuss the limitations of each analytic technique.
- Compare and contrast the various analytic techniques.
- Discuss existing clinical applications for each analytic technique.
- Describe the operation and component parts of the following instruments: spectrophotometer, atomic absorption spectrometer, fluorometer, osmometer, ion-selective electrode, and pH electrode.
- Outline the quality assurance and preventive maintenance procedures involved with the following instruments: spectrophotometer, fluorometer, osmometer, ion-selective electrode, and pH electrode.

For additional student resources, please visit thePoint®
at http://thepoint.lww.com

Analytic techniques and instrumentation provide the foundation for all measurements made in a modern clinical chemistry laboratory. The majority of techniques fall into one of four basic disciplines within the field of analytic chemistry: spectrometry (including **spectrophotometry, atomic absorption**, and mass spectrometry [MS]); luminescence (including fluorescence and **chemiluminescence**); electroanalytic methods (including **electrophoresis**, potentiometry, and amperometry); and chromatography (including gas, liquid, and thin layer). Due to the rapid growth and increased utilization in clinical laboratories, chromatography and MS will be covered separately in Chapter 6.

SPECTROPHOTOMETRY

The instruments that measure electromagnetic radiation have several concepts and components in common. Shared instrumental components are discussed in some detail in a later section. Photometric instruments measure light intensity without consideration of wavelength. Most instruments today use filters (photometers), prisms, or gratings (spectrometers) to select (isolate) a narrow range of the incident wavelength. Radiant energy that passes through an object will be partially reflected, absorbed, and transmitted.

Electromagnetic radiation is described as photons of energy traveling in waves. The relationship between wavelength and energy E is described by Planck's formula:

$$E = h\nu \qquad \text{(Eq. 5-1)}$$

where h is a constant $(6.62 \times 10^{-27}$ erg sec), known as Planck constant, and ν is frequency. Because the frequency of a wave is inversely proportional to the wavelength, it follows that the energy of electromagnetic radiation is inversely proportional to wavelength. Figure 5.1A shows

this relationship. Electromagnetic radiation includes a spectrum of energy from short-wavelength, highly energetic gamma rays and x-rays on the left in Figure 5.1B to long-wavelength radiofrequencies on the right. Visible light falls in between, with the color violet at 400 nm and red at 700 nm wavelengths being the approximate limits of the visible spectrum.

The instruments discussed in this section measure either absorption or emission of radiant energy to determine the concentration of atoms or molecules. The two phenomena, absorption and emission, are closely related. For a ray of electromagnetic radiation to be absorbed, it must have the same frequency as a rotational or vibrational frequency in the atom or molecule that it strikes. Levels of energy that are absorbed move in discrete steps, and any particular type of molecule or atom will absorb only certain energies and not others. When energy is absorbed, valence electrons move to an orbital with a higher energy level. Following energy absorption, the excited electron will fall back to the ground state by emitting a discrete amount of energy in the form of a characteristic wavelength of radiant energy.

Absorption or emission of energy by atoms results in a line spectrum. Because of the relative complexity of molecules, they absorb or emit a bank of energy over a large region. Light emitted by incandescent solids (tungsten or deuterium) is in a continuum. The three types of spectra are shown in Figure 5.2.[1-3]

Beer Law

The relationship between absorption of light by a solution and the concentration of that solution has been described by Beer and others. Beer law states that the concentration of a substance is directly proportional to the amount of light absorbed or inversely proportional to the logarithm of the transmitted light. Percent transmittance (%T) and absorbance (A) are related photometric terms that are explained in this section.

Figure 5.3A shows a beam of monochromatic light entering a solution. Some of the light is absorbed. The remainder passes through, strikes a light detector, and is converted to an electric signal. Percent transmittance

FIGURE 5.1 Electromagnetic radiation—relationship of energy and wavelength.

FIGURE 5.2 Characteristic absorption or emission spectra. (Adapted from Coiner D. *Basic Concepts in Laboratory Instrumentation*. Bethesda, MD: ASMT Education and Research Fund; 1975-1979.)

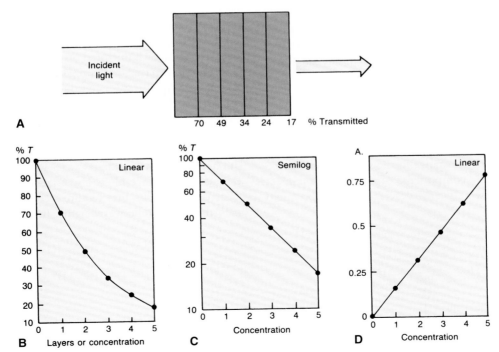

% Transmittance = $\dfrac{T}{I}$ × 100

Defined as 100% *T*

A   Blank

% *T* = $\dfrac{\text{Sample beam signal}}{\text{Blank beam signal}}$ × 100

B   Sample

FIGURE 5.3 Percent transmittance (%*T*) defined.

is the ratio of the radiant energy transmitted (*T*) divided by the radiant energy incident on the sample (*I*). All light absorbed or blocked results in 0% *T*. A level of 100% *T* is obtained if no light is absorbed. In practice, the solvent without the constituent of interest is placed in the light path, as in Figure 5.3B. Most of the light is transmitted, but a small amount is absorbed by the solvent and cuvette or is reflected away from the detector. The electrical readout of the instrument is set arbitrarily at 100% *T*, while the light is passing through a "blank" or reference. The sample containing absorbing molecules to be measured is placed in the

light path. The difference in amount of light transmitted by the blank and that transmitted by the sample is due only to the presence of the compound being measured. The %*T* measured by commercial spectrophotometers is the ratio of the sample transmitted beam divided by the blank transmitted beam.

Equal thicknesses of an absorbing material will absorb a constant fraction of the energy incident upon the layers. For example, in a tube containing layers of solution (Fig. 5.4A), the first layer transmits 70% of the light incident upon it. The second layer will, in turn, transmit 70% of the light incident upon it. Thus, 70% of 70% (49%) is transmitted by the second layer. The third layer transmits 70% of 49%, or 34% of the original light. Continuing on, successive layers transmit 24% and 17%, respectively. The %*T* values, when plotted on linear graph paper, yield the curve shown in Figure 5.4B. Considering each equal layer as many monomolecular layers, we can translate layers of material to concentration. If semilog graph paper is used to plot the same figures, a straight line is obtained (Fig. 5.4C), indicating that, as concentration increases, %*T* decreases in a logarithmic manner.

Absorbance *A* is the amount of light absorbed. It cannot be measured directly by a spectrophotometer but rather is mathematically derived from %*T* as follows:

$$\%T = \frac{I}{I_0} \times 100 \qquad \text{(Eq. 5-2)}$$

where I_0 is the incident light and *I* is the transmitted light.

A

Incident light

70 49 34 24 17   % Transmitted

B   Layers or concentration

C   Concentration

D   Concentration

FIGURE 5.4 (A) Percent of original incident light transmitted by equal layers of light-absorbing solution. **(B)** Percent *T* versus concentration on linear graph paper. **(C)** Percent *T* versus concentration on semilog graph paper. **(D)** *A* versus concentration on linear graph paper.

Absorbance is defined as follows:

$$A = -\log(I/I_0) = \log(100\%) - \log\%T$$
$$= 2 - \log\%T \qquad \text{(Eq. 5-3)}$$

According to Beer law, absorbance is directly proportional to concentration (Fig. 5.4D):

$$A = \varepsilon \times b \times c \qquad \text{(Eq. 5-4)}$$

where ε = molar absorptivity, the fraction of a specific wavelength of light absorbed by a given type of molecule; b is the length of light path through the solution; and c is the concentration of absorbing molecules.

Absorptivity depends on the molecular structure and the way in which the absorbing molecules react with different energies. For any particular molecular type, absorptivity changes as wavelength of radiation changes. The amount of light absorbed at a particular wavelength depends on the molecular and ion types present and may vary with concentration, pH, or temperature.

Because the path length and molar absorptivity are constant for a given wavelength,

$$A \sim c \qquad \text{(Eq. 5-5)}$$

Unknown concentrations are determined from a calibration curve that plots absorbance at a specific wavelength versus concentration for standards of known concentration. For calibration curves that are linear and have a zero y-intercept, unknown concentrations can be determined from a single calibrator. Not all calibration curves result in straight lines. Deviations from linearity are typically observed at high absorbances. The stray light within an instrument will ultimately limit the maximum absorbance that a spectrophotometer can achieve, typically 2.0 absorbance units.

Spectrophotometric Instruments

A spectrophotometer is used to measure the light transmitted by a solution to determine the concentration of the light-absorbing substance in the solution. Figure 5.5 illustrates the basic components of a single-beam spectrophotometer, which are described in subsequent sections.

Components of a Spectrophotometer
Light Source

The most common source of light for work in the visible and near-infrared regions is the incandescent tungsten or tungsten-iodide lamp. Only about 15% of radiant energy emitted falls in the visible region, with most emitted as near-infrared.[1-3] Often, a heat-absorbing filter is inserted between the lamp and the sample to absorb the infrared radiation.

The lamps most commonly used for ultraviolet (UV) work are the deuterium discharge lamp and the mercury arc lamp. Deuterium provides continuous emission down to 165 nm. Low-pressure mercury lamps emit a sharp line spectrum, with both UV and visible lines. Medium and high-pressure mercury lamps emit a continuum from UV to the mid-visible region. The most important factors for a light source are range, spectral distribution within the range, the source of radiant production, stability of the radiant energy, and temperature.

Monochromators

Isolation of individual wavelengths of light is an important and necessary function of a monochromator. The degree of wavelength isolation is a function of the type of device used and the width of entrance and exit slits. The bandpass of a monochromator defines the range of wavelengths transmitted and is calculated as width at half the maximum transmittance (Fig. 5.6).

Numerous devices are used for obtaining monochromatic light. The least expensive are colored glass filters. These filters usually pass a relatively wide band of radiant energy and have a low transmittance of the selected wavelength. Although not precise, they are simple and inexpensive.

Interference filters produce monochromatic light based on the principle of constructive interference of waves. Two pieces of glass, each mirrored on one side, are separated by a transparent spacer that is precisely one-half the desired wavelength. Light waves enter one side of the filter and are reflected at the second surface. Wavelengths that are twice the space between the two glass surfaces will reflect back and forth, reinforcing others of the same wavelengths and finally passing on through. Other wavelengths will cancel out because of phase differences (destructive interference). Because interference filters also transmit multiples of the desired wavelengths, they require accessory filters to eliminate these harmonic wavelengths. Interference filters can

FIGURE 5.5 Single-beam spectrophotometer.

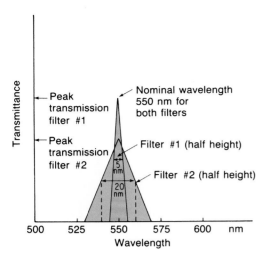

FIGURE 5.6 Spectral transmittance of two monochromators with band pass at half height of 5 and 20 nm.

be constructed to pass a very narrow range of wavelengths with good efficiency.

The simple glass prism is another type of monochromator. A narrow beam of light focused on a prism is refracted as it enters the denser glass. Short wavelengths are refracted more than long wavelengths, resulting in dispersion of white light into a continuous spectrum. The prism can be rotated, allowing only the desired wavelength to pass through an exit slit.

Diffraction gratings are most commonly used as monochromators. A diffraction grating consists of many parallel grooves (15,000 or 30,000 per inch) etched onto a polished surface. Diffraction, the separation of light into component wavelengths, is based on the principle that wavelengths bend as they pass a sharp corner. The degree of bending depends on the wavelength. As the wavelengths move past the corners, wave fronts are formed. Those that are in phase reinforce one another, whereas those not in phase cancel out and disappear. This results in complete spectra. Gratings with very fine line rulings produce a widely dispersed spectrum. They produce linear spectra, called orders, in both directions from the entrance slit. Because the multiple spectra have a tendency to cause stray light problems, accessory filters are used.

Sample Cell

The next component of the basic spectrophotometer is the sample cell or cuvette, which typically has a flat surface. The light path must be kept constant to have absorbance proportional to concentration. This is easily checked by preparing a colored solution to read midscale when using the wavelength of maximum absorption. Each cuvette to be tested is filled, readings are taken, and results are compared against an acceptable tolerance (e.g., $\pm 0.25\%$ T). Cuvettes are sold in matched sets. Square cuvettes have plane-parallel optical surfaces and a constant light path. Cuvettes with scratched optical surfaces scatter light and should be discarded. Inexpensive glass cuvettes can be used for applications in the visible range, but they absorb light in the UV region. Quartz cuvettes enable transmission of light and are used when substances absorb in this region (e.g., NADH at 340 nm).

Photodetectors

The purpose of the detector is to convert the transmitted radiant energy into an equivalent amount of electrical energy. The least expensive of the devices is known as a barrier-layer cell, or photocell. The photocell is composed of a film of light-sensitive material, frequently selenium, on a plate of iron. Over the light-sensitive material is a thin, transparent layer of silver. When exposed to light, electrons in the light-sensitive material are excited and released to flow to the highly conductive silver. In comparison with the silver, a moderate resistance opposes the electron flow toward the iron, forming a hypothetical barrier to flow in that direction. Consequently, this cell generates its own electromotive force, which can be measured. The produced current is proportional to the incident radiation. Photocells require no external voltage source but rely on internal electron transfer to produce a current in an external circuit. Because of their low internal resistance, the output of electrical energy is not easily amplified. Consequently, this type of detector is used mainly in filter photometers with a wide bandpass, producing a fairly high level of illumination so that there is no need to amplify the signal. The photocell is inexpensive and durable; however, it is temperature sensitive and nonlinear at very low and very high levels of illumination.

A phototube (Fig. 5.7) is similar to a barrier-layer cell in that it has photosensitive material that gives off electrons when light energy strikes it. It differs in that an outside voltage is required for operation. Phototubes contain a negatively charged cathode and a positively charged anode enclosed in a glass case. The cathode is composed of a material (e.g., rubidium or lithium) that acts as a resistor in the dark but emits electrons when exposed to light. The emitted electrons jump over to the positively charged anode, where they are collected and return through an external, measurable circuit.

FIGURE 5.7 Phototube drawing and schematic.

The cathode usually has a large surface area. Varying the cathode material changes the wavelength at which the phototube gives its highest response. The photocurrent is linear, with the intensity of the light striking the cathode as long as the voltage between the cathode and the anode remains constant. A vacuum within the tubes avoids scattering of the photoelectrons by collision with gas molecules.

The third major type of light detector is the photomultiplier (PM) tube, which detects and amplifies radiant energy. As shown in Figure 5.8, incident light strikes the coated cathode, emitting electrons. The electrons are attracted to a series of anodes, known as dynodes, each having a successively higher positive voltage. These dynodes are of a material that gives off many secondary electrons when hit by single electrons. Initial electron emission at the cathode triggers a multiple cascade of electrons within the PM tube itself. Because of this amplification, the PM tube is 200 times more sensitive than the phototube. PM tubes are used in instruments designed to be extremely sensitive to very low light levels and light flashes of very short duration. The accumulation of electrons striking the anode produces a current signal, measured in amperes, that is proportional to the initial intensity of the light. The analog signal is converted first to a voltage and then to a digital signal through the use of an analog-to-digital converter. Digital signals are processed electronically to produce absorbance readings.

In a photodiode, absorption of radiant energy by a reverse-biased pn-junction diode (pn, positive–negative) produces a photocurrent that is proportional to the incident radiant power. Although photodiodes are not as sensitive as PM tubes because of the lack of internal amplification, their excellent linearity (six to seven decades of radiant power), speed, and small size make them useful in applications where light levels are adequate.[4] Photodiode array (PDA) detectors are available in integrated circuits containing 256 to 2,048 photodiodes in a linear arrangement. A linear array is shown in Figure 5.8. Each photodiode responds to a specific wavelength, and as a result, a complete UV/visible spectrum can be obtained in less than 1 second. Resolution is 1 to 2 nm and depends on the number of discrete elements. In spectrophotometers using PDA detectors, the grating is

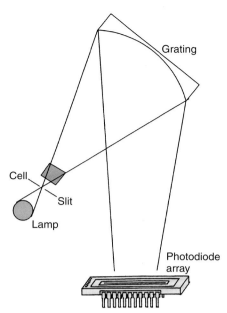

FIGURE 5.9 Photodiode array spectrophotometer illustrating the placement of the sample cuvette before the monochromator.

positioned after the sample cuvette and disperses the transmitted radiation onto the PDA detector (Fig. 5.9).

For single-beam spectrophotometers, the absorbance reading from the sample must be blanked using an appropriate reference solution that does not contain the compound of interest. Double-beam spectrophotometers permit automatic correction of sample and reference absorbance, as shown in Figure 5.10. Because the intensities of light sources vary as a function of wavelength, double-beam spectrophotometers are necessary when the absorption spectrum for a sample is to be obtained. Computerized, continuous zeroing, single-beam spectrophotometers have replaced most double-beam spectrophotometers.

Spectrophotometer Quality Assurance

Performing at least the following checks should validate instrument function: wavelength accuracy, stray light, and linearity. Wavelength accuracy means that the wavelength indicated on the control dial is the actual wavelength of light passed by the monochromator. It is most commonly checked using standard absorbing solutions or filters with absorbance maxima of known wavelength. Didymium or holmium oxide in glass is stable and frequently used as filters. The filter is placed in the light path, and the wavelength control is set at the wavelength at which maximal absorbance is expected. The wavelength control is then rotated in either direction to locate the actual wavelength that has maximal absorbance. If these two wavelengths do not match, the optics must be adjusted to calibrate the monochromator correctly.

Some instruments with narrow bandpass use a mercury vapor lamp to verify wavelength accuracy. The mercury lamp is substituted for the usual light source, and the spectrum is scanned to locate mercury emission lines. The wavelength indicated on the control is compared with

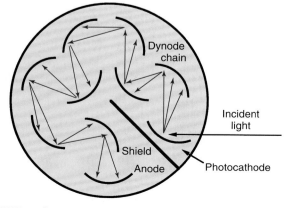

FIGURE 5.8 Dynode chain in a photomultiplier.

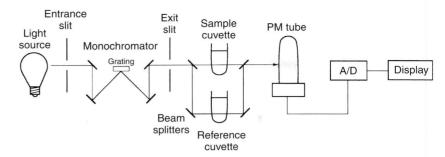

FIGURE 5.10 Double-beam spectrophotometer.

known mercury emission peaks to determine the accuracy of the wavelength indicator control.

Stray light refers to any wavelengths outside the band transmitted by the monochromator. Figure 5.11 shows the performance of a spectrophotometer to measure high absorbance in the presence of stray light. The most common causes of stray light are reflection of light from scratches on optical surfaces or from dust particles anywhere in the light path and higher order spectra produced by diffraction gratings. The major effect is absorbance error, especially in the high absorbance range. Stray light is detected by using cutoff filters, which eliminate all radiation at wavelengths beyond the one of interest. To check for stray light in the near-UV region, for example, a filter that does not transmit in the region of 200 to 400 nm is inserted. If the instrument reading is greater than 0% T, stray light is present. Certain liquids, such as $NiSO_4$, $NaNO_2$, and acetone, absorb strongly at short wavelengths and can be used to detect stray light in the UV range.

Linearity is demonstrated when a change in concentration results in a straight line calibration curve, as discussed under Beer law. Colored solutions may be carefully diluted and used to check linearity, using the wavelength of maximal absorbance for that color. Sealed sets of different colors and concentrations are available commercially. They should be labeled with expected absorbance for a given bandpass instrument. Less than expected absorbance is an indication of stray light or of a bandpass that is wider than specified. Sets of neutral-density filters to check linearity over a range of wavelengths are also commercially available.

FIGURE 5.11 Spectrophotometer's ability to measure high absorbance with stray light. (*A*) No stray light, with no deviation from the actual absorbance. (*B*) Some stray light within the instrument showing deviations from the actual at high absorbance. (*C*) A higher degree of stray light showing further deviation from the actual absorbance.

Atomic Absorption Spectrophotometer

The atomic absorption spectrophotometer is used to measure concentration by detecting the absorption of electromagnetic radiation by atoms rather than by molecules. The basic components are shown in Figure 5.12. The usual light source, known as a hollow-cathode lamp, consists of an evacuated gas-tight chamber containing an anode, a cylindrical cathode, and an inert gas, such as helium or argon. When voltage is applied, the filler gas is ionized. Ions attracted to the cathode collide with the metal, knock atoms off, and cause the metal atoms to be excited. When they return to the ground state, light energy is emitted that is characteristic of the metal in the cathode. Generally, a separate lamp is required for each metal (e.g., a copper hollow-cathode lamp is used to measure this metal).

Electrodeless discharge lamps are a relatively new light source for atomic absorption spectrophotometers. A bulb is filled with argon and the element to be tested. A radio-frequency generator around the bulb supplies the energy to excite the element, causing a characteristic emission spectrum of the element.

The analyzed sample must contain the reduced metal in the atomic vaporized state. Commonly, this is done by using the heat of a flame to break the chemical bonds and form free, unexcited atoms. The flame is the sample cell in this instrument, rather than a cuvette. There are various designs; however, the most common burner is the premix long-path burner. The sample, in solution, is aspirated as a spray into a chamber, where it is mixed with air and fuel. This mixture passes through baffles, where large drops fall and are drained off. Only fine droplets reach the flame. The burner is a long, narrow slit, to permit a longer path length for absorption of incident radiation. Light from the hollow-cathode lamp passes through the sample of ground state atoms in the flame. The amount of light absorbed is proportional to the concentration. When a ground state atom absorbs light energy, an excited atom is produced. The excited atom then returns to the ground state, emitting light of the same energy as it absorbed. The flame sample thus contains a dynamic population of ground state and excited atoms, both absorbing and emitting radiant energy. The emitted energy from the flame will go in all directions, and it will be a steady emission. Because the purpose of the instrument is to measure the amount of light absorbed, the light detector must be able to distinguish between the light beam emitted by the hollow-cathode lamp and that emitted by excited atoms in the flame. To do this, the hollow-cathode

FIGURE 5.12 Single-beam atomic absorption spectrophotometer—basic components.

light beam is modulated by inserting a mechanical rotating chopper between the light and the flame or by pulsing the electric supply to the lamp. Because the light beam being absorbed enters the sample in pulses, the transmitted light will also be in pulses. There will be less light in the transmitted pulses because part of it will be absorbed. There are, therefore, two light signals from the flame—an alternating signal from the hollow-cathode lamp and a direct signal from the flame emission. The measuring circuit is tuned to the modulated frequency. Interference from the constant flame emission is electronically eliminated by accepting only the pulsed signal from the hollow cathode.

The monochromator is used to isolate the desired emission line from other lamp emission lines. In addition, it serves to protect the photodetector from excessive light emanating from flame emissions. A PM tube is the usual light detector.

Flameless atomic absorption requires an instrument modification that uses an electric furnace to break chemical bonds (electrothermal atomization). A tiny graphite cylinder holds the sample, either liquid or solid. An electric current passes through the cylinder walls, evaporates the solvent, ashes the sample, and, finally, heats the unit to incandescence to atomize the sample. This instrument, like the spectrophotometer, is used to determine the amount of light absorbed. Again, Beer law is used for calculating concentration. A major problem is that background correction is considerably more necessary and critical for electrothermal techniques than for flame-based atomic absorption methods. Currently, the most common approach uses a deuterium lamp as a secondary source and measures the difference between the two absorbance signals. However, there has also been extensive development of background correction techniques based on the Zeeman effect.[1] The presence of an intense static magnetic field will cause the wavelength of the emitted radiation to split into several components. This shift in wavelength is the Zeeman effect.

Atomic absorption spectrophotometry is sensitive and precise. It is routinely used to measure concentration of trace metals that are not easily excited. It is generally more sensitive than flame emission because the vast majority of atoms produced in the usual propane or air-acetylene flame remain in the ground state available for light absorption. It is accurate, precise, and specific. One disadvantage, however, is the inability of the flame to dissociate samples into free atoms. For example, phosphate may interfere with calcium analysis by formation of calcium phosphate. This may be overcome by adding cations that compete with calcium for phosphate. Routinely, lanthanum or strontium is added to samples to form stable complexes with phosphate. Another possible problem is the ionization of atoms following dissociation by the flame, which can be decreased by reducing the flame temperature. Matrix interference, due to the enhancement of light absorption by atoms in organic solvents or formation of solid droplets as the solvent evaporates in the flame, can be another source of error. This interference may be overcome by pretreatment of the sample by extraction.[5]

Recently, inductively coupled plasma (ICP) has been used to increase sensitivity for atomic emission. The torch, an argon plasma maintained by the interaction of a radiofrequency field and an ionized argon gas, is reported to have used temperatures between 5,500 and 8,000 K. Complete atomization of elements is thought to occur at these temperatures. Use of ICP as a source is recommended for determinations involving refractory elements such as uranium, zirconium, and boron. ICP with MS detection is the most sensitive and specific assay technique for all elements on the periodic chart. Atomic absorption spectrophotometry is used less frequently because of this newer technology.

Flame Photometry

The flame emission photometer, which measures light emitted by excited atoms, was widely used to determine concentration of Na^+, K^+, or Li^+. With the development of ion-selective electrodes for these analytes, flame photometers are no longer routinely used in clinical chemistry laboratories. The reader should refer to previous editions of this book for discussion of this technique.

Fluorometry

As seen with the spectrophotometer, light entering a solution may pass mainly through or may be absorbed partly or entirely, depending on the concentration and the wavelength entering that particular solution. Whenever absorption occurs, there is a transfer of energy to the medium. Each molecular type possesses a series of electronic energy levels and can pass from a lower energy level to a higher energy level only by absorbing an integral unit (quantum) of light that is equal in energy to the difference between the two energy states. There are additional energy levels owing to rotation or vibration of molecular parts. The excited state lasts about 10^{-5} seconds before the electron loses energy and returns to the ground state. Energy is lost by collision, heat loss, transfer to other molecules, and emission of radiant energy. Because the molecules are excited by absorption of radiant energy and lose energy by multiple interactions, the radiant energy emitted is less than the absorbed energy. The difference between the maximum wavelengths, excitation, and emitted fluorescence is called Stokes shift. Both excitation (absorption) and fluorescence (emission) energies are characteristic for a given molecular type; for example, Figure 5.13 shows the absorption and fluorescence spectra of quinine in sulfuric acid. The dashed line on the left shows the short-wavelength excitation energy that is maximally absorbed, whereas the solid line on the right is the longer wavelength (less energy) fluorescent spectrum.

Basic Instrumentation

Filter fluorometers measure the concentrations of solutions that contain fluorescing molecules. A basic instrument is shown in Figure 5.14. The source emits short-wavelength high-energy excitation light. A mechanical attenuator controls light intensity. The primary filter, placed between the radiation source and the sample, selects the wavelength that is best absorbed by the solution to be measured. The fluorescing

FIGURE 5.13 Absorption and fluorescence spectra of quinine in 0.1 N sulfuric acid. (Adapted from Coiner D. *Basic Concepts in Laboratory Instrumentation*. Bethesda, MD: ASMT Education and Research Fund; 1975-1979.)

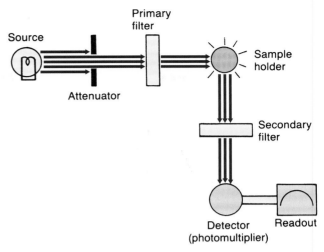

FIGURE 5.14 Basic filter fluorometer. (Adapted from Coiner D. *Basic Concepts in Laboratory Instrumentation*. Bethesda, MD: ASMT Education and Research Fund; 1975-1979.)

sample in the cuvette emits radiant energy in all directions. The detector (placed at right angles to the sample cell) and a secondary filter that passes the longer wavelengths of fluorescent light prevent incident light from striking the photodetector. The electrical output of the photodetector is proportional to the intensity of fluorescent energy. In spectrofluorometers, the filters are replaced by a grating monochromator.

Gas discharge lamps (mercury and xenon arc) are the most frequently used sources of excitation radiant energy. Incandescent tungsten lamps are seldom used because they release little energy in the UV region. Mercury vapor lamps are commonly used in filter fluorometers. Mercury emits a characteristic line spectrum. Resonance lines at 365 to 366 nm are commonly used. Energy at wavelengths other than the resonance lines is provided by coating the inner surface of the lamp with a material that absorbs the 254-nm mercury radiation and emits a broad band of longer wavelengths. Most spectrofluorometers use a high-pressure xenon lamp. Xenon has a good continuum, which is necessary for determining the excitation spectra.

Monochromator fluorometers use gratings for isolation of incident radiation. Light detectors are almost exclusively PM tubes because of their higher sensitivity to low light intensities. Double-beam instruments are used to compensate for instability due to electric power fluctuation.

Fluorescence concentration measurements are related to molar absorptivity of the compound, intensity of the incident radiation, quantum efficiency of the energy emitted per quantum absorbed, and length of the light path. In dilute solutions with instrument parameters held constant, fluorescence is directly proportional to concentration. Generally, a linear response will be obtained until the concentration of the fluorescent species is so high that the sample begins to absorb significant amounts of excitation light. A curve demonstrating nonlinearity as concentration increases is shown in Figure 5.15. The solution must absorb less than 5% of the exciting radiation for a linear response

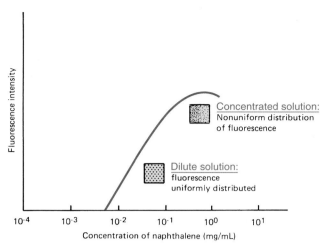

FIGURE 5.15 Dependence of fluorescence on the concentration of fluorophore. (Adapted from Guilbault GG. *Practical Fluorescence, Theory, Methods and Techniques*. New York, NY: Marcel Dekker; 1973.)

to occur.[6] As with all quantitative measurements, a standard curve must be prepared to demonstrate that the concentration used falls in a linear range.

In fluorescence polarization, radiant energy is polarized in a single plane. When the sample (fluorophore) is excited, it emits polarized light along the same plane as the incident light if the fluorophore does not rotate in solution (i.e., it is attached or bound to a large molecule). In contrast, a small molecule emits depolarized light because it will rotate out of the plane of polarization during its excitation lifetime. This technique is widely used for the detection of therapeutic and abused drugs. In the procedure, the sample analyte is allowed to compete with a fluorophore-labeled analyte for a limited antibody to the analyte. The lower the concentration of the sample analyte, the higher the macromolecular antibody–analyte–fluorophore formed and the lower the depolarization of the radiant light.

Advantages and Disadvantages of Fluorometry

Fluorometry has two advantages over conventional spectrophotometry: specificity and sensitivity. Fluorometry increases specificity by selecting the optimal wavelength for both absorption and fluorescence, rather than just the absorption wavelength seen with spectrophotometry.

Fluorometry is approximately 1,000 times more sensitive than most spectrophotometric methods.[6] One reason is because the emitted radiation is measured directly; it can be increased simply by increasing the intensity of the exciting radiant energy. In addition, fluorescence measures the amount of light intensity present over a zero background. In absorbance, however, the quantity of the absorbed light is measured indirectly as the difference between the transmitted beams. At low concentrations, the small difference between 100% T and the transmitted beam is difficult to measure accurately and precisely, limiting the sensitivity.

The biggest disadvantage is that fluorescence is very sensitive to environmental changes. Changes in pH affect

availability of electrons, and temperature changes the probability of loss of energy by collision rather than fluorescence. Contaminating chemicals or a change of solvents may change the structure. UV light used for excitation can cause photochemical changes. Any decrease in fluorescence resulting from any of these possibilities is known as quenching. Because so many factors may change the intensity or spectra of fluorescence, extreme care is mandatory in analytic technique and instrument maintenance.

Chemiluminescence

In chemiluminescence reactions, part of the chemical energy generated produces excited intermediates that decay to a ground state with the emission of photons.[7] The emitted radiation is measured with a PM tube, and the signal is related to analyte concentration. Chemiluminescence is different from fluorescence in that no excitation radiation is required and no monochromators are needed because the chemiluminescence arises from one species. Most importantly, chemiluminescence reactions are oxidation reactions of luminol, acridinium esters, and dioxetanes characterized by a rapid increase in intensity of emitted light followed by a gradual decay. Usually, the signal is taken as the integral of the entire peak. Enhanced chemiluminescence techniques increase the chemiluminescence efficiency by including an enhancer system in the reaction of a chemiluminescent agent with an enzyme. The time course for the light intensity is much longer (60 minutes) than that for conventional chemiluminescent reactions, which last for about 30 seconds (Fig. 5.16).

Advantages of chemiluminescence assays include subpicomolar detection limits, speed (with flash-type reactions, light is only measured for 10 seconds), ease of use (most assays are one-step procedures), and simple instrumentation.[7] The main disadvantage is that impurities can cause a background signal that degrades the sensitivity and specificity.

Turbidity and Nephelometry

Turbidimetric measurements are made with a spectrophotometer to determine the concentration of particulate matter in a sample. The amount of light blocked by a suspension

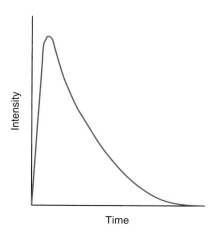

FIGURE 5.16 Representative intensity-versus-time curve for a transient chemiluminescence signal.

of particles depends not only on concentration but also on size. Because particles tend to aggregate and settle out of suspension, sample handling becomes critical. Instrument operation is the same as for any spectrophotometer.

Nephelometry is similar, except that light scattered by the small particles is measured at an angle to the beam incident on the cuvette. Figure 5.17 demonstrates two possible optical arrangements for a nephelometer. Light scattering depends on wavelength and particle size. For macromolecules with a size close to or larger than the wavelength of incident light, sensitivity is increased by measuring the forward light scatter.[8] Instruments are available with detectors placed at various forward angles, as well as at 90° to the incident light. Monochromatic light obtains uniform scatter and minimizes sample heating. Certain instruments use light amplification by stimulated emission of radiation (laser) as a source of monochromatic light; however, any monochromator may be used.

Measuring light scatter at an angle other than 180° that is employed in turbidimetry minimizes error from colored solutions and increases sensitivity. Because both methods depend on particle size, some instruments quantitate initial change in light scatter rather than total scatter. Reagents must be free of any particles, and cuvettes must be free of any scratches.

Laser Applications

Laser is based on the interaction of radiant energy with suitably excited atoms or molecules. The interaction leads to stimulated emission of radiation. The wavelength, direction of propagation, phase, and plane of polarization of the emitted light are the same as those of the incident radiation. Laser light is polarized and coherent and has narrow spectral width and small cross-sectional area with low divergence. The radiant emission can be very powerful and either continuous or pulsating.

Laser light can serve as the source of incident energy in a spectrometer or nephelometer. Some lasers produce bandwidths of a few kilohertz in both the visible and infrared regions, making these applications about three to six orders more sensitive than conventional spectrometers.[9]

Laser spectrometry can also be used for the determination of structure and identification of samples, as well as for diagnosis. Quantitation of samples depends on the spectrometer used. An example of the clinical application of laser is the hematology and flow cytometer analyzers for the differential analysis of white blood cells.[10]

ELECTROCHEMISTRY

Electrochemistry is the basis for many types of analyses are used in the clinical laboratory, including potentiometry, amperometry, coulometry, and polarography. The two basic electrochemical cells involved in these analyses are galvanic and electrolytic cells.

Galvanic and Electrolytic Cells

An electrochemical cell can be set up as shown in Figure 5.18. It consists of two half-cells and a salt bridge, which can be a piece of filter paper saturated with electrolytes. Instead of two beakers as shown, the electrodes can be immersed in a single, large beaker containing a salt solution. In such a setup, the solution serves as the salt bridge.

In a galvanic cell, as the electrodes are connected, there is spontaneous flow of electrons from the electrode with the lower electron affinity (oxidation; e.g., silver). These electrons pass through the external meter to the cathode (reduction), where OH^- ions are liberated. This reaction continues until one of the chemical components is depleted, at which point, the cell is "dead" and cannot produce electrical energy to the external meter.

Current may be forced to flow through the dead cell only by applying an external electromotive force E. This is called an electrolytic cell. In short, a galvanic cell can be built from an electrolytic cell. When the external E is turned off, accumulated products at the electrodes will spontaneously produce current in the opposite direction of the electrolytic cell.

Half-Cells

It is impossible to measure the electrochemical activity of one half-cell; two reactions must be coupled and one reaction compared with the other. To rate half-cell reactions, a specific electrode reaction is arbitrarily assigned 0.00 V. Every other reaction coupled with this arbitrary zero reaction is either positive or negative, depending on the relative affinity for electrons. The electrode defined as 0.00 V is the standard hydrogen electrode: H_2 gas at 1 atmosphere (atm). The hydrogen gas in contact with H^+ in solution develops a potential. The hydrogen electrode coupled with a zinc half-cell is cathodic, with the reaction $2H^+ + 2e^- \rightarrow H_2$, because H_2 has a greater affinity than does Zn for electrons. Cu, however, has a greater affinity than H_2 for electrons, and

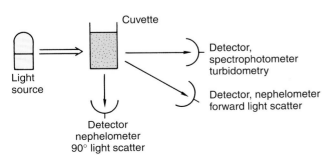

FIGURE 5.17 Nephelometer versus spectrophotometer—optical arrangements.

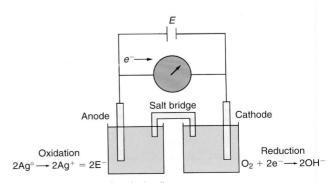

FIGURE 5.18 Electrochemical cell.

TABLE 5.1 **Standard Reduction Potentials**

	Potential, V
$Zn^{2+} + 2e \leftrightarrow Z$	−0.7628
$Cr^{2+} + 2e \leftrightarrow Cr$	−0.913
$Ni^{2+} + 2e \leftrightarrow Ni$	−0.257
$2H^+ + 2e \leftrightarrow H_2$	0.000
$Cu^{2+} + 2e \leftrightarrow Cu$	0.3419
$Ag^+ + e \leftrightarrow Ag$	0.7996

Data presented are examples from Lide DR. *CRC Handbook of Chemistry and Physics*. 93rd ed. Boca Raton, FL: CRC Press; 2012-2013.

thus the anodic reaction $H_2 \rightarrow 2H^+ + 2e^-$ occurs when coupled to the Cu-electrode half-cell.

The potential generated by the hydrogen-gas electrode is used to rate the electrode potential of metals in 1 mol/L solution. Reduction potentials for certain metals are shown in Table 5.1.[11] A hydrogen electrode is used to determine the accuracy of reference and indicator electrodes, the stability of standard solutions, and the potentials of liquid junctions.

Ion-Selective Electrodes

Potentiometric methods of analysis involve the direct measurement of electrical potential due to the activity of free ions. **Ion-selective electrodes** (ISEs) are designed to be sensitive toward individual ions.

pH Electrodes

An ISE universally used in the clinical laboratory is the pH electrode. The basic components of a pH meter are shown in Figure 5.19.

Indicator Electrode

The pH electrode consists of a silver wire coated with AgCl, immersed into an internal solution of 0.1 mmol/L HCl, and placed into a tube containing a special glass membrane tip. This membrane is only sensitive to hydrogen ions (H^+). Glass membranes that are selectively sensitive to H^+ consist of spe-

cific quantities of lithium, cesium, lanthanum, barium, or aluminum oxides in silicate. When the pH electrode is placed into the test solution, movement of H^+ near the tip of the electrode produces a potential difference between the internal solution and the test solution, which is measured as pH and read by a voltmeter. The combination pH electrode also contains a built-in reference electrode, either Ag/AgCl or calomel (Hg/Hg_2Cl_2) immersed in a solution of saturated KCl.

The specially formulated glass continually dissolves from the surface. The present concept of the selective mechanism that causes the formation of electromotive force at the glass surface is that an ion-exchange process is involved. Cationic exchange occurs only in the gel layer—there is no penetration of H^+ through the glass. Although the glass is constantly dissolving, the process is slow, and the glass tip generally lasts for several years. pH electrodes are highly selective for H^+; however, other cations in high concentration interfere, the most common of which is sodium. Electrode manufacturers should list the concentration of interfering cations that may cause error in pH determinations.

Reference Electrode

The reference electrode commonly used is the calomel electrode. Calomel, a paste of predominantly mercurous chloride, is in direct contact with metallic mercury in an electrolyte solution of potassium chloride. As long as the electrolyte concentration and the temperature remain constant, a stable voltage is generated at the interface of the mercury and its salt. A cable connected to the mercury leads to the voltmeter. The filling hole is needed for adding potassium chloride solution. A tiny opening at the bottom is required for completion of electric contact between the reference and indicator electrodes. The liquid junction consists of a fiber or ceramic plug that allows a small flow of electrolyte filling solution.

Construction varies, but all reference electrodes must generate a stable electrical potential. Reference electrodes generally consist of a metal and its salt in contact with a solution containing the same anion. Mercury/mercurous chloride, as in this example, is a frequently used reference electrode; the disadvantage is that it is slow to reach a new stable voltage following temperature change and it is unstable above 80°C.[1,2] Ag/AgCl is another common reference electrode. It can be used at high temperatures, up to 275°C, and the AgCl-coated Ag wire makes a more compact electrode than that of mercury. In measurements in which chloride contamination must be avoided, a mercury sulfate and potassium sulfate reference electrode may be used.

Liquid Junctions

Electrical connection between the indicator and reference electrodes is achieved by allowing a slow flow of electrolyte from the tip of the reference electrode. A junction potential is always set up at the boundary between two dissimilar solutions because of positive and negative ions diffusing across the boundary at unequal rates. The resultant junction potential may increase or decrease the potential of the reference electrode. Therefore, it is important that the junc-

FIGURE 5.19 Necessary components of a pH meter.

tion potential be kept to a minimum reproducible value when the reference electrode is in solution.

KCl is a commonly used filling solution because K^+ and Cl^- have nearly the same mobilities. When KCl is used as the filling solution for Ag/AgCl electrodes, the addition of AgCl is required to prevent dissolution of the AgCl salt. One way of producing a lower junction potential is to mix K^+, Na^+, NO_3^-, and Cl^- in appropriate ratios.

Readout Meter

Electromotive force produced by the reference and indicator electrodes is in the millivolt range. Zero potential for the cell indicates that each electrode half-cell is generating the same voltage, assuming there is no liquid junction potential. The isopotential is that potential at which a temperature change has no effect on the response of the electrical cell. Manufacturers generally achieve this by making the midscale (pH 7.0) correspond to 0 V at all temperatures. They use an internal buffer whose pH changes due to temperature compensate for the changes in the internal and external reference electrodes.

Nernst Equation

The electromotive force generated because of H^+ at the glass tip is described by Nernst equation, which is shown in a simplified form:

$$\varepsilon = \Delta pH \times \frac{RT \ln 10}{F} = \Delta pH \times 0.059\ V \quad (Eq.\ 5\text{-}6)$$

where ε is the electromotive force of the cell, F is the Faraday constant (96,500 C/mol), R is the molar gas constant, and T is temperature, in Kelvin.

As the temperature increases, H^+ activity increases and the potential generated increases. Most pH meters have a temperature compensation knob that amplifies the millivolt response when the meter is on pH function. pH units on the meter scale are usually printed for use at room temperature. On the voltmeter, 59.16 is read as 1 pH unit change. The temperature compensation changes the millivolt response to compensate for changes due to temperature from 54.2 at 0°C to 66.10 at 60°C. However, most pH meters are manufactured for greatest accuracy in the 10°C to 60°C range.

Calibration

The steps necessary to standardize a pH meter are fairly straightforward. First, balance the system with the electrodes in a buffer with a 7.0 pH. The balance or intercept control shifts the entire slope, as shown in Figure 5.20. Next, replace the buffer with one of a different pH. If the meter does not register the correct pH, amplification of the response changes the slope to match that predicted by Nernst equation. If the instrument does not have a slope control, the temperature compensator performs the same function.

pH Combination Electrode

The most commonly used pH electrode has both the indicator and reference electrodes combined in one small probe,

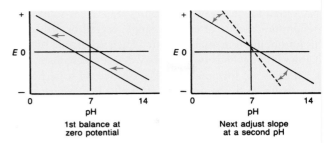

FIGURE 5.20 pH meter calibration. (Adapted from Willard HH, Merritt LL, Dean JA, et al. *Instrumental Methods of Analysis*. Belmont, CA: Wadsworth; 1981.)

which is convenient when small samples are tested. It consists of an Ag/AgCl internal reference electrode sealed in a narrow glass cylinder with a pH-sensitive glass tip. The reference electrode is an Ag/AgCl wire wrapped around the indicator electrode. The outer glass envelope is filled with KCl and has a tiny pore near the tip of the liquid junction. The solution to be measured must completely cover the glass tip. Examples of other ISEs are shown in Figure 5.21. The reference electrode, electrometer, and calibration system described for pH measurements are applicable to all ISEs.

There are three major ISE types: inert metal electrodes in contact with a redox couple, metal electrodes that participate in a redox reaction, and membrane electrodes. The membrane can be solid material (e.g., glass), liquid (e.g., ion-exchange electrodes), or special membrane (e.g., compound electrodes), such as gas-sensing and enzyme electrodes.

The standard hydrogen electrode is an example of an inert metal electrode. The Ag/AgCl electrode is an example of the second type. The electrode process $AgCl + e^- \rightarrow Ag^+ + Cl^-$ produces an electrical potential proportional to chloride ion (Cl^-) activity. When Cl^- is held constant, the electrode is used as a reference electrode. The electrode in contact with varying Cl^- concentrations is used as an indicator electrode to measure Cl^- concentration.

The H^+-sensitive gel layer of the glass pH electrode is considered a membrane. A change in the glass formulation makes the membrane more sensitive to sodium ions

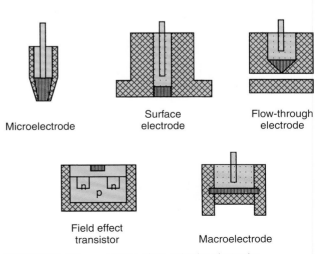

FIGURE 5.21 Other examples of ion-selective electrodes.

(Na^+) than to H^+, creating a sodium ISE. Other solid-state membranes consist of either a single crystal or fine crystals immobilized in an inert matrix such as silicone rubber. Conduction depends on a vacancy defect mechanism, and the crystals are formulated to be selective for a particular size, shape, and change—for example, F^--selective electrodes of LaF_3, Cl^--sensitive electrodes with AgCl crystals, and AgBr electrodes for the detection of Br^-.

The calcium ISE is a liquid membrane electrode. An ion-selective carrier, such as dioctylphenyl phosphonate dissolved in an inert water-insoluble solvent, diffuses through a porous membrane. Because the solvent is insoluble in water, the test sample cannot cross the membrane, but calcium ions (Ca^{2+}) are exchanged. The Ag/AgCl internal reference in a filling solution of $CaCl_2$ is in contact with the carrier by means of the membrane.

Potassium-selective liquid membranes use the antibiotic valinomycin as the ion-selective carrier. Valinomycin membranes show great selectivity for K^+. Liquid membrane electrodes are recharged every few months to replace the liquid ion exchanger membrane and the porous membrane.

Gas-Sensing Electrodes

Gas electrodes are similar to pH glass electrodes but are designed to detect specific gases (e.g., CO_2 and NH_3) in solutions and are usually separated from the solution by a thin, gas-permeable hydrophobic membrane. Figure 5.22 shows a schematic illustration of the pCO_2 electrode. The membrane in contact with the solution is permeable only to CO_2, which diffuses into a thin film of sodium bicarbonate solution. The pH of the bicarbonate solution is changed as follows:

$$CO_2 + H_2O \leftrightarrow H_2CO_3 \leftrightarrow H^+ + HCO_3^- \quad \text{(Eq. 5-7)}$$

The change in pH of the HCO_3^- is detected by a pH electrode. The pCO_2 electrode is widely used in clinical laboratories as a component of instruments for measuring serum electrolytes and blood gases.

In the NH_3 gas electrode, the bicarbonate solution is replaced by ammonium chloride solution, and the membrane

is permeable only to NH_3 gas. As in the pCO_2 electrode, NH_3 changes the pH of NH_4Cl as follows:

$$NH_3 + H_2O \leftrightarrow NH_4^+ + OH^- \quad \text{(Eq. 5-8)}$$

The amount of OH^- produced varies linearly with the log of the partial pressure of NH_3 in the sample.

Other gas-sensing electrodes function on the basis of an amperometric principle—that is, measurement of the current flowing through an electrochemical cell at a constant applied electrical potential to the electrodes. Examples are the determination of pO_2, glucose, and peroxidase.

The chemical reactions of the pO_2 electrode (Clark electrode), an electrochemical cell with a platinum cathode and an Ag/AgCl anode, are illustrated in Figure 5.18. The electrical potential at the cathode is set to -0.65 V and will not conduct current without oxygen in the sample. The membrane is permeable to oxygen, which diffuses through to the platinum cathode. Current passes through the cell and is proportional to the pO_2 in the test sample.

Glucose determination is based on the reduction in pO_2 during glucose oxidase reaction with glucose and oxygen. Unlike the pCO_2 electrode, the peroxidase electrode has a polarized platinum anode and its potential is set to $+0.6$ V. Current flows through the system when peroxide is oxidized at the anode as follows:

$$H_2O_2 \rightarrow 2H^+ + 2e^- + O_2 \quad \text{(Eq. 5-9)}$$

Enzyme Electrodes

The various ISEs may be covered by immobilized enzymes that can catalyze a specific chemical reaction. Selection of the ISE is determined by the reaction product of the immobilized enzyme. Examples include urease, which is used for the detection of urea, and glucose oxidase, which is used for glucose detection. A urea electrode must have an ISE that is selective for NH_4^+ or NH_3, whereas glucose oxidase is used in combination with a pH electrode.

Coulometric Chloridometers and Anodic Stripping Voltammetry

Chloride ISEs have largely replaced coulometric titrations for the determination of chloride in body fluids. Anodic stripping voltammetry was widely used for the analysis of lead and is best measured by electrothermal (graphite furnace) atomic absorption spectroscopy or, preferably, inductively coupled plasma-mass spectrometry (ICP-MS).

ELECTROPHORESIS

Electrophoresis is the migration of charged solutes or particles in an electrical field. Iontophoresis refers to the migration of small ions, whereas zone electrophoresis is the migration of charged macromolecules in a porous support medium such as paper, cellulose acetate, or agarose gel film.

FIGURE 5.22 The pCO_2 electrode.

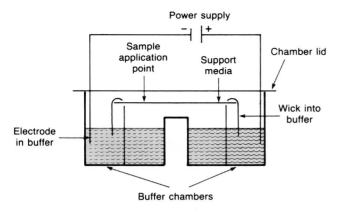

FIGURE 5.23 Electrophoresis apparatus—basic components.

An electrophoretogram is the result of zone electrophoresis and consists of sharply separated zones of a macromolecule. In a clinical laboratory, the macromolecules of interest are proteins in serum, urine, cerebrospinal fluid (CSF), and other biologic body fluids and erythrocytes and tissue.

Electrophoresis consists of five components: the driving force (electrical power), the support medium, the buffer, the sample, and the detecting system. A typical electrophoretic apparatus is illustrated in Figure 5.23.

Charged particles migrate toward the opposite charged electrode. The velocity of migration is controlled by the net charge of the particle, the size and shape of the particle, the strength of the electric field, chemical and physical properties of the supporting medium, and the electrophoretic temperature. The rate of mobility[12] of the molecule (μ) is given by

$$\mu = \frac{Q}{K} \leftrightarrow r \leftrightarrow n \qquad \text{(Eq. 5-10)}$$

where Q is net charge of the particle, K is a constant, r is the ionic radius of the particle, and n is the viscosity of the buffer.

From the equation, the rate of migration is directly proportional to the net charge of the particle and inversely proportional to its size and the viscosity of the buffer.

Procedure

The sample is soaked in hydrated support for approximately 5 minutes. The support is put into the electrophoresis chamber, which was previously filled with the buffer. Sufficient buffer must be added to the chamber to maintain contact with the support. Electrophoresis is carried out by applying a constant voltage or constant current for a specific time. The support is then removed and placed in a fixative or rapidly dried to prevent diffusion of the sample. This is followed by staining the zones with an appropriate dye. The uptake of dye by the sample is proportional to sample concentration. After excess dye is washed away, the supporting medium may need to be placed in a clearing agent. Otherwise, it is completely dried.

Power Supply

Power supplies operating at either constant current or constant voltage are available commercially. In electrophoresis, heat is produced when current flows through a medium that has resistance, resulting in an increase in thermal agitation of the dissolved solute (ions) and leading to a decrease in resistance and an increase in current. The increase leads to increases in heat and evaporation of water from the buffer, increasing the ionic concentration of the buffer and subsequent further increases in the current. The migration rate can be kept constant by using a power supply with constant current. This is true because, as electrophoresis progresses, a decrease in resistance as a result of heat produced also decreases the voltage.

Buffers

Two buffer properties that affect the charge of ampholytes are pH and ionic strength. The ions carry the applied electric current and allow the buffer to maintain constant pH during electrophoresis. An ampholyte is a molecule, such as protein, whose net charge can be either positive or negative. If the buffer is more acidic than the isoelectric point (pI) of the ampholyte, it binds H^+, becomes positively charged, and migrates toward the cathode. If the buffer is more basic than the pI, the ampholyte loses H^+, becomes negatively charged, and migrates toward the anode. A particle without a net charge will not migrate, remaining at the point of application. During electrophoresis, ions cluster around a migrating particle. The higher the ionic concentration, the higher the size of the ionic cloud and the lower the mobility of the particle. Greater ionic strength produces sharper protein-band separation but leads to increased heat production. This may cause denaturation of heat-labile proteins. Consequently, the optimal buffer concentration should be determined for any electrophoretic system. Generally, the most widely used buffers are made of monovalent ions because their ionic strength and molality are equal.

Support Materials
Cellulose Acetate

Paper electrophoresis use has been replaced by cellulose acetate or agarose gel in clinical laboratories. Cellulose is acetylated to form cellulose acetate by treating it with acetic anhydride. Cellulose acetate, a dry, brittle film composed of about 80% air space, is produced commercially. When the film is soaked in buffer, the air spaces fill with electrolyte and the film becomes pliable. After electrophoresis and staining, cellulose acetate can be made transparent for densitometer quantitation. The dried transparent film can be stored for long periods. Cellulose acetate prepared to reduce electroendosmosis is available commercially. Cellulose acetate is also used in isoelectric focusing.

Agarose Gel

Agarose gel is another widely used supporting medium. Used as a purified fraction of agar, it is neutral and, therefore, does not produce electroendosmosis. After electrophoresis and staining, it is detained (cleared), dried, and scanned with a densitometer. The dried gel can be stored indefinitely. Agarose gel electrophoresis requires small amounts of sample (~2 mL); it does not bind protein and, therefore, migration is not affected.

Polyacrylamide Gel

Polyacrylamide gel electrophoresis involves separation of protein on the basis of charge and molecular size. Layers of gel with different pore sizes are used. The gel is prepared before electrophoresis in a tube-shaped electrophoresis cell. The small-pore separation gel is at the bottom, followed by a large-pore spacer gel and, finally, another large-pore gel containing the sample. Each layer of gel is allowed to form a gelatin before the next gel is poured over it. At the start of electrophoresis, the protein molecules move freely through the spacer gel to its boundary with the separation gel, which slows their movement. This allows for concentration of the sample before separation by the small-pore gel. Polyacrylamide gel electrophoresis separates serum proteins into 20 or more fractions rather than the usual 6 fractions separated by cellulose acetate or agarose. It is widely used to study individual proteins (e.g., isoenzymes).

Starch Gel

Starch gel electrophoresis separates proteins on the basis of surface charge and molecular size, as does polyacrylamide gel. The procedure is not widely used because of technical difficulty in preparing the gel.

Treatment and Application of Sample

Serum contains a high concentration of protein, especially albumin, and therefore, serum specimens are routinely diluted with buffer before electrophoresis. In contrast, urine and CSF are usually concentrated. Hemoglobin hemolysate is used without further concentration. Generally, preparation of a sample is done according to the suggestion of the manufacturer of the electrophoretic supplies.

Cellulose acetate and agarose gel electrophoresis require approximately 2 to 5 μL of sample. These are the most common routine electrophoreses performed in clinical laboratories. Because most commercially manufactured plates come with a thin plastic template that has small slots through which samples are applied, overloading of agarose gel with sample is not a frequent problem. After serum is allowed to diffuse into the gel for approximately 5 minutes, the template is blotted to remove excess serum before being removed from the gel surface. Sample is applied to cellulose acetate with a twin-wire applicator designed to transfer a small amount.

Detection and Quantitation

Separated protein fractions are stained to reveal their locations. Different stains come with different plates from different manufacturers. The simplest way to accomplish detection is visualization under UV light, whereas densitometry is the most common and reliable way for quantitation. Most densitometers will automatically integrate the area under a peak, and the result is printed as percentage

FIGURE 5.24 Densitometer—basic components.

of the total. A schematic illustration of a densitometer is shown in Figure 5.24.

Electroendosmosis

The movement of buffer ions and solvent relative to the fixed support is called endosmosis or electroendosmosis. Support media, such as paper, cellulose acetate, and agar gel, take on a negative charge from adsorption of hydroxyl ions. When current is applied to the electrophoresis system, the hydroxyl ions remain fixed while the free positive ions move toward the cathode. The ions are highly hydrated, resulting in net cathodic movement of solvent. Molecules that are nearly neutral are swept toward the cathode with the solvent. Support media such as agarose and acrylamide gel are essentially neutral, eliminating electroendosmosis. The position of proteins in any electrophoresis separation depends not only on the nature of the protein but also on all other technical variables.

Isoelectric Focusing

Isoelectric focusing is a modification of electrophoresis. An apparatus is used similar to that shown in Figure 5.25. Charged proteins migrate through a support medium that has a continuous pH gradient. Individual proteins move in the electric field until they reach a pH equal to their isoelectric point, at which point they have no charge and cease to move.

Capillary Electrophoresis

In capillary electrophoresis (CE), separation is performed in narrow-bore fused silica capillaries (inner diameter

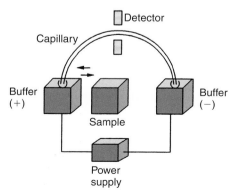

FIGURE 5.25 Schematic of capillary electrophoresis instrumentation. Sample is loaded on the capillary by replacing the anode buffer reservoir with the sample reservoir. (Adapted from Heiger DN. *High-Performance Capillary Electrophoresis*. Waldbronn, Germany: Hewlett-Packard; 1992.)

FIGURE 5.26 Differential solute migration superimposed on electro-osmotic flow in capillary zone electrophoresis. (Adapted from Heiger DN. *High-Performance Capillary Electrophoresis*. Waldbronn, Germany: Hewlett-Packard; 1992.)

25 to 75 μm). Usually, the capillaries are only filled with buffer, although gel media can also be used. A CE instrumentation schematic is shown in Figure 5.25. Initially, the capillary is filled with buffer and then the sample is loaded; applying an electric field performs the separation. Detection can be made near the other end of the capillary directly through the capillary wall.[13]

A fundamental CE concept is the electro-osmotic flow (EOF). EOF is the bulk flow of liquid toward the cathode upon application of an electric field, and it is superimposed on electrophoretic migration. EOF controls the amount of time solutes remain in the capillary. Cations migrate fastest because both EOF and electrophoretic attraction are toward the cathode; neutral molecules are all carried by the EOF but are not separated from each other; and anions move slowest because, although they are carried to the cathode by the EOF, they are attracted to the anode and repelled by the cathode (Fig. 5.26). Widely used for monitoring separated analytes, UV-visible detection is performed directly on the capillary; however, sensitivity is poor because of the small dimensions of the capillary, resulting in a short path length. Fluorescence, laser-induced fluorescence, and chemiluminescence detection can be used for higher sensitivity.

CE has been used for the separation, quantitation, and determination of molecular weights of proteins and peptides; for the analysis of polymerase chain reaction products; and for the analysis of inorganic ions, organic acids, pharmaceuticals, optical isomers, and drugs of abuse in serum and urine.[14] While traditionally serum protein electrophoresis (Chapter 11) for the diagnosis of plasma cell dyscrasias has been performed using polyacrylamide gel electrophoresis, CE has now become widely used for this analysis due to its faster run time and its relative automation.

Two-Dimensional Electrophoresis

This electrophoresis assay combines two different electrophoresis dimensions to separate proteins from complex matrices such as serum or tissue. In the first dimension, proteins are resolved according to their isoelectric points (pIs), using immobilized pH gradients. Commercial gradients are available in a variety of pH ranges. In the second dimension,

proteins are separated according to their relative size (molecular weight), using sodium dodecyl sulfate–polyacrylamide gel electrophoresis. A schematic of this is shown in Figure 5.27. Gels can be run under denaturing or nondenaturing conditions (e.g., for the maintenance of enzyme activity) and visualized by a variety of techniques, including the use of colorimetric dyes (e.g., Coomassie blue or silver stain) and radiographic, fluorometric, or chemiluminescence of appropriately labeled polypeptides. These latter techniques are considerably more sensitive than the colorimetric dyes.

OSMOMETRY

An osmometer is used to measure the concentration of solute particles in a solution. The mathematic definition is

FIGURE 5.27 Hypothetical example of a two-dimensional electrophoretogram from a patient with a disease (*panel 1*) compared with a normal subject (*panel 2*). The patient exhibits a protein (*oval*) that is not expressed in the normal subject. This protein might be a potential marker for this disease. (Gels courtesy of Kendrick Laboratories, Madison, WI.)

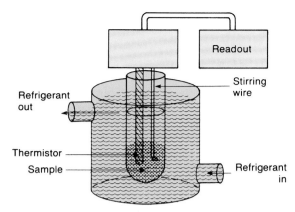

FIGURE 5.28 Freezing point osmometer. (Adapted from Coiner D. *Basic Concepts in Laboratory Instrumentation*. Bethesda, MD: ASMT Education and Research Fund; 1975-1979.)

$$\text{Osmolality} = \varphi \times n \times C \qquad \text{(Eq. 5-11)}$$

where ϕ is the osmotic coefficient, n is the number of dissociable particles (ions) per molecule in the solution, and C is the concentration in moles per kilogram of solvent.

The osmotic coefficient is an experimentally derived factor to correct for the fact that some of the molecules, even in a highly dissociated compound, exist as molecules rather than as ions.

The four physical properties of a solution that change with variations in the number of dissolved particles in the solvent are osmotic pressure, vapor pressure, boiling point, and freezing point. Osmometers measure osmolality indirectly by measuring one of these colligative properties, which change proportionally with osmotic pressure. Osmometers in clinical use measure either freezing point depression or vapor pressure depression; results are expressed in milliosmolal per kilogram (mOsm/kg) units.

Freezing Point Osmometer

Figure 5.28 illustrates the basic components of a freezing point osmometer. The sample in a small tube is lowered into a chamber with cold refrigerant circulating from a cooling unit. A thermistor is immersed in the sample. To measure temperature, a wire is used to gently stir the sample until it is cooled to several degrees below its freezing point. It is possible to cool water to as low as −40°C and still have liquid water, provided no crystals or particulate matter is present. This is referred to as a supercooled solution. Vigorous agitation when the sample is supercooled results in rapid freezing. Freezing can also be started by "seeding" a supercooled solution with crystals. When the supercooled solution starts to freeze as a result of the rapid stirring, a slush is formed and the solution actually warms to its freezing point temperature. The slush, an equilibrium of liquid and ice crystals, will remain at the freezing point temperature until the sample freezes solid and drops below its freezing point.

Impurities in a solvent will lower the temperature at which freezing or melting occurs by reducing the bonding forces between solvent molecules so that the molecules break away from each other and exist as a fluid at a lower temperature. The decrease in the freezing point temperature is proportional to the number of dissolved particles present.

The thermistor is a material that has less resistance when the temperature increases. The readout uses a Wheatstone bridge circuit that detects temperature change as proportional to change in thermistor resistance. Freezing point depression is proportional to the number of solute particles. Standards of known concentration are used to calibrate the instruments in mOsm/kg.

SURFACE PLASMON RESONANCE

A rather novel optical technique that is emerging into the clinical laboratory is surface plasmon resonance or SPR. This technique enables the study of the binding of ligands to surface receptors such as membrane proteins in real time. Figure 5.29A illustrates a schematic diagram of SPR using the "Kretschmann" geometry while Figure 5.29B illustrates a typical plot of binding affinity as reflected by a change in refractive index versus time. A light source passes through a prism and onto a back side of a sensor chip containing a metal such as gold and reflects off the back of the chip onto

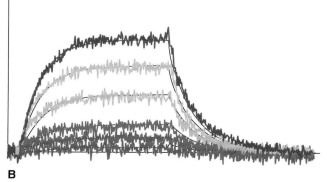

FIGURE 5.29 Schematic of surface plasmon resonance spectroscopy. **(A)** Block diagram of the SPR sensor. **(B)** Output demonstrating the kinetics of analyte binding to the sensor. (Figures courtesy of Bio-Rad Laboratories, Hercules, CA. See text for details.)

a detector. At the proper angle of light, the light is absorbed by the electrons in the metal causing a resonance. This decreases the amount of light reaching the detector. SPR can be used to measure interactions between immobilized antibodies and freely circulating analytes (or vice versa). In a clinical research setting, SPR is being used for the analysis of low molecular weight compounds, proteins and biomarkers, hormones, nucleic acids, circulating antibodies, and infectious microorganisms from biological matrices.[15] The analytical sensitivity of SPR is similar to that of conventional immunoassays. The costs for developing and using SPR may be less expensive since there are no labels involved. Moreover, sensors can be placed into an array for multiplexing purposes.

For additional student resources, please visit **thePoint** at http://thepoint.lww.com

---

questions

1. Which of the following is *not* necessary for obtaining the spectrum of a compound from 190 to 500 nm?
   a. Tungsten light source
   b. Deuterium light source
   c. Double-beam spectrophotometer
   d. Quartz cuvettes
   e. Photomultiplier

2. Stray light in a spectrophotometer places limits on
   a. Upper range of linearity
   b. Sensitivity
   c. Photometric accuracy below 0.1 absorbance units
   d. Ability to measure in the UV range
   e. Use of a grating monochromator

3. Which of the following light sources is used in atomic absorption spectrophotometry?
   a. Hollow-cathode lamp
   b. Xenon arc lamp
   c. Tungsten light
   d. Deuterium lamp
   e. Laser

4. Which of the following is true concerning fluorometry?
   a. Fluorescence is an inherently more sensitive technique than absorption.
   b. Emission wavelengths are always set at lower wavelengths than excitation.
   c. The detector is always placed at right angles to the excitation beam.
   d. All compounds undergo fluorescence.
   e. Fluorometers require special detectors.

5. Which of the following techniques has the highest potential sensitivity?
   a. Chemiluminescence
   b. Fluorescence
   c. Turbidimetry
   d. Nephelometry
   e. Phosphorescence

6. Which electrochemical assay measures current at fixed potential?
   a. Amperometry
   b. Anodic stripping voltammetry
   c. Coulometry
   d. Analysis with ISEs
   e. Electrophoresis

7. Which of the following refers to the movement of buffer ions and solvent relative to the fixed support?
   a. Electroendosmosis
   b. Isoelectric focusing
   c. Iontophoresis
   d. Zone electrophoresis
   e. Plasmapheresis

8. Reverse-phase liquid chromatography refers to
   a. A polar mobile phase and nonpolar stationary phase
   b. A nonpolar mobile phase and polar stationary phase
   c. Distribution between two liquid phases
   d. Size used to separate solutes instead of charge
   e. Charge used to separate solutes instead of size

9. Which of the following is *not* an advantage of CE?
   a. Multiple samples can be assayed simultaneously on one injection.
   b. Very small sample size.
   c. Rapid analysis.
   d. Use of traditional detectors.
   e. Cations, neutrals, and anions move in the same direction at different rates.

10. Tandem mass spectrometers
    a. Are two mass spectrometers placed in series with each other
    b. Are two mass spectrometers placed in parallel with each other
    c. Require use of a gas chromatograph
    d. Require use of an electrospray interface
    e. Do not require an ionization source

(continues on page 120)

review questions (continued)

11. Which of the following is *false* concerning the principles of point-of-care testing devices?
    a. Devices do not require quality control testing.
    b. They use principles that are identical to laboratory-based instrumentation.
    c. Biosensors have enabled miniaturization particularly amendable for point-of-care testing.
    d. Onboard microcomputers control instrument functions and data reduction.
    e. Whole blood analysis is the preferred specimen.

12. Which is the most sensitive detector for spectrophotometry?
    a. Photomultiplier.
    b. Phototube.
    c. Electron multiplier.
    d. Photodiode array.
    e. All are equally sensitive.

13. Which of the following is Beer law?
    a. $A = \varepsilon \times b \times c$
    b. $\%T = I/I_0 \times 100$
    c. $E = h\nu$
    d. $\varepsilon = \Delta\text{pH} \times 0.59 \text{ V}$
    e. $\text{Osmolality} = \varphi \times n \times C$

14. Which of the following correctly ranks electromagnetic radiation from low energy to high energy?
    a. Microwaves, infrared, visible, UV, x-rays, gamma, cosmic
    b. Cosmic, gamma, x-rays, UV, visible, infrared, microwaves
    c. UV, visible, infrared, microwaves, x-rays, cosmic, gamma
    d. UV, visible, infrared, cosmic, gamma, microwaves, x-rays
    e. Visible, UV, infrared, cosmic, gamma, microwaves, x-rays

15. What is the purpose of the chopper in an atomic absorption spectrophotometer?
    a. Correct for the amount of light emitted by the flame
    b. Correct for the fluctuating intensity of the light source
    c. Correct for the fluctuating sensitivity of the detector
    d. Correct for differences in the aspiration rate of the sample
    e. Correct for the presence of stray light

16. Which of the following best describes the process of fluorescence?
    a. Molecules emit a photon at lower energy when excited electrons return to the ground state.
    b. Atoms emit a photon when the electrons are excited.
    c. Molecules emit a photon when the electrons are excited.
    d. Molecules emit a photon at the same energy when excited electrons return to the ground state.
    e. Molecules emit a photon at higher energy when excited electrons return to the ground state.

17. Which is most accurate concerning ISEs?
    a. Gas-specific membranes are necessary for oxygen and carbon dioxide electrodes.
    b. The pH electrode uses a solid-state membrane.
    c. The calcium electrode does not require a reference electrode.
    d. The sodium electrode uses an ion-selective carrier (valinomycin).
    e. The ISE for urea uses immobilized urease.

18. Which of the following regarding MS is *false*?
    a. Mass spectrometers can be used to sequence DNA.
    b. Ions are formed by the bombardment of electrons.
    c. Quadrupole and ion trap sectors separate ions according to their mass-to-charge ratio.
    d. Each chemical compound has a unique mass spectrum.
    e. MS detects for gas and liquid chromatography.

19. Which of the following is not an objective of proteomics research?
    a. Identifying specific gene mutations
    b. Identifying novel proteins as potential new biomarkers for disease
    c. Identifying posttranslational modifications of proteins
    d. Understanding the mechanism of diseases
    e. Determining which genes are expressed and which genes are dormant

20. Which of the following procedures is not currently or routinely used for point-of-care testing devices?
    a. Polymerase chain reaction
    b. Immunochromatography
    c. Biosensors
    d. Colorimetric detection
    e. Electrochemical detection

references

1. Christian GD, O'Reilly JE. *Instrumental Analysis*. 2nd ed. Boston, MA: Allyn and Bacon; 1986.
2. Willard HH, Merritt LL, Dean JA, et al. *Instrumental Methods of Analysis*. Belmont, CA: Wadsworth; 1981.
3. Coiner D. *Basic Concepts in Laboratory Instrumentation*. Bethesda, MD: ASMT Education and Research Fund; 1975-1979.
4. Ingle JD, Crouch SR. *Spectrochemical Analysis*. Upper Saddle River, NJ: Prentice-Hall; 1988.
5. Holland JF, Enke CG, Allison J, et al. Mass spectrometry on the chromatographic time scale: realistic expectations. *Anal Chem*. 1983;55:997A.
6. Guilbault GG. *Practical Fluorescence, Theory, Methods and Techniques*. New York, NY: Marcel Dekker; 1973.
7. Kricka LJ. Chemiluminescent and bioluminescent techniques. *Clin Chem*. 1991;37:1472.
8. Wild D. *The Immunoassay Handbook*. London, UK: Macmillan Press; 1994.
9. Svelto O. *Principles of Lasers*. 2nd ed. New York, NY: Plenum Press; 1982.
10. *Coulter Hematology Analyzer: Multidimensional Leukocyte Differential Analysis*. Vol. 11(1). Miami, FL: Beckman Coulter; 1989.
11. Weast RC. *CRC Handbook of Chemistry and Physics*. 61st ed. Cleveland, OH: CRC Press; 1981.
12. Burtis CA. *Tietz Textbook of Clinical Chemistry*. 2nd ed. Philadelphia, PA: WB Saunders; 1993.
13. Heiger DN. *High-Performance Capillary Electrophoresis: An Introduction*. 2nd ed. Waldbronn, Germany: Hewlett-Packard; 1992.
14. Monnig CA, Kennedy RT. Capillary electrophoresis. *Anal Chem*. 1994;66:280R.
15. Mariani S, Minunni M. Surface plasmon resonance applications in clinical analysis. *Anal Bioanal Chem*. 2014;406:2303-2323.

6

Chromatography and Mass Spectrometry

JULIA C. DREES, MATTHEW S. PETRIE, and ALAN H. B. WU

chapter outline

chapter objectives

*Upon completion of this chapter, the clinical laboratorian should be able to do the
following:*

- Explain the general principles of each analytic method.
- Discuss the limitations of each analytic technique.
- Compare and contrast the various analytic techniques.
- Discuss existing clinical applications for each analytic technique.
- Describe the operation and component parts of the following instruments: mass
  spectrometer and gas chromatograph.
- Outline the quality assurance and preventive maintenance procedures involved with
  the following instruments: mass spectrometer and gas chromatograph.

For additional student resources, please visit the Point®
at http://thepoint.lww.com

Over the past several decades, the number of analytes measured in clinical laboratories has increased dramatically. This has been accompanied by an equally high demand for technologies that can accurately measure a large variety of compounds. Liquid or gas chromatography (GC) coupled to **mass spectrometry** (MS) has long been considered the gold standard for most testing due to its high sensitivity and specificity. In this chapter, we will discuss how these high-complexity instruments operate and, in turn, how they are utilized in the modern clinical laboratory.

CHROMATOGRAPHY

Chromatography refers to the group of techniques used to separate complex mixtures on the basis of different physical interactions between the individual compounds and the stationary phase of the system. The basic components in any chromatographic technique are the mobile phase (gas or liquid), which carries the complex mixture (sample); the stationary phase (solid or liquid), through which the mobile phase flows; the column holding the stationary phase; and the separated components (eluate).

Modes of Separation
Adsorption
Adsorption chromatography, also known as liquid–solid chromatography, is based on the competition between the sample and the mobile phase for adsorptive sites on the solid stationary phase. There is an equilibrium of solute molecules being adsorbed to the solid surface and desorbed and dissolved in the mobile phase. The molecules that are most soluble in the mobile phase move fastest; the least soluble move slowest. Thus, a mixture is typically separated into classes according to polar functional groups. The stationary phase can be acidic polar (e.g., silica gel), basic polar (e.g., alumina), or nonpolar (e.g., charcoal). The mobile phase can be a single solvent or a mixture of two or more solvents, depending on the analytes to be desorbed. Liquid–solid chromatography is not widely used in clinical laboratories because of technical problems with the preparation of a stationary phase that has homogeneous distribution of absorption sites.

Partition
Partition chromatography is also referred to as liquid–liquid chromatography. Separation of solute is based on relative solubility in an organic (nonpolar) solvent and an aqueous (polar) solvent. In its simplest form, partition (extraction) is performed in a separatory funnel. Molecules containing polar and nonpolar groups in an aqueous solution are added to an immiscible organic solvent. After vigorous shaking, the two phases are allowed to separate. Polar molecules remain in the aqueous solvent; nonpolar molecules are extracted in the organic solvent. This results in the partitioning of the solute molecules into two separate phases.

The ratio of the concentration of the solute in the two liquids is known as the partition coefficient:

$$K = \frac{\text{solute in stationary phase}}{\text{solute in mobile phase}} \quad \text{(Eq. 6-1)}$$

Modern partition chromatography uses pseudoliquid stationary phases that are chemically bonded to the support or high-molecular-weight polymers that are insoluble in the mobile phase.[1] Partition systems are considered normal phase when the mobile solvent is less polar than the stationary solvent and reverse phase when the mobile solvent is more polar.

Partition chromatography is applicable to any substance that may be distributed between two liquid phases. Because ionic compounds are generally soluble only in water, partition chromatography works best with nonionic compounds.

Steric Exclusion
Steric exclusion, a variation of liquid–solid chromatography, is used to separate solute molecules on the basis of size and shape. The chromatographic column is packed with porous material, as shown in Figure 6.1. A sample containing different-sized molecules moves down the column dissolved in the mobile solvent. Small molecules enter the pores in the packing and are momentarily trapped. Large molecules are excluded from the small pores and so move quickly between the particles. Intermediate-sized molecules are partially restricted from entering the pores and, therefore, move through the column at an intermediate rate that is between those of the large and small molecules.

Early methods used hydrophilic beads of cross-linked dextran, polyacrylamide, or agarose, which formed a gel when soaked in water. This method was termed gel filtration. A similar separation process using hydrophobic gel beads of polystyrene with a nonaqueous mobile phase was

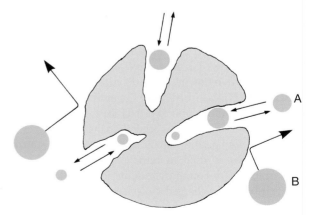

FIGURE 6.1 Pictorial concept of steric exclusion chromatography. Separation of sample components by their ability to permeate pore structure of column-packing material. Smaller molecules (*A*) permeating the interstitial pores; large excluded molecules (*B*). (Adapted from Parris NA. *Instrumental Liquid Chromatography: A Practical Manual on High Performance Liquid Chromatographic Methods*. New York, NY: Elsevier; 1976.)

Cation-exchange resin

A

Anion-exchange resin

B

FIGURE 6.2 Chemical equilibrium of ion-exchange resins. **(A)** Cation-exchange resin. **(B)** Anion-exchange resin.

FIGURE 6.3 Thin-layer chromatography plate in chromatographic chamber.

called gel permeation chromatography. Current porous packing uses rigid inorganic materials such as silica or glass. The term steric exclusion includes all these variations. Pore size is controlled by the manufacturer, and packing materials can be purchased with different pore sizes, depending on the size of the molecules being separated.

Ion-Exchange Chromatography

In ion-exchange chromatography, solute mixtures are separated by virtue of the magnitude and charge of ionic species. The stationary phase is a resin, consisting of large polymers of substituted benzene, silicates, or cellulose derivatives, with charged functional groups. The resin is insoluble in water, and the functional groups are immobilized as side chains on resin beads that are used to fill the chromatographic column. Figure 6.2A shows a resin with sulfonate functional groups. Hydrogen[+] ions are loosely held and free to react. This is an example of a cation-exchange resin. When a cation such as Na^+ comes in contact with these functional groups, an equilibrium is formed, following the law of mass action. Because there are many sulfonate groups, Na^+ is effectively and completely removed from solution. The Na^+ concentrated on the resin column can be eluted from the resin by pouring acid through the column, driving the equilibrium to the left.

Anion-exchange resins are made with exchangeable hydroxyl ions such as the diethylamine functional group illustrated in Figure 6.2B. They are used like cation-exchange resins, except that hydroxyl ions are exchanged for anions. The example shows Cl^- in sample solution exchanged for OH^- from the resin functional group. Anion and cation resins mixed together (mixed-bed resin) are used to deionize water. The displaced protons and hydroxyl ions combine to form water. Ionic functional groups other than the illustrated examples are used for specific analytic applications. Ion-exchange chromatography is used to remove interfering substances from a solution, to concentrate dilute ion solutions, and to separate mixtures of charged molecules, such as amino acids. Changing pH and ionic concentration of the mobile phase allows separation of mixtures of organic and inorganic ions.

Chromatographic Procedures

Thin-Layer Chromatography

Thin-layer chromatography (TLC) is a variant of column chromatography. A thin layer of sorbent, such as alumina,

silica gel, cellulose, or cross-linked dextran, is uniformly coated on a glass or plastic plate. Each sample to be analyzed is applied as a spot near one edge of the plate, as shown in Figure 6.3. The mobile phase (solvent) is usually placed in a closed container until the atmosphere is saturated with solvent vapor. One edge of the plate is placed in the solvent, as shown. The solvent migrates up the thin layer by capillary action, dissolving and carrying sample molecules. Separation can be achieved by any of the four processes previously described, depending on the sorbent (thin layer) and solvent chosen. After the solvent reaches a predetermined height, the plate is removed and dried. Sample components are identified by comparison with standards on the same plate. The distance a component migrates, compared with the distance the solvent front moves, is called the retention factor, R_f:

$$R_f = \frac{\text{distance leading edge of component moves}}{\text{total distance solvent front moves}} \quad \text{(Eq. 6-2)}$$

Each sample component R_f is compared with the R_f of standards. Using Figure 6.3 as an example, standard A has an R_f value of 0.4, standard B has an R_f value of 0.6, and standard C has an R_f value of 0.8. The first unknown contains A and C, because the R_f values are the same. This ratio is valid only for separations run under identical conditions. Because R_f values may overlap for some components, further identifying information is obtained by spraying different stains on the dried plate and comparing colors of the standards.

TLC is most commonly used as a semiquantitative screening test. Technique refinement has resulted in the development of semiautomated equipment and the ability to quantitate separated compounds. For example, sample applicators apply precise amounts of sample extracts in concise areas. Plates prepared with uniform sorbent thickness, finer particles, and new solvent systems have resulted in the technique of high-performance thin-layer chromatography (HPTLC).[2] Absorbance of each developed spot is measured using a densitometer, and the concentration is calculated by comparison with a reference standard chromatographed under identical conditions.

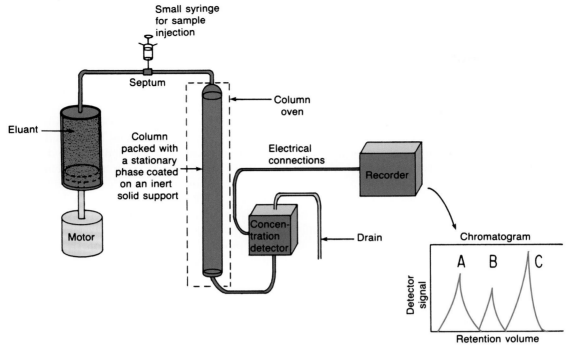

FIGURE 6.4 High-performance liquid chromatography basic components. (Adapted from Bender GT. *Chemical Instrumentation: A Laboratory Manual Based on Clinical Chemistry*. Philadelphia, PA: WB Saunders; 1972.)

High-Performance Liquid Chromatography

Modern **high-performance liquid chromatography** (HPLC) uses pressure for fast separations, controlled temperature, in-line detectors, and gradient elution techniques.[3,4] Figure 6.4 illustrates the basic components.

Pumps

A pump forces the mobile phase through the column at a much greater velocity than that accomplished by gravity flow columns and includes pneumatic, syringe, reciprocating, or hydraulic amplifier pumps. The most widely used pump today is the mechanical reciprocating pump, which is used as a multihead pump with two or more reciprocating pistons. During pumping, the pistons operate out of phase (180° for two heads, 120° for three heads) to provide constant flow. Pneumatic pumps are used for preoperative purposes; hydraulic amplifier pumps are no longer commonly used.

Columns

The stationary phase is packed into long stainless steel columns. HPLC is usually run at ambient temperatures, although columns can be put in an oven and heated to enhance the rate of partition. Fine, uniform column packing results in much less band broadening but requires pressure to force the mobile phase through. The packing can also be pellicular (an inert core with a porous layer), inert and small particles, or macroporous particles. The most common material used for column packing is silica gel. It is very stable and can be used in different ways. It can be used as solid packing in liquid–solid chromatography or coated with a solvent, which serves as the stationary phase (liquid–liquid). As a result of the short lifetime of coated particles, molecules of the mobile-phase liquid are now bonded to the surface of silica particles.

Reversed-phase HPLC is now popular; the stationary phase is nonpolar molecules (e.g., octadecyl C-18 hydrocarbon) bonded to silica gel particles. For this type of column packing, the mobile phase commonly used is acetonitrile, methanol, water, or any combination of solvents. A reversed-phase column can be used to separate ionic, nonionic, and ionizable samples. A buffer is used to produce the desired ionic characteristics and pH for separation of the analyte. Column packings vary in size (3 to 20 mm), using smaller particles mostly for analytic separations and larger ones for preparative separations.

Sample Injectors

A small syringe can be used to introduce the sample into the path of the mobile phase that carries it into the column (Fig. 6.4). The best and most widely used method, however, is the loop injector. The sample is introduced into a fixed-volume loop. When the loop is switched, the sample is placed in the path of the flowing mobile phase and flushed onto the column. Loop injectors have high reproducibility and are used at high pressures. Many HPLC instruments have loop injectors that can be programmed for automatic injection of samples. When the sample size is less than the volume of the loop, the syringe containing the sample is often filled with the mobile phase to the volume of the loop before filling the loop. This prevents the possibility of air being forced through the column because such a practice may reduce the lifetime of the column-packing material.

Detectors

Modern HPLC detectors monitor the eluate as it leaves the column and, ideally, produce an electronic signal proportional to the concentration of each separated component. Spectrophotometers that detect absorbances of visible or UV light are most commonly used. Photodiode array (PDA) and other rapid scanning detectors are also used for spectral comparisons and compound identification and purity. These detectors have been used for drug analyses in urine. Obtaining a UV scan of a compound as it elutes from a column can provide important information as to its identity. Unknowns can be compared against library spectra in a similar manner to MS. Unlike gas chromatography/MS, which requires volatilization of targeted compounds, liquid chromatography (LC)/PDA enables direct injection of aqueous urine samples.

Because many biologic substances fluoresce strongly, fluorescence detectors are also used, involving the same principles discussed in the section on spectrophotometric measurements. Another common HPLC detector is the amperometric or electrochemical detector, which measures current produced when the analyte of interest is either oxidized or reduced at some fixed potential set between a pair of electrodes.

An MS can also be used as a detector, as described later.

Recorders

The recorder is used to record detector signal versus the time the mobile phase passed through the instrument, starting from the time of sample injection. The graph is called a chromatogram (Fig. 6.5). The retention time is used to identify compounds when compared with standard retention times run under identical conditions. Peak area is proportional to concentration of the compounds that produced the peaks.

When the elution strength of the mobile phase is constant throughout the separation, it is called isocratic elution. For samples containing compounds of widely differing relative compositions, the choice of solvent is a compromise. Early eluting compounds may have retention times close to zero, producing a poor separation (resolution), as shown in Figure 6.5A. Basic compounds often have low retention times because C-18 columns cannot tolerate high pH mobile phases. The addition of cation-pairing reagents to the mobile phase (e.g., octane sulfonic acid) can result in better retention of negatively charged compounds onto the column.

The late-eluting compounds may have long retention times, producing broad bands resulting in decreased sensitivity. In some cases, certain components of a sample may have such a

FIGURE 6.5 Chromatograms. **(A)** Isocratic ion-exchange separation mobile phase contains 0.055 mol/L NaNO$_3$. **(B)** Gradient elution mobile phase gradient from 0.01 to 0.1 mol/L NaNO$_3$ at 2% per minute. **(C)** Gradient elution—5% per minute. (Adapted from Horváth C. *High Performance Liquid Chromatography, Advances and Perspectives*. New York, NY: Academic Press; 1980.)

FIGURE 6.6 Gas–liquid chromatography basic components. (Adapted from Bender GT. *Chemical Instrumentation: A Laboratory Manual Based on Clinical Chemistry*. Philadelphia, PA: WB Saunders; 1972.)

great affinity for the stationary phase that they do not elute at all. Gradient elution is an HPLC technique that can be used to overcome this problem. The composition of the mobile phase is varied to provide a continual increase in the solvent strength of the mobile phase entering the column (Fig. 6.5B). The same gradient elution can be performed with a faster change in concentration of the mobile phase (Fig. 6.5C).

Gas Chromatography

Gas chromatography is used to separate mixtures of compounds that are volatile or can be made volatile.[5] GC may be gas–solid chromatography, with a solid stationary phase, or gas–liquid chromatography (GLC), with a nonvolatile liquid stationary phase. GLC is commonly used in clinical laboratories. Figure 6.6 illustrates the basic components of a GC system. The setup is similar to HPLC, except that the mobile phase is a gas and samples are partitioned between a gaseous mobile phase and a liquid stationary phase. The carrier gas can be nitrogen, helium, or argon. The selection of a carrier gas is determined by the detector used in the instrument. The instrument can be operated at a constant temperature or programmed to run at different temperatures if a sample has components with different volatilities. This is analogous to gradient elution described for HPLC.

The sample, which is injected through a septum, must be injected as a gas or the temperature of the injection port must be above the boiling point of the components so that they vaporize upon injection. Sample vapor is swept through the column partially as a gas and partially dissolved in the liquid phase. Volatile compounds that are present mainly in the gas phase will have a low partition coefficient and will move quickly through the column. Compounds with higher boiling points will move slowly through the column. The effluent passes through a detector that produces an electric signal proportional to the concentration of the volatile components. As in HPLC, the chromatogram is used both to identify the compounds by the retention time and to determine their concentration by the area under the peak.

Columns

GLC columns are generally made of glass or stainless steel and are available in a variety of coil configurations and sizes. Packed columns are filled with inert particles such as diatomaceous earth or porous polymer or glass beads coated with a nonvolatile liquid (stationary) phase. These columns are usually 1/8 to 1/4 inch wide and 3 to 12 ft long. Capillary wall-coated open tubular columns have inside diameters in the range of 0.25 to 0.50 mm and are up to 60 m long. The liquid layer is coated on the walls of the column. A solid support coated with a liquid stationary phase may in turn be coated on column walls. The liquid stationary phase must be nonvolatile at the temperatures used, must be thermally stable, and must not react chemically with the solutes to be separated. The stationary phase is termed nonselective when separation is primarily based on relative volatility of the compounds. Selective liquid phases are used to separate polar compounds based on relative polarity (as in liquid–liquid chromatography).

Detectors

Although there are many types of detectors, only thermal conductivity (TC) and flame ionization detectors are discussed because they are the most stable (Fig. 6.7). TC detectors

A

B

FIGURE 6.7 (A) Schematic diagram of a thermal conductivity detector. **(B)** Schematic diagram of a flame ionization detector. (Adapted from Tietz NW, ed. *Fundamentals of Clinical Chemistry*. Philadelphia, PA: WB Saunders; 1987).

Mass Spectrometer Components

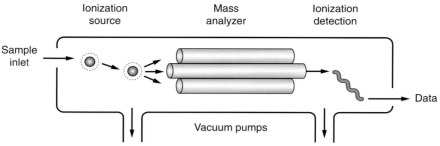

FIGURE 6.8 The components of a mass spectrometer. In this case, the ionization source pictured is electrospray ionization and the mass analyzer is a quadrupole.

contain wires (filaments) that change electrical resistance with change in temperature. The filaments form opposite arms of a Wheatstone bridge and are heated electrically to raise their temperature. Helium, which has a high TC, is usually the carrier gas. Carrier gas from the reference column flows steadily across one filament, cooling it slightly. Carrier gas and separated compounds from the sample column flow across the other filament. The sample components usually have a lower TC, increasing the temperature and resistance of the sample filament. The change in resistance results in an unbalanced bridge circuit. The electrical change is amplified and fed to the recorder. The electrical change is proportional to the concentration of the analyte. Flame ionization detectors are widely used in the clinical laboratory. They are more sensitive than TC detectors. The column effluent is fed into a small hydrogen flame burning in excess air or atmospheric oxygen. The flame jet and a collector electrode around the flame have opposite potentials. As the sample burns, ions form and move to the charged collector. Thus, a current proportional to the concentration of the ions is formed and fed to the recorder.

MASS SPECTROMETRY

Definitive identification of samples eluting from GC or HPLC columns is possible when an MS is used as a detector.[6] The coupled techniques, GC/MS and LC/MS, have powerful analytic capabilities with widespread clinical applications. The sample in an MS is first volatilized and then ionized to form charged molecular ions and fragments that are separated according to their mass-to-charge (m/z) ratio; the sample is then measured by a detector, which gives the intensity of the ion current for each species. These steps take place in the four basic components that are standard in all MSs: the sample inlet, ionization source, mass analyzer, and ion detector (Fig. 6.8). Ultimately, molecule identification is based on the formation of characteristic fragments. Figure 6.9 illustrates the mass spectrum of Δ9-carboxytetrahydrocannabinol, a metabolite of marijuana.

Sample Introduction and Ionization

Direct infusion is commonly used to interface a GC or LC with an MS; however, the challenge of introducing a liquid sample from an LC column into an MS was a significant barrier until recent technological advances in ionization techniques.

Electron Ionization

The most common form of ionization used in GC/MS is electron ionization (EI). This method requires a source of electrons in the form of a filament to which an electric potential is applied, typically at 70 eV.[7] The molecules in the source are bombarded with high-energy electrons, resulting

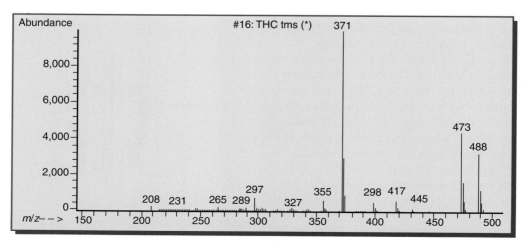

FIGURE 6.9 Mass spectrum of the trimethylsilane derivative of Δ9-carboxytetrahydrocannabinol (marijuana metabolite).

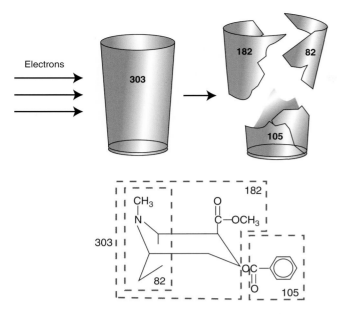

FIGURE 6.10 Electron bombardment breaks cocaine into fragments, with number and size quantified. Unlike the illustrative glass tumbler, the result of mass fragmentation of cocaine or other chemical compounds is both predictable and reproducible, especially with electron ionization.

in the formation of charged molecular ions and fragments. Molecules break down into characteristic fragments according to their molecular structure (Fig. 6.10). The ions formed and their relative proportions are reproducible and can be used for qualitative identification of the compound. Since most instruments use the same 70 eV potential, the fragmentation of molecules on different days and different instruments is remarkably similar, allowing the comparison of unknown spectra to spectra in a published reference library.[7]

Atmospheric Pressure Ionization

Unlike EI in GC/MS, most LC/MS ionization techniques are conducted at atmospheric pressure. As such, the ion source of this type of instrument is not included in the high-vacuum region of the instrument. Two types of ionization for

LC/MS will be discussed here: electrospray ionization (ESI) and atmospheric pressure chemical ionization (APCI), while matrix-assisted laser desorption ionization (MALDI) will be discussed later in the section on proteomics. ESI and APCI also differ from EI in that they are "soft" ionization techniques that leave the molecular ion largely intact in the source. Many LC/MS techniques employ technologies after the source, in the mass analyzer, to fragment molecules and generate the daughter or fragment ions used in identification. However, ionization techniques used in LC/MS produce fragments and therefore mass spectra that are somewhat less reproducible between instruments than EI used in GC/MS. This may prove to limit the utility of reference library spectra produced in other instruments.

Electrospray Ionization

Thanks to its wide mass range and high sensitivity, ESI can be applied to a wide range of biological macromolecules in addition to small molecules and has become the most common ionization source for LC/MS. ESI involves passing the LC effluent through a capillary to which a voltage has been applied. The energy is transferred to the solvent droplets, which become charged.[7] Evaporation of the solvent through heat and gas causes the droplets to decrease in size, which increases the charge density on the surface. Eventually, the Coulombic repulsion of like charges leads to the ejection of ions from the droplet (Fig. 6.11).[8] The individually charged molecules are drawn into the MS for mass analysis. ESI is adept at forming singly charged small molecules, but larger molecules can also be ionized using this method. Larger molecules such as proteins become multiply charged in ESI, and since MSs measure the m/z, even these large molecules can be observed in an instrument with a relatively small mass range (Fig. 6.12).[8]

Atmospheric Pressure Chemical Ionization

Another important ionization source is APCI, which is similar to ESI in that the liquid from LC is introduced directly into the ionization source. However, the droplets are not charged and the source contains a heated vaporizer to allow rapid desolvation of the drops.[8] A high voltage is applied to a

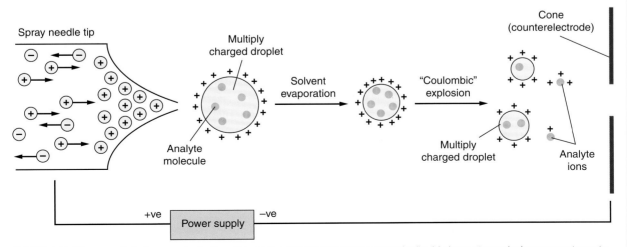

FIGURE 6.11 Diagram of electrospray ionization, the most common ionization source for liquid chromatography/mass spectrometry.

FIGURE 6.12 A theoretical protein with a molecular weight of 10,000 can be multiply charged, which will generate numerous peaks. A mass spectrometer with a relatively small mass range can still detect the multiply charged ions since the *m/z* is reduced.

corona discharge needle, which emits a cloud of electrons to ionize compounds after they are converted to the gas phase.

Mass Analyzer

The actual measuring of the *m/z* occurs when the gas phase ions pass into the mass analyzer. Mass analyzers generate electric fields that can manipulate the charged molecules to sort them according to their *m/z*.

Quadrupole

A diagram of a quadrupole MS is shown in Figure 6.13. The quadrupole is the most common mass analyzer in use today. The electric field on the two sets of diagonally opposed rods allows only ions of a single selected *m/z* value to pass through the analyzer to the detector. All other ions are deflected into the rods. The rods can be scanned from low to high mass to allow ions of increasing mass to form stable sinusoidal orbits and traverse the filtering sector. This technique will generate a full-scan mass spectrum. Alternatively, specific masses can be selected to monitor a few target analytes. This technique is called selected ion monitoring (SIM) and it allows for a longer dwell time (time spent monitoring a single ion) and therefore higher sensitivity.[7] A full scan provides more information than does SIM since ions not specifically selected in

SIM are not detected. Therefore, a full scan would be preferable for general unknown screening while SIM analysis is more suitable for target compound analysis.

Ion Trap

The ion trap can be thought of as a modified quadrupole. A linear ion trap employs a stopping potential on the end electrodes to confine ions along the two-dimensional axis of the quadrupoles. In a three-dimensional ion trap, the four rods, instead of being arranged parallel to each other, form a three-dimensional sphere in which ions are "trapped." In all ion traps, after a period of accumulation, the electric field adjusts to selectively destabilize the trapped ions, which are mass-selectively ejected from the cavity to the detector based on their *m/z*.[7] The unique feature of ion trap MSs is that they trap and store ions generated over time, effectively concentrating the ions of interest and yielding a greater sensitivity.

Tandem Mass Spectrometry

Tandem MSs (GC/MS/MS and LC/MS/MS) can be used for greater selectivity and lower detection limits. A common form of MS/MS is to link three quadrupoles in series; such an instrument is referred to as a triple quad (Fig. 6.14). Generally, each quadrupole has a separate function.[8] Following an appropriate ionization method, the first

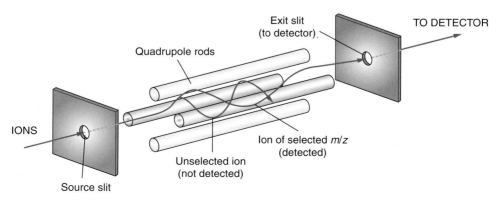

FIGURE 6.13 Single quadrupole mass spectrometer.

GC / MS / MS

FIGURE 6.14 Triple quadrupole mass spectrometer.

quadrupole (Q1) is used to scan across a preset *m/z* range and select an ion of interest. The second quadrupole (Q2) functions as a collision cell. In a process called collision-induced dissociation, the ions are accelerated to high kinetic energy and allowed to collide with neutral gas molecules (usually nitrogen, helium, or argon) to fragment the ions. The single ion that passed through the first analyzer is called the precursor (or parent) ion while the ions formed during

fragmentation of the precursor ions are called product (or daughter) ions. The third quadrupole (Q3) serves to analyze the product ions generated in Q2. This last quadrupole can be set to scan all of the product ions to produce a full product ion scan or to selectively allow one or more of these product ions through to the detector in a process called selected reaction monitoring. Various scanning modes commonly used in a triple quad are shown in Figure 6.15.

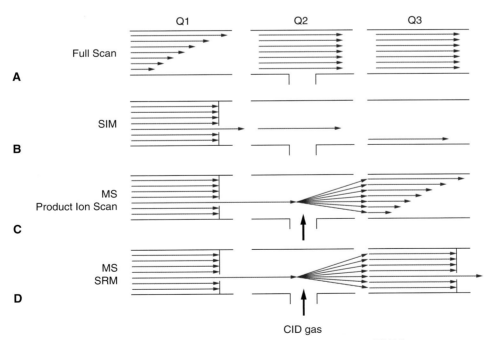

FIGURE 6.15 Scanning modes used in a triple quadrupole mass spectrometer. **(A)** Full-scan mass spectrometry (MS) detects all ions. **(B)** Selected ion monitoring (SIM) detects ions of one selected *m/z*. **(C)** Product ion scans select ions of one *m/z* in Q1 to pass onto Q2, the collision cell, where the ion is fragmented. All ion fragments are allowed to pass through to the detector. **(D)** Selected reaction monitoring (SRM) is similar to the product ion scan, but only fragments of one selected *m/z* are allowed to pass onto the detector. Both **(C)** and **(D)** are examples of tandem mass spectrometry (MS/MS). CID, collision-induced dissociation.

In some triple quad instruments, the third quadrupole can also function as a linear ion trap to add further sensitivity to MS/MS.

High-Resolution MS

Newer technologies utilizing high-resolution mass spectrometers based on time-of-flight (TOF) or Orbitrap (Thermo Fisher) technologies have gained popularity in recent years. These instruments can measure large numbers of analytes simultaneously in complex biological matrices and have been particularly useful for drug screening applications.[9] Compared with traditional or "nominal resolution" mass spectrometers that determine masses to approximately 0.5 Da, high-resolution instruments such as TOF and Orbitrap mass spectrometers operate at resolutions that allow the exact mass of an unknown compound to be calculated to approximately 0.001 to 0.0001 Da. The resolution of a mass spectrometer is defined as the mass of a given compound divided by the width of the corresponding peak and is commonly designated by the term full width at half maximum (FWHM) (Fig. 6.16A). TOF mass spectrometers achieve resolutions of 10,000 to 50,000 FWHM utilizing the principle that given the same kinetic energy, lighter ions travel faster than heavier ions. By measuring the time taken for an ion to traverse the flight tube and hit the detector, the m/z ratio can be calculated (Fig. 6.16B). Orbitrap mass spectrometers operate on a different principle. With Orbitrap instruments, ions are injected tangentially to the electric field between the outer barrel-like electrode and the inner spindle-like electrode and the stable orbit achieved is proportional to the m/z value (Fig. 6.16C). Orbitrap mass spectrometers can achieve 100,000 to 250,000 FWHM.

Detector

The most common means of detecting ions employs an electron multiplier (Fig. 6.17). In this detector, a series of dynodes with increasing potentials are linked. When ions strike the first dynode surface, electrons are emitted. These electrons are attracted to the next dynode where more secondary electrons are emitted due to the higher potential of

FIGURE 6.16 **(A)** Pictorial representation of the full width at half maximum (FWHM) definition of mass resolution. (Reprinted with permission from Thermo Fisher Scientific.) **(B)** Diagram of the principle of time-of-flight (TOF) mass spectrometers. (Reprinted with permission, http://msr.dom.wustl.edu/Research/MALDI_TOF_Mass_Spec_and_Proteomics/Time-of-Flight_Mass_Spectrometry_Fundamentals.htm) **(C)** Diagram of Orbitrap mass spectrometry. (Reprinted with permission from Thermo Fisher Scientific.)

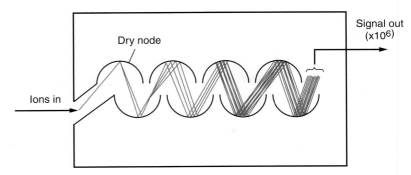

FIGURE 6.17 Diagram of an electron multiplier detector in a mass spectrometer.

subsequent dynodes. A cascade of electrons is formed by the end of the chain of dynodes, resulting in overall signal amplification on the order of 1 million or greater.[8]

APPLICATIONS OF MS IN THE CLINICAL LABORATORY

Small Molecule Analysis

Mass spectrometers coupled to GC or LC can be used not only for the identification and quantitation of compounds but also for structural information and molecular weight determination (high-resolution MS).[10] GC/MS systems are widely used for measuring drugs of abuse in urine toxicology confirmations. Drugs and metabolites must be extracted from body fluids and typically reacted with derivatizing reagents to form compounds that are more volatile for the GC process. Computerized libraries and matching algorithms are available within the instrument to compare mass spectral results of an unknown substance obtained from a sample to the reference library.

Increasingly, LC/MS (including LC/MS/MS) technology is taking its place alongside GC/MS in clinical laboratories. LC offers a number of advantages over GC. Typically, LC requires less extensive extraction procedures and derivatization is rarely used, saving time and expense. Solid-phase extraction columns can be incorporated directly into the injector for online purifications (Fig. 6.18) In addition, polar and heat-labile compounds fare better in LC.[7] However; the chromatography itself in LC can be somewhat less robust than in GC, resulting in wider peaks and more variable retention times and potentially requiring maintenance that is more frequent. Another disadvantage of LC/MS is the less reproducible mass spectra, as mentioned earlier. One drawback to implementing LC or GC/MS in clinical laboratories is the long run times associated with the chromatographic separation. For low-volume testing, this is not an issue; however, for medium- or high-volume testing, it remains a significant challenge. To overcome this, laboratories can utilize technologies such as ultra-performance liquid chromatography (UPLC) or multiplexing. With UPLC, both the column and the pumps are robust enough to handle very high pressures (>600 bar), allowing faster flow rates, which in turn dramatically reduces the run time.

For very high-volume testing, several HPLC (or UPLC) pumps can be connected to a single mass spectrometer, which is referred to as multiplexing. This technology works because analyte peaks are only typically approximately 5 to 30 seconds in width, and in theory, that is the only time the LC flow needs to be in-line with the mass spectrometer. LC separations typically require much longer gradients for good resolution, and additionally, the column must be equilibrated before the next run, which takes several minutes. In multiplexing, the LC pumps are staggered so that once the peak of interest has been analyzed by the mass spectrometer, the flow is diverted to waste. At that point, the flow from the next LC pump is placed in-line with the mass spectrometer and the cycle repeats. Multiplexing can reduce the run time by a factor of the number of LC pumps and is well suited for high-volume targeted analysis but not for untargeted screening. For example, if the total run

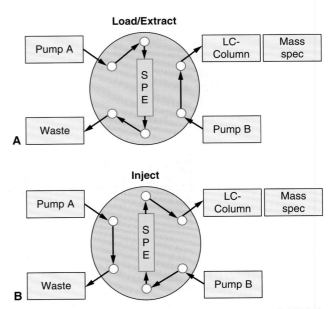

FIGURE 6.18 Diagram of an online extraction method for LC-MS/MS. An LC injector is depicted. **(A)** In the "load/extract" position, samples are loaded using pump A onto the extraction column while the LC mobile phase is directed to the main analytical column using pump B. **(B)** In the "inject" position, the LC mobile is directed using pump B through the extraction column eluting any compounds directly to the main analytical column. SPE = solid phase extraction column.

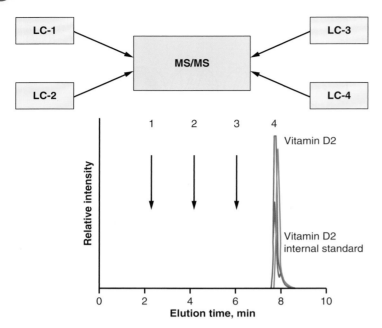

FIGURE 6.19 Multiplexing of four liquid chromatograms into one mass spectrometer. See text for details.

time with a single LC pump takes 8 minutes, then a system with four multiplexed LC pumps would take only 2 minutes to measure the same analyte (see Fig. 6.19). Utilizing technologies such as UPLC and multiplexing has allowed clinical laboratories to measure very high-volume analytes using MS.

High-resolution mass spectrometry has applications in unknown toxicology analysis whereby the drug or metabolite is unknown to the testing laboratory. With soft ionization (i.e., minimal fragmentation of the parent ion), high-resolution MS enables putative identification of drugs by identifying the compounds molecular weight to three or four decimal points. From this information, the exact molecular formula can be deduced and a search of the literature can uncover compounds that have that molecular formula. By definition, these compounds are stereo- or structure isomers of each other. Figure 6.20 shows the chemical formula of three compounds that have the same *nominal* molecular weight of m/z 285 but

different *exact* molecular weights. Using high-resolution mass spectrometry, the three compounds can be differentiated from each other. This feature is particularly useful for identification of "designer drugs." These are drugs that have similar pharmacologic activity but differ from well-known drugs with the substitution of a functional group. "Bath salts" are a group of designer amines that are currently being abused and are difficult to detect using conventional targeted mass spectrometric techniques. Designer fentanyl compounds have been produced for many years.

Besides its use in toxicology, LC/MS also has great potential for measuring low-level and mixed-polarity analytes such as vitamin D, testosterone, and immunosuppressant drugs due to its superior sensitivity and specificity over immunoassays. In addition, LC/MS has the advantage of being able to detect multiple analytes (such as a panel of drugs or a series of metabolites) in one run. LC/MS is free from the antibody interferences seen in immunoassays, although LC/MS has its own type of

FIGURE 6.20 Chemical structure of **(A)** morphine, $C_{17}H_{19}NO_3$, m/w 285.3377; **(B)** 7-aminoclonazepam (clonazepam metabolite), $C_{15}H_{12}ClNO_3$, m/z 285.7283; and **(C)** pentazocine, $C_{19}H_{27}NO$, m/z 285.2093.

interference in the form of ion suppression. This effect is seen when a co-eluting chemical in the sample prevents a compound of interest from being ionized, thereby reducing or eliminating its signal. LC/MS also requires highly skilled operators and is not nearly as automated as immunoassay instruments.

Mass Spectrometry in Proteomics and Pathogen Identification

The next generation of biomarkers for human diseases will be discovered using techniques found within the research fields of genomics and proteomics. Genomics uses the known sequences of the entire human genome for determining the role of genetics in certain human diseases. Proteomics is the investigation of the protein products encoded by these genes. Protein expression is equal to and, in many cases, more important for disease detection than genomics because these products determine what is currently occurring within a cell, rather than the genes, which indicate what a cell might be capable of performing. Moreover, many (posttranslational) changes can occur to the protein, as influenced by other proteins and enzymes that cannot be easily predicted by knowledge at the genomic level. A "shotgun" approach is often used in the discovery of new biochemical markers. The proteins from samples (e.g., serum, urine, and tissue extract) from normal individuals are compared with those derived from patients with the disease being studied. Before being analyzed on the mass spectrometer, the complex mixture of proteins must first be separated using chromatographic techniques. Proteins can be trypsin digested and separated by HPLC or techniques such as two-dimensional electrophoresis (Chapter 5) can be used to separate proteins into individual spots or bands.

Proteins that only appear in either the normal or diseased specimens are further studied. For proteomic analysis, computer programs are available that digitally compare gels to determine spots or areas that are different. When candidate proteins have been found, the spots can be isolated and subjected to traditional trypsin digestion followed by HPLC-MS/MS or to MALDI-TOF MS (see below) to identify the protein and possibly any posttranslational modifications that may have occurred. Using this approach, the researcher does not have any preconceptions or biases as to what directions or particular proteins to look for.

MALDI-TOF

MALDI-TOF MS is used for the analysis of biomolecules, such as peptides and proteins. Protein samples, such as those isolated from a two-dimensional electrophoretogram, are mixed with an appropriate matrix solvent and spotted onto a stainless steel plate. The solvent is dried and the plate is introduced into the vacuum system of the MALDI-TOF analyzer. As shown in Figure 6.21, a laser pulse irradiates the sample, causing desorption and ionization of both the matrix and the sample. Because the

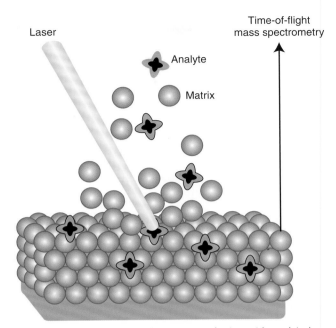

FIGURE 6.21 Sample desorption process prior to matrix-assisted laser desorption ionization time-of-flight (MALDI-TOF) analysis. (Diagram courtesy of Stanford Research Systems, Sunnyvale, CA.)

monitored mass spectral range is high (>500 Da), the ionization of the low-molecular-weight matrix can be readily distinguished from high-molecular-weight peptides and proteins and does not interfere with the assay of the protein. Ions from the sample are focused into the mass spectrometer. The time required for an ion with a given mass to reach the detector is a nonlinear function of the mass, with larger ions requiring more time than smaller ions. The molecular weight of the proteins acquired by mass spectrum is used to determine the identity of the sample and is helpful in determining posttranslational modifications that may have occurred. For very large proteins, samples can be pretreated with trypsin, which cleaves peptide bonds after lysine and arginine, to produce lower-molecular-weight fragments that can then be measured. The detection limit of this assay is about 10^{-15} to 10^{-18} mol.

Pathogen Identification

Although MS has primarily been utilized in chemistry and toxicology sections for the analysis of small molecules and proteins, high-resolution MS can be used for the identification of pathogens in modern microbiology laboratories.[11] Isolated bacterial or fungal colonies can be directly spotted onto the MALDI plate and ionized, which results in a protein "fingerprint" of the species. This protein "fingerprint" is composed of mainly ribosomal proteins and can be compared with a digital database of species (Fig. 6.22). Because MALDI-TOF MS requires inexpensive reagents and only takes 5 to 10 minutes per run, it is significantly cheaper and faster than traditional automated biochemical identification techniques. Another

FIGURE 6.22 Matrix-assisted laser desorption ionization time-of-flight (MALDI-TOF) spectral fingerprints of five different bacterial species. (Adapted from Carbonnelle E, Mesquita C, Bille E, et al. *Clin Biochem.* 2011;44:104–109.)

application of high-resolution MS for pathogen identification is the Abbott PLEX-ID polymerase chain reaction (PCR)/TOF, which combines the sensitivity of PCR and specificity and rapid turnaround time of ESI-TOF MS. In this application, PCR is used to amplify DNA from the unknown pathogen and ESI-TOF MS is used to calculate exact masses of these PCR-generated DNA fragments. From the exact masses, the number of purine and pyrimidine nucleotide bases (As, Ts, Gs, and Cs) can be determined. The unique purine and pyrimidine nucleotide composition of the PCR-generated fragments can then be compared with a preexisting digital library in order to identify the unknown pathogen. Unlike MALDI-TOF and traditional automated identification platforms, which required the organism to be cultured, PCR/ESI-TOF can be used directly from patient specimens.

Mass Spectrometry at the Point of Care

Analytical instrumentation for mass spectrometry is advancing to the point that desktop or even handheld instruments will be available in the near future. This will enable testing of important analytes at bedside. One area that has received attention is the use of portable mass

spectrometry to analyze biopsy specimens intraoperatively. Results of such testing may determine if a surgeon has removed all of the tumorous tissue and can terminate the surgery or if the doctor has to continue the procedure to search for more tumor. In order for this application to be useful, testing must be rapid and the equipment small and simple enough to be useful in the operating room itself. In a study conducted at the Brigham and Women's Hospital in Boston, investigators analyzed tissue sections removed from patients with a glioma.[12] These investigators used desorption ESI mass spectrometry to identify 2-hydroxyglutarate, a metabolite found in high concentrations in brain tumors that exhibit mutations in isocitrate dehydrogenase. Mass spectrometry instrumentation was brought into the operating room and the analysis was conducted during the surgery itself. This work is made possible through the use of desorption ambient ionization, a method that introduces samples directly into a mass spectrometry without extraction. Figure 6.23 shows a block diagram of the Direct Analysis in Real Time (DART) ionization system, one of the ambient ionization technologies. DART has been used for the analysis of pharmaceutical, plants, and food analysis.

FIGURE 6.23 Schematic of the Direct Analysis in Real Time ionization instrumentation for ambient temperature mass spectrometry. (Used with permission from Ion Sense, Inc. Saugus, MA.)

For additional student resources, please visit the Point® at http://thepoint.lww.com

questions

1. Which of the following statements is TRUE?
   a. Partition chromatography is most appropriate for identifying analytes that may be distributed between two liquid phases.
   b. Steric exclusion chromatography is best suited for separating analytes based on their solubility in the mobile solvent.
   c. In liquid–solid chromatography, the stationary phase separates analytes based on size, shape, and polarity.
   d. Ion-exchange chromatography has a resin phase that is soluble to water, and separation of the mixture is based on magnitude and charge of ionic species.
   e. The partition coefficient is measured and compared with standards in thin-layer chromatography.

2. In high-performance thin-layer chromatography (HPTLC), developed bands are compared with reference standard concentrations. Each band is measured by:
   a. Mass spectrometer
   b. Densitometer
   c. Ruler
   d. Biuret protein assay
   e. Two-dimensional electrophoresis

3. In which of the following components of a chromatography instrument does selective separation of a mixture occur?
   a. Sample injection port
   b. Column
   c. Spectrometer
   d. Quadrupole
   e. Mass analyzer

4. True or False? In chromatography, the stationary phase is always of a solid matrix.

5. Mass spectrometry identifies analytes based on:
   a. Mass-to-charge ratio
   b. Retention factor
   c. Density of the band
   d. Molecular weight
   e. Solubility in the mobile phase

6. Drugs of abuse are typically measured by:
   a. Thin-layer chromatography
   b. Liquid–liquid chromatography
   c. Gas–liquid chromatography
   d. Steric exclusion chromatography
   e. HPLC

(continues on page 138)

review questions (continued)

7. PCR/ESI-TOF has the distinct advantage in pathogen identification because:
   a. It requires the patient sample to be cultured and then analysis can be performed

b. It can be used directly from patient specimens
c. It uses the protein "fingerprint" to identify the pathogen.

references

1. Parris NA. *Instrumental Liquid Chromatography: A Practical Manual on High Performance Liquid Chromatographic Methods.* New York, NY: Elsevier; 1976.
2. Jurk H. *Thin-Layer Chromatography. Reagents and Detection Methods.* Vol. 1a. Weinheim, Germany: Verlagsgesellschaft; 1990.
3. Bender GT. *Chemical Instrumentation: A Laboratory Manual Based on Clinical Chemistry.* Philadelphia, PA: WB Saunders; 1972.
4. Horváth C. *High Performance Liquid Chromatography, Advances and Perspectives.* New York, NY: Academic Press; 1980.
5. Constantin E, Schnell A. *Mass Spectrometry.* New York, NY: Ellis Horwood; 1990.
6. Kebarle E, Liang T. From ions in solution to ions in the gas phase. *Anal Chem.* 1993;65:972A.
7. Karasek FW, Clement RE. *Basic Gas Chromatography: Mass Spectrometry.* New York, NY: Elsevier; 1988.
8. Levine B. *Principles of Forensic Toxicology.* Washington, DC: AACC Press; 2006.
9. Jiwan JL, Wallemacq P, Hérent MF. HPLC—high resolution mass spectrometry in clinical laboratory? *Clin Biochem.* 2011;44:136–147.
10. Siuzdak, G. *The Expanding Role of Mass Spectrometry in Biotechnology.* San Diego, CA: MCC Press; 2006.
11. Carbonnelle E, Mesquita C, Bille E, et al. MALDI-TOF mass spectrometry tools for bacterial identification in clinical microbiology laboratory. *Clin Biochem.* 2011;44:104–109.
12. Santagata S, Eberlin LS, Norton I, et al. Intraoperative mass spectrometry mapping of an onco-metabolite to guide brain tumor surgery. *Proc Natl Acad Sci U S A.* 2014;111:11121–11126.

7

Principles of Clinical Chemistry Automation

RYAN W. GREER and JOELY A. STRASESKI

chapter outline

key terms

chapter objectives

Upon completion of this chapter, the clinical laboratorian should be able to do the following:

- Define the following terms: automation, channel, continuous flow, discrete analysis, dwell time, flag, random access, and throughput.
- Discuss the history of the development of automated analyzers in the clinical chemistry laboratory.
- List four driving forces behind the development of new automated analyzers.
- Name three basic approaches to sample analysis used by automated analyzers.
- Explain the major steps in automated analysis.
- Provide examples of commercially available discrete chemistry analyzers and modular systems.
- Compare the different approaches to automated analysis used by instrument manufacturers.
- Discriminate between an open versus a closed reagent system.
- Relate three considerations in the selection of an automated analyzer.
- Explain the concept of total laboratory automation.
- Differentiate the three phases of the laboratory testing process.
- Discuss future trends in automated analyzer development.

For additional student resources, please visit thePoint® at http://thepoint.lww.com

The modern clinical chemistry laboratory uses a high degree of automation. Many steps in the analytic process that were previously performed manually can now be performed automatically, permitting the operator to focus on manual processes and increasing both efficiency and capacity. The analytic process can be divided into three major phases—preanalytic, analytic, and postanalytic—corresponding to sample processing, chemical analysis, and data management, respectively. Substantial improvements have occurred in all three areas during the past decade. Five major diagnostic vendors sell automated analyzers and reagents. These vendors are continually refining their products to make them more functional and user friendly. The analytic phase is the most automated, and more research and development efforts are focusing on increasing automation of the preanalytic and postanalytic processes.

HISTORY OF AUTOMATED ANALYZERS

Following the introduction of the first automated analyzer by Technicon in 1957, automated instruments proliferated from many manufacturers.[1] This first "AutoAnalyzer" (AA) was a continuous flow, single-**channel**, sequential batch analyzer capable of providing a single test result on approximately 40 samples per hour. The next generation of Technicon instruments to be developed was the Simultaneous Multiple Analyzer (SMA) series. SMA-6 and SMA-12 were analyzers with multiple channels (for different tests), working synchronously to produce 6 or 12 test results simultaneously at the rate of 360 or 720 tests per hour. It was not until the mid-1960s that these continuous flow analyzers had any significant competition in the marketplace.

In 1970, the first commercial centrifugal analyzer was introduced as a spin-off technology from NASA outer space research. Dr. Norman Anderson developed a prototype in 1967 at the Oak Ridge National Laboratory as an alternative to continuous flow technology, which had significant carryover problems and costly reagent waste. He wanted to perform analyses in parallel and also take advantage of advances in computer technology. The second generation of these instruments (1975) was more successful as a result of miniaturization of computers and advances in the polymer industry for high-grade, optical plastic cuvettes.

The next major development that revolutionized clinical chemistry instrumentation occurred in 1970 with the introduction of the Automatic Clinical Analyzer (ACA) (DuPont [now Siemens]). It was the first noncontinuous flow, discrete analyzer as well as the first instrument to have **random access** capabilities, whereby stat specimens could be analyzed out of sequence on an as-needed basis. Plastic test packs, positive patient identification, and infrequent calibration were among the unique features of the ACA. Other major milestones were the introduction of thin film analysis technology in 1976 and the production of the Kodak Ektachem (now VITROS) Analyzer (now Ortho-Clinical Diagnostics) in 1978. This instrument was the first to use microsample volumes and reagents on slides for dry chemistry analysis and to incorporate computer technology extensively into its design and use.

Since 1980, several primarily discrete analyzers have been developed that incorporate such characteristics as ion-selective electrodes (ISEs), fiberoptics, polychromatic analysis, continually more sophisticated computer hardware and software for data handling, and larger test menus. The popular and more successful analyzers using these and other technologies since 1980 are Astra (now Synchron) analyzers (Beckman Coulter), which extensively used ISEs; Paramax (no longer available), which introduced primary tube sampling; and the Hitachi analyzers (Boehringer-Mannheim, now Roche Diagnostics), with reusable reaction disks and fixed diode arrays for spectral mapping. Automated systems that are commonly used in clinical chemistry laboratories today are Aeroset and ARCHITECT analyzers (Abbott Diagnostics), Advia analyzers (Siemens), Synchron analyzers (Beckman Coulter), Dimension analyzers (Siemens), VITROS analyzers (Ortho-Clinical Diagnostics), and several Roche analyzer lines.

Many manufacturers of these instrument systems have adopted the more successful features and technologies of other instruments, where possible, to make each generation of their product more competitive in the marketplace. The differences among the manufacturers' instruments, operating principles, and technologies are less distinct now than they were in the beginning years of laboratory automation.

DRIVING FORCES TOWARD MORE AUTOMATION

Since 1995, the pace of changes with current routine chemistry analyzers and the introduction of new ones have slowed considerably, compared with the first half of the 1990s. Certainly, analyzers are faster and easier to use as a result of continual reengineering and electronic refinements. Methods are more precise, sensitive, and specific, although some of the same principles are found in today's instruments as in earlier models. Manufacturers have worked successfully toward automation with "walk-away" capabilities and minimal operator intervention.[2] Manufacturers have also responded to the physicians' desire to bring laboratory testing closer to the patient. The introduction of small, portable, easy-to-operate benchtop analyzers in physician office laboratories, as well as in surgical and critical care units that demand immediate laboratory results, has resulted in a hugely successful domain of point-of-care (POC) analyzers.[3] Another specialty area with a rapidly developing arsenal of analyzers is immunochemistry. Immunologic techniques for assaying drugs, specific proteins, tumor markers, and hormones have evolved to an increased level of automation. Instruments that use techniques such as fluorescence polarization immunoassay, nephelometry, and competitive and noncompetitive immunoassay with chemiluminescent detection have become popular in laboratories.

FIGURE 7.1 Modular chemistry/immunoassay analyzers. **(A)** Siemens Dimension Vista 500. (Photograph courtesy of Siemens.) **(B)** Roche MODULAR *ANALYTICS*. (Photograph courtesy of Roche Diagnostics.) **(C)** Abbott ARCHITECT ci8200. (Photograph courtesy of Abbott Diagnostics.) **(D)** Beckman Coulter Synchron LXi 725. (Photograph courtesy of Beckman Coulter.)

The most recent milestone in chemistry analyzer development has been the combination of chemistry and immunoassay into a single **modular analyzer**. The Dimension RxL analyzer with a heterogeneous immunoassay module was introduced in 1997. This design permits further workstation consolidation with consequent improvements in operational efficiency and further reductions in turnaround time. Modular analyzers combining chemistry and immunoassay capabilities are now available from several vendors that meet the needs of mid- and high-volume laboratories (Fig. 7.1).

Other forces are also driving the market toward more focused automation. Higher volume of testing and faster turnaround time have resulted in fewer and more centralized core laboratories performing more comprehensive testing.[4] The use of laboratory panels or profiles has declined, with more diagnostically directed individual tests as dictated by recent policy changes from Medicare and Medicaid. Researchers have known for many years that chemistry panels only occasionally lead to new diagnoses in patients who appear healthy.[5] The expectation of quality results with higher accuracy and precision is ever present with the regulatory standards set by the Clinical Laboratory Improvement Amendments, the

Joint Commission (formerly the Joint Commission on Accreditation of Healthcare Organizations), the College of American Pathologists, and others. Intense competition among instrument manufacturers has driven automation into more sophisticated analyzers with creative technologies and unique features. Furthermore, escalating costs have spurred healthcare reform and, more specifically, managed care and capitation environments within which laboratories are forced to operate.

BASIC APPROACHES TO AUTOMATION

There are many advantages to automating procedures. One purpose is to increase the number of tests performed by one laboratorian in a given period. Labor is an expensive commodity in clinical laboratories. Through mechanization, the labor component devoted to any single test is minimized, and this effectively lowers the cost per test. A second purpose is to minimize the variation in results from one laboratorian to another. By reproducing the components in a procedure as identically as possible, the coefficient of variation is lowered, and reproducibility is increased. Accuracy is then not dependent on the skill or workload of a particular operator on a particular day. This allows better comparison of results from day to day and week to week. Automation, however, cannot correct for deficiencies inherent in methodology. A third advantage is gained because automation eliminates the potential errors of manual analyses such as volumetric pipetting steps, calculation of results, and transcription of results. A fourth advantage accrues because instruments can use very small amounts of samples and reagents. This allows less blood to be drawn from each patient, and the use of small amounts of reagents decreases the cost of consumables. In addition, automation facilitates better space utilization thru consolidation.

There are three basic approaches with instruments: continuous flow, centrifugal analysis, and discrete analysis. All three can use batch analysis (i.e., large number of specimens in one run), but only discrete analyzers offer random access, or stat, capabilities.

In **continuous flow**, liquids (reagents, diluents, and samples) are pumped through a system of continuous tubing. Samples are introduced in a sequential manner, following each other through the same network. A series of air bubbles at regular intervals serve as separating and cleaning media. Continuous flow, therefore, resolves the major consideration of uniformity in the performance of tests because each sample follows the same reaction path. Continuous flow also assists the laboratory that needs to run many samples requiring the same procedure. The more sophisticated continuous flow analyzers used parallel single channels to run multiple tests on each sample—for example, SMA. The major drawbacks that contributed to the eventual demise of traditional continuous flow analyzers (i.e., AA and SMA) in the marketplace were significant carryover problems and wasteful use of continuously flowing reagents. Technicon's (now Siemens) answer to these problems was a noncontinuous flow discrete analyzer (the RA1000), using random access fluid (a hydrofluorocarbon liquid to reduce surface tension between samples/reagents and their tubing) and, thereby, reducing carryover. Later, the Chem 1 was developed by Technicon to use Teflon tubing and Teflon oil, virtually eliminating carryover problems. The Chem 1 was a continuous flow analyzer but only remotely comparable to the original continuous flow principle.

Centrifugal analysis uses the force generated by centrifugation to transfer and then contain liquids in separate cuvettes for measurement at the perimeter of a spinning **rotor**. Centrifugal analyzers are most capable of running multiple samples, one test at a time, in a batch. Batch analysis is their major advantage because reactions in all cuvettes are read virtually simultaneously, taking no longer to run a full rotor of about 30 samples than it would take to run a few. Laboratories with a high workload of individual tests for routine batch analysis may use these instruments. Again, each cuvette must be uniformly matched to each other to maintain quality handling of each sample. The Cobas-Bio (Roche Diagnostics), with a xenon flash lamp and longitudinal cuvettes,[6] and the IL Monarch, with a fully integrated walk-away design, are two of the more successful centrifugal analyzers.

Discrete analysis is the separation of each sample and accompanying reagents in a separate container. Discrete analyzers have the capability of running multiple tests one sample at a time or multiple samples one test at a time. They are the most popular and versatile analyzers and have almost completely replaced continuous flow and centrifugal analyzers. However, because each sample is in a separate reaction container, uniformity of quality must be maintained in each cuvette so that a particular sample's quality is not affected by the particular space that it occupies. The analyzers listed in Table 7.1 are examples of current discrete analyzers with random access capabilities.

STEPS IN AUTOMATED ANALYSIS

In clinical chemistry, **automation** is the mechanization of the steps in a procedure. Manufacturers design their instruments to mimic manual techniques. The major processes performed by an automated analyzer can be divided into specimen identification and preparation, chemical reaction, and data collection and analysis. An overview of these processes is provided in Table 7.2.

Each step of automated analysis is explained in this section, and several different applications are discussed. Several instruments have been chosen because they have components that represent either common features used in chemistry instrumentation or a unique method of automating a step in a procedure. None of the representative instruments is completely described, but rather the important components are described in the text as examples.

Specimen Preparation and Identification
Preparation of the sample for analysis has been and remains a manual process in most laboratories. The

clotting time (if using serum), centrifugation, and the transferring of the sample to an analyzer cup (unless using primary tube sampling) cause delay and expense in the testing process. One alternative to manual preparation is to automate this process by using **robotics**, or front-end automation, to "handle" the specimen through these steps and load the specimen onto the analyzer. Another option is to bypass the specimen preparation altogether by using whole blood for analysis—for example, Abbott-Vision. Robotics for specimen preparation has already become a reality in some clinical laboratories in the United States and other countries. Another approach is to use a plasma separator tube and perform primary tube sampling with heparin plasma. This eliminates the need both to wait for the sample to clot and to aliquot the sample. More discussion about preanalytic specimen processing, or front-end automation, appears later in this chapter.

The sample must be properly identified, and its location in the analyzer must be monitored throughout the test. The simplest means of identifying a sample is by placing a manually labeled sample cup in a numbered analysis position on the analyzer, in accordance with a manually prepared worksheet or a computer-generated load list. The most sophisticated approach that is commonly used today employs a **bar code** label affixed to the primary collection tube. This label contains patient demographics and also may include test requests.

The bar code–labeled tubes are then transferred to the loading zone of the analyzer, where the bar code is scanned and the information is stored in the computer's memory. The analyzer is then capable of monitoring all functions of identification, test orders and parameters, and sample position. Certain analyzers may take test requests downloaded from the laboratory information system (LIS) and run them when the appropriate sample is identified and ready to be pipetted.

Specimen Measurement and Delivery
Most instruments use either circular carousels or rectangular racks as specimen containers for holding disposable sample cups or primary sample tubes in the loading or pipetting zone of the analyzer. These cups or tubes hold standards, controls, and patient specimens to be pipetted into the reaction chambers of the analyzers. The slots in the trays or racks are usually numbered to aid in sample identification. The trays or racks move automatically in one-position steps at preselected speeds. The speed determines the number of specimens to be analyzed per hour. As a convenience, the instrument can determine the slot number containing the last sample and terminate the analysis after that sample. The instrument's microprocessor holds the number of samples in memory and aspirates only in positions containing samples.

On the VITROS analyzer, sample cup trays are quadrants that hold 10 samples each in cups with conical bottoms.

TABLE 7.1　Summary of Features for Selected Mid- and High-Volume Clinical Chemistry Analyzers

	Mid Volume					High Volume				
	Abbott Diagnostics Architect c8000	Beckman Coulter Inc. UniCel DxC 600i	Ortho-Clinical Diagnostics VITROS 350	Roche Diagnostics Cobas 6000	Siemens Healthcare Diagnostics Inc. Dimension Vista 500	Abbott Diagnostics Architect c16000	Beckman Coulter, Inc. UniCel DxC 680i	Ortho-Clinical Diagnostics VITROS 5,1 FS	Roche Diagnostics Cobas 8000	Siemens Healthcare Diagnostics Inc. Dimension Vista 1500
First year sold in the United States	2003	2006	2005	2006	2009	2007	2009	2004	2010	2006
Throughput (tests per hour, depends on test mix)	133–200	900	40–60	85–300	83–166	1,800	1400	600–700	8,400	1500
No. of assays onboard simultaneously	58	89	60	88	>100	68	115	125	88	>100
No. of open channels	220	100	—	40	10	220	100	20	40	10
No. of ion-selective electrode channels	3	5	3	3	3	3	5	3	3	3
Minimum sample volume aspirated (µL)	2	3	6	1.5	50	2	3	2	1.5	50 µL
Dedicated pediatric sample cup/dead volume (µL)	Yes/50	Yes/–	No/35	Yes/50	No/10	Yes/50	Yes/20	No/35	Yes/50	No/10–20 µL
Short sample/clot detection	Yes/Yes	Yes/Yes	Yes/Yes	Yes/Yes	Yes/Yes	Yes/Yes	Yes/Yes	Yes/Yes	Yes/Yes	Yes/Yes
Index measurements	Yes	Yes	No	Yes	Yes	Yes	Yes	Yes	Yes	Yes
Onboard test automatic inventory	Yes	Yes	Yes	Yes	Yes	Yes	Yes	Yes	Yes	Yes
Remote troubleshooting by modem	Yes	Yes	No	Yes	Yes	Yes	Yes	Yes	Yes	Yes

Information obtained from Dabkowski B. Vendors toil and tinker to refine chemistry analyzers. *CAP Today.* 2011;July:56–71 and directly from vendors.

TABLE 7.2 Summary of Chemistry Analyzer Operations

Identification and Preparation

1. Sample identification	This is usually done by reading the bar code. This information can also be entered manually
2. Determine test(s) to perform	The LIS communicates to the analyzer, which test(s) have been ordered

Chemical Reaction

3. Reagent systems and delivery	One or more reagents can be dispensed into the reaction cuvette
4. Specimen measurement and delivery	A small aliquot of the sample is introduced into the reaction cuvette
5. Chemical reaction phase	The sample and reagents are mixed and incubated
6. Measurement phase	Optical readings may be initiated before or after all reagents have been added
7. Signal processing and data handling	The analyte concentration is estimated from a calibration curve that is stored in the analyzer
8. Send result(s) to LIS	The analyzer communicates results for the ordered tests to the LIS

Operations generally occur in the order listed from 1 to 8. However, there may be slight variations in the order. Some steps may be deleted or duplicated. Most analyzers have the capability to dilute the sample and repeat the testing process if the analyte concentration exceeds the linear range of the assay.

The four quadrants fit on a tray carrier (Fig. 7.2). Although the tray carrier accommodates only 40 samples, more trays of samples can be programmed and then loaded in place of completed trays while tests on other trays are in progress. A disposable sample tip is hand loaded adjacent to each sample cup on the tray. Roche/Hitachi analyzers can use five-position racks to hold samples (Fig. 7.3). A modular analyzer can accommodate as many as 60 of these racks at one time.

Nearly all contemporary chemistry analyzers sample from primary collection tubes, or for limited volume samples, there are microsample tubes. The tubes are placed in either racks or carousels. Bar code labels for each sample, which include the patient name and identification number, can be printed on demand by the operator (Fig. 7.4). This allows samples to be loaded in any order. The Dimension analyzers make use of a continuous belt of flexible, disposable plastic cuvettes carried through the analyzer's water bath on a main drive track. The cuvettes are loaded onto the analyzer from a continuous spool. These cuvettes index through the instrument at the rate of one every 5 seconds

and are cut into sections or groups as required. A schematic of the Dimension RxL cuvette production and reading system is shown in Figure 7.5. Exposure of the sample to air can lead to sample evaporation and produce errors in analysis. Evaporation of the sample may be significant and may cause the concentration of the constituents being analyzed to rise 50% in 4 hours.[7] Instruments measuring electrolytes, the carbon dioxide present in the samples, will be lost to the atmosphere, resulting in low carbon dioxide values. Manufacturers have devised a variety of mechanisms to minimize this effect—for example, lid covers for trays and individual caps that can be pierced, which includes **closed-tube sampling** from primary collection tubes.[8]

The actual measurement of each aliquot for each test must be accurate. This is generally accomplished through aspiration of the sample into a **probe**. When the discrete instrument is in operation, the probe automatically dips into each sample cup and aspirates a portion of the liquid. After a preset, computer-controlled time interval, the probe quickly rises from the cup. Sampling probes on instruments using specific sampling cups are programmed or adjusted to reach a prescribed depth in those cups to

FIGURE 7.2 VITROS. The four quadrant trays, each holding ten samples, fit on a tray carrier. (Photograph courtesy of Ortho-Clinical Diagnostics.)

FIGURE 7.3 Roche/Hitachi five-position rack.

FIGURE 7.4 Sample collection tubes are identified with bar code labels. (Photograph courtesy of Siemens.)

maximize the use of available sample. Those analyzers capable of aspirating sample from primary collection tubes usually have a parallel liquid level–sensing probe

that will control entry of the sampling probe to a minimal depth below the surface of the serum, allowing full aliquot aspiration while avoiding clogging of the probe with serum separator gel or clot (Fig. 7.6).

In continuous flow analyzers, when the sample probe rises from the cup, air is aspirated for a specified time to produce a bubble in between sample and reagent plugs of liquid. Then the probe descends into a container where wash solution is drawn into the probe and through the system. The wash solution is usually deionized water, possibly with a surfactant added. Remembering that all samples follow the same reaction path, the necessity for the wash solution between samples becomes obvious. Immersion of the probe into the wash reservoir cleanses the outside, whereas aspiration of an aliquot of solution cleanses the lumen. The reservoir is continually replenished with an excess of fresh solution. The wash aliquot, plus the previously mentioned air bubble, maintains sample integrity and minimizes sample carryover.

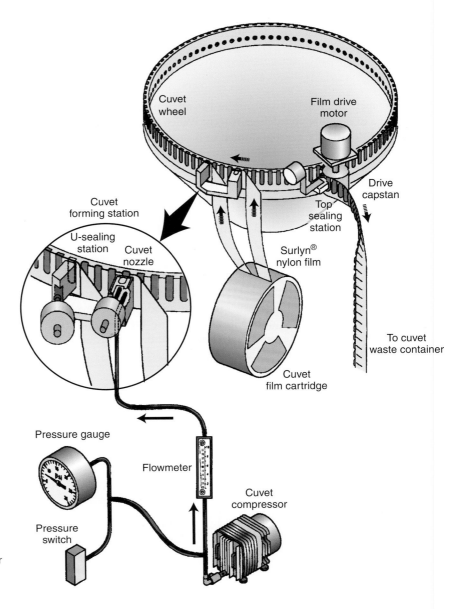

FIGURE 7.5 Analyzer production system for sealed cuvettes. (Photograph courtesy of Siemens.)

FIGURE 7.6 Dual sample probes of a chemistry analyzer. Note the liquid level sensor to the left of probes. (Photograph courtesy of Roche Diagnostics.)

Certain pipetters use a disposable tip and an air displacement syringe to measure and deliver reagent. When this is used, the pipetter may be reprogrammed to measure sample and reagent for batches of different tests comparatively easily. Besides eliminating the effort of priming the reagent delivery system with the new solution, no reagent is wasted or contaminated because nothing but the pipette tip contacts it.

The cleaning of the probe and tubing after each dispensing to minimize the carryover of one sample into the next is a concern for many instruments. In some systems, the reagent or diluent is also dispersed into the cuvette through the same tubing and probe. Deionized water may be dispensed into the cuvette after the sample to produce a specified dilution of the sample and also to rinse the dispensing system. In the Technicon RA1000, a random access fluid is the separation medium. The fluorocarbon fluid is a viscous, inert, immiscible, nonwetting substance that coats the delivery system. The coating on the sides of the delivery system prevents carryover due to the wetting of the surfaces and, forming a plug of the solution between samples, prevents carryover by diffusion. A small amount (10 μL) of this fluid is dispensed into the cuvette with the sample. Surface tension leaves a coating of the fluid in the dispensing system.

If a separate probe or tip is used for each sample and discarded after use, as in the VITROS, the issue of carryover is a moot point. VITROS has a unique sample dispensing system. A proboscis presses into a tip on the sample tray, picks it up, and moves over the specimen to aspirate the volume required for the tests programmed for that sample. The tip is then moved over to the slide-metering block. When a slide is in position to receive an aliquot, the proboscis is lowered so that a dispensed 10-μL drop touches the slide, where it is absorbed from the nonwetting tip. A stepper motor-driven piston controls aspiration and drop formation. The precision of dispensing is specified at ±5%.

In several discrete systems, the probe is attached by means of nonwettable tubing to precision syringes. The syringes draw a specified amount of sample into the probe and tubing. Then the probe is positioned over a cuvette and the sample is dispensed. The Hitachi 736 used two sample probes to simultaneously aspirate a double volume of sample in each probe immersed in one specimen container and, thereby, deliver sample into four individual test channels, all in one operational step (Fig. 7.7). The loaded probes pass through a fine mist shower bath before delivery to wash off any sample residue adhering to the outer surface of the probes. After delivery, the probes move to a rinse bath station for cleaning the inside and outside surfaces of the probes.

Many chemistry analyzers use computer-controlled stepping motors to drive both the sampling and washout syringes. Every few seconds, the sampling probe enters a specimen container, withdraws the required volume, moves to the cuvette, and dispenses the aliquot with a volume of water to wash the probe. The washout volume is adjusted to yield the final reaction volume. If a procedure's range of linearity is exceeded, the system will

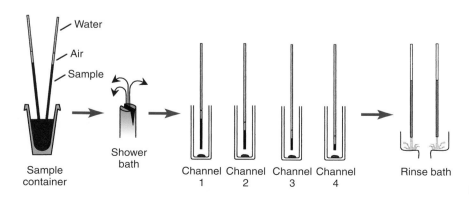

FIGURE 7.7 Sampling operation of the Hitachi 736 analyzer. (Courtesy of Roche Diagnostics.)

retrieve the original sample tube, repeat the test using one-fourth the original sample volume for the repeat test, and calculate a new result, taking the dilution into consideration.

Economy of sample size is a major consideration in developing automated procedures, but methodologies have limitations to maintain proper levels of sensitivity and specificity. The factors governing sample and reagent measurement are interdependent. Generally, if sample size is reduced, then either the size of the reaction cuvette and final reaction volume must be decreased or the reagent concentration must be increased to ensure sufficient color development for accurate photometric readings.

Reagent Systems and Delivery

Reagents may be classified as liquid or dry systems for use with automated analyzers. Liquid reagents may be purchased in bulk volume containers or in unit dose packaging as a convenience for stat testing on some analyzers. Dry reagents are packaged in various forms. They may be bottled as lyophilized powder, which requires reconstitution with water or a buffer. Unless the manufacturer provides the diluent, the water quality available in the laboratory is important. A second and unique type of dry reagent is the multilayered **dry chemistry slide** for the VITROS analyzer (rebranded in 2001 as the VITROS MicroSlide technology). These slides have microscopically thin layers of dry reagents mounted on a plastic support. The slides are approximately the size and thickness of a postage stamp.

Reagent handling varies according to instrument capabilities and methodologies. Many test procedures use sensitive, short-lived working reagents; so contemporary analyzers use a variety of techniques to preserve them. One technique is to keep all reagents refrigerated until the moment of need and then quickly preincubate them to reaction temperature or store them in a refrigerated compartment on the analyzer that feeds directly to the dispensing area. Another means of preservation is to provide reagents in a dried, tablet form and reconstitute them when the test is to be run. A third is to manufacture the reagent in two stable components that will be combined at the moment of reaction. If this approach is used, the first component also may be used as a diluent for the sample. The various manufacturers often use combinations of these reagent-handling techniques.

Reagents also must be dispensed and measured accurately. Many instruments use bulk reagents to decrease the preparation and changing of reagents. Instruments that do not use bulk reagents have unique reagent packaging. In continuous flow analyzers, reagents and diluents are supplied from bulk containers into which tubing is suspended. The inside diameter, or bore, of the tubing governs the amount of fluid that will be dispensed. A proportioning pump, along with a manifold, continuously and precisely introduces, proportions, and pumps liquids and air bubbles throughout the continuous flow system.

To deliver reagents, many discrete analyzers use techniques similar to those used to measure and deliver the samples. Syringes, driven by a stepping motor, pipette the reagents into reaction containers. Piston-driven pumps, connected by tubing, may also dispense reagents. Another technique for delivering reagents to reaction containers uses pressurized reagent bottles connected by tubing to dispensing valves. The computer controls the opening and closing of the valves. The fill volume of reagent into the reaction container is determined by the precise amount of time the valve remains open.

The Vitros analyzers use slides to contain their entire reagent chemistry system. Multiple layers on the slide are backed by a clear polyester support. The coating itself is sandwiched in a plastic mount. There are three or more layers: (1) a spreading layer, which accepts the sample; (2) one or more central layers, which can alter the aliquot; and (3) an indicator layer, where the analyte of interest may be quantified (Fig. 7.8). The number of layers varies depending on the assay to be performed. The color developed in the indicator layer varies with the concentration of the analyte in the sample. Physical or chemical reactions can occur in one layer, with the product of these reactions proceeding to another layer, where subsequent reactions can occur. Each layer may offer a unique environment and the possibility to carry out a reaction comparable to that offered in a chemistry assay or it may promote an entirely different activity that does not occur in the liquid phase. The ability to create multiple reaction sites allows the possibility of

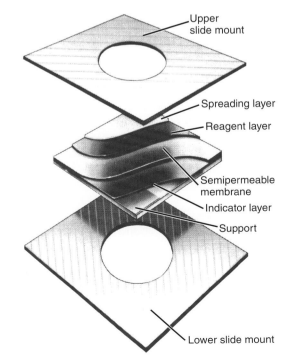

FIGURE 7.8 VITROS slide with multiple layers contains the entire reagent chemistry system. (Courtesy of Ortho-Clinical Diagnostics.)

FIGURE 7.9 Wash stations on a chemistry analyzer perform the following: (1) aspirate reaction waste and dispense water, (2) aspirate and dispense rinse water, (3) aspirate rinse water and dispense water for measurement of cell blank, and (4) aspirate cell blank water to dryness. (Photograph courtesy of Roche Diagnostics.)

manipulating and detecting compounds in ways not possible in solution chemistries. Interfering materials can be left behind or altered in upper layers.

Chemical Reaction Phase

This phase consists of mixing, separation, incubation, and reaction time. In most discrete analyzers, the chemical reactants are held in individual moving containers that are either disposable or reusable. These reaction containers also function as the cuvettes for optical analysis. If the cuvettes are reusable, then wash stations are set up immediately after the read stations to clean and dry these containers (Fig. 7.9). This arrangement allows the analyzer to operate continuously without replacing cuvettes. Examples of this approach include ADVIA Centaur (Siemens), ARCHITECT (Abbott Diagnostics), Cobas (Roche Diagnostics), and UniCel DxC Synchron (Beckman Coulter) analyzers. Alternatively, the reactants may be placed in a stationary reaction chamber in which a flow-through process of the reaction mixture occurs before and after the optical reading.

Mixing

A vital component of each procedure is the adequate mixing of the reagents and sample. Instrument manufacturers go to great lengths to ensure complete mixing. Nonuniform mixtures can result in noise in continuous flow analysis and in poor precision in discrete analysis.

Mixing was accomplished in continuous flow analyzers (e.g., the Chem 1) through the use of coiled tubing. When the reagent and sample stream go through coiled loops, the liquid rotates and tumbles in each loop. The differential rate of liquids falling through one another produces mixing in the coil.

RA1000 used a rapid start–stop action of the reaction tray. This causes a sloshing action against the walls of the cuvettes, which mixes the components. Centrifugal analyzers may use a start–stop sequence of rotation or bubbling of air through the sample and reagent to mix them while these solutions are moving from transfer disk to rotor. This process of transferring and mixing occurs in just a few seconds. The centrifugal force is responsible for the mixing as it pushes sample from its compartment, over a partition into a reagent-filled compartment and, finally, into the cuvette space at the perimeter of the rotor.

In the VITROS MicroSlide technology, the spreading layer provides a structure that permits a rapid and uniform spreading of the sample over the reagent layer(s) for even color development.

Most automated wet chemistry analyzers use stirring paddles that dip into the reaction container for a few seconds to stir sample and reagents, after which they return to a wash reservoir (Fig. 7.10). Other instruments use forceful dispensing to accomplish mixing.

Separation

In chemical reactions, undesirable constituents that will interfere with an analysis may need to be separated from the sample before the other reagents are introduced into the system. Protein causes major interference in many analyses. One approach without separating protein is to use a very high reagent-to-sample ratio (the sample is highly diluted) so that any turbidity caused by precipitated protein is not sensed by the spectrophotometer. Another approach is to shorten the reaction time to eliminate slower-reacting interferents.

FIGURE 7.10 Stirring paddles on a chemistry analyzer. (Photograph courtesy of Roche Diagnostics.)

In the older continuous flow systems, a dialyzer was the separation or filtering module. It performed the equivalent of the manual procedures of precipitation, centrifugation, and filtration, using a fine-pore cellophane membrane. In the VITROS MicroSlide technology, the spreading layer of the slide not only traps cells, crystals, and other small particulate matter but also retains large molecules, such as protein. In essence, what passes through the spreading layer is a protein-free filtrate.

Most contemporary discrete analyzers have no automated methodology by which to separate interfering substances from the reaction mixture. Therefore, methods have been chosen that have few interferences or that have known interferences that can be compensated for by the instrument (e.g., using correction formulas).

Incubation

A heating bath in discrete or continuous flow systems maintains the required temperature of the reaction mixture and provides the delay necessary to allow complete color development. The principal components of the heating bath are the heat transfer medium (i.e., water or air), the heating element, and the thermoregulator. A thermometer is located in the heating compartment of an analyzer and is monitored by the system's computer. On many discrete analyzer systems, the multicuvettes incubate in a water bath maintained at a constant temperature of usually 37°C.

Slide technology incubates colorimetric slides at 37°C. There is a precondition station to bring the temperature of each slide close to 37°C before it enters the incubator. The incubator moves the slides at 12-second intervals in such a manner that each slide is at the incubator exit four times during the 5-minute incubation time. This feature is used for two-point rate methods and enables the first point reading to be taken part way through the incubation time. Potentiometric slides are held at 25°C. The slides are kept at this temperature for 3 minutes to ensure stability before reading.

Reaction Time

Before the optical reading by the spectrophotometer, the reaction time may depend on the rate of transport through the system to the "read" station, timed reagent additions with moving or stationary reaction chambers, or a combination of both processes. An environment conducive to the completion of the reaction must be maintained for a sufficient length of time before spectrophotometric analysis of the product is made. Time is a definite limitation. To sustain the advantage of speedy multiple analyses, the instrument must produce results as quickly as possible.

It is possible to monitor not only completion of a reaction but also the rate at which the reaction is proceeding. The instrument may delay the measurement for a predetermined time or may present the reaction mixtures for measurement at constant intervals of time. Use of rate reactions may have two advantages: the total analysis time is shortened and interfering chromogens that react slowly may be negated. Reaction rate is controlled by temperature;

therefore, the reagent, timing, and spectrophotometric functions must be coordinated to work in harmony with the chosen temperature. The environment of the cuvettes is maintained at a constant temperature by a liquid bath, containing water or some other fluid with good heat transfer properties, in which the cuvettes move.

Measurement Phase

After the reaction is completed, the formed products must be quantified. Almost all available systems for measurement have been used, such as ultraviolet, fluorescent, and flame photometry; ion-specific electrodes; gamma counters; and luminometers. Still, the most common is visible and ultraviolet light spectrophotometry, although adaptations of traditional fluorescence measurement, such as fluorescence polarization, chemiluminescence, and bioluminescence, have become popular. The Abbott AxSYM, for example, is a popular instrument for drug analysis that uses fluorescence polarization to measure immunoassay reactions.

Analyzers that measure light require a monochromator to achieve the desired component wavelength. Traditionally, analyzers have used filters or filter wheels to separate light. The old AAs used filters that were manually placed in position in the light path. Many instruments still use rotating filter wheels that are microprocessor controlled so that the appropriate filter is positioned in the light path. However, newer and more sophisticated systems offer the higher resolution afforded by diffraction gratings to achieve light separation into its component colors. Many instruments now use such monochromators with either a mechanically rotating grating or a fixed grating that spreads its component wavelengths onto a fixed array of photo diodes—for example, Hitachi analyzers (Fig. 7.11). This latter grating arrangement, as well as rotating filter wheels, easily

FIGURE 7.11 Photometer for a chemistry analyzer. Fixed diffraction grating separates light into specific wavelengths and reflects them onto a fixed array of 11 specific photodetectors. Photometer has no moving parts. (Courtesy of Roche Diagnostics.)

accommodates polychromatic light analysis, which offers improved sensitivity and specificity over monochromatic measurement. By recording optical readings at different wavelengths, the instrument's computer can then use these data to correct for reaction mixture interferences that may occur at adjacent, as well as desired, wavelengths.

Many newer instruments use fiberoptics as a medium to transport light signals from remote read stations back to a central monochromator detector box for analysis of these signals. The fiberoptic cables, or "light pipes" as they are sometimes called, are attached from multiple remote stations where the reaction mixtures reside to a centralized monochromator/detector unit that, in conjunction with the computer, sequences and analyzes a large volume of light signals from multiple reactions.

The containers holding the reaction mixture also play a vital role in the measurement phase. In most discrete wet chemistry analyzers, the cuvette used for analysis is also the reaction vessel in which the entire procedure has occurred. The reagent volume and, therefore, sample size, speed of analysis, and sensitivity of measurement are some aspects influenced by the method of analysis. A beam of light is focused through the container holding the reaction mixture. The amount of light that exits from the container is dictated primarily by the absorbance of light by the reaction mixture. The exiting light strikes a photodetector, which converts the light into electrical energy. Filters and light-focusing components permit the desired light wavelength to reach the photodetector. The photometer continuously senses the sample photodetector output voltage and, as is the process in most analyzers, compares it with a reference output voltage. The electrical impulses are sent to a read-out device, such as a printer or computer, for storage and retrieval.

Centrifugal analysis measurement occurs while the rotor is rotating at a constant speed of approximately 1,000 rpm. Consecutive readings are taken of the sample, the dark current (readings between cuvettes), and the reference cuvette. Each cuvette passes through the light source every few milliseconds. After all the data points have been determined, centrifugation stops, and the results are printed. The rotor is removed from the analyzer and discarded. For endpoint analyses, an initial absorbance is measured before the constituents have had time to react, usually a few seconds, and is considered a blank measurement. After enough time has elapsed for the reaction to be completed, another absorbance reading is taken. For rate analyses, the initial absorbance is measured, and then a lag time is allowed (preset into the instrument for each analysis). For each assay, several data points are determined at a programmed time interval. The instrument monitors the absorbance measurements at each data point and calculates a result.

Slide technology depends on reflectance spectrophotometry, as opposed to traditional transmittance photometry, to provide a quantitative result. The amount of chromogen in the indicator layer is read after light passes through the indicator layer, which is reflected from the bottom of a pigment-containing layer (usually the spreading layer), and is returned through the indicator layer to a light detector. For colorimetric determinations, the light source is a tungsten–halogen lamp. The beam focuses on a filter wheel holding up to eight interference filters, which are separated by a dark space. The beam is focused at a 45° angle to the bottom surface of the slide, and a silicon photodiode detects the portion of the beam that reflects down. Three readings are taken for the computer to derive reflectance density. The three recorded signals taken are (1) the filter wheel blocking the beam, (2) reflectance of a reference white surface with the programmed filter in the beam, and (3) reflectance of the slide with the selected filter in the beam (Fig. 7.12).

After a slide is read, it is shuttled back in the direction from which it came, where a trap door allows it to drop into a waste bin. If the reading was the first for a two-point rate test, the trap door remains closed, and the slide reenters the incubator.

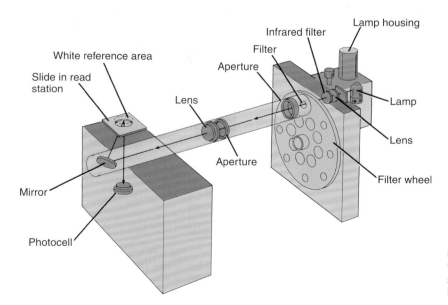

FIGURE 7.12 Components of the system for making colorimetric determinations with slide technology. (Courtesy of Ortho-Clinical Diagnostics.)

There are a number of fully automated, random access immunoassay systems, which use chemiluminescence or electrochemiluminescence technology for reaction analysis. In chemiluminescence assays, quantification of an analyte is based on emission of light resulting from a chemical reaction.[9] The principles of chemiluminescent immunoassays are similar to those of radioimmunoassay and immunoradiometric assay, except that an acridinium ester is used as the tracer and paramagnetic particles are used as the solid phase. Sample, tracer, and paramagnetic particle reagent are added and incubated in disposable plastic cuvettes, depending on the assay protocol. After incubation, magnetic separation and washing of the particles are performed automatically. The cuvettes are then transported into a light-sealed luminometer chamber, where appropriate reagents are added to initiate the chemiluminescent reaction. On injection of the reagents into the sample cuvette, the system luminometer detects the chemiluminescent signal. Luminometers are similar to gamma counters in that they use a photomultiplier tube detector; however, unlike gamma counters, luminometers do not require a crystal to convert gamma rays to light photons. Light photons from the sample are detected directly, converted to electrical pulses, and then counted.

Signal Processing and Data Handling

Because most automated instruments print the results in reportable form, accurate calibration is essential to obtaining accurate information. There are many variables that may enter into the use of calibration standards. The matrices of the standards and unknowns may be different. Depending on the methodology, this may or may not present problems. If secondary standards are used to calibrate an instrument, the methods used to derive the standard's constituent values should be known. Standards containing more than one analyte per vial may cause interference problems. Because there are no primary standards available for enzymes, either secondary standards or calibration factors based on the molar extinction coefficients of the products of the reactions may be used.

Many times, a laboratory will have more than one instrument capable of measuring a constituent. Unless there are different normal ranges published for each method, the instruments should be calibrated so that the results are comparable. The advantage of calibrating an automated instrument is the long-term stability of the standard curve, which requires only monitoring with controls on a daily basis. Some analyzers use low- and high-concentration standards at the beginning of each run and then use the absorbances of the reactions produced by the standards to produce a standard curve electronically for each run. Other instruments are self-calibrating after analyzing standard solutions.

The original continuous flow analyzers used six standards assayed at the beginning of each run to produce a calibration curve for that particular batch. Now, continuous flow analyzers use a single-level calibrator to calibrate each run with water used to establish the baseline.

The centrifugal analyzer uses standards pipetted into designated cuvettes in each run for endpoint analyses. After the delta absorbance for each sample has been obtained, the computer calculates the results by determining a constant for each standard. The constants are derived by dividing the concentration of the standard (preentered into the computer) by the delta absorbance and averaging the constants for each of the standards to obtain a factor. The concentration of each control and unknown is determined by multiplying the delta absorbance of the unknown by the factor. If the concentration of an unknown exceeds the range of the standards, the result is printed with a **flag**. Enzyme activity is derived by a linear regression fit of the delta absorbance versus time. The slope of the produced line is multiplied by the enzyme factor (preentered) to calculate the activity.

Slide technology requires more sophisticated calculations to produce results. The calibration materials require a protein-based matrix because of the necessity for the calibrators to behave as serum when reacting with the various layers of the slides. Calibrator fluids are bovine serum based, and the concentration of each analyte is determined by reference methods. Endpoint tests require three calibrator fluids, blank-requiring tests need four calibrator fluids, and enzyme methods require three calibrators. Colorimetric tests use spline fits to produce the standardization. In enzyme analysis, a curve-fitting algorithm estimates the change in reflection density per unit time. This is converted to either absorbance or transmission-density change per unit time. Then, a quadratic equation converts the change in transmission density to volume activity (U/L) for each assay.

Most automated analyzers retain the calibrations for each lot of a particular method until the laboratorian programs the instrument for recalibration. Instrument calibration is initiated or verified by assaying a minimum of three levels of primary standards or, in the case of enzymes, reference samples. The values obtained are compared with the known concentrations by using linear regression, with the x-axis representing the expected values and the y-axis representing the mean of the values obtained. The slope (scale factor) and y-intercept (offset) are the adjustable parameters. On earlier models of this instrument, the parameters were determined and entered manually into the instrument computer by the operator; however, on later, more automated models, the instrument performs calibration automatically on operator's request. After calibration has been performed and the chemical or electrical analysis of the specimen is either in progress or completed, the instrument's computer goes into data acquisition and calculation mode. The process may involve signal averaging, which may entail hundreds of data pulses per second, as with a centrifugal analyzer, and blanking and correction formulas for interferents that are programmed into the computer for calculation of results.

All advanced automated instruments have some method of reporting printed results with a link to sample identification. In sophisticated systems, the demographic sample information is entered in the instrument's computer together with the tests required. Then the sample identification is printed with the test results. Most laboratories use bar code labels printed by the LIS to identify sample. Bar code–labeled samples can be loaded directly on the analyzer without the need to enter identifying information manually. Microprocessors control the tests, reagents, and timing, while verifying the bar code for each sample. This is the link between the results reported and the specimen identification. Even the simplest of systems sequentially number the test results to provide a connection with the samples.

Because most instruments now have either a built-in or attached video monitor, the sophisticated software programs that come with the instrument can be displayed for determining the status of different aspects of the testing process. Computerized monitoring is available for such parameters as reaction and instrument linearity, quality control data with various options for statistical display and interpretation, short sample sensing with flags on the printout, abnormal patient results flagged, clot detection, reaction vessel or test chamber temperature, and reagent inventories. The printer can also display patients' results as well as various warnings previously mentioned. Most instrument manufacturers offer computer software for preventive maintenance schedules and algorithms for diagnostic troubleshooting. Some manufacturers also install phone modems on the analyzer for a direct communication link between the instrument and their service center for instant troubleshooting and diagnosis of problems.

SELECTION OF AUTOMATED ANALYZERS

Each manufacturer's approach to automation is unique. The instruments being evaluated should be rated according to previously identified needs. One laboratory may need a stat analyzer, whereas another's need may be a batch analyzer for high-test volumes. When considering cost, the price of the instrument and, even more importantly, the total cost of consumables are significant. The high capital cost of an instrument may actually be small when divided by the large number of samples to be processed. It is also important to calculate the total cost per test for each instrument that is considered. Moreover, a break-even analysis to study the relationship of fixed costs, variable costs, and profits can be helpful in analyzing the financial justification and economic impact on a laboratory. Of course, the mode of acquisition, that is, purchase, lease, rental, and so on, must also be factored into this analysis. The variable cost of consumables will increase as more tests are performed or samples are analyzed. The ability to use reagents produced by more than one supplier (open vs. closed reagent systems) can provide a laboratory with the ability to customize testing and, possibly, save money. The labor component also

should be evaluated. With the large number of instruments available on the market, the goal is to find the right instrument for each situation.[10]

Another major concern toward the selection of an instrument is its analytic capabilities. What are the instrument's performance characteristics for accuracy, precision, linearity, specificity, and sensitivity (which may be method dependent), calibration stability, and stability of reagents (both shelf life and onboard or reconstituted)? The best way to verify these performance characteristics of an analyzer before making a decision on an instrument is to see it in operation. Ideally, if a manufacturer will place an instrument in the prospective buyer's laboratory on a trial basis, then its analytic performance can be evaluated to the customer's satisfaction with studies to verify accuracy, precision, and linearity. At the same time, laboratory personnel can observe such design features as its test menus, true walk-away capability, user friendliness, and the space that the instrument and its consumables occupies in their laboratory.

Clinical chemistry instrumentation provides speed and precision for assays that would otherwise be performed manually. The chosen methodologies and adherence to the requirements of the assay provide accuracy. No one may assume that the result produced is the correct value. Automated methods must be evaluated completely before being accepted as routine. It is important to understand how each instrument actually works.

TOTAL LABORATORY AUTOMATION

The pressures of healthcare reform and managed care have caused increasing interest in improving productivity of the preanalytic and postanalytic phases of laboratory testing.[11] As for the analytic process itself, routine analyzers in clinical chemistry today have nearly all the mechanization they need. The next generation of automation will replicate the Japanese practice of "black box" labs, in which the sample goes in at one end and the printed result comes out the other end.[12] Much effort has been expended during the past decade on the development of automated "front-end" feeding of the sample into the analytic "box" and computerized/automated management of the data that come out the back end of the box. There have been many developments in the three phases of the laboratory testing process—that is, preanalytic (sample processing), analytic (chemical analyses), and postanalytic (data management)—as they merge closer into an integrated **total laboratory automation (TLA)** system. Automation equipment vendors are developing open architecture components that provide more flexibility in automation implementation.[13] An example of a commercial TLA system is shown in Figure 7.13.

Preanalytic Phase (Sample Processing)

The sample-handling protocol currently available on all major chemistry analyzers is to use the original specimen collection tube (primary tube sampling) of any size (after

FIGURE 7.13 Schematic of total laboratory automation system. (Courtesy of Labotix Automation.)

plasma or serum separation) as the sample cup on the analyzer and to use bar code readers, also on the analyzer, to identify the specimen. An automated process is gradually replacing manual handling and presentation of the sample to the analyzer. Increasing efficiency while decreasing costs has been a major impetus for laboratories to start integrating some aspects of TLA into their operations. Conceptually, TLA refers to automated devices and robots integrated with existing analyzers to perform all phases of laboratory testing. Most attention to date has been devoted to development of the front-end systems that can identify and label specimens, centrifuge the specimen and prepare aliquots, and sort and deliver samples to the analyzer or to storage.[14] Back-end systems may include removal of specimens from the analyzer and transport to storage, retrieval from storage for retesting, realiquoting, or disposal, as well as comprehensive management of the data from the analyzer and interfacing with the LIS.

Dr. Sasaki[15] installed the first fully automated clinical laboratory in the world at Koshi Medical School in Japan; since then, the concept has gradually, but steadily, become a reality in the United States. The University of Nebraska and the University of Virginia have been pioneers for TLA system development. In 1992, a prototype of a laboratory automation platform was developed at the University of Nebraska, the key components being a conveyance system, bar-coded specimens, a computer software package to control specimen movement and tracking, and coordination of robots with the instruments as work cells.[16] Some of the first automated laboratories in the United States have reported their experiences with front-end automation with a wealth of information for others interested in the technology.[17,18]

The first hospital laboratory to install an automated system was the University of Virginia Hospital in Charlottesville in 1995. Their Medical Automation Research Center cooperated with Johnson & Johnson and Coulter Corporation to use a VITROS 950 attached to a Coulter/IDS "U" lane for direct sampling from a specimen conveyor without using intervening robotics.[19] The first commercially available turnkey system was the Hitachi Clinical Laboratory Automation System (Boehringer-Mannheim Diagnostics; now Roche Diagnostics). It couples the Hitachi line of analyzers to a conveyor belt system to provide a completely operational system with all interfaces.[20]

Robotics and front-end automation are changing the face of the clinical laboratory.[21] Much of the benefit derivable from TLA can be realized merely by automating the front end. The planning, implementation, and performance evaluation of an automated transport and sorting system by a large reference laboratory have been described in detail.[22,23] Several instrument manufacturers are currently working on or are already marketing interfacing front-end devices together with software for their own chemistry analyzers. Johnson & Johnson introduced the VITROS 950 AT (Automation Technology) system in 1995 with an open architecture design to allow laboratories to select from many front-end automation systems rather than being locked into a proprietary interface. A Lab-Track interface is now available on the Dimension RxL (Siemens) that is compatible with major laboratory automation vendors and allows for direct sampling from a track system. Also, the technology now exists for microcentrifugal separators to be integrated into clinical chemistry analyzers.[24] Several other systems are now on the market, including the Advia LabCell system

TABLE 7.3 **Summary of Features for Selected Laboratory Automation Systems and Workcells**

	Abbott Diagnostics "Accelerator APS"	Beckman Coulter "Power Processor"	Roche Diagnostics Corp. "Modular Pre-Analytics"	Siemens Healthcare Diagnostics "Advia Workcell"
First year sold in the United States	2005	1998	2003	2002
Preanalytical processor/total laboratory automation	Yes/Yes	Yes/Yes	Yes/Yes	Yes/Yes
Automated centrifugation available	Yes	Yes	Yes	Yes
Automated input/accessioning available	Yes	Yes	Yes	Yes
Automated decapping available	Yes	Yes	Yes	Yes
Automated sorting available	Yes	Yes	Yes	Yes
Automated aliquoting available	No	Yes	Yes	No
Automated recapper or sealer available	Sealer	Sealer	Recapper	No
Automated storage and retrieval available	Yes	Yes	Yes	Yes

Information obtained from Aller R. *CAP Today.* 2011;September:20–40.

(Siemens), which uses a modular approach to automation. The Power Processor Core System (Beckman Coulter) performs sorting, centrifugation, and cap removal. The enGen Series Automation System (Ortho-Clinical Diagnostics) provides sorting, centrifugation, uncapping, and sample archiving functions and interface directly with a VITROS 950 AT analyzer. The instruments listed in Table 7.3 are examples of current TLA solutions offered commercially. Much of the benefit of TLA is derived from automation of the front-end processing steps. Therefore, several manufacturers have developed stand-alone automated front-end processing systems. The Genesis FE500 (Tecan) is an example of a stand-alone front-end system that can centrifuge, uncap, aliquot into a labeled pour-off tube, and sort into analyzer racks. Systems with similar functionality are available from Labotix, Motoman, and PVT. An example of one such system is shown in Figure 7.14. Stand-alone automated sample uncappers and recappers are available from PVT and Sarstedt. These latter devices are less flexible than the complete stand-alone front-end systems and require samples to be presented to them in racks that will work with a single analyzer. Some laboratories have taken a modular approach with devices for only certain automated functions. Ciba-Corning Clinical Laboratories installed Coulter/IDS

FIGURE 7.14 Schematic of preanalytic automation system. (Courtesy of Labotix Automation.)

robotic systems in several regional laboratories.[19] Recently, a thawing–mixing work cell that is compatible with a track system in a referral laboratory has been described.[25] The bottom line is that robotics and front-end automation are here to stay. As more and more clinical laboratories reengineer for TLA, they are building core laboratories containing all of their automated analyzers as the necessary first step to more easily link the different instruments into one TLA system.[26]

Analytic Phase (Chemical Analyses)

There have been changes and improvements that are now common to many general chemistry analyzers. They include ever smaller microsampling and reagent dispensing with multiple additions possible from randomly replaced reagents; expanded onboard and total test menus, especially drugs and hormones; accelerated reaction times with chemistries for faster throughput and lower dwell time; higher resolution optics with grating monochromators and diode arrays for polychromatic analysis; improved flow through electrodes; enhanced user-friendly interactive software for quality control, maintenance, and diagnostics; integrated modems for online troubleshooting; LIS-interfacing data management systems; reduced frequencies of calibration and controls; automated modes for calibration, dilution, rerun, and maintenance; as well as ergonomic and physical design improvements for operator ease, serviceability, and maintenance reduction. The features and specifications of five mid- and five high-volume systems are summarized in Table 7.1. One main advantage of modular chemistry analyzers is scalability. As workload increases, additional modules can be added to increase throughput. A schematic of the MODULAR *ANALYTICS* system (Roche) is shown in Figure 7.15. This system can accommodate from one to four D, P, or E modules. This provides flexibility to adapt to changing workloads. Chemistry and immunoassay testing can be combined, obviating the need to split samples. Repeat testing can be accomplished automatically using the rerun buffer, which holds the samples until all testing is completed.

Postanalytic Phase (Data Management)

Although most of the attention in recent years in TLA concept has been devoted to front-end systems for sample handling, several manufacturers have been developing

and enhancing back-end handling of data. Bidirectional communication between the analyzer(s) and the host computer or LIS has become an absolutely essential link to request tests and enter patient demographics, automatically transfer this customized information to the analyzer(s), as well as post the results in the patient's record. Evaluation and management of data from the time of analysis until posting have become more sophisticated and automated with the integration of work station managers into the entire communication system.[27] Most data management devices are personal computer–based modules with manufacturers' proprietary software that interfaces with one or more of their analyzers and the host LIS. They offer automated management of quality control data with storage and evaluation of quality control results against the laboratory's predefined quality control perimeters with multiple plotting, displaying, and reporting capabilities. Review and editing of patient results before verification and transmission to the host are enhanced by user-defined perimeters for reportable range limits, panic value limits, delta checks, and quality control comparisons for clinical change, repeat testing, and algorithm analysis. Reagent inventory and quality control, along with monitoring of instrument functions, are also managed by the workstation's software. Most LIS vendors have interfacing software available for all the major chemistry analyzers.

Some data handling needs associated with automation cannot be adequately handled by most current LISs. For example, most current analyzers are capable of assessing the degree of sample hemolysis, icterus, and lipemia (see Table 7.1). However, making this information available and useful to either the clinician or laboratorian in an automated fashion requires additional manipulation of the data. Ideally, the tests ordered on the sample, the threshold for interference of each test by each of the three agents, and whether the interference is positive or negative need to be determined. In the case of lipemia, the results for affected tests need to be held until the sample can be clarified and the tests rerun. It is difficult or impossible for the current LISs to perform this latter task. There is a need for a "gap-filler" between the instrument and the LIS. One company, Data Innovations, has developed a system called Instrument Manager, which links the analyzer to the LIS and provides the ability for the user to define rules for release of information to the LIS. In addition, flags can be displayed to the instrument operator to perform additional operations, such as sample clarification and reanalysis. The ability to fully automate data review using rules-based analysis is a key factor in moving toward TLA. The use of "autoverification" capabilities found with many postanalytic LISs has contributed to a significant reduction in result turnaround time.

FUTURE TRENDS IN AUTOMATION

Clinical chemistry automation continues to evolve at a rapid pace in the 21st century. With most of the same forces driving the automation market as those discussed in this

FIGURE 7.15 Schematic drawing of Roche MODULAR *ANALYTICS* system. (Courtesy of Roche Diagnostics.)

chapter, analyzers will continue to perform more cost effectively and efficiently. More integration and miniaturization of components and systems will persist to accommodate more sophisticated portable analyzers for the successful POC testing market. Effective communications among all automation stakeholders for a given project are key to successful implementation.[28]

More new tests for expanded menus will be developed, with a mixture of measurement techniques used on the analyzers to include more immunoassays and polymerase chain reaction–based assays. Spectral mapping, or multiple wavelength monitoring, with high-resolution photometers in analyzers, will be routine for all specimens and tests as more instruments are designed with the monochromator device in the light path after the cuvette, not before. Spectral mapping capabilities will allow simultaneous analysis of multiple chemistry analytes in the same reaction vessel. This will have a tremendous impact on throughput and turnaround time of test results. Mass spectrometry and capillary electrophoresis will be used more extensively in clinical laboratories for identification and quantification of elements and compounds in extremely small concentrations. In the coming years, more system and workflow integration will occur with robotics and data management for more inclusive TLA.[29] To accomplish this, more companies will form alliances to place their instrumentation products in the laboratories. The incorporation of artificial intelligence into analytic systems will evolve, using both experts systems and neural networks.[30,31] This will greatly advance the technologies of robotics, digital processing of data, computer-assisted diagnosis, and data integration with electronic patient records.

Finally, technologic advances in chip technology and biosensors will accelerate the development of noninvasive, in vivo testing.[32–34] Transcutaneous monitoring is already available with some blood gases. "True" or dynamic values from in vivo monitoring of constituents in blood and other body fluids will revolutionize laboratory medicine as we know it today.

For additional student resources, please visit **the Point®** at **http://thepoint.lww.com**

---

questions

1. Which of the following is NOT a driving force for more automation?
  a. Increased use of chemistry panels
  b. High-volume testing
  c. Fast turnaround time
  d. Expectation of high-quality, accurate results

2. Which of the following approaches to analyzer automation can use mixing paddles to stir?
  a. Discrete analysis
  b. Centrifugal analysis
  c. Continuous flow
  d. Dry chemistry slide analysis

3. Which of the following types of analyzers offers random access capabilities?
  a. Discrete analyzers
  b. Continuous flow analyzers
  c. Centrifugal analyzers
  d. None of these

4. All of the following are primary considerations in the selection of an automated chemistry analyzer EXCEPT
  a. How reagents are added or mixed
  b. The cost of consumables
  c. Total instrument cost
  d. The labor component

5. An example of a modular integrated chemistry/immunoassay analyzer would be the
  a. Aeroset
  b. Dimension Vista 3000 T
  c. Paramax
  d. VITROS

6. *Dwell time* refers to the
  a. Time between initiation of a test and the completion of the analysis
  b. Number of tests an instrument can handle in a specified time
  c. Ability of an instrument to perform a defined workload in a specified time
  d. None of these

7. The first commercial centrifugal analyzer was introduced in what year?
  a. 1970
  b. 1957
  c. 1967
  d. 1976

8. All of the following are advantages to automation EXCEPT
  a. Correction for deficiencies inherent in methodologies
  b. Increased number of tests performed
  c. Minimized labor component
  d. Use of small amounts of samples and reagents in comparison to manual procedures

review questions (continued)

9. Which of the following steps in automation generally remains a manual process in most laboratories?
   a. Preparation of the sample
   b. Specimen measurement and delivery
   c. Reagent delivery
   d. Chemical reaction phase

10. Which of the following chemistry analyzers uses slides to contain the entire reagent system?
   a. VITROS analyzers
   b. ACA analyzers
   c. Synchron analyzers
   d. None of these

11. Reflectance spectrometry uses which of the following?
   a. Luminometer
   b. Tungsten–halogen lamp
   c. Photomultiplier tube
   d. UV lamp
   e. Thermometer to monitor temperature in reaction vessel

12. Modifications in microsampling and reagent dispensing improve which of the following phases in clinical testing?
   a. Physician ordering phase
   b. Preanalytical phase
   c. Analytical phase
   d. Postanalytical phase
   e. All of the above phases

13. Bidirectional communication between the chemistry analyzer and the laboratory information system has had the greatest impact on which of the following phases of clinical testing?
   a. Preanalytical
   b. Analytical
   c. Postanalytical
   d. All of the above
   e. None of the above

references

1. Hodnett J. Automated analyzers have surpassed the test of time. *Adv Med Lab*. 1994;6:8.
2. Schoeff LE, Williams RH. *Principles of Laboratory Instruments*. St. Louis, MO: Mosby–Year Book; 1993.
3. Jacobs E, Simson E. Point of care testing and laboratory automation: the total picture of diagnostic testing at the beginning of the next century. *Clin Lab News*. 1999;25(12):12–14.
4. Boyce N. Why hospitals are moving to core labs. *Clin Lab News*. 1996;22:1–2.
5. Boyce N. Why labs should discourage routine testing. *Clin Lab News*. 1996;22:1, 9.
6. Eisenwiener H, Keller M. Absorbance measurement in cuvettes lying longitudinal to the light beam. *Clin Chem*. 1979;25:117–121.
7. Burtis CA. Factors influencing evaporation from sample cups, and assessment of their effect on analytic error. *Clin Chem*. 1975;21:1907–1917.
8. Burtis CA, Watson JS. Design and evaluation of an anti-evaporative cover for use with liquid containers. *Clin Chem*. 1992;38:768–775.
9. Dudley RF. Chemiluminescence immunoassay: an alternative to RIA. *Lab Med*. 1990;21:216.
10. Haboush L. Lab equipment management strategies: balancing costs and quality. *Clin Lab News*. 1997;23:20–21.
11. Schoeff L. Clinical instrumentation (general chemistry analyzers). *Anal Chem*. 1997;69:200R–203R.
12. Ringel M. National survey results: automation is everywhere. *MLO Med Lab Obs*. 1996;28:38–43.
13. Douglas L. Redefining automation: perspectives on today's clinical laboratory. *Clin Lab News*. 1997;23:48–49.
14. Felder R. Front-end automation. In: Kost G, ed. *Handbook of Clinical Laboratory Automation and Robotics*. New York, NY: Wiley; 1995.
15. Sasaki M. A fully automated clinical laboratory. *Lab Inform Mgmt*. 1993;21:159–168.
16. Markin R, Sasaki M. A laboratory automation platform: the next robotic step. *MLO Med Lab Obs*. 1992;24:24–29.
17. Bauer S, Teplitz C. Total laboratory automation: a view of the 21st century. *MLO Med Lab Obs*. 1995;27:22–25.
18. Bauer S, Teplitz C. Laboratory automation, part 2. Total lab automation: system design. *MLO Med Lab Obs*. 1995;27:44–50.
19. Felder R. Cost justifying laboratory automation. *Clin Lab News*. 1996;22:10–11, 17.
20. Felder R. Laboratory automation: strategies and possibilities. *Clin Lab News*. 1996;22:10–11.
21. Boyd J, Felder R, Savory J. Robotics and the changing face of the clinical laboratory. *Clin Chem*. 1996;42:1901–1910.
22. Hawker CD, Garr SB, Hamilton LT, et al. Automated transport and sorting system in a large reference laboratory: part 1. Evaluation of needs and alternatives and development of a plan. *Clin Chem*. 2002;48:1751–1760.
23. Hawker CD, Roberts WL, Garr SB, et al. Automated transport and sorting system in a large reference laboratory: part 2. Implementation of the system and performance measures over three years. *Clin Chem*. 2002;48:1761–1767.
24. Richardson P, Molloy J, Ravenhall R, et al. High speed centrifugal separator for rapid online sample clarification in biotechnology. *J Biotechnol*. 1996;49:111–118.
25. Hawker CD, Roberts WL, DaSilva A, et al. Development and validation of an automated thawing and mixing workcell. *Clin Chem*. 2007;53:2209–2211.
26. Zenie F. Re-engineering the laboratory. *J Automat Chem*. 1996;18:135–141.
27. Saboe T. Managing laboratory automation. *J Automat Chem*. 1995;17:83–88.

28. Fisher JA. Laboratory automation: communicating with all stakeholders is the key to success. *Clin Lab News.* 2000;26(7):38–40.

29. Brzezicki L. Workflow integration: does it make sense for your lab? *Adv Lab.* 1996;23:57–62.

30. Place J, Truchaud A, Ozawa K, et al. Use of artificial intelligence in analytical systems for the clinical laboratory. *J Automat Chem.* 1995;17:1–15.

31. Boyce N. Neural networks in the lab: new hope or just hype? *Clin Lab News.* 1997;23:2–3.

32. Boyce N. Tiny "lab chips" with huge potential? *Clin Lab News.* 1996;22:21.

33. Rosen S. Biosensors: where do we go from here? *MLO Med Lab Obs.* 1995;27:24–29.

34. Aller RD. Chemistry analyzers branching out. *CAP Today.* 2002;16(7):84–106.

8

Immunochemical Techniques

ALAN H. B. WU

chapter outline

chapter objectives

Upon completion of this chapter, the clinical laboratorian should be able to do the following:

State the principle of each of the following methods:
- Double diffusion
- Radial immunodiffusion
- Immunoelectrophoresis
- Immunofixation electrophoresis
- Nephelometry
- Turbidimetry
- Competitive immunoassay
- Noncompetitive immunoassay
- Immunoblot
- Direct immunocytochemistry
- Indirect immunocytochemistry
- Immunophenotyping by flow cytometry
- Compare and contrast the general types of labels used in immunoassays.
- Classify an immunoassay, given its format, as homogeneous or heterogeneous, competitive or noncompetitive, and by its label.
- Explain how the concentration of the analyte in the test sample is related to the amount of bound labeled reagent for competitive and noncompetitive immunoassays.
- Describe the three methods used to separate unbound labeled reagent from bound labeled reagent.
- Describe the data reduction in the classic competitive radioimmunoassay.
- Compare and contrast EMIT, DELFIA, MEIA, RIA, FPIA, ELISA, CEDIA, ICON, and OIA methodologies.

key terms

Affinity
Antibody
Antigen
Avidity
Competitive immunoassay
Counterimmunoelectrophoresis
Cross-reactivity
Direct immunofluorescence (DIF)
Enzyme-linked immunosorbent
   assays (ELISAs)
Epitope
Flow cytometry
Hapten (Hp)
Heterogeneous immunoassay
Homogeneous immunoassay
Immunoblot
Immunocytochemistry
Immunoelectrophoresis (IEP)
Immunofixation electrophoresis
   (IFE)
Immunohistochemistry
Monoclonal
Nephelometry
Noncompetitive immunoassay
Polyclonal
Prozone
Radial immunodiffusion (RID)
Rocket technique
Solid phase
Tracer
Turbidimetry
Western blot

> For additional student resources, please visit thePoint®
> at http://thepoint.lww.com

Immunoassays were first developed by Dr. Rosalyn Yallow and colleagues in 1959, who developed a radioimmunoassay (RIA) for the measurement of insulin.[1] Dr. Yallow went on to share the Nobel Prize in physiology or medicine for this discovery in 1977. Today, immunoassays are one of the essential analytical techniques used in clinical chemistry laboratories for the measurement of proteins, hormones, metabolites, therapeutic drugs, drugs of abuse, cells, and even nucleic acids from serum, plasma, whole blood, tissues, and organs. Instrumentation has undergone tremendous advancement from manual RIA to totally automated analyzers capable of random access, high throughput, and wide menu options. Despite these advancements, the basic principle of how immunoassays work remains largely unchanged, a half century later.

This chapter introduces the generic analytic methods used in many areas of the clinical laboratory—the binding of **antibody** (Ab) to **antigen** (Ag) for the specific and sensitive detection of an analyte. In immunoassays, an Ag binds to an Ab. The Ag–Ab interactions may involve unlabeled reactants in less analytically sensitive techniques or a labeled reactant in more sensitive techniques. The design, label, and detection system combine to create many different assays, which enable the measurement of a wide range of molecules. This chapter reviews the concepts of binding, describes the nature of the reagents used, and discusses basic assay design of selected techniques used in the clinical laboratory; as such, it is intended to be an overview rather than an exhaustive review.

IMMUNOASSAYS
General Considerations
In an immunoassay, an Ab molecule recognizes and binds to an *Ag*. The molecule of interest may be either an Ag or an Ab. This binding is related to the concentration of each reactant, the specificity of the Ab for the Ag, the **affinity** and **avidity** for the pair, and the environmental conditions. Although this chapter focuses on immunoassays that use an Ab molecule as the binding reagent, other assays such as receptor assays and competitive binding protein assays use receptor proteins or transport proteins as the binding reagent, respectively. The same principles apply to these assays. An Ab molecule is an immunoglobulin (Ig) with a functional domain known as F(ab); this area of the Ig protein binds to a site on the Ag. An Ag is relatively large and complex and usually has multiple sites that can bind to antibodies (Abs) with different specificities; each site on the Ag is referred to as an antigenic determinant or **epitope.** Some confusion exists in the terminology used: some immunologists refer to an *immunogen* as the molecule that induces the biologic response and synthesis of Ab, and some use *Ag* to refer to that which binds to Ab. However, all agree that the antigenic site to which an F(ab) can bind is the epitope.

The degree of binding is an important consideration in an immunoassay. The binding of an Ab to an Ag is directly related to the affinity and avidity of the Ab for the epitope, as well as the concentration of the Ab and epitope. Under standard conditions, the **affinity** of an Ab is measured using a **hapten (Hp)** because the Hp is a low molecular weight Ag considered to have only one epitope. The affinity for the Hp is related to the likelihood to bind or to the degree of complementary nature of each. The reversible reaction is summarized in Equation 8-1:

$$\text{Hapten + antibody} \rightleftharpoons \text{hapten − antibody complex} \quad \text{(Eq. 8-1)}$$

The binding between an Hp and the Ab obeys the law of mass action and is expressed mathematically in Equation 8-2:

$$K_a = \frac{k_1}{k_2} = \frac{[\text{Hp} - \text{Ab}]}{[\text{Hp}][\text{Ab}]} \quad \text{(Eq. 8-2)}$$

K_a is the affinity or equilibrium constant and represents the reciprocal of the concentration of free Hp when 50% of the binding sites are occupied. The greater the affinity of the Hp for the Ab, the smaller is the concentration of Hp needed to saturate 50% of the binding sites of the Ab. For example, if the affinity constant of a **monoclonal** antibody (MAb) is 3×10^{11} L/mol, it means that an Hp concentration of 3×10^{-11} mol/L is needed to occupy half of the binding sites. Typically, the affinity constant of Abs used in immunoassay procedures ranges from 10^9 to 10^{11} L/mol, whereas the affinity constant for transport proteins ranges from 10^7 to 10^8 L/mol and the affinity for receptors ranges from 10^8 to 10^{11} L/mol.

As with all chemical (molecular) reactions, the initial concentrations of the reactants and the products affect the extent of complex binding. In immunoassays, the reaction moves forward (to the right) (Eq. 8-1) when the concentration of reactants (Ag and Ab) exceeds the concentration of the product (Ag–Ab complex) and when there is a favorable affinity constant.

The forces that bring an antigenic determinant and an Ab together are noncovalent, reversible bonds that result from the cumulative effects of hydrophobic, hydrophilic, and hydrogen bonding and van der Waals forces. The most important factor that affects the cumulative strength of bonding is the goodness (or closeness) of fit between the Ab and the Ag. The strength of most of these interactive forces is inversely related to the distance between the interactive sites. The closer the Ab and Ag can physically approach one another, the greater are the attractive forces.

After the Ag–Ab complex is formed, the likelihood of separation (which is inversely related to the tightness of bonding) is referred to as *avidity*. The avidity represents a value-added phenomenon in which the strength of binding of all Ab–epitope pairs exceeds the sum of single Ab–epitope binding. In general, the stronger the affinity and avidity, the greater is the possibility of **cross-reactivity**.

The specificity of an Ab is most often described by the Ag that induced the Ab production, the homologous Ag. Ideally, this Ab would react only with that Ag. However, an Ab can react with an Ag that is structurally similar to the homologous Ag; this is referred to as *cross-reactivity*. Considering that an antigenic determinant can be five or six amino acids or one immunodominant sugar, it is not surprising that Ag similarity is common. The greater the similarity between the cross-reacting Ag and the homologous Ag, the stronger is the bond with the Ab.[2] Reagent Ab production is achieved by polyclonal or monoclonal techniques. In **polyclonal** Ab production, the stimulating Ag is injected in an animal responsive to the Ag; the animal detects this foreign Ag and mounts an immune response to eliminate the Ag. If part of this immune response includes strong Ab production, then blood is collected and Ab is harvested, characterized, and purified to yield the commercial antiserum reagent. This polyclonal Ab reagent is a mixture of Ab specificities. Some Abs react with the stimulating epitopes and some are endogenous to the host. Multiple Abs directed against the multiple epitopes on the Ag are present and can cross-link the multivalent Ag. Polyclonal Abs are often used as "capture" Abs in sandwich or indirect immunoassays.

In contrast, an immortal cell line produces *monoclonal* Abs; each line produces one specific Ab. This method developed as an extension of the hybridoma work published by Kohler and Milstein in 1975.[3] The process begins by selecting cells with the qualities that will allow the synthesis of a homogeneous Ab. First, a host (commonly, a mouse) is immunized with an Ag (the one to which an Ab is desired); later, the sensitized lymphocytes of the spleen are harvested. Second, an immortal cell line (usually a nonsecretory mouse myeloma cell line that is hypoxanthine guanine phosphoribosyltransferase deficient) is required to ensure that continuous propagation in vitro is viable. These cells are then mixed in the presence of a fusion agent, such as polyethylene glycol, which promotes the fusion of two cells to form a hybridoma. In a selective growth medium, only the hybrid cells will survive. B cells have a limited natural life span in vitro and cannot survive, and the unfused myeloma cells cannot survive due to their enzyme deficiency. If the viable fused cells synthesize Ab, then the specificity and isotype of the Ab are evaluated. MAb reagent is commercially produced by growing the hybridoma in tissue culture or in compatible animals. An important feature of MAb reagent is that the Ab is homogeneous (a single Ab, not a mixture of Abs). Therefore, it recognizes only one epitope on a multivalent Ag and cannot cross-link a multivalent Ag.

Unlabeled Immunoassays
Immune Precipitation in Gel

In one of the simplest unlabeled immunoassays introduced into the clinical laboratory, unlabeled Ab was layered on top of unlabeled Ag (both in the fluid phase); during the incubation period, the Ab and Ag diffused and the presence of precipitation was recorded. The precipitation occurred because each Ab recognized an epitope and the

FIGURE 8.1 Precipitin curve showing the amount of precipitate versus antigen concentration. The concentration of the antibody (from the assay kit) is constant. Note that one signal can be produced by two different analyte concentrations (*arrows*). A similar curve is observed for the hook effect seen in two-site sandwich immunoassays.

multivalent Ags were cross-linked by multiple Abs. When the Ag–Ab complex is of sufficient size, the interaction with water is limited so that the complex becomes insoluble and precipitates.

It has been observed that if the concentration of Ag is increased while the concentration of Ab remains constant, the amount of precipitate formed is related to the ratio of Ab to Ag. As shown in Figure 8.1, there is an optimal ratio of the concentration of Ab to the concentration of Ag that results in the maximal precipitation; this is the zone of equivalence. If the amount of Ag exceeds the amount of Abs supplied by the test kit, cross-linking is decreased (Fig. 8.2), no precipitation is formed, and the assay is in **prozone**. Although originally described with precipitation reactions, this concept applies in particular to immunonephelometry for the measurement of specific proteins, in which the ratio of Ab to Ag is critical. For these types of calibration curves, a single signal from the reaction can be produced by two different Ag concentrations (see *arrows* of Fig. 8.1). Therefore, accurate results require dilution of the sample to move the result out of the prozone area and into the area of assay linearity.

Precipitation reactions in gel are not as commonly performed in the clinical laboratory today. Gel is dilute agarose (typically <1%) dissolved in an aqueous buffer. This provides a semisolid medium through which soluble Ag and Ab can easily pass. Precipitated immune complexes are easier to discern in gel versus a liquid suspension. Immune precipitation methods in gel can be classified as passive methods or those using electrophoresis and are summarized in Table 8.1. The simplest and least sensitive method is double diffusion (the Ouchterlony technique).[4] Agarose is placed on a solid surface and allowed to solidify. Wells are cut into the agarose. A common template is six Ab wells, surrounding a single Ag well in the center. Soluble Ag and soluble Ab are added to separate wells and diffusion occurs. The intensity and pattern of the precipitation band are

FIGURE 8.2 Antibody (Ab)–antigen (Ag) reactions. **Top left**: Ab excess condition. **Top right**: Ag excess condition. Both of these conditions lead to the formation of soluble complexes. **Bottom**: Bioequivalence leading to the formation of an insoluble "lattice" complex, detectable by immunonephelometry. (Used with permission from Immunology, Chapter 7, Immunoglobulins-antigen-Antibody Reactions. Microbiology and Immunology On-Line, University of South Carolina School of Medicine.)

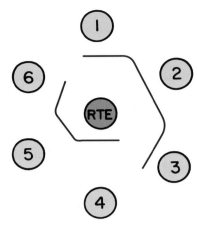

FIGURE 8.3 A schematic demonstrating the pattern of identity. The center well contains the antigen, rabbit thymus extract (RTE). *Well 1* is filled with a serum known to contain Sm antibody. Test sera are in *wells 2* and *3*; the pattern of identity, the smooth continuous line between the three wells, confirms the presence of Sm antibody in the test sera. *Well 4* is filled with a serum known to contain U1-ribonucleoprotein (RNP) antibody. Test sera in *wells 5* and *6* also contain U1-RNP antibody, confirmed by the pattern of identity between the known serum and the test sera.

interpreted. As shown in Figure 8.3, the precipitin band of an unknown sample is compared with the precipitin band of a sample known to contain the Ab. A pattern of identity confirms the presence of the Ab in the unknown sample. Patterns of partial identity and nonidentity are ambiguous. This technique can be used to detect Abs associated with autoimmune diseases, such as Sm and ribonucleoprotein detected in systemic lupus erythematosus, SSA and SSB in Sjögren's syndrome, and Scl-70 in progressive systemic sclerosis. However, most of these Abs are also detected using enzyme-linked immunoassays or multiplex bead array systems (e.g., Luminex Corp).

The single-diffusion technique, **radial immunodiffusion** (RID), is an immune precipitation method used to quantitate protein (the Ag). In this method, monospecific antiserum is added to the liquefied agarose; then, the agarose is poured into a plate and cooled. Wells are cut into the solidified agarose. Multiple standards, one or more quality control samples, and patient samples are added to the wells. The Ag diffuses from the well in all directions, binds to the soluble Ab in the agarose, and forms a complex seen as a concentric precipitin ring. The diameter of the ring is related to the concentration of the Ag that diffused from the well. A standard curve is constructed to determine the concentration in the quality control and patient samples. The usable analytic range is between the lowest and highest standards. If the ring is greater than the highest standard, the sample should be diluted and retested. If the ring is less than the lowest standard, the sample should be run on a low-level plate. Two variations exist: the endpoint (Mancini) method[5] and the kinetic (Fahey-McKelvey) method.[6] The endpoint method requires that all Ag diffuse from the well and the concentration of the Ag is related to the square of the diameter of the precipitin ring; the standard curve is plotted and a line of the best fit is computed. To ensure that all of the Ag has diffused, the incubation time is 48 to 72 hours, depending on the molecular weight of the Ag; for example, IgG quantitation requires 48 hours, and IgM requires 72 hours. In contrast, the kinetic method requires that all rings be measured at a fixed time of 18 hours; a sample with a greater concentration will diffuse at a faster rate and will be larger at a fixed time. The diameter of the precipitin ring is plotted against the Ag concentration on a logarithmic scale. For those performing

TABLE 8.1 Immune Precipitation Methods

Gel

Passive

Double diffusion (Ouchterlony technique)
Single diffusion (radial immunodiffusion)

Electrophoresis

Counterimmunoelectrophoresis
Immunoelectrophoresis
Immunofixation electrophoresis
Rocket electrophoresis

Soluble Phase

Turbidimetry
Nephelometry

RID, the endpoint method is favored because of its stability and indifference to temperature variations; however, turnaround time is longer compared with the kinetic method.

Counterimmunoelectrophoresis is an immune precipitation method that uses an electrical field to cause the Ag and Ab to migrate toward each other. Two parallel lines of wells are cut into agarose; Ab is placed in one line and Ag is placed in the other. Ab will migrate to the cathode and the Ag to the anode; a precipitin line forms where they meet. This qualitative test is useful to detect bacterial Ags in cerebrospinal fluid and other fluids when a rapid laboratory response is needed.

Immunoelectrophoresis (IEP) and **immunofixation electrophoresis (IFE)** are two methods used in the clinical laboratory to characterize monoclonal proteins in serum and urine. In 1964, Grabar and Burtin[7] published methods for examining serum proteins using electrophoresis coupled with immunochemical reactions in agarose. Serum proteins are electrophoretically separated, and then, reagent Ab is placed in a trough running parallel to the separated proteins. The Ab reagent and separated serum proteins diffuse; when the reagent Ab recognizes the serum protein and the reaction is in the zone of equivalence, a precipitin arc is seen. The agarose plate is stained (typically, with a protein stain such as Amido black 10), destained, and dried to enhance the readability of precipitin arcs, especially weak arcs. The size, shape, density, and location of the arcs aid in the interpretation of the protein. All interpretation is made by comparing the arcs of the patient sample with the arcs of the quality control sample, a normal human serum. Because IEP is used to evaluate a monoclonal gammopathy, the heavy chain class and light chain type must be determined. To evaluate the most common monoclonal proteins, the following antisera are used: antihuman whole serum (which contains a mixture of Abs against the major serum proteins), antihuman IgG (γ-chain specific), antihuman IgM (μ-chain specific), antihuman IgA (α-chain specific), antihuman λ (λ-chain specific), and antihuman k (k-chain specific). The test turnaround time and the subtlety in interpretation have discouraged the use of IEP as the primary method to evaluate MAbs.

IFE has replaced IEP in essentially all clinical laboratories.[8] A serum, urine, or cerebrospinal fluid sample is placed in all six lanes of an agarose gel and electrophoresed to separate the proteins. Cellulose acetate (or some other porous material) is saturated with Ab reagent and then applied to one lane of the separated protein. If the Ab reagent recognizes the protein, an insoluble complex is formed. After staining and drying of the agarose film, interpretation is based on the migration and appearance of bands. As shown in Figure 8.4, the monoclonal protein will appear as a discrete band (with both a heavy and a light chain monospecific antiserum occurring at the same position). Polyclonal proteins will appear as a diffuse band. The concentration of patient sample may need adjustment to ensure the reaction is in the zone of equivalence.

The **rocket technique** (Laurell technique, or electroimmunoassay) is also an immune precipitation method.[9,10]

FIGURE 8.4 Immunofixation electrophoresis. **(A)** IgG k monoclonal immunoglobulin. **(B)** IgA λ monoclonal immunoglobulin with free λ light chains. **(C)** IgG λ and IgM k biclonal immunoglobulins. **(D)** Diffuse IgA heavy chain band without a corresponding light chain.

In this quantitative technique, reagent Ab is mixed with agarose; Ag is placed in the well and electrophoresed. As the Ag moves through the agarose, it reacts with the reagent Ab and forms a "rocket," with stronger precipitation along the edges. The height of the rocket is proportional to the concentration of Ag present; the concentration is determined based on a calibration curve. The narrow range of linearity may require dilution or concentration of the unknown sample.

Detection of Fluid-Phase Ag–Ab Complexes

A different strategy to quantitate Ag–Ab complexes is to use an instrument to detect the soluble Ag–Ab complexes as they interact with light. When Ag and Ab combine, complexes are formed that act as particles in suspension and thus can scatter light. The size of the particles determines the type of scatter that will dominate when the solution interacts with nearly monochromatic light.[11] When the particle, such as albumin or IgG, is relatively small compared with the wavelength of incident light, the particle will scatter light symmetrically, both forward and backward. A minimum of scattered light is detectable at 90° from the incident light. Larger molecules and Ag–Ab complexes have diameters that approach the wavelength of incident light and scatter light with a greater intensity in the forward direction. The wavelength of light is selected based on its ability to be scattered in a forward direction and the ability of the Ag–Ab complexes to absorb the wavelength of light.

Turbidimetry measures the light transmitted and **nephelometry** measures the light scattered. Turbidimeters (spectrophotometers or colorimeters) are designed to measure the light passing through a solution so the photodetector is placed at an angle of 180° from the incident light. If light scattering is insignificant, turbidity can be expressed as "optical density," which is directly related to the concentration of suspended particles and path length. Nephelometers measure light at an angle other than 180° from the incident light; most measure forward light scattered at less than

90° because the sensitivity is increased (see Chapter 5). The relative concentration of the Ab reagent and Ag is critical to ensure that the size of the complex generated is best detected by the nephelometer or turbidimeter and that the immune reaction is not in the prozone region. Therefore, it may be important to test more than one dilution of the patient sample, to monitor the presence of excess Ab, or to add additional antiserum and monitor the peak rate. Specific protein analyzers that use immunonephelometry as the detection scheme have automated sample dilution protocols in order to find an optimum Ag concentration to produce measurable precipitants.

For both turbidimetry and nephelometry, all reagents and sera must be free of particles that could scatter the light. Pretreatment of serum with polyethylene glycol, a non-ionic, hydrophilic polymer, enhances the Ag–Ab interaction. Because the polymer is more hydrophilic than the Ag or Ab, water is attracted from the Ag and Ab to the polyethylene glycol. This results in a faster rate and greater quantity of Ag–Ab complex formation.

Both methods can be performed in an endpoint or a kinetic mode. In the endpoint mode, a measurement is taken at the beginning of the reaction (the background signal) and one is taken at a set time later in the reaction (plateau or endpoint signal); the concentration is determined using a calibration curve. In the kinetic mode, the rate of complex formation is continuously monitored and the peak rate is determined. The peak rate is directly related to the concentration of the Ag, although this is not necessarily linear. Thus, a calibration curve is required to determine concentration in unknown samples.

In general, turbidimetry is less sensitive of an analytical technique than nephelometry. In the former case, the decrease in the amount of light due to scattering is measured relative to the intensity of the reference blank, that is, no sample, equivalent to 100% transmittance. If the sample concentration of the analyte is high, a large precipitate is formed resulting in a significant decrease in the amount of light that can easily be measured by turbidimetry. If, however, the amount of precipitate is small due to a low sample concentration, the amount of light decreased is minimal and the instrument must measure the difference between two high-intensity light signals. Because in turbidimetry the amount of light is measured at an angle of 90°, the reference blank produces no signal (no light scattering). When a microprecipitate is formed, the light-scattered signal is more analytically discernible when measured against a dark reference baseline.

Labeled Immunoassays
General Considerations
In all labeled immunoassays, a reagent (Ag or Ab) is usually labeled by attaching a particle or molecule that will better detect lower concentrations of Ag–Ab complexes. Therefore, the label improves analytic sensitivity. All assays have a binding reagent, which can bind to the Ag or ligand. If the binding reagent is an Ab, the assay is an immunoassay. If the binding agent is a receptor (e.g., estrogen or progesterone receptor), the assay is a receptor assay. If the binding reagent is a transport protein (e.g., thyroxine-binding globulin or transcortin), the assay may be called competitive protein-binding assay. Immunoassays are used today almost exclusively, with two notable exceptions: estrogen and progesterone receptor assays and the thyroid hormone–binding ratio, which uses thyroxine-binding globulin.

Immunoassays may be described based on the label—which reactant is labeled, the relative concentration and source of the Ab, the method used to separate free from bound labeled reagents, the signal that is measured, and the method used to assign the concentration of the analyte in the sample. Immunoassay design, therefore, has many variables to consider, leading to diverse assays.

Labels
The simplest way to identify an assay is by the label used. Table 8.2 lists the commonly used labels and the methods used to detect the label.

TABLE 8.2 Labels and Detection Methods

Immunoassay	Common Label	Detection Method
RIA	^{3}H	Liquid scintillation counter
	^{125}I	Gamma counter
EIA	Horseradish peroxidase	Photometer, fluorometer, luminometer
	Alkaline phosphatase	Photometer, fluorometer, luminometer
	β-D-Galactosidase	Fluorometer, luminometer
	Glucose-6-phosphate dehydrogenase	Photometer, luminometer
CLA	Isoluminol derivative	Luminometer
	Acridinium esters	Luminometer
FIA	Fluorescein	Fluorometer
	Europium	Fluorometer
	Phycobiliproteins	Fluorometer
	Rhodamine B	Fluorometer
	Umbelliferone	Fluorometer

CLA, chemiluminescent assay; EIA, enzyme immunoassay; FIA, fluorescent immunoassay; RIA, radioimmunoassay.

Radioactive Labels

The original immunoassays made use of radionuclides, and atoms with unstable nuclei that spontaneously emit radiation are radioactive and referred to as radionuclides. These have largely been replaced by nonisotopic labels. Therefore, the discussion of radiolabels has been omitted in this edition of *Clinical Chemistry*. The reader is referred to previous version of this text for historic information of radioactive labels.

Enzyme Labels

Enzymes are commonly used to label the Ag/Hp or Ab.[12,13] Horseradish peroxidase (HRP), alkaline phosphatase (ALP), and glucose-7-phosphate dehydrogenase are used most often. Enzymes are biologic catalysts that increase the rate of conversion of substrate to product and are not consumed by the reaction. As such, an enzyme can catalyze many substrate molecules, amplifying the amount of product generated. The enzyme activity may be monitored directly by measuring the product formed or by measuring the effect of the product on a coupled reaction. Depending on the substrate used, the product can be photometric, fluorometric, or chemiluminescent. For example, a typical photometric reaction using HRP-labeled Ab (Ab-HRP) and the substrate (a peroxide) generates the product (oxygen). The oxygen can then oxidize a reduced chromogen (reduced orthophenylenediamine [OPD]) to produce a colored compound (oxidized OPD), which is measured using a photometer:

$$Ab - HRP + peroxide \rightarrow Ab = HRP + O_2$$
$$O_2 + reduced\ OPD \rightarrow oxidized\ OPD + H_2O \quad (Eq.\ 8\text{-}3)$$

Fluorescent Labels

Fluorescent labels (fluorochromes or fluorophores) are compounds that absorb radiant energy of one wavelength and emit radiant energy of a longer wavelength in less than 10^{-4} seconds. Generally, the emitted light is detected at an angle of 90° from the path of excitation light using a fluorometer or a modified spectrophotometer. The difference between the excitation wavelength and emission wavelength (Stokes shift) usually ranges between 20 and 80 nm for most fluorochromes. Some fluorescence immunoassays simply substitute a fluorescent label (such as fluorescein) for an enzyme label and quantitate the fluorescence.[14] Another approach, time-resolved fluorescence immunoassay, uses a highly efficient fluorescent label, such as europium chelate,[15] which fluoresces approximately 1,000 times slower than the natural background fluorescence and has a wide Stokes shift. The delay allows the fluorescent label to be detected with minimal interference from background fluorescence. The long Stokes shift facilitates measurement of emission radiation while excluding the excitation radiation. The resulting assay is highly sensitive and time resolved, with minimized background fluorescence.

Luminescent Labels

Luminescent labels emit a photon of light as the result of an electrical, biochemical, or chemical reaction.[16,17] Some organic compounds become excited when oxidized and emit light as they revert to the ground state. Oxidants include hydrogen peroxide, hypochlorite, or oxygen. Sometimes, a catalyst is needed, such as peroxidase, ALP, or metal ions.

Luminol, the first chemiluminescent label used in immunoassays, is a cyclic diacylhydrazide that emits light energy under alkaline conditions in the presence of peroxide and peroxidase. Because peroxidase can serve as the catalyst, assays may use this enzyme as the label; the chemiluminogenic substrate, luminol, will produce light that is directly proportional to the amount of peroxidase present (Eq. 8-4):

$$Luminol + 2H_2O_2 + OH^- \xrightarrow{Peroxidase}$$
$$3\text{-aminophthalate} + light\ (425\ nm) \quad (Eq.\ 8\text{-}4)$$

A popular chemiluminescent label, acridinium esters, is a triple-ringed organic molecule linked by an ester bond to an organic chain. In the presence of hydrogen peroxide and under alkaline conditions, the ester bond is broken and an unstable molecule (*N*-methylacridone) remains. Light is emitted as the unstable molecule reverts to its more stable ground state:

$$Acridinium\ ester + 2H_2O_2 + OH^- \rightarrow$$
$$N\text{-methylacridone} + CO_2 + H_2O + \quad (Eq.\ 8\text{-}5)$$
$$light\ (430\ nm)$$

ALP commonly conjugated to an Ab has been used in automated immunoassay analyzers to produce some of the most sensitive chemiluminescent assays. ALP catalyzes adamantyl 1,2-dioxetane aryl phosphate substrates to release light at 477 nm. The detection limit approaches 1 zmol, or approximately 602 enzyme molecules.[18,19]

Assay Design

Competitive Immunoassays

The earliest immunoassay was a **competitive immunoassay** in which the radiolabeled Ag (A*; also called the **tracer**) competed with unlabeled Ag for a limited number of binding sites (Ab) (Fig. 8.5). The proportion of Ag and Ag* binding with the Ab is related to the Ag and Ag* concentration and requires limited Ab in the reaction. In the competitive assay, the Ag* concentration is constant and limited. As the concentration of Ag increases, more binds to the Ab, resulting in less binding of Ag*. These limited reagent assays were very sensitive because low concentrations of unlabeled Ag yielded a large measurable signal from the bound labeled Ag. If the competitive assay is designed to reach equilibrium, the incubation times are often long.

The Ag–Ab reaction can be accomplished in one step when labeled antigen (Ag*), unlabeled antigen (Ag), and reagent antibody (Ab) are simultaneously incubated together to yield bound labeled antigen (Ag*Ab), bound

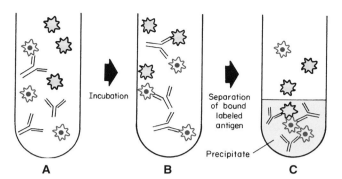

FIGURE 8.5 Competitive labeled immunoassay. During simultaneous incubation, labeled antigen and unlabeled antigen compete for the antibody-binding sites. The bound label in the precipitate is frequently measured.

unlabeled antigen (AgAb), and free label (Ag*), as shown in Figure 8.5 and Equation 8-6:

$$
\begin{aligned}
&\text{Ag}^*\,(\text{fixed reagent}) + \text{Ag} + \text{Ab} \\
&(\text{limited reagent}) \rightarrow \text{Ag}^*\text{Ab} + \text{AgAb} + \text{Ag}^*
\end{aligned}
\qquad \text{(Eq. 8-6)}
$$

A generic, heterogeneous, competitive simultaneous assay begins by pipetting the test sample (quality control, calibrator, or patient) into test tubes. Next, labeled Ag and Ab reagents are added. After incubation and separation of free labeled (unbound) Ag, the bound labeled Ag is measured.

Alternatively, the competitive assay may be accomplished in sequential steps. First, labeled Ag is incubated with the reagent Ab and then labeled Ag is added. After a longer incubation time and a separation step, the bound labeled Ag is measured. This approach increases the analytic sensitivity of the assay.

Consider the example in Table 8.3. A relatively small, yet constant, number of Ab combining sites is available to combine with a relatively large, constant amount of Ag* (tracer) and calibrators with known Ag concentrations. Because the amount of tracer and Ab is constant, the only variable in the test system is the amount of unlabeled Ag. As the concentration of unlabeled Ag increases, the concentration (or percentage) of free tracer increases.

By using multiple calibrators, a dose–response curve is established. As the concentration of unlabeled Ag increases, the concentration of tracer that binds to the Ab decreases. In the example presented in Table 8.3, if the amount of unlabeled Ag is zero, maximum tracer will combine with the Ab. When no unlabeled Ag is present, maximum binding by the tracer is possible; this is referred to as B_0, B_{max}, maximum binding, or the zero standard. When the amount of unlabeled Ag is the same as the tracer, each will bind equally to the Ab. As the concentration of Ag increases in a competitive assay, the amount of tracer that complexes with the binding reagent decreases. If the tracer is of low molecular weight, free tracer is often measured. If the tracer is of high molecular weight, the bound tracer is measured. The data may be plotted in one of three ways: bound/free versus the arithmetic dose of unlabeled Ag, percentage bound versus the log dose of unlabeled Ag, and logit bound/B_0 versus the log dose of the unlabeled Ag (Fig. 8.6).

TABLE 8.3	Competitive Binding Assay Example						
AG	+	AG*	+	AB	→	AGAB +	AG*AB +	AG*

CONCENTRATION OF REACTANTS			CONCENTRATION OF PRODUCTS		
AG	AG*	AB	AGAB	AG*AB	AG*
0	200	100	0	100	100
50	200	100	20	80	120
100	200	100	34	66	134
200	200	100	50	50	150
400	200	100	66	34	166

SAMPLE CALCULATIONS

Dose of [Ag]	% B	B/F
0	$\dfrac{100}{200} = 50$	$\dfrac{100}{100} = 1$
50	$\dfrac{80}{200} = 40$	$\dfrac{80}{120} = 67$
100	$\dfrac{66}{200} = 33$	$\dfrac{66}{134} = 33$
200	$\dfrac{50}{200} = 25$	$\dfrac{50}{150} = 33$
400	$\dfrac{34}{200} = 17$	$\dfrac{34}{166} = 20$

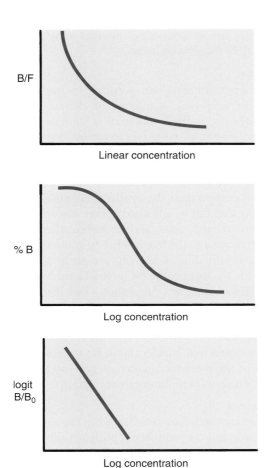

FIGURE 8.6 Dose–response curves in a competitive assay. B, bound labeled antigen; F, free labeled antigen; B_0, maximum binding; % B, $B/B_0 \times 100$.

FIGURE 8.7 Dose–response curve in a noncompetitive immunoassay. CPM, counts per minute.

The bound fraction can be expressed in several different formats. Bound/free is CPM of the bound fraction compared with the CPM of the free fraction. Percent bound (% B) is the CPM of the bound fraction compared with the CPM of maximum binding of the tracer (B_0) multiplied by 100. Logit B/B_0 transformation is the natural log of $(B/B_0)/(1 - B/B_0)$. When B/B_0 is plotted on the ordinate and the log dose of the unlabeled Ag is plotted on the abscissa, a straight line with a negative slope is produced using linear regression.

It is important to remember that the best type of curve-fitting technique is determined by experiment and that there is no assurance that a logit-log plot of the data will always generate a straight line. To determine the best method, several different methods of data plotting should be tried when a new assay is introduced. Every time the assay is performed, a dose–response curve should be prepared to check the performance of the assay. The relative error for all RIA dose–response curves is minimal when $B/B_0 = 0.5$ and increases at both high and low concentrations of the plot. As shown in the plot of B/B_0 versus log of the Ag concentration (Fig. 8.8), a relatively large change in the concentration at either end of the curve produces little change in the B/B_0 value. Patient values derived from a

B/B_0 value greater than 0.9 or less than 0.1 should be interpreted with caution. When the same data are displayed using the logit-log plot, it is easy to overlook the error at either end of the straight line.

Noncompetitive Immunoassays
Sometimes known as immunometric assays, **noncompetitive immunoassays** use a labeled reagent Ab to detect the Ag. Excess labeled Ab is required to ensure that the labeled Ab reagent does not limit the reaction. The concentration of the Ag is directly proportional to the bound labeled Ab as shown in Figure 8.7. The relationship is linear up to a limit and then is subject to the high-dose hook effect.

In the sandwich assay to detect Ag (also known as an Ag capture assay), immobilized unlabeled Ab captures the Ag. After washing to remove unreacted molecules, the labeled detector Ab is added. After another washing to remove free labeled detector Ab, the signal from the bound labeled Ab is proportional to the Ag captured. This format relies on the ability of the Ab reagent to react with a single epitope on the Ag. The specificity and quantity of MAbs have allowed the rapid expansion of diverse assays. A schematic is shown in Figure 8.8.

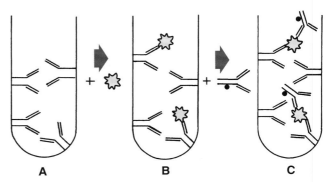

FIGURE 8.8 Two-site noncompetitive sandwich assay to detect antigen. Immobilized antibody captures the antigen. Then, labeled antibody is added, binds to the captured antigen, and is detected.

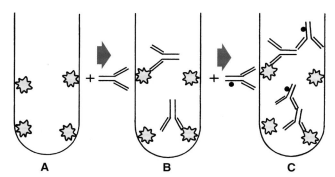

FIGURE 8.9 Two-site noncompetitive sandwich assay to detect antibody. Immobilized antigen captures the antibody. Then, labeled antibody is added, binds to the captured antibody, and is detected.

The sandwich assay is another noncompetitive assay used to detect Ab, in which the immobilized Ag captures specific Ab. After washing, the labeled detector Ab is added and binds to the captured Ab. The amount of bound labeled Ab is directly proportional to the amount of specific Ab present (Fig. 8.9). This assay can be modified to determine the Ig class of the specific Ab present in serum. For example, if the detector Ab was labeled and monospecific (e.g., rabbit antihuman IgM [μ-chain specific]), it would detect and quantitate only human IgM captured by the immobilized Ag.

Separation Techniques

All immunoassays require that free labeled reactant be distinguished from bound labeled reactant. In *heterogeneous assays*, physical separation is necessary and is achieved by adsorption, precipitation, or interaction with a **solid phase** as listed in Table 8.4. The better the separation of bound from free reactant, the more reliable the assay will be. This is in contrast to *homogeneous assays*, in which the activity or expression of the label depends on whether the labeled

reactant is free or bound. No physical separation step is needed in homogeneous assays.

Adsorption

Adsorption techniques use particles to trap small Ags, labeled or unlabeled. A mixture of charcoal and crosslinked dextran is used. Charcoal is porous and readily combines with small molecules to remove them from solution; dextran prevents nonspecific protein binding to the charcoal. The size of the dextran influences the size of the molecule that can be adsorbed; the lower the molecular weight of dextran used, the smaller is the molecular weight of free Ag that can be adsorbed. Other adsorbents include silica, ion exchange resin, and Sephadex. After adsorption and centrifugation, the free labeled Ag is found in the precipitate. The binding of the capture Ab to paramagnetic particles is the most common method used by automated immunoassay analyzers. Separation takes place by applying a powerful magnet, thereby adhering bound analytes to each reaction chamber (Fig. 8.10). Unbound constituents and labels are removed by aspiration. Thereafter, the magnet is removed that enables the pellet to reconstitute and additional reagents added in order to generate the analytical signal (usually a chemiluminescent reaction).

Precipitation

Nonimmune precipitation occurs when the environment is altered, affecting the solubility of protein. Compounds such as ammonium sulfate, sodium sulfate, polyethylene glycol, and ethanol precipitate protein nonspecifically; both free Ab and Ag–Ab complexes will precipitate. Ammonium sulfate and sodium sulfate "salt out" free globulins and Ag–Ab complexes. Ethanol denatures protein and Ag–Ab complexes, causing precipitation. Polyethylene glycol precipitates larger protein molecules with or without the Ag attached. Ideally, after centrifugation, all bound labeled Ag will be in the precipitate, leaving free labeled Ag in the supernatant.

TABLE 8.4	**Characteristics of Separation Techniques**	
Separation Technique	**Example**	**Action**
Adsorption	Charcoal and dextran	Traps free labeled antigen
	Silica	Separation by centrifugation
	Ion exchange resin	
	Sephadex	
Precipitation		
Nonimmune	Ethanol	Denatures bound labeled antigen
	Ammonium sulfate	Separation by centrifugation
	Sodium sulfate	
	Polyethylene glycol	
Immune	Second antibody	Primary antibody is recognized and forms an insoluble complex
	Staphylococcal protein A	
Solid phase	Polystyrene	Separation by centrifugation
	Membranes	One reactant is adsorbed or covalently attached to the inert surface
	Magnetized particles	Separation by washing

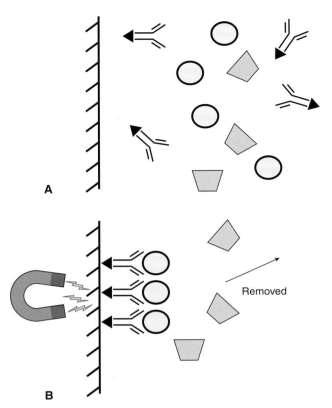

FIGURE 8.10 Separation by paramagnetic particles. **(A)** Addition of sample containing the analyte (*circle*) and other constituent (*rhomboid*) to a capture antibody containing a paramagnetic particle (*solid triangle*). **(B)** Application of a magnet to adhere capture antibodies and analyte to the side of the reaction chamber. The unbound constituent is removed by aspiration. Removal of the magnet and addition of signal antibody facilitate measurement (not shown).

Soluble Ag–Ab complexes can be precipitated by a second Ab that recognizes the primary Ab in the soluble complex. The result is a larger complex that becomes insoluble and precipitates. Centrifugation is again used to aid in the separation. This immune precipitation method is also known as the double-Ab or second-Ab method. For example, in a growth hormone assay, the primary or Ag-specific Ab produced in a rabbit recognizes growth hormone. The second Ab, produced in a sheep or goat, would recognize rabbit Ab. Labeled Ag–Ab complexes, unlabeled Ag–Ab complexes, and free primary Abs are precipitated by the second Ab. This separation method is more specific than nonimmune precipitation because only the primary Ab is precipitated. A similar separation occurs when staphylococcal protein A (SPA) replaces the second Ab. SPA binds to human IgG causing precipitation.

Solid Phase
The use of a *solid phase* to immobilize reagent Ab or Ag provides a method to separate free from bound labeled reactant after washing. The solid-phase support is an inert surface to which reagent Ag or Ab is attached. The solid-phase support may be, but is not limited to, polystyrene surfaces, membranes, and magnetic beads. The immobilized Ag or Ab may

be adsorbed or covalently bound to the solid-phase support; covalent linkage prevents spontaneous release of the immobilized Ag or Ab. Immunoassays using solid-phase separation are easier to perform and to automate and require less manipulation and time to perform than other immunoassays. However, a relatively large amount of reagent Ab or Ag is required to coat the solid-phase surface, and consistent coverage of the solid phase is difficult to achieve.

Interferences with Sandwich Immunoassays
While an advantage of sandwich-type immunoassays is the production of linear calibration curves (Fig. 8.1), the disadvantage is that these assays are subjected to false-positive and false-negative interferences. Normally, the target analyte is required for the production of a positive analytical signal (Fig. 8.11A). If, however, the sample contains unusual Abs, such as human antimouse antibodies (HAMA) or heterophile Abs, they can bind to both the capture and labeled Abs producing an analytical signal in the absence of the analyte (Fig. 8.11B). Individuals who are exposed to mouse Ags can develop HAMA Abs that recognize monoclonal Abs derived from murine cell lines as Ags.[20] Heterophile Abs are formed from patients who have autoimmune disease and other disorders.[21] Although the principle is different, the "hook" effect is similar to the prozone effect in that excess concentrations of the Ag from the sample reduce the analytical signal.[22] As shown in Figure 8.12, excess Ag binds to free labeled Ab, prohibiting the labeled Ab to bind to the capture Ab (via the analyte), and the resulting signal is reduced after the wash step. Analytes that are present in very low and high concentrations, such as human chorionic gonadotropin (hCG) during the first trimester of pregnancy, are subjected to the hook effect. Commercial assays must be designed to either be immune to the hook effect or produce some warning flag to the analyst that the sample must be diluted in order to obtain an accurate result. In anticipation of the need for sample dilution, some laboratories automatically perform dilutions of a sample from a patient known to have high analyte values (e.g., hCG during pregnancy).

FIGURE 8.11 Heterophile or human antimouse interference. **(A)** Analytical signal in the presence of the analyte. The capture antibody (*left*), attached to a solid support, binds to the analyte (*circle*) at one epitope of the analyte. The labeled antibody (*right*) is added and binds to the analyte at a second analyte epitope. **(B)** False-positive signal in the presence of an interfering antibody. The interfering antibody (*gray middle*) binds to both the capture (*left*) and label (*right*) antibodies, forming a "sandwich" in the absence of the analyte causing a false-positive signal.

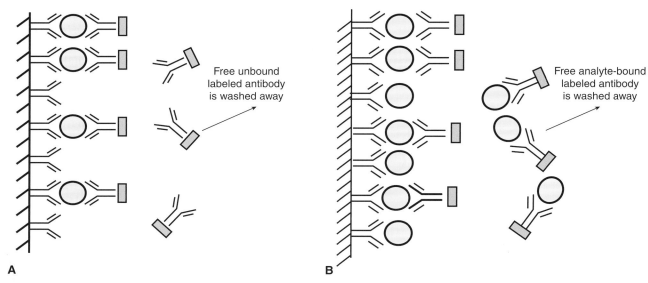

A **B**

FIGURE 8.12 The hook effect. **(A)** Analytical signal in the presence of the analyte at a concentration that is within the dynamic range of the assay. There is an excess amount of capture (*left*) and labeled (*right*) antibodies such that all analytes are bound (none are free in solution). Excess free unbound labeled antibody is washed away, and the resulting signal is proportional to the number of captured labeled antibody (4 units in this example). **(B)** Analytical signal in the presence of the analyte at a concentration that is above the dynamic range of the assay. All of the capture antibody is bound with the analyte. The excess antigen is found free in solution and binds to excess labeled antibody found free in solution. These labeled antibodies cannot bind to the analyte-bound capture antibody because the site is already occupied with the analyte. The free analyte-bound labeled antibody is washed away. This leaves 4 units remaining, the same number as in example A despite the much higher analyte concentration.

There have been recent advances in monoclonal antibody techniques to improve performance. Figure 8.1 shows the structure of a mouse (A) and human (B) antibody. A "chimeric antibody" (C) is an engineered antibody whereby the antigen recognition site (Fab) originates from the mouse, while the constant portion contain sequences that are from the human species. A "humanized" antibody (D) contains small segments from the mouse but sufficient in number to recognize the foreign antigen. Use of chimeric and humanized antibodies minimizes or eliminates HAMA and heterophile antibody interferences, because these atypical antibodies bind to the Fc portion of the antibodies used as reagents in immunoassays (Fig. 8.13).

Examples of Labeled Immunoassays

Particle-enhanced turbidimetric inhibition immunoassay is a homogeneous competitive immunoassay in which low molecular weight Hps bound to particles compete with unlabeled analyte for the specific Ab. The extent of particle agglutination is inversely proportional to the concentration of unlabeled analyte and is assessed by measuring the change in transmitted light.[23]

Enzyme-linked immunosorbent assays (ELISAs), a popular group of **heterogeneous immunoassays**, have an enzyme label and use a solid phase as the separation technique. Four formats are available: a competitive assay using labeled Ag, a competitive assay using labeled Ab, a noncompetitive assay to detect Ag, and a noncompetitive assay to detect Ab. ELISAs are widely used in clinical research as there are commercial assays available to hundreds of analytes. If the analyte has clinical value, an automated version would be made available to the clinical laboratory scientist.

If the assay is only used for research purposes, for example, cytokine analysis, then ELISAs are the technique of choice because they can be easily produced by the manufacturers and most research laboratories have ELISA plate readers. The disadvantage of ELISAs is that they typically use enzyme or fluorescence detection, which is not as sensitive as chemiluminescence or radiodetection. The assays are more labor

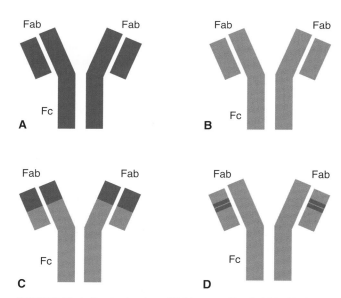

FIGURE 8.13 Antibody structure. **(A)** Mouse antibody (all in *blue*). **(B)** Human antibody (all in *brown*). **(C)** Chimeric antibody. The Fab portion is derived from the mouse (in *blue*). The Fc portion is human (in *brown*). **(D)** Humanized antibody. Parts of the Fab portion is derived from the mouse (*blue stripes*) but retains recognition against the antigen. The Fc portion is human (*brown*).

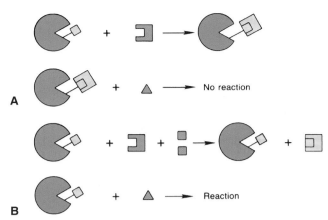

FIGURE 8.14 Enzyme-multiplied immunoassay technique. **(A)** When enzyme-labeled antigen is bound to the antibody, the enzyme activity is inhibited. **(B)** Free patient antigen binds to the antibody and prevents antibody binding to the labeled antigen. The substrate indicates the amount of free labeled antigen.

intensive than modern clinical assays, although some laboratories have automated plate washing and reading stations to improve workflow if there is a high volume of testing needed.

One of the earliest **homogeneous assays** was enzyme-multiplied immunoassay technique (EMIT), an enzyme immunoassay (Siemens Healthcare Corp).[24] As shown in Figure 8.14, the reactants in most test systems include an enzyme-labeled Ag (commonly, a low molecular weight analyte, such as a drug), an Ab directed against the Ag, the substrate, and test Ag. The enzyme is catalytically active when the labeled Ag is free (not bound to the Ab). It is thought that when the Ab combines with the labeled Ag, the Ab sterically hinders the enzyme. The conformational changes that occur during Ag–Ab interaction inhibit the enzyme activity. In this homogeneous assay, the unlabeled Ag in the sample competes with the labeled Ag for the Ab-binding sites; as the concentration of unlabeled Ag increases, less enzyme-labeled Ag can bind to the Ab. Therefore, more labeled Ag is free, and the enzymatic activity is greater.

Cloned enzyme donor immunoassays (CEDIAs) are competitive, homogeneous assays in which the genetically engineered label is β-galactosidase (Microgenics Corp).[25] The enzyme is in two inactive pieces: the enzyme acceptor and the enzyme donor. When these two pieces bind together, enzyme activity is restored. In the assay, the Ag labeled with the enzyme donor and the unlabeled Ag in the sample compete for specific Ab-binding sites. When the Ab binds to the labeled Ag, the enzyme acceptor cannot bind to the enzyme donor; therefore, the enzyme is not restored and the enzyme is inactive. More unlabeled Ag in the sample results in more enzyme activity.

Microparticle capture enzyme immunoassay (MEIA) is an automated assay available on the AxSYM Analyzer (Abbott Laboratories). The microparticles serve as the solid phase, and a glass fiber matrix separates the bound labeled reagent. Both competitive and noncompetitive assays are available. Although the label is an enzyme (ALP), the substrate (4-methylumbelliferyl phosphate) is fluorogenic.

Solid-phase fluorescence immunoassays are analogous to the ELISA methods except that the label fluoresces. Of particular note is FIAX (BioWhittaker). In this assay, fluid-phase unlabeled Ag is captured by Ab on the solid phase; after washing, the detector Ab (with a fluorescent label attached) reacts with the solid-phase captured Ag.

Particle concentration fluorescence immunoassay is a heterogeneous, competitive immunoassay in which particles are used to localize the reaction and concentrate the fluorescence. Labeled Ag and unlabeled Ag in the sample compete for Ab bound to polystyrene particles. The particles are trapped and the fluorescence is measured. The assay can also be designed so that labeled Ab and unlabeled Ab compete for Ag fixed onto particles.

Fluorescence excitation transfer immunoassay is a competitive, **homogeneous immunoassay** using two fluorophores (such as fluorescein and rhodamine).[26] When the two labels are in close proximity, the emitted light from fluorescein will be absorbed by rhodamine. Thus, the emission from fluorescein is quenched. Fluorescein-labeled Ag and unlabeled Ag compete for rhodamine-labeled Ab. More unlabeled Ag lessens the amount of fluorescein-labeled Ag that binds; therefore, more fluorescence is present (less quenching).

Substrate-level fluorescence immunoassay is another competitive, homogeneous assay. This time, the Hp is labeled with a substrate; when catalyzed by an appropriate enzyme, fluorescent product is generated. Substrate-labeled Hp and unlabeled Hp in the sample compete with Ab; the bound labeled Hp cannot be catalyzed by the enzyme.

Fluorescence polarization immunoassay (FPIA) is another assay that uses a fluorescent label.[27] This homogeneous immunoassay uses polarized light to excite the fluorescent label. Polarized light is created when light passes through special filters and consists of parallel light waves oriented in one plane. When polarized light is used to excite a fluorescent label, the emitted light could be polarized or depolarized. Small molecules, such as free fluorescent-labeled Hp, rotate rapidly and randomly, interrupting the polarized light. Larger molecules, such as those created when the fluorescent-labeled Hp binds to an Ab, rotate more slowly and emit polarized light parallel to the excitation polarized light. The polarized light is measured at a 90° angle compared with the path of the excitation light. In a competitive FPIA, fluorescent-labeled Hp and unlabeled Hp in the sample compete for limited Ab sites. When no unlabeled Hp is present, the labeled Hp binds maximally to the Ab, creating large complexes that rotate slowly and emit a high level of polarized light. When Hp is present, it competes with the labeled Hp for the Ab sites; as the Hp concentration increases, more labeled Hp is displaced and is free. The free labeled Hp rotates rapidly and emits less polarized light. The degree of labeled Hp displacement is inversely related to the amount of unlabeled Hp present.

Dissociation-enhanced lanthanide fluoroimmunoassay (DELFIA) is an automated system (Thermo Fisher Scientific) that measures time-delayed fluorescence from the label europium. The assay can be designed as a competitive, heterogeneous assay or a noncompetitive (sandwich), heterogeneous assay.[28]

The classic RIA is a heterogeneous, competitive assay with a tracer.[1] When bound tracer is measured, the signal from the label (CPM) is inversely related to the concentration of the unlabeled Ag in the sample.

Rapid Immunoassay for Point of Care Testing

The sensitivity and specificity of automated labeled assays and the trend for decentralized laboratory testing have led to the development of assays that are easy to use, simple (many classified as waived or moderately complex related to the Clinical Laboratory Improvement Amendments of 1988), fast, and site neutral and require no instrumentation. Those discussed here are representative of currently available commercial kits; however, this discussion is not intended to be exhaustive. Three categories of rapid immunoassays emerge: (1) latex particles for visualization of the reaction, (2) fluid flow and labeled reactant, and (3) changes in a physical or chemical property following Ag–Ab binding.

The earliest rapid tests were those in which a latex particle suspension was added to the sample; if the immunoreactive component attached to the particle recognized its counterpart in the sample, macroscopic agglutination occurred. Colored latex particles are now available to facilitate reading the reaction.

Self-contained devices that use the liquid nature of the specimen have evolved. In flowthrough systems, a capture reagent is immobilized onto a membrane, the solid phase. The porous nature of the membranes increases the surface area to which the capture reagent can bind. The more capture reagent that binds to the membrane, the greater is the potential assay sensitivity. After the capture reagent binds to the membrane, other binding sites are saturated with a nonreactive blocking chemical to reduce nonspecific binding by substances in the patient sample. In the assay, the sample containing the analyte is allowed to pass through the membrane and the analyte is bound to the capture reagent. Commonly, the liquid is attracted through the membrane by an absorbent material. The analyte is detected by a labeled reactant, as well as the signal from the labeled reactant.

The next step in the development of self-contained, single-use devices was to incorporate internal controls. One scheme to detect hCG, the ImmunoConcentration Assay (ICON, Hybritech),[29] creates three zones in which specifically treated particles are deposited. In the assay zone, particles are coated with reagent Ab specific for the assay; in the negative control zone, particles are coated with nonimmune Ab; and in the positive control zone, particles are coated with an immune complex specific for the assay. The patient sample (serum or urine) passes through the membrane, and the analyte is captured by the specific reagent Ab in the assay zone. Next, a labeled Ab passes through the membrane, which fixes to the specific immune complex formed in the assay zone or the positive control zone. Following color development, a positive reaction is noted when the assay and positive zones are colored.

A second homogeneous immunoassay involves the tangential flow of fluid across a membrane. The fluid dissolves and binds to the dried capture reagent; the complex flows to the detection area, where it is concentrated and viewed.

A third homogeneous immunoassay, enzyme immunochromatography, involves vertical flow of fluid along a membrane.[30] This is quantitative and does not require any instrumentation. A dry paper strip with immobilized Ab is immersed in a solution of unlabeled analyte and an enzyme-labeled analyte; the liquid migrates up the strip by capillary action. As the labeled and unlabeled analyte migrate, they compete and bind to the immobilized Ab. A finite amount of labeled and unlabeled analyte mixture is absorbed. The migration distance of the labeled analyte is visualized when the strip reacts with a substrate reagent and develops a colored reaction product. Comparing the migration distance of the sample with the calibrator allows the concentration of the unlabeled ligand to be assigned.

The next generation of rapid immunoassays involves change in physical or chemical properties after an Ag–Ab interaction occurs. One example is the optical immunoassay (OIA).[31] A silicon wafer is used to support a thin film of optical coating; this is then topped with the capture Ab. Sample is applied directly to the device. If an Ag–Ab complex forms, the thickness of the optical surface increases and changes the optical path of light. The color changes from gold to purple. Some studies suggest that this method has better analytic sensitivity than immunoassays, which rely on the fluid flow.

There is great commercial interest in developing high sensitive immunoassays for certain analytes such as cardiac troponin. Figure 8.15 illustrates one "lab-on-a-chip" concept.

Immunoblots

Most assays described this far are designed to measure a single analyte. In some circumstances, it is beneficial to separate multiple Ags by electrophoresis so as to be able to simultaneously detect multiple serum Abs. The **Western blot** is a transfer technique used to detect specific Abs. As shown in Figure 8.16, multiple protein Ags (such as those associated with the human immunodeficiency virus) are isolated, denatured, and separated by sodium dodecyl sulfate–polyacrylamide gel electrophoresis (SDS-PAGE). SDS denatures the protein and adds an overall negative charge proportional to the molecular weight of the protein. The PAGE of SDS-treated proteins allows the separation of protein based on molecular weight. The separated proteins are then transferred to a new medium (e.g., nylon, nitrocellulose, or polyvinylidene difluoride membrane). The separated proteins will be fixed on the new medium and may be stained to assure separation. Each lane on the membrane is then incubated with patient or control sample. The Ab recognizes and binds to the Ag, forming an insoluble complex. After washing, a labeled Ab reagent detects the complex. Depending on the label, it may yield a photometric, fluorescent, or chemiluminescent product that appears as a band. The bands from the patient sample are compared

FIGURE 8.15 Point of care immunoassay using "lab-on-a-chip" design. **(A)** The device takes a single drop of blood and displays the results in less than 15 minutes. **(B)** A U-shaped capillary is fitted above the chip with a membrane filter on one inlet and a dried sphere containing magnetic beads on the other. The membrane filter traps the whole blood cells, while the plasma is wicked into the capillary. The plasma travels down and back up the capillary to the dry sphere, which dissolves and releases its magnetic beads onto the chip below. **(C)** Specifically bound magnetic beads are tethered to the surface of the chip through an immunological bond relying on the capture of cardiac troponin. Magnetic separation forces are generated by passing current through wires embedded in proximity to the bead sensors. The nonspecifically bound magnetic beads are pulled away from the sensors by the on-chip generated magnetic forces. Magnetic beads remaining in the detection area are counted by the embedded sensor. The latter determines digitally (i.e., 1 or 0) if a bead is present by thresholding the signal from the bead. Each sensor can detect 1 magnetic bead. (Figure used with permission from Xip.)

with those from the control containing Ab that will react with known Ags. Molecular weight markers are also separated and stained to provide a guide for interpretation of molecular weight.

Immunocytochemistry and Immunohistochemistry

When Ab reagents are used to detect Ags in cells or tissue, the methods are known as **immunocytochemistry** and **immunohistochemistry**, respectively. When the Ag is an integral part of the cell or tissue, this is direct testing. A second strategy, indirect testing, uses cells or tissue as a substrate (the source of Ag) to capture serum Ab; this complex is then detected using a labeled Ab reagent.

Fluorescent labels are most commonly used in immunocytochemistry and immunohistochemistry. When used to microscopically identify bacteria or constituents in tissue (e.g., immune complexes deposited in vivo), the method is

A HIV reference strain protein extract

B SDS-PAGE electrophoresis

Separated proteins transferred

C

D Overlay with serum sample

E Overlay with antihuman Ig-HRP

F Patient antibody visualized

FIGURE 8.16 Immunoblot (Western blot) to detect antibodies to human immunodeficiency virus (HIV) antigens. **(A)** The HIV is disrupted and extracted to generate its antigens. **(B)** The HIV antigens are separated by sodium dodecyl sulfate–polyacrylamide gel electrophoresis (SDS-PAGE). **(C)** The separated antigens are visualized and then transferred to a membrane. **(D)** Each lane of the membrane is overlaid with a patient or control serum. **(E)** After incubation and washing, a labeled antibody reagent is overlaid onto all lanes. **(F)** The bound labeled antibody is detected. Ig, immunoglobulin; HRP, horseradish peroxidase.

called **direct immunofluorescence (DIF)** or direct fluorescence assay (DFA). A specially configured fluorescence microscope is necessary. Appropriate wavelengths of light are selected by a filter monochromator to excite the fluorescent label; the fluorescent label emits light of a second wavelength that is selected for viewing by a second filter monochromator. Examples of DFA include detection of *Treponema pallidum* in lesional fluid or detection of immune complexes in glomerulonephritis associated with Goodpasture's syndrome and lupus nephritis.

When a fluorescent label is used in indirect testing, this is *indirect immunofluorescence (IIF)* or an indirect immunofluorescence assay (IFA). The substrate is placed on a microscopic slide, serum is overlaid and allowed to react with the Ag, and the bound Ab is detected by the labeled antihuman globulin reagent. The slide is viewed using a fluorescence microscope. The most common IFA performed in the clinical laboratory detects Abs to nuclear Ags. Both the titer and

pattern of fluorescence provide useful information to diagnose connective tissue disease. Other autoantibodies and Abs to infectious disease can be detected by IFA.

Immunophenotyping

An important and more recent advance in immunocytochemistry is the use of a flow cytometer to detect intracellular and cell surface Ags. This technique, *immunophenotyping*, is used to classify cell lineage and identify the stage of cell maturation. In particular, immunophenotyping aids in the diagnosis of leukemias and lymphomas. Differentiating between acute myelogenous leukemia and acute lymphoblastic leukemia is difficult morphologically and requires additional information to identify the phenotypically expressed molecules. In lymphoid leukemias and lymphomas, identification of tumor cells as either T or B lymphocytes can be an important predictor of clinical outcome. Another application is to determine the CD4/CD8 ratio (the ratio of the number of helper T lymphocytes to cytotoxic T lymphocytes) and, more recently, the absolute number of CD4-positive (CD4+) cells. This is the standard method to diagnose infection and to initiate and monitor treatment, although viral load quantitation is considered by many to be a better marker.

Immunophenotyping begins with a living cell suspension. The cells may come from peripheral blood, bone marrow, or solid tissue. Leukocytes or mononuclear cells can be isolated using density gradient separation (centrifugation through Ficoll-Hypaque) or by red blood cell lysis. Tissue, such as lymph node and bone marrow, requires mechanical removal of cells from the tissue to collect a cell suspension. Based on patient history and type of specimen, a panel of fluorochrome-labeled MAbs is used. Fluorochromes commonly used in immunophenotyping include fluorescein isothiocyanate, phycoerythrin, peridinin chlorophyll, CY-5, allophycocyanin, and tetramethylrhodamine isothiocyanate. An aliquot of the cell suspension is incubated with one or more MAbs, depending on the design of the flow cytometer. If the cell expresses the Ag, then the labeled MAb binds and the fluorescent label can be detected. **Flow cytometry** is based on cells transported under fluidic pressure passing one by one through a laser beam. The forward light scatter, side light scatter, and light emitted from fluorescent labels are detected by photomultiplier tubes. Forward light scatter is related to the size of the cell, and side light scatter is related to the granularity of the cell. When these two parameters are used together in a scattergram (two-parameter histogram), the desired cell population can be electronically selected. This cell population is also evaluated for emission from the labeled MAb. For a single parameter, the frequency of cells versus the intensity of fluorescence (the channel number) is recorded and displayed as a single-parameter histogram. Alternatively, if two parameters are evaluated on the same cell, then a scattergram is generated that diagrams the expression of two Ags simultaneously. By using a panel of MAbs, the cell can be identified and the relative or absolute number of the cell can be determined.

Future Directions for Immunoassays

For many years, immunoassays have occupied an irreplaceable space within the clinical laboratory due to the attributes of this technology. Automated immunoassay analyzers are prevalent and will continue to have a major role in clinical testing. Newer instrumentation has focused on the integration of chemistry and immunochemistry within a single testing platform (e.g., Dimension Vista, Siemens Healthcare Corp.). These instruments have advantages to "stand-alone" chemistry analyzers for testing analytes that require spectrophotometry, electrochemistry, and immunoassays on a single sample.

Aptamers are oligonucleotides that have been designed and engineered to bind to specific analytes and offer an alternative to Abs used in immunoassays.[32] Aptamers may be easier to develop than Abs and may offer some advantages regarding analyte specificity. However, aptamers have not yet been adopted into routine clinical practice.

Advancements in mass spectrometry have begun to challenge immunoassays in a few areas for the measurement of low molecular weight analytes including hormones, therapeutic drug monitoring (i.e., immunosuppressants), inborn errors of metabolism, and vitamin D.[33] Liquid chromatography/mass spectrometry (LC/MS) offers the advantages of high analytical sensitivity, freedom from matrix effects, and multianalyte analysis. However, LC/MS instruments are expensive and require a high degree of operator expertise; therefore, implementation has been limited to larger academic hospitals.

For additional student resources, please visit thePoint® at http://thepoint.lww.com

questions

1. The strength of binding between an antigen and antibody is related to the
- **a.** Goodness of fit between the epitope and the F(ab)
- **b.** Concentration of antigen and antibody
- **c.** Source of antibody production, because monoclonal antibodies bind better
- **d.** Specificity of the antibody

2. In monoclonal antibody production, the specificity of the antibody is determined by the
- **a.** Sensitized B lymphocytes
- **b.** Myeloma cell line
- **c.** Sensitized T lymphocytes
- **d.** Selective growth medium

3. Which unlabeled immune precipitation method in gel is used to quantitate a serum protein?
- **a.** Radial immunodiffusion
- **b.** Double diffusion
- **c.** Counterimmunoelectrophoresis
- **d.** Immunofixation electrophoresis

4. In immunofixation electrophoresis, discrete bands appear at the same electrophoretic location, one reacted with antihuman IgA (α-chain–specific) reagent, and the other reacted with antihuman λ reagent. This is best described as
- **a.** An IgA λ monoclonal protein
- **b.** An IgA λ polyclonal protein
- **c.** IgA biclonal proteins
- **d.** Cross-reactivity

5. In nephelometry, the antigen–antibody complex formation is enhanced in the presence of
- **a.** Polyethylene glycol
- **b.** High ionic strength saline solution
- **c.** Normal saline
- **d.** Complement

6. Which homogeneous immunoassay relies on inhibiting the activity of the enzyme label when bound to antibody reagent to eliminate separating free labeled from bound labeled reagent?
- **a.** EMIT
- **b.** CEDIA
- **c.** MEIA
- **d.** ELISA

7. In flow cytometry, the side scatter is related to the
- **a.** Granularity of the cell
- **b.** DNA content of the cell
- **c.** Size of the cell
- **d.** Number of cells in G_0 and G_1

8. You analyze the DNA content on a sample of breast tissue for suspected malignancy using flow cytometry and get the following results: DI = 2.5 and % cells in S phase = 29%. Based on these results you can conclude
- **a.** These results are likely indicative of a malignant breast tumor
- **b.** This is normal breast tissue
- **c.** These results are consistent with a mostly diploid population
- **d.** The results are not consistent with one another; no information is gained

9. The nucleic acid technique in which RNA is converted to cDNA, which is then amplified, is known as
- **a.** RT-PCR
- **b.** PCR
- **c.** RFLP
- **d.** In situ hybridization

references

1. Berson SA, Yalow RS. Assay of plasma insulin in human subjects by immunological methods. *Nature.* 1959;184:1648–1649.
2. Sheehan C. An overview of antigen–antibody interaction and its detection. In: Sheehan C, ed. *Clinical Immunology: Principles and Laboratory Diagnosis.* 2nd ed. Philadelphia, PA: Lippincott-Raven Publishers; 1997:109.
3. Kohler G, Milstein C. Continuous cultures of fused cells secreting antibody of predefined specificity. *Nature.* 1975;256:495.
4. Ouchterlony O. Antigen–antibody reactions in gel. *Acta Pathol Microbiol Scand.* 1949;26:507.
5. Mancini G, Carbonara AO, Heremans JF. Immunochemical quantitation of antigens by single radial immunodiffusion. *Immunochemistry.* 1965;2:235.
6. Fahey JL, McKelvey EM. Quantitative determination of serum immunoglobulins in antibody-agar plates. *J Immunol.* 1965;98:84.
7. Grabar P, Burtin P. *Immunoelectrophoresis.* Amsterdam: Elsevier; 1964.
8. Alper CC, Johnson AM. Immunofixation electrophoresis: a technique for the study of protein polymorphism. *Vox Sang.* 1969;17:445.
9. Laurell CB. Quantitative estimation of proteins by electrophoresis in agarose gel containing antibodies. *Anal Biochem.* 1966;15:45.
10. Laurell CB. Electroimmunoassay. *Scand J Clin Lab Invest.* 1972;29(suppl 124):21.
11. Kusnetz J, Mansberg HP. Optical considerations: nephelometry. In: Ritchie RF, ed. *Automated Immunoanalysis. Part 1.* New York: Marcel Dekker; 1978.
12. Engvall E, Perlmann P. Enzyme-linked immunosorbent assay (ELISA). Quantitative assay of immunoglobulin G. *Immunochemistry.* 1971;8:871.
13. Van Weemen BK, Schuurs AHWM. Immunoassay using antigen-enzyme conjugates. *FEBS Lett.* 1971;15:232.
14. Nakamura RM, Bylund DJ. Fluorescence immunoassays. In: Rose NR, deMarcario EC, Folds JD, et al., eds. *Manual of Clinical Laboratory Immunology.* 5th ed. Washington, DC: ASM Press; 1997:39.
15. Diamandis EP, Evangelista A, Pollack A, et al. Time-resolved fluoroimmunoassays with europium chelates as labels. *Am Clin Lab.* 1989;8(8):26.
16. Kricka LJ. Chemiluminescent and bioluminescent techniques. *Clin Chem.* 1991;37:1472.
17. Kricka LJ. Selected strategies for improving sensitivity and reliability of immunoassays. *Clin Chem.* 1994;40:347.
18. Bronstein I, Juo RR, Voyta JC. Novel chemiluminescent adamantyl 1,2-dioxetane enzyme substrates. In: Stanley PE, Kricka LJ, eds. *Bioluminescence and Chemiluminescence: Current Status.* Chichester: Wiley; 1991:73.
19. Edwards B, Sparks A, Voyta JC, et al. New chemiluminescent dioxetane enzyme substrates. In: Campbell AK, Kricka LJ, Stanley PE, eds. *Bioluminescence and Chemiluminescence: Fundamentals and Applied Aspects.* Chichester: Wiley; 1994:56-59.
20. Kricka L. Human anti-animal antibody interferences in immunological assays. *Clin Chem.* 1999;45:942.
21. Kaplan IV, Levinson SS. When is a heterophile antibody not a heterophile antibody? When it is an antibody against a specific immunogen. *Clin Chem.* 1999;45:616.
22. Butch AW. Dilution protocols for detection of hook effects/ prozone phenomenon. *Clin Chem.* 2000;46:1719.
23. Litchfield WJ. Shell-core particles for the turbidimetric immunoassays. In: Ngo TT, ed. *Nonisotopic Immunoassay.* New York: Plenum Press; 1988.
24. Rubenstein KE, Schneider RS, Ullman EF. "Homogeneous" enzyme immunoassay. A new immunochemical technique. *Biochem Biophys Res Commun.* 1972;47:846.
25. Henderson DR, Freidman SB, Harris JD, et al. CEDIA, a new homogeneous immunoassay system. *Clin Chem.* 1986;32:1637.
26. Ullman EF, Schwartzberg M, Rubinstein KD. Fluorescent excitation transfer assay: a general method for determination of antigen. *J Biol Chem.* 1976;251:4172.
27. Dandliker WB, Kelly RJ, Dandiker BJ, et al. Fluorescence polarization immunoassay: theory and experimental methods. *Immunochemistry.* 1973;10:219.
28. Diamandis EP. Immunoassays with time-resolved fluorescence spectroscopy: principles and applications. *Clin Biochem.* 1988;21:139.
29. Valkirs GE, Barton R. ImmunoConcentration: a new format for solid-phase immunoassays. *Clin Chem.* 1985;31:1427.
30. Rubenstein AS, Hostler RD, White CC, et al. Particle entrapment: application to ICON immunoassay. *Clin Chem.* 1986;32:1072.
31. Harbeck RJ, Teague J, Crossen GR, et al. Novel, rapid optical immunoassay technique for detection of group A streptococci from pharyngeal specimens: comparison with standard culture methods. *J Clin Microbiol.* 1993;31:839.
32. Min K, Cho M, Han S, et al. A simple and direct electrochemical detection of interferon-gamma using its RNA and DNA aptamers. *Biosens Bioelectron.* 2008;23:1819.
33. Grebe SKG, Singh RJ. LC–MS/MS in the clinical laboratory—where to from here? *Clin Biochem Rev.* 2011;32:5–31.

9

Molecular Theory and Techniques

SHASHI MEHTA

chapter outline

Nucleic Acid–Based Techniques
Nucleic Acid Chemistry
Nucleic Acid Extraction
Hybridization Techniques
DNA Sequencing
DNA Chip Technology

Target Amplification
Probe Amplification
Signal Amplification
Nucleic Acid Probe Applications
Questions
References

chapter objectives

Upon completion of this chapter, the clinical laboratorian should be able to do the following:

- Explain the principles of hybridization.
- State the principle of each of the following methods:
- DNA sequencing
- Polymerase chain reaction
- Transcription-based amplification system
- Southern blot
- In situ hybridization
- Restriction fragment length polymorphism
- Describe the three types of amplification assays and list examples of each type of assay.
- Describe the process of dideoxy sequencing.
- Describe the principle of fluorescence resonance energy transfer as it is used in a real-time polymerase chain reaction assay.

key terms

Amplicon
Anneal
Branched chain signal amplification (bDNA) system
Deoxyribonucleic acid (DNA)
Dideoxynucleotides
DNA sequencing
Hybridization
In situ hybridization
Ligase chain reaction (LCR)
Messenger RNA (mRNA)
Northern blot
Nucleic acid probe
Nucleic acid sequence–based amplification (NASBA)
Polymerase chain reaction (PCR)
Restriction fragment length polymorphism
Reverse transcriptase polymerase chain reaction (RT-PCR)
Ribonucleic acid (RNA)
Self-sustained sequence replication
Southern blot
Strand displacement amplification (SDA)
Transcription-mediated amplification (TMA)

For additional student resources, please visit thePoint
at http://thepoint.lww.com

Molecular techniques, assays that target nucleic acid instead of protein, are the latest development in clinical laboratory testing. This chapter introduces molecular techniques that at their core consist of the binding of a nucleic acid to its complementary target nucleic acid sequence. The target nucleic acid may or may not be amplified prior to detection and/or quantitation. Thus, nucleic acid–based methods are designed to detect changes at the **deoxyribonucleic acid (DNA)** or **ribonucleic acid (RNA)** level rather than to detect a synthesized gene product, such as a protein detected in immunoassays. Molecular techniques used in the clinical laboratory to identify unique nucleic acid sequences include enzymatic cleavage of nucleic acids, gel electrophoresis, enzymatic amplification of target sequences, and hybridization with nucleic acid probes. This chapter reviews the concepts of binding, describes the nature of the reagents used, discusses basic assay design of selected techniques used in the clinical laboratory, and illustrates the importance of single nucleotide polymorphism (SNP) and DNA sequence; as such, it is intended to be an overview rather than an exhaustive review.

NUCLEIC ACID–BASED TECHNIQUES

Molecular testing is a rapidly expanding area in the clinical laboratory. Research laboratories have used these techniques for many years; however, U.S. Food and Drug Administration (FDA)–approved assays for the detection and quantitation of DNA and RNA in clinical samples have only developed within the past 10 to 15 years. Key quality issues to be addressed in any clinical DNA-based assays include sample quality and preparation, sensitivity of reagents to inactivating contaminants, amplification bias and variability, selection of appropriate controls, restriction enzyme efficiency, and reproducibility and cross-contamination of amplification reactions. Nucleic acids store all genetic information and direct the synthesis of specific proteins. By evaluating nucleic acids, insight into cellular changes may be recognized before specific protein products are detectable. Genetically based diseases, presence of infectious organisms, differences between individuals for forensic and transplantation purposes, and altered cell growth regulation are areas that have been investigated using nucleic acid hybridization. The most recent development is the use of molecular arrays (up to 10^5 to 10^6 probes per single array) for high-speed analysis of multiple ligands, analysis of gene expression, and determination of mutations with possible therapeutic implications.

Nucleic Acid Chemistry

DNA stores human genetic information and directs the amino acid sequence of peptides and proteins. It is composed of two strands of nucleotides; each strand is a polymer of deoxyribose molecules linked by strong 3′–5′ phosphodiester bonds that join the 3′ hydroxyl group of one sugar to the 5′ phosphate group of a second sugar. A purine or pyrimidine base is also attached to each sugar. The two strands are arranged in a double helix, with the bases pointing toward the center. The strands are antiparallel, so that the 3′–5′-end of one strand bonds with a strand in the 5′ → 3′ direction. Because the phosphate esters are strong acids and dissociated at neutral pH, the strand has a negative charge that is proportional to its length. The purine bases (adenine [A] and thymine [T]) and the pyrimidine bases (cytosine [C] and guanine [G]) maintain the double helix by forming hydrogen bonds between base pairs as shown in Figure 9.1. Adenine pairs with thymine with two hydrogen bonds and cytosine pairs with guanine with three hydrogen bonds. The strands are complementary due to the fixed manner in which the base pairs bond.

Under physiologic conditions, the helical structure of double-stranded DNA (dsDNA) is stable due to the numerous, although weak, hydrogen bonds between base pairs and the hydrophobic interaction between the bases in the center of the helix. However, the weak bonds can be broken in vitro by changing environmental conditions; the strands are denatured and separate from each other. Once denatured, the negative charge of each strand causes the strands to repel each other. The two complementary strands can

FIGURE 9.1 DNA molecule. The double helix of the DNA is shown along with details of how the bases, sugars, and phosphates connect to form the structure of the molecule. DNA is a double-stranded molecule twisted into a helix (think of a spiral staircase). Each spiraling strand, composed of a sugar–phosphate backbone and attached bases, is connected to a complementary strand by noncovalent hydrogen bonding between paired bases. The bases are adenine (A), thymine (T), cytosine (C), and guanine (G). A and T are connected by two hydrogen bonds. G and C are connected by three hydrogen bonds.

be reassociated or reannealed if the conditions change and favor this process. The renaturation will follow the rules of base pairing so the original DNA molecule is recovered.

RNA is also present in human cells and is chemically similar to DNA. RNA differs from DNA in three ways: (1) ribose replaces deoxyribose as the sugar; (2) uracil replaces thymine as a purine base; and (3) RNA is single stranded. DNA and RNA work together to synthesize proteins. Genomic dsDNA is enzymatically split into its two strands, one of which serves as the template for the synthesis of complementary **messenger RNA (mRNA)**. As mRNA is released from the template DNA, the DNA strands reanneal. The mRNA specifies the amino acid to be added to the peptide chain by transfer RNA, which transports the amino acid to the ribosome, where peptide chain elongates.

This discussion of protein synthesis highlights that physiologically, DNA is routinely denatured, binds to RNA, and reanneals to reestablish the original DNA, always following base pair rules. These processes form the foundation of nucleic acid **hybridization** assays in which complementary strands of nucleic acid from unrelated sources bind together to form a hybrid or *duplex*. Molecular testing in the clinical laboratory consists of two major areas: (1) the use of DNA probes to directly detect or characterize a specific target and (2) the use of nucleic acid amplification technologies to detect or characterize a specific target DNA or RNA. Procedures that use probes include solid-phase assays (capture hybridization and Southern and Northern blotting), solution-based assays (protection assays and hybrid capture assays), and in situ hybridization assays. Amplification procedures include nucleic acid amplification (polymerase chain reaction [PCR], nucleic acid–based sequence amplification, transcription-mediated amplification [TMA], and strand displacement amplification [SDA]), probe amplification (ligase chain reaction [LCR]), and signal amplification (branched chain DNA assay).

Nucleic Acid Extraction

Nucleic acid extraction requires the release of DNA or RNA from the cell followed by its purification and quantitation. Nucleic acid can be extracted from a variety of specimens that include whole blood, serum, plasma, bone marrow, cerebrospinal fluid, urine, cultured cells, amniotic fluid, and paraffin-embedded tissue.[1,2] The extracted DNA or RNA needs to be free of each other and also proteins, lipids, carbohydrates, and other contaminants. A commercial kit–based liquid and solid phase and automated methods have been utilized to obtain nucleic acids for hybridization techniques described in this chapter.

In liquid phase, DNA extraction detergent such as sodium dodecyl sulfate liberates DNA and proteins, which are digested by protease or salt precipitated and removed. The lipids and protein remnants can also be removed by organic extraction with phenol and chloroform. The isolated nucleic acid from free nucleus and other cellular contents is then purified by precipitation with cold ethanol. In solid-phase nucleic acid extraction method, DNA is reversibly absorbed onto coated silica onto either filters or magnetic beads at higher ionic strength solutions. The contaminants are washed away in the presence of chaotropic salts and alcohol. The DNA is then eluted by changing to low ionic strength buffer solutions and reprecipitated with cold ethanol. The purpose of these extraction methods is to isolate target nucleic acid, remove inhibitors, and concentrate nucleic acids.

There are commercial QIAamp/DNeasy kits available for extractions of genomic DNA. The buffer formulation is altered in these kits to favor genomic DNA rather than RNA binding (however, some RNA will copurify unless RNase is added during the procedure). These kits may be directed to samples that have a matrix (e.g., collagen, plant cell wall, and gram-positive bacterial cell wall), samples that have a membrane but are not embedded within a matrix (cell culture, blood, and *Escherichia coli*), and samples that have neither a matrix nor cell membrane (viruses, extracellular DNA in urine, or cell culture). These kits differ by the proteases included or by the addition of carrier nucleic acid to compensate for low concentrations.

The extracted nucleic acids are subjected to spectrophotometric evaluations at 260 and 280 nm for quantitation and determination of purity. The quantity of DNA and RNA is approximated by using the following estimation:

$$DNA\,(\mu g\,/\,mL) = OD \times dilution\ factor \times 50$$
$$RNA\,(\mu g\,/\,mL) = OD \times dilution\ factor \times 40$$

The amount of nucleic acid purity can also be assessed by calculating a ratio of optical densities at 260 nm divided by 280 nm since absorbance at 280 nm provides an estimation of protein contamination. The absorbance at 280 nm is due to amino acids tyrosine, tryptophan, and phenylalanine present in protein. The ratio of greater than 1.8 in a clinical specimen is considered to be of an acceptable purity.

For clinical assays, it is important to determine the nucleic acid degradation in an extracted specimen due to either extraction or storage. This is of concern especially for RNA preparations due to environmental presence of RNAse. The degradation is determined by ethidium bromide staining of the agarose gel electrophoresis aliquot of the extracted specimen. A DNA of good purity runs as a high molecular weight band at the origin, whereas degraded DNA will run smeared as many fragments of molecular weight bands. A high-purity RNA of eukaryotic cells demonstrates two bands of 28S and 18S.

The factors to consider for the nucleic acid extractions are usually the specimen, sample volume needed for hybridization procedures, purity, size of the nucleic acid to be isolated, ease of operation, and potential for high throughput in clinical laboratories. A number of automated workstations for nucleic acid extractions are commercially available. Many of these automated workstations can work with anticoagulated blood, which is fresh or frozen or tissue specimens, and isolate DNA or RNA in less than 1 hour.

The automated isolation procedures for total RNA in some instances require the addition of genomic DNA-binding agent prior to sample loading in the automated workstation.

Hybridization Techniques

A **nucleic acid probe** is a short strand of DNA or RNA of a known sequence that is well characterized and complementary for the base sequence on the test target. Probes may be fragments of genomic nucleic acids, cloned DNA (or RNA), or synthetic DNA. The genomic nucleic acids are isolated from purified organisms. Some probes are molecularly cloned in a bacterial host. First, the sequence of DNA to be used as the probe must be isolated using bacterial restriction endonucleases to cut the DNA at a specific base sequence. The desired base sequence (the probe) is inserted into a plasmid vector, circular dsDNA. The vector with the insert is incorporated into a host cell, such as *E. coli*, where the vector replicates. The replicated desired base sequence is then isolated and purified. For short DNA segments, an oligonucleotide probe can be synthesized using an automated process; if the amino acid sequence of the protein is known, it is possible to determine the base sequence based on amino acid sequence.

The principle of hybridization is based on the reversible complementary base pairing of nucleotides. A strand of DNA (or RNA) can base-pair with a complementary oligonucleotide sequence by hydrogen bonding. The process of hybridization is controlled by the solution buffer, temperature, and the presence or absence of denaturant. High stringency conditions that include low salt concentrations, high temperatures, and the presence of denaturant such as formamide can only accept perfect complementary sequences to base-pair and hybridize. These conditions can be altered to low stringency by lowering the temperature, increasing the salt concentration, and the addition of denaturant to base-pair mismatched sequences.

In a hybridization reaction, the probe must be detected. The probe can be labeled directly with a radionuclide (such as ^{32}P), enzyme, or biotin. ^{32}P is detected by autoradiography when the radioactive label exposes x-ray film wherever the probe is located. If the probe is directly labeled with an enzyme, an appropriate substrate must be added to generate a colorimetric, fluorescent, or chemiluminescent product. Biotin-labeled probes can bind to avidin, which is complexed to an enzyme (e.g., alkaline phosphatase and horseradish peroxidase); the enzyme activity can then be detected. Alternatively, the biotinylated probe can be detected by a labeled avidin antibody reagent.

The probe techniques to be discussed are listed in Table 9.1. Hybridization can take place either in a solid support medium or in solution.

Solid Support Hybridization

Dot blot and sandwich hybridization assays are the simplest types of solid support hybridization assays.[3] In the dot blot assay, clinical samples are applied directly to a membrane surface. The membrane is heated to denature or separate

TABLE 9.1	Probe Techniques

Unamplified
Southern blot
Northern blot
In situ hybridization
Restriction fragment length polymorphism

Target Amplification
Polymerase chain reaction
Reverse transcriptase polymerase chain reaction
Transcription-based amplification systems
Transcription-mediated amplification
Nucleic acid sequence–based amplification
Strand displacement assay

Probe Amplification
Ligase chain reaction

Signal Amplification
Branched DNA assay

DNA strands, and then, labeled probes are added. After careful washing to remove any unhybridized probe, the presence of the remaining probe is detected by autoradiography or enzyme assays. A positive result indicates the presence of a specific sequence of interest. This permits qualitative testing of a clinical specimen because it only indicates the presence or absence of a particular genetic sequence. It is much easier to handle multiple samples in this manner.[4] However, there may be difficulty with the interpretation of weak positive reactions because there can be background interference.[3]

Sandwich hybridization is a modification of the dot blot procedure. It was designed to overcome some of the background problems associated with the use of unpurified samples.[5] The technique uses two probes, one of which is bound to the membrane and serves to capture target sample DNA. The second probe **anneals** to a different site on the target DNA, and it has a label for detection. The sample nucleic acid is thus sandwiched in between the capture probe on the membrane and the signal-generating probe.[5] Because of the fact that two hybridization events must take place, specificity is increased. Sandwich hybridization assays have been developed using microtiter plates instead of membranes, which has made the procedure more adaptable to automation.[5]

A classic method for DNA analysis, attributed to E. M. Southern, is the **Southern blot**.[6] In this method, DNA is extracted from a sample using a phenolic reagent and then enzymatically digested using restriction endonucleases to produce DNA fragments. These fragments are then separated by agarose gel electrophoresis. The separated DNA fragments are denatured and transferred to a solid support medium—most commonly, nitrocellulose or a charged nylon membrane. The transfer occurs by the capillary action of a salt solution, transferring DNA to the membrane or using an electric current to transfer the DNA. When the DNA is on the membrane, a labeled probe is added that binds to the complementary base sequence and appears as a band. In a similar method, the **Northern blot**, RNA is extracted, digested, electrophoresed, blotted, and finally probed.

Restriction fragment length polymorphism (RFLP) is a technique that evaluates differences in genomic DNA sequences.[7] This technique can help establish identity or nonidentity in forensic or paternity testing or to identify a gene associated with a disease. Genomic DNA is extracted from a sample (e.g., peripheral blood leukocytes) and is purified and quantitated. A restriction endonuclease, which cleaves DNA sequences at a specific site, is added. If there is a mutation or change in the DNA sequence, this may cause the length of the DNA fragment to be different from usual. Southern blotting can be used to identify the different lengths of the DNA fragments. A labeled specific probe could be used to identify a specific aberration. **Polymerase chain reaction (PCR)** can be used to amplify the target DNA sequence before RFLP analysis.

Solution Hybridization

Hybridization assays can also be performed in a solution phase. In this type of setting, both the target nucleic acid and the probe are free to interact in a reaction mixture, resulting in increased sensitivity compared with that of solid support hybridization. It also requires a smaller amount of sample, although the sensitivity is improved when target DNA is extracted and purified.[8]

For solution hybridizations, the probe must be single stranded and incapable of self-annealing.[4] Several unique detection methods exist. In one of these, an S1 nuclease is added to the reaction mix. This will only digest unannealed or single-stranded DNA, leaving the hybrids intact. dsDNA can then be recovered by precipitation with trichloroacetic acid or by binding it to hydroxyapatite columns.[4,9]

A second and less technically difficult means of solution hybridization is the hybridization protection assay. For this assay, a chemiluminescent acridinium ester is attached to a probe. After the hybridization reaction takes place, the solution is subjected to alkaline hydrolysis, which hydrolyzes the chemiluminescent ester if the probe is not attached to the target molecule. If the probe is attached to the target DNA, the ester is protected from hydrolysis. Probes that remain bound to a specific target sequence give off light when exposed to a chemical trigger such as hydrogen peroxide at the end of the assay.

Digene Hybrid Capture 2 (Digene Corp., Gaithersburg, MD) assay for the detection of human papillomavirus (HPV) is a solution-phase hybridization assay that uses an antibody specific for DNA/RNA hybrids to "capture" and detect the hybrids that are formed during the solution hybridization of HPV DNA in the sample with an unlabeled RNA probe.

Solution-phase hybridization assays are fairly adaptable to automation, especially those using chemiluminescent labels. Assays can be performed in a few hours.[4] However, low positive reactions are difficult to interpret because of the possibility of cross-reacting target molecules.[10]

In situ hybridization is performed on cells, tissue, or chromosomes that are fixed on a microscope slide.[11] After the DNA is heat denatured, a labeled probe is added and will hybridize the target sequence after the slide is cooled. Colorimetric or fluorescent products are generally used. One strength of this method is the morphologic context in which the localization of target DNA is viewed.

DNA Sequencing

DNA sequencing is considered the "gold standard" for many molecular applications from mutation detection to genotyping, but it requires proper methodology and interpretation to prevent misinterpretation. The sequence should be analyzed on both DNA strands to provide even greater accuracy. Patient sequences are compared with known reference sequences to detect mutations. Most sequencing strategies include PCR amplification as the first step to amplify the region of interest to be sequenced. The sequencing reaction itself is based on the dideoxy chain termination reaction developed by Sanger and colleagues in 1977.[12] This reaction generates fragments of newly synthesized DNA, which upon incorporation of one of four **dideoxynucleotides** halts synthesis of the new DNA. The fragments are of varying lengths due to incorporation of the dideoxynucleotides. These nucleotides lack the 3'- and 2'-hydroxyl (OH) group on the pentose ring, and because DNA chain elongation requires the addition of deoxynucleotides to the 3'-OH group, incorporation of the dideoxynucleotide terminates chain length. Varying lengths of DNA are synthesized, all with a dideoxynucleotide at the end. The reaction mixture is then run on a gel, separating the various DNA fragments by size, and the sequence is read directly from the gel. The most commonly used form of this sequencing method in the clinical laboratory uses "cycle sequencing," which is similar to a PCR in that the steps involved include denaturation, annealing of a primer, chain extension, and termination by varying the temperature of the reaction. The newly generated fragments are tagged with a fluorescent dye and separated, based upon size, by denaturing gel or capillary electrophoresis and detected by fluorescence detectors as the fragments pass through the detector. Using this automated method with capillary electrophoresis, about 600 base pairs can be sequenced in a 2½-hour period (Fig. 9.2). DNA sequencing is most commonly used to detect mutations. For example, in infectious disease, testing such as sequencing of the human immunodeficiency virus (HIV) for drug resistance and of the hepatitis C virus (HCV) is used to establish appropriate therapy and treatment decisions.

Pyrosequencing[1,2] is a relatively new technique for a short to moderate sequence analysis that is based on the release of pyrophosphate during DNA synthesis as each dNTP (deoxyribonucleotide triphosphate) is incorporated with elongation of DNA. In this method, after primer annealing to template strand and with subsequent addition of the complementary dNTPs toward the 3'-end by DNA polymerase, PPi (pyrophosphate) is released as the nucleotide forms a phosphodiester bond with the primer.

FIGURE 9.2 Sanger dideoxy DNA sequencing. The region of interest is first amplified using polymerase chain reaction. Sequence-specific primers then hybridize with the denatured amplicons, followed by extension of the new strand by DNA polymerase. At various points in the DNA extension, a dideoxy base (ddA, ddG, ddT, or ddC) is incorporated, which stops further extension of DNA. This results in a mixture of newly synthesized products of various lengths. Each dideoxy terminator base is labeled with a specific fluorescent tag, which can be detected with a fluorescent detector. The fragments are separated based upon their size, and fluorescence is read on each strand, resulting in the sequence of the DNA.

Sulfurylase and its substrate adenosine 5′-phosphosulfate then convert PPi to ATP, which subsequently transforms luciferin to oxyluciferin by luciferase. This conversion of oxyluciferin generates a luminescent signal proportional to the amount of ATP. The light signal is detected by a charge-coupled device and seen as a peak in a pyrogram. The number of nucleotides incorporated is proportional to the height of each peak observed. Apyrase degrades unincorporated nucleotides and ATP. When degradation is completed, another nucleotide is added. As the complementary DNA (cDNA) is synthesized, the nucleotide sequence is determined from the signal peaks in real time by built-in computer software. The technique does not require gel electrophoretic separation of ddNTPs (dideoxyribonucleoside triphosphate), DNA fragments, and radioactive or fluorescent labels. The pyrosequencing technique is useful for the detection of SNP and has been applied in the diagnosis of infectious diseases and human leukocyte antigen typing.

Next-Generation Sequencing
Sanger developed biochemical sequencing methods are now replaced by a new technology where fragmented DNA is sequenced in massively parallel reactions with the use of oligonucleotide adapters. This next-generation sequencing

(NGS) can generate a whole genome or exome (coding region) sequence. There are a variety of commercial instruments available for NGS that utilizes sequencing-by-synthesis chemistries. These instruments utilize an extremely sensitive CCD camera to detect light emitted from the reaction.

Roche developed FLX+ 454 Genome Sequencer uses PCR amplification cycle products on an etched glass fiber with beads. The generation of a pyrophosphate group emits light after the introduction of a known unlabeled nucleotide one at a time. The light signal identifies the incorporation of the base in an extended DNA strand. HiSeq 2000 System developed by Illumina utilizes reversible specific detectable fluorescent dye–based nucleotide terminator. The amplification process provides enhanced light signal with every PCR cycle. This method has a very high throughput that can read in the order of gigabases in a short period of time. MiSeq also developed by Illumina is a smaller version of HiSeq, but with similar throughput. In contrast, Personal Genome Machine by Ion Torrent builds on an amplified cDNA library. A new DNA fragment in this technology is synthesized from a template provided by the library with a detection that relies on the changes in pH due to the release of a H+ ion during nucleotide incorporation.

DNA Chip Technology
Previously, genetic studies examined individual gene expression by Northern blotting or polymorphisms by gel-based restriction digests and sequence analysis, but with advances in microchips and bead-based array technologies, high-throughput analysis of genetic variation is now possible. Biochips, also called microarrays, are very small devices used to examine DNA, RNA, and other substances. These chips allow thousands of biological reactions to be performed at once.[13] Typically, a biochip consists of a small rectangular solid surface that is made of glass or silicon with short DNA or RNA probes anchored to the surface.[14] The number of probes on a biochip surface can vary from 10 to 20 up to hundreds of thousands.[13,14] Usually, the nucleic acid in the sample is amplified before analysis. After amplification, the sample, labeled with a fluorescent tag, is loaded onto the chip. Hybridization occurs on the surface of the chip, allowing thousands of hybridization reactions to occur at one time. Unbound strands of the target sample are then washed away. The fluorescent tagged hybridized samples are detected using a fluorescent detector.[13] The intensity of the fluorescent signal at a particular location is proportional to the sequence homology at a particular locus. Complete sequence matches result in bright fluorescence, while single-base mismatches result in a dimmer signal, indicative of a point mutation. Because most SNPs are silent and have no apparent functional consequence, the challenge is to identify the set of SNPs that are directly related to or cause disease. Detection of point mutations can be used for classification of leukemias, molecular staging of tumors, and characterization of microbial agents.[15]

One prime example is the determination of genes associated with drug resistance in HIV testing. Identification of such genes guides the physician in selecting a proper drug regimen for a particular patient.

Microarrays

In this technology, thousands of known unlabeled 5 to 50 bp DNA sequence probes are immobilized on a solid support to which clinical specimens are incubated for hybridization. The solid support can be a silicon chip or a nylon membrane that holds different probes at a specific location allowing multitudes of hybridization reactions. Microarrays (1) are clinically used to detect genetic polymorphism and disease-specific spectrum of mutations simultaneously (2) can perform comparative genomic hybridization to evaluate genomic gains and losses and determine molecular karyotype.

Currently, Affymetrix, Inc., has developed GeneChips, proprietary, high-density microarrays that contain 10,000 to 400,000 different short DNA probes on a 1.2-cm × 1.2-cm glass wafer. GeneChips are available for HIV-1 genotyping,[15] human *p53* tumor suppressor gene mutation analysis, and human cytochrome *p450* gene mutation analysis, with other GeneChips currently under development.

Target Amplification

Target amplification systems are in vitro methods for the enzymatic replication of a target molecule to levels at which it can be readily detected.[8] This allows the target sequence to be identified and further characterized. There are numerous different types of target amplification. Examples include PCR, **transcription-mediated amplification (TMA)**, SDA, and **nucleic acid sequence–based amplification (NASBA)**. Of these, PCR (Table 9.1) is by far the best known and most widely used technique in clinical laboratories.[16] However, the other non-PCR methods have become more popular in recent years.

The PCR, developed by K. B. Mullis of Cetus Company,[17,18] is an amplified hybridization technique that enzymatically synthesizes millions of identical copies of the target DNA to increase the analytic sensitivity. The test reaction mixture (Table 9.2) includes the test DNA sample (lysed cells or tissue enzymatically digested with RNase and proteinase and then extracted), oligonucleotide primers (Table 9.3), thermostable DNA polymerase (e.g., *Taq* polymerase, from *Thermus aquaticus*), and nucleotide triphosphates (ATP,

TABLE 9.2	**Real-Time Polymerase Chain Reaction Components**

Taq POLYMERASE
Primers
Probe are used in real-time PCR master mix solutions.
Magnesium salts
Nucleic acid bases
Buffers, other salts, additives, water
DNA or RNA template
Reverse transcriptase if RNA template is used
PCR, polymerase chain reaction

TABLE 9.3	**Primers**

A single-stranded DNA or RNA that can hybridize to a single-stranded template DNA and provide a free 3′-hydroxyl end to which DNA polymerase can add deoxynucleotides to synthesize a chain of DNA complementary to the template DNA

They are short nucleic acid sequences, one forward and one reverse that functions as a starting point for addition of nucleotides.

Sequences are complementary to target regions.

Target regions are typically 60–200 bases apart.

T_m of the primers are 58°C–60°C (lower than the probe so they anneal after the probe anneals).

They "prime" DNA synthesis by *Taq* polymerase during polymerase chain reaction.

GTP, CTP, and TTP) in a buffer. The process, shown in Figure 9.3, begins by heating the target DNA to denature it and then separating the strands. Two oligonucleotide primers (probes) that recognize the edges of the target DNA are added and anneal to the target DNA. Thermostable DNA

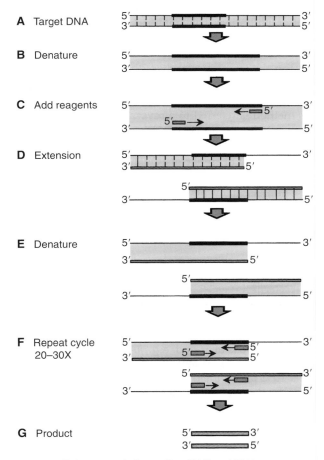

FIGURE 9.3 Polymerase chain reaction. **(A)** Target DNA sequence is indicated by the *bold line*. **(B)** Double-stranded DNA is denatured (separated) by heating. **(C)** Reagents are added, and the primer binds to the target DNA sequence. **(D)** Polymerase extends the primers. **(E–G)** Heating, annealing of the primer, and extension are repeated.

TABLE 9.4 *Taq* Polymerase

Is a thermostable enzyme
5′–3′ polymerase activity
Some modified versions must be heat activated (usually 5–10 min) to eliminate false priming at start of PCR.
Magnesium salts are needed for polymerase and nuclease activities of *Taq* polymerase. Higher Mg concentrations increase nuclease activity (5–9 mM) and must be optimized in real-time PCRs.

PCR, polymerase chain reaction.

polymerase and nucleotide triphosphates extend the primer. The process of heat denaturation, cooling to allow the primers to anneal and heating again to extend the primers, is repeated manyfold (15 to 30 times or more). PCR is an exponential amplification reaction in which after n cycles, there is $(1 + x)^n$ times as much target as was present initially, where x is the mean efficiency of the reaction for each cycle. Theoretically, as few as 20 cycles would yield approximately 1 million times the amount of target DNA initially present. However, in reality, the theoretical maxima are never reached and more cycles are necessary to achieve such levels of amplification. The amplified target DNA sequences, known as **amplicons**, can be analyzed by gel electrophoresis, Southern blot, sequencing, or directly labeled probes.

When the target is microbial RNA or mRNA, the RNA must be enzymatically converted to DNA by reverse transcriptase; the product, cDNA, can then be analyzed by PCR. This method is referred to a **reverse transcriptase polymerase chain reaction (RT-PCR)**. Initially, PCR was a qualitative assay, but assays have been developed that allowed for quantitation of amplicons. Quantitative RT-PCR is used to measure viral loads in HIV- and HCV-infected patients. These numbers allow physicians to determine disease status and evaluate efficacy of antiviral treatments.

The latest PCR innovation is the development of "real-time" RT-PCR, which allows for direct measurement of amplicon accumulation during the exponential phase of the reaction. Two important findings led to the discovery of real-time PCR: (1) finding that the *Taq* polymerase (Table 9.4) possesses 5′ → 3′ exonuclease activity[19,20] and (2) the construction of dual-labeled oligonucleotide probes that emit a fluorescence signal only on cleavage, based on the principle of *fluorescence resonance energy transfer (FRET)*.[21] FRET involves the nonradioactive transfer of energy from a donor molecule to an acceptor molecule. Probe-based (Table 9.5) systems, such as TaqMan probes,[22] molecular beacons,[23] and scorpion primers,[24] rely on the close proximity of donor fluorophores and nonfluorophore acceptor molecules (quenchers) in the unhybridized probe, so that little or no signal is generated as the fluorescence of the donor is quenched by the acceptor. Upon hybridization to the target, the fluorophore and quencher become separated through either conformational changes (molecular beacons and scorpion primers) or enzymatic cleavage of the fluorophore from the quencher as a result of the 5′ to 3′ nuclease activity of *Taq* polymerase. Real-time detection occurs when the fluorescence emission of the reporter probe (driven by the accumulation of amplicons) is monitored cycle by cycle. The results are available immediately and, more importantly, there is no manipulation of the postamplification sample, reducing the chance of contaminating other samples with amplified products. A typical post RT-PCR sigmoidal curve is demonstrated in Figure 9.4. The threshold cycle (C_T) is defined as the value at which the sample fluorescence crosses the threshold. A standard chart of the target copy number against C_T can provide a reference plot for quantitation of the unknown target in samples.

A variety of controls (as shown in Table 9.6) are run in a PCR reaction to ensure that all added reagents are working, the target is not degraded due to either improper handling or contamination, and a quantitation of the desired target can be assessed.

PCR is limited by expense, the need for special thermocyclers, potential aerosol contamination from one sample

TABLE 9.5 Probes

It is a defined RNA or DNA fragment, usually 20–35 bases long.
Reporter dye at 5′-end, e.g., FAM™, TET™, and TAMRA™
Quencher dye is at 3′-end, e.g., TAMRA™ and QSY7™
3′ end blocked to prevent extension during PCR.
T_m is 10°C above the primers, so the probe anneals first.
Reporter dye and quencher dye are in close proximity in the intact probe.
Energy from the reporter dye is transferred to quencher dye.
There is suppression of reporter fluorescence with an intact probe.
Probe sequence is complementary to target sequence.
During PCR, if the target is present, the probe specifically anneals before the primers anneal.
5′–3′ nuclease activity of *Taq* polymerase cleaves the annealed probe into fragments, which are displaced from the target.
The reporter dye is no longer in close proximity to quencher dye; fluorescence not suppressed.
Fluorescence is then emitted by reporter dye and increases with each PCR cycle.

PCR, polymerase chain reaction.

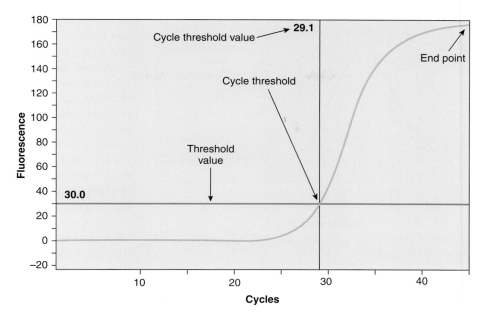

FIGURE 9.4 The plot of fluorescence observed in real time (x-axis) and numbers of cycles completed (y-axis). The graph demonstrates a typical polymerase chain reaction run analysis.

to another, nonspecific annealing, and degree of stringency. Stringency is related to the stability of the bonding between target DNA or RNA and the probe and is based on the degree of match and the length of the probe. Stability of the duplex is strongly influenced by temperature, pH, and ionic strength of the hybridization solution. Under low-stringency conditions (low temperature or increased ionic strength), imperfect binding occurs as indicated earlier.

Additionally, DNA melt curve analysis has been extremely useful. DNA melting temperature (T_m) is defined as the temperature at which 50% of the DNA is double stranded and 50% is single stranded. Each PCR product or amplicon has its own specific melting temperature and is determined by its G–C content, the number of base pair mismatches, and the ionic strength of the solution. T_m can be used (1) to determine the purity of amplification product, (2) to identify amplification products, and (3) to optimize the assay annealing temperature. The melting curve analysis is accomplished by slowly raising the temperature at the end of the PCR run followed by the continuous fluorescence measurements at 2°C increments.[1,25] DNA melt temperature analysis has been successfully used for

determination of single point mutations. Figure 9.5 shows the hybridization followed by melt curve determination of the amplified product with a primer set complementary to wild-type target gene with a strong binding. The homozygous mutant shows a lower melt temperature and heterozygous allele indicates two melt temperatures corresponding to homozygous wild type and mutant.

The melting curve analysis is useful in detection of single point mutations or difference.

Transcription-Based Amplification

Other techniques have evolved to overcome some of these shortcomings, to standardize methods for use in clinical laboratories, or to provide new proprietary approaches. Amplification of the target, probe, and signal has been described. The classic target amplification method, PCR, increases the number of target nucleic acids so that simple signal detection systems can be used. Another target amplification method is **self-sustained sequence replication** or *transcription-based amplification system (TAS)*, which detects target RNA and involves continuous isothermic cycles of reverse transcription.[26,27] The first non-PCR nucleic

TABLE 9.6	**Controls Used in a PCR Reaction and Its Purpose**
Positive Control	A known target sample—to confirm amplification
No Template Control (NTC)	All added reagents except target DNA or RNA—to rule out contamination and false-positive results
Exogenous Control	An irrelevant target with corresponding set of primers are amplified simultaneously with the desired target and its primer set—to ensure that the reaction mix was working.
Endogenous Control	A primer set for housekeeping gene that is present in the specimen for amplification in the same reaction mix—to determine if the extraction procedure was working.
Standard Markers	DNA ladder to determine the molecular weight of the amplified product
Known Target Controls	Used at different concentrations and run in separate wells—to generate standard curve for quantitation of the target

FIGURE 9.5 Hybridization followed by melt curve determination of the amplified product.

acid amplification method developed was a TAS by Kwoh et al. in 1989 that amplified an RNA target.[28] The principle of the reaction was a two-step process that involved generation of cDNA from the target RNA followed by reverse transcription of the cDNA template into multiple copies of RNA. Multiple cycles result in amplification of the target (Fig. 9.6). From this system, two other non-PCR target amplification methods have been developed that are currently used in

clinical assays: NASBA and TMA. The advantages of these two methods are that they are both isothermal reactions that do not require the use of a thermal cycler.

Strand displacement amplification (SDA) was originally developed and patented by Becton Dickinson, Inc. (Franklin Lakes, NJ), in 1991.[29,30] One set of primers incorporates a specific restriction enzyme site that is later attacked by an endonuclease. The resulting "nick" created in only one strand by the restriction enzyme allows for displacement of the amplified strands that then, in turn, serve as targets for further amplification and nick digestion. A modified deoxynucleotide (dATPαS; one of the oxygen molecules in the triphosphate moiety has been replaced with sulfur) is used to synthesize a double-stranded, hemiphosphorothioated DNA recognition site for the restriction enzyme cleavage that allows only single-strand nicking of the unmodified strand instead of cutting through both strands. Becton Dickinson currently markets this methodology under the label BD ProbeTec, and it is FDA approved for the detection of *Legionella pneumophila*, with a combination kit for *Chlamydia trachomatis* and *Neisseria gonorrhoeae*.[31]

Probe Amplification

Rather than directly amplifying the target, there are several techniques that amplify the detection molecule or probe itself. The LCR is an example of this technique. The **ligase**

FIGURE 9.6 Transcription-based amplification systems. Non–polymerase chain reaction (PCR) method of amplifying RNA targets. Nucleic acid sequence–based amplification (NASBA) and transcription-mediated amplification (TMA) are based upon this methodology; NASBA uses three enzymes (reverse transcriptase, RNase H, and T7 DNA-dependent RNA polymerase), while TMA only uses RNA polymerase and a reverse transcriptase with inherent RNase H activity. Initial steps in the procedure involve generation of complementary DNAs (cDNAs) from the target RNA using primers (which incorporate a T7 RNA polymerase binding site) **(A** and **B)**. RNase H then destroys the initial strands of target RNA from the RNA cDNA hybrids **(C)**. The cDNA then serves as template for the generation of double-stranded cDNA, with one strand (containing the T7 binding site) serving as the template for reverse transcription and synthesis of multiple copies of RNA using the T7 RNA polymerase **(D)**. The RNAs then serve as templates for more cDNA templates to be made, and the cycles continue **(E)**.

chain reaction (LCR) is a probe amplification technique that uses two pairs of labeled probes that are complementary for two, short-target DNA sequences in close proximity.[32] After hybridization, the DNA ligase interprets the break between the ends as a nick and links the probe pairs.

Signal Amplification

Signal amplification methods are designed to increase the signal strength by increasing the concentration of the label. This technique uses multiple probes and several simultaneous hybridization steps. It has been compared to decorating a Christmas tree, and it involves several sandwich hybridizations. In the first step, target-specific oligonucleotide probes capture the target sequence to a solid support. Then, a second set of target-specific probes called extenders hybridize to adjoining sequences and act as binding sites for a large piece called the branched amplification multimer. Each branch of the amplification multimer has multiple side branches capable of binding numerous (up to 10,000) enzyme-labeled oligonucleotides onto each target molecule (Fig. 9.7). Perhaps the best known of the signal amplification systems is the **branched chain signal amplification (bDNA) system** originally developed by Chiron Corporation and now sold through Siemens Healthcare Diagnostics (Tarrytown, NJ).[33] The most recent bDNA system has high specificity and can provide quantitative detection over a range of several orders of magnitude (10^2 to 10^5 copies/mL).[5,34] Branched chain systems are well suited for the detection of nucleic acid target with sequence heterogeneity, such as HCV and HIV, because if one or two of the capture or extender probes fail to hybridize, the signal-generating capacity is not lost as a result of the presence of several remaining probe complexes. Additionally, the need for several independent probe-target hybridization events provides a great deal of specificity. The danger of false-positive results caused by carryover of target material is decreased because the target itself is not amplified. However, nonspecific localization of reagents can result in background amplification.[5] Assays for hepatitis B virus, HCV, HIV-1, and cytomegalovirus have been developed using this method.[34] This system is also used to quantitate HIV-1 with a lower limit of detection at 75 copies/mL.[31] It has been validated for the quantitation of viral load testing of all the subtypes. Therefore, this technique can be used for quantitation and to help monitor the therapeutic response.

Nucleic Acid Probe Applications

Nucleic acid probes are used to detect infectious organisms; to detect gene rearrangements, chromosomal translocations, or chromosomal breakage; to detect changes in oncogenes and tumor suppressor factors; to aid in prenatal diagnosis of an inherited disease or carrier status; to identify polymorphic markers used to establish identity or nonidentity; and to aid in donor selection. Nucleic acid probes are useful in identifying microorganisms in a patient specimen or confirming an organism isolated in culture. Probes are currently available to confirm *Mycobacterium* sp., *Legionella* sp., *Salmonella*, diarrheagenic *E. coli* strains, *Shigella*, and *Campylobacter* sp. Probes also are available to identify fungi such as *Blastomyces dermatitidis*, *Coccidioides immitis*, *Cryptococcus neoformans*, and *Histoplasma capsulatum*. Direct identification of microorganisms in patient specimens includes *Chlamydia trachomatis*, *N. gonorrhoeae*, cytomegalovirus, Epstein-Barr virus, and herpes simplex virus. In addition, viral load testing for HIV and HCV is detected using probe technology. Detection of multidrug-resistant strains of *Mycobacterium tuberculosis* may lead to more timely public health control measures. Identification of genes for antimicrobial resistance in other organisms will help in more effective treatment for severe infections.[35] HCV genotyping and pretreatment viral load testing in newly diagnosed infections provide the physician with valuable information to determine therapy regimens.[36] HIV viral load testing can play a role in the diagnosis of HIV in neonates born to HIV-infected mothers as well as in the diagnosis of acute HIV infections, which are defined as the period after exposure to the virus but before seroconversion.[37]

Table 9.7 summarizes target and signal amplification techniques currently used in clinical diagnosis. A detailed review of all these techniques is beyond the scope of this chapter.

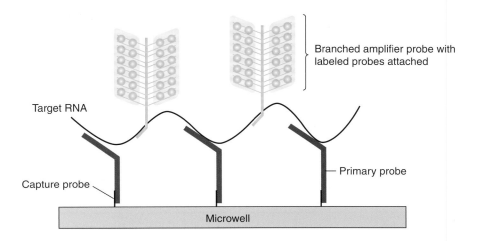

FIGURE 9.7 Branched chain amplification. Several different probes are used to amplify the signal rather than the target DNA itself. The first probe captures the target. Amplifier 1 binds in a different place and forms the base for amplifier 2, the branched chain. Amplifier 3 contains the signal.

Branched amplifier probe with labeled probes attached

Target RNA

Primary probe

Capture probe

Microwell

TABLE 9.7   **Target and Signal Amplification Techniques**

Target Amplification Techniques
- Single enzymes or multiple enzymes synthesize copies of target nucleic acid sequences.[2]
- Usually, two oligonucleotide primers bind to complementary sequences on the target.
- Can produce >10^8 copies of target sequences within hours
- Sensitive to false-positives or contamination
- Below is a list of some of the commonly available diagnostic methods and its characteristics.

Transcription-Mediated Amplification	• RNA is the target. • Makes complementary DNA (cDNA) • Utilizes two enzymes: reverse transcriptase with RNAse H activity and RNA polymerase • Products are chemiluminescent and detected by hybridization protection assay. • Gen-Probe Platform for HIV/HCV assay
Nucleic Acid Sequence–Based Amplification	• RNA is the target. • Makes complementary DNA (cDNA) • Utilizes three enzymes: reverse transcriptase, RNAse H, and T7 RNA polymerase • Products are detected by electrochemiluminescent. • NASBA platform for clinical detection of retroviruses
Strand Displacement Assay (SDA)	• DNA is the target. • Uses amplification and bumper primers • Target is altered with a restriction enzyme site. • Product is a double-stranded DNA. • BD Platform for *N. gonorrhoeae* detection

Signal Amplification Techniques
- Enhanced visibility of the target
- Designed to amplify a probe signal
- Detected signal is directly proportional to the concentration of available target.
- Below is a list of some of the commonly available diagnostic methods and its characteristics.

Branched Chain DNA	• RNA is the target and hybridizes to immobilized probes. • Utilizes extender probes and preamplifiers • No DNA synthesis and amplification to avoid carry-over contamination • Chemiluminescent detection with alkaline phosphatase system • HCV viral load detection
Hybrid Capture Method	• Target DNA is hybridized with complementary RNA probe. • Antibody-based capture of DNA/RNA hybrids • Chemiluminescent detection with alkaline phosphatase system • Detection of human papillomavirus

Gene rearrangement studies by Southern blot are helpful to distinguish between T- and B-lymphocyte lineage.[38] Also, the chromosome translocation associated with most follicular, non-Hodgkin's lymphomas and certain diffuse, large-cell lymphomas has been detected and monitored. The Philadelphia chromosome in chronic myelogenous leukemia is associated with the translocation that results in the detection of the *bcr/abl* fusion gene.[39] Other mutations associated with hematologic and solid tumors are being described daily.

Prenatal diagnosis of genetic diseases such as sickle cell anemia, cystic fibrosis,[40] Huntington's chorea,[41] Duchenne-type muscular dystrophy,[42] and von Willebrand's disease[43] has been made possible using probe technology. In addition, the carrier status in Duchenne-type muscular dystrophy and von Willebrand's disease can be determined.

PCR has been used to detect major histocompatibility complex class I and class II polymorphism.[44] The increased accuracy of detecting differences in the genes, rather than the gene product, has been used to improve transplant compatibility.

Recent developments in microfluidics is advancing the molecular diagnostic techniques from laboratory to point of care testing requiring microchip-based platform and integrated sample processing and detection. While it is difficult to miniaturize, all the steps required in an isothermal PCR detection method requiring at least a source of heat one-step assays have been introduced by GeneXpert, Enigma Diagnostics, DxNA, Spartan RX platform, and Iquum analyzers. These are single-step assays still requiring small portable instruments with on-demand individual cartridge-based STAT assays for infectious diseases and mutations. The turnaround time of diagnosis in these instruments is from 20 to 70 minutes.

questions

1. True or False? Molecular arrays typically contain a single probe for high-throughput analysis of gene expression or determination of mutations in patient samples.

2. Which of the following is LEAST likely to affect the purification of genomic DNA for analysis in molecular methods?
   a. Sample volume required for hybridization
   b. Size of the nucleic acid to be isolated
   c. Presence of RNA in the sample
   d. Presence of protein in the sample
   e. Presence of deoxyribose

3. Why is it important to add RNase to the patient sample when isolating genomic DNA?
   a. RNase serves as an enzymatic tag on DNA probes.
   b. RNase will remove excess collagen from the patient sample.
   c. RNase will transport the amino acid to the ribosome, where the peptide chain elongates.
   d. RNase clones DNA to RNA.
   e. RNase digests RNA in the patient sample that could copurify with genomic DNA.

4. All of the following describe a nucleic acid probe except:
   a. Short strand of DNA of a known sequence
   b. Short strand of RNA of a known sequence
   c. Can be cloned in bacteria
   d. Can be inserted into a plasmid vector
   e. Can be labeled with avidin

5. Of the following, which is a common example of solid support hybridization?
   a. Southern blot

b. Chemiluminescence
c. Hybridization protection assay
d. Digene Hybrid Capture 2
e. In situ hybridization

6. When sequencing DNA, _____ stops DNA synthesis in polymerase chain reaction amplification.
   a. Dideoxynucleotides
   b. DNA polymerase
   c. Insertion of thymine
   d. 3'-OH group
   e. Pyrophosphates

7. One of the most common clinical applications for identifying SNPs in patients is:
   a. SNPs have been useful in optimizing the treatment of HIV.
   b. SNPs have been useful in diagnosing metabolic syndrome.
   c. SNPs have been used to facilitate transcription-mediated amplification.
   d. Currently, there are no clinical applications for the identification of SNPs as these are silent and have no apparent function.
   e. SNPs are added to the patient sample during polymerase amplification reactions to create the complimentary nucleic acid sequence.

8. The development of "real-time" PCR was driven by:
   a. Learning that Taq polymerase that has 5'- to 3' exonuclease activity
   b. The development of a dot blot hybridization methods
   c. The development of chain ligase reaction
   d. The ability to volatilize a sample in a nebulizer
   e. The development of scorpion primers

references

1. Buckingham L. *Molecular Diagnostics: Fundamentals, Methods and Clinical Applications.* 2nd ed. Philadelphia, PA: F.A. Davis and Company; 2012.
2. Ronaghi M. Pyrosequencing sheds light on DNA sequencing. *Genome Res.* 2001;11:3–11.
3. Parslow TG. Molecular genetic techniques for clinical analysis of the immune system. In: Stites DP, Terr AI, Parslow TG, eds. *Medical Immunology.* 9th ed. Stamford, CT: Appleton & Lange; 1997:309–318.
4. Podzorski RP. Molecular methods. In: Detrick B, Hamilton RG, Folds JD, et al., eds. *Manual of Molecular and Clinical Laboratory Immunology.* 7th ed. Washington, DC: American Society for Microbiology; 2006:26–52.

5. Lo DYM, Chiu RWK. Principles of molecular biology. In: Burtis CA, Ashwood ER, Bruns DE, eds. *Tietz Textbook of Clinical Chemistry and Molecular Diagnostics.* 4th ed. St. Louis, MO: Elsevier Saunders; 2006:1393–1406.
6. Southern EM. Detection of specific sequences among DNA fragments separated by gel electrophoresis. *J Mol Biol.* 1975;98:503.
7. Saiki RK, Scharf S, Faloona F, et al. Enzymatic amplification of beta-globulin genomic sequences and restriction site analysis for diagnosis of sickle cell anemia. *Science.* 1985;230:1350–1354.
8. Tenover FC, Unger ER. Nucleic acid probes for detection and identification of infectious agents. In: Persing DH, Smith TF,

Tenover FC, et al., eds. *Diagnostic Molecular Microbiology: Principles and Applications.* Washington, DC: American Society for Microbiology; 1993:3–25.

9. Hansen CA. Clinical applications of molecular biology in diagnostic hematology. *Lab Med.* 1993;24:562.

10. Unger ER, Piper MA. Molecular diagnostics: basic principles and techniques. In: Henry JB, ed. *Clinical Diagnosis and Management by Laboratory Methods.* 20th ed. Philadelphia, PA: WB Saunders; 2001:1275–1295.

11. Hankin RC. In situ hybridization: principles and applications. *Lab Med.* 1992;23:764.

12. Sanger F, Nicklen S, Coulson AR. DNA sequencing with chain terminating inhibitors. *Proc Natl Acad Sci U S A.* 1977;74:5463.

13. Friedrich MJ. New chip on the block. *Lab Med.* 1996;30:180.

14. Check W. Clinical microbiology eyes nucleic acid-based technologies. *ASM News.* 1998;64:84.

15. Vahey M, Nau ME, Barrick S, et al. Performance of the Affymetrix GeneChip HIV PRT 440 platform for antiretroviral drug resistance genotyping of human immunodeficiency virus type 1 clades and viral isolates with length polymorphisms. *J Clin Microbiol.* 1999;37:2533.

16. Forbes BA, Sahm DF, Weissfeld AS. *Bailey and Scott's Diagnostic Microbiology.* 10th ed. St. Louis, MO: Mosby; 1998:188–207.

17. Mullis KB, Faloona FA. Specific synthesis of DNA in vitro via a polymerase-catalyzed chain reaction. *Methods Enzymol.* 1987;155:335.

18. Mullis KB. The unusual origin of the polymerase chain reaction. *Sci Am.* 1990;262:56.

19. Foy CA, Parkes HC. Emerging homogenous DNA-based technologies in the clinical laboratory. *Clin Chem.* 2001;47:990.

20. Holland PA, Abramson RD, Watson R, et al. Detection of specific polymerase chain reaction by utilizing the 5′ to 3′ exonuclease activity of *Thermus aquaticus* DNA polymerase. *Proc Natl Acad Sci U S A.* 1991;88:7276.

21. Szollosi J, Damjanovich S, Matyus L. Application of fluorescence resonance energy transfer in the clinical laboratory: routine and research. *Cytometry.* 1998;15:159.

22. Livak K, Flood S, Marmaro J, et al. Oligonucleotides with fluorescent dyes at opposite ends provide a quenched probe system useful for detecting PCR product and nucleic acid hybridization. *PCR Methods Appl.* 1995;4:357.

23. Tyagi S, Kramer F. Molecular beacons: probes that fluoresce upon hybridization. *Nat Biotechnol.* 1996;14:303.

24. Whicombe D, Theaker J, Guy S, et al. Detection of PCR products using self-probing amplicons and fluorescence. *Nat Biotechnol.* 1999;17:804.

25. Coleman WB, Tsongalis GJ. *Molecular Diagnostics for the Clinical Laboratorian.* 2nd ed. Totowa, NJ: Humana Press; 2006.

26. Guatelli JC, Whitfield KM, Kwoh DY, et al. Isothermal in vitro amplification of nucleic acids by a multienzyme reaction modeled after retroviral replication. *Proc Natl Acad Sci U S A.* 1990;87:1874.

27. Fahy E, Kwoh DY, Gingeras TR. Self-sustained sequence replication (3SR): an isothermal transcription-based amplification system alternative to PCR. *PCR Methods Appl.* 1991;1:25.

28. Kwoh DY, Davis GR, Whitfield KM, et al. Transcription-based amplification system and detection of amplified human immunodeficiency virus type 1 with a bead-based sandwich hybridization format. *Proc Natl Acad Sci U S A.* 1989;86:1173–1177.

29. Little MC, Andrews J, Moore R, et al. Strand displacement amplification and homogenous real-time detection incorporated in a second-generation DNA probe system, BDProbe TecET. *Clin Chem.* 1999;45:777–784.

30. Walker G, Fraiser M, Schram J, et al. Strand displacement amplification: an isothermal in vitro DNA amplification technique. *Nucleic Acids Res.* 1992;20:1691–1696.

31. BD ProbeTec™ ET System. http://www.bd.com/ds/product-Center/MD-ProbetecEt.asp. Accessed July 31, 2012.

32. Barany F. Genetic disease detection and DNA amplification using cloned thermostable ligase. *Proc Natl Acad Sci U S A.* 1991;88:189.

33. Wiedbrauk DL. Molecular methods for virus detection. *Lab Med.* 1992;23:737.

34. Persing DH. In vitro nucleic acid amplification techniques. In: Persing DH, Smith TF, Tenover FC, et al., eds. *Diagnostic Molecular Microbiology: Principles and Applications.* Washington, DC: American Society for Microbiology; 1993:51–87.

35. Mitchell PS, Persing DH. Current trends in molecular microbiology. *Lab Med.* 1999;30:263.

36. Zein NN. Clinical significance of hepatitis C virus genotypes. *Clin Microbiol Rev.* 2000;13:223–235.

37. Ferreira-Gonzalez A, Versalovic J, Habecbu S, et al. Molecular methods in diagnosis and monitoring of infectious diseases. In: Bruns DE, Ashwood ER, Burtis CA, eds. *Fundamentals of Molecular Diagnostics.* St. Louis, MO: Saunders Elsevier; 2007:171–196.

38. Farkas DH. The Southern blot: application to the B- and T-cell gene rearrangement test. *Lab Med.* 1992;23:723.

39. Ni H, Blajchman MA. Understanding the polymerase chain reaction. *Transfus Med Rev.* 1994;8:242.

40. Gasparini P, Novelli G, Savoia A, et al. First-trimester prenatal diagnosis of cystic fibrosis using the polymerase chain reaction: report of eight cases. *Prenat Diagn.* 1989;9:349.

41. Thies U, Zuhlke C, Bockel B, et al. Prenatal diagnosis of Huntington's disease (HD): experience with six cases and PCR. *Prenat Diagn.* 1992;12:1055.

42. Clemens PR, Fenwick RG, Chamberlain JS, et al. Carrier detection and prenatal diagnosis in Duchenne and Becker muscular dystrophy families, using dinucleotide repeat polymorphism. *Am J Hum Genet.* 1991;49:951.

43. Peake IR, Bowen D, Bignell P. Family studies and prenatal diagnosis in severe von Willebrand disease by polymerase chain reaction amplification of variable number tandem repeat region of the von Willebrand factor gene. *Blood.* 1990;76:555.

44. Erlich H, Tugawan T, Begovich AB, et al. HLA-DR, DQ, and DP typing using PCR amplification and immobilized probes. *Eur J Immunogenet.* 1991;18:33.

10

Point-of-Care Testing

HEATHER CROOKSTON

chapter outline

key terms

chapter objectives

Upon completion of this chapter, the clinical laboratorian should be able to do the following:

- Define point-of-care testing (POCT).
- Explain what basic structure is required to manage a POCT program.
- Explain the nuts and bolts process of implementing a POC test.
- State the basic principles behind common POC applications.

For additional student resources, please visit thePoint®
at http://thepoint.lww.com

INTRODUCTION

Point-of-care testing (POCT) is defined as "those analytical patient-testing activities provided within the institution, but performed outside the physical facilities of the clinical laboratories."[1] POCT is also known by many names including "near-patient testing,"[2] "extra-laboratory analyses,"[3] "ancillary testing," "bedside testing,"[4] "physician's office testing,"[5] and "alternative site testing." A convenience for the patient and physician, POCT brings the laboratory to the patient. POCT is increasingly being used not only in the emergency department, operating rooms, and intensive care units (ICUs) but also in the clinics, physician offices, nursing homes, pediatric units, pharmacies, counseling centers, and ambulances. Advances in medical, analytical, and engineering technologies in the last two decades led to the appearance of a large number of portable measurement devices for a variety of the different analytes. These include tests for electrolytes, glucose, hemoglobin A1c, urinalysis, pregnancy, drugs of abuse, therapeutic drug monitoring, occult blood, blood gases, coagulation tests, enzymes, and cardiac markers. POCT is also available for infectious diseases such as HIV, gonorrhea, syphilis, streptococcus, influenza, fungal infections, and tuberculosis.

POCT offers several advantages compared with central laboratory testing (Table 10.1). The major advantage of POCT is faster delivery of results. POCT is designed to work with the flow of patient management and care, allowing physicians to order and perform the test and immediately make a medical decision.

Smaller sample volume allows POCT use in neonatal and pediatric population and is preferred for those undersized patients requiring frequent testing. The overall cost of patient care is arguably smaller due to improved patient workflows. Testing near the patient requires fewer steps than transporting a specimen to the laboratory, processing, aliquoting, testing, and communicating results back to clinical staff, all of which may reduce preanalytical and postanalytical laboratory-related errors. Portability of POCT allows for increased access to testing in a wider variety of sites, for example, rural areas, accident sites, areas with limited infrastructure and personnel, and locations with underserved populations. One example of the latter is the

TABLE 10.1 Potential Advantages and Disadvantages of POCT[a]

Advantages	Disadvantages
Convenience for both the attending physician/nurse and patient	POCT is significantly more expensive than the cost of central laboratory testing due to the higher disposable and reagent costs of the POCT analyzers
Reduced turnaround time for test results to expedite medical decision making in operating rooms, emergency department, and intensive care units	Maintenance of quality control and quality assurance is difficult as anyone can run the analysis, in the absence of operator lockout
Reduction in clinic visits, hospital admissions, and length of hospital stay due to faster laboratory services	Management of POCT is challenging—there are numerous operators to train, multiple sites to manage, and hundreds of POC tests to validate
Better patient management due to improved visibility and interaction with a patient	Preanalytic, analytic, and postanalytic issues are not recognized easily as tests are performed by nonlaboratory individuals
Decreased manpower needs associated with test requesting and reporting, especially for patients necessitating tests several times a day (e.g., glucose determination)	Interindividual variability in POCT results may be greater when compared with central laboratory testing
Fingerstick POCT is less traumatic for a patient as smaller sample volume is required	Difficulties with documentation of test results, billing, and regulatory compliance
Reduced risk of preanalytical errors due to absence of transporting a specimen to a core laboratory, processing, aliquoting, testing, and communicating results back to clinical staff. Reduced risk of sample deterioration	Proper integration of test result into the patient's electronic medical record may be more difficult if tested on a device that does not automatically interface
Improved patient outcome	
Improved cost of overall patient care	Managing reagent supply and storage at multiple sites can be problematic
	Central laboratory test results and POCT results are not always comparable due to differences in specimen types, technology, interfering substances, etc
Wide menu of POC analytes for specimens that do not require processing	
Availability to a wider variety of sites (e.g., rural areas, areas with limited infrastructure/personnel, and sites with underserved populations)	

[a]POCT, point-of-care testing.

use of a portable POCT to test for tuberculosis in the risk populations in low-income countries.[6]

Although POCT offers many advantages, there are some negative aspects of POCT (Table 10.1). On a cost per test basis, POCT is more expensive than the cost of central laboratory testing as a result of the higher disposable and reagent costs of the POCT analyzers. End users may be able to counterbalance these increased costs by gaining efficiencies in improved patient workflows and increased patient satisfaction. Additionally, quality of results is a concern because POCT is usually performed by nonlaboratory personnel who may include nurses, physicians, emergency medical technicians, pharmacists, medics, patients, and medical office assistants. End users with multiple responsibilities and limited laboratory training may not appreciate the value of laboratory quality control (QC) in ensuring quality test results.

LABORATORY REGULATIONS

Accreditation

In the United States, laboratory testing for patient care (with limited exceptions) requires a Clinical Laboratory Improvement Amendments (CLIA) certificate. CLIA was enacted by Congress and established quality standards for all laboratory testing, thereby ensuring the accuracy, reliability, and timeliness of patient test results regardless of where the test was performed.[7] The requirements are based on the complexity of the test and not the type of laboratory where the testing is performed (POC or central laboratory). All laboratories performing POCT must be certified under one of the five types of CLIA certificates listed in Table 10.2. The CLIA certificate must be appropriate for the testing that is performed in the laboratory (i.e., appropriate complexity). In addition to the federal program, state departments of public health or public organizations may apply for "deemed" status, which allows these organizations to perform laboratory accreditation and inspections.

POCT Complexity

Tests are classified based on their complexity. The Food and Drug Administration (FDA) uses several criteria to assign complexity to any test, and the three categories are "waived" tests, **moderate-complexity tests**, and **high-complexity tests. Waived tests** are a category of tests defined by CLIA, such as dipstick tests, urine pregnancy tests, and blood glucose monitoring devices, which are subject to the lowest level of regulation and are cleared by the FDA for home uses. They employ methodologies that are so simple and accurate as to render the likelihood of erroneous results negligible and pose almost no risk of harm to the patient if the test is performed incorrectly. A full list of currently waived tests can be found on the FDA website (http://www.accessdata.fda.gov/scripts/cdrh/cfdocs/cfClia/testswaived.cfm). Laboratories performing nonwaived tests (moderate-complexity tests and high-complexity tests) must fulfill all the requirements for personnel qualifications, proficiency testing and inspections, quality assurance and QCs, and patient test management.

The fourth category of POCT is *provider-performed microscopy procedures*, or *PPMPs*, which is a subcategory of moderate-complexity testing. These tests involve the use of a microscope, limited to bright-field or phase-contrast microscopy. Generally, the specimens are labile and cannot survive transport to a clinical laboratory. Only licensed physicians, dentists, and midlevel practitioners may perform PPMP. There are usually no QC materials available for PPMP; however, the individual performing PPMP endures the certification process and participates in proficiency testing.

To determine to which category POC test or procedure belongs, refer to the following searchable and continuously renewable FDA-approved test menu: http://www.accessdata.fda.gov/scripts/cdrh/cfdocs/cfClia/search.cfm.

IMPLEMENTATION

Establishing Need

When establishing a POCT site, the approach and steps in the implementation will be different in nearly every case insofar as organizational culture, and the financial situation of any given institution may vary greatly. However, there

TABLE 10.2	**Types of CLIA Certificates**[a]
Certificate of Waiver	Issued to a laboratory to perform only waived tests
Certificate of Registration	Issued to a laboratory that enables the entity to conduct moderate- or high-complexity laboratory testing or both until the entity is determined by survey to be in compliance with CLIA regulations
Certificate for PPMPs	Issued to a laboratory in which a physician, midlevel practitioner, or dentist performs no tests other than the microscopy procedures
	Permits the laboratory to also perform waived tests
Certificate of Compliance	Issued to a laboratory after an inspection that finds the laboratory to be in compliance with all applicable CLIA requirements
Certificate of Accreditation	Issued to a laboratory on the basis of the laboratory's accreditation by an accreditation organization approved by the Health Care Finance Administration

CLIA, Clinical Laboratory Improvement Amendments; POCT, point-of-care testing; PPMP, provider-performed microscopy procedure.
[a]Clinical Laboratory Improvement Act. How to Obtain a CLIA Certificate of Waiver, http://www.cms.gov/Regulations-and-Guidance/Legislation/CLIA/downloads//howobtaincertificateofwaiver.pdf

BOX 10.1 Questions to Ask When Implementing POCT

- Which test is required and in which specific area? How is the service currently provided, and is this a means to resolve a problem?
- What is the expected annual test volume?
- What clinical question is being asked when requesting this test?
- What clinical decision is likely to be made and action to be taken upon receipt of the result?
- How will POCT increase patient satisfaction?
- Are personnel competent to perform the POCT? Are facilities available to perform the test and store equipment, reagents, and documentation?

- Will a change in practice be required?
- Can central laboratory deliver the required service? How do POCT cost, reference ranges, accuracy, and precision compare to similar tests in a laboratory?
- Are available POCT analyzers user friendly? Can POCT analyzers interface with an LIS and a patient electronic medical record?
- Are both internal and external QC materials available?
- Does the company providing POCT analyzers and reagents offer a reliable support service?

are some common guidelines to implementation that apply to nearly every case. Support of the organization must be present to evaluate the requests for POCT. Typically, a multidisciplinary committee consisting of laboratory staff, physicians, nursing representatives, and hospital/laboratory administration is formed to create a structure for receiving and establishing criteria for approving requests for POCT. Before implementing a POCT service, an interdisciplinary committee should address the questions similar to those listed in Box 10.1. The decision to establish POCT program is made after justifying the clinical need, cost comparisons, and the analytic performance requirements. Other factors should also be considered, including space, any previous track record of regulatory compliance, personnel who will be performing the testing, and metrics to determine if the POCT implementation is successful.

POCT Implementation Protocol

After making the decision to implement POCT, the responsible party selects the method of choice and begins validation. Desirable characteristics of POCT analyzers include ease of use, method accuracy and comparability to the main laboratory method, portability, durability, low maintenance, simple QC, QC lockout features, simple sample handling requirements, bar code patient and operator identification capabilities, and the ability to interface with a laboratory information system (LIS). The manufacturer should aid in providing minimum acceptability requirements, instrument manuals, package inserts for reagents and QCs, materials safety data sheet, and training materials. The manufacture also typically assists with instrumentation setup and validation studies. Method validation should confirm the manufacturer's specifications, and a *procedure/ policy* should be written for each test. This should not be simply a collection of materials obtained from a manufacturer; rather, these documents should aid in the development of an easy-to-follow, simple, and concise procedure. The procedure should include information on the principle of the method; personnel qualifications; specimen, reagents, supplies, and equipment requirements; QC and calibrations; patient-testing procedure; reference ranges;

reporting limits; and interfering substances if applicable. All required regulatory or certifying standards should be in place prior to initiating patient testing (Box 10.2).

Personnel Requirements

For a POC program with moderate-complexity tests, unlike for those POC programs with Certificate of Waiver or certificate for PPMP, institutions are required to have a certain organizational and administrative structure where staff has established qualifications, competency, and experience. The *director of laboratory* is usually a Ph.D. scientist, or a physician with at least 1 year of experience directing a laboratory with 20 continuing medical education credits,[8] or a person with a bachelor's degree with 2 years' laboratory experience plus 2 years of supervising experience. Responsibilities of a director are very broad and include policy making, ensuring compliance with regulatory standards, and administrative duties. Importantly, the director is responsible for the analytic performance of all tests. The director must make technical decisions based on a constant monitoring of ongoing proficiency, accuracy, and precision. Such individuals should be a liaison between the clinicians, hospital administration, and laboratory personnel.

Each laboratory performing moderate-complexity tests must have a technical and a clinical consultant. The *technical consultant* is responsible for scientific oversight of the POCT, while the *clinical consultant* is required to provide clinical and medical advice. The director of a POCT program, the technical consultant, and the clinical consultant may be the same person.

Even though the implementation of the POCT program may be done differently depending on an institution, the entity responsible for quality management of the POCT program is always the laboratory. It is useful, therefore, for a laboratory to have a person supervising the POCT program, so a *POCT coordinator (POCC)* fulfills this role. The POCC monitors day-to-day activities of *testing personnel*, and it is the responsibility of the POCC to coordinate POC patient testing and facilitate compliance with procedures and policies and regulatory requirements. The POCC develops a training program for testing personnel and

BOX 10.2 Point-of-Care Checklist

1. *Quality management*

   The POC program has a written QM program as well as organizational system setting forth levels of authority, responsibility, and accountability. There is a documented system to address unusual patient results or instrument troubleshooting. There is a written procedure for each POCT.

2. *Specimen handling*

   There is a documented procedure describing methods for patient identification and preparation, as well as for specimen collection, accessioning, and preservation before testing. There is a procedure for entering POCT results into the permanent medical record of a patient. Reference intervals should be established.

3. *Reagents*

   All reagents should be stored and labeled as recommended by the manufacturer.

4. *Instruments and equipment*

   Equipment must be evaluated and scheduled for a regular maintenance, as required by the manufacturer.

5. *Personnel*

   The director of the POCT program is a physician or a doctoral scientist. The testing personnel have adequate, specific training to ensure competence, and this must be documented.

6. *Quality Control and Calibration*

   Calibrations and quality controls are run at regular intervals (at least daily). Acceptable limits are defined for control procedures, and there are documented corrective actions when control results exceed defined acceptability limits. Upper and lower limits of the analytical measurement range (AMR) for each analyte are defined.

7. *Safety*

   There is a program to assure that the safety of patients and health care personnel is not compromised by POCT.

Adapted from the College of American Pathologists Point-of-Care-Testing Checklist 01.04.2012 (http://www.cap.org).

ensures documentation of competency training. The POCC also oversees completion of proficiency testing programs, performs on-site review of patient testing, QC, and maintenance logs and reports problems and regulatory noncompliance to appropriate management personnel.

Even though the laboratory is responsible for the POCT policies and procedures, it is the clinical staff that does the actual testing. Fostering a partnership between the operators and laboratory will help solve problems that may arise during the testing process. In this decentralized testing model, the specifics of how training is performed, how competency records are maintained, and how reagents are ordered may be different for each institution. The laboratory should monitor POC areas and ensure consistent feedback is provided regarding compliance with any applicable regulations. However, before any testing is initiated, clarifying individual roles and expectations is key to the success of the program.

QUALITY MANAGEMENT

Accuracy Requirements

Understanding how accurate the results need to be in the context of how the test will be used clinically is important before any patient testing is initiated. Ideally, a POC test will provide equivalent results with those from the central laboratory. If this were the case, depending on a clinical situation, physicians would have an option to choose either test and achieve the same clinical outcome. Unfortunately, despite the ongoing harmonization and **standardization** efforts, currently, there are still accuracy and imprecision concerns with some POCT. One example is the ongoing accuracy and precision problems with glucose meters.

Authors of one study applied simulation modeling to relate performance characteristics of glucose analyzers to error rates in insulin dosage.[9] Interestingly, glucose meters that met existing POCT quality specifications allowed a large fraction of administered insulin doses to differ from the intended doses. In addition, two landmark studies on tight glycemic controls gave completely different outcomes.[10,11] While one study showed that tight glycemic controls and the following intensive insulin therapy reduce morbidity and mortality among critically ill patients in the surgical ICU,[10] authors of another study found that intensive glucose control increased mortality among adults in the ICU.[11] There has been a considerable debate in the laboratory medicine literature that the difference in these two studies' outcome was due to the test method.[12–14] Due to complaints about glucose meter inaccuracy, the FDA is currently developing new standards for glucose meter accuracy.

QC and Proficiency Testing

The purpose of a quality management program is to ensure quality test results. A thorough validation should verify the analytical performance and any applicable limitations with the assay. Ongoing daily QC will alert the operator to any reagent or instrument issues. Some devices have both internal and external QC, both of which have distinctly different roles. Internal QC, which is also referred to as onboard QC, internal checks, electronic QC, or intelligent QC,[15] is performed at specific time intervals or at least daily. Internal QC ensures the electronics of the device are performing as expected or, if a manual test, the integrity of the specific test system. Some instruments automate QC and/or calibration, which is helpful for regulatory compliance. This also ensures the instrument is ready to perform quality testing at all times. Another important feature is to tie QC performance requirements to test availability. If QC has not been performed as required and is unsatisfactory, the instrument does not allow patient testing until corrective action has taken place. This is known as QC lockout.

The entire testing process should be checked periodically according to the manufacturer and regulatory requirements by running an external QC. Here, a control sample is introduced to the test system in the same manner as a patient sample. Another form of external QC is proficiency testing, where blind samples are sent to participating laboratories to perform testing. In the United States, results from one laboratory are compared with the results from the laboratories using the same method (peer group).

Quality management programs also need to ensure that the operators are competent to perform testing. After initial training, ongoing assessment of their performance is required. This is commonly called the recertification process. Careful control of personnel records is an important part of the quality management program and may be managed at the POCT site or directly by the laboratory. Some POCT programs will allow "super users" (supervisors, managers, or POCC) to track training renewal dates and to lockout operators whose training has expired.

The greatest source of error in POCT is the preanalytical error. While the above features are necessary for any POCT program, it is more difficult to identify errors arising from poor specimen, for example, sample contamination, dilution, circulating interference (lipemia, icterus, and hemolysis), and proper specimen source (arterial, venous, and fingerstick). For this reason, careful assessment of an area's compliance in proper specimen collection and handling is needed prior to implementing testing.

Preventing postanalytic errors in reporting can be achieved more reliably with **connectivity**. With the aid of bar codes, modern technology has improved patient identification and decreased transcription errors in many health care applications. However, linear bar code identification methods are not fail-safe.[16] Hospitals should work with laboratories, pharmacy, radiology, and admissions to standardize scanning and printing specifications across a system. Careful control and tight specifications of bar code scanning and printing equipment will minimize the misidentification threat to patient safety.

Total-system POCT quality assurance is thus the combination of several QC mechanisms:

- A mechanism to perform a thorough systems validation
- Reliable, user-friendly POCT device
- Training of POCT operators
- Competency assessment of all individuals involved in POCT
- QC testing and monitoring
- Proficiency testing
- Connectivity and bar-coding technologies

POC APPLICATIONS

POCT makes up nearly 30% of the total in vitro diagnostics market in the United States.[17] A wide variety of POCT devices can be loosely classified into a single-use system, handheld device, benchtop device, or the wearable device (Box 10.3). POCT devices are designed with a consideration for the operators who may have little to no laboratory training. Handheld devices are getting smaller and more ergonomic with every generation. A variety of analytical principles used in a laboratory have also been implemented in POCT devices, including the following:

- Reflectance
- Electrochemistry, electrical impedance
- Light scattering/optical motion
- Immunoturbidimetry
- Lateral flow, flow-through, or solid phase immunoassays
- Spectrophotometry, multiwavelength spectrophotometry
- Fluorescence, time-resolved fluorescence
- Polymerase chain reaction

Contemporary POCT analyzers are capable of delivering test results in less than a minute using a single-step protocol

---

BOX 10.3 Types of POCT Analyzers

1. Single-use, qualitative, or semiquantitative cartridge/strip tests
   - Urine and blood chemistry
   - Infectious disease agents, cardiac markers, hCG

2. Single-use quantitative cartridge/strip tests with a reader device
   - Glucose
   - Blood chemistry
   - Coagulation
   - Cardiac markers, drugs, C-reactive protein (CRP), allergy, fertility tests

- *Chlamydia*
- HbA1c, urine albumin
- Blood chemistry
- pH, blood gases, electrolytes, metabolites

3. Multiple-use quantitative cartridge/benchtop devices
   - Hemoglobin species, bilirubin
   - pH, blood gases, electrolytes, metabolites
   - Cardiac markers, drugs, CRP
   - Complete blood count

Modified from the *Tietz Textbook of Clinical Chemistry and Molecular Diagnostics.* 5th ed. Table 20-1.

on a variety of unprocessed specimens such as whole blood, cerebrospinal fluid, urine, and stool specimens. Ideally, the results of POCT should meet the analytical specifications that are "fit-for-purpose" and should be comparable to those of the central laboratory.

Glucose testing is the highest volume POCT. These are devices with single-use cartridges or strips that use the reflectance or electrochemistry analytical principles for glucose measurement. Hemoglobin A1c testing is also rapidly increasing, although we are yet to see a device that measures both glucose and hemoglobin A1c. Both of these tests should not be used for a tight glucose control at bedside but rather employed as monitoring procedures because of the cases of hypoglycemia as well as cases of erroneous POCT measurements due to interfering substances.[18,19]

Mature POCT areas employ tests for the measurements of urine and blood chemistry, coagulation testing, pH and blood gases, hemoglobin and bilirubin, and complete blood count. Other areas of POCT that are rapidly evolving are intraoperative immunoassay of parathyroid hormone, creatinine and cardiac markers in emergency departments, and infectious diseases (HIV).

INFORMATICS AND POCT

Capturing patient ID, operator ID, reference range, and the result documentation in the permanent record can be challenging without connectivity. Due to the number of interfaces that would be required, POCT analyzers are usually connected with LIS via a docking station and/or data management (DM) system that can connect to multiple POCT devices from different manufacturers through a single interface connection to the LIS/hospital information system (HIS) for all data transmissions. This creates an additional step to entering test result into LIS and later to the patient medical record.

With a multitude of POCT devices, it is not practical to have a separate device–LIS interfacing system for each device. Accordingly, the Connectivity Industry Consortium (CIC) represented by more than 30 instrument manufacturers, information technology companies, and end users has developed a set of standards to ensure POCT device bidirectionality, device connection commonality, commercial software intraoperability and security, and regulatory compliance. The developed standards govern the communication between the POCT devices and the DM as well as the actual interface between the DM and the LIS. The standards have been adopted by the

National Committee for Clinical Laboratory Standards (now the Clinical and Laboratory Standards Institute or CLSI).[20,21] Prior to the CIC, each vendor developed its own proprietary means of communicating data from POCT devices, with different physical connections, the wiring, and even the language and communication format or protocol. Nowadays, the CIS standards are becoming widely accepted by vendors and by users who necessitate a more universal POCT connectivity.

According to the CLSI guidelines,[21] certain patient information should always accompany the patient test result across the POCT device, the DM, the LIS, and the medical records. These include:

- Patient, sample, operator, and device identifiers
- Date and time of specimen collection and analysis
- Type of specimen
- Test requested and test result with appropriate units
- Error messages and action messages

These obligatory information items might also be accompanied by additional information such as reference intervals, calibrator/reagent/QC detail (e.g., lot number and expiration date), and specific comments and alerts.

In the course of selecting a POCT device, consideration must be given to the type of data output a POCT device provides. These include visual readings, printers, display screens, Ethernet and RS232 ports, modems, infrared beams, and radio signals. Preference is usually given to a device that is suitable for an already developed POCT connectivity system of an institution, which also makes the training of operators easier. Additionally, the connectivity communication system between a device and the DM can be unidirectional (one-way) or bidirectional (two-way). One-way connectivity allows the DM to only read information from the POCT device, while the two-way connectivity also lets the DM to upload data to the POCT devices. This is especially helpful in the POC system with multiple devices insofar as the DM can update information (e.g., lists of valid operators, reagent lot information, and patient information) for all POCT devices simultaneously.

Integration of POCT results with LIS and medical records allows for better management of such diseases as diabetes mellitus and hyperlipidemia and also in critical situations such as glycemic control in intensive care, management of heart failure, and assistance with dosing of anticoagulants. In these particular instances, the wireless connectivity of POCT devices in conjunction with docking stations is in great demand.

For additional student resources, please visit the**Point** at http://thepoint.lww.com

questions

1. A CLIA waived test requires that operators
   a. Must follow manufacturer's instructions
   b. Must have annual competence assessment
   c. Must perform proficiency testing
   d. Must perform QC daily

2. Quality control lockout
   a. Prevents quality control from being recorded when outside 2 standard deviations
   b. Prevents testing when quality control has not been performed
   c. Prevents operators from changing quality control records
   d. Prevents the wrong quality control material to be used for a particular test

3. EQC per CLIA means
   a. Equivalent
   b. Electronic
   c. External
   d. Essential

4. For laboratories with a provider-performed microscopy procedure CLIA certificate, which of the following would NOT be approved?
   a. Urinalysis
   b. Semen analysis
   c. Hematology differential
   d. Wet prep

5. Connectivity for POCT provides the ability to
   a. Charge meters at docking stations on the hospital units
   b. Accept barcode patient identification
   c. Perform electronic quality control
   d. Transmit patient results to the medical record
   e. Prevent password sharing for operator identification

6. Which of the following specimens is NOT used for a waived POC test?
   a. Urine
   b. Whole blood
   c. Plasma
   d. Eye fluid

7. Competency for nonwaived testing
   a. Is required for the CLIA director
   b. Is NOT required for physicians in their specialty
   c. Should be performed and documented annually for all operators
   d. Should be performed and documented initially after 6 months, then annually thereafter

references

1. CAP Commission on Laboratory Accreditation, Laboratory Accreditation Program. *Point-of-Care Testing Checklist*. Northfield, IL: CAP; April 2012.
2. Crook M. *Handbook of Near-Patient Testing*. London, UK: Greenwich Medical Media Limited; 1999:1–116.
3. Price CP. Quality assurance of extra-laboratory analyses. In: Marks V, Alberti KG, eds. *Clinical Biochemistry Nearer the Patient II*. London, UK: Bailliere Tindall; 1987:166–178.
4. Oliver G. *On Bedside Testing*. London, UK: HK Lewis; 1884:1–128.
5. Mass D. Consulting to physician office laboratories. In: Snyder JR, Wilkinson DS, eds. *Management in Laboratory Medicine*. 3rd ed. New York: Lippincott; 1998: 443–450.
6. Boehme CC, Nabeta P, Hillemann D, et al. Rapid molecular detection of tuberculosis and rifampin resistance. *N Engl J Med*. 2010;363:1005–1015.
7. U.S. Department of Health and Human Services. Medicare, Medicaid and CLIA Programs. Regulations implementing the Clinical Laboratory Improvement Amendments of 1988 (CLIA): final rule. *Fed Regist*. 1992;57:7002–7186.
8. A List of CME Courses for Laboratory Directors of Moderate Complexity Laboratories: http://www.cms.gov/Regulations-and-Guidance/Legislation/CLIA/ CME_Courses_for_Laboratory_Directors_of_Moderate_Complexity_Laboratories.html. Accessed July 30, 2012.
9. Boyd JC, Bruns DE. Quality specifications for glucose meters: assessment by simulation modeling of errors in insulin dose. *Clin Chem*. 2001;47(2):209–214.
10. van den Berghe G, Wouters P, Weekers F, et al. Intensive insulin therapy in critically ill patients. *N Engl J Med*. 2001;345(19):1359–1367.
11. NICE-SUGAR Study Investigators; Finfer S, Chittock DR, et al. Intensive versus conventional glucose control in critically ill patients. *N Engl J Med*. 2009;360:1283–1297.
12. Cembrowski GS, Tran DV, Slater-MacLean L, et al. Could susceptibility to low hematocrit interference have compromised the results of the NICE-SUGAR trial? *Clin Chem*. 2010;56(7):1193–1195.
13. Mahoney JJ, Maguire P, Ellison JM, et al. Response to Cembrowski et al. regarding "Could susceptibility to low hematocrit interference have compromised the results of the NICE-SUGAR trial?". *Clin Chem*. 2010;56(10):1643; author reply 1643–1644.
14. Hoedemaekers CW, Klein Gunnewiek JM, Van der Hoeven JG. Point-of-care glucose measurement systems should be used with great caution in critically ill intensive care unit patients. *Crit Care Med*. 2010;38(1):339; author reply 339–340.

15. Gill JP, Shephard M. The conduct of quality control and quality assurance testing for POCT outside the laboratory. *Clin Biochem Rev.* 2010;31(3):85–88.

16. Snyder ML, Carter A, Jenkins K, et al. Patient mis-identification caused by errors in standard barcode technology. *Clin Chem.* 2010;56(10):1554–1560.

17. Kalorama Information Worldwide Point of Care Diagnostics. http://www.kaloramainformation.com/. Accessed July 30, 2012.

18. Hoedemaekers CW, Klein Gunnewiek JM, Prinsen MA, et al. Accuracy of bedside glucose measurement from three glucometers in critically ill patients. *Crit Care Med.* 2008;36:3062–3066.

19. Eastham JH, Mason D, Barnes DL, et al. Prevalence of interfering substances with point-of-care glucose testing in a community hospital. *Am J Health Syst Pharm.* 2009;66:167–170.

20. Clinical Laboratory Standards Institute. *Point-of-Care Connectivity: Approved Standard.* 2nd ed. CLSI Document POCT01-A2. Wayne, PA: CLSI; 2006.

21. Clinical Laboratory Standards Institute. *Implementation Guide of POCT01 for Healthcare Providers: Approved Guideline.* CLSI Document POCT02-A. Wayne, PA: CLSI; 2008.

PART two

Clinical Correlations and Analytic Procedures

chapter outline

11

Amino Acids and Proteins

TAKARA L. BLAMIRES

chapter objectives

Upon completion of this chapter, the clinical laboratorian should be able to do the following:

- Identify essential and nonessential amino acids required for protein synthesis.
- Describe the basic structure and general properties of amino acids.
- Discuss general characteristics of the following aminoacidopathies, including the metabolic defect in each and procedures commonly used for detection:
  - Phenylketonuria
  - Tyrosinemia
  - Alkaptonuria
  - Maple syrup urine disease
  - Isovaleric acidemia
  - Homocystinuria
  - Citrullinemia
  - Argininosuccinic aciduria
  - Cystinuria
- Describe the basic structure and general properties of amino acids and proteins, including both conjugated and simple proteins.
- Outline basic protein synthesis and catabolism.
- Discuss the function and clinical significance of the following proteins:
  - Prealbumin
  - Albumin
  - Myoglobin
  - Cardiac troponin
  - Brain Natriuretic Peptide
  - Fibronectin
  - Adiponectin
  - β-Trace protein
  - Cross-linked C-telopeptides
  - Cystatin C
  - Amyloid
- Discuss the function and clinical significance of the following globulins:
  - α_1-Antitrypsin
  - α_1-Fetoprotein

(continues on page 204)

key terms

Aminoacidopathies
Amino acid
Conjugated protein
Denaturation
Globulins
Hyperproteinemia
Hypoproteinemia
Isoelectric point (p*I*)
Nitrogen balance
Peptide bond
Polypeptide
Protein
Proteinuria
Simple protein

For additional student resources, please visit thePoint® at http://thepoint.lww.com

chapter objectives (continued)

- α₁-Acid glycoprotein
- α₁-Antichymotrypsin
- Inter-α-trypsin inhibitor
- Gc-globulin
- Haptoglobin
- Ceruloplasmin
- α₂-Macroglobulin
- Transferrin
- Hemopexin
- Lipoproteins
- β₂-Microglobulin
- Complement
- Fibrinogen
- C-reactive protein
- High-sensitivity C-reactive protein
- Immunoglobulin
- Discuss at least five general causes of abnormal serum or plasma protein concentrations.
- List the reference intervals for serum or plasma total protein and albumin and discuss nonpathologic factors that influence their concentrations.
- Describe common methodologies used in the analysis of total protein, albumin, and protein fractionation including structural characteristics or chemical properties that are relevant to each measurement and the clinical usage of each.
- Identify the five fractions (zones) of a serum protein electrophoresis using the routine method and identify proteins that migrate into each zone.
- Given a densitometric scan of a patient serum protein electrophoresis, correlate the pattern with associated disease states.
- Describe the principle of the methods used for both qualitative and quantitative determination and identification of urine proteins.
- Discuss the use of cerebrospinal fluid protein measurements in evaluation of diseases affecting the central nervous system.

AMINO ACIDS

Overview

Amino acids are the building blocks of proteins. The content and arrangement of amino acids in a specific protein are determined by the sequence of bases in the gene that encodes for that protein. Cellular growth, repair, and maintenance are all dependent on amino acids. The chemical properties of the amino acids in a specific protein determine its biologic activity.[1] Proteins catalyze almost all reactions in living cells, controlling virtually all cellular processes.

Basic Structure

A single amino acid contains at least one amino group and one carboxyl functional group. The N-terminal end of the amino group (–NH₂) and the C-terminal end of the carboxyl group (–COOH) are bonded to the α-carbon forming an amino acid. The basic structure of an amino acid is depicted in Figure 11.1. Amino acids differ from one another by the chemical composition of their R group (side chains). The R groups found on the 20 different amino acids used in building proteins are shown in Table 11.1. The amino group of one amino acid can be linked with the carboxyl group of another amino acid forming a **peptide bond** (Fig. 11.2). When a chain of amino acids is linked by peptide bonds, it is known as a **polypeptide**, and a large polypeptide constitutes a **protein**. Proteins found in human serum range from 100 to 150 amino acids in the length of their polypeptide chains.

FIGURE 11.1 General structure of an α-amino acid.

TABLE 11.1   **Amino Acids Required in the Synthesis of Proteins**

Amino Acid	R	Amino Acid	R
Glycine (Gly)	—H	Glutamine (Gln)	$-CH_2-CH_2-\overset{\overset{\displaystyle O}{\|\|}}{C}-NH_2$
Alanine (Ala)	$-CH_3$	Serine (Ser)	$\overset{\displaystyle OH}{\underset{\displaystyle}{\|}}$ $-CH_2$
Valine (Val)[a]	$-\overset{\displaystyle CH_3}{\underset{\displaystyle}{\|}}$ $-CH-CH_3$	Threonine (Thr)[a]	$\overset{\displaystyle OH}{\underset{\displaystyle}{\|}}$ $-CH-CH_3$
Leucine (Leu)[a]	$-CH_2-\overset{\displaystyle CH_3}{\underset{\displaystyle}{\|}}CH-CH_3$	Tyrosine (Tyr)	$-CH_2-\bigcirc-OH$
Isoleucine (Ile)[a]	$-\overset{\displaystyle CH_3}{\underset{\displaystyle}{\|}}CH-CH_2-CH_3$	Lysine (Lys)[a]	$-CH_2-CH_2-CH_2-CH_2-NH_2$
Cysteine (Cys)	$-CH_2-SH$	Arginine (Arg)	$-CH_2-CH_2-CH_2-\overset{\displaystyle}{N}-\overset{\overset{\displaystyle NH_2}{\|}}{C}-NH_2$
Methionine (Met)[a]	$-CH_2-CH_2-S-CH_3$	Histidine (His)	$-CH_2$ imidazole
Tryptophan (Trp)[a]	$-CH_2$ indole	Aspartic acid (Asp)	$-CH_2-COOH$
Phenylalanine (Phe)[a]	$-CH_2-\bigcirc$	Glutamate (Glu)	$-CH_2-CH_2-COOH$
Asparagine (Asn)	$-CH_2-\overset{\overset{\displaystyle O}{\|\|}}{C}-NH_2$	Proline (Pro)[a,b]	pyrrolidine-COOH

The R group is the group attached to the α carbon.
[a]Nutritionally essential.
[b]Exception to attachment of R group is proline.

Metabolism

About half of the 20 amino acids required by humans for protein synthesis cannot be synthesized in vivo at a rapid enough rate to support growth. These nutritionally essential amino acids must be supplied by the diet in the form of proteins. Under normal circumstances, proteolytic enzymes, such as pepsin and trypsin, completely digest dietary proteins into their constituent amino acids. The amino acids are then rapidly absorbed from the intestine into the bloodstream and become part of the body's pool of amino acids. Amino acids are also released by catabolism of body proteins to be used for energy or synthesis of new proteins.

The essential amino acids are arginine, histidine, isoleucine, leucine, lysine, methionine, phenylalanine, threonine, tryptophan, and valine. Arginine may also be classified as semiessential as dietary supplementation is required in

$$NH_2-\overset{\overset{\displaystyle R_1}{\|}}{\underset{\underset{\displaystyle H}{\|}}{C}}-COOH \ + \ NH_2-\overset{\overset{\displaystyle R_2}{\|}}{\underset{\underset{\displaystyle H}{\|}}{C}}-COOH \ \xrightarrow{-H_2O} \ NH_2-\overset{\overset{\displaystyle R_1}{\|}}{\underset{\underset{\displaystyle H}{\|}}{C}}-\overset{\overset{\displaystyle O}{\|\|}}{C}-\overset{\displaystyle}{\underset{\underset{\displaystyle H}{\|}}{N}}-\overset{\overset{\displaystyle R_2}{\|}}{\underset{\underset{\displaystyle H}{\|}}{C}}-COOH$$

Peptide bond

FIGURE 11.2 Formation of a dipeptide.

youth, but adults can synthesize adequate amounts to meet the body's needs. The human body can synthesize sufficient amounts of alanine, asparagine, aspartic acid, cysteine, glutamic acid, glutamine, glycine, proline, serine, and tyrosine. Because additional dietary intake of these amino acids is unnecessary, they are classified as nonessential amino acids. However, some nonessential amino acids are produced from essential ones and a deficiency in the essential amino acid may require supplementation of the nonessential amino acid. For example, tyrosine, a nonessential amino acid, is produced from phenylalanine, an essential amino acid. If the diet is deficient in phenylalanine, tyrosine will also be deficient and may require additional dietary intake.

Amino acids are primarily used in the synthesis of body proteins such as plasma, intracellular, and structural proteins; however, they are also used in the synthesis of nonprotein nitrogen-containing compounds such as purines, pyrimidines, porphyrins, creatine, histamine, thyroxine, epinephrine, and coenzyme NAD. In addition, proteins provide up to 20% of the total energy required daily by the body. To be utilized as an energy source, proteins must first be broken down into their constituent amino acids. The amino group is then removed from the amino acid by either deamination or transamination. The ammonium ion that is produced during deamination of the amino acids is converted into urea via the urea cycle in the liver.[2] The resultant ketoacid enters into a common metabolic pathway with carbohydrates and fats to be converted into useable energy. Glucogenic amino acids generate precursors of glucose, such as pyruvate or citric acid cycle intermediates. Examples include alanine, which can be deaminated to pyruvate; arginine, which is converted to α-ketoglutarate; and aspartic acid, which is converted to oxaloacetate. Ketogenic amino acids, such as leucine and lysine, are degraded to acetyl-CoA or acetoacetyl-CoA and form ketone bodies. Isoleucine, phenylalanine, tryptophan, tyrosine, and threonine are both ketogenic and glucogenic.

Essential Amino Acids
Arginine (Arg)
Arginine is a complex amino acid often found at the catalytic (active) site in proteins and enzymes due to its amine-containing side chain. Arginine plays an important role in cell division, wound healing, stimulation of protein synthesis, immune function, and the release of hormones. One important role of arginine is the conversion of ammonia, which is highly toxic, into urea, which can be safely excreted via the urinary system.

Histidine (His)
Histidine is one of the basic by pH amino acids due to its imidazole side chain. Histidine is needed to help grow and repair body tissues and to maintain the myelin sheaths that protect nerve cells and is the direct precursor of histamine, which is involved in immune response. It also plays an important role in the manufacturing of red and white blood cells and in protecting the body from heavy metal

toxicity and is an important source of carbon atoms in the synthesis of purines for DNA and RNA synthesis.

Isoleucine (Ile), Leucine (Leu), and Valine (Val)
Isoleucine, leucine, and valine are branched-chain amino acids that are collectively referred to as the branched-chain amino acid group. These branched-chain amino acids promote healing of muscle tissue, skin, and bones; help regulate blood glucose concentrations; and maintain energy levels. Additionally, isoleucine plays an important role in hemoglobin formation, whereas leucine is necessary for optimal growth in infants. Leucine and valine also aid in maintaining the nitrogen balance in adults. Valine is used in treatments for muscle, mental, and emotional problems such as insomnia and anxiety, as well as liver and gallbladder disease.

Lysine (Lys)
Lysine has a net positive charge, which makes it one of three basic, by charge, amino acids. It plays a role in the production of antibodies and lowering triglyceride levels. Lysine also helps in the absorption and conservation of calcium and plays an important role in the formation of collagen, a component of cartilage and connective tissue.

Methionine (Met)
Methionine is an important amino acid that helps to initiate translation of messenger RNA (mRNA) by being the first amino acid incorporated into the N-terminal position of all proteins.[3] Methionine is a source of sulfur, which is required for normal metabolism and growth. Methionine also assists in the breakdown of fats, helps to detoxify lead and other heavy metals, helps diminish muscle weakness, and prevents brittle hair. Methionine reacts with adenosine triphosphate (ATP) in the synthesis of many important substances, including epinephrine and choline.

Phenylalanine (Phe)
Phenylalanine is classified as a nonpolar amino acid because of the hydrophobic nature of its benzyl side chain. It promotes alertness and vitality, elevates mood, decreases pain, aids in memory and learning, and is used to treat arthritis and depression. Phenylalanine uses an active transport channel to cross the blood–brain barrier and is used by the brain to produce norepinephrine, a neurotransmitter that transmits signals between nerve cells. In large quantities, phenylalanine can interfere with production of serotonin, another neurotransmitter. Phenylalanine is the direct metabolic precursor of tyrosine, and deficiency of phenylalanine will also result in a deficiency of tyrosine.

Threonine (Thr)
Threonine is an alcohol-containing amino acid that is an important component in the formation of collagen, elastin (a connective tissue protein), and tooth enamel. It is also important in the production of neurotransmitters and health of the nervous system. Threonine helps maintain proper protein balance in the body and aids liver function, metabolism, and assimilation.

Tryptophan (Trp)

Tryptophan is a metabolic precursor for serotonin, melatonin (a neurohormone), and niacin (a vitamin). Tryptophan is a natural relaxant that helps alleviate insomnia by inducing sleep, soothes anxiety, and reduces depression. It is used in the treatment of migraine headaches, aids in weight control by reducing appetite, and helps control hyperactivity in children.

Nonessential Amino Acids

Alanine (Ala)

Alanine is one of the simplest amino acids and is a product of the breakdown of DNA or the dipeptides, anserine and carnosine. It is also formed as a result of glucose metabolism (glycolysis) in muscle tissue and the conversion of pyruvate, a pivotal compound in carbohydrate metabolism.[4] Alanine plays a major role in the transfer of nitrogen from peripheral tissues to the liver for processing and excretion and strengthens the immune system through production of antibodies. Alanine also helps in reducing the buildup of toxic substances released when muscle protein is broken down quickly to meet the energy demands of the body.

Asparagine (Asn)

Asparagine is derived from aspartic acid and ATP through transamidation, which is the transfer of an amide group from one compound to another.[4] Asparagine is one of the principal and most abundant amino acids involved in the transport of nitrogen. It is required by the nervous system and plays an important role in the synthesis of ammonia; however, a primary function of asparagine is in the conversion of one amino acid into another via amination or transamination. Amination is the process by which an amine group is introduced into an organic molecule, and transamination is the transfer of an amino acid to an α-ketoacid.

Aspartic Acid (Asp)

Aspartic acid, or aspartate, is synthesized from oxaloacetate through transamination. An important role of aspartic acid is as the precursor for several other amino acids. Amino acids that are synthesized from aspartic acid include asparagine, arginine, lysine, methionine, threonine, isoleucine, and several nucleotides. Aspartic acid is a metabolite in the citric acid cycle and the urea cycle. It also participates in the generation of glucose from nonsugar substrates, which is known as gluconeogenesis.

Cysteine (Cys)

Cysteine is classified as a nonessential amino acid; however, infants, the elderly, and individuals with certain metabolic diseases or intestinal absorption issues may require supplementation. Cysteine should not be confused with cystine as they are two different amino acids. However, cysteine is named after cystine as it is an oxidized dimer of cysteine.[5] Cysteine is potentially toxic, so it is absorbed during digestion as cystine, which is more stable in the gastrointestinal tract and less toxic. Cystine is transported to cells, where it is reduced to two cysteine molecules upon cell entry.

Cysteine can also be synthesized in vivo from the essential amino acid methionine through a series of enzymatic reactions. Cysteine is an important structural and functional component of many proteins and enzymes and has significant antioxidant properties.

Glutamic Acid (Glu)

Glutamic acid, or glutamate, is synthesized from the transamination of a number of amino acids such as alanine and aspartic acid. When an amino group is added to glutamic acid, it forms another important amino acid, glutamine. Glutamic acid is one of two amino acids that have a net negative charge by pH, making it a very polar molecule. Glutamic acid serves as a neurotransmitter, and its dysregulation has been linked to epileptic seizures. It is also important in the metabolism of sugars and fats and aids in the transport of potassium into spinal fluid.

Glutamine (Gln)

Glutamine is the most abundant amino acid in the body and is synthesized from glutamic acid. Glutamine has many important functions including renal maintenance of the acid–base balance, providing fuel for a healthy digestive tract,[6] and acting as the basis of the building blocks for synthesis of RNA and DNA. Glutamine is also a source of cellular energy and aids in immune function. Another vital role of glutamine is the transport of ammonia to the liver for metabolism. Ammonia is a by-product of protein breakdown. It is transported to the liver where it is converted into urea and excreted by the kidneys. Studies have shown glutamine to be useful in the treatment of serious illnesses, injury, trauma, burns, cancer treatment–related side effects, and wound healing for postoperative patients.[7]

Glycine (Gly)

Glycine is synthesized from another nonessential amino acid, serine. Glycine is essential for synthesis of nucleic acids, bile acids, proteins, peptides, purines, ATP, porphyrins, hemoglobin, glutathione, creatine, bile salts, glucose, glycogen, and other amino acids. The liver utilizes glycine in the detoxification of compounds and in the synthesis of bile acids. Glycine is also an inhibitory neurotransmitter in the central nervous system (CNS) and a metal complexing agent. Additionally, glycine retards muscle degeneration, improves glycogen storage, and promotes healing.

Proline (Pro)

Proline is produced from glutamine and is the precursor for hydroxyproline. Hydroxyproline is manufactured into collagen, tendons, ligaments, and cardiac tissue. Proline is involved in wound healing, especially that of cartilage, and in the strengthening of joints, tendons, and cardiac tissue. It also works in tandem with vitamin C to promote healthy connective tissues.

Serine (Ser)

Serine is synthesized from 3-phosphoglycerate, which is an intermediate in glycolysis. Serine is needed for the proper metabolism of lipids and fatty acids and plays an important role in the body's synthetic pathways for pyrimidines, purines, creatine, and porphyrins. It is highly concentrated in all cell membranes, is a component of the protective myelin sheaths surrounding nerve fibers, and aids in the production of antibodies for the maintenance of a healthy immune system.

Tyrosine (Tyr)

Tyrosine is metabolically synthesized from phenylalanine. Tyrosine is a precursor of the adrenal hormones epinephrine, norepinephrine, and dopamine and thyroid hormones including thyroxine. It is important in overall metabolism and aiding in function of the adrenal glands, thyroid, and pituitary glands. Tyrosine stimulates metabolism and the nervous system and acts as a mood elevator, making it useful in the treatment of chronic fatigue, narcolepsy, anxiety, depression, low sex drive, allergies, and headaches.

Recently Identified Amino Acids

Selenocysteine (Sec)

Selenocysteine is recognized as the 21st amino acid, but unlike other amino acids present in proteins, it is not coded for directly in the genetic code. Selenocysteine is encoded by a UGA codon, which is normally a stop codon; however, like the other amino acids used by cells, selenocysteine has a specialized transfer RNA (tRNA). Selenocysteine was named as an amino acid in 2002 and was found to be the selenium analogue of cysteine, in which a selenium atom replaces sulfur. Selenocysteine is present in several enzymes, such as formate dehydrogenases, glycine reductases, and some hydrogenases. It has been discovered that HIV-1 encodes a functional selenoprotein, and patients with HIV infection have been shown to have a lower-than-average blood plasma selenium level.[8,9]

Pyrrolysine (Pyl)

Pyrrolysine is the 22nd naturally occurring genetically encoded amino acid used by some prokaryotes and single-celled microorganisms in enzymes that are part of their methane-producing metabolism. This lysine derivative is encoded by the UAG codon, normally a stop codon, possibly modified by the presence of a specific downstream sequence forcing the incorporation of pyrrolysine instead of terminating translation.[10] This amino acid is not present in humans.

Aminoacidopathies

Aminoacidopathies are a class of inherited errors of metabolism in which there is an enzyme defect that inhibits the body's ability to metabolize certain amino acids. The abnormalities exist either in the activity of a specific enzyme in the metabolic pathway or in the membrane transport system for the amino acids. Aminoacidopathies cause severe medical complications, such as brain damage, due to the accumulation of toxic amino acids or their by-products in the blood and tissues. Due to the severity of these complications, many states require newborn screening tests to aid in early diagnosis and initiation of therapies. Phenylketonuria

(PKU) is one of the most well-known aminoacidopathies and was the first newborn screening test introduced in the early 1960s. Now, some states require screening tests for up to 26 amino acids,[11] and more than 100 diseases have been identified that result from inherited errors of amino acid metabolism.

Phenylketonuria

PKU is inherited as an autosomal recessive trait and occurs in about 1 in 15,000 births in the United States. The metabolic defect in the classic form of PKU is an absence of activity of the enzyme phenylalanine hydroxylase (PAH) due to mutations in the *PAH* gene. PAH catalyzes the conversion of phenylalanine to tyrosine as illustrated in Figure 11.3. In the newborn, the upper limit of normal for phenylalanine concentration in the blood is 120 µmol/L (2 mg/dL).[12] In the absence of PAH activity, phenylalanine concentrations are usually greater than 1,200 µmol/L and in untreated classic PKU, blood concentrations as high as 2.4 mmol/L can be found. Chronically elevated blood concentrations of phenylalanine and its metabolites, such as phenylpyruvic acid, phenylpyruvate (also known as phenylketone), and phenyllactic acid, can cause significant and permanent brain damage.

FIGURE 11.3 Metabolism of phenylalanine and tyrosine.

Phenylalanine and its metabolites are found in both the blood and urine of patients with PKU and cause the urine to have a characteristic "musty" or "mousy" odor. Partial deficiencies of PAH activity are typically classified as mild PKU and result in phenylalanine concentrations between 600 to 1,200 µmol/L. Patients with phenylalanine concentrations in the range of 180 to 600 µmol/L with no accompanying accumulation of phenylketones are classified as having non-PKU mild hyperphenylalaninemia.

In infants and children with this inherited defect, retarded mental development and microcephaly occur as a result of the toxic effects of phenylalanine or its metabolic by-products on the brain. Brain damage can be avoided if the disease is detected at birth and the infant is maintained on a diet containing very low levels of phenylalanine. Women with untreated PKU during pregnancy almost always have infants who are microcephalic and mentally retarded. However, fetal effects of maternal PKU are preventable if the mother maintains a phenylalanine-restricted diet before conception and throughout pregnancy.

Hyperphenylalaninemia can also be the result of a deficiency in the enzymes needed for regeneration and synthesis of tetrahydrobiopterin (BH_4). BH_4 is a cofactor required for the enzymatic hydroxylation of phenylalanine, tyrosine, and tryptophan. Deficiency of BH_4 results in elevated blood concentrations of phenylalanine and deficient production of neurotransmitters from tyrosine and tryptophan. Although cofactor defects account for only 1% to 5% of all cases of hyperphenylalaninemia, they must be differentiated from PKU so that appropriate treatment with the active cofactor along with the neurotransmitter precursors L-DOPA and 5-OH tryptophan can be initiated.[13]

Screening for PKU is now required in all states in the United States, and blood is collected at about 3 days of age. If the screening test is abnormal, other tests are performed to confirm or exclude PKU. Once diagnosed as PKU, the goal of treatment is to maintain the blood concentration of phenylalanine between 120 and 600 µmol/L (2 and 10 mg/dL) through diet modification. Phenylalanine is still required for normal growth; therefore, a diet with some phenylalanine is recommended, but in much lower amounts than a typical diet contains. High-protein foods, such as meat, fish, poultry, eggs, cheese, and milk, should be avoided, and calculated amounts of cereals, starches, fruits, and vegetables, along with a milk substitute, are usually recommended.

In 2007, the U.S. Food and Drug Administration (FDA) approved sapropterin dihydrochloride (Kuvan®), the first drug to help manage PKU.[14] The drug helps reduce phenylalanine concentrations by increasing the activity of the PAH enzyme. This drug is only effective for patients that have some PAH activity, who continue to follow a phenylalanine-restricted diet and have their phenylalanine levels monitored.

The Guthrie test is a semiquantitative, bacterial inhibition assay for phenylalanine based on the ability of phenylalanine to facilitate bacterial growth in a culture medium despite the presence of a growth inhibitor. To perform the Guthrie test, an agar gel plate containing β-2-thienylalanine, a growth inhibitor, is inoculated with *Bacillus subtilis*. Blood is collected from the newborn onto a piece of filter paper, and a small disk is punched out of the filter paper and placed on the inoculated agar plate. The β-2-thienylalanine present in the agar inhibits bacterial growth; however, in the presence of phenylalanine leached from the impregnated filter paper disk, inhibition is overcome and bacteria grow around the disk. The Guthrie test is sensitive enough to detect serum phenylalanine concentrations of 180 µmol/L (3 mg/dL). The test has been widely used throughout North America and Europe as one of the core newborn screening tests since the late 1960s. In recent years, this test has been replaced in many areas by newer techniques, such as high-performance liquid chromatography (HPLC) and tandem mass spectrometry (MS/MS).

Another screening test for PKU involves a microfluorometric assay for the direct measurement of phenylalanine in dried blood filter disks. In contrast to the Guthrie test, this method yields quantitative results, is more adaptable to automation, and is not affected by the presence of antibiotics. The procedure is based on the fluorescence of a complex formed by phenylalanine, ninhydrin, and copper in the presence of a dipeptide. The test requires pretreatment of the dried blood filter disk with trichloroacetic acid (TCA). The extract is then added to a microtiter plate with a mixture of ninhydrin, succinate, and leucylalanine in the presence of copper tartrate. The fluorescence of the complex is measured using excitation/emission wavelengths of 360 and 530 nm, respectively.[15]

Positive screening results for PKU must be verified by another method. One rapid diagnostic procedure for neonatal PKU uses microwave-assisted silylation followed by gas chromatography–mass spectrometry (GC/MS). In this procedure, amino acids are extracted from neonatal blood samples, rapidly derived with *N,O-bis*(trimethylsilyl)-trifluoroacetamide under microwave irradiation, and the derivatives are analyzed by GC/MS.

The reference method for quantitative serum phenylalanine is HPLC; however, MS/MS is now considered to be the gold standard for detecting a variety of congenital diseases in newborns. Mass spectrometry is an analytical technique that measures the mass-to-charge ratio of charged particles.[16] It is most commonly used to identify the composition of a specimen by generating a mass spectrum representing the masses of the specimen's components. Patients with PKU generally demonstrate an increase in phenylalanine concentrations and a decrease in tyrosine concentrations. Using MS/MS, both analytes can be quantitated, and a ratio of phenylalanine to tyrosine (Phe/Tyr) can be calculated. Using the ratio between the analytes rather than individual concentrations increases the specificity of the measurement and lowers the false-positive rate for PKU to less than 0.01%. MS/MS methods have greater sensitivity allowing detection of lower concentrations of phenylalanine and earlier diagnosis of PKU, sometimes as early as the first day of life. Most newborn screening MS/MS methods have the ability to detect more than 25 different genetic disorders with a single specimen so this technology is rapidly replacing the multiple procedures currently used in newborn screening programs when the laboratory can support MS/MS testing.

Prenatal diagnosis and detection of carrier status in families with PKU are now available using DNA analysis as PKU results from multiple independent mutations (>400 identified) at the PAH locus.

Tyrosinemia

Tyrosinemia is another inherited autosomal recessive aminoacidopathy. This inborn metabolic disorder of tyrosine catabolism is characterized by the excretion of tyrosine and its catabolites in urine or tyrosinuria. There are three types of tyrosinemia each caused by deficiencies of different enzymes in the metabolic pathway of tyrosine.

Type I tyrosinemia is the most severe form occurring in about 1 in 100,000 births worldwide. This form of tyrosinemia is caused by a mutation in the *FAH* gene, which codes for the enzyme fumarylacetoacetate hydrolase (FAH). FAH is the last of five enzymes required for metabolism of tyrosine. Symptoms of type I tyrosinemia generally manifest in the first few months of life and include failure to thrive, diarrhea, vomiting, jaundice, a cabbage-like odor, distended abdomen, swelling of the legs, and an increased predisposition for bleeding. Type I tyrosinemia can lead to liver and kidney failure, problems affecting the nervous system such as peripheral neuropathy, and an increased risk of liver cancer later in life. Untreated, patients with type I tyrosinemia typically do not live past the age of ten.

Type II tyrosinemia is caused by a mutation in the *TAT* gene, which leads to a deficiency of the enzyme tyrosine aminotransferase (TAT). Type II tyrosinemia occurs in less than 1 in 250,000 births worldwide. TAT is the first enzyme of the five enzymes required for the conversion of tyrosine to smaller molecules that are excreted by the kidneys or used in energy-producing reactions. About half of the individuals with type II tyrosinemia have impaired mental development. Other symptoms manifest in the eyes and skin including abnormal light sensitivity (photophobia), eye pain and redness, and painful skin lesions on the palms and soles of the feet.

Type III tyrosinemia is a rare disorder with only a few cases having been reported worldwide. It is caused by a mutation in the *HPD* gene that results in deficiency of the enzyme 4-hydroxyphenylpyruvate dioxygenase (HPD). HPD is the second enzyme of the cascade required for tyrosine metabolism and is found mainly in the liver, with lesser amounts found in the kidneys. Patients with type III tyrosinemia typically have impaired mental development, seizures, and some intermittent loss of balance and coordination.

Diagnostic criteria for tyrosinemia include an elevated tyrosine blood concentration using MS/MS and an elevated concentration of succinylacetone.[17] Succinylacetone is a toxic metabolite that forms when tyrosine cannot be metabolized through the appropriate enzymatic pathway. Succinylacetone can cause severe damage to the liver and kidneys resulting in the need for a full or partial liver transplant. The treatment for tyrosinemia is generally a low-protein diet, but may also include medications such as nitisinone (NTBC). Nitisinone prevents the formation of maleylacetoacetic acid and fumarylacetoacetic acid, which can be converted to succinylacetone. Since nitisinone's first use for treatment of tyrosinemia in 1991, it has replaced liver transplantation as the first-line treatment for this rare condition.

Alkaptonuria

Alkaptonuria is another inherited autosomal recessive amino acid disorder with an occurrence of about 1 in 250,000 births worldwide. A mutation in the *HGD* gene leads to a deficiency of the enzyme homogentisate oxidase (HGD), which is required for proper metabolism of tyrosine and phenylalanine. As a result of this enzyme deficiency, patients with alkaptonuria have elevated concentrations of homogentisic acid (HGA) in the blood, deposit HGA in connective tissues, and excrete HGA in their urine. Patients with alkaptonuria typically do not present with symptoms until their third decade of life. Over time, HGA is deposited in the cartilage of the ears, nose, and tendons of the extremities and results in a dark blue-black pigmentation known as ochronosis. Small dark spots on the sclera of the eye may also be seen. HGA also accumulates in the cartilage of joints, such as the hips, and causes an arthritis-like degeneration, which is frequently the first symptom reported by patients. HGA is excreted through the renal system and is found in the urine of patients with alkaptonuria. If the urine specimen is allowed to mix with air, it will eventually result in a brownish-black color due to oxidization of HGA.

The ferric chloride test may be performed as a rapid screen for the presence of HGA in urine. When ferric chloride is added to an aliquot of urine that contains HGA, it will turn black due to the interaction with the phenol group. Patients with alkaptonuria may be prescribed high-dose vitamin C supplementation as this vitamin has been shown to slow down the accumulation of HGA in the cartilage, which may slow the progression of arthritis.

Maple Syrup Urine Disease

Maple syrup urine disease (MSUD) results from an absence or greatly reduced activity of a complex of enzymes known as branched-chain α-ketoacid decarboxylase (BCKD). This deficiency is inherited in an autosomal recessive pattern and is the result of a mutation in the *BCKDHA*, *BCKDHB*, or *DBT* genes. Deficiency of the BCKD complex inhibits the normal metabolism of the three essential branched-chain amino acids leucine, isoleucine, and valine. MSUD has been part of several state newborn screening programs since the mid-1970s, with a reported occurrence of 1 in 185,000 births worldwide. The most striking feature of this hereditary disease is the characteristic "maple syrup" or "burnt sugar" odor of the urine, breath, and skin of patients with MSUD. This characteristic odor is the result of the accumulation of the branched-chain amino acids and their corresponding ketoacids in the blood, urine, and cerebrospinal fluid (CSF).

Newborns with MSUD typically develop lethargy, vomiting, lack of appetite, and signs of failure to thrive within a week of birth. Elevated concentrations of leucine, isoleucine, valine, and their associated ketoacids can be toxic to the brain and may result in muscle rigidity, stupor, and respiratory irregularities. Undiagnosed and untreated, the disease can progress to cause severe mental retardation, seizures, acidosis, and hypoglycemia and can lead to death. If diagnosed early on, MSUD can be controlled by restricting dietary proteins to minimize leucine, isoleucine, and valine.

A modified Guthrie test can be used to screen for MSUD. An agar gel plate containing 4-azaleucine, another growth inhibitor, is inoculated with *Bacillus subtilis*. A small disk is punched out of filter paper that contains blood from the newborn and is placed on the inoculated agar plate. The 4-azaleucine present in the agar inhibits bacterial growth; however, in the presence of the branched-chain amino acids leached from the impregnated filter paper disk, inhibition is overcome and bacteria grow around the disk. A microfluorometric assay for the three branched-chain amino acids uses a filter paper specimen treated with a solvent mixture of methanol and acetone to denature the hemoglobin. Leucine dehydrogenase is added to an aliquot of the extract, and the fluorescence of the NADH produced in the subsequent reaction is measured at 450 nm, with an excitation wavelength of 360 nm.[18] A leucine concentration greater than 4 mg/dL is indicative of MSUD. MS/MS is also being used in screening and quantitative testing for MSUD. Prenatal diagnosis of MSUD is made by testing the decarboxylase enzyme concentration in cells cultured from amniotic fluid.

Isovaleric Acidemia

Isovaleric acidemia (IVA) is an autosomal recessive disorder caused by mutation of the *IVD* gene, which codes for isovaleryl-CoA dehydrogenase (IVD). IVD plays an important role in the metabolism of leucine.

Isovaleric acidemia occurs in approximately 1 in 250,000 births in the United States. Some people with gene mutations that cause isovaleric acidemia are asymptomatic and never experience any signs or symptoms of the condition. For those patients with IVA that are not asymptomatic, a characteristic feature of IVA is a distinctive odor of sweaty feet caused by the buildup of isovaleric acid. Other clinical manifestations of this disorder may become apparent as early as a few days after birth and include failure to thrive, vomiting, and lethargy. Health problems related to IVA range from very mild to life threatening, such as seizures and coma, but, when severe, can result in permanent damage to the brain and nervous system and possible death.

Treatment for IVA includes a protein-restrictive diet to lower the levels of accumulating isovaleric acid, which is toxic to the central nervous system. Oral administration of glycine and carnitine supplementation may be prescribed because they interact with isovaleric acid to form nontoxic, readily excreted products.

If IVA is suspected, the urine of newborns can be screened for isovaleric acid using MS/MS or chromatography. Laboratory results for patients with IVA reveal metabolic acidosis, mild-to-moderate ketonuria, hyperammonemia, thrombocytopenia, and neutropenia.

Homocystinuria

Homocystinuria is yet another inherited autosomal recessive disorder of amino acid metabolism. Mutations in the *CBS*, *MTHFR*, *MTR*, *MTRR*, and *MMADHC* can result in homocystinuria. The most common form of homocystinuria is the result of a mutation in the *CBS* gene and occurs in about 1 in 200,000 births worldwide. This mutation results in a deficiency of the enzyme cystathionine β-synthase, which is necessary for metabolism of methionine. This deficiency results in elevated plasma and urine concentrations of methionine and of the precursor homocysteine. Symptoms associated with this form of homocystinuria include nearsightedness; dislocation of the lens in the eye, caused by the lack of cysteine synthesis essential for collagen formation; osteoporosis; and, frequently, mental retardation.[19]

Treatment includes dietary restriction of proteins to reduce concentrations of methionine as well as high doses of vitamin B_6. Those who do not respond to this treatment may need trimethylglycine and folic acid supplementation.

Newborn screening for homocystinuria may also be performed using a modified Guthrie test. In this form of the test, L-methionine sulfoximine is utilized as the bacterial growth inhibitor and increased plasma methionine levels will result in bacterial growth. HPLC and MS/MS methods are commonly used as confirmatory methods, and a methionine concentration greater than 2 mg/dL indicates homocystinuria. Alternatively, urinary total homocysteine concentrations can be measured using liquid chromatography–tandem mass spectrometry (LC-MS/MS).[20]

Citrullinemia

Citrullinemia belongs to a class of genetic diseases called urea cycle disorders. In the urea cycle, excess nitrogen, generated during protein metabolism, is used in the formation of urea, which can be safely excreted in urine. Citrullinemia is inherited in an autosomal recessive pattern and occurs in two forms.

Type I citrullinemia is the result of a mutation in the *ASS1* gene. This gene codes for synthesis of the enzyme argininosuccinic acid synthetase (ASS). A deficiency of ASS leads to an accumulation of the amino acid citrulline as well as ammonia in the blood due to impaired conversion of ammonia into urea for excretion. Type I citrullinemia is the most common form occurring in about 1 in 57,000 births worldwide. In affected infants, clinical symptoms include lack of appetite, failure to thrive, vomiting, lethargy, seizures, and coma as toxic ammonia builds up in the body. If not treated promptly, severe brain damage or death may occur.

Type II citrullinemia is caused by a mutation in the *SLC25A13* gene that codes for production of the transport protein citrin. Citrin helps transport molecules inside the cell that are used in the production and breakdown of simple sugars, production of proteins, and the urea cycle. In type II citrullinemia, cells are prevented from making citrin, which inhibits the urea cycle and disrupts the production of proteins and nucleotides. The resulting accumulation of ammonia and other toxic substances leads to confusion, restlessness, memory loss, personality changes, seizures, and coma.

Treatment of citrullinemia includes a high-caloric, protein-restrictive diet; arginine supplementation, and administration of sodium benzoate and sodium phenylacetate.

Argininosuccinic Aciduria

Argininosuccinic aciduria (ASA) is another urea cycle amino acid disorder that is inherited in an autosomal recessive pattern and is the result of a mutation in the *ASL* gene. ASA occurs in approximately 1 in 70,000 births worldwide. Infants with argininosuccinic acidemia lack the enzyme argininosuccinic acid lyase (ASL), which plays a role in the conversion of ammonia into urea. When ASL is deficient, the urea cycle cannot proceed normally and nitrogen accumulates in the blood in the form of ammonia. Ammonia is especially damaging to the nervous system and can result in seizures as well as possible coma. Clinical symptoms of ASA typically develop within the first few days of life and begin with lethargy and unwillingness to eat.

Treatment of ASA is similar to that for citrullinemia and includes a high-calorie, protein-restrictive diet; arginine supplementation; and administration of sodium benzoate and sodium phenylacetate. It should be noted that newborn screening tests cannot differentiate citrullinemia from argininosuccinic acidemia.[21]

Cystinuria

Cystinuria is an inherited autosomal recessive disorder, occurring in approximately 1 in 10,000 births worldwide, which is caused by mutations in the *SLC3A1* and *SLC7A9* genes. These genes code for the synthesis of a protein complex found in the kidneys that is responsible for the reabsorption of cystine from urine. Cystinuria is characterized by inadequate reabsorption of cystine during urine formation in the kidneys resulting in an elevated concentration of cystine. When saturated, cystine can precipitate out of the urine and form stones in the kidneys, ureters, or bladder. Kidney stones often recur throughout a patient's lifetime and are responsible for the symptoms of the disease, including hematuria, flank pain, and, frequently, urinary tract infections.

Treatment for cystinuria is generally aimed at preventing the formation of cystine stones. This may be accomplished by increasing the patient's fluid intake to 4 L/day, which serves to increase the volume of urine, reduce the concentration of cystine, and minimize the likelihood of it precipitating and forming stones. When a high fluid intake does not reduce the formation of stones, penicillamine may be prescribed. Penicillamine forms a more soluble complex with cystine, which prevents it from precipitating and forming stones. Once stones have formed, percutaneous

nephrolithotripsy may be performed as an alternative to surgery to remove the kidney stones.

Cystinuria can be diagnosed by testing the urine for cystine using cyanide nitroprusside, which produces a red-purple color on reaction with sulfhydryl groups. False-positive results as a result of homocysteine must be ruled out. Patients with cystinuria also excrete elevated concentrations of lysine, arginine, and ornithine. These amino acids are more soluble in urine and generally do not lead to stone formation; however, ion exchange chromatography can be used for quantitative analysis, which may aid in the diagnosis of cystinuria.

Methods of Analysis

Blood samples for amino acid analysis should be drawn after at least 6 to 8 hours of fasting to avoid the effect of absorbed amino acids originating from dietary proteins. The sample is collected in a heparin tube with the plasma promptly removed from the cells, taking care not to aspirate the platelet and white cell layer to prevent contamination with platelet or leukocyte amino acids. White blood cell levels of aspartic acid and glutamic acid, for example, are about 100 times higher than those in plasma; hemolysis is unacceptable for the same reason. Deproteinization should be performed within 30 minutes of sample collection, and analysis should be performed immediately or the sample frozen at −20°C to −40°C.

Urinary amino acid analysis can be performed on a random specimen for screening purposes. For quantitation, a 24-hour urine specimen preserved with thymol or organic solvents is required. Amniotic fluid may also be analyzed.

For amino acid screening, the method of choice is thin-layer chromatography. The application of either one- or two-dimensional separations depends on the purpose of the analysis. If searching for a particular category of amino acids, such as branched-chain amino acids or a single amino acid, usually, a one-dimensional separation is sufficient. For more general screening, two-dimensional chromatography is essential. The amino acids migrate along one solvent front, and then the chromatogram is rotated 90° and a second solvent migration performed. A variety of solvents have been used, including butanol, acetic acid, water and ethanol, and ammonia and water mixtures. The chromatogram is viewed by staining with ninhydrin, which gives most amino acids a blue color. Amino acids can also be separated and quantitated by ion exchange chromatography, an HPLC reversed-phase system equipped with fluorescence detection,[22] or capillary electrophoresis. As discussed, another technique that provides a highly specific and sensitive method for the measurement of amino acids is MS/MS.[23]

PROTEINS

Overview

Proteins play key roles in every cell throughout the human body. Some of their major functions include catalyzing biochemical reactions as enzymes, transporting metals such as iron and copper, acting as receptors for hormones, providing structure and support to cells, and participating in immune response as antibodies. From these few examples of their numerous functions, it is easy to see that proteins are truly the physical basis of life.[24]

Basic Structure

Proteins consist of the elements carbon, oxygen, hydrogen, nitrogen, and sulfur. It is the fact that proteins contain nitrogen that sets them apart from pure carbohydrates and lipids, which do not contain nitrogen atoms. Proteins are polymers built from one or more unbranched chains of amino acids. A typical protein contains 200 to 300 amino acids, but some are much smaller (peptides) and some are much larger (e.g., titin, in muscle). Proteins are considered macromolecules and range in molecular mass from approximately 6,000 Daltons for insulin to several million Daltons for some structural proteins.

There are four distinct levels of a protein's structure: primary, secondary, tertiary, and quaternary. *Primary structure* represents the number and types of amino acids in the specific amino acid sequence. In order to function properly, proteins must have the correct sequence of amino acids. For example, when the amino acid valine is substituted for glutamic acid in the α-chain of hemoglobin A, hemoglobin S is formed, which results in sickle cell anemia.

Secondary structure refers to commonly formed structures stabilized by hydrogen bonds between the amino acids within the protein. Common secondary structures are the α-helix, β-pleated sheet, and turns, with most serum proteins forming a helix.[25] Secondary structures add new properties to a protein such as strength and flexibility (Fig. 11.4).

Tertiary structure refers to the overall shape, or conformation, of the protein molecule. The conformation is known as the *fold*, or the spatial relationship of the secondary structures to one another. Tertiary structures are three dimensional and result from the interaction of side chains, which are stabilized through the hydrophobic effect, ionic attraction, hydrogen bonds, and disulfide bonds. The function and physical and chemical properties of a protein are related to its tertiary structure.[26]

FIGURE 11.4 Secondary structure of proteins.

Quaternary structure is the shape or structure that results from the interaction of more than one protein molecule, or protein subunits, held together by noncovalent forces such as hydrogen bonds and electrostatic interactions.

General Chemical Properties

The structure of a protein directly affects its chemical properties. Proteins contain many ionizable groups on the side chains of their amino acids as well as on their N- and C-terminal ends. As a result, proteins can be positively and negatively charged. The side chains of lysine, arginine, and histidine include basic groups, and acidic groups are found on the side chains of glutamate, aspartic acid, cysteine, and tyrosine. The acid or base groups that are not involved in the peptide bond can exist in different charged forms depending on the pH of the surrounding environment (Fig. 11.5). The pH of the solution, the pK_a of the side chain, and the side chain's environment influence the charge on each side chain. The relationship between pH, pK_a, and charge for individual amino acids can be described by the Henderson-Hasselbalch equation:

$$pH = pK_a + \log \frac{[\text{conjugate base}]}{[\text{conjugate acid}]} \quad \text{(Eq. 11-1)}$$

In general terms, as the pH of a solution increases, becoming more alkaline, deprotonation of the acidic and basic groups occurs; carboxyl groups are converted to carboxylate anions (R–COOH to R–COO⁻) and ammonium groups are converted to amino groups (R–NH₃+ to R–NH₂). The pH at which an amino acid or protein has no net charge is known as its **isoelectric point (p*I*)**. When the pH is greater than the p*I*, the protein has a net negative charge, and when the pH is less than the p*I*, the protein has a net positive charge. Therefore, the p*I* is the point at which the number of positively charged groups equals the number of negatively charged groups in a protein. If a protein is placed in a solution that has a pH greater than the p*I*, the protein will be negatively charged. If the protein is placed in a solution that has a pH less than the p*I*, the protein will be positively charged. Proteins differ in their p*I* values, but for most proteins it occurs in the pH range of 5.5 to 8. Because proteins carry different net charges depending on the pH, the difference in net charge at a given pH is the basis for several procedures used to separate and quantify proteins.

The net charge on the surface of a protein depends on the number and type of amino acids it contains as well as the pH of its environment. A protein's solubility is dependent on the charge on its surface with its lowest solubility at its p*I* where the positive and negative charges balance and the net charge is zero. If there is a charge at the protein surface, the protein is referred to as hydrophilic and prefers to interact with water rather than with other protein molecules making it more soluble. The solubility of proteins in blood requires a pH in the range of 7.35 to 7.45. Without a net surface charge, the protein is less soluble and protein–protein interactions and precipitation are more likely.

FIGURE 11.5 Charged states of amino acids.

Some laboratory methods rely on the solubility of proteins to separate and quantify them.

When the secondary, tertiary, or quaternary structure of a protein is disturbed, the protein may lose its functional and chemical characteristics. This loss of its native, or naturally occurring, folded structure is called **denaturation**. Denaturation can be caused by heat, hydrolysis by strong acid or alkali, enzymatic action, exposure to urea or other substances, or exposure to ultraviolet light.

Synthesis

Most plasma proteins are synthesized in the liver and secreted by the hepatocyte into circulation. Immunoglobulins are an exception because they are synthesized in plasma cells. It is the information encoded in genes that provides each protein with its own unique amino acid sequence. The amino acid sequence of a polypeptide chain is determined by a corresponding sequence of bases (guanine, cytosine, adenine, and thymine) in the DNA contained in the specific gene. This genetic code is a set of three nucleotides known as codons, with each three-nucleotide combination standing for a specific amino acid. Because DNA contains four nucleotides, the total number of possible codons is 64; therefore, some redundancy in the genetic code allows for some amino acids to be specified by more than one codon. Double-stranded DNA unfolds in the nucleus, and one strand is used as a template for the formation of a complementary strand of mRNA in a process known as *transcription*. The mRNA is manufactured in the cell nucleus and then translocated across the nuclear membrane into the cytoplasm for *translation*.

In the process of translation, the mRNA strand is used as a template for protein synthesis by the ribosome. The mRNA is loaded onto the ribosome and is read three nucleotides at a time by matching each codon to its base pairing anticodon located on a tRNA molecule. tRNA is a short chain of RNA that occurs freely in the cytoplasm. Each amino acid has a specific tRNA that contains three bases corresponding to the three bases in the mRNA. The tRNA carries its particular amino acid to the ribosome and attaches to the mRNA in accordance with the matching codon. As each new tRNA brings in the next amino acid, the preceding amino acid is transferred onto the amino group of the new amino acid and enzymes located in the ribosomes form a peptide bond. The tRNA is released into the cytoplasm, where it can pick up another amino acid, and the cycle repeats. In this manner, the amino acids are aligned in sequence and joined together. This process continues until the mRNA message is read and all amino acids are in the specific sequence to form the polypeptide chain. When the terminal codon is reached, the peptide chain is detached and the ribosome and mRNA dissociate. Figure 11.6 illustrates basic protein synthesis.

Protein synthesis occurs at a rate of approximately two to six peptide bonds per second. Intracellular proteins are generally synthesized on free ribosomes, whereas proteins made by the liver for secretion are made on ribosomes attached to the rough endoplasmic reticulum. In some tissues, hormones, such as thyroxine, growth hormone, insulin, and testosterone, may assist in controlling protein synthesis.

Catabolism and Nitrogen Balance

Unlike fats and carbohydrates, nitrogen has no designated storage, and dietary proteins play an essential role in providing all the essential amino acids. Insufficient dietary quantities of even one amino acid can quickly limit

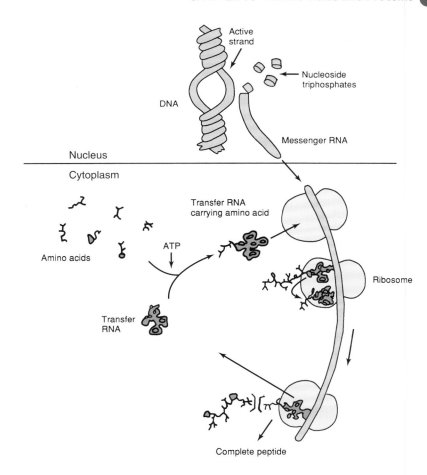

FIGURE 11.6 Schematic summary of protein synthesis.

synthesis of many essential proteins.[27] Most proteins in the body are repetitively synthesized and then degraded allowing for efficient recycling of amino acids. A balance exists between protein synthesis (anabolism) and protein breakdown (catabolism) and the turnover totals about 125 to 220 g of protein each day, with the rate of individual proteins varying widely. For example, plasma proteins and most intracellular proteins are rapidly degraded, having half-lives of hours or days, whereas some of the structural proteins, such as collagen, are metabolically stable and have half-lives of years. In health, **nitrogen balance** is maintained by equal intake and excretion of amino acids. Pregnant women, growing children, and adults recovering from major illness are often in positive nitrogen balance, which means that their nitrogen intake exceeds their loss as net protein synthesis proceeds. When more nitrogen is excreted than is incorporated into the body, an individual is in negative nitrogen balance. A negative nitrogen balance may occur in conditions in which there is excessive tissue destruction, such as burns, wasting diseases, continual high fevers, or starvation.

The breakdown of protein occurs in the digestive tract and kidneys, but primarily in the liver. Nitrogen elimination begins intracellularly with protein degradation. There are two main routes for converting intracellular proteins to free amino acids: a lysosomal pathway and a cytosolic pathway.

The central reactions that remove amino acid nitrogen from the body are known as *transaminations*. Transaminations involve moving an α-amino group from a donor α-amino acid to the keto carbon of an acceptor α-ketoacid. These reversible reactions are catalyzed by a group of intracellular enzymes known as *transaminases* and result in the production of ammonia and ketoacids. The ammonia is converted to urea by the urea cycle in hepatocytes, which is excreted in the urine. The ketoacids are oxidized by means of the citric acid cycle and are converted into glucose or fat.

Classification

From 2003 to 2005, the Human Plasma Proteome Project directed by the Human Plasma Proteome Organization (HUPO) prepared and distributed reference specimens of human serum and plasma to 55 participating laboratories worldwide. Some of the long-term goals of this project are the comprehensive analysis of plasma and serum protein constituents in humans and their physiologic, pathologic, and pharmacologic applications. Protocols used combinations of depletion, fractionation, mass spectrometry, and immunoassay methods linked via search engines and annotation groups to gene and protein databases. A new human plasma proteome database was created with, obviously, much work yet to be done.[28] The findings from the collaborative project and from laboratory-specific ancillary projects were published in a special issue of *Proteomics*, "Exploring the Human Plasma Proteome" in August 2005.

Generally speaking, proteins do everything in the living cell.[29] Proteins are responsible for many different functions within cells so they are commonly classified by the function(s) they perform.

Enzymes

Enzymes are proteins that catalyze biochemical reactions. They are normally found intracellularly, but are released into the bloodstream as a result of tissue damage, making enzyme measurements an important diagnostic tool. Transaminases, dehydrogenases, and phosphatases are just a few examples of enzyme groups that are routinely tested in the clinical laboratory to evaluate possible tissue damage.

Hormones

Hormones are chemical messenger proteins that control the action(s) of specific cells or organs. Hormones directly affect growth and development, metabolism, sexual function, reproduction, and behavior. Examples of hormones that are commonly tested in the clinical laboratory in blood, urine, or saliva are insulin, testosterone, growth hormone, follicle-stimulating hormone, and cortisol.

Transport Proteins

Many proteins are involved in the transport of ions, small molecules, or macromolecules, such as hormones, vitamins, minerals, and lipids, across a biologic membrane. Examples of commonly measured transport proteins are hemoglobin, albumin, ceruloplasmin, haptoglobin, and transferrin.

Immunoglobulins

Immunoglobulins or antibodies are proteins that are produced by B cells (lymphocytes) in the bone marrow. Immunoglobulins mediate the humoral immune response to identify and neutralize foreign antigens. Examples of immunoglobulins of clinical importance are IgG, IgM, IgE, and IgA.

Structural Proteins

Fibrous proteins provide structure to many cells and tissues throughout the body, such as muscle, tendons, and bone matrix. Collagen, elastin, and keratin are examples of structural proteins.

Storage Proteins

Storage proteins serve as reservoirs for metal ions and amino acids so they can be stored without causing harm and released later. Ferritin is a commonly measured protein that stores iron for later use in the manufacture of hemoglobin.

Energy Source

Some proteins serve as an energy source for tissues and muscle. Creatine is one example of an energy source protein as it helps to supply energy to cells throughout the body, but is primarily found in muscle tissue.

TABLE 11.2	**Functions of Proteins**

Energy—tissue nutrition
Osmotic force—maintenance of water distribution between cells and tissue, interstitial compartments, and the vascular system of the body
Acid–base balance—participation as buffers to maintain pH
Transport—metabolic substances
Antibodies—part of immune defense system
Hormones—hormones and receptors
Structure—connective tissue
Enzymes—catalysts
Hemostasis—participation in coagulation of blood

Osmotic Force

Some proteins function in the distribution of water throughout the compartments of the body. Their colloid osmotic force, due to their size, does not allow proteins to cross the capillary membranes. As a result, water is absorbed from the tissue into the venous portion of the capillary. When the concentration of plasma proteins is significantly decreased, the concomitant decrease in the plasma colloidal osmotic (oncotic) pressure results in increased levels of interstitial fluid and edema. This often occurs in renal disease when proteins are inappropriately excreted in urine and plasma protein concentrations are decreased.

Protein functions are summarized in Table 11.2.

Proteins may also be classified according to their structure. **Simple proteins** contain peptide chains composed of only amino acids. Simple proteins may be globular or fibrous in shape. Globular proteins are globe-like and have symmetrical proteins that are soluble in water. Globular proteins function as transporters, enzymes, and messengers. Examples of globular proteins are albumin, hemoglobin, and the immunoglobulins, IgG, IgA, and IgM. Fibrous proteins form long protein filaments or subunits, are asymmetrical and usually inert, and are generally water insoluble due to their hydrophobic R groups. Fibrous proteins provide structure to cells, such as connective tissues, tendons, bone, and muscle. Examples of fibrous proteins include troponin and collagen. **Conjugated proteins** consist of a protein and a nonprotein. The nonamino part of a conjugated protein is generally referred to as the prosthetic group. The prosthetic group may be a lipid, carbohydrate, porphyrin, metal, etc. It is the prosthetic group that defines the characteristics of a conjugated protein. Examples of conjugated proteins are metalloproteins, glycoproteins, lipoproteins, and nucleoproteins. Metalloproteins have a metal ion attached to the protein, either directly, as in ferritin, which contains iron, and ceruloplasmin, which contains copper, or as a complex metal such as hemoglobin and flavoproteins. Lipoproteins are composed of a protein and a lipid such as cholesterol or triglyceride; examples of lipoproteins include high-density lipoproteins (HDLs) and low-density lipoproteins (LDLs). There are several terms used to describe conjugated proteins that are bound to carbohydrates. Generally, molecules with a composition of 10% to 40% carbohydrate are referred to as glycoproteins. Examples of glycoproteins are haptoglobin and α_1-antitrypsin. When the percentage of carbohydrate is greater than 40%, the protein conjugate is referred to as a mucoprotein or proteoglycan. An example of a mucoprotein is mucin, which is a lubricant that protects body surfaces from friction or erosion. Increased mucin production occurs in many adenocarcinomas, including cancer of the pancreas, lung, breast, ovary, and colon. Moreover, mucins are also being investigated for their potential as diagnostic markers.[30] Nucleoproteins are those proteins that are combined with nucleic acids. Chromatin is an example of a nucleoprotein as it is a complex of DNA and protein that makes up chromosomes.

Several databases have been developed to aid in the identification of proteins based on their structure. The Structural Classification of Proteins (SCOP) database was created to provide a detailed and comprehensive description of the structural domains of proteins based on similarities in their amino acid sequences and three-dimensional structures. SCOP utilizes four levels of structural classification: class, fold, superfamily, and family. Originally published in 1995, SCOP is usually updated at least annually by Alexei G. Murzin et al., upon whose expertise the classification rests.[31] The Families of Structurally Similar Proteins (FSSP), also known as Fold classification, is based on the structure–structure alignment of proteins and a three-dimensional comparison of protein structures in the Protein Data Bank. Alignments and classification are updated continuously by the Dali (Distance matrix ALIgnment) server, which is an automatic server that makes a three-dimensional comparison of protein structures.[32]

PLASMA PROTEINS

Plasma proteins are the most commonly analyzed proteins in the clinical laboratory and can be divided into two major groups: albumin and **globulins**. There are four major types of globulins with specific properties and functions. Analysis of blood specimens will typically include four protein measurements: total protein, albumin, globulins, and the albumin-to-globulin (A/G) ratio; however, there are many other clinically important proteins that may be measured when indicated by clinical presentation. Some of the more significant plasma proteins and their function, structure, and relation to disease states are discussed below. The characteristics of select plasma proteins are listed in Table 11.3.

Prealbumin

Prealbumin, or transthyretin, is so named because it migrates before albumin in classic serum protein electrophoresis (SPE). It can also be separated using high-resolution electrophoresis (HRE) or immunoelectrophoresis techniques. Prealbumin is a transport protein for the thyroid hormones, thyroxine (T_4), and triiodothyronine (T_3). Prealbumin also forms a complex with retinol-binding protein to transport

retinol (vitamin A) and is rich in the amino acid tryptophan. Serum and plasma prealbumin concentrations may be decreased in hepatic damage due to decreased protein synthesis, during an acute-phase inflammatory response, or as a result of tissue necrosis. A low prealbumin may also indicate poor nutritional status. Diets deficient in protein may not provide sufficient amino acids for adequate protein synthesis by the liver resulting in decreased plasma concentrations of prealbumin, albumin, and β-globulins. Prealbumin has a half-life of approximately 2 days, so blood concentrations of prealbumin decrease faster than do those of other proteins with a longer half-life when protein synthesis is inhibited. Blood concentrations of prealbumin may be increased in patients receiving steroid therapy, who have issues with alcohol abuse, or who are in chronic renal failure.

Albumin

Albumin is synthesized in the liver at a rate of 9 to 12 g/day and is the most abundant protein in the plasma. Albumin also exists in the extravascular (interstitial) space. The total amount of extravascular albumin exceeds the total intravascular amount by about 30%; however, the concentration of albumin in plasma (albumin mass/plasma volume) is much greater than its concentration in the interstitial space. Albumin leaves the bloodstream at a rate of 4% to 5% of the total intravascular albumin concentration per hour. This rate of movement is known as the *transcapillary escape rate*, which measures systemic capillary efflux of albumin. Albumin is responsible for nearly 80% of the colloid osmotic pressure (COP) of the intravascular fluid, which maintains the appropriate fluid balance in the tissue. Albumin also buffers pH and is a negative acute-phase reactant protein.

A primary function of albumin is its capacity to bind and transport various substances in the blood. There are four binding sites on albumin that have varying specificities for different substances. Albumin is involved in the transport of thyroid hormones, unconjugated bilirubin, fat-soluble hormones, iron, fatty acids, calcium (Ca^{2+}), magnesium (Mg^{2+}), and many drugs such as salicylic acid (aspirin). Albumin also binds certain dyes, which is the basis for many of the methods used for quantitation of albumin.

Several recent studies have focused on the clinical applications of glycated (or glycosylated) albumin as a more sensitive indicator of short-term hyperglycemic control than glycated hemoglobin. Glycated hemoglobin represents trends in blood glucose over a period of 3 months or approximately 120 days, which is the life span of red blood cells. As the half-life of serum albumin is 20 days, glycated albumin represents serum glucose patterns approximating 1 month. Affinity chromatographic methods based on specific interaction of boronic acids with glycated proteins have been applied to determine serum concentrations of glycated albumin.[33]

Decreased blood concentrations of albumin are most commonly associated with an acute inflammatory response as albumin is a negative acute-phase reactant. Liver and kidney disease may also result in low blood albumin concentrations.

TABLE 11.3   Characteristics of Selected Plasma Proteins

	Reference Value (Adult, g/L)	Molecular Mass (Da)	Isoelectric Point, p/	Electrophoretic Mobility pH 8.6	
Prealbumin	0.1–0.4	55,000	4.7	7.6	Indicator of nutrition; binds thyroid hormones and retinol-binding protein
Albumin	35–55	66,300	4.9	5.9	Binds bilirubin, steroids, fatty acids; major contributor to oncotic pressure
α_1-Globulins					
α_1-Antitrypsin	2–4	53,000	4.0	5.4	Acute-phase reactant; protease inhibitor
α_1-Fetoprotein	1×10^5	76,000	2.7	6.1	Principal fetal protein. Elevated levels indicate risk for spina bifida.
α_1-Acid glycoprotein (orosomucoid)	0.55–1.4	44,000		5.2	Acute-phase reactant, may be related to immune response
α_1-Lipoprotein	2.5–3.9	200,000		4.4–5.4	Transports lipids (HDL)
α_1-Antichymotrypsin	0.3–0.6	68,000		Inter α	Inhibits serine proteinases
Inter-α–trypsin inhibitor	0.2–0.7	160,000		Inter α	Inhibits serine proteinases
Gc-globulin	0.2–0.55	59,000		Inter α	Transports vitamin D and binds actin
α_2-GLOBULINS HAPTOGLOBINS					
Type 1-1	1.0–2.2	100,000		4.5	Acute-phase reactant; binds hemoglobin
Type 2-1	1.6–3.0	200,000	4.1	3.5–4.0	Binds hemoglobin
Type 2-2	1.2–1.6	400,000		3.5–4.0	Binds hemoglobin
Ceruloplasmin	0.15–0.60	134,000	4.4	4.6	Acute-phase reactant, oxidase activity; contains copper
α_2-Macroglobulin	1.5–4.2	725,000	5.4	4.2	Inhibits proteases
β-GLOBULINS					
Pre-β lipoprotein	1.5–2.3	250,000		3.4–4.3	Transports lipids (primarily VLDL triglyceride)
Transferrin	2.04–3.60	76,000	5.9	3.1	Transports iron
Hemopexin	0.5–1.0	57,000–80,000		3.1	Binds heme
β-Lipoprotein	2.5–4.4	3,000,000		3.1	Transports lipids (primarily LDL cholesterol)
β_2-Microglobulin (B2M)	0.001–0.002	11,800		β_2	Component of leukocyte antigen (HLA) molecules
C4 complement	0.20–0.65	206,000		0.8–1.4	Immune response
C3 complement	0.55–1.80	180,000		0.8–1.4	Immune response
C1q complement	0.15	400,000			Immune response
Fibrinogen	2.0–4.5	341,000	5.8	2.1	Precursor of fibrin clot
CRP	0.01	118,000	6.2		Acute-phase reactant, motivates phagocytosis in inflammatory disease
γ-GLOBULINS					
Immunoglobulin G	8.0–12.0	150,000	5.8–7.3	0.5–2.6	Antibodies
Immunoglobulin A	0.7–3.12	180,000		2.1	Antibodies (in secretions)
Immunoglobulin M	0.5–2.80	900,000		2.1	Antibodies (early response)
Immunoglobulin D	0.005–0.2	170,000		1.9	Antibodies
Immunoglobulin E	6×10^4	190,000		2.3	Antibodies (reagins, allergy)

HDL, high-density lipoproteins; VLDL, very-low-density lipoprotein; HLA, human leukocyte antigen; CRP, C-reactive protein.

The liver is a primary site for protein synthesis, and damage to hepatocytes, such as in liver cirrhosis, may result in decreased protein synthesis. Note that an increase in globulins occurs in early liver cirrhosis, which balances the loss in albumin to give a total protein concentration within acceptable limits. Albumin is normally excreted in very small amounts by the kidneys; however, increased renal loss of albumin commonly occurs in renal disease. This increased excretion occurs when the glomerulus no longer restricts the passage of proteins from the blood into the ultrafiltrate as occurs in nephrotic syndrome. Low albumin concentrations may also be the result of malnutrition and malabsorption in which an inadequate ingestion of proteins or amino acid-rich foods results in decreased protein synthesis by the liver. Less commonly, low blood albumin concentrations occur as a result of hypothyroidism, burns or exfoliative dermatitis, dilution by excessive intake (polydipsia), or infusion of liquids (intravenously). Albumin may be redistributed by hemodilution, increased capillary permeability, or decreased lymph clearance. In sepsis, there is a profound reduction in plasma albumin associated with marked fluid shifts. Mutations resulting from an autosomal recessive trait can cause an absence of albumin, known as analbuminemia, or presence of albumin that has unusual molecular characteristics, which is referred to as bisalbuminemia. Bisalbuminemia is demonstrated by the presence of two albumin bands during electrophoresis instead of the single band usually observed. Both analbuminemia and bisalbuminemia are rare.

Abnormally high albumin concentrations are seldom clinically important and are generally associated with dehydration or excessive albumin infusion.[34]

Globulins

The globulin group of proteins consists of α_1, α_2, β, and γ fractions. Each fraction consists of a number of different proteins with individual functions. Select examples of globulins from each of the fractions are discussed below.

α_1-Antitrypsin

α_1-Antitrypsin is a glycoprotein synthesized mainly in the liver. Its main function is in the inhibition of the protease, neutrophil elastase. Neutrophil elastase is released from leukocytes during an infection, but can also destroy alveoli leading to emphysema if not inhibited by α_1-antitrypsin. Mutations in the *SERPINA1* gene can lead to a deficiency of α_1-antitrypsin protein or an abnormal form of the protein that does not properly control neutrophil elastase. The abnormal form of α_1-antitrypsin can also accumulate in the liver causing cirrhosis. α_1-Antitrypsin is a positive acute-phase reactant; therefore, increased levels of α_1-antitrypsin are seen in inflammatory reactions as well as in pregnancy and contraceptive use. Several phenotypes of α_1-antitrypsin deficiency have been identified. The most common phenotype is MM (allele *Pi*^M) and is associated with normal α_1-antitrypsin activity. Other alleles are *Pi*^S, Pi^Z, Pi^F, and *Pi* (null). The homozygous phenotype ZZ individual is at greatest risk for developing hepatic and pulmonary disease

from α_1-antitrypsin deficiency. Replacement therapy using purified α_1-antitrypsin protein from pooled plasma can dramatically slow disease progression. It is also recommended that individuals with α_1-antitrypsin deficiency do not smoke.

Decreased α_1-antitrypsin levels are most often identified in the clinical laboratory by the lack of an α_1-globulin band on serum protein electrophoresis because α_1-antitrypsin accounts for approximately 90% of the α_1-globulin fraction, which migrates immediately following albumin. Quantitative methods used to confirm α_1-antitrypsin deficiency are radial immunodiffusion and automated immunonephelometric assays. Phenotyping may also be performed using immunofixation techniques.[35]

α_1-Fetoprotein

α_1-Fetoprotein (AFP) is synthesized in utero by the developing embryo and fetus and then by the parenchymal cells of the liver. AFP concentrations decrease gradually after birth, reaching adult concentrations by 8 to 12 months of age. The physiologic function of AFP in adults has not been completely identified, but it has been proposed that α_1-fetoprotein protects the developing fetus from immunologic attack by the mother. Conditions associated with an elevated AFP concentration include spina bifida, neural tube defects, abdominal wall defects, anencephaly, general fetal distress, and the presence of twins. Low levels of maternal AFP indicate an increased risk for trisomy 21 (Down syndrome) and trisomy 18 (Edwards syndrome).

AFP screening is performed between 15 and 20 weeks gestation when maternal AFP increases gradually; therefore, interpretation requires accurate dating of the pregnancy. Measurements of AFP can be affected by laboratory-specific technique, which can result in difficulty comparing absolute results between centers. AFP levels are also affected by maternal weight, race, and diabetes; therefore, test results need to be adjusted for these variables. To account for these maternal variables, the multiple of the median or MoM is utilized. MoM is a reflection of an individual patient's value compared with the median. MoM is calculated by dividing the patient's AFP value by the median reference value for that gestational age. Most screening laboratories use 2.0 MoM as the upper limit and 0.5 MoM as the lower limit of normal for maternal serum. The methods commonly used for AFP determinations are radioimmunoassay (RIA) and enzyme-labeled immunoassay (EIA). Maternal screening tests have been established as a triple or quadruple test group using a mathematical calculation involving the concentrations of AFP, human chorionic gonadotropin (hCG), unconjugated estriol, and inhibin A. These calculations are used to determine a numerical risk for chromosomal abnormalities in the fetus, which can be compared with an established cutoff. The interpretation of these test results should be provided by a genetic counselor or clinician to aid parents and their physicians in making decisions about the management of the pregnancy.

AFP may also be used as a tumor marker and is fractionated by affinity electrophoresis into three isoforms

(L1, L2, and L3) based on their reactivity with the lectin *Lens culinaris* agglutinin (LCA). AFP-L3 is now being considered as a tumor marker for the North American population for screening chronic liver disease patients for hepatocellular carcinoma (HCC). Results for AFP-L3 are reported as a ratio of LCA-reactive AFP to total AFP (AFP-L3%). Studies have shown that AFP-L3% test results of greater than 10% are associated with a sevenfold increase in the risk of developing HCC within the next 21 months.[36] AFP's utility as a tumor marker will be discussed further in Chapter 32.

α_1-Acid Glycoprotein

α_1-Acid glycoprotein (AAG), or orosomucoid, is a major plasma glycoprotein that is negatively charged even in acidic solutions lending to its name. This protein is produced by the liver and is a positive acute-phase reactant. The possibility that AAG regulates immune responses has been suggested by several findings.[37] There is a strong similarity in the amino acid sequences between AAG and immunoglobulin. AAG elevates following stress, inflammation, tissue damage, acute myocardial infarction (AMI), trauma, pregnancy, cancer, pneumonia, rheumatoid arthritis, and surgery. Serum AAG concentrations are also used in diagnosis and evaluation of neonatal bacterial infections. In the past decade, the binding of drugs to this plasma protein has become increasingly important in regard to drug action, distribution, and disposition. The analytic methods used most commonly for the determination of AAG are radial immunodiffusion, immunoturbidity, and nephelometry. Immunofixation techniques have been used to study inherited variants. The reference interval for healthy individuals is 50 to 120 mg/dL.

CASE STUDY 11.1

Immediately following the birth of a baby girl, the attending physician requested a protein electrophoretic examination of the mother's serum. This was done on a sample that was obtained on the mother's admission to the hospital the previous day. An electrophoretic examination was also performed on the cord blood specimen. Laboratory reports are shown in Case Study Table 11.1.1.

CASE STUDY TABLE 11.1.1 Electrophoresis Values

Test	Results for Maternal Serum	Results for Cord Blood	Adult Reference Interval
Albumin	4.2 g/dL	3.5 g/dL	3.5–5.0 g/dL
α_1-Globulins	0.3 g/dL	0.0 g/dL	0.1–0.4 g/dL
α_2-Globulins	1.2 g/dL	0.4 g/dL	0.3–0.8 g/dL
β-Globulins	1.3 g/dL	0.7 g/dL	0.6–1.1 g/dL
γ-Globulins	1.3 g/dL	1.0 g/dL	0.5–1.7 g/dL

The appearance of the mother's electrophoretic pattern was within that expected for a healthy person. The electrophoretic pattern of the cord blood serum resembled the one shown in Figure 11.8C.

Questions

1. What protein fraction is abnormal in the cord blood serum?

2. An abnormality in this fraction is most often associated with what disease?

3. What other test(s) may be done to confirm this abnormality?

α_1-Antichymotrypsin

α_1-Antichymotrypsin is an α-globulin glycoprotein that is a member of the serine proteinase inhibitor (serpin) family. It inhibits the activity of the enzymes cathepsin G, pancreatic elastase, mast cell chymase, and chymotrypsin by cleaving them into a different shape (conformation). α_1-Antichymotrypsin is produced in the liver and is a positive acute-phase protein that increases during inflammation. Deficiency of this protein has been associated with liver disease due to decreased synthesis. Mutations in α_1-antichymotrypsin have been identified in patients with Parkinson's disease and chronic obstructive pulmonary disease. α_1-Antichymotrypsin is also associated with the pathogenesis of Alzheimer's disease as it is an integral component of the amyloid deposits in Alzheimer's disease.[38]

Inter-α-Trypsin Inhibitor

Inter-α-trypsin inhibitors (ITIs) are a family of serine protease inhibitors, assembled from two precursor proteins: a light chain and one or two heavy chains. While there is only one type of light chain, there are five different homologous heavy chains (ITIHs). ITIH molecules have been shown to play a particularly important role in inflammation and carcinogenesis.[39] Elevations in ITIs are often seen in inflammatory disorders.

Gc-Globulin

Gc-globulin (Gc) is also known as group-specific component or vitamin D–binding protein. Gc-globulin is mainly synthesized by hepatocytes and is the major carrier protein for vitamin D and its metabolites. It also transports components such as fatty acids and endotoxins. Gc binds actin released from cells upon injury, and the Gc–actin complexes are rapidly cleared from the circulation, thereby preventing the harmful effects of actin filaments in blood vessels. The resulting decrease in Gc concentration makes it usable as a prognostic indicator of survival of patients with significant tissue injury after trauma and among patients with hepatic failure.[40] Gc may be of importance for bone formation and in the immune system as it can act as a cochemotactic factor in facilitating chemotaxis of neutrophils and monocytes.

Due to genetic polymorphism in the Gc gene, which are codominant alleles, three major electrophoretic variants of Gc exist, Gc2, Gc1s, and Gc1f. Elevations of Gc-globulin are seen in the third trimester of pregnancy and in patients taking estrogen oral contraceptives. Severe liver disease and protein-losing syndromes are associated with low concentrations. Immunonephelometry is the method of choice for Gc measurements in the clinical laboratory.

Haptoglobin

Haptoglobin (Hp) is an α_2-glycoprotein synthesized in the liver and is a tetramer consisting of two α and two β chains. Haptoglobin is a positive acute-phase protein that increases in many inflammatory diseases, such as ulcerative colitis, acute rheumatic disease, acute myocardial infarction, and severe infection. Increases are also seen in conditions such as burns and nephrotic syndrome when large amounts of fluid and lower-molecular-weight proteins are lost; however, haptoglobin measurements are not generally used to diagnose or monitor either of these conditions. The primary function of haptoglobin is to bind free hemoglobin to prevent the loss of its constituent, iron, into the urine. When haptoglobin and hemoglobin attach, the reticulo-endothelial cells, predominantly in the spleen, remove the haptoglobin–hemoglobin complex from circulation so the hemoglobin constituents, iron and amino acids, can be recycled and haptoglobin is destroyed.

Haptoglobin concentrations are primarily used to evaluate possible hemolytic anemia and to distinguish it from anemias due to other causes. Patients with anemia typically have an increased reticulocyte count, decreased red blood cell count, decreased hemoglobin, and decreased hematocrit. Patients with a hemolytic anemia will also have a decreased haptoglobin concentration due to its destruction by the reticuloendothelial system. If the haptoglobin concentration is normal and the reticulocyte count is increased, it is likely the anemia is due to destruction of red bloods in organs such as the spleen and liver. Since the hemoglobin is not released into the bloodstream, it will not bind to haptoglobin, and haptoglobin concentrations will be within the reference interval. If the haptoglobin concentration and the reticulocyte count are within the reference interval, it is likely the anemia is not due to red blood cell breakdown. If haptoglobin concentrations are decreased without any sign of hemolytic anemia, it is possible the liver is not producing adequate amounts of haptoglobin.

An individual's haptoglobin phenotype has been reported as an independent risk factor for cardiovascular disease (CVD) in patients with type 2 diabetes mellitus.[41] Three phenotypes of haptoglobin are found in humans: Hp1-1, Hp2-1, and Hp2-2. Homozygous Hp1-1 yields one band during electrophoresis. Peptide chains form polymers with each other and with haptoglobin 1 chains to provide the other two electrophoretic patterns, which have been designated as Hp2-1 and Hp2-2 phenotypes.

Radial immunodiffusion and immunonephelometric methods have been used for the quantitative determination of haptoglobin.

Ceruloplasmin

Ceruloplasmin is a copper-containing, α_2-glycoprotein enzyme that is synthesized in the liver. Ceruloplasmin is a positive acute-phase reactant and is frequently elevated in inflammation, severe infection, and tissue damage and may be increased with some cancers. Ceruloplasmin may also be increased during pregnancy and in patients who are taking estrogen, oral contraceptives, and medications such as carbamazepine, phenobarbital, and valproic acid. Ninety percent or more of total serum copper is bound to ceruloplasmin with the remaining ten percent bound to albumin.

Ceruloplasmin is primarily measured along with blood and urine copper tests to aid in the diagnosis of Wilson's disease. Wilson's is an autosomal recessive inherited disorder associated with decreased concentrations of ceruloplasmin, typically 0.1 g/L, and excess storage of copper in the liver, brain, and other organs, which results in hepatic cirrhosis and neurologic damage. In Wilson's disease, the total serum copper concentration is decreased, but the urinary excretion of copper is increased. Copper is also deposited in the cornea, producing the characteristic Kayser-Fleischer rings. Low ceruloplasmin is also seen in malnutrition, malabsorption, severe liver disease, nephrotic syndrome, and Menkes' syndrome, in which a decreased absorption of copper results in a decrease in ceruloplasmin and distinctive "kinky hair."

The early analytic method of ceruloplasmin determination was based on its copper oxidase activity. Most assays today use immunochemical methods including radial immunodiffusion and nephelometry.

α_2-Macroglobulin

α_2-Macroglobulin is a tetramer of four identical subunits that is synthesized by the liver and is a major component of the α_2 band in protein electrophoresis. α_2-Macroglobulin inhibits proteases such as trypsin, thrombin, kallikrein, and plasmin by means of a bait region that can entrap proteinases. Entrapment reduces the accessibility of the proteinase functional sites, particularly to large molecules, but it does not completely inactivate them. After binding with and inhibiting proteases, α_2-macroglobulin is removed by the reticuloendothelial system.

In nephrosis, concentrations of serum α_2-macroglobulin may increase tenfold because its large size inhibits filtration at the renal glomeruli, which makes measurement of α_2-macroglobulin useful in evaluation of renal disease. Increased concentrations may also be seen in patients with diabetes or liver disease as well as patients using contraceptive medications. During pregnancy, serum α_2-macroglobulin concentrations may increase by 20%.

The analytic methods used for measurement of α_2-macroglobulin are radial immunodiffusion, immunonephelometry, enzyme-linked immunosorbent assay (ELISA), and latex agglutination immunoassay.

Transferrin

Transferrin, or siderophilin, is a negative acute-phase glycoprotein synthesized by the liver. It is the major component of the β-globulin fraction on protein electrophoresis and plays an important role in the transport of iron. Transferrin binds and transports iron to its storage sites, such as the liver, where it is incorporated into apoferritin, another protein, to form ferritin. Transferrin also carries iron to other sites, such as the bone marrow, that synthesize hemoglobin and other iron-containing compounds. Although iron bound to transferrin represents less than 0.1% (4 mg) of the total body iron, dynamically, it is the most important iron pool. Transferrin also prevents iron from being inappropriately deposited in tissues during temporary increases in absorbed iron or free iron.

Transferrin concentrations are routinely measured to determine the cause of anemia, to gauge iron metabolism, and to determine the iron-carrying capacity of the blood. In iron deficiency anemia, transferrin concentrations are abnormally elevated as a compensation mechanism.

Low transferrin concentrations can impair hemoglobin production and lead to anemia. A deficiency of plasma transferrin may also result in the inappropriate accumulation and precipitation of iron in tissues as hemosiderin. An increase of iron bound to transferrin is found in a hereditary disorder of iron metabolism, known as hemochromatosis, in which excess iron is deposited in the tissue, especially the liver and the pancreas. This disorder is associated with bronze skin, cirrhosis, diabetes mellitus, and low plasma transferrin levels.

Because transferrin is made in the liver, transferrin is low in liver disease or when there is not enough protein in the diet.[42] A decreased transferrin concentration can also be due to excessive loss through the kidneys in protein-losing disorders such as nephrotic syndrome. Many conditions, including infection, inflammation, and malignancy, can decrease transferrin levels as it is a negative acute-phase protein.

Atransferrinemia is inherited as an autosomal recessive trait due to mutation of both transferrin genes, with a resulting absence of transferrin. It is characterized by anemia and iron deposition (hemosiderosis) in the liver and heart and damage to the heart can lead to heart failure. This disease can be effectively treated by plasma infusions of transferrin.

The analytic methods used for the quantitation of transferrin are immunodiffusion and immunonephelometry. Total iron-binding capacity (TIBC) is typically measured along with serum iron to evaluate either iron deficiency or iron overload. The iron concentration divided by TIBC gives the transferrin saturation, which is a more useful indicator of iron status than iron or TIBC alone. In iron deficiency, total serum iron is low, but TIBC is increased, and transferrin saturation becomes very low. In iron overload, total serum iron is high and TIBC is low or normal, causing transferrin saturation to increase. It is customary to test for transferrin, rather than TIBC, when evaluating nutritional status or liver function.

Hemopexin

The parenchymal cells of the liver synthesize hemopexin, which migrates electrophoretically in the β-globulin region and is an acute-phase reactant. The main function of hemopexin is to bind with free heme, which causes oxidative damage. When free heme (ferroprotoporphyrin IX) is formed during the breakdown of hemoglobin, myoglobin, or catalase, it binds to hemopexin in a 1:1 ratio. The heme–hemopexin complex is carried to the liver, where the complex is destroyed and heme components are recycled. In this manner, hemopexin preserves the body's iron and amino acid stores. Because hemopexin is destroyed during this process, low hemopexin concentrations are diagnostic of hemolytic anemia. Increased concentrations of hemopexin are found in inflammation, diabetes mellitus, Duchenne-type muscular dystrophy, and some malignancies, especially melanomas. Hemopexin determinations are performed by radial immunodiffusion.[43]

Lipoproteins

Lipoproteins are complexes of proteins and lipids whose function is to transport cholesterol, triglycerides, and phospholipids in the bloodstream. Lipoproteins are subclassified according to their apolipoprotein and lipid content into chylomicrons, very-low-density lipoproteins (VLDL), intermediate-density lipoproteins (IDL), low-density lipoproteins (LDL), and high-density lipoproteins (HDL). In high-resolution electrophoresis, HDL migrates between the albumin and α₁-globulin zone, VLDL migrates at the beginning of the β-globulin fraction (pre-β), and LDL appears as a separate band in the β-globulin region. A detailed discussion of the structure, function, and laboratory methods used to measure lipoproteins can be found in Chapter 15.

β₂-Microglobulin

β₂-Microglobulin (B2M) is the light chain component of the major histocompatibility complex or human leukocyte antigen (HLA). This protein is found on the surface of most nucleated cells and is present in high concentrations on lymphocytes. Because of its small size (molecular weight, 11,800 kDa), B2M is filtered by the renal glomerulus, but is almost completely reabsorbed and catabolized in the proximal tubules. Elevated serum levels are the result of impaired clearance by the kidney or overproduction of the protein that occurs in a number of inflammatory diseases, such as rheumatoid arthritis and systemic lupus erythematosus (SLE). In patients with human immunodeficiency virus, a high B2M level in the absence of renal failure indicates a large lymphocyte turnover rate, suggesting the virus is killing lymphocytes. B2M may sometimes be seen on high-resolution electrophoresis, but because of its low concentration, it is usually measured by immunoassay.

Complement

The complement system is a natural defense mechanism that protects the human body from infections. These proteins are synthesized in the liver as single polypeptide chains and circulate in the blood as nonfunctional precursors. Complement C3 is the most abundant complement protein in the human serum, with complement C4 being the second most abundant. In the classic pathway, activation of these proteins begins when the first complement factor, C1q, binds to an antigen–antibody complex. Each complement protein (C2–C9) is then activated sequentially and can bind to the membrane of the cell to which the antigen–antibody complex is bound, leading to lysis of the cell. An alternate pathway for complement activation is known as the properdin pathway. In this pathway, early components are bypassed and the process begins with C3. This pathway is triggered by different substances and does not require the presence of an antibody; however, the lytic attack on the cell membrane follows the same sequence of C5 to C9.

Increased levels of both C3 and C4 are linked to acute inflammatory disease and tissue inflammation. Decreased levels of C3 are typically associated with autoimmune disease, neonatal respiratory distress syndrome, bacteremia, tissue injury, and chronic hepatitis. Complement C3 has been found to be important in the pathogenesis of age-related macular degeneration, and this finding further underscores the influence of the complement pathway in the pathogenesis of this disease.[44] Decreased levels of C4 are seen in disseminated intravascular coagulation (DIC), acute glomerulonephritis, chronic hepatitis, and SLE. Inherited deficiencies of individual complement proteins have also been described.

C3 and C4 are the most commonly measured in the clinical laboratory. Complement C3 is used as a screening test because of its pivotal position in both the classic and alternative pathway. C3 concentrations, however, are not the most sensitive indicator of classic pathway activation and a decreased complement C4 concentration is frequently found to be a more sensitive measure of mild classic pathway activation. Methods for measuring complement include nephelometric immunoassay and turbidimetry.

Fibrinogen

Fibrinogen is one of the largest proteins in blood plasma. It is synthesized in the liver and is classified as a glycoprotein because it has considerable carbohydrate content. The function of fibrinogen is to form a fibrin clot when activated by thrombin; therefore, all fibrinogen is virtually removed in the clotting process and should not be present in serum specimens. Fibrinogen is a positive acute-phase reactant and increases significantly during an inflammatory process. Fibrinogen levels also rise with pregnancy and the use of oral contraceptives. Decreased values generally reflect extensive coagulation, during which fibrinogen is consumed.

Fibrinogen is a clottable protein and its measurement in the laboratory is determined by analyzing clot formation. The concentration of fibrinogen is proportional to the time required to form a clot after the addition of thrombin to citrated plasma. Fibrin split products, which are degradation products of fibrinogen and fibrin, are determined by immunoassay methods such as radial immunodiffusion, nephelometry, and RIA. On plasma electrophoresis, fibrinogen can be seen as a small, distinct band between the β- and γ-globulin regions and indicates use of plasma instead of serum.

C-Reactive Protein

C-reactive protein (CRP) is synthesized in the liver and is one of the first acute-phase proteins to rise in response to inflammatory disease. CRP received its name because it precipitates with the C substance, a polysaccharide of pneumococci. CRP rises sharply whenever there is tissue inflammation. Inflammation has been demonstrated through many studies to be important in the development of atherosclerosis, which is the fatty deposit that accumulates in the inner lining of arteries. Atherosclerosis, in addition to being a disease of lipid accumulation, also represents a chronic inflammatory process causing an elevated CRP. Elevated levels of CRP stimulate the production of tissue factor, which initiates coagulation, activates complement, and binds to LDL in the atherosclerotic plaque. As a result, CRP concentrations are measured during the evaluation of arteriosclerosis and risk for cardiovascular disease. Major factors that promote atherosclerosis such as cigarette smoking, hypertension, plaque-causing lipoproteins, and hyperglycemia are well established.[45] These risk factors contribute to the activation of cells involved in the inflammatory process and contribute to the formation of plaque along the arterial wall. They may also contribute to plaque breaking off the artery wall, resulting in the formation of a blood clot. Interventions such as weight loss, diet, exercise, and smoking cessation and administration of pharmacologic agents such as statins all lead to reduced CRP levels and reduced vascular risk.

The American Heart Association and the Centers for Disease Control and Prevention published a joint scientific statement in 2003 on the use of inflammatory markers in clinical and public health practice. This statement was developed after systematically reviewing the evidence of association between inflammatory markers (mainly CRP) and coronary heart disease and stroke.[46] Most studies to date have focused on heart disease, but new research shows that having CRP in the high-normal range may also be associated with other diseases such as colon cancer, complications of diabetes, obesity, and the risk of developing type 2 diabetes mellitus.[47] According to these studies, individuals with CRP levels greater than 3 mg/L have four to six times greater risk for development of diabetes than individuals with lower levels of CRP. Part of the link between heart disease and diabetes is due to inflammation.

CRP is not tissue specific, but does have value as a general indicator of inflammation. Normally, there are minimal amounts of CRP in blood. A high or increasing amount of CRP suggests an acute infection or inflammation. A result above 1 mg/dL is usually considered high for CRP, and most infections and inflammations result in CRP levels above 10 mg/dL. In cases of inflammatory rheumatic diseases, such as rheumatoid arthritis and SLE, CRP is used to assess the effectiveness of treatment and monitor periods of disease eruption. However, even in known cases of inflammatory disease, a low CRP concentration is possible and is not indicative of the absence of inflammation. CRP is also significantly elevated in acute rheumatic fever, bacterial infections, myocardial infarctions, carcinomatosis, gout, and viral infections. CRP is generally measured by immunologic methods, including nephelometry and EIA and traditional methods have a sensitivity of approximately 3 to 5 mg/L.

High-Sensitivity CRP

High-sensitivity CRP (hsCRP) is the C-reactive protein, but is named for a monoclonal antibody–based test methodology that can detect CRP at levels below 1 mg/L. The hsCRP test is most commonly used to determine risk of CVD. Concentrations of less than 1 mg/L, 1 to 3 mg/L, and greater than 3 mg/L correspond to low, moderate, and high-risk groups, respectively, for future cardiovascular events.[48] High levels of hsCRP consistently predict recurrent coronary events in patients with unstable angina and AMI. Elevated hsCRP concentrations are also associated with lower survival rates in these patients. Some studies also suggest that higher concentrations of hsCRP may increase the risk that an artery will reclose after it has been opened with balloon angioplasty. A more detailed discussion of cardiovascular risk factors can be found in Chapter 26.

Immunoglobulins

The immunoglobulins (Igs), or antibodies, are glycoproteins composed of 82% to 96% protein and 4% to 18% carbohydrate. They are produced by white blood cells, known as B cells, that confer humoral immunity. These proteins consist of two identical heavy (H) chains and two identical light (L) chains linked by two disulfide bonds. They can be in the form of a monomer with one unit, a dimer with two units, or a pentamer with five units. There are five classes (isotopes) of immunoglobulins, IgG, IgA, IgM, IgD, and IgE, based on the type of heavy chain they possess; their heavy chains are γ, α, μ, δ, and ε, respectively. There are two types of light chains, kappa (k) and lambda (λ) chains. For example, IgG has two γ-type heavy chains and two identical light chains, either k or λ. Each heavy chain has two regions, the constant region and the variable region. The constant region is identical in all antibodies of the same isotype, but differs in antibodies of different isotypes. The variable region of the heavy chain differs in antibodies produced by different B cells, but is the same for all antibodies produced by a single B cell or B-cell clone. The ratio of k to λ chains is 2:1, which is sometimes used as a marker of immune abnormalities.

The N-terminal regions of the heavy and light chains exhibit highly variable amino acid composition referred to as VH and VL, respectively. This variable region is involved in antigen binding. Similarly, to the variable region, the constant domains of light and heavy chains are referred to as CL and CH, respectively. The constant regions are involved in complement binding, placental passage, and binding to cell membranes.

Genes for the variable regions contain three distinct types of segments encoded in the human genome. For example, the immunoglobulin heavy chain region contains 65 *Variable* (V) genes plus 27 *Diversity* (D) genes and six functional *Joining* (J) genes.[49] The light chains also possess numerous V and J genes, but do not have D genes. By the mechanism of DNA rearrangement of these regional genes, it is possible to generate an antibody repertoire of more than 10^7 possible combinations. V(D)J recombination is a genetic mechanism that randomly selects and assembles segments of genes encoding specific proteins, which generates a diverse repertoire of T-cell receptor and immunoglobulin molecules. These molecules are necessary for the recognition of diverse antigens from bacterial, viral, and parasitic invaders and from dysfunctional cells such as tumor cells.[50]

Immunoglobulin class switching, or isotype switching, is a biologic mechanism that changes an antibody from one class to another. For example, an isotype IgM could be changed to an isotype IgG. This process occurs after activation of the B cell, which allows the cell to produce different classes of antibody. Only the constant region of the antibody heavy chain changes during class switching. Because the variable region does not change, class switching does not affect the antigens that are bound by the antibody. Instead, the antibody retains affinity for the same antigens, but can interact with different effector molecules, which are regulatory molecules that bind to a protein and alter their activity.[51]

The antibody molecule has a "Y" shape, with the tip being the site that binds antigen, and, therefore, recognizes specific foreign objects. This region of the antibody is called the Fab (fragment, antigen binding) region. It is composed of one constant and one variable domain from each heavy and light chain of the antibody. The base of the Y is called the Fc, or fragment, crystallisable, region and is composed of two heavy chains that contribute two or three constant domains depending on the class of the antibody.[52] By binding to specific proteins, the Fc region ensures that each antibody generates an appropriate immune response for a given antigen. The Fc region also binds to various cell receptors, such as Fc receptors, and other immune molecules, such as complement proteins. By doing this, it mediates different physiologic effects including opsonization, cell lysis, and degranulation of mast cells, basophils, and eosinophils.[53]

IgG is the most abundant class of antibodies found in blood plasma and lymph. IgG antibodies act on bacteria, fungi, viruses, and foreign particles by agglutination, opsonization, and complement activation and by neutralizing toxins. IgG is increased in liver disease, infections, IgG myeloma, parasitic disease, and many rheumatic diseases. Decreased IgG levels are associated with acquired immunodeficiency, an increased susceptibility to infections, hereditary deficiency, protein-losing states, and non-IgG myeloma. Immunoglobulins are not synthesized to any extent by the developing fetus; however, IgG can cross the placenta so any IgG present in a newborn's serum was synthesized by the mother.

IgA is the main immunoglobulin found in mucous secretions, including tears, saliva, colostrum, vaginal fluid, and secretions from the respiratory and gastrointestinal mucosa, and is also found in small amounts in blood. It exists in two isotypes, IgA1 (90%) and IgA2 (10%). IgA1 is found in serum and is made by bone marrow B cells, while IgA2 is made by B cells located in the mucosa. IgA is also classified based upon location, serum IgA and secretory IgA. Secretory IgAs are polymers of two to four IgA monomers linked by two additional chains, one being the J chain (Joining chain), which is a polypeptide-containing cysteine and completely different structurally from other immunoglobulin chains. Secretory IgA is resistant to enzyme degradation and remains active in the digestive and respiratory tracts to provide antibody protection in body secretions. Increases in serum IgA are found in liver disease, infections, and autoimmune diseases, while decreases are found in depressed protein synthesis and immunodeficiency.

IgM is the first antibody to appear in response to antigenic stimulation and is present in B cells. IgM is a pentamer and contains a J chain, which also makes it an important secretory immunoglobulin. Anti-A and anti-B IgM antibodies occur naturally as part of the ABO blood grouping system. Increased IgM concentration is found in toxoplasmosis, primary biliary cirrhosis, cytomegalovirus, rubella, herpes, syphilis, and various bacterial and fungal diseases. A monoclonal increase in IgM antibodies is seen in Waldenström's macroglobulinemia as a spike in the vicinity of the late β zone on protein electrophoresis. Decreases are seen in protein-losing conditions and hereditary immunodeficiency. IgM cannot cross the placenta, but it is the only immunoglobulin synthesized by the neonate.

IgD molecules are present on the surface of most, but not all, B cells early in their development though little IgD is ever released into the circulation. IgD may help regulate B-cell function; however, the specific function of circulating IgD is largely unknown. Its concentration is typically increased in infections, liver disease, and connective tissue disorders.[54]

IgE is produced by B cells and plasma cells and is associated with allergic and anaphylactic reactions. In contrast to other immunoglobulins, the concentration of IgE in the circulation is very low. An elevated IgE concentration is not diagnostic of any single condition, but elevated IgE levels are observed in many inflammatory and infectious diseases, including asthma and hay fever. Monoclonal increases are seen in IgE myeloma, but are rare.

The immunoglobulins have been determined using radial immunodiffusion, nephelometry, turbidimetry, electrochemiluminescent immunoassay (ECLIA), and RIA. Fluorescent immunoassay techniques and immunonephelometric assays have also been used, and solid-phase displacement RIAs, double-antibody RIAs, solid-phase sandwich RIAs, and nephelometry are all used to measure IgE.[55] Monoclonal increases are seen on serum protein electrophoresis (SPE) patterns as spikes.

CASE STUDY 11.2

Victoria and Rusty were worried about their infant Bailey since his first trip to the hospital at 3 weeks of age. At that time, he had a temperature of 103°F and a runny nose. The emergency department physician examined the infant, but determined the child was suffering from a common cold, probably brought home by his older siblings, and that all would be fine. Since then Bailey's health has not improved and he has experienced an unusual number of bacterial infections. The antibiotics that Bailey's pediatrician prescribed have cleared up the bacterial respiratory infections, but the infection seems to recur.

Bailey is now back at the hospital with pneumonia and his physician has ordered a number of laboratory tests as he is now worried about Bailey's immune system. The studies show that Bailey has normal levels of B cells and T cells, with his immunoglobulin levels and hematology results listed in Case Study Table 11.2.1.

CASE STUDY TABLE 11.2.1 Laboratory Results

Test	Result	Reference Interval
Hematocrit	35%	6 mo–2 y: 30.9–37.0%
Hemoglobin	11.9 g/dL	6 mo–2 y: 10.3–12.4 g/dL
White blood cell count	$14.0 \times 10^3/\mu L$	6 mo–2 y: 6.2–14.5 × $10^3/\mu L$
IgG	153 mg/dL	1–3 y: 507–1,407 mg/dL
IgM	576 mg/dL	1–3 y: 18–171 mg/dL
IgA	11 mg/dL	1–3 y: 63–298 mg/dL
IgD	0 mg/dL	Newborn to adult: 0–8 mg/dL
IgE	1 kIU/L	1–3 y: <90 kIU/L
Total protein	8.7 g/dL	1 y: 5.4–7.5 g/dL
Albumin	3.8 g/dL	1–3 y: 3.4–4.2 g/dL

Questions

1. Which immunoglobulin type(s) are abnormal in this patient's serum?

2. How do the laboratory results correlate with recurring bacterial infections?

3. How does isotype switching explain the lack of IgG, IgA, and IgE in this patient's serum?

OTHER PROTEINS OF CLINICAL SIGNIFICANCE

Myoglobin

Myoglobin is a single-chain globular protein of 153 amino acids, containing a heme prosthetic group. Myoglobin is the primary oxygen-carrying protein found in striated skeletal and cardiac muscle, accounting for approximately 2% of total muscle protein. Most myoglobin found in cells is dissolved in the cytoplasm. It can reversibly bind oxygen similarly to the hemoglobin molecule, but myoglobin requires a very low oxygen tension to release the bound oxygen.

As a cardiac biomarker, myoglobin has been used in conjunction with troponin to help diagnose or rule out an acute myocardial infarction, or heart attack. When striated muscle is damaged, myoglobin is released into the bloodstream resulting in elevated blood concentrations. Following an acute myocardial infarction, blood concentrations of myoglobin elevate within 2 to 3 hours and reach peak concentrations within 8 to 12 hours. Myoglobin is a small molecule freely filtered by the kidneys so blood concentrations return to normal within 18 to 30 hours after the AMI. Because of the early appearance and rapid clearance of myoglobin, it is also a useful marker for monitoring the success or failure of reperfusion. Although the diagnostic sensitivity of myoglobin elevations following an AMI is reported to be between 75% and 100%, myoglobin is not specific to cardiac tissue. Elevations are also seen in conditions affecting muscle tissue, such as progressive muscular dystrophy and crush injuries in which skeletal muscle is damaged. Myoglobin is a nephrotoxin, and in severe muscle injury, concentrations of myoglobin may raise very quickly causing damage to the kidneys. Renal failure can also elevate blood concentrations of serum myoglobin due to impaired filtration at the glomerulus. Table 11.4 lists some causes of serum myoglobin elevation.

Latex agglutination, ELISA, immunonephelometry, ECLIA, and fluoroimmunoassays are most commonly used in the clinical laboratory for myoglobin measurement, but a qualitative spot test using immunochromatography is also available.

Cardiac Troponin

Cardiac troponin (cTn) represents a complex of regulatory proteins that include troponin C (TnC), troponin I (cTnI), and troponin T (cTnT) that are specific to cardiac muscle. Cardiac troponins are considered the "gold standard" for diagnosis of acute coronary syndrome (ACS) in which the blood supply to the heart muscle is suddenly impeded. It is

recommended that cTn be measured in all patients presenting with symptoms suggestive of ACS, in conjunction with physical examination and electrocardiogram.[56] Because of the specificity of cTn for myocardial damage, a single blood cTn measurement above the decision limit, along with clinical evidence, is indicative of myocardial injury.

The American College of Cardiology and the European Society of Cardiology in conjunction with the National Academy of Clinical Biochemistry recommend the use of a decision limit for myocardial injury at the 99th percentile of the reference population for cTnT and cTnI.[57] Although it is acceptable to use the manufacturer's decision limits, each laboratory should, if possible, define its own cutoff value based on its reference population and, ideally, not exceed a total imprecision of 10% at the diagnostic cutoff. Normal blood concentrations of cTnI are generally below 10 ng/mL and may rise tenfold following an AMI. cTn testing may be ordered by itself or in conjunction with other cardiac biomarkers, such as creatine kinase (CK), CK-MB, and myoglobin. cTnI and cTnT tests are quickly replacing total CK and CK-MB measurements because they are more specific to cardiac tissue and remain elevated in circulation for a longer period of time.[57] Following an AMI, blood concentrations of cardiac troponins elevate within 3 to 12 hours of onset, reach peak concentrations within 12 to 24 hours, and remain elevated for 1 to 3 weeks. If CK, CK-MB, and myoglobin concentrations are normal, but troponin is elevated, it is possible that damage to the heart was minor or that the injury took place more than 24 hours in the past. If the initial troponin measurement is within the reference interval, but subsequent (6- and 12-hour specimens) troponin results are elevated, then damage to the heart likely occurred a couple of hours prior to the initial specimen collection and blood concentrations had not yet significantly elevated. When CK is elevated, but troponin is within the reference interval, it is likely that symptoms are present due to a cause other than AMI, such as skeletal muscle injury.

Cardiac troponins can be measured using ELISA or immunoenzymometric assays using two monoclonal antibodies directed against different epitopes, or antigenic determinants, on the protein. A more detailed discussion of cardiac markers can be found in Chapter 26.

Brain Natriuretic Peptide and N-Terminal–Brain Natriuretic Peptide

Natriuretic peptides are a family of structurally related hormones that include atrial natriuretic peptide (ANP), B-type (or brain) natriuretic peptide (BNP), C-type natriuretic peptide (CNP), and dendroaspis natriuretic peptide (DNP). B-type natriuretic peptides are produced initially as a 134–amino acid prepropeptide, which is cleaved into proBNP108, a precursor molecule stored in myocytes. Upon release, proBNP108 is cleaved by the protease, furin, into N-terminal (NT)-proBNP, a 76–amino acid biologically inert portion, and BNP, which is biologically active. NT-proBNP and BNP are found in greatest concentration in the left ventricular myocardium, but are also detectable in atrial tissue and the myocardium of the right ventricle.

TABLE 11.4   Causes of Myoglobin Elevations

Acute myocardial infarction
Angina without infarction
Rhabdomyolysis
Muscle trauma
Renal failure
Myopathies
Vigorous exercise
Intramuscular injections
Open heart surgery
Seizures (tonic–clonic)
Electric shock
Arterial thrombosis
Certain toxins

The natriuretic peptides are neurohormones that affect body fluid homeostasis, through natriuresis and diuresis, and blood pressure, through decreased angiotensin II and norepinephrine synthesis. Both are major components in the pathology of congestive heart failure, which is why BNP has become a popular marker for congestive heart failure.[58]

Laboratory methods for measurement of BNP and NT-proBNP include RIA, microparticle enzyme immunoassay (MEIA), and ECLIA.

Fibronectin

Fibronectin is a glycoprotein composed of two nearly identical subunits. Although fibronectin is the product of a single gene, the resulting protein can exist in multiple forms due to splicing of a single pre-mRNA. The variants demonstrate a wide variety of cellular interactions including roles in cell adhesion, tissue differentiation, growth, and wound healing. These proteins are found in plasma and on cell surfaces and can be synthesized by hepatocytes, endothelial cells, peritoneal macrophages, and fibroblasts.

Fetal fibronectin (fFN) is used to help predict the short-term risk of premature delivery. fFN is produced at the boundary between the amniotic sac and the lining of the uterus; it is thought that fFN helps maintain the integrity of this boundary and adherence of the placenta to the uterus. fFN is normally detectable in amniotic fluid and placental tissue during early pregnancy, but in a normal pregnancy, it is not detectable after 24 weeks' gestation. Elevated fFN concentrations between 22 and 36 weeks gestation reflect a disturbance at the uteroplacental junction and are associated with an increased risk of preterm labor and delivery.

Adiponectin

Adiponectin is a 247–amino acid hormone composed of an N-terminal collagen-like domain and a C-terminal globular domain produced by adipocytes. Adiponectin exists in trimers, hexamers, and multimers in the blood. Recent studies have shown an inverse correlation between body mass index and adiponectin values. Lower levels of adiponectin correlate with an increased risk of heart disease, type 2 diabetes mellitus, metabolic syndrome, and obesity.[59]

β-Trace Protein

β-Trace protein (BTP), or prostaglandin D synthase, is a 168–amino acid, low-molecular-mass protein in the lipocalin protein family. Recently, blood BTP measurements were established as an accurate marker of cerebrospinal fluid leakage and have also been used as a potential marker in detecting impaired renal function though BTP is no more sensitive than cystatin C.[60] BTP serum values correlate significantly with serum cystatin C, glomerular filtration rate, and urine microproteins, but BTP is not a diagnostically efficient test for evaluation of the glomerular filtration rate. One benefit of BTP measurement is that BTP concentrations, in contrast to cystatin C concentrations, are not influenced by glucocorticoid therapy. BTP is also being evaluated as a promising marker in the diagnosis of perilymphatic fluid fistulas.

Cross-Linked C-Telopeptides

Cross-linked C-telopeptides (CTXs) are proteolytic fragments of collagen I formed during bone turnover, and their presence in serum and urine is a biochemical marker of bone resorption. Bone resorption rates increase at menopause resulting in elevated blood CTX concentrations. After 3 to 6 months of antiresorptive therapy, CTX concentrations drop 35% to 55% compared to baseline concentrations. There are a few limitations in measuring CTX concentrations, which include the need to establish a baseline value as well as the variability in CTX concentrations due to a patient's diet, exercise, diurnal variation, etc. CTX measurements cannot replace bone mineral density testing in the diagnosis of osteoporosis; however, CTX testing is useful in monitoring response to antiresorptive therapy as it is noninvasive and can be repeated often. ECLIA technology is used to measure CTX in the laboratory.

Cystatin C

Cystatin C, a low-molecular-mass protein with 120 amino acids, is a cysteine proteinase inhibitor. It is freely filtered by the glomerulus and almost completely reabsorbed and catabolized by the proximal tubular cells. Cystatin C was recently proposed as a new sensitive endogenous serum marker for the glomerular filtration rate because it is produced and destroyed at a fairly constant rate. When the glomerular filtration rate is reduced, blood concentrations of substances removed by them, such as cystatin C and creatinine, increase and are an indication of impaired renal function. Unlike creatinine, which has been traditionally used in determinations of glomerular function, cystatin C concentrations are not affected by muscle mass, gender, age, or race nor are they generally affected by most drugs, infections, diet, or inflammation. In some facilities, cystatin C may be used as an alternative to creatinine and creatinine clearance testing to screen for and monitor kidney dysfunction. While there are ongoing studies supporting the use of cystatin C, there is still a degree of uncertainty about when and how it should be used.[61] It may be useful in cases where creatinine measurement is not appropriate, such as in patients with cirrhosis, obesity, malnutrition, or who have a reduced muscle mass. In addition to kidney dysfunction, cystatin C has been associated with an increased risk of cardiovascular disease and heart failure in the elderly.[62] Cystatin C measurements may be performed by particle-enhanced immunoturbidimetric or immunonephelometric methods.

Amyloid

Amyloids are insoluble fibrous protein aggregates formed due to an alteration in their secondary structure known as β-pleated sheets. Amyloidosis refers to conditions in which amyloids are abnormally deposited in organs and tissues, including the heart and blood vessels, brain and peripheral nerves, kidneys, liver, spleen, and intestines, causing localized or widespread organ failure. Amyloidosis can be inherited secondary to diseases that cause overabundant or abnormal protein production, such as chronic infections, malignancies, and rheumatologic disorders.

Amyloid β42 (Aβ42) and Tau protein tests are not routinely performed, but may be used to aid in the differential diagnosis of Alzheimer's disease from other forms of dementia. Abnormal forms of Tau, a brain phosphoprotein, make up part of the structure of neurofibrillary tangles (twisted protein fragments that clog nerve cells), while Aβ42, which is formed from β amyloid precursor protein, is associated with the creation of senile plaques. Tau protein and Aβ42 tests are performed primarily in research settings on cerebrospinal fluid. In a symptomatic patient, a low Aβ42 concentration along with an elevated Tau concentration indicates an increased likelihood of developing Alzheimer's disease, but it does not mean the patient will absolutely develop Alzheimer's. If a symptomatic patient has normal levels of Aβ42 and Tau proteins, the cause of dementia is not likely to be related to Alzheimer's disease.

CASE STUDY 11.3

A 76-year-old woman was admitted to the hospital with gangrene of her right toe. She was disoriented and had difficulty finding the right words to express herself. On evaluation, it was revealed she lived alone and was responsible for her own cooking. A daughter who lived in the area said her mother was a poor eater, even with much encouragement. An ECG, performed on admission, showed possible ectopic rhythm with occasional premature supraventricular contractions. The cardiologist suspected a possible inferior myocardial infarction of undetermined age. Laboratory results are shown in Case Study Table 11.3.1.

CASE STUDY TABLE 11.3.1 Laboratory Results

Day 1—Baseline

Test	Results	Reference Interval
CK total	187 U/L	40–325 U/L
CK-MB mass	6 µg/L	<8 µg/L
Troponin I	16.3 µg/L	0–2 µg/L
NT-proBNP	60 pmol/L	2–50 pmol/L
Prealbumin	15 mg/dL	17–42 mg/dL
Albumin	2.7 g/dL	3.7–4.9 g/dL

Day 1—5 Hours Later

Test	Results	Reference Interval
CK total	180 U/L	40–325 U/L
CK-MB mass	5.4 µg/L	<8 µg/L
Troponin I	17.5 µg/L	0–2 µg/L
NT-proBNP	100.5 pmol/L	2–50 pmol/L

Day 2

Test	Results	Reference Interval
CK total	177 U/L	40–325 U/L
CK-MB mass	4.5 µg/L	<8 µg/L
Troponin I	13.7 µg/L	0–2 µg/L
NT-proBNP	143 pmol/L	2–50 pmol/L
Myoglobin	>500 µg/L	<76 µg/L

Questions

1. What is the clinical significance of the troponin I results for this patient?

2. What condition(s) presented in the scenario would correlate with the low prealbumin value?

3. What is a possible explanation for the patient's elevated myoglobin?

TOTAL PROTEIN ABNORMALITIES

Total protein measurements include all plasma proteins and are used in the evaluation of nutritional status, kidney disease, liver disease, and many other conditions. If total protein results are abnormal, further testing must be performed to identify which protein fraction is abnormal so that a specific diagnosis can be made.

Hypoproteinemia

Hypoproteinemia, a total protein concentration below the reference interval, occurs in any condition where a negative nitrogen balance exists. General causes of hypoproteinemia include excessive loss, decreased synthesis, and increased protein catabolism. Excessive loss of plasma proteins may occur as a result of renal disease in which increased glomerular permeability allows inappropriate passage of proteins into the glomerular ultrafiltrate for excretion. Plasma proteins may also be lost due to leakage into the gastrointestinal tract during inflammation of the digestive system, through loss of blood in open wounds, internal bleeding, or extensive burns. Hypoproteinemia may be the result of decreased intake of proteins and amino acids, because of malnutrition, maldigestion, or malabsorption, as seen in sprue. Inadequate dietary proteins may result in a deficiency of essential amino acids and impaired protein synthesis. Liver disease can also cause low serum protein concentrations as the liver is a primary site for protein synthesis. Inherited immunodeficiency disorders, in which antibody production is diminished, also result in decreased blood total protein concentrations. Accelerated catabolism of proteins, as might occur in burns, trauma, or other injuries, is another cause of hypoproteinemia.

Hyperproteinemia

Hyperproteinemia, or an increase in total plasma proteins, is not associated with disease state, but is commonly the result of dehydration. In dehydration, excessive water is lost from the vascular system, but proteins, due to their size, remain within the blood vessels. Although the absolute quantity of proteins in the blood remains unchanged, the concentration appears elevated due to a decreased volume of water, which is the solvent. Dehydration results from a variety of conditions, including vomiting, diarrhea, excessive sweating, diabetic acidosis, and hypoaldosteronism.

In addition to dehydration, hyperproteinemia may be the result of excessive production, primarily of the γ-globulins. These disorders are characterized by the appearance of a monoclonal protein or paraprotein in the serum, which often appears in the urine as well. Monoclonal proteins are intact immunoglobulin molecules or, occasionally, k or λ light chains only. Many disorders, including chronic inflammatory states, collagen vascular disorders, and other neoplasms, may be associated with paraproteins. Waldenström's macroglobulinemia is a rare type of slow-growing, non-Hodgkin lymphoma associated with IgM paraprotein; however, the most well-known monoclonal disorder is multiple myeloma, in which neoplastic plasma cells proliferate in the bone marrow. Paraproteins in multiple myeloma may reach serum concentrations of several grams per deciliter and are usually IgG, IgA, or k or λ light chains.

Polyclonal increases in immunoglobulins, which would be represented by increases in both k and λ light chains, are seen in the serum and urine in many chronic diseases. Table 11.5 summarizes disease states affecting total protein concentrations with their relative changes in albumin and globulin fractions.

METHODS OF ANALYSIS

Total Nitrogen

A total nitrogen determination measures all chemically bound nitrogen in the specimen and can be performed on various sample types, but is most commonly performed using plasma. Both protein and nonprotein nitrogen compounds, such as urea and creatinine, are measured and reported as the blood urea nitrogen (BUN) concentration. Total nitrogen concentrations are useful in assessing causes of nitrogen imbalance and in monitoring the nitrogen nutritional status of patients receiving total parenteral nutrition, such as individuals with neurologic injuries who are sustained on intravenous fluids for an extended period of time.

The most common method for total nitrogen analysis uses chemiluminescence.[62] The specimen, in the presence of oxygen, is heated to a high temperature ($1,100 \pm 20°C$) causing all the chemically bound nitrogen to be oxidized to nitric oxide. The nitric oxide is then mixed with ozone (O_3) to form an excited nitrogen dioxide molecule (NO_2). When this molecule decays to its ground state, it emits chemiluminescent light, which can be detected, amplified, and converted to an electronic signal proportional to the total nitrogen content in the specimen.

Total Protein

The specimen most often used to determine total protein concentration is serum rather than plasma. A fasting specimen is not generally required; however, lipemia may interfere with some of the methods. Hemolyzed specimens are unacceptable because the release of red blood cell proteins into the serum can falsely elevate the total protein result.

Total protein concentrations are lower at birth, but reach adult levels by 3 years of age. The reference interval

TABLE 11.5	Protein Levels in Selected Disease States		
Total Protein	**Albumin**	**Globulin**	**Disease**
N, ↓	↓	↑	Hepatic damage • Cirrhosis β-γ bridging • Hepatitis ↑ γ-globulins • Obstructive jaundice ↑ α₂-, β-globulins Burns, trauma Infections • Acute ↑ α₁-, α₂-globulins • Chronic ↑ α₁-, α₂-, γ-globulins
↓	↓	N	Malabsorption Inadequate diet Nephrotic syndrome ↑ α₂-, β-globulins; ↓ γ-globulins
↓	N	↓	Immunodeficiency syndromes
↓	↓	↓	Salt retention syndrome
↑	↑	↑	Dehydration
↑	N	↑	Multiple myeloma Monoclonal and polyclonal gammopathies

↑, increased; ↓, decreased; N, normal levels.

Method	Principle	Comment
Kjeldahl	Digestion of protein; measurement of nitrogen content	Reference method; assume average nitrogen content of 16%
Biuret	Formation of violet-colored chelate between Cu^{2+} ions and peptide bonds	Routine method; requires at least two peptide bonds and an alkaline medium
Dye binding	Protein binds to dye and causes a spectral shift in the absorbance maximum of the dye	Research use

Refractometry is a rapid, simple method, but is not commonly used for total protein analysis.[63]

for serum total protein is 6.5 to 8.3 g/dL (65 to 83 g/L) for adults; however, when patients are drawn in a recumbent position, the reference interval is 6.0 to 7.8 g/dL (60 to 78 g/L) due to reduction in serum albumin and fluid shift toward the extracellular compartments. Albumin concentrations decrease with age and lower total protein concentrations are also seen in pregnancy. Methods for the determination of total protein are described below and summarized in Table 11.6.

Kjeldahl

The classic method for quantitation of total protein is the Kjeldahl method, which measures the amount of nitrogen in the specimen. Serum proteins are precipitated with an organic acid, such as trichloroacetic acid (TCA) or tungstic acid, and the nonprotein nitrogen is removed with the supernatant. The protein pellet is then digested in sulfuric acid (H_2SO_4) with heat (340°C to 360°C) and a catalyst, such as cupric sulfate ($CuSO_4$), to accelerate the reaction. Potassium sulfate (K_2SO_4) is also introduced to increase the boiling point, which improves the efficiency of the digestion step. Sulfuric acid oxidizes carbon, hydrogen, and sulfur found in proteins to carbon dioxide (CO_2), carbon monoxide (CO), water, and sulfur dioxide (SO_2). Nitrogen in the protein is converted to ammonium bisulfite (NH_4HSO_4), which is then measured by adding alkali and distilling the ammonia into a standard boric acid solution. The ammonium borate ($NH_4H_2BO_3$) formed is then titrated with a standard solution of hydrochloric acid (HCl) to determine the amount of nitrogen in the original specimen.

This method is no longer routinely used in the clinical laboratory because it is time consuming and relies on some assumptions that are not always true. In this method, proteins are assumed to contain an average mass of 16% nitrogen; however, the actual nitrogen content of serum proteins varies from 15.1% to 16.8%. Therefore, error is introduced if the protein standard in use differs in composition from the serum specimen to be analyzed because the percentage of nitrogen content will not be the same. The method also requires the assumption that no clinically significant proteins are lost in the precipitation step.

Biuret

The biuret procedure is the most widely used method for the determination of total protein and is recommended by the International Federation of Clinical Chemistry expert panel. This reaction is based on the principle that in an alkaline medium and the presence of at least two peptide bonds, cupric ions (Cu^{2+}) will complex with groups involved in the peptide bond to form a violet-colored chelate. The reagent also contains sodium potassium tartrate, which forms a complex with cupric ions to prevent their precipitation in the alkaline solution, and potassium iodide, which acts as an antioxidant. The absorbance of the colored chelate is measured at 540 nm using a spectrophotometer. The color and resultant absorbance are proportional to the number of peptide bonds present and reflect the total protein concentration of the specimen. The color of the reaction varies from a pink to a reddish violet color because when small peptides react, the color of the chelate has a different shade than that seen with larger peptides. Lipemic specimens should not be used with this method as they are considered an interferent.[64]

Dye Binding

Dye-binding methods are based on the ability of most serum proteins to bind dyes, although the affinity with which they bind may vary. Bromophenol blue, Ponceau S, amido black 10B, lissamine green, and Coomassie brilliant blue are commonly used to stain protein bands after electrophoresis. One dye-binding method, Coomassie brilliant blue 250, relies on the binding of Coomassie brilliant blue 250 to protein, which causes a shift in the absorbance maximum of the dye from 465 to 595 nm. The resulting increase in absorbance at 595 is used to determine the total protein concentration of the specimen. Although dye-binding methods are simple and fast, the unequal dye-binding response of individual proteins requires caution when using this type of method with the complex mixture of proteins found in human serum.

Fractionation, Identification, and Quantitation of Specific Proteins

When evaluating total serum protein concentrations, it may be clinically useful to determine the albumin and globulin fractions and compare them as a ratio (A/G ratio). To determine the A/G ratio, total protein and albumin concentrations are measured, and then the concentration of globulins can be calculated by subtracting the albumin concentration from the total protein concentration (globulins = total protein – albumin). The A/G ratio is calculated by dividing the albumin concentration by the calculated globulin concentration (A/G = albumin/globulins). A decreased A/G ratio may be the result of decreased albumin or increased globulins. Low serum albumin concentrations may be the result of decreased protein synthesis by the liver or renal loss of proteins as might occur in diseases of the kidneys. Globulins may be elevated due to conditions such as multiple myeloma, chronic inflammatory disorders, and rheumatoid arthritis. An elevated A/G ratio may be associated with decreased globulin synthesis. The following are methods for measuring protein fractions.

Salt Fractionation

In salt fractionation, globulins are separated from albumin by a precipitation process using sodium salt. Addition of the salt causes the globulins to precipitate out of solution. The albumin that remains in solution in the supernatant is then measured by any of the routine total protein methods. Salt fractionation is not routinely used because simpler and more direct methods are available that react specifically with albumin.

Albumin

The most widely used methods for determining albumin are dye-binding procedures. The pH of the solution is adjusted so that albumin is positively charged and binds to an anionic dye by electrostatic forces. When bound to albumin, the dye has a different absorption maximum than the free dye. The concentration of albumin is calculated by measuring the absorbance of the albumin–dye complex, which is proportional to the specimen's albumin concentration. A variety of dyes have been used, including methyl orange, 2,4′-hydroxyazobenzene-benzoic acid (HABA), bromocresol green (BCG), and bromocresol purple (BCP). Methyl orange is not specific for albumin and β-lipoproteins and some α_1- and α_2-globulins will bind to this dye, which could result in falsely elevated values. HABA is more specific for albumin, but several compounds, such as salicylates (aspirin), penicillin, conjugated bilirubin, and sulfonamides, interfere with the binding of albumin to HABA, which can result in falsely low values. BCG is not affected by interfering substances such as bilirubin and salicylates; however, hemoglobin binds to BCG and can lead to falsely high albumin values. For example, for every 100 mg/dL of hemoglobin, albumin is increased by 0.1 g/dL.[65] BCG has been reported to overestimate low albumin values in patients when accompanied by an elevated α-globulin fraction, such as occurs in nephrotic syndrome or end-stage renal disease.[66] It has also been found that α-globulins react with BCG, giving a color intensity that is approximately one-third of the reaction seen with albumin. The specificity of the reaction for albumin can be improved by taking absorbance readings within a short, standardized interval (<5 minutes) as α-globulins contribute significantly at longer incubations.[67]

BCP binds specifically to albumin and is not subject to most interferences, but does appear to be affected by the presence of bilirubin. BCP is precise and exhibits excellent correlation with immunodiffusion reference methods; however, BCP is not without its disadvantages. In patients with renal insufficiency, the BCP method has been found to underestimate the serum albumin.[68] The serum of these patients appears to contain either a substance tightly bound to albumin or a structurally altered albumin that inhibits binding with BCP. Both BCG and BCP methods are used to quantitate albumin, but BCP is commonly preferred. Albumin methods are summarized in Table 11.7.

Total Globulins

Another approach to protein fractionation is the measurement of total globulins. The total protein and globulin concentrations are measured and albumin is calculated by subtracting the globulin result from total protein

Method	Principle	Comment
TABLE 11.7	**Albumin Methods**	
Salt precipitation	Globulins are precipitated in high salt concentrations; albumin in supernatant is quantitated by biuret reaction.	Labor intensive
DYE BINDING		
Methyl orange	Albumin binds to dye; causes shift in absorption maximum	Nonspecific for albumin
HABA [2,4′-hydroxyazobenzene-benzoic acid]	Albumin binds to dye; causes shift in absorption maximum	Many interference (salicylates, bilirubin)
BCG (bromocresol green)	Albumin binds to dye; causes shift in absorption maximum	Sensitive; overestimates low albumin levels; most commonly used dye
BCP (bromocresol purple)	Albumin binds to dye; causes shift in absorption maximum	Specific, sensitive, precise
Electrophoresis	Proteins separated based on electric charge	Accurate; gives overview of relative changes in different protein fractions

(albumin = total protein − globulin). The total globulin concentration in serum is determined by a direct colorimetric method using glyoxylic acid. Glyoxylic acid, in the presence of Cu^{2+} and an acid medium, such as acetic acid and H_2SO_4, combines with tryptophan found in globulins to produce a purple color. Albumin has approximately 0.2% tryptophan compared with the 2% to 3% found in serum globulins. The measurement of globulins based on their tryptophan content has never come into common use because of the ease and simplicity of the dye-binding methods for albumin.

Electrophoresis

When an abnormality in the total protein or albumin concentration is found, protein electrophoresis may be performed. Electrophoresis separates proteins on the basis of their electric charge and density. Proteins, when placed in an electric current, will move according to their charge, which is determined by the pH of the surrounding buffer. At a pH greater than their pI, the protein is negatively charged (anion) and will migrate toward the anode, which is the positive terminal. At a pH less than their pI, the protein will be positively charged (cation) and will migrate toward the negatively charged terminal, the cathode. The speed of migration can be estimated from the difference between the pI of the protein and the pH of the buffer. The greater the difference between the pH of the buffer and the pI, the greater the magnitude of the net charge of that protein and the faster it will move in the electric field. In addition to the charge of the protein, the velocity of the migration also depends on the electric field strength, reaction temperature, composition, pH and ionic strength of the buffer; and the size and shape of the protein. The electrophoretic mobility (μ) of a specific protein may be calculated using the following equation where s is the distance traveled in centimeters, t is time of migration in seconds, and F is the field strength in V/cm.

$$\mu = \frac{(s/t)}{F} \qquad \text{(Eq. 11-2)}$$

Historically, electrophoresis used an aqueous medium and was called *moving boundary electrophoresis*. Later, paper was used as a solid medium in a process known as *zone electrophoresis*. Cellulose acetate and agarose gel are commonly used support media in today's clinical laboratories.

Serum Protein Electrophoresis

In the standard performance of serum protein electrophoresis (SPE), serum specimens are applied close to the cathode end of a support medium that is saturated with an alkaline buffer (pH 8.6). The support medium is connected to two electrodes and a current is passed through the medium to separate the proteins. All major serum proteins carry a net negative charge at pH 8.6 and migrate toward the positive terminal, the anode. Using standard SPE methods, serum proteins separate into five bands in the following order: albumin travels farthest toward the anode followed by α_1-globulins, α_2-globulins, β-globulins, and γ-globulins.

FIGURE 11.7 Serum protein electrophoretic patterns on agarose and cellulose acetate. **(A)** Agarose gel—note the monoclonal γ-globulin. **(B)** Cellulose acetate. (Courtesy of Department of Laboratory Medicine, The University of Texas M.D. Anderson Hospital, Drs. Liu, Fritsche, and Trujillo and Ms. McClure, Supervisor.)

The width of the protein band in a particular fraction depends on the concentration of proteins present in that fraction; homogeneous protein gives a narrow band.

After separation, the protein fractions are fixed by immersing the support medium in an acid solution, such as acetic acid, to denature the proteins and immobilize them. In order to visualize the bands, the proteins are then stained. A variety of dyes have been used including Ponceau S, amido black, and Coomassie brilliant blue. Typical cellulose acetate electrophoretic patterns are shown in Figure 11.7A, and Figure 11.7B shows the patterns obtained using agarose gel as the support medium.

The fixed and stained medium is then placed in a scanning densitometer. The pattern on the membrane moves past a slit through which light is transmitted to a phototube to record the absorbance of the dye bound tin each protein fraction. The absorbances are normally recorded on a strip-chart recorder to obtain a pattern of the fractions (Fig. 11.8).

Many scanning densitometers compute the area under the absorbance curve for each band and report the percentage of total dye that appears in each fraction. The concentration is then calculated as a percentage of the total protein that was determined by one of the total protein methods, such as the biuret procedure.

Measurements of the bound dye may also be made by cutting out the separated bands from the membrane and eluting the dye from each band in 0.1 mol/L sodium hydroxide (NaOH). The absorbances are added to obtain the total absorbance, and the percentage of the total absorbance found in each fraction is then calculated.

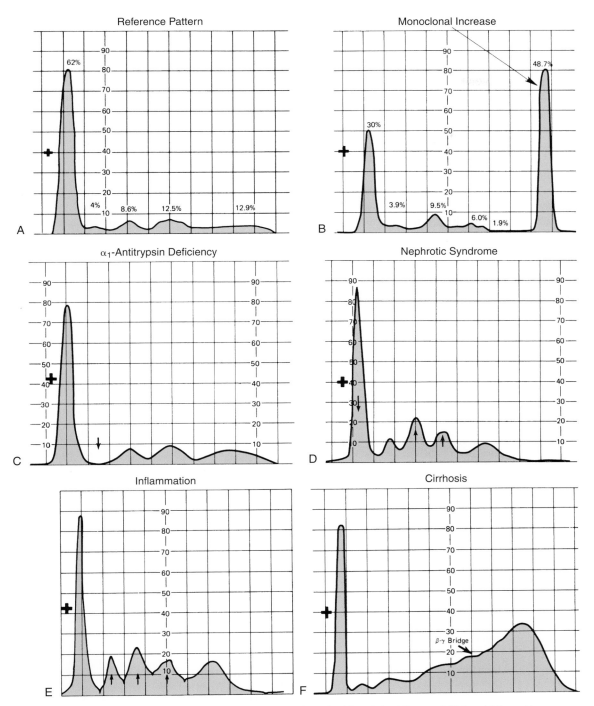

FIGURE 11.8 Selected densitometric patterns of protein electrophoresis. Albumin is at the anodal (+) end followed by α₁-, α₂-, β-, and γ-globulin fractions. *Arrows* indicate decrease or increase in fractions. **(A)** Reference pattern (agarose). **(B)** Monoclonal increase in γ area (agarose). **(C)** α₁-Antitrypsin deficiency (cellulose acetate). **(D)** Nephrotic syndrome (cellulose acetate). **(E)** Inflammation (cellulose acetate). **(F)** Cirrhosis (cellulose acetate). (**A** and **B** are courtesy of Drs. Liu and Fritsche and Jose Trujillo, Director, and Ms. McClure of the Department of Laboratory Medicine, The University of Texas M.D. Anderson Hospital. Others are courtesy of Dr. Wu of the Hermann Hospital Laboratory/The University of Texas Medical School.)

A reference serum control is processed with each electrophoretic run (Fig. 11.8A). Reference values for each fraction are as follows:

Albumin, 53% to 65% of the total protein (3.5 to 5.0 g/dL)
α₁-Globulin, 2.5% to 5% (0.1 to 0.3 g/dL)

α₂-Globulin, 7% to 13% (0.6 to 1.0 g/dL)
β-Globulin, 8% to 14% (0.7 to 1.1 g/dL)
γ-Globulin, 12% to 22% (0.8 to 1.6 g/dL)

Inadvertent use of plasma specimens will result in a narrow band between the β and γ regions because of the presence of fibrinogen. The presence of free hemoglobin can cause a small band in the late α_2 or early β zone, and the presence of hemoglobin–haptoglobin complexes will cause a small band in the α_2 zone. The biggest advantage of electrophoresis compared with the quantitation of specific proteins is the overview it provides. The electrophoretic pattern can give information about the relative increases and decreases within the protein population, as well as information about the homogeneity of a fraction.

Probably the most significant finding from an electrophoretic pattern is monoclonal immunoglobulin disease. The densitometric scan shows a sharp peak if the increase in immunoglobulins is a result of a monoclonal increase (Fig. 11.8B). A spike in the γ, β, or, sometimes, α_2 region signals the need for examination of the immunoglobulins and observation for clinical signs of myelomatosis. A deficiency of the predominant immunoglobulin, IgG, is seen as a much paler stain in the γ area. Another significant finding is a decrease in α_1-antitrypsin (Fig. 11.8C).

In nephrotic syndrome, the patient loses serum albumin and low-molecular-weight proteins in the urine and some IgG is also lost. At the same time, an increase occurs in α_2-macroglobulin, β-lipoprotein, complement components, and haptoglobin. These two events lead to a dramatic decrease in the relative amount of albumin and a significant increase in the relative amounts of α_2-globulin and β-globulin fractions (Fig. 11.8D).

Inflammatory conditions result in a decrease in albumin and an increase in the α_1-globulins (AAG and α_1-antitrypsin), α_2-globulins (ceruloplasmin and haptoglobin), and β-globulin band (CRP) (Fig. 11.8E). This pattern, also called an acute-phase reactant pattern, is seen in trauma, burns, infarction, malignancy, and liver disease. Positive acute-phase reactants are increased in the serum within days following trauma or exposure to inflammatory agents and negative acute-phase reactants such as albumin are markedly decreased. Fibrinogen, haptoglobin, ceruloplasmin, and amyloid increase severalfold, whereas CRP and α_2-macroglobulin increase several hundredfold. Chronic infections also produce a decrease in albumin, but demonstrate a corresponding increase in globulins in the γ fraction as well as the α_1, α_2, and β fractions.

The electrophoretic pattern of serum proteins in liver disease shows a relative decrease in serum albumin and a relative increase in γ-globulins. In the pattern for cirrhosis of the liver, there are some fast-moving γ-globulins that prevent resolution of the β- and γ-globulin bands. This is known as the β–γ bridge of cirrhosis (Fig. 11.8F).

In infectious hepatitis, the γ-globulin fraction rises with increasing hepatocellular damage. In obstructive jaundice, there is an increase in the α_2- and β-globulins. Also noted in obstructive jaundice is an increased concentration of lipoprotein, which is an indicator of its biliary origin. This is especially the case when there is little or no decrease of serum albumin.

CASE STUDY 11.4

A 60-year-old woman with a history of rheumatoid arthritis, smoking of 60 packs/y, chronic obstructive pulmonary disease, and treated hypertension underwent a screening colonoscopy and then felt poorly for a week. She saw her family physician, who referred her to the local hospital for additional tests. Her creatinine and BUN concentrations 2 weeks after the colonoscopy were 4.6 and 46 mg/dL, respectively, and a baseline serum creatinine from a previous physician's office visit was 0.9 mg/dL. Laboratory results from the hospital visit are shown in Case Study Table 11.4.1.

CASE STUDY TABLE 11.4.1 Laboratory Results

Test	Results	Reference Interval
Creatinine	3.7 mg/dL	Women <1.2 mg/dL
BUN	35 mg/dL	5–20 mg/dL
Creatinine clearance	12.5 mL/min	75–115 mL/min
C3	148 mg/dL	80–200 mg/dL
C4	19 mg/dL	15–80 mg/dL
Albumin	4.1 g/dL	3.5–5.0 g/dL
Calcium	9 mg/dL	8–10 mg/dL
Phosphorous	4.6 mg/dL	2.5–4.5 mg/dL
Cryoglobulin screen	Negative	
Serum protein electrophoresis—polyclonal hypergammaglobulinemia with no monoclonal immunoglobulin spike identified		
Urine protein electrophoresis—protein 15.9 mg/dL with normal immunofixation electrophoresis		
Urine sediment—no RBCs, 4–8 WBCs per high power field, granular, and hyaline casts noted		

Questions

1. What disease state is the most likely explanation for the patient's laboratory results?

2. What is the significance of the polyclonal hypergammaglobulinemia with no monoclonal immunoglobulin spike identified on SPE?

3. Is the patient's urine protein normal?

High-Resolution Protein Electrophoresis

Standard SPE separates proteins into five distinct bands, but by modifying the electrophoretic parameters, proteins can be further separated into as many as twelve bands. High-resolution protein electrophoresis (HRE) uses a

Normal HRE Pattern

1 2 3 4   5   6   7 8 9 10   11   12

Zones	Serum proteins found in zones
1. PREALBUMIN ZONE	-Prealbumin
2. ALBUMIN ZONE	-Albumin
3. ALBUMIN-α_1 INTERZONE	-α-Lipoprotein (α-Fetoprotein)
4. α_1 ZONE	-α_1-Antitrypsin, α_1-Acid glycoprotein
5. α_1-α_2 INTERZONE	-Gc-globulin, inter-α-trypsin inhibitor, α_1-antichymotrypsin
6. α_2 ZONE	-α_2-Macroglobulin, Haptoglobin
7. α_2-β_1 INTERZONE	-Cold insoluble globulin, (Hemoglobin)
8. β_1 ZONE	-Transferrin
9. β_1-β_2 INTERZONE	-β-Lipoprotein
10. β_2 ZONE	-C3
11. γ_1 ZONE	-IgA (Fibrinogen), IgM (Monoclonal Igs, light chains)
12. γ_2 ZONE	-IgC (C-reactive protein) (Monoclonal Igs, light chains)

Proteins listed in ( ) are normally found in too low a concentration to be visible in a normal pattern.

FIGURE 11.9 High-resolution electrophoretic (HRE) pattern of serum. (Courtesy of Helena Laboratories, Beaumont, TX.)

higher voltage coupled with a cooling system in the electrophoretic apparatus and a more concentrated buffer. The support medium most commonly used is agarose gel. To obtain HRE patterns, specimens are applied on the agarose gel, electrophoresed in a chamber cooled by a gel block, stained, and then visually inspected. Each band is compared with the same band on a reference pattern for color density, appearance, migration rates, and appearance of abnormal bands or regions of density. A normal serum HRE pattern is shown in Figure 11.9. As with SPE, the patterns may be scanned with a densitometer to obtain semiquantitative estimates of the protein found in each band. HRE is particularly useful in detecting small monoclonal bands and differentiating unusual bands or prominent increases of normal bands that can be confused with a monoclonal gammopathy.[69]

Capillary Electrophoresis

Capillary electrophoresis is a collection of techniques in which the separation of molecules takes place in silica capillaries. The capillaries are typically 30 to 50 cm long with an internal diameter between 25 and 100 µm. The capillaries are filled with a conducting solution, usually an aqueous buffer, the detection end of the capillary is grounded, and the sample injection end is connected to a high-voltage power supply. When a positive voltage is applied, the positively charged buffer molecules flow to the detection end, which is negative relative to the injection end. The net flow of the buffer is called electro-osmotic flow (EOF). When a specimen is injected, all molecules have a tendency to move toward the negatively charged detector end of the capillary due to EOF. However, the negatively charged molecules in the specimen also have a tendency to migrate back toward the positively charged injector end; this is referred to as *electrophoretic mobility*. EOF is usually stronger than electrophoretic mobility and all ions migrate to the detector end, but with different net mobilities based on their differences in size and charge. The separated molecules are detected by their absorbance as they pass through a small window near the detection end of the capillary. Use of the capillaries allows heat to be effectively dissipated, which means that higher operating voltages can be used and, therefore, analysis times are faster. Additionally, the required specimen volume is quite small (nanoliters).

Isoelectric Focusing

Isoelectric focusing (IEF) is zone electrophoresis that separates proteins on the basis of their p*I*. IEF uses polyacrylamide or agarose gel mediums, which contain a pH gradient. The pH gradient is established by the incorporation of small polyanions and polycations in the gel. In the presence of an electric field, the varying pIs of the polyions cause them to seek their place in the gradient and to remain there. The pH gradient may range from 3.5 to 10. When a protein is electrophoresed in the gel, it migrates to a place on the gel where the pH is the same as its p*I*. The protein becomes focused there because, if it should diffuse in either direction, it leaves its p*I* and gains a net charge. When this occurs, the electric current once again carries it back to its point of no charge, or its p*I*.

The clinical applications of IEF include phenotyping of α_1-antitrypsin deficiencies, determination of genetic variants of enzymes and hemoglobins, detection of paraproteins in serum, oligoclonal bands in CSF, and isoenzyme determinations.

Immunochemical Methods

Specific proteins may be identified by immunochemical assays in which the reaction of the antigenic protein and its antibody is measured. Methods using various modifications of this principle include radial immunodiffusion, immunoelectrophoresis, immunofixation electrophoresis (Fig. 11.10), electroimmunodiffusion, immunoturbidimetry, and immunonephelometry. A more detailed discussion of these techniques can be found in Chapter 8.

Normal IFE electrophoresis

IFE electrophoresis showing IgA λmonoclonal band

IFE electrophoresis showing IgM κmonoclonal band

FIGURE 11.10 Patterns of immunofixation electrophoresis (IFE).

PROTEINS IN OTHER BODY FLUIDS

The development of a disease-oriented database for proteins found in body fluids has been stimulated by the development of computers capable of handling large amounts of data and the development of high-resolution methods for the quantitative analysis of proteins in body fluids.[70]

Body fluids now being studied for their protein content include blood, urine, cerebrospinal fluid, tears, and peritoneal, pleural, seminal, and vaginal fluids. This section focuses on discussion of the protein content of urine and CSF.

Urinary Protein

Urinary proteins are plasma proteins originating from the kidney and urinary tract or from other sources such as the vagina and prostate. Plasma proteins appear in the urine when they have passed through the renal glomerulus and have not been reabsorbed by the renal tubules. Qualitative testing for **proteinuria** is commonly

performed using a reagent test strip. These methods are based on the change of an indicator dye in the presence of protein, known as the *protein error of indicators*. In an acidic pH, an indicator that is yellow in the absence of protein progresses through various shades of green and finally to blue as the concentration of protein increases. A protein concentration of 6 mg/dL or greater produces a color change.

Most quantitative assays require timed urine collections of 12 to 24 hours to account for diurnal variation. To perform a timed urine collection, the patient is instructed to completely empty their bladder and discard this initial void. Subsequent voids are collected into a large container for the next 24 hours. At the end of the 24-hour period, the bladder is completely emptied and their final void is included in the collection. The total volume of the timed specimen is measured and recorded. Results for urinary protein are generally reported in terms of the mass of protein excreted during a 24-hour period by calculating the amount of protein present in the total volume of urine collected during that time.

There are several precipitation methods for the determination of total protein in urine and other body fluids, including the measurement of turbidity when urinary proteins are mixed with an anionic organic acid such as sulfosalicylic acid, TCA, or benzethonium chloride. These methods are sensitive, but the reagent does not react equally with each protein fraction. This is particularly true of sulfosalicylic acid, which produces four times more turbidity with albumin than with α-globulin.

One quantitative method for urine proteins consists of precipitation of the proteins, dissolution of the protein precipitate, and color formation with biuret reagent. Another procedure for measuring urinary protein uses the Folin-Ciocalteu reagent, which is a phosphotungstomolybdic acid solution, frequently called phenol reagent because it oxidizes phenolic compounds. The reagent changes color from yellow to blue during reaction with tyrosine, tryptophan, and histidine residues in protein. This method is about ten times more sensitive than the biuret method. Lowry et al. increased the sensitivity of the Folin-Ciocalteu reaction by incorporating a biuret reaction as the initial step. After the cupric ions bind to the peptide bonds, the Folin-Ciocalteu reagent is added. As the Cu^{2+}–protein complex is oxidized, the reagent is reduced, forming the chromogens tungsten blue and molybdenum blue. This increased the sensitivity a hundredfold greater than that of the biuret method alone. Another modification uses a pyrogallol red–molybdate complex that reacts with protein to produce a blue–purple complex.

Dye-binding methods using Coomassie brilliant blue and Ponceau S have also been used to determine the quantitative total protein content of urine; however, dye-binding assays are not sensitive enough for urine microalbumin (MAU) testing, making immunochemical assays the most widely used MAU methods.[71] These immunoassays include immunoturbidimetry, immunofluorescence,

TABLE 11.8 Urine Protein Methods

Method	Principle	Comment
Turbidimetric methods (sulfosalicylic acid, trichloroacetic acid, or benzethonium chloride)	Proteins are precipitated as fine particles; turbidity is measured spectrophotometrically	Rapid, easy to use; unequal sensitivity for individual protein
Biuret	Proteins are concentrated by precipitation, redissolved in alkali, then reacted with Cu^{2+}; Cu^{2+} forms colored complex with peptide bonds.	Accurate
Folin-Lowry	Initial biuret reaction; oxidation of tyrosine, tryptophan, and histidine residues by Folin phenol reagent (mixture of phosphotungstic and phosphomolybdic acids): measurement of resultant blue color	Very sensitive
Dye binding (Coomassie blue, Ponceau S)	Protein binds to dye, causes shift in absorption maximum	Limited linearity; unequal sensitivity for individual proteins

ELISA, RIA, and zone immunoelectrophoresis. Table 11.8 summarizes the various methods for measurement of urinary total protein.

The reference values or intervals for urinary proteins are highly method dependent, ranging from 100 to 250 mg every 24 hours. Turbidimetric procedures are most frequently used today because of their ease of use, speed, and sensitivity. Immunochemical, chromatographic, and liquid chromatography–mass spectrometry methods for quantifying urine albumin are also being used. Even a fluorescence resonance energy transfer assay for point-of-care testing of urinary albumin has been developed.[72]

CASE STUDY 11.5

A male patient aged 47 years came to the clinic after a minor work accident. He works as a painter and had fallen off a 12-foot scaffold and hurt his ankle. He had a complicated medical history that included severe diabetes, diagnosed a decade earlier, with peripheral neuropathy and retinopathy; chronic renal insufficiency; hypertension for the past 20 years; and hyperlipidemia. At this clinic visit, the patient was noted to have mild hepatomegaly. The patient's blood showed a normochromic normocytic anemia. An SPE with immunofixation demonstrated a monoclonal IgGk of less than 100 mg/dL. Urine protein electrophoresis (UPE) with immunofixation was negative for light chains (Bence Jones protein). Although his ankle was not sprained, the patient continued to have breathing problems over the next several months and returned to the clinic often. Among many other tests, a follow-up SPE and a UPE with immunofixation were performed. The results are shown below.

Questions

1. What does the presence of the monoclonal IgGk band indicate?
2. What further information is obtained from the UPE?
3. Was this patient's SPE finding consistent with his complicated medical history?

CSF Protein

CSF is formed in the choroid plexus of the ventricles of the brain by ultrafiltration of blood plasma. Total protein and glucose measurements are routinely performed on CSF in addition to a differential cell count, culture, and sensitivity studies. The reference interval for CSF total protein for patients between 10 and 40 years of age is 15 to 45 mg/dL.

An abnormally increased CSF total protein is generally associated with conditions in which there is increased permeability of the capillary endothelial barrier through which ultrafiltration occurs. Examples of such conditions include bacterial, viral, and fungal meningitis; traumatic lumbar puncture; multiple sclerosis; obstruction; neoplasm; disk herniation; and cerebral infarction. The degree of permeability of the blood–brain barrier can be evaluated by measuring the CSF albumin and comparing it with simultaneous measurement of serum albumin. Albumin is used as the reference protein for permeability because it is not synthesized to any degree in the central nervous system. The reference interval for the CSF-to-serum albumin ratio is 2.7 to 7.3; a value above the reference interval may indicate damage to the blood–brain barrier. Low CSF protein values are found in hyperthyroidism and when fluid is leaking from the central nervous system.

CASE STUDY 11.6

A 55-year-old man with no history of illness suffered a blow to the head. He was unconscious when admitted to the hospital and remained in that state until his death 15 days later. A nasogastric tube was inserted to administer the required nutrients (protein, carbohydrates, fat, minerals, and vitamins). The total water intake was 1,500 mL/d. Starting on day 5, his blood pressure gradually fell. The 24-hour urine volumes recorded from an indwelling catheter are listed below:

Day After Admission	Urine Volume (mL/24 h)
6	1,500
8	1,300
10	1,200
12	1,100
14	900

The patient's hemoglobin and hematocrit were elevated. Laboratory results for blood chemistry analysis on day 13 and are shown in Case Study Table 11.6.1.

CASE STUDY TABLE 11.6.1 Laboratory Results

Test	Results	Reference Intervals
Total protein	9.4 g/dL	6.5–8.3 g/dL
Albumin	6.0 g/dL	3.5–5.0 g/dL
Blood urea nitrogen (BUN)	80 mg/dL	5–20 mg/dL
Sodium	175 mmol/L	136–145 mmol/L
Potassium	4.0 mmol/L	3.5–5.1 mmol/L
Chloride	134 mmol/L	98–107 mmol/L

Questions

1. What is the most likely explanation for the elevated total protein concentration?
2. What other results support this conclusion?
3. Why is the blood urea nitrogen result elevated?

The total CSF protein may be determined by more sensitive chemical or spectrophotometric methods referred to earlier in the discussion on urinary proteins. The most frequently used procedures are turbidimetric using TCA, sulfosalicylic acid with sodium sulfate, or benzethonium chloride. Dye-binding methods (e.g., Coomassie brilliant blue), a kinetic biuret reaction, and the Lowry method using a Folin phenol reagent are also available.

Although total protein concentrations in the CSF are informative, diagnosis of specific disorders often requires measurement of individual protein fractions. The pattern of proteins present can be visualized best by electrophoresis of a concentrated CSF specimen. A normal CSF pattern shows prealbumin, a prominent albumin band, α_1-globulin composed predominantly of α_1-antitrypsin, an α_2 band consisting primarily of haptoglobin and ceruloplasmin, a β_1 band composed principally of transferrin, and a CSF-specific transferrin that is deficient in carbohydrate, referred to as τ protein, in the β_2 zone. The globulin present in the γ band is typically IgG with a small amount of IgA.

CASE STUDY 11.7

An 84-year-old woman resident of a nursing home was admitted to the hospital for treatment of lower back pain resulting from a fall. Radiologic examination revealed a vertebral compression fracture. Because she demonstrated signs of general deterioration, further medical evaluation was performed. A neurologic examination and CT scan were normal. Serologic examinations for collagen vascular disease were also negative, although the CRP showed a modest increase. Serum protein electrophoresis was done to rule out multiple myeloma. The serum protein fractions were as follows: albumin, 3.2 g/dL; α₁-globulins, 0.31 g/dL; α₂-globulins, 1.59 g/dL (elevated in a tight band); β-globulins, 0.72 g/dL; and γ-globulins, 0.96 g/dL.

Questions

1. What would the next step be in the evaluation of this patient?

2. Given the following additional result (haptoglobin: 416 mg/dL), what condition would explain her abnormal protein electrophoresis pattern?

3. What other proteins would you expect to be abnormal?

Normal CSF protein electrophoresis

3 X Oligoclonal bands in CSF protein electrophoresis

FIGURE 11.11 Patterns of cerebrospinal fluid (CSF) protein electrophoresis.

Electrophoretic patterns of CSF from patients who have multiple sclerosis demonstrate multiple, distinct oligoclonal bands in the γ zone (Fig. 11.11). The presence of discrete bands in the γ region of CSF that are not also present in the serum is consistent with production of IgG in the CSF. These bands cannot be seen on routine cellulose acetate electrophoresis, but require a high-resolution technique using agarose. More than 90% of patients with multiple sclerosis demonstrate the presence of oligoclonal bands, although oligoclonal bands have also been found in inflammatory conditions and infectious neurologic diseases, such as Guillain-Barre syndrome, bacterial meningitis, viral encephalitis, subacute sclerosing panencephalitis, and neurosyphilis.[73]

To differentiate elevated CSF IgG concentrations due to local CNS production from leakage of plasma into the CSF, the laboratory may compare CSF and serum IgG concentrations with reference to albumin in a value known as the IgG index. A CSF IgG-to-albumin ratio higher than that of serum (raised IgG index) is indicative of local CNS production of IgG. A serum IgG-to-albumin ratio much higher than that of CSF (low IgG index) is suggestive of hypergammaglobulinemia or low serum albumin. The reference range for IgG index is 0.26 to 0.70. To identify the source of the elevated CSF IgG levels, the IgG-albumin index can be calculated as follows:

$$\text{CSF IgG index} = \frac{\text{CSF IgG (mg/dL)} \times \text{serum albumin (g/dL)}}{\text{serum IgG (g/dL)} \times \text{CSF albumin (mg/dL)}} \quad \text{(Eq. 11-3)}$$

The CSF albumin concentration corrects for increased permeability. Another index to aid in discriminating the source of IgG in the CSF is the IgG synthesis rate calculation using the formula of Tourtellotte et al.[74] The reference interval for the synthesis rate is −9.9 to +3.3 mg/d.

In the investigation of multiple sclerosis, myelin basic proteins present in the CSF are also assayed because these proteins can provide an index of active demyelination. Myelin basic proteins are constituents of myelin, the sheath

that surrounds many of the CNS axons. In very active demyelination, concentrations of myelin basic proteins of 17 to 100 ng/mL are found using RIA. In slow demyelination, values of 6 to 16 ng/mL occur, and in remission, the values are less than 4 ng/mL. In addition to multiple sclerosis, other conditions that induce CNS demyelination and elevated concentrations of myelin basic protein include meningoencephalitis, SLE, diabetes mellitus, and chronic renal failure.

CASE STUDY 11.8

A 36-year-old woman complained of intermittent blurred vision and numbness and weakness in her left leg that had persisted for longer than 3 weeks. On examination, vertical nystagmus (involuntary back-and-forth or circular movements of eyes) was noted on upward gaze. CSF was drawn and the specimen was clear and colorless with normal cell count. The CSF total protein level was 49 mg/dL with an IgG of 8.1 mg/dL. Electrophoresis of the patient's serum and CSF revealed the following pattern: more than two oligoclonal bands in CSF (seen in Fig. 11.7) and a polyclonal pattern on SPE.

Questions

1. What is the significance of the CSF protein bands indicated by the arrows?

2. What conditions would produce this type of CSF protein electrophoresis pattern?

3. What other tests would be helpful in the investigation of this patient's diagnosis?

4. What laboratory test can be useful for monitoring the course of this patient's condition?

For additional student resources, please visit thePoint® at http://thepoint.lww.com

questions

1. Which of the following acute-phase reactant proteins *decreases* during inflammation?
   a. Transferrin
   b. α_1-Antitrypsin
   c. Haptoglobin
   d. Fibrinogen

2. Which of the following refers to the three-dimensional spatial configuration of a single polypeptide chain determined by disulfide linkages, hydrogen bonds, electrostatic attractions, and van der Waals forces?
   a. Primary structure
   b. Secondary structure
   c. Tertiary structure
   d. Quaternary structure

3. Which of the following plasma proteins is primarily responsible for maintaining in vivo colloidal osmotic pressure?
   a. Albumin
   b. Hemoglobin
   c. Fibrinogen
   d. α_2-Macroglobulin

4. Which of the following best describes a *peptide bond*?
   a. An amino group and carboxyl group bonded to an alpha-carbon
   b. A double carbon bond between the alpha-carbons of two amino acids
   c. An amino group bonded to a carboxyl group of another amino acid
   d. Two carboxyl groups bonded to the alpha-carbon of an amino acid

5. Which of the following results would correlate best with malnutrition and a poor protein–caloric status?
   a. Decreased prealbumin
   b. Decreased γ-globulins
   c. Elevated ceruloplasmin
   d. Elevated α_1-fetoprotein

6. Which of the following conditions would correlate best with a normal level of myoglobin?
   a. Multiple myeloma
   b. Acute myocardial infarction
   c. Acute renal failure
   d. Skeletal muscle injury

7. An immunofixation protein electrophoresis is performed on serum from a patient with the most common type of multiple myeloma. The resulting pattern would most likely reveal which of the following?
   a. An IgG monoclonal band
   b. Oligoclonal bands
   c. Significant β–γ bridging
   d. An IgM monoclonal band

8. Which of the following would indicate a plasma specimen was used for protein electrophoresis instead of serum?
   a. A small peak between the β- and γ-globulins
   b. A broad increase in the γ-globulin fraction
   c. A bridge between the α_1- and α_2-globulins
   d. A significantly decreased albumin peak

9. Which of the following conditions would correlate best with the serum proteink electrophoresis results below?
   albumin: decreased
   α_1-globulins: increased
   α_2-globulins: increased
   β-globulins: normal
   γ-globulins: normal
   a. Acute inflammation
   b. Chronic liver cirrhosis
   c. Nephrotic syndrome
   d. Monoclonal gammopathy

10. Which of the following conditions would correlate best with the presence of distinct oligoclonal bands in the γ-zone on CSF protein electrophoresis?
    a. Multiple sclerosis
    b. Multiple myeloma
    c. Bacterial meningitis
    d. Myoglobinemia

11. When a protein is dissolved in a buffer solution that is more alkaline than its pI and an electric current is passed through the solution, the protein will act as:
    a. An anion and migrate to the anode
    b. A cation and migrate to the cathode
    c. An anion and migrate to the cathode
    d. An uncharged particle and will not move

review questions (continued)

12. Which of the following conditions would correlate best with an elevated serum total protein with high levels of both albumin and globulins?
   a. Dehydration
   b. Myocardial infarction
   c. Glomerulonephritis
   d. Liver cirrhosis

13. Which of the following urine total protein results would correlate best with a patient with nephrotic syndrome?
   a. Normal
   b. Lower than normal
   c. Higher than normal
   d. Similar to levels in CSF total protein levels

14. Isoelectric focusing is used to phenotype α_1-antitrypsin deficiencies. When protein is electrophoresed, it migrates to which of the following?
   a. The site where the pH is the same as its pI.
   b. The site where the mass of the protein correlates with the pI.
   c. The site where the protein's net charge exceeds the pI.
   d. The site where the protein's net charge is less than the pI.

15. A CSF–serum albumin ratio of 9.8 was reported. How is this best interpreted?
   a. This ratio is in the normal range for the patient.
   b. The blood–brain barrier may be compromised.
   c. It is biologically impossible to achieve this value.
   d. This is diagnostic of fungal meningitis.

16. Which of the following CSF proteins would be measured when investigating active demyelination in multiple sclerosis?
   a. CSF–serum albumin ratio
   b. α_1-Antitrypsin
   c. Myelin basic protein
   d. Immunoglobulin G

references

1. Baldwin A, Lapointe M. The chemistry of amino acids. The Biology Project; 2004. www.biology.arizona.edu/biochemistry/problem_sets/aa/aa.html. Accessed August 21, 2012.
2. Brosnan J. Interorgan amino acid transport and its regulation. *J Nutr.* 2003;133(6 suppl 1):2068S–2072S.
3. Nelson DL, Cox MM. *Lehninger's Principles of Biochemistry.* 3rd ed. New York, NY: Worth Publishing; 2000.
4. IUPAC-IUBMB Joint Commission on Biochemical Nomenclature. Nomenclature and symbolism for amino acids and peptides. Recommendations on organic & biochemical nomenclature, symbols & terminology etc. www.iupac.org/publications/pac/1984/pdf/5605x0595.pdf. Accessed May 17, 2007.
5. Wear JE, Keevil BG. Measurement of cystine in urine by liquid chromatography–tandem mass spectrometry. *Clin Chem.* 2005;51:787–789.
6. Boza JJ, Dangin M, Moennoz D, et al. Free and protein-bound glutamine have identical splanchnic extraction in healthy human volunteers. *Am J Physiol Gastrointest Liver Physiol.* 2001;281:267–274.
7. Morlion BJ, Stehle P, Wachtler P, et al. Total parenteral nutrition with glutamine dipeptide after major abdominal surgery: a randomized, double-blind, controlled study. *Ann Surg.* 1998;227:302–308.
8. Francesconi KA, Pannier F. Selenium metabolites in urine: a critical overview of past work and current status. *Clin Chem.* 2004;50:2240–2253.
9. Gill M, Gupta S, Zichittella L. Selenocysteine: the 21st amino acid. www.albany.edu/faculty/cs812/bio366/selenocysteine_ppt.pdf. Accessed October 4, 2008.
10. Atkins JF, Gesteland R. Biochemistry. The 22nd amino acid. *Science.* 2002;296:1409–1410.
11. National Newborn Screening and Genetics Resource Center. Current newborn conditions by state. http://genes-r-us.uthscsa.edu. Accessed August 21, 2012.
12. Chace DH, Millington DS, Terada N, et al. Rapid diagnosis of phenylketonuria by quantitative analysis for phenylalanine and tyrosine in neonatal blood spots by tandem mass spectrometry. *Clin Chem.* 1993;39:66–71.
13. Williams RA, Mamotte CDS, Burnett JR. Phenylketonuria: an inborn error of phenylalanine metabolism. *Clin Biochem Rev.* 2008;29(1):31–41. PMCID: PMC2423317.
14. Food and Drug Administration (FDA). FDA approves Kuvan for treatment of phenylketonuria (PKU). http://www.fda.gov/bbs/topics/news/2007/new01761.html. Accessed December 13, 2007.
15. Yamaguchi A, Mizushima Y, Fukushi M, et al. Microassay system for newborn screening for phenylketonuria, maple syrup urine disease, homocystinuria, histidinemia and galactosemia with use of a fluorometric microplate reader. *Screening.* 1992;1:49.
16. Sparkman OD. *Mass Spectrometry Desk Reference.* Pittsburgh, PA: Global View; 2000.
17. Pass KA, Morrissey M. Enhancing newborn screening for tyrosinemia type I. *Clin Chem.* 2008;54:627–629.
18. Oglesbee D, Sanders KA, Lacey JM, et al. Second-tier test for quantification of alloisoleucine and branched-chain amino acids in dried blood spots to improve newborn screening for maple syrup urine disease (MSUD). *Clin Chem.* 2008;54:542–549.
19. Picker JD, Levy HL. Homocystinuria caused by cystathionine beta-synthase deficiency. In: *GeneReviews at GeneTests: Medical Genetics Information Resource (Database Online)* (*Updated March 29, 2006*); 1997–2008. Copyright University of Washington, Seattle. http://www.genetests.org. Accessed April 2, 2008.

20. Magera MJ, Lacey JM, Casetta B, et al. Method for the determination of total homocysteine in plasma and urine by stable isotope dilution and electrospray tandem mass spectrometry. *Clin Chem.* 1999;45:1517–1522.

21. Thoene JG. Citrullinemia type I. In: *GeneReviews at GeneTests: Medical Genetics Information Resource (Database Online) (Updated December 22, 2006)*; 1997–2008. Copyright University of Washington, Seattle. http://www.genetests.org. Accessed April 2, 2008.

22. Turnell DC, Cooper JD. Rapid assay for amino acids in serum or urine by pre-column derivatization and reversed-phase liquid chromatography. *Clin Chem.* 1982;28:527–531.

23. Chace DH. Use of tandem mass spectrometry for multianalyte screening of dried blood specimens from newborns. *Clin Chem.* 2003;49:1797–1817.

24. Kimball J. *Biology.* 6th ed. Dubuque, IA: William C. Brown; 1995.

25. Proteins: introduction. http://www.elmhurst.edu/~chm/vchembook/565proteins.html. Accessed October 2, 2008.

26. Proteins, peptides, and amino acids. http://www.cem.msu.edu/~reusch/VirtualText/proteins.htm. Accessed October 2, 2008.

27. Branden C, Tooze J. *Introduction to Protein Structure.* 2nd ed. New York, NY: Garland Publishing; 1999.

28. Omenn GS, States DJ, Adamski M, et al. Overview of the HUPO Plasma Proteome Project: results from the pilot phase with 35 collaborating laboratories and multiple analytical groups, generating a core dataset of 3020 proteins and a publicly-available database. *Proteomics.* 2005;5:3226–3245.

29. Petsko GA, Ringe D. *Protein Structure and Function.* London, UK: New Science Press in association with Sinauer Associates and Blackwell Science; 2003:180.

30. Singh AP, Moniaux N, Chauhan SC, et al. Inhibition of MUC4 expression suppresses pancreatic tumor cell growth and metastasis. *Cancer Res.* 2004;64:622–630.

31. Lo Conte L, Brenner SE, Hubbard TJ, et al. SCOP database in 2002: refinements accommodate structural genomics. *Nucleic Acids Res.* 2002;30:264–267.

32. Holm L, Ouzounis C, Sander C, et al. A database of protein structure families with common folding motifs. *Protein Sci.* 1992;1:1691–1698.

33. Kazuyoshi I, Yuichiro S, Yukie K, et al. Determination of glycated albumin by enzyme-linked boronate immunoassay (ELBIA). *Clin Chem.* 1998;44:256–263.

34. Albumin: the test sample. http://labtestsonline.org/understanding/analytes/albumin/sample.html. Accessed October 2, 2008.

35. Technical Bulletin. *Alpha-1-Antitrypsin Deficiency, Genotyping: DNA Test for the S and Z Alleles and Protein Measurement.* Salt Lake City, UT: ARUP Laboratories; 2007.

36. Technical Bulletin. *AFP-L3% in Serum (Includes Total Alpha Fetoprotein): For Risk Assessment of Hepatocellular Carcinoma in Patients with Chronic Liver Disease.* Salt Lake City, UT: ARUP Laboratories; 2007.

37. Israili ZH, Dayton PG. Human alpha-1-glycoprotein and its interactions with drugs. *Drug Metab Rev.* 2001;3:161–235.

38. Nilsson LNG, Bales KR, DiCarlo G, et al. α-1-Antichymotrypsin promotes β-sheet amyloid plaque deposition in a transgenic mouse model of Alzheimer's disease. *J Neurosci.* 2001;21:1444–1451.

39. Hamm A, Veeck J, Bektas N, et al. Frequent expression loss of Inter-alpha-trypsin inhibitor heavy chain (ITIH) genes in multiple human solid tumors: a systematic expression analysis. *BMC Cancer.* 2008;8:25.

40. Lis Lauridsen A, Vestergaard P, Nexo E. Mean serum concentration of vitamin D-binding protein (Gc globulin) is related to the Gc phenotype in women. *Clin Chem.* 2001;47:753–756.

41. Levy A. Haptoglobin phenotype and prevalent coronary heart disease in the Framingham offspring cohort. *Atherosclerosis.* 2003;172:361–365.

42. TIBC and transferrin. http://labtestsonline.org/understanding/analytes/tibc/glance.html. Accessed October 2, 2008.

43. Tolosano E, Altruda F. Hemopexin: structure, function, and regulation. *DNA Cell Biol.* 2002;21:297–306.

44. Yates JR, Sepp T, Matharu BK, et al. Complement C3 variant and the risk of age-related macular degeneration. *N Engl J Med.* 2007;357:553–561.

45. Wong SS. Strategic utilization of cardiac markers for the diagnosis of acute myocardial infarction. *Ann Clin Lab Sci.* 1996;26:301.

46. Ridker PM. Clinical application of C-reactive protein for cardiovascular disease detection and prevention. *Circulation.* 2003;107:363–369.

47. King DE, Mainous AG, Buchanan TA, et al. C-reactive protein and glycemic control in adults with diabetes. *Diabetes Care.* 2003;26:1535–1539.

48. Ridker PM. C-reactive protein: a simple test to help predict risk of heart attack and stroke. *Circulation.* 2003;108:e81.

49. Matsuda F, Ishii K, Bourvagnet P, et al. The complete nucleotide sequence of the human immunoglobulin heavy chain variable region locus. *J Exp Med.* 1998;188:2151–2162.

50. Abbas AK, Lichtman AH. *Cellular and Molecular Immunology.* 5th ed. Philadelphia, PA: WB Saunders; 2003.

51. Tangye SG, Ferguson A, Avery DT, et al. Isotype switching by human B cells is division-associated and regulated by cytokines. *J Immunol.* 2002;169:4298–4306.

52. Janeway CA Jr, Travers P, Walport M, et al. *Immunobiology.* 5th ed. New York, NY: Garland Publishing; 2001.

53. Woof J, Burton D. Human antibody-Fc receptor interactions illuminated by crystal structures. *Nat Rev Immunol.* 2004;4:89–99.

54. Preud'homme JL, Petit I, Barra A, et al. Structural and functional properties of membrane and secreted IgD. *Mol Immunol.* 2000;37:871–887.

55. Winter WE, Hardt MS, Fuhrman S. Immunoglobulin E: importance in parasitic infections and hypersensitivity responses. *Arch Pathol Lab Med.* 2000;124:1382–1385.

56. Chiu A, Chan W-K, Cheng S-H, et al. Troponin-I, myoglobin, and mass concentration of creatine kinase-MB in acute myocardial infarction. *QJM.* 1999;92:711–718.

57. Morrow DA, Cannon CP, Jesse RL, et al. National Academy of Clinical Biochemistry Laboratory Medicine Practice Guidelines: clinical characteristics and utilization of biochemical markers in acute coronary syndromes. *Clin Chem.* 2007;53:552–574.

58. Sakhuja R, Januzzi JL. NT-proBNP: a new test for diagnosis, prognosis and management of congestive heart failure. *Cardiology.* 2004;1(1):148–149.

59. Nakamura Y, Shimada K, Fukuda D, et al. Implications of plasma concentrations of adiponectin in patients with coronary artery disease. *Heart.* 2004;90:528–533.

60. Huber AR, Risch L. Recent developments in the evaluation of glomerular filtration rate: is there a place for beta-trace? *Clin Chem.* 2005;51:1329–1330.

61. Shlipak MG, Sarnak MJ, Katz R, et al. Cystatin C and the risk of death and cardiovascular events among elderly persons. *N Engl J Med.* 2005;352:2049–2060.

62. Peters T Jr, Biamonte ET, Doumas BT. Protein (total) in serum, urine, cerebrospinal fluid, albumin in serum. In: Faulkner WR, Meites S, eds. *Selected Methods in Clinical Chemistry*. Vol. 9. Washington, DC: American Association for Clinical Chemistry; 1982:317.

63. Reichert TS-METER. *Total Solids Refractometer Model 1310400A Instruction Manual*. Depew, NY: Reichert, Inc. 2003 [publication 10400A-101 Rev. D].

64. Chromy V, Fischer J. Photometric determination of total protein in lipemic serum. *Clin Chem*. 1977;23:754.

65. Doumas BT, Watson WA, Biggs HG. Albumin standards and the measurement of serum albumin with bromocresol green. *Clin Chim Acta*. 1971;31:87.

66. Speicher CE, Widish JR, Gaudot FJ, et al. An evaluation of the overestimation of serum albumin by bromocresol green. *Am J Clin Pathol*. 1978;69:347.

67. Gustafsson JEC. Improved specificity of serum albumin determination and estimation of acute phase reactants by use of the bromocresol green reaction. *Clin Chem*. 1976;22:616.

68. Clase CM, St Pierre MW, Churchill DN. Conversion between bromocresol green- and bromocresol purple-measured albumin in renal disease. *Nephrol Dial Transplant*. 2001;16:1925–1929.

69. Keren D. High resolution electrophoresis aids detection of gammopathies. *Clin Chem News*. 1989;14:26–29.

70. Merril CR, Goldstein MP, Myrick JE, et al. The Protein Disease Database of human body fluids: I. Rationale for the development of this database. *Appl Theor Electrophor*. 1995;5:49–54.

71. Choi S, Choi EY, Kim HS, et al. On-site quantification of human urinary albumin by a fluorescence immunoassay. *Clin Chem*. 2004;50:1052–1055.

72. Qin Q-P, Peltola O, Pettersson K. Time-resolved fluorescence resonance energy transfer assay for point-of-care testing of urinary albumin. *Clin Chem*. 2003;49:1105–1113.

73. Fact Sheet Immunopathology. CSF electrophoresis and the detection of oligoclonal bands. *Inst Clin Pathol Med Res*. 2002 [9/02 0119].

74. Tourtellotte WW, Staugaitis SM, Walsh MJ, et al. The basis of intra-blood-brain-barrier IgG synthesis. *Ann Neurol*. 1985;17:21–27.

12

Nonprotein Nitrogen Compounds

ELIZABETH L. FRANK

key terms

Ammonia
Azotemia
Coupled enzymatic method
Creatine
Creatinine
Creatinine clearance
Estimated glomerular filtration rate
Glomerular filtration rate (GFR)
Gout
Hyperammonemia
Hyperuricemia
Hypouricemia
Postrenal
Prerenal
Protein-free filtrate
Reabsorption
Secretion
Urea
Urea nitrogen/creatinine ratio
Uremia or uremic syndrome
Uric acid

chapter objectives

Upon completion of this chapter, the clinical laboratorian should be able to do the following:

• List the nonprotein nitrogen components of the blood and recognize their chemical structures and relative physiologic concentrations.
• Describe the biosynthesis and excretion of urea, uric acid, creatinine, creatine, and ammonia.
• State the specimen collection, transport, and storage requirements necessary for determinations of urea, uric acid, creatinine, creatine, and ammonia.
• Discuss commonly used methods for the determination of urea, uric acid, creatinine, creatine, and ammonia in plasma and urine. Identify sources of error and variability in these methods and describe the effects on the clinical utility of the laboratory measurements.
• Recognize the reference intervals for urea, uric acid, creatinine, and ammonia in plasma and urine. State the effects of age and gender on these values.
• Perform calculations to convert laboratory results between systems of measurement.
• Describe the major pathological conditions associated with increased and decreased plasma concentrations of urea, uric acid, creatinine, creatine, and ammonia.
• Describe the use of the urea nitrogen/creatinine ratio to distinguish prerenal, renal, and postrenal causes of uremia.
• Relate the solubility of uric acid to the pathologic consequences of increased plasma uric acid.

> **For additional student resources, please visit** the**Point**®
> **at http://thepoint.lww.com**

chapter objectives (continued)

- Explain the use and limitations of serum creatinine for calculations of estimated glomerular filtration rate.
- Describe the toxic effects related to an increased plasma ammonia concentration.
- Suggest possible clinical conditions associated with test results, given patient values for urea, uric acid, creatinine, and ammonia and supporting clinical history.

The term nonprotein nitrogen (NPN) originated in the early days of clinical chemistry when analytic methodology required removal of protein from a specimen before analysis. The concentration of nitrogen-containing compounds in this protein-free filtrate was quantified spectrophotometrically by converting nitrogen to **ammonia** and subsequent reaction with Nessler's reagent ($K_2[HgI_4]$) to produce a yellow color.[1] The method was technically difficult but provided an accurate determination of total NPN concentration. Although determination of total urinary nitrogen is of value in the assessment of nitrogen balance for nutritional management,[2] more useful clinical information is obtained by analyzing a patient's specimen for individual nitrogen-containing compounds.

Numerous compounds of clinical interest are included in the NPN fraction of plasma and urine. The most abundant of these are listed in Table 12.1.[3] The majority of these compounds arise from the catabolism of proteins and nucleic acids. The biochemistry, clinical utility, and analytical methods for measurement of the NPN compounds urea, uric acid, creatinine, creatine, and ammonia are presented in this chapter.

UREA

The NPN compound present in highest concentration in the blood is **urea** (Fig. 12.1). Urea is the major excretory product of protein metabolism.[4] It is formed in the liver from amino groups ($-NH_2$) and free ammonia generated during protein catabolism.[5] This enzymatically catalyzed process is termed the urea cycle. Since historic assays for urea were based on the measurement of nitrogen, the term blood urea nitrogen (BUN) has been used to refer to urea determination. Urea nitrogen (urea N) is a more appropriate term.[6]

Biochemistry

Protein metabolism produces amino acids that can be oxidized to produce energy or stored as fat and glycogen. These processes release nitrogen, which is converted to urea and excreted as a waste product. Following synthesis in the liver, urea is carried in the blood to the kidney, where it is readily filtered from the plasma by the glomerulus. Most of the urea in the glomerular filtrate is excreted in the urine, although some urea is reabsorbed by passive diffusion during passage of the filtrate through the renal tubules. The amount reabsorbed depends on the urine flow rate and extent of hydration. Small quantities of urea ($<10\%$ of the total) are excreted through the gastrointestinal (GI) tract and skin. The concentration of urea in the plasma is determined by the protein content of the diet, the rate of protein catabolism, and renal function and perfusion.[7]

Clinical Application

Measurement of urea is used to evaluate renal function, to assess hydration status, to determine nitrogen balance, to aid in the diagnosis of renal disease, and to verify adequacy of dialysis.[4]

Measurements of urea were originally performed on a protein-free filtrate of whole blood and based on measuring the amount of nitrogen. Current analytic methods have retained this custom, and urea is often reported in terms of nitrogen concentration rather than urea concentration. Urea N concentration can be converted to urea concentration by multiplying by 2.14, as follows:

$$\frac{1\,mg\;urea\;N}{dL} \times \frac{1\,mmol\;N}{14\,mg\;N} \times \frac{1\,mmol\;urea}{2\,mmol\;N} \times \frac{60\,mg\;urea}{1\,mmol\;urea} = \frac{2.14\,mg\;urea}{dL} \quad \text{(Eq. 12-1)}$$

In the International System of Units (SI), urea is reported in units of millimoles per liter. Urea N concentration in

TABLE 12.1	**Clinically Significant Nonprotein Nitrogen Compounds**	
Compound	**Approximate Plasma Concentration (% of Total NPN)**	**Approximate Urine Concentration (% of Excreted Nitrogen)**
Urea	45–50	86.0
Amino acids	25	—
Uric acid	10	1.7
Creatinine	5	4.5
Creatine	1–2	—
Ammonia	0.2	2.8

FIGURE 12.1 Structure of urea.

GLDH = glutamate dehydrogenase (EC 1.4.1.3)

FIGURE 12.2 Enzymatic assay for urea.

milligrams per deciliter may be converted to urea concentration in millimoles per liter by multiplying by 0.36.[8]

Analytical Methods

Several analytic approaches have been used to assay urea. Enzymatic methods are used most frequently in clinical laboratories.[9] The enzyme urease (urea amidohydrolase, EC 3.5.1.5) catalyzes hydrolysis of urea in the sample, and the ammonium ion (NH_4^+) produced in the reaction is quantified.[10] The most common method couples the urease reaction with glutamate dehydrogenase (GLDH, EC 1.4.1.3), and the rate of disappearance of nicotinamide adenine dinucleotide (reduced, NADH) at 340 nm is measured (Fig. 12.2).[11]

Ammonium from the urease reaction can also be measured by the color change associated with a pH indicator. This approach has been incorporated into instruments using liquid reagents, a multilayer film format, and reagent strips.[12–14] A method that uses an electrode to measure the rate of increase in conductivity as ammonium ions are produced from urea is in use in approximately 15% of laboratories in the United States.[9,15] Because the rate of change in conductivity is measured, ammonia contamination is not a problem as it is in other methods.

A reference method using isotope dilution mass spectrometry (IDMS) has been developed.[16] Analytic methods are summarized in Table 12.2.

Specimen Requirements

Urea concentration may be measured in plasma, serum, or urine. If plasma is collected, ammonium ions and high concentrations of sodium citrate and sodium fluoride must be avoided; citrate and fluoride inhibit urease.[8] Although the protein content of the diet influences urea concentration, the effect of a single protein-containing meal is minimal and a fasting sample is not required usually. A nonhemolyzed sample is recommended. Urea is susceptible to bacterial decomposition, so specimens (particularly urine) that cannot be analyzed within a few hours should be refrigerated. Timed urine specimens should be refrigerated during the collection period. Methods for plasma or serum may require modification for use with urine specimens because of high urea concentration and the presence of endogenous ammonia.[8]

Reference Intervals

Urea Nitrogen[8]		
Adult		
Plasma or serum	6–20 mg/dL	2.1–7.1 mmol/L
Urine, 24 h	12–20 g/d	0.43–0.71 mol urea/d

Pathophysiology

An elevated concentration of urea in the blood is called **azotemia**. Very high plasma urea concentration accompanied by renal failure is called **uremia** or the **uremic syndrome**. This condition is eventually fatal if not treated by dialysis or transplantation. Conditions causing increased plasma urea are classified according to the cause into three main categories: **prerenal**, renal, and **postrenal**.[7]

Prerenal azotemia is a result of reduced renal blood flow. Less blood is delivered to the kidney; consequently, less urea is filtered. Causative factors include congestive heart failure, shock, hemorrhage, dehydration, and other factors resulting in a significant decrease in blood volume. The amount of protein metabolism also induces prerenal changes in blood urea concentration. A high-protein diet or increased

TABLE 12.2	Summary of Analytic Methods—Urea	
Enzymatic Methods		
Methods use a similar first step—catalyzed by urease	Enzymatic production of ammonium ion (NH_4^+) from urea	See Figure 12.2.
GLDH-coupled enzymatic	Enzymatic reaction of NH_4^+, 2-oxoglutarate, and NADH to form glutamate and NAD+	Used on many automated instruments; best as a kinetic measurement
Indicator dye	NH_4^+ + pH indicator → color change	Used in automated systems, multilayer film reagents, and dry reagent strips
Conductometric	Conversion of unionized urea to NH_4^+ and CO_3^{2-} results in increased conductivity.	Specific and rapid
Other Methods		
Isotope dilution mass spectrometry	Detection of characteristic fragments following ionization; quantification using isotopically labeled compound	Proposed reference method

TABLE 12.3	Causes of Abnormal Plasma Urea Concentration
Increased Concentration	
Prerenal	Congestive heart failure
	Shock, hemorrhage
	Dehydration
	Increased protein catabolism
	High-protein diet
Renal	Acute and chronic renal failure
	Renal disease, including glomerular nephritis and tubular necrosis
Postrenal	Urinary tract obstruction
Decreased Concentration	
	Low protein intake
	Severe vomiting and diarrhea
	Liver disease
	Pregnancy

protein catabolism, such as occurs in stress, fever, major illness, corticosteroid therapy, and GI hemorrhage, may increase the urea concentration.

Decreased renal function causes an increase in plasma urea concentration as a result of compromised urea excretion. Renal causes of elevated urea include acute and chronic renal failure, glomerular nephritis, tubular necrosis, and other intrinsic renal disease (see Chapter 27). Postrenal azotemia can be due to obstruction of urine flow anywhere in the urinary tract by renal calculi, tumors of the bladder or prostate, or severe infection.

The major causes of decreased plasma urea concentration include low protein intake and severe liver disease. Plasma urea concentration is decreased during late pregnancy and in infancy as a result of increased protein synthesis. The conditions affecting plasma urea concentration are summarized in Table 12.3.

Differentiation of the cause of abnormal urea concentration is aided by calculation of the **urea nitrogen/creatinine (urea N/creatinine) ratio**, which is normally 10:1 to 20:1. Prerenal conditions tend to elevate plasma urea, whereas plasma creatinine remains normal, causing a high urea N/creatinine ratio. A high urea N/creatinine ratio with an elevated creatinine is usually seen in postrenal conditions. A low urea N/creatinine ratio is observed in conditions associated with decreased urea production, such as low protein intake, acute tubular necrosis, and severe liver disease.[7]

CASE STUDY 12.1

A 65-year-old man was first admitted for treatment of chronic obstructive lung disease, renal insufficiency, and significant cardiomegaly. Pertinent laboratory data on admission (5/31) are shown in Case Study Table 12.1.1.

CASE STUDY TABLE 12.1.1 Laboratory Results— First Admission

Test	5/31	6/3	6/7
Urea N (mg/dL)	45	24	11
Creatinine (mg/dL)	1.8	1.3	0.9
Urea N/creatinine	25	18.5	12.2
pH	7.22	7.50	
pCO_2 (mm Hg)	74.4	48.7	
pO_2 (mm Hg)	32.8	57.6	
O_2 sat (%)	51.3	91.0	

Because of severe respiratory distress, the patient was transferred to the intensive care unit, placed on a respirator, and given diuretics and intravenous (IV) fluids to promote diuresis. This treatment brought about a significant improvement in both cardiac output and renal function, as shown by laboratory results several days later (6/3). After 2 additional days on a respirator with IV therapy, the patient's renal function had returned to normal and, at discharge, his laboratory results were within normal limits (6/7).

The patient was readmitted 6 months later because of the increasing inability of his family to arouse him. On admission, he was shown to have a tremendously enlarged heart with severe pulmonary disease, heart failure, and probable renal failure. Laboratory studies on admission were as shown in Case Study Table 12.1.2. Numerous attempts were made to improve the patient's cardiac and pulmonary function, all to no avail, and the patient died 4 days later.

CASE STUDY TABLE 12.1.2 Laboratory Results— Second Admission

Urea N (mg/dL)	90
Creatinine (mg/dL)	3.9
Uric acid (mg/dL)	12.0
Urea N/creatinine	23
pH	7.35
pCO_2 (mm Hg)	59.9
pO_2 (mm Hg)	34.6
O_2 sat (%)	63.7

Question

1. What is the most likely cause of the patient's elevated urea nitrogen? Which data support your conclusion?

URIC ACID

Uric acid is the product of catabolism of the purine nucleic acids.[17] Although it is filtered by the glomerulus and secreted by the distal tubules into the urine, most uric acid is reabsorbed in the proximal tubules and reused.[18] Uric acid is relatively insoluble in plasma and, at high concentrations, can be deposited in the joints and tissue, causing painful inflammation.

Biochemistry

Purines, such as adenine and guanine from the breakdown of ingested nucleic acids or from tissue destruction, are converted into uric acid, primarily in the liver. Uric acid is transported in the plasma from the liver to the kidney, where it is filtered by the glomerulus. **Reabsorption** of 98% to 100% of the uric acid from the glomerular filtrate occurs in the proximal tubules. Small amounts of uric acid are secreted by the distal tubules into the urine. Renal excretion accounts for about 70% of uric acid elimination; the remainder passes into the GI tract and is degraded by bacterial enzymes.[18]

Nearly all of the uric acid in plasma is present as monosodium urate. At the pH of plasma (pH ~ 7), urate is relatively insoluble; at concentrations greater than 6.8 mg/dL, the plasma is saturated. As a result, urate crystals may form and precipitate in the tissues. In acidic urine (pH < 5.75), uric acid is the predominant species and uric acid crystals may form.[18]

Clinical Application

Uric acid is measured to confirm diagnosis and monitor treatment of **gout**, to prevent uric acid nephropathy during chemotherapeutic treatment, to assess inherited disorders of purine metabolism, to detect kidney dysfunction, and to assist in the diagnosis of renal calculi.[19]

Analytical Methods

In higher primates, such as humans and apes, uric acid is the final breakdown product of purine metabolism.[4] Most other mammals have the ability to catabolize purines to allantoin, a more water-soluble end product. This reaction is shown in Figure 12.3. Uric acid is readily oxidized to allantoin and, therefore, can function as a reducing agent in chemical reactions. This property was exploited in early analytic procedures for the determination of uric acid. The most common method of this type is the Caraway method, which is based on the oxidation of uric acid in a **protein-free filtrate**, with subsequent reduction of phosphotungstic acid in alkaline solution to tungsten blue.[20] The method lacks specificity.

Methods using uricase (urate oxidase, EC 1.7.3.3), the enzyme that catalyzes the oxidation of uric acid to allantoin, are more specific and are used almost exclusively in clinical laboratories. The simplest of these methods measures the differential absorption of uric acid and allantoin at 293 nm.[21] The difference in absorbance before and after incubation with uricase is proportional to the uric acid concentration. Proteins can cause high background absorbance, reducing sensitivity; hemoglobin and xanthine can cause negative interference.[22]

Coupled enzyme methods measure the hydrogen peroxide produced as uric acid is converted to allantoin.[23,24] Peroxidase or catalase (EC 1.11.1.6) is used to catalyze a chemical indicator reaction. The color produced is proportional to the quantity of uric acid in the specimen. Enzymatic methods of this kind have been adapted for use on traditional wet chemistry analyzers and for dry chemistry slide analyzers. Bilirubin and ascorbic acid, which destroy peroxide, if present in sufficient quantity, can interfere. Commercial reagent preparations often include potassium ferricyanide and ascorbate oxidase to minimize these interferences.

HPLC (high-performance liquid chromatography) methods, typically using UV detection, have been developed.[25] IDMS has been proposed as a candidate reference method.[26,27] Analytic methods are summarized in Table 12.4.

Specimen Requirements

Uric acid may be measured in heparinized plasma, serum, or urine. Serum should be removed from cells as quickly as possible to prevent dilution by intracellular contents. Diet may affect uric acid concentration overall, but a recent meal has no significant effect and a fasting specimen is unnecessary. Gross lipemia should be avoided. High bilirubin concentration may falsely decrease results obtained by peroxidase methods. Significant hemolysis, with concomitant glutathione release, may result in low values. Drugs such as salicylates and thiazides have been shown to increase values for uric acid.[28]

Uric acid is stable in plasma or serum after red blood cells have been removed. Serum samples may be stored refrigerated for 3 to 5 days. Ethylenediaminetetraacetic acid (EDTA) or fluoride additives should not be used for

FIGURE 12.3 Conversion of uric acid to allantoin.

TABLE 12.4 | **Summary of Analytic Methods—Uric Acid**

Chemical Methods		
Phosphotungstic acid	In carbonate solution (Na_2CO_3/OH^-), uric acid + $H_3PW_{12}O_{40}$ + O_2 → allantoin + tungsten blue + CO_2	Nonspecific; requires protein removal
Enzymatic Methods		
Similar first step—catalyzed by uricase	Enzymatic production of allantoin from uric acid	See Figure 12.3. Very specific
Coupled enzymatic—peroxidase	H_2O_2 + indicator dye → colored compound	Readily automated; reducing agents interfere
Spectrophotometric	Decrease in absorbance at 293 nm measured	Hemoglobin and xanthine interfere
Other Methods		
Isotope dilution mass spectrometry	Detection of characteristic fragments following ionization; quantification using isotopically labeled compound	Proposed reference method

specimens that will be tested by a uricase method. Urine collections must be alkaline (pH 8).[8]

Reference Intervals

Uric Acid (Uricase Method)[8]			
Adult	**Plasma or Serum**		
Male		3.5–7.2 mg/dL	0.21–0.43 mmol/L
Female		2.6–6.0 mg/dL	0.16–0.36 mmol/L
Child		2.0–5.5 mg/dL	0.12–0.33 mmol/L
Adult	Urine, 24 h	250–750 mg/d	1.5–4.4 mmol/d

Results expressed in conventional units of milligrams per deciliter can be converted to SI units using the molecular mass of uric acid (168 g/mol).

Pathophysiology

Abnormally increased plasma uric acid concentration is found in gout, increased catabolism of nucleic acids, and renal disease.[18] Gout is a disease found primarily in men and is usually first diagnosed between 30 and 50 years of age. Affected individuals have pain and inflammation of the joints caused by precipitation of sodium urates. In 25% to 30% of these patients, **hyperuricemia** is a result of overproduction of uric acid, although hyperuricemia may be exacerbated by a purine-rich diet, drugs, and alcohol. Plasma uric acid concentration in affected individuals is usually greater than 6.0 mg/dL. Patients with gout are susceptible to the formation of renal calculi, although not all persons with abnormally high serum urate concentrations develop this complication. In women, urate concentration rises after menopause. Postmenopausal women may develop hyperuricemia and gout. In severe cases, deposits of crystalline uric acid and urates called tophi form in tissue, causing deformities.[18]

Another common cause of elevated plasma uric acid concentration is increased metabolism of cell nuclei, as occurs in patients on chemotherapy for such proliferative diseases as leukemia, lymphoma, multiple myeloma, and polycythemia. Monitoring uric acid concentration in these patients is important to avoid nephrotoxicity. Allopurinol,

which inhibits xanthine oxidase (EC 1.1.3.22), an enzyme in the uric acid synthesis pathway, is used for treatment.

Patients with hemolytic or megaloblastic anemia may exhibit elevated uric acid concentration. Increased urate concentrations may be found following ingestion of a diet rich in purines (e.g., liver, kidney, sweetbreads, and shellfish) or as a result of increased tissue catabolism due to inadequate dietary intake (starvation).[18]

Inherited disorders of purine metabolism are associated with significant increases in physiological uric acid concentrations.[18] Lesch-Nyhan syndrome is an X-linked genetic disorder (seen only in males) caused by the complete deficiency of hypoxanthine–guanine phosphoribosyltransferase (EC 2.4.2.8), an important enzyme in the biosynthesis of purines. Lack of this enzyme prevents the reutilization of purine bases in the nucleotide salvage pathway and results in increased de novo synthesis of purine nucleotides and high plasma and urine concentrations of uric acid. Neurologic symptoms, mental retardation, and self-mutilation characterize this extremely rare disease. Mutations in the first enzyme in the purine synthesis pathway, phosphoribosylpyrophosphate synthetase (EC 2.7.6.1), also cause elevated uric acid concentration. Increased uric acid is found secondary to glycogen storage disease (deficiency of glucose-6-phosphatase, EC 3.1.3.9) and fructose intolerance (deficiency of fructose-1-phosphate aldolase, EC 2.1.2.13). Metabolites such as lactate and triglycerides are produced in excess and compete with urate for renal excretion in these diseases.

Hyperuricemia as a result of decreased uric acid excretion is a common feature of toxemia of pregnancy (preeclampsia) and lactic acidosis presumably as a result of competition for binding sites in the renal tubules. Chronic renal disease causes elevated uric acid concentration because filtration and **secretion** are impaired.

Uric acid nephrolithiasis, the formation of kidney stones (renal calculi), may occur due to a variety of predisposing factors and conditions.[29] In acidic urine, the relatively insoluble uric acid precipitates to form calculi, which can cause intense flank pain. The stones may be dissolved by alkalinization of the urine or treated by increased fluid intake and administration of xanthine oxidase inhibitors to reduce uric acid production.

Hypouricemia is less common than hyperuricemia and is usually secondary to severe liver disease or defective tubular reabsorption, as in Fanconi syndrome (a disorder of reabsorption in the proximal convoluted tubules of the kidney).[30] Decreased plasma uric acid can be caused by chemotherapy with 6-mercaptopurine or azathioprine, inhibitors of de novo purine synthesis, and as a result of overtreatment with allopurinol. Some studies have shown an association between low uric acid concentrations and neurodegenerative conditions such as Alzheimer's and Parkinson's diseases.[31]

Conditions known to affect plasma urate concentrations are shown in Table 12.5.

CREATININE/CREATINE

Creatinine is formed from **creatine** and creatine phosphate in muscle and is excreted into the plasma at a constant rate related to muscle mass. Plasma creatinine is inversely related to **glomerular filtration rate (GFR)** and, although an imperfect measure, it is commonly used to assess renal filtration function.[6]

Biochemistry
Creatine is synthesized primarily in the liver from arginine, glycine, and methionine.[5] It is then transported to other tissues, such as muscle, where it is converted to creatine phosphate, which serves as a high-energy source. Creatine

phosphate loses phosphoric acid and creatine loses water to form the cyclic compound, creatinine, which diffuses into the plasma and is excreted in the urine. The structures and relationship of these compounds are shown in Figure 12.4.

Creatinine is released into the circulation at a relatively constant rate that has been shown to be proportional to an individual's muscle mass. It is removed from the circulation by glomerular filtration and excreted in the urine. Small amounts of creatinine are secreted by the proximal tubule and reabsorbed by the renal tubules.[6] Daily creatinine excretion is reasonably stable.

Clinical Application
Measurement of creatinine concentration is used to determine the sufficiency of kidney function, to determine the severity of kidney damage, and to monitor the progression of kidney disease.[32]

Plasma creatinine concentration is a function of relative muscle mass, the rate of creatine turnover, and renal function. The amount of creatinine in the bloodstream is reasonably stable, although the protein content of the diet does influence the plasma concentration. Because of the constancy of endogenous production, urinary creatinine excretion has been used as a measure of the completeness of 24-hour urine collections in a given individual, although the uncertainty associated with this practice may exceed that introduced by use of the urine volume and collection time for standardization.[33] Urinary constituents may be expressed as a ratio to creatinine quantity rather than as mass excreted per day.

Creatinine clearance (CrCl), a measure of the amount of creatinine eliminated from the blood by the kidneys, and GFR are used to gauge renal function.[34] The GFR is the volume of plasma filtered (V) by the glomerulus per unit of time (t):

$$\text{GFR} = \frac{V}{t} \tag{Eq. 12-2}$$

Assuming a substance, S, can be measured and is freely filtered at the glomerulus and neither secreted nor reabsorbed by the tubules, the volume of plasma filtered would be equal to the mass of S filtered (M_S) divided by its plasma concentration (P_S):

$$V = \frac{M_S}{P_S} \tag{Eq. 12-3}$$

The mass of S filtered is equal to the product of its urine concentration (U_S) and the urine volume (V_U):

$$M_S = U_S V_S \tag{Eq. 12-4}$$

If the urine and plasma concentrations of S, the volume of urine collected, and the time over which the sample was collected are known, the GFR can be calculated:

$$\text{GFR} = \frac{U_S V_U}{P_S t} \tag{Eq. 12-5}$$

TABLE 12.5	Causes of Abnormal Plasma Uric Acid Concentration

Increased Concentration
Gout
Treatment of myeloproliferative disease with cytotoxic
    drugs
Hemolytic and proliferative processes
Purine-rich diet
Increased tissue catabolism or starvation
Enzyme deficiencies
    Lesch-Nyhan syndrome (hypoxanthine guanine
        phosphoribosyltransferase deficiency)
    Phosphoribosylpyrophosphate synthetase
        deficiency
    Glycogen storage disease type I (glucose-6-phos-
        phatase deficiency)
    Fructose intolerance (fructose-1-phosphate aldolase
        deficiency)
Toxemia of pregnancy
Lactic acidosis
Chronic renal disease
Drugs and poisons

Decreased Concentration
Liver disease
Defective tubular reabsorption (Fanconi syndrome)
Chemotherapy with azathioprine or
    6-mercaptopurine
Overtreatment with allopurinol

CK = creatine kinase (EC 2.7.3.2)

FIGURE 12.4 Interconversion of creatine, creatine phosphate, and creatinine.

The clearance of a substance is the volume of plasma from which that substance is removed per unit time. The formula for CrCl is given as follows, where U_{Cr} is urine creatinine concentration and P_{Cr} is plasma creatinine concentration:

$$CrCl = \frac{U_{Cr} V_U}{P_{Cr} t} \quad \text{(Eq. 12-6)}$$

CrCl is usually reported in units of mL/min and can be corrected for body surface area (see Chapter 27). CrCl overestimates GFR because a small amount of creatinine is reabsorbed by the renal tubules and up to 10% of urine creatinine is secreted by the tubules. However, CrCl provides a reasonable approximation of GFR.[34]

The observed relationship between plasma creatinine and GFR and relatively constant plasma creatinine concentrations should make the analyte a good endogenous filtration marker. However, measurement of plasma creatinine does not provide sufficient sensitivity for the detection of mild renal dysfunction. Measured creatinine concentration used in combination with other variables in one of several empirically determined equations provides a better assessment of renal disease, in part because the equations estimate GFR, not CrCl.

Clinical laboratories have been strongly encouraged to report an estimated GFR when serum creatinine is ordered as a means to increase identification of kidney disease and improve patient care.[35] Initially, the abbreviated Modification of Diet in Renal Disease (MDRD) equation was advocated.[36] The equation includes four variables—serum

creatinine concentration, age, gender (sex), and ethnicity—and makes the assumption that all filtered creatinine is excreted. The MDRD equation is most useful when serum creatinine results are produced in an assay that has been calibrated to be traceable to an IDMS method.[37]

When serum creatinine is measured using an IDMS-traceable method, the MDRD equation for **estimated glomerular filtration rate (eGFR)** is

$$eGFR\ (mL/min/1.73\,m^2) = 175 \times (S_{Cr})^{-1.154} \times (age)^{-0.203} \times (0.742\,if\,female) \times (1.210\,if\,African-American) \quad \text{(Eq. 12-7)}$$

where S_{cr} is serum (plasma) creatinine concentration in mg/dL and age is in years.[38] Results are normalized to a standard body surface area (1.73 m²). The equation is valid for individuals older than 18 years and younger than 70 years.[37] The formula was developed with data from nonhospitalized patients known to have chronic kidney disease and is reasonably accurate for this population, although eGFR values greater than 60 mL/min/1.73 m² calculated using this equation are negatively biased and should not be reported.

Effectiveness of the equation in other populations is being investigated and alternate equations have been proposed.[39] The Chronic Kidney Disease Epidemiology (CKD-EPI) Collaboration published an equation developed using results from healthy adults and adults with chronic kidney disease.[40] The CKD-EPI equation is used to report higher values (>60 mL/min/1.73 m²) for adults 18 years and older.

A modified Schwartz equation has been developed to calculate eGFR in the pediatric population.[41] The equation is

$$eGFR \left(mL/min/1.73m^2 \right) = (0.41 \times height)/S_{cr}$$

(Eq. 12-8)

Height is measured in cm and S_{cr} is serum (plasma) creatinine concentration in mg/dL. The equation can be used to calculate eGFR for children younger than 18 years old. The original Schwartz equation overestimates the GFR by 20% to 40% for creatinine concentrations measured by a traceable method.[35]

Analytical Methods
Creatinine
The methods most frequently used to measure creatinine are based on the Jaffe reaction first described in 1886.[42] In this reaction, creatinine reacts with picric acid in alkaline solution to form a red-orange chromogen. The reaction was adopted for the measurement of blood creatinine by Folin and Wu in 1919.[43] The reaction is nonspecific and subject to positive interference by a large number of compounds, including acetoacetate, acetone, ascorbate, glucose, and pyruvate. More accurate results are obtained when creatinine in a protein-free

filtrate is adsorbed onto Fuller's earth (aluminum magnesium silicate) or Lloyd's reagent (sodium aluminum silicate), then eluted and reacted with alkaline picrate.[44] This method is time consuming and not readily automated; it is not routinely used.

Two approaches have been used to increase the specificity of assay methods for creatinine: a kinetic Jaffe method and reaction with various enzymes. In the kinetic Jaffe method, serum is mixed with alkaline picrate and the rate of change in absorbance is measured.[45] Although this method eliminates some of the nonspecific reactants, it is subject to interference by α-keto acids and cephalosporins.[46] Bilirubin and hemoglobin may cause a negative bias, probably a result of their destruction in the strong base used. The kinetic Jaffe method is used routinely despite these problems because it is inexpensive, rapid, and easy to perform.

In an effort to enhance the specificity of the Jaffe reaction, several **coupled enzymatic methods** have been developed.[47,48] The method using creatininase (creatinine amidohydrolase, EC 3.5.2.10), creatinase (creatine amidinohydrolase, EC 3.5.3.3), sarcosine oxidase (EC 1.5.3.1), and peroxidase (EC 1.11.1.7) was adapted for use on a dry slide analyzer.[49]

IDMS is used as a reference method.[37] Assays used on automated analyzers are designated as "traceable" (calibrated) to an IDMS method. Analytic methods for creatinine are summarized in Table 12.6.

TABLE 12.6 Summary of Analytic Methods—Creatinine

Chemical Methods Based on Jaffe Reaction

Jaffe reaction	In alkaline solution, creatinine + picrate → red-orange complex	
Jaffe kinetic	Jaffe reaction performed directly on sample; detection of color formation timed to avoid interference of noncreatinine chromogens	Positive bias from α-keto acids and cephalosporins; requires automated equipment for precision
Jaffe with adsorbent	Creatinine in protein-free filtrate adsorbed onto Fuller's earth (aluminum magnesium silicate), then reacted with alkaline picrate to form colored complex	Adsorbent improves specificity; previously considered reference method
Jaffe without adsorbent	Creatinine in protein-free filtrate reacts with alkaline picrate to form colored complex	Positive bias from ascorbic acid, glucose, glutathione, α-keto acids, uric acid, and cephalosporins

Enzymatic Methods

Creatininase–H_2O_2	In a series of enzymatically catalyzed reactions, creatinine is hydrolyzed to creatine, which is converted to sarcosine and urea. Sarcosine is oxidized to glycine, CH_2O, and H_2O_2. Peroxidase-catalyzed oxidation of a colorless substrate produces a colored product + H_2O	Adapted for use as dry slide method; potential to replace Jaffe; no interference from acetoacetate or cephalosporins; some positive bias due to lidocaine
Creatininase–CK	In a series of reactions catalyzed by the enzymes creatininase, creatine kinase, pyruvate kinase, and lactate dehydrogenase, NAD^+ is produced and measured as a decrease in absorbance	Lacks sensitivity; not used widely

Other Methods

Isotope dilution mass spectrometry	Detection of characteristic fragments following ionization; quantification using isotopically labeled compound	Highly specific; accepted reference method

Specimen Requirements

Creatinine may be measured in plasma, serum, or urine. Hemolyzed and icteric samples should be avoided, particularly if a Jaffe method is used. Lipemic samples may produce erroneous results in some methods. A fasting sample is not required, although high-protein ingestion may transiently elevate serum concentrations. Urine should be refrigerated after collection or frozen if longer storage than 4 days is required.[8]

Sources of Error

Ascorbate, glucose, α-keto acids, and uric acid may increase creatinine concentration measured by the Jaffe reaction, especially at temperatures above 30°C. This interference is significantly decreased when kinetic measurement is applied. Depending on the concentration of reactants and measuring time, interference from α-keto acids may persist in kinetic Jaffe methods. Some of these substances interfere in enzymatic methods for creatinine measurement. Bilirubin causes a negative bias in both Jaffe and enzymatic methods. Ascorbate will interfere in enzymatic methods that use peroxidase as a reagent.[8]

Patients taking cephalosporin antibiotics may have falsely elevated results when the Jaffe reaction is used. Other drugs have been shown to increase creatinine results. Dopamine, in particular, is known to affect both enzymatic and Jaffe methods. Lidocaine causes a positive bias in some enzymatic methods.[28]

Creatine

The traditional method for creatine measurement relies on the analysis of the sample using an endpoint Jaffe method for creatinine before and after it is heated in acid solution. Heating converts creatine to creatinine and the difference between the two sample measurements is the creatine concentration. High temperatures may result in the formation of additional chromogens and the precision of this method is poor. Several enzymatic methods have been developed; one is the creatininase assay. The initial enzyme is omitted and creatine kinase (EC 2.7.3.2), pyruvate kinase (EC 2.1.7.40), and lactate dehydrogenase (EC 1.1.1.27) are coupled to produce a measurable colored product.[50] Creatine can be measured by HPLC.[51]

CASE STUDY 12.2

A 3-year-old girl was admitted with a diagnosis of acute lymphocytic leukemia. Her admitting laboratory data are shown in Case Study Table 12.2.1. After admission, she was treated by administration of packed red cells, 2 units of platelets, IV fluids, and allopurinol. On the second hospital day, chemotherapy was begun, using IV vincristine and prednisone and intrathecal injections of methotrexate, prednisone, and cytosine arabinoside. She was discharged for home care 5 days later. She was continued on prednisone and allopurinol at home. She received additional chemotherapy 1 month later (11/1) and again on 11/14. On 12/6, she was readmitted because she had painful sores in her mouth and was unable to eat.

Questions

1. How would you explain the significant elevations of uric acid on admission?
2. Which two factors are responsible for the normal concentrations of uric acid seen in subsequent admissions?
3. Which is the most likely cause of the abnormally low concentration of urea nitrogen observed on 12/6? Which other laboratory test would confirm your suspicions?

CASE STUDY TABLE 12.2.1 Laboratory Results

	10/1	10/2	10/3	10/4	11/14	12/6	6/20
Urea N (mg/dL)	12.0	a	a	15	4.0	2.0	a
Creatinine (mg/dL)	0.7	a	a	1.0	0.7	a	0.7
Uric acid (mg/dL)	12.0	9.2	4.0	1.9	2.3	a	3.1
WBC (mm³)	56,300	a	a		3,700	2,800	3,700	a

[a]Indicates test not performed.

Reference Intervals

Reference intervals vary with assay type, age, and gender.[8] Creatinine concentration decreases with age beginning in the 5th decade of life.

Creatinine			
Adult	Plasma or Serum	Jaffe Method	Enzymatic Method
Male		0.9–1.3 mg/dL (80–115 µmol/L)	0.6–1.1 mg/dL (53–97 µmol/L)
Female		0.6–1.1 mg/dL (53–97 µmol/L)	0.5–0.8 mg/dL (44–71 µmol/L)
Child		0.3–0.7 mg/dL (27–62 µmol/L)	0.0–0.6 mg/dL (0–53 µmol/L)
Adult Male	Urine, 24 h	800–2,000 mg/d (7.1–17.7 mmol/d)	
Female		600–1,800 mg/d (5.3–15.9 mmol/d)	

Pathophysiology
Creatinine
Elevated creatinine concentration is associated with abnormal renal function, especially as it relates to glomerular function. Plasma concentration of creatinine is inversely proportional to the clearance of creatinine. Therefore, when plasma creatinine concentration is elevated, GFR is decreased, indicating renal damage. Plasma creatinine is a relatively insensitive marker and may not be measurably increased until renal function has deteriorated more than 50%.[6]

CASE STUDY 12.3

An 80-year-old woman was admitted with a diagnosis of hypertension, congestive heart failure, anemia, possible diabetes, and chronic renal failure. She was treated with diuretics and IV fluids and released 4 days later. Her laboratory results are shown in Case Study Table 12.3.1.

Five months later, she was readmitted for treatment of repeated bouts of dyspnea. She was placed on a special diet and medication to control her hypertension and was discharged. Medical staff believed that she had not been taking her medication as prescribed, and she was counseled regarding the importance of regular doses.

Questions
1. What is the most probable cause of the patient's elevated urea nitrogen? Which data support your conclusion?
2. Note that this patient's admitting diagnosis is "possible diabetes." If the patient had truly been diabetic, with an elevated blood glucose and a positive acetone, what effect would this have had on the measured values of creatinine? Explain.

CASE STUDY TABLE 12.3.1 Laboratory Results

	First Admission	Second Admission		
	2/11	2/15	7/26	7/28
Urea N (mg/dL)	58	a	a	61
Creatinine (mg/dL)	6.2	6.2	6.4	6.0
Uric acid (mg/dL)	10.0	a	a	9.2
Urea N/ creatinine	9.4	a	a	10.1
Glucose (mg/dL)	86	80	113	a

[a]Indicates test not performed.

Creatine
In muscle disease such as muscular dystrophy, poliomyelitis, hyperthyroidism, and trauma, both plasma creatine and urinary creatinine are often elevated. Plasma creatinine concentrations are usually normal in these patients. Measurement of creatine kinase is used typically for the diagnosis of muscle disease because analytic methods for creatine are not readily available in most clinical laboratories. Plasma creatine concentration is not elevated in renal disease.[6]

AMMONIA
Ammonia is produced in the deamination of amino acids during protein metabolism.[5] It is removed from the circulation and converted to urea in the liver. Free ammonia is toxic; however, ammonia is present in the plasma in low concentrations.

Biochemistry
Ammonia (NH_3) is produced in the catabolism of amino acids and by bacterial metabolism in the lumen of the intestine.[52] Some endogenous ammonia results from anaerobic metabolic reactions that occur in skeletal muscle during exercise. Ammonia is consumed by the parenchymal cells of the liver in the Krebs-Henseleit or urea cycle to produce urea, a nontoxic compound that is excreted in the urine. At normal physiologic pH, most ammonia in the blood exists as ammonium ion (NH_4^+). Figure 12.5 shows the pH-dependent equilibrium between NH_3 and NH_4^+. Ammonia is excreted as ammonium ion by the kidney and acts to buffer urine.[53]

Clinical Application
Clinical conditions in which blood ammonia concentration provides useful information are hepatic failure, Reye's syndrome, and inherited deficiencies of urea cycle enzymes. Severe liver disease is the most common cause of disturbed ammonia metabolism. The monitoring of blood ammonia may be used to determine prognosis, although correlation between the extent of hepatic encephalopathy and plasma ammonia concentration is not always consistent. Arterial ammonia concentration is a better indicator of the severity of disease.[54,55]

Reye's syndrome, occurring most commonly in children, is a serious disease that can be fatal. Frequently, the disease is preceded by a viral infection and the administration of aspirin. Reye's syndrome is an acute metabolic disorder of the liver, and autopsy findings show severe fatty infiltration of that organ.[56] Blood ammonia concentration can be correlated with both the severity of the disease and

$$NH_4^+ + H_2O \rightleftharpoons NH_3 + H_3O^+$$

FIGURE 12.5 Interconversion of ammonium ion and ammonia.

prognosis. Survival reaches 100% if plasma NH_3 concentration remains below five times normal.[57]

Ammonia is of use in the diagnosis of inherited deficiency of urea cycle enzymes. Testing should be considered for any neonate with unexplained nausea, vomiting, or neurological deterioration associated with feeding.[58]

Assay of blood ammonia can be used to monitor hyperalimentation therapy and measurement of urine ammonia can be used to confirm the ability of the kidneys to produce ammonia.[8]

Analytical Methods

The accurate laboratory measurement of ammonia in plasma is complicated by its low concentration, instability, and pervasive contamination. Two approaches have been used for the measurement of plasma ammonia. One is a two-step approach in which ammonia is isolated from the sample and then assayed. The second involves direct measurement of ammonia by an enzymatic method or ion-selective electrode. Assays detect NH_3 or NH_4^+.

One of the first analytic methods for ammonia, developed by Conway in 1935, exploited the volatility of ammonia to separate the compound in a microdiffusion chamber.[59] Ammonia gas from the sample diffuses into a separate compartment and is absorbed in a solution containing a pH indicator. The amount of ammonia is determined by titration.

Ammonia can be measured by an enzymatic method using GLDH. This method is convenient and the most common technique used currently.[60] The decrease in absorbance at 340 nm as nicotinamide adenine dinucleotide phosphate (reduced, NADPH) is consumed in the reaction is proportional to the ammonia concentration in the specimen. NADPH is the preferred coenzyme because it is used specifically by GLDH; NADH will participate in reactions of other endogenous substrates, such as pyruvate. Adenosine diphosphate is added to the reaction mixture to increase the rate of the reaction and to stabilize GLDH.[61] This method is used on many automated systems and is available as a prepared kit from numerous manufacturers.

A dry slide automated system uses a thin-film colorimetric assay.[62] In this method, ammonia reacts with an indicator to produce a colored compound that is detected spectrophotometrically. Direct measurement using an ion-selective electrode has been developed.[63] The electrode measures the change in pH of a solution of ammonium chloride as ammonia diffuses across a semipermeable membrane. Analytic methods for ammonia are summarized in Table 12.7.

Specimen Requirements

Careful specimen handling is extremely important for plasma ammonia assays. Whole blood ammonia concentration increases rapidly following specimen collection because of in vitro amino acid deamination. Venous blood should be obtained without trauma and placed on ice immediately. Heparin and EDTA are suitable anticoagulants. Commercial collection containers should be evaluated for ammonia interference before a new lot is put into use. Samples should be centrifuged at 0 to 4°C within 20 minutes of collection and the plasma removed. Specimens should be assayed as soon as possible or frozen. Frozen plasma is stable for several days at −20°C. Erythrocytes contain two to three times as much ammonia as plasma; hemolysis should be avoided.

Cigarette smoking by the patient is a significant source of ammonia contamination. It is recommended that patients do not smoke for several hours before a specimen is collected.[8]

Many substances influence the in vivo ammonia concentration.[8,22] Ammonium salts, asparaginase, barbiturates, diuretics, ethanol, hyperalimentation, narcotic analgesics, and some other drugs may increase ammonia in plasma. Diphenhydramine, *Lactobacillus acidophilus*, lactulose, levodopa, and several antibiotics decrease concentrations. Glucose at concentrations greater than 600 mg/dL (33 mmol/L) interferes in dry slide methods.

Sources of Error

Ammonia contamination is a potential problem in the laboratory measurement of ammonia. Precautions must be taken to minimize contamination in the laboratory in which the assay is performed. Elimination of sources of ammonia contamination can significantly improve the accuracy of ammonia assay results. Sources of contamination include tobacco smoke, urine, and ammonia in detergents, glassware, reagents, and water.

The ammonia content of serum-based control material is unstable. Frozen aliquots of human serum albumin containing known amounts of ammonium chloride or ammonium sulfate may be used. Solutions containing known amounts of ammonium sulfate are commercially available.

TABLE 12.7   Summary of Analytic Methods—Ammonia

Chemical Methods		
Ion-selective electrode	Diffusion of NH_3 through selective membrane into NH_4Cl causes a pH change, which is measured potentiometrically	Good accuracy and precision; membrane stability may be a problem.
Spectrophotometric	NH_3 + bromophenol blue → blue color	
Enzymatic Methods		
Catalyzed by GLDH	Enzymatic reaction of NH_4^+, 2-oxoglutarate, and NADPH to form glutamate and $NADP^+$, which is detected spectrophotometrically	Most common on automated instruments; accurate and precise

Reference Intervals

Values obtained vary somewhat with the method used.[8] Higher concentrations are seen in newborns.

Ammonia			
Adult	Plasma	19–60 µg/dL	11–35 µmol/L
Urine, 24 h	140–1,500 mg N/d	10–107 mmol N/d	
Child (10 d to 2 y)	Plasma	68–136 µg/dL	40–80 µmol/L

Pathophysiology

In severe liver disease in which there is significant collateral circulation (as in cirrhosis) or if parenchymal liver cell function is severely impaired, ammonia is not removed from the circulation and blood concentration increases. High concentrations of NH_3 are neurotoxic and often associated with encephalopathy. Ammonia alters metabolic processes in the brain, which results in accumulation of toxic species, and impairs astrocyte function.[54,64]

Hyperammonemia is associated with inherited deficiency of urea cycle enzymes.[58] Measurement of plasma ammonia is important in the diagnosis and monitoring of these inherited metabolic disorders (see Chapter 35).

For additional student resources, please visit the**Point** at http://thepoint.lww.com

questions

1. Which one of the following is not an NPN substance?
   a. Allantoin
   b. Ammonia
   c. Creatinine
   d. Urea

2. Which compound constitutes nearly half of the NPN substances in the blood?
   a. Ammonia
   b. Creatine
   c. Urea
   d. Uric acid

3. A technologist reports urea N of 9 mg/dL. What is the urea concentration for this sample?
   a. 3.2 mg/dL
   b. 4.2 mg/dL
   c. 18.0 mg/dL
   d. 19.3 mg/dL

4. Which blood collection tube additive can be used to collect a specimen for measurement of urea?
   a. Ammonium
   b. Lithium heparin
   c. Sodium citrate
   d. Sodium fluoride

5. In the clinical laboratory, urea N is measured most often using
   a. Conductivity
   b. Enzymatic reactions
   c. Isotope dilution mass spectrometry
   d. Multilayer film formats

6. Elevated blood urea concentration is termed
   a. Azotemia
   b. BUN
   c. Uremia
   d. Uremic syndrome

7. Prerenal azotemia is caused by
   a. Acute renal failure
   b. Chronic renal failure
   c. Congestive heart failure
   d. Urinary tract obstruction

8. A technologist obtains a urea N value of 61 mg/dL and a serum creatinine value of 2.5 mg/dL on a patient. These results indicate
   a. Congestive heart failure
   b. Dehydration
   c. Glomerular nephritis
   d. Urinary tract obstruction

9. Uric acid is the final product of
   a. Allantoin metabolism
   b. Amino acid metabolism
   c. Purine metabolism
   d. The urea cycle

10. Sources of error in measurement of uric acid include
    a. Assay interference
    b. Competition from alternate purine substrates
    c. Narrow spectrophotometer bandwidth
    d. Nonspecific enzyme activity

review questions (continued)

11. Which condition is not associated with elevated plasma uric acid concentration?
   a. Allopurinol overtreatment
   b. Gout
   c. Lesch-Nyhan syndrome
   d. Renal disease

12. Complete deficiency of hypoxanthine–guanine phosphoribosyltransferase results in which disease?
   a. Allantoinism
   b. Glycogen storage disease
   c. Lesch-Nyhan syndrome
   d. Megaloblastic anemia

13. Uric acid nephrolithiasis refers to
   a. Acidification of the urine to dissolve renal calculi
   b. Formation of renal calculi composed of uric acid
   c. Precipitation of urates in the urinary tract
   d. Saturation of the kidney with uric acid

14. A 45-year-old male presents to the emergency department complaining of intense joint pain. The previous night the patient experienced similar pain accompanied by inflammation and redness of his wrists and large toe. The physician on-call orders testing for serum uric acid concentration. Which laboratory results and diagnosis are consistent with the physician's assessment? The reference interval for uric acid is 3.5 to 7.2 mg/dL.
   a. Uric acid 1.9 mg/dL; Fanconi syndrome
   b. Uric acid 1.0 mg/dL; hereditary xanthinuria
   c. Uric acid 9.1 mg/dL; alcoholism
   d. Uric acid 9.1 mg/dL; gout

15. Which statement describes creatinine biosynthesis accurately?
   a. Creatine is phosphorylated in the liver to form phosphocreatinine.
   b. Creatine phosphate undergoes spontaneous cyclization to form creatinine.
   c. Creatinine is formed from creatine and creatine phosphate in the liver.
   d. Creatinine is synthesized from arginine, glycine, and methionine in the liver.

16. Substances known to increase results when measuring creatinine by the Jaffe reaction include all of the following EXCEPT
   a. Ascorbic acid
   b. Bilirubin
   c. Glucose
   d. α-Keto acids

17. In the Jaffe reaction, a red-orange chromogen is formed when creatinine reacts with
   a. Aluminum magnesium silicate
   b. Creatininase
   c. Phosphocreatine
   d. Picric acid

18. Creatinine excretion typically
   a. Decreases from childhood to middle age
   b. Does not vary with age and sex
   c. Is higher for females than for males
   d. Is highest for adult men aged 18 to 50 years

19. Use of serum creatinine to calculate GFR
   a. Is discouraged because the calculations are complex
   b. Is encouraged as a means to identify kidney disease and improve patient care
   c. Requires hospitalization of the patient for specimen collection
   d. Requires simultaneous measurement of creatinine in a 24-hour urine collection

20. Which factor must be considered for calculation of creatinine clearance using the MDRD equation?
   a. Certification of body mass index
   b. Documentation of specimen collection time
   c. Identification of ethnicity
   d. Verification that the patient was fasting

21. Which situation would be expected to falsely increase measured blood ammonia concentration?
   a. The patient smoked two cigarettes 15 minutes prior to phlebotomy.
   b. The patient was fasting for 8 hours before blood collection.
   c. The patient ate a steak dinner the night before the specimen was collected.
   d. The specimen was placed on ice immediately after collection.

22. Although arterial blood is the recommended specimen for determination of this analyte, it is seldom used.
   a. Ammonia
   b. Creatine
   c. Urea
   d. Uric acid

23. Toxic effects of elevated blood ammonia concentration include
   a. Decreased renal function
   b. Hemorrhage and dehydration
   c. Mental status changes and coma
   d. Pain and inflammation of peripheral joints

(continues on page 258)

review questions (continued)

24. Ammonia concentrations are measured to evaluate
  a. Acid–base status
  b. Glomerular filtration
  c. Hepatic encephalopathy
  d. Renal failure

25. Ammonia concentration correlates with disease severity and prognosis for
  a. Astrocytosis
  b. Inherited deficiencies of urea cycle enzymes
  c. Neurological deterioration
  d. Reye's syndrome

references

1. Gentzkow CJ. An accurate method for determination of blood urea nitrogen by direct nesslerization. *J Biol Chem.* 1942;143:531–544.
2. Matthews DE. Proteins and amino acids. In: Shils ME, ed. *Modern Nutrition in Health and Disease.* 10th ed. Philadelphia, PA: Lippincott Williams & Wilkins; 2006:23–61.
3. Montgomery R, Conway TW, Spector AA, et al. *Biochemistry: a Case-Oriented Approach.* 6th ed. St. Louis, MO: Mosby; 1996.
4. Oh MS. Evaluation of renal function, water, electrolytes and acid-base balance. In: McPherson RA, Pincus MR, eds. *Henry's Clinical Diagnosis and Management by Laboratory Methods.* 22nd ed. Philadelphia, PA: Saunders Elsevier; 2011:169–192.
5. Coomes MW. Amino acid metabolism. In: Devlin TM, ed. *Textbook of Biochemistry with Clinical Correlations.* 6th ed. Hoboken, NJ: Wiley-Liss; 2006;743–787.
6. Lamb EJ, Price CP. Kidney function tests. In: Burtis CA, Ashwood ER, Bruns DE, eds. *Tietz Textbook of Clinical Chemistry and Molecular Diagnostics.* 5th ed. St. Louis, MO: Elsevier Saunders; 2012;669–707.
7. Winter WE. The kidney. In: Laposata M, ed. *Laboratory Medicine: the Diagnosis of Disease in the Clinical Laboratory.* 2nd ed. New York: McGraw-Hill Education; 2014. Accessmedicine.mhmedical.com. Accessed February 2016.
8. Wu AHB. *Tietz Clinical Guide to Laboratory Tests.* 4th ed. St. Louis, MO: WB Saunders; 2006.
9. SURVEYS 2015: C-B Chemistry/Therapeutic Drug Monitoring and U-B Urine Chemistry. Northfield, IL: College of American Pathologists; 2015.
10. Berthelot MPE. Violet d'aniline. *Repert Chim Appl.* 1859;1:284.
11. Talke H, Schubert GE. Enzymatic urea determination in the blood and serum in the warburg optical test. *Klin Wochenschr.* 1965;43:174–175.
12. Orsonneau J, Massoubre C, Cabanes M, et al. Simple and sensitive determination of urea in serum and urine. *Clin Chem.* 1992;38:619–623.
13. Ohkubo A, Kamei S, Yamanaka M, et al. Multilayer-film analysis for urea nitrogen in blood, serum, or plasma. *Clin Chem.* 1984;30:1222–1225.
14. Akai T, Naka K, Yoshikawa C, et al. Salivary urea nitrogen as an index to renal function: a test-strip method. *Clin Chem.* 1983;29:1825–1827.
15. Paulson G, Ray R, Sternberg J. A rate sensing approach to urea measurement. *Clin Chem.* 1971;17:644.
16. Kessler A, Siekmann L. Measurement of urea in human serum by isotope dilution mass spectrometry: a reference procedure. *Clin Chem.* 1999;45:1523–1529.
17. Cory JG. Purine and pyrimidine nucleotide metabolism. In: Devlin TM, ed. *Textbook of Biochemistry with Clinical Correlations.* 6th ed. Hoboken, NJ: Wiley-Liss; 2006:789–822.
18. Burns CM, Wortmann RL. Disorders of purine and pyrimidine metabolism. In: Kasper DL, Fauci AS, Hauser SL, Longo DL, Jameson JL, Loscalzo J, eds. *Harrison's Principles of Internal Medicine.* 19th ed. New York: McGraw-Hill Medical; 2015. http://accessmedicine.mhmedical.com. Accessed February 2016.
19. Uric acid. Lab Tests Online. https://labtestsonline.org/understanding/analytes/uric-acid. Reviewed June 25, 2013. Accessed February 2016.
20. Caraway WT, Hald PM. Uric acid. In: Seligson D, ed. *Standard Methods of Clinical Chemistry.* Vol. 4. New York, NY: Academic Press; 1963:239–247.
21. Feichtmeier TV, Wrenn HT. Direct determination of uric acid using uricase. *Am J Clin Pathol.* 1955;25:833–839.
22. Young DS. *Effects of Preanalytical Variables on Clinical Laboratory Tests.* 3rd ed. Washington, DC: American Association for Clinical Chemistry Press; 2007.
23. Gochman N, Schmitz JM. Automated determination of uric acid with use of a uricase-peroxidase system. *Clin Chem.* 1971;17:1154–1159.
24. Kageyama N. A direct colorimetric determination of uric acid in serum and urine with uricase-catalase system. *Clin Chim Acta.* 1971;31:421–426.
25. Cooper N, Khosravan R, Erdmann C, et al. Quantification of uric acid, xanthine and hypoxanthine in human serum by HPLC for pharmacodynamic studies. *J Chromatogr B.* 2006;837:1–10.
26. Ellerbe P, Cohen A, Welch MJ, et al. Determination of serum uric acid by isotope dilution mass spectrometry as a new candidate reference method. *Anal Chem.* 1990;62:2173–2177.
27. Dai X, Fang X, Zhang C, et al. Determination of serum uric acid using high-performance liquid chromatography (HPLC)/isotope dilution mass spectrometry (ID-MS) as a candidate reference method. *J Chromatogr B Analyt Technol Biomed Life Sci.* 2007;857:287–295.
28. Young DS. *AACC Effects on Clinical Laboratory Tests: Drugs, Disease, Herbs and Natural Products.* www.clinfx.com. Published 2013. Accessed February 2016.
29. Uric acid nephrolithiasis. http://www.uptodate.com. Updated January 7, 2016. Accessed February 2016.
30. Medical Dictionary: MedlinePlus. U.S. National Library of Medicine. https://www.nlm.nih.gov/medlineplus/mplusdictionary.html. Page updated April 18, 2012. Accessed February 2016.
31. Kutzing MK, Firestein BL. Altered uric acid levels and disease states. *J Pharmacol Exp Ther.* 2008;324:1–7.

32. Creatinine. Lab Tests Online. https://labtestsonline.org/understanding/analytes/creatinine. Reviewed August 31, 2015. Accessed February 2016.

33. Garde AH, Hansen AM, Kristiansen J, et al. Comparison of uncertainties related to standardization of urine samples with volume and creatinine concentration. *Ann Occup Hyg.* 2004;48:171–179.

34. Assessment of Kidney Function. http://www.uptodate.com. Updated August 27, 2014. Accessed February 2016.

35. National Kidney Disease Education Program. http://www.niddk.nih.gov/health-information/health-communication-programs/nkdep. Accessed February 2016.

36. Levey AS, Coresh J, Balk E, et al. National kidney foundation practice guidelines for chronic kidney disease: evaluation, classification, and stratification. *Ann Intern Med.* 2003;139:137–147.

37. Myers GL, Miller WG, Coresh J, et al. Recommendations for improving serum creatinine measurement: a report from the Laboratory Working Group of the National Kidney Disease Education Program. *Clin Chem.* 2006;52:5–18.

38. Levey AS, Coresh J, Greene T, et al. Expressing the modification of diet in renal disease study equation for estimating glomerular filtration rate with standardized serum creatinine vales. *Clin Chem.* 2007;53:766–772.

39. Miller WG. Glomerular filtration rate: the importance of standardized serum creatinine in detecting kidney disease. *Clin Lab News.* 2011;37:10–12.

40. Levey AS, Stevens LA, Schmid CH, et al. A new equation to estimate glomerular filtration rate. *Ann Intern Med.* 2009;150:604–612.

41. Schwartz GJ, Munoz A, Schneider MF, et al. New equations to estimate GFR in children with CKD. *J Am Soc Nephrol.* 2009;20:629–637.

42. Jaffe M. Uber den niederschlag welchen pikrinsaure in normalen harn erzeugt und uber eine neue reaktion des kreatinins. *Z Physiol Chem.* 1886;10:391.

43. Folin O, Wu H. System of blood analysis. *J Biol Chem.* 1919;31:81.

44. Haeckel R. Assay of creatinine in serum with use of Fuller's earth to remove interferents. *Clin Chem.* 1981;27:179–183.

45. Larsen K. Creatinine assay by a reaction kinetic principle. *Clin Chim Acta.* 1972;41:209–217.

46. Bowers LD, Wong ET. Kinetic serum creatinine assays. II. A critical evaluation and review. *Clin Chem.* 1980;26:555–561.

47. Moss GA, Bondar RJL, Buzzelli DM. Kinetic enzymatic method for determining serum creatinine. *Clin Chem.* 1975;21:1422–1426.

48. Fossati P, Prencipe L, Berti G. Enzymic creatinine assay: a new colorimetric method based on hydrogen peroxide measurement. *Clin Chem.* 1983;29:1494–1496.

49. Creatinine Test Methodology. *Kodak Ektachem Clinical Chemistry Products.* Rochester, NY: Eastman Kodak Company; 1992: Pub No MP2-49.

50. Beyer C. Creatine measurement in serum and urine with an automated enzymatic method. *Clin Chem.* 1993;39:1613–1619.

51. Smith-Palmer T. Separation methods applicable to urinary creatine and creatinine. *J Chromatogr B Analyt Technol Biomed Life Sci.* 2002;781:93–106.

52. Dufour DR. Liver disease. In: Burtis CA, Ashwood ER, Bruns DE, eds. *Tietz Textbook of Clinical Chemistry and Molecular Diagnostics.* 5th ed. St. Louis, MO: Elsevier Saunders; 2012:1637–1693.

53. Hood JL, Scott MG. Physiology and disorders of water, electrolyte, and acid-base metabolism. In: Burtis CA, Ashwood ER, Bruns DE, eds. *Tietz Textbook of Clinical Chemistry and Molecular Diagnostics.* 5th ed. St. Louis, MO: Elsevier Saunders; 2012:1609–1635.

54. Pincus MR, Tierno PM, Fenelus M, et al. Evaluation of liver function. In: McPherson RA, Pincus MR, eds. *Henry's Clinical Diagnosis and Management by Laboratory Methods.* 22nd ed. Philadelphia, PA: Elsevier Saunders; 2011:296–311.

55. Bhatia V, Singh R, Acharya SK. Predictive value of arterial ammonia for complications and outcome in acute liver failure. *Gut.* 2006;55:98–104.

56. Acute toxic-metabolic encephalopathy in children. http://www.uptodate.com. Updated June 22, 2015. Accessed February 2016.

57. Fitzgerald JF, Clark JH, Angelides AG, et al. The prognostic significance of peak ammonia levels in Reye's syndrome. *Pediatrics.* 1982;70:997–1000.

58. Pasquali M, Longo N. Newborn screening and inborn errors of metabolism. In: Burtis CA, Ashwood ER, Bruns DE, eds. *Tietz Textbook of Clinical Chemistry and Molecular Diagnostics.* 5th ed. St. Louis, MO: Elsevier Saunders; 2012:2045–2082.

59. Conway EJ, O'Malley E. Microdiffusion methods: ammonia and urea using buffered absorbents (revised methods for ranges greater than 10 µg N). *Biochem J.* 1942;36:655–661.

60. Mondzac A, Ehrlich GE, Seegmiller JE. An enzymatic determination of ammonia in biological fluids. *J Lab Clin Med.* 1965;66:526–531.

61. *Ammonia Test Methodology. Roche/Hitachi Products.* Indianapolis, IN: Roche Diagnostics Corporation; 2001.

62. VITROS AMON Slides. *Instructions for Use. VITROS Chemistry Products.* Rochester, NY: Ortho-Clinical Diagnostics; 2002:Pub No MP2–90.

63. Willems D, Steenssens W. Ammonia determined in plasma with a selective electrode. *Clin Chem.* 1988;34:2372.

64. Albrecht J, Zielinska M, Norenberg MD. Glutamine as a mediator of ammonia neurotoxicity: A critical appraisal. *Biochem Pharmacol.* 2010;80:1303–1308.

chapter outline

key terms

chapter objectives

Upon completion of this chapter, the clinical laboratorian should be able to do the following:

• Define the term enzyme, including physical composition and structure.
• Classify enzymes according to the International Union of Biochemistry.
• Discuss the different factors affecting the rate of an enzymatic reaction.
• Explain enzyme kinetics including zero-order and first-order kinetics.
• Explain why the measurement of serum enzyme concentrations is clinically useful.
• Discuss which enzymes are useful in the diagnosis of various disorders, including cardiac, hepatic, bone, and muscle malignancies and acute pancreatitis.
• Discuss the tissue sources, diagnostic significance, clinical assays, and the sources of error for the following enzymes: creatine kinase, lactate dehydrogenase, aspartate aminotransferase, alanine aminotransferase, alkaline phosphatase, acid phosphatase, γ-glutamyltransferase, amylase, lipase, cholinesterase, and glucose-6-phosphate dehydrogenase.
• Evaluate patient serum enzyme concentrations in relation to disease states.
• Discus the clinical importance for detecting macroenzymes.
• Discuss the role of enzymes in drug metabolism.

For additional student resources, please visit thePoint at http://thepoint.lww.com

Enzymes are specific biologic proteins that catalyze biochemical reactions without altering the equilibrium point of the reaction or being consumed or changed in composition. The other substances in the reaction are converted to products. The catalyzed reactions are frequently specific and essential to physiologic functions, such as the hydration of carbon dioxide, nerve conduction, muscle contraction, nutrient degradation, and energy use. Found in all body tissue, enzymes frequently appear in the serum following cellular injury or, sometimes, in smaller amounts, from degraded cells. Certain enzymes, such as those that facilitate coagulation, are specific to plasma and, therefore, are present in significant concentrations in plasma. Plasma or serum enzyme levels are often useful in the diagnosis of particular diseases or physiologic abnormalities. This chapter discusses the general properties and principles of enzymes, aspects relating to the clinical diagnostic significance of specific physiologic enzymes, and assay methods for those enzymes.

GENERAL PROPERTIES AND DEFINITIONS

Enzymes catalyze many specific physiologic reactions. These reactions are facilitated by the enzyme structure and several other factors. As a protein, each enzyme contains a specific amino acid sequence (*primary structure*), with the resultant polypeptide chains twisting (*secondary structure*), which then folds (*tertiary structure*) and results in structural cavities. If an enzyme contains more than one polypeptide unit, the *quaternary structure* refers to the spatial relationships between the subunits. Each enzyme contains an *active site*, often a water-free cavity, where the substance on which the enzyme acts (the *substrate*) interacts with particular charged amino acid residues. An *allosteric site*—a cavity other than the active site—may bind regulator molecules and, thereby, be significant to the basic enzyme structure.

Even though a particular enzyme maintains the same catalytic function throughout the body, that enzyme may exist in different forms within the same individual. The different forms may be differentiated from each other based on certain physical properties, such as electrophoretic mobility, solubility, or resistance to inactivation. The term **isoenzyme** is generally used when discussing such enzymes; however, the International Union of Biochemistry (IUB) suggests restricting this term to multiple forms of genetic origin. An **isoform** results when an enzyme is subject to posttranslational modifications. Isoenzymes and isoforms contribute to heterogeneity in properties and function of enzymes.

In addition to the basic enzyme structure, a nonprotein molecule, called a **cofactor**, may be necessary for enzyme activity. Inorganic cofactors, such as chloride or magnesium ions, are called **activators**. A **coenzyme** is an organic cofactor, such as nicotinamide adenine dinucleotide (NAD). When bound tightly to the enzyme, the coenzyme is called a *prosthetic group*. The enzyme portion (**apoenzyme**), with its respective coenzyme, forms a complete and active system, a **holoenzyme**.

Some enzymes, mostly digestive enzymes, are originally secreted from the organ of production in a structurally inactive form, called a *proenzyme* or **zymogen**. Other enzymes later alter the structure of the proenzyme to make active sites available by hydrolyzing specific amino acid residues. This mechanism prevents digestive enzymes from digesting their place of synthesis.

ENZYME CLASSIFICATION AND NOMENCLATURE

To standardize enzyme nomenclature, the Enzyme Commission (EC) of the IUB adopted a classification system in 1961; the standards were revised in 1972 and 1978. The IUB system assigns a *systematic name* to each enzyme, defining the substrate acted on, the reaction catalyzed, and, possibly, the name of any coenzyme involved in the reaction. Because many systematic names are lengthy, a more usable, trivial, *recommended name* is also assigned by the IUB system.[1]

In addition to naming enzymes, the IUB system identifies each enzyme by an EC numerical code containing four digits separated by decimal points. The first digit places the enzyme in one of the following six classes:

1. **Oxidoreductases.** Catalyze an oxidation–reduction reaction between two substrates
2. **Transferases.** Catalyze the transfer of a group other than hydrogen from one substrate to another
3. **Hydrolases.** Catalyze hydrolysis of various bonds
4. **Lyases.** Catalyze removal of groups from substrates without hydrolysis; the product contains double bonds
5. **Isomerases.** Catalyze the interconversion of geometric, optical, or positional isomers
6. **Ligases.** Catalyze the joining of two substrate molecules, coupled with breaking of the pyrophosphate bond in adenosine triphosphate (ATP) or a similar compound

The second and third digits of the EC code number represent the subclass and sub-subclass of the enzyme, respectively, divisions that are made according to criteria specific to the enzymes in the class. The final number is the serial number specific to each enzyme in a sub-subclass. Table 13.1 provides the EC code numbers, as well as the systematic and recommended names, for enzymes frequently measured in the clinical laboratory.

Table 13.1 also lists common and standard abbreviations for commonly analyzed enzymes. Without IUB recommendation, capital letters have been used as a convenience to identify enzymes. The common abbreviations, sometimes developed from previously accepted names for the enzymes, were used until the standard abbreviations listed in the table were developed.[2,3] These standard abbreviations are used in the United States and are used later in this chapter to indicate specific enzymes.

TABLE 13.1 **Classification of Frequently Quantitated Enzymes**

Class	Recommended Name	Common Abbreviation	Standard Abbreviation	EC Code No.	Systematic Name
Oxidoreductases	Lactate dehydrogenase	LDH	LDH	1.1.1.27	L-Lactate:NAD⁺ oxidoreductase
	Glucose-6-phosphate dehydrogenase	G-6-PDH	G-6-PD	1.1.1.49	D-Glucose-6-phosphate:NADP⁺ 1-oxidoreductase
	Glutamate dehydrogenase	GLD	GLD	1.4.1.3	L-Glutamate:NAD(P) oxidoreductase, deaminase
Transferases	Aspartate aminotransferase	GOT (glutamate oxaloacetate transaminase)	AST	2.6.1.1	L-Aspartate:2-oxoglutarate aminotransferase
	Alanine aminotransferase	GPT (glutamate transaminase)	ALT	2.6.1.2	L-Alanine:2-oxoglutarate aminotransferase
	Creatine kinase	CPK (creatine phosphokinase)	CK	2.7.3.2	ATP:creatine N-phosphotransferase
	γ-Glutamyl-transferase	GGTP	GGT	2.3.2.2	(5-Glutamyl)peptide: amino acid-5-glutamyltransferase
	Glutathione-S-transferase	α-GST	GST	2.5.1.18	Glutathione transferase
	Glycogen phosphorylase	GP	GP	2.4.1.1	1,4-D-Glucan: orthophosphate α-D-glucosyltransferase
	Pyruvate kinase	PK	PK	2.7.1.40	Pyruvate kinase
Hydrolases	Alkaline phosphatase	ALP	ALP	3.1.3.1	Orthophosphoric monoester phosphohydrolase (alkaline optimum)
	Acid phosphatase	ACP	ACP	3.1.3.2	Orthophosphoric monoester phosphohydrolase (acid optimum)
	α-Amylase	AMY	AMS	3.2.1.1	1,4-D-Glucan glucanohydrolase
	Cholinesterase	PCHE	CHE	3.1.1.8	Acetylcholine acylhydrolase
	Chymotrypsin	CHY	CHY	3.4.21.1	Chymotrypsin
	Elastase-1	E1	E1	3.4.21.36	Elastase
	5-Nucleotidase	NTP	NTP	3.1.3.5	5′-Ribonucleotide phosphohydrolase
	Triacylglycerol lipase		LPS	3.1.1.3	Triacylglycerol acylhydrolase
	Trypsin	TRY	TRY	3.4.21.4	Trypsin
Lyases	Aldolase	ALD	ALD	4.1.2.13	D-D-Fructose-1,6-bisdiphosphate D-glyceraldehyde-3-phosphate-lyase
Isomerases	Triosephosphate isomerase	TPI	TPI	5.3.1.1	Triosephosphate isomerase
Ligase	Glutathione synthetase	GSH-S	GSH-S	6.3.2.3	Glutathione synthase

Adapted from Competence Assurance, ASMT. *Enzymology, An Educational Program*. Bethesda, MD: RMI Corporation; 1980.

ENZYME KINETICS

Catalytic Mechanism of Enzymes

There are some chemical reactions that may occur at a slow rate if there is not enough kinetic energy to drive the reaction to the formation of products (uncatalyzed reaction). Other chemical reactions may occur spontaneously if the free energy or available kinetic energy is higher for the reactants than for the products. The reaction then proceeds toward the lower energy if a sufficient number of the reactant molecules possess enough excess energy to break their chemical bonds and collide to form new bonds. The excess energy, called **activation energy**, is the energy required to raise all molecules in 1 mole of a compound

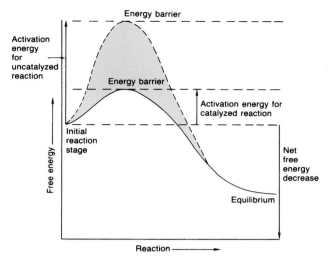

FIGURE 13.1 Energy versus progression of reaction, indicating the energy barrier that the substrate must surpass to react with and without enzyme catalysis. The enzyme considerably reduces the free energy needed to activate the reaction.

at a certain temperature to the transition state at the peak of the energy barrier. At the transition state, each molecule is equally likely to either participate in product formation or remain an unreacted molecule. Reactants possessing enough energy to overcome the energy barrier participate in product formation.

One way to provide more energy for a reaction is to increase the temperature, which will increase intermolecular collisions; however, this does not normally occur physiologically. Enzymes catalyze physiologic reactions by lowering the activation energy level that the reactants (*substrates*) must reach for the reaction to occur (Fig. 13.1). The reaction may then occur more readily to a state of equilibrium in which there is no net forward or reverse reaction, even though the equilibrium constant of the reaction is not altered. The extent to which the reaction progresses depends on the number of substrate molecules that pass the energy barrier.

The general relationship among enzyme, substrate, and product may be represented as follows:

$$\textbf{E} + \textbf{S} \rightarrow \textbf{ES} \rightarrow \textbf{E} + \textbf{P} \qquad \text{(Eq. 13-1)}$$

where E is enzyme, S is substrate, ES is enzyme–substrate complex, and P is product.

The ES complex is a physical binding of a substrate to the active site of an enzyme. The structural arrangement of amino acid residues within the enzyme makes the three-dimensional active site available. At times, the binding of ligand drives a rearrangement to make the active site. The transition state for the ES complex has a lower energy of activation than the transition state of S alone, so that the reaction proceeds after the complex is formed. An actual reaction may involve several substrates and products.

Different enzymes are specific to substrates in different extents or respects. Certain enzymes exhibit *absolute specificity*, meaning that the enzyme combines with only one substrate and catalyzes only the one corresponding reaction. Other enzymes are *group specific* because they combine with all substrates containing a particular chemical group, such as a phosphate ester. Still other enzymes are specific to chemical bonds and thereby exhibit *bond specificity*.

Stereoisomeric specificity refers to enzymes that predominantly combine with only one optical isomer of a certain compound. In addition, an enzyme may bind more than one molecule of substrate, and this may occur in a cooperative fashion. Binding of one substrate molecule, therefore, may facilitate binding of additional substrate molecules.

Factors That Influence Enzymatic Reactions

Substrate Concentration

The rate at which an enzymatic reaction proceeds and whether the forward or reverse reaction occurs depend on several reaction conditions. One major influence on enzymatic reactions is substrate concentration. In 1913, Michaelis and Menten hypothesized the role of substrate concentration in formation of the **enzyme–substrate (ES) complex**. According to their hypothesis, represented in Figure 13.2, the substrate readily binds to free enzyme at a low substrate concentration. The reaction rate steadily increases when more substrate is added, with the amount of enzyme exceeding the amount of substrate. When this occurs, the reaction is following **first-order kinetics** because the reaction rate is directly proportional to substrate concentration. Eventually, when the substrate concentration is high enough to saturate all available enzyme, the reaction velocity has reached its maximum. When product is formed, the resultant free enzyme immediately combines with excess free substrate. The reaction is in

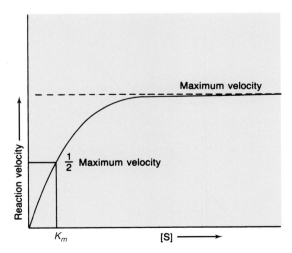

FIGURE 13.2 Michaelis-Menten curve of velocity versus substrate concentration for enzymatic reaction. K_m is the substrate concentration at which the reaction velocity is half of the maximum level.

zero-order kinetics, and the reaction rate depends only on enzyme concentration.

The **Michaelis-Menten constant** (K_m), derived from the theory of Michaelis and Menten, is a constant for a specific enzyme and substrate under defined reaction conditions and is an expression of the relationship between the velocity of an enzymatic reaction and substrate concentration. The assumptions are made that equilibrium among E, S, ES, and P is established rapidly and that the E + P → ES reaction is negligible. The rate-limiting step is the formation of product and enzyme from the ES complex. Then, maximum velocity is fixed, and the reaction rate is a function of only the enzyme concentration. As designated in Figure 13.2, K_m is specifically the substrate concentration at which the enzyme yields half the possible maximum velocity. Therefore, K_m indicates the amount of substrate needed for a particular enzymatic reaction.

The Michaelis-Menten hypothesis of the relationship between reaction velocity and substrate concentration can be represented mathematically as follows:

$$V = \frac{V_{max}[S]}{K_m + [S]} \quad \text{(Eq. 13-2)}$$

where V is measured velocity of reaction, V_{max} is maximum velocity, [S] is substrate concentration, and K_m is Michaelis-Menten constant of enzyme for specific substrate.

Theoretically, V_{max} and then K_m could be determined from the plot in Figure 13.2. However, V_{max} is difficult to determine from the hyperbolic plot and often not actually achieved in enzymatic reactions because enzymes may not function optimally in the presence of excessive substrate. A more accurate and convenient determination of V_{max} and K_m may be made through a Lineweaver-Burk plot, a double-reciprocal plot of the Michaelis-Menten constant, which yields a straight line (Fig. 13.3). The reciprocal is taken of

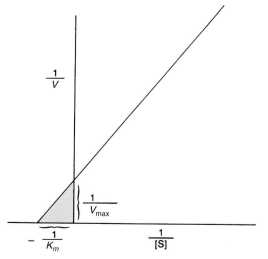

FIGURE 13.3 Lineweaver-Burk transformation of Michaelis-Menten curve. V_{max} is the reciprocal of the x-intercept of the straight line. K_m is the negative reciprocal of the x-intercept of the same line.

both the substrate concentration and the velocity of an enzymatic reaction. The equation becomes

$$\frac{1}{V} = \frac{K_m}{V_{max}} \frac{1}{[S]} + \frac{1}{V_{max}} \quad \text{(Eq. 13-3)}$$

Enzyme Concentration

Because enzymes catalyze physiologic reactions, the enzyme concentration affects the rate of the catalyzed reaction. As long as the substrate concentration exceeds the enzyme concentration, the velocity of the reaction is proportional to the enzyme concentration. The higher the enzyme level, the faster the reaction will proceed because more enzyme is present to bind with the substrate.

pH

Enzymes are proteins that carry net molecular charges. Changes in pH may denature an enzyme or influence its ionic state, resulting in structural changes or a change in the charge on an amino acid residue in the active site. Hence, each enzyme operates within a specific pH range and maximally at a specific pH. Most physiologic enzymatic reactions occur in the pH range of 7.0 to 8.0, but some enzymes are active in wider pH ranges than others. In the laboratory, the pH for a reaction is carefully controlled at the optimal pH by means of appropriate buffer solutions.

Temperature

Increasing temperature usually increases the rate of a chemical reaction by increasing the movement of molecules, the rate at which intermolecular collisions occur, and the energy available for the reaction. This is the case with enzymatic reactions until the temperature is high enough to denature the protein composition of the enzyme. For each 10 degree increase in temperature, the rate of the reaction will approximately double until, of course, the protein is denatured.

Each enzyme functions optimally at a particular temperature, which is influenced by other reaction variables, especially the total time for the reaction. The optimal temperature is usually close to that of the physiologic environment of the enzyme; however, some denaturation may occur at the human physiologic temperature of 37°C. The rate of denaturation increases as the temperature increases and is usually significant at 40°C to 50°C.

Because low temperatures render enzymes reversibly inactive, many serum or plasma specimens for enzyme measurement are refrigerated or frozen to prevent activity loss until analysis. Storage procedures may vary from enzyme to enzyme because of individual stability characteristics. Repeated freezing and thawing, however, tends to denature protein and should be avoided.

Because of their temperature sensitivity, enzymes should be analyzed under strictly controlled temperature conditions. Incubation temperatures should be accurate within ±0.1°C. Laboratories usually attempt to establish an analysis temperature for routine enzyme measurement of 25°C,

30°C, or 37°C. Attempts to establish a universal temperature for enzyme analysis have been unsuccessful and, therefore, reference ranges for enzyme levels may vary significantly among laboratories. In the United States, however, 37°C is most commonly used.

Cofactors

Cofactors are nonprotein entities that must bind to particular enzymes before a reaction occurs. Common *activators* (inorganic cofactors) are metallic (Ca^{2+}, Fe^{2+}, Mg^{2+}, Mn^{2+}, Zn^{2+}, and K^+) and nonmetallic (Br^- and Cl^-). The activator may be essential for the reaction or may only enhance the reaction rate in proportion with concentration to the point at which the excess activator begins to inhibit the reaction. Activators function by alternating the spatial configuration of the enzyme for proper substrate binding, linking substrate to the enzyme or coenzyme, or undergoing oxidation or reduction.

Some common coenzymes (organic cofactors) are nucleotide phosphates and vitamins. Coenzymes serve as second substrates for enzymatic reactions. When bound tightly to the enzyme, coenzymes are called *prosthetic groups.* For example, NAD as a cofactor may be reduced to nicotinamide adenine dinucleotide phosphate (NADP) in a reaction in which the primary substrate is oxidized. Increasing coenzyme concentration will increase the velocity of an enzymatic reaction in a manner synonymous with increasing substrate concentration. When quantitating an enzyme that requires a particular cofactor, that cofactor should always be provided in excess so that the extent of the reaction does not depend on the concentration of the cofactor.

Inhibitors

Enzymatic reactions may not progress normally if a particular substance, an *inhibitor*, interferes with the reaction. *Competitive inhibitors* physically bind to the active site of an enzyme and compete with the substrate for the active site.

With a substrate concentration significantly higher than the concentration of the inhibitor, the inhibition is reversible because the substrate is more likely than the inhibitor to bind the active site and the enzyme has not been destroyed.

A *noncompetitive inhibitor* binds an enzyme at a place other than the active site and may be reversible in the respect that some naturally present metabolic substances combine reversibly with certain enzymes. Noncompetitive inhibition also may be *irreversible* if the inhibitor destroys part of the enzyme involved in catalytic activity. Because the inhibitor binds the enzyme independently from the substrate, increasing substrate concentration does not reverse the inhibition.

Uncompetitive inhibition is another kind of inhibition in which the inhibitor binds to the ES complex—increasing substrate concentration results in more ES complexes to which the inhibitor binds and, thereby, increases the inhibition. The enzyme–substrate–inhibitor complex does not yield product. Lastly, a *mixed inhibitor* has the ability to bind to either the E or ES complex at a different site from the substrate active site.

Each of the four types of inhibition are unique with respect to effects on the V_{max} and K_m of enzymatic reactions (Fig. 13.4). In competitive inhibition, the effect of the inhibitor can be counteracted by adding excess substrate to bind the enzyme. The amount of the inhibitor is then negligible by comparison, and the reaction will proceed at a slower rate but to the same maximum velocity as an uninhibited reaction. The K_m is a constant for each enzyme and cannot be altered. However, because the amount of substrate needed to achieve a particular velocity is higher in the presence of a competing inhibitor, the K_m appears to increase when exhibiting the effect of the inhibitor.

The substrate and inhibitor, commonly a metallic ion, may bind an enzyme simultaneously in noncompetitive inhibition. The inhibitor may inactivate either an ES

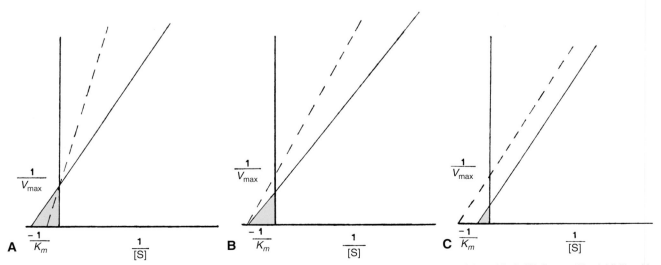

FIGURE 13.4 Normal Lineweaver-Burk plot (*solid line*) compared with each type of enzyme inhibition (*dotted line*). **(A)** Competitive inhibition V_{max} unaltered; K_m appears increased. **(B)** Noncompetitive inhibition V_{max} decreased; K_m unchanged. **(C)** Uncompetitive inhibition V_{max} decreased; K_m appears decreased.

complex or just the enzyme by causing structural changes in the enzyme. Even if the inhibitor binds reversibly and does not inactivate the enzyme, the presence of the inhibitor when it is bound to the enzyme slows the rate of the reaction. Thus, for noncompetitive inhibition, the maximum reaction velocity cannot be achieved. Increasing substrate levels has no influence on the binding of a noncompetitive inhibitor, so the K_m is unchanged.

Because uncompetitive inhibition requires the formation of an ES complex, increasing substrate concentration increases inhibition. Therefore, maximum velocity equal to that of an uninhibited reaction cannot be achieved, and the K_m appears to be decreased.

In addition, mixed inhibitors have the potential to interfere with substrate binding and enzyme catalysis. Consequently, the apparent V_{max} may decrease, and the apparent Km may decrease or increase.

Measurement of Enzyme Activity

Because enzymes are usually present in very small quantities in biologic fluids and often difficult to isolate from similar compounds, a convenient method of enzyme quantitation is measurement of catalytic activity. Activity is then related to concentration. Common methods might photometrically measure an increase in product concentration, a decrease in substrate concentration, a decrease in coenzyme concentration, or an increase in the concentration of an altered coenzyme.

If the amount of substrate and any coenzyme is in excess in an enzymatic reaction, the amount of substrate or coenzyme used, or product or altered coenzyme formed, will depend only on the amount of enzyme present to catalyze the reaction. Enzyme concentrations, therefore, are always performed in zero-order kinetics, with the substrate in sufficient excess to ensure that no more than 20% of the available substrate is converted to product. Any coenzymes also must be in excess. NADH is a coenzyme frequently measured in the laboratory. NADH absorbs light at 340 nm, whereas NAD does not, and a change in absorbance at 340 nm is easily measured.

In specific laboratory methodologies, substances other than substrate or coenzyme are necessary and must be present in excess. NAD or NADH is often convenient as a reagent for a *coupled enzyme* assay when neither NAD nor NADH is a coenzyme for the reaction. In other coupled enzyme assays, more than one enzyme is added in excess as a reagent and multiple reactions are catalyzed. After the enzyme under analysis catalyzes its specific reaction, a product of that reaction becomes the substrate on which an intermediate *auxiliary enzyme* acts. A product of the intermediate reaction becomes the substrate for the final reaction, which is catalyzed by an *indicator enzyme* and commonly involves the conversion of NAD to NADH or vice versa.

When performing an enzyme quantitation in zero-order kinetics, inhibitors must not be present and other variables that may influence the rate of the reaction must be carefully controlled. A constant pH should be maintained by means of an appropriate buffer solution. The temperature should be constant within ±0.1°C throughout the assay at a temperature at which the enzyme is active (usually, 25°C, 30°C, or 37°C).

During the progress of the reaction, the period for the analysis also must be carefully selected. When the enzyme is initially introduced to the reactants and the excess substrate is steadily combining with available enzyme, the reaction rate rises. After the enzyme is saturated, the rates of product formation, release of enzyme, and recombination with more substrate proceed linearly. After a time, usually 6 to 8 minutes after reaction initiation, the reaction rate decreases as the substrate is depleted, the reverse reaction is occurring appreciably, and the product begins to inhibit the reaction. Hence, enzyme quantitations must be performed during the linear phase of the reaction.

One of two general methods may be used to measure the extent of an enzymatic reaction: (1) fixed-time and (2) continuous-monitoring or kinetic assay. In the *fixed-time method*, the reactants are combined, the reaction proceeds for a designated time, the reaction is stopped (usually by inactivating the enzyme with a weak acid), and a measurement is made of the amount of reaction that has occurred. The reaction is assumed to be linear over the reaction time; the larger the reaction, the more enzyme is present.

In *continuous-monitoring* or **kinetic assays**, multiple measurements, usually of absorbance change, are made during the reaction, either at specific time intervals (usually every 30 or 60 seconds) or continuously by a continuous-recording spectrophotometer. These assays are advantageous over fixed-time methods because the linearity of the reaction may be more adequately verified. If absorbance is measured at intervals, several data points are necessary to increase the accuracy of linearity assessment. Continuous measurements are preferred because any deviation from linearity is readily observable.

The most common cause of deviation from linearity occurs when the enzyme is so elevated that all substrate is used early in the reaction time. For the remainder of the reaction, the rate change is minimal, with the implication that the coenzyme concentration is very low. With continuous monitoring, the laboratorian may observe a sudden decrease in the reaction rate (deviation from zero-order kinetics) of a particular determination and may repeat the determination using less patient sample. The decrease in the amount of patient sample operates as a dilution, and the answer obtained may be multiplied by the dilution factor to obtain the final answer. The sample itself is not diluted so that the diluent cannot interfere with the reaction. (Sample dilution with saline may be necessary to minimize negative effects in analysis caused by hemolysis or lipemia.) Enzyme activity measurements may not be accurate if storage conditions compromise integrity of the protein, if enzyme inhibitors are present, or if necessary cofactors are not present.

Calculation of Enzyme Activity

When enzymes are quantified relative to their activity rather than a direct measurement of concentration, the units used to report enzyme levels are *activity units*. The definition for the activity unit must consider variables that may alter results (e.g., pH, temperature, substrate). Historically, specific method developers frequently established their own units for reporting results and often named the units after themselves (i.e., Bodansky and King units). To standardize the system of reporting quantitative results, the EC defined the **international unit (IU)** as the amount of enzyme that will catalyze the reaction of 1 μmol of substrate per minute under specified conditions of temperature, pH, substrates, and activators. Since specified conditions may vary among laboratories, reference values are still often laboratory specific. Enzyme concentration is usually expressed in units per liter (IU/L). The unit of enzyme activity recognized by the International System of Units (Système International d'Unités [SI]) is the katal (mol/s). The mole is the unit for substrate concentration, and the unit of time is the second. Enzyme concentration is then expressed as katals per liter (kat/L) (1.0 IU = 17 nkat).

When enzymes are quantitated by measuring the increase or decrease of NADH at 340 nm, the molar absorptivity $(6.22 \times 10^3 \text{ mol/L})$ of NADH is used to calculate enzyme activity.

Measurement of Enzyme Mass

Immunoassay methodologies that quantify enzyme concentration by mass are also available and are routinely used for quantification of some enzymes, such as creatine kinase (CK)-MB. Immunoassays may overestimate active enzyme as a result of possible cross-reactivity with inactive enzymes, such as zymogens, inactive isoenzymes, macroenzymes, or partially digested enzyme. The relationship between enzyme activity and enzyme quantity is generally linear but should be determined for each enzyme. Enzymes may also be determined and quantified by electrophoretic techniques, which provide resolution of isoenzymes and isoforms.

Ensuring the accuracy of enzyme measurements has long been a concern of laboratorians. The Clinical Laboratory Improvement Amendment of 1988 (CLIA '88) has established guidelines for quality control and proficiency testing for all laboratories. Problems with quality control materials for enzyme testing have been a significant issue. Differences between clinical specimens and control sera include species of origin of the enzyme, integrity of the molecular species, isoenzyme forms, matrix of the solution, addition of preservatives, and lyophilization processes. Many studies have been conducted to ensure accurate enzyme measurements and good quality control materials.[4]

Enzymes as Reagents

Enzymes may be used as reagents to measure many nonenzymatic constituents in serum. For example, glucose, cholesterol, and uric acid are frequently quantified by means of enzymatic reactions, which measure the concentration of the analyte due to the specificity of the enzyme. Enzymes are also used as reagents for methods to quantify analytes that are substrates for the corresponding enzyme. One example, lactate dehydrogenase (LDH), may be a reagent when lactate or pyruvate concentrations are evaluated. For such methods, the enzyme is added in excess in a quantity sufficient to provide a complete reaction in a short period.

Immobilized enzymes are chemically bonded to adsorbents, such as agarose or certain types of cellulose, by azide groups, diazo, and triazine. The enzymes act as recoverable reagents. When substrate is passed through the preparation, the product is retrieved and analyzed, and the enzyme is present and free to react with more substrate. Immobilized enzymes are convenient for batch analyses and are more stable than enzymes in a solution. Enzymes are also commonly used as reagents in competitive and noncompetitive immunoassays, such as those used to measure human immunodeficiency virus (HIV) antibodies, therapeutic drugs, and cancer antigens. Commonly used enzymes include horseradish peroxidase, alkaline phosphatase (ALP), glucose-6-phosphate dehydrogenase, and β-galactosidase. The enzyme in these assays functions as an indicator that reflects either the presence or absence of the analyte.

ENZYMES OF CLINICAL SIGNIFICANCE

Table 13.2 lists the commonly analyzed enzymes, including their systematic names and clinical significance. Each enzyme is discussed in this chapter with respect to tissue source, diagnostic significance, assay method, source of error, and reference range.

CASE STUDY 13.1

A 57-year-old moderately overweight Caucasian male visits his family physician with a symptom of "indigestion" of 5 days' duration. He has also had bouts of sweating, malaise, and headache. His blood pressure is 140/105 mm Hg; his family history includes a father with diabetes who died at age 62 of AMI secondary to diabetes mellitus. An electrocardiogram revealed changes from one performed 6 months earlier. The results of the patient's blood work are as follows:

CK	129 U/L	(30–60)
CK-MB	4%	(<6%)
LDH	280 U/L	(100–225)
LDH	Isoenzymes	LDH-1 > LDH-2
AST	35 U/L	(5–30)

Questions

1. Can a diagnosis of AMI be ruled out in this patient?
2. What further cardiac markers should be run on this patient?
3. Should this patient be admitted to the hospital?

TABLE 13.2 Major Enzymes of Clinical Significance

Enzyme	Clinical Significance
Acid phosphatase (ACP)	Prostatic carcinoma
Alanine aminotransferase (ALT)	Hepatic disorder
Aldolase (ALD)	Skeletal muscle disorder
Alkaline phosphatase (ALP)	Hepatic disorder
	Bone disorder
Amylase (AMY)	Acute pancreatitis
Angiotensin-converting enzyme (ACE)	Blood pressure regulation
Aspartate aminotransferase (AST)	Myocardial infarction
	Hepatic disorder
	Skeletal muscle disorder
Chymotrypsin (CHY)	Chronic pancreatitis insufficiency
Creatine kinase (CK)	Myocardial infarction
	Skeletal muscle disorder
Elastase-1 (E1)	Chronic pancreatitis insufficiency
Glucose-6-phosphate dehydrogenase (G-6-PD)	Drug-induced hemolytic anemia
Glutamate dehydrogenase (GLD)	Hepatic disorder
γ-Glutamyltransferase (GGT)	Hepatic disorder
Glutathione-S-transferase (GST)	Hepatic disorder
Glycogen phosphorylase (GP)	Acute myocardial infarction
Lactate dehydrogenase (LDH)	Myocardial infarction
	Hepatic disorder
	Hemolysis
	Carcinoma
Lipase (LPS)	Acute pancreatitis
5'-Nucleotidase	Hepatic disorder
Pseudocholinesterase (PChE)	Organophosphate poisoning
	Genetic variants
	Hepatic disorder
	Suxamethonium sensitivity
Pyruvate kinase (PK)	Hemolytic anemia
Trypsin (TRY)	Acute pancreatitis

Creatine Kinase

CK is an enzyme with a molecular weight of approximately 82,000 that is generally associated with ATP regeneration in contractile or transport systems. Its predominant physiologic function occurs in muscle cells, where it is involved in the storage of high-energy creatine phosphate. Every contraction cycle of muscle results in creatine phosphate use, with the production of ATP. This results in relatively constant levels of muscle ATP. The reversible reaction catalyzed by CK is shown in Equation 13-4.

$$\text{Creatine} + ATP \xrightleftharpoons{CK} \text{Creatine phosphate} + \text{ADP}$$

(Eq. 13-4)

Tissue Source

CK is widely distributed in tissue, with highest activities found in skeletal muscle, heart muscle, and brain tissue. CK is present in much smaller quantities in other tissue sources, including the bladder, placenta, gastrointestinal tract, thyroid, uterus, kidney, lung, prostate, spleen, liver, and pancreas.

Diagnostic Significance

Due to the high concentrations of CK in muscle tissue, CK levels are frequently elevated in disorders of cardiac and skeletal muscle (myocardial infarction [MI], rhabdomyolysis, and muscular dystrophy). The CK level is considered a sensitive indicator of acute myocardial infarction (AMI) and muscular dystrophy, particularly the Duchenne type. Extreme elevations of CK occur in Duchenne-type muscular dystrophy, with values reaching 50 to 100 times the upper limit of normal (ULN). Although total CK levels are sensitive indicators of these disorders, they are not entirely specific indicators inasmuch as CK elevation is found in various other abnormal cardiac and skeletal muscle conditions. Levels of CK also vary with muscle mass and, therefore, may depend on gender, race, degree of physical conditioning, and age.

Elevated CK levels are also occasionally seen in central nervous system disorders such as cerebrovascular accident, seizures, nerve degeneration, and central nervous system shock. Damage to the blood–brain barrier must occur to allow enzyme release to the peripheral circulation.

TABLE 13.3		Creatine Kinase Isoenzymes— Tissue Localization and Sources of Elevation
Isoenzyme	**Tissue**	**Condition**
CK-MM	Heart	Myocardial infarction
	Skeletal muscle	Skeletal muscle disorder
		Muscular dystrophy
		Polymyositis
		Hypothyroidism
		Malignant hyperthermia
		Physical activity
		Intramuscular injection
CK-MB	Heart	Myocardial infarction
	Skeletal muscle	Myocardial injury
		Ischemia
		Angina
		Inflammatory heart disease
		Cardiac surgery
		Duchenne-type muscular dystrophy
		Polymyositis
		Malignant hyperthermia
		Reye's syndrome
		Rocky Mountain spotted fever
		Carbon monoxide poisoning
CK-BB	Brain	Central nervous system shock
	Bladder	Anoxic encephalopathy
	Lung	Cerebrovascular accident
	Prostate	Seizure
	Uterus	Placental or uterine trauma
	Colon	Carcinoma
	Stomach	Reye's syndrome
	Thyroid	Carbon monoxide poisoning
		Malignant hyperthermia
		Acute and chronic renal failure

FIGURE 13.5 Electrophoretic migration pattern of normal and atypical CK isoenzymes.

On electrophoretic separation, CK-BB will migrate fastest toward the anode and is therefore called *CK-1*. CK-BB is followed by CK-MB (*CK-2*) and, finally, by CK-MM (*CK-3*), exhibiting the slowest mobility (Fig. 13.5). Table 13.3 indicates the tissue localization of the isoenzymes and the major conditions associated with elevated levels. Separation of CK isoforms may also by visualized by high-voltage electrophoretic separation. Isoforms occur following cleavage of the carboxyl-terminal amino acid from the M subunit by serum carboxypeptidase N. Three isoforms have been described for CK-MM and two isoforms for CK-MB; the clinical significance is not well established.

The major isoenzyme in the sera of healthy people is the MM form. Values for the MB isoenzyme range from undetectable to trace (<6% of total CK). It also appears that CK-BB is present in small quantities in the sera of healthy people; however, the presence of CK-BB in serum depends on the method of detection. Most techniques cannot detect CK-BB in normal serum.

CK-MM is the major isoenzyme fraction found in striated muscle and normal serum. Skeletal muscle contains almost entirely CK-MM, with a small amount of CK-MB. The majority of CK activity in heart muscle is also attributed to CK-MM, with approximately 20% a result of CK-MB.[7] Normal serum consists of approximately 94% to 100% CK-MM. Injury to both cardiac and skeletal muscle accounts for the majority of cases of CK-MM elevations (Table 13.3). Hypothyroidism results in CK-MM elevations because of the involvement of muscle tissue (increased membrane permeability), the effect of thyroid hormone on enzyme activity, and, possibly, the slower clearance of CK as a result of slower metabolism.

Mild to strenuous activity may contribute to elevated CK levels, as may intramuscular injections. In physical activity, the extent of elevation is variable. However, the degree of exercise in relation to the exercise capacity of the individual is the most important factor in determining the degree of elevation.[8] Patients who are physically well conditioned show lesser degrees of elevation than do patients who are less conditioned. Levels may be elevated for as long as 48 hours following exercise. CK elevations are generally less than five times ULN following intramuscular injections and usually not apparent after 48 hours, although elevations may persist for 1 week. The predominant isoenzyme is CK-MM.

The quantity of CK-BB in the tissue (Table 13.3) is usually small. The small quantity, coupled with its relatively short half-life (1 to 5 hours), results in CK-BB activities that are generally low and transient and not usually

Other pathophysiologic conditions in which elevated CK levels occur are hypothyroidism, malignant hyperpyrexia, and Reye's syndrome. Table 13.3 lists the major disorders associated with abnormal CK levels. Serum CK levels and CK/progesterone ratio have been useful in the diagnosis of ectopic pregnancies.[5] Total serum CK levels have also been used as an early diagnostic tool to identify patients with *Vibrio vulnificus* infections.[6]

Because enzyme elevation is found in numerous disorders, the separation of total CK into its various isoenzyme fractions is considered a more specific indicator of various disorders than total levels. Typically, the clinical relevance of CK activity depends more on isoenzyme fractionation than on total levels.

CK occurs as a dimer consisting of two subunits that can be separated readily into three distinct molecular forms. The three isoenzymes have been designated as CK-BB (brain type), CK-MB (hybrid type), and CK-MM (muscle type).

measurable when tissue damage occurs. Highest concentrations are found in the central nervous system, the gastrointestinal tract, and the uterus during pregnancy. Although brain tissue has high concentrations of CK, serum rarely contains CK-BB of brain origin. Because of its molecular size (80,000), its passage across the blood–brain barrier is hindered. However, when extensive damage to the brain has occurred, significant amounts of CK-BB can sometimes be detected in the serum. It has been observed that CK-BB may be significantly elevated in patients with carcinoma of various organs. It has been found in association with untreated prostatic carcinoma and other adenocarcinomas. These findings indicate that CK-BB may be a useful tumor-associated marker.[9] The most common causes of CK-BB elevations are central nervous system damage, tumors, childbirth, and the presence of macro-CK, an enzyme–immunoglobulin complex. In most of these cases, the CK-BB level is greater than 5 U/L, usually in the range of 10 to 50 U/L. Other conditions listed in Table 13.3 usually show CK-BB activity below 10 U/L.[10]

The value of CK isoenzyme separation can be found principally in detection of myocardial damage. Cardiac tissue contains significant quantities of CK-MB, approximately 20% of all CK-MB. Whereas CK-MB is found in small quantities in other tissue, myocardium is essentially the only tissue from which CK-MB enters the serum in significant quantities. Demonstration of elevated levels of CK-MB, greater than or equal to 6% of the total CK, is considered a good indicator of myocardial damage, particularly AMI. Other nonenzyme proteins, called troponins, have been found to be even more specific and may elevate in the absence of CK-MB elevations. Following MI, the CK-MB levels begin to rise within 4 to 8 hours, peak at 12 to 24 hours, and return to normal levels within 48 to 72 hours.

This time frame must be considered when interpreting CK-MB levels.

CK-MB activity has been observed in other cardiac disorders (Table 13.3). Therefore, increased quantities are not entirely specific for AMI but probably reflect some degree of ischemic heart damage. Consequently, troponin is the preferred marker to detect MI because it is the most sensitive and specific for myocardial damage. The specificity of CK-MB levels in the diagnosis of AMI can be increased if interpreted in conjunction with LDH isoenzymes and/or troponins and if measured sequentially over a 48-hour period to detect the typical rise and fall of enzyme activity seen in AMI (Fig. 13.6). The MB isoenzyme also has been detected in the sera of patients with noncardiac disorders. CK-MB levels found in these conditions probably represent leakage from skeletal muscle, although in Duchenne-type muscular dystrophy, there may be some cardiac involvement as well. CK-MB levels in Reye's syndrome also may reflect myocardial damage. Despite the findings of CK-MB levels in disorders other than MI, its presence still remains a significant indicator of AMI.[11] The typical time course of CK-MB elevation following AMI is not found in other conditions.

Nonenzyme proteins (troponin I and troponin T) have been used as a more sensitive and specific marker of myocardial damage. These proteins are released into the bloodstream earlier and persist longer than CK and its isoenzyme CK-MB. More information on these protein markers of AMI can be found in Chapters 10 and 26.

Numerous reports have been made describing the appearance of unusual CK isoenzyme bands displaying electrophoretic properties that differ from the three major isoenzyme fractions[12–16] (Fig. 13.5). These atypical forms are generally of two types and are referred to as macro-CK and mitochondrial CK.

FIGURE 13.6 Time–activity curves of enzymes in myocardial infarction for AST, CK, CK-MB, and LDH. CK, specifically the MB fraction, increases initially, followed by AST and LDH. LDH is elevated the longest. All enzymes usually return to normal within 10 days.

Macro-CK appears to migrate to a position midway between CK-MM and CK-MB. This type of macro-CK largely comprises CK-BB complexed with immunoglobulin. In most instances, the associated immunoglobulin is IgG, although a complex with IgA also has been described. The term *macro-CK* has also been used to describe complexes of lipoproteins with CK-MM. The incidence of macro-CK in sera ranges from 0.8% to 1.6%. Currently, no specific disorder is associated with its presence, although it appears to be age and sex related, occurring most frequently in women older than age 50.

Mitochondrial CK (CK-Mi) is bound to the exterior surface of the inner mitochondrial membranes of muscle, brain, and liver. It migrates to a point cathodal to CK-MM and exists as a dimeric molecule of two identical subunits. It occurs in serum in both the dimeric state and in the form of oligomeric aggregates of high molecular weight (350,000). CK-Mi is not present in normal serum and is typically not present following MI. The incidence of CK-Mi ranges from 0.8% to 1.7%. For it to be detected in serum, extensive tissue damage must occur, causing breakdown of the mitochondrion and cell wall. Its presence does not correlate with any specific disease state but appears to be an indicator of severe illness. CK-Mi has been detected in cases of malignant tumor and cardiac abnormalities.

In view of the indefinite correlation between these atypical CK forms and a specific disease state, it appears that their significance relates primarily to the methods used for detecting CK-MB. In certain analytic procedures, these atypical forms may be measured as CK-MB, resulting in erroneously high CK-MB levels.

Methods used for measurement of CK isoenzymes include electrophoresis, ion-exchange chromatography, and several immunoassays, including radioimmunoassay (RIA) and immunoinhibition methods. Although mass methods are more sensitive and preferred for quantitation of CK-MB, electrophoresis has been the reference method. The electrophoretic properties of the CK isoenzymes are shown in Figure 13.5. Generally, the technique consists of performing electrophoresis on the sample, measuring the reaction using an overlay technique and then visualizing the bands under ultraviolet light. With electrophoresis, the atypical bands can be separated, allowing their detection apart from the three major bands. Often a strongly fluorescent band appears, which migrates in close proximity to the CK-BB form. The exact nature of this fluorescence is unknown, but it has been attributed to the binding of fluorescent drugs or bilirubin by albumin.

In addition to visualizing atypical CK bands, other advantages of electrophoresis methods include detecting an unsatisfactory separation and allowing visualization of adenylate kinase (AK). AK is an enzyme released from erythrocytes in hemolyzed samples and appearing as a band cathodal to CK-MM. AK may interfere with chemical or immunoinhibition methods, causing a falsely elevated CK or CK-MB value.

Ion-exchange chromatography has the potential for being more sensitive and precise than electrophoretic procedures performed with good technique. On an unsatisfactory column, however, CK-MM may merge into CK-MB and CK-BB may be eluted with CK-MB. Also, macro-CK may elute with CK-MB.

Antibodies against both the M and B subunits have been used to determine CK-MB activity. Anti-M inhibits all M activity but not B activity. CK activity is measured before and after inhibition. Activity remaining after M inhibition is a result of the B subunit of both MB and BB activity. The residual activity after inhibition is multiplied by 2 to account for MB activity (50% inhibited). The major disadvantage of this method is that it detects BB activity, which, although not normally detectable, will cause falsely elevated MB results when BB is present. In addition, the atypical forms of CK-Mi and macro-CK are not inhibited by anti-M antibodies and also may cause erroneous results for MB activity.

Immunoassays detect CK-MB reliably with minimal cross-reactivity. Immunoassays measure the concentration of enzyme protein rather than enzymatic activity and can, therefore, detect enzymatically inactive CK-MB. This leads to the possibility of permitting detection of infarction earlier than other methods. A double-antibody immunoinhibition assay is also available. This technique allows differentiation of MB activity due to AK and the atypical isoenzymes, resulting in a more specific analytic procedure for CK-MB.[17] Point-of-care assay systems for CM-MB are available but not as widely used as those for troponins.

Assay Enzyme Activity

As indicated by Equation 13-4, CK catalyzes both forward and reverse reactions involving phosphorylation of creatine or ADP. Typically, for analysis of CK activity, this reaction is coupled with other enzyme systems, and a change in absorbance at 340 nm is determined. The forward reaction is coupled with the pyruvate kinase–LDH–NADH system and proceeds according to Equation 13-5:

$$\text{Creatine} + \text{ATP} \underset{}{\overset{CK}{\rightleftharpoons}} \text{Creatine phosphate} + \text{ADP}$$
$$\text{ADP} + \text{phosphoenolpyruvate} \underset{}{\overset{PK}{\rightleftharpoons}} \text{Pyruvate} + \text{ATP}$$
$$\text{Pyruvate} + \text{NADH} + \text{H}^+ \underset{}{\overset{LD}{\rightleftharpoons}} \text{Lactate} + \text{NAD}^+$$

(Eq. 13-5)

The reverse reaction is coupled with the hexokinase–glucose-6-phosphate dehydrogenase–NADP system, as indicated in Equation 13-6:

$$\text{Creatine phosphate} + \text{ADP} \underset{}{\overset{CK}{\rightleftharpoons}} \text{Creatine ADP}$$
$$\text{ATP} + \text{glucose} \underset{}{\overset{KH}{\rightleftharpoons}} \text{ADP} + \text{glucose-6-phosphate}$$
$$\text{Glucose 6-phosphate} + \text{NADPH}^+ \overset{G\text{-}6\text{-}PD}{\rightleftharpoons}$$
$$\text{6-phosphogluconate} + \text{NADPH}$$

(Eq. 13-6)

The reverse reaction proposed by Oliver and modified by Rosalki is the most commonly performed method in the clinical laboratory.[13] The reaction proceeds two to six times faster than the forward reaction, depending on the assay conditions, and there is less interference from side reactions. The optimal pH for the reverse reaction is 6.8; for the forward reaction, it is 9.0.

CK activity in serum is unstable, being rapidly inactivated because of oxidation of sulfhydryl groups. Inactivation can be partially reversed by the addition of sulfhydryl compounds to the assay reagent. Compounds such as *N*-acetylcysteine, mercaptoethanol, thioglycerol, and dithiothreitol are among those used.

Source of Error

Hemolysis of serum samples may be a source of elevated CK activity. Erythrocytes are virtually devoid of CK; however, they are rich in AK activity. AK reacts with ADP to produce ATP, which is then available to participate in the assay reaction, causing falsely elevated CK levels. This interference can occur with hemolysis of greater than 320 mg/L hemoglobin, which releases sufficient AK to exhaust the AK inhibitors in the reagent. Trace hemolysis causes little, if any, CK elevation. Serum should be stored in a dark place because CK is inactivated by light. Activity can be restored after storage in the dark at 4°C for 7 days or at −20°C for 1 month when the assay is conducted using a sulfhydryl activator.[18] Because of the effect of muscular activity and muscle mass on CK levels, it should be noted that people who are physically well trained tend to have elevated baseline levels and that patients who are bedridden for prolonged periods may have decreased CK activity.

Reference Range

Total CK:

Male, 46–171 U/L (37°C)
Female, 34–145 U/L (37°C)
CK-MB: <5% total CK

The higher values in males are attributed to increased muscle mass. Note that enzyme reference ranges are subject to variation, depending on the method used and the assay conditions.

Lactate Dehydrogenase

LDH is an enzyme that catalyzes the interconversion of lactic and pyruvic acids. It is a hydrogen transfer enzyme that uses the coenzyme NAD^+ according to Equation 13-7:

$$\underset{\text{Lactate}}{\overset{\displaystyle CH_3}{\underset{\displaystyle COOH}{\overset{\displaystyle |}{\underset{\displaystyle |}{HC-OH}}}}} + NAD^+ \underset{}{\overset{LD}{\rightleftharpoons}} \underset{\text{Pyruvate}}{\overset{\displaystyle CH_3}{\underset{\displaystyle COOH}{\overset{\displaystyle |}{\underset{\displaystyle |}{C=O}}}}} + NADH + H^+$$

(Eq. 13-7)

Tissue Source

LDH is widely distributed in the body. High activities are found in the heart, liver, skeletal muscle, kidney, and erythrocytes; lesser amounts are found in the lung, smooth muscle, and brain.

Diagnostic Significance

Because of its widespread activity in numerous body tissue, LDH is elevated in a variety of disorders. Increased levels are found in cardiac, hepatic, skeletal muscle, and renal diseases, as well as in several hematologic and neoplastic disorders. The highest levels of total LDH are seen in pernicious anemia and hemolytic disorders. Intramedullary destruction of erythroblasts causes elevation as a result of the high concentration of LDH in erythrocytes. Liver disorders, such as viral hepatitis and cirrhosis, show slight elevations of two to three times ULN. AMI and pulmonary infarct also show slight elevations of approximately the same degree (2 to 3× ULN). In AMI, LDH levels begin to rise within 12 to 24 hours, reach peak levels within 48 to 72 hours, and may remain elevated for 10 days. Skeletal muscle disorders and some leukemias contribute to increased LDH levels. Marked elevations can be observed in most patients with acute lymphoblastic leukemia in particular.

Because of the many conditions that contribute to increased activity, an elevated total LDH value is a rather nonspecific finding. LDH assays, therefore, assume more clinical significance when separated into isoenzyme fractions. The enzyme can be separated into five major fractions, each comprising four subunits. It has a molecular weight of 128,000 Da. Each isoenzyme comprises four polypeptide chains with a molecular weight of 32,000 Da each. Two different polypeptide chains, designated H (heart) and M (muscle), combine in five arrangements to yield the five major isoenzyme fractions. Table 13.4 indicates the tissue localization of the LDH isoenzymes and the major disorders associated with elevated levels. LDH-1 migrates most quickly toward the anode, followed in sequence by the other fractions, with LDH-5 migrating the slowest.

In the sera of healthy individuals, the major isoenzyme fraction is LDH-2, followed by LDH-1, LDH-3, LDH-4, and LDH-5 (for the isoenzyme ranges, see Table 13.5). LDH-1 and LDH-2 are present to approximately the same extent in the tissues listed in Table 13.4. However, cardiac tissue and red blood cells contain a higher concentration of LDH-1. Therefore, in conditions involving cardiac necrosis (AMI) and intravascular hemolysis, the serum levels of LDH-1 will increase to a point at which they are present in greater concentration than LDH-2, resulting in a condition known as the **LDH flipped pattern** (LDH-1 > LDH-2).[19] This flipped pattern is suggestive of AMI. However, LDH is not specific to cardiac tissue and is not a preferred marker of diagnosis of AMI. LDH-1/LDH-2 ratios greater than 1 also may be observed in hemolyzed serum samples.[20] Elevations of LDH-3 occur most frequently with pulmonary involvement and are also observed in patients with various carcinomas. The LDH-4 and LDH-5 isoenzymes are found primarily in liver and skeletal muscle tissue, with LDH-5 being the predominant fraction in these tissues. LDH-5 levels have greatest clinical significance in the detection of hepatic disorders, particularly intrahepatic disorders. Disorders of skeletal muscle will reveal elevated LDH-5 levels, as depicted in the muscular dystrophies.

TABLE 13.4	Lactate Dehydrogenase (LDH) Isoenzymes—Tissue Localization and Sources of Elevation	
Isoenzyme	Tissue	Disorder
LDH-1 (HHHH)	Heart	Myocardial infarction
	Red blood cells	Hemolytic anemia
LDH-2 (HHHM)	Heart	Megaloblastic anemia
	Red blood cells	Acute renal infarct
		Hemolyzed specimen
LDH-3 (HHMM)	Lung	Pulmonary embolism
	Lymphocytes	Extensive
	Spleen	Pulmonary pneumonia
	Pancreas	Lymphocytosis
		Acute pancreatitis
		Carcinoma
LDH-4 (HMMM)	Liver	Hepatic injury or inflammation
LDH-5 (MMMM)	Skeletal muscle	Skeletal muscle injury

A sixth LDH isoenzyme has been identified, which migrates cathodic to LDH-5.[21–23] LDH-6 is alcohol dehydrogenase. In reporting studies, LDH-6 has been present in patients with arteriosclerotic cardiovascular failure. It is believed that its appearance signifies a grave prognosis and impending death. LDH-5 is elevated concurrently with the appearance of LDH-6, probably representing hepatic congestion due to cardiovascular disease. It is suggested, therefore, that LDH-6 may reflect liver injury secondary to severe circulatory insufficiency.

LDH has been shown to complex with immunoglobulins and to reveal atypical bands on electrophoresis. LDH complexed with IgA and IgG usually migrates between LDH-3 and LDH-4. This macromolecular complex is not associated with any specific clinical abnormality.

Analysis of LDH isoenzymes can be accomplished by electrophoresis, by immunoinhibition or chemical inhibition methods, or by differences in substrate affinity. Because of limited clinical utility, such tests are not commonly used. The electrophoretic procedure has been widely used historically. After electrophoretic separation, the isoenzymes can be detected either fluorometrically or colorimetrically.

TABLE 13.5	Lactate Dehydrogenase (LDH) Isoenzymes as a Percentage of Total LDH
Isoenzyme	%
LDH-1	14–26
LDH-2	29–39
LDH-3	20–26
LDH-4	8–16
LDH-5	6–16

Source: Lott JA, Stang JM. Serum enzymes and isoenzymes in the diagnosis and differential diagnosis of myocardial ischemia and necrosis. *Clin Chem.* 1980;26:1241.

LDH can use other substrates in addition to lactate, such as α-hydroxybutyrate. The H subunits have a greater affinity for α-hydroxybutyrate than to the M subunits. This has led to the use of this substrate in an attempt to measure the LDH-1 activity, which consists entirely of H subunits. The chemical assay, known as the measurement of α-hydroxybutyrate dehydrogenase (α-HBD) activity, is outlined in Equation 13-8.

(Eq. 13-8)

α-HBD is not a separate and distinct enzyme but is considered to represent the LDH-1 activity of total LDH. However, α-HBD activity is not entirely specific for the LDH-1 fraction because LDH-2, LDH-3, and LDH-4 also contain varying amounts of the H subunit. HBD activity is increased in those conditions in which the LDH-1 and LDH-2 fractions are increased.

LDH is commonly used to measure lactic and pyruvic acids or as a coupled reaction.

Assay for Enzyme Activity

LDH catalyzes the interconversion of lactic and pyruvic acids using the coenzyme NAD^+. The reaction sequence is outlined in Equation 13-9:

$$Lactate + NAD^+ \rightleftharpoons Pyruvate + NADH + H^+$$

(Eq. 13-9)

The reaction can proceed in either a forward (lactate [L]) or reverse (pyruvate [P]) direction. Both reactions have been used in clinical assays. The rate of the reverse reaction is approximately three times faster, allowing smaller sample volumes and shorter reaction times. However, the reverse reaction is more susceptible to substrate exhaustion and loss of linearity. The optimal pH for the forward reaction is 8.3 to 8.9; for the reverse reaction, it is 7.1 to 7.4.

Source of Error

Erythrocytes contain an LDH concentration approximately 100 to 150 times that found in serum. Therefore, any degree of hemolysis should render a sample unacceptable for analysis. LDH activity is unstable in serum regardless of the temperature at which it is stored. If the sample cannot be analyzed immediately, it should be stored at 25°C and analyzed within 48 hours. LDH-5 is the most labile isoenzyme. Loss of activity occurs more quickly at 4°C than at 25°C. Serum samples for LDH isoenzyme analysis should be stored at 25°C and analyzed within 24 hours of collection.

Reference Range

LDH, 125–220 U/L (37°C)

Aspartate Aminotransferase

Aspartate aminotransferase (AST) is an enzyme belonging to the class of **transferases**. It is commonly referred to as a *transaminase* and is involved in the transfer of an amino group between aspartate and α-keto acids. The older terminology, *serum glutamic-oxaloacetic transaminase* (*SGOT*, or *GOT*), may also be used. Pyridoxal phosphate functions as a coenzyme. The reaction proceeds according to Equation 13-10:

(Eq. 13-10)

The transamination reaction is important in intermediary metabolism because of its function in the synthesis and degradation of amino acids. The ketoacids formed by the reaction are ultimately oxidized by the tricarboxylic acid cycle to provide a source of energy.

Tissue Source

AST is widely distributed in human tissue. The highest concentrations are found in cardiac tissue, liver, and skeletal muscle, with smaller amounts found in the kidney, pancreas, and erythrocytes.

Diagnostic Significance

The clinical use of AST is limited mainly to the evaluation of hepatocellular disorders and skeletal muscle involvement. In AMI, AST levels begin to rise within 6 to 8 hours, peak at 24 hours, and generally return to normal within 5 days. However, because of the wide tissue distribution, AST levels are not useful in the diagnosis of AMI.

AST elevations are frequently seen in pulmonary embolism. Following congestive heart failure, AST levels also may be increased, probably reflecting liver involvement as a result of inadequate blood supply to that organ. AST levels are highest in acute hepatocellular disorders. In viral hepatitis, levels may reach 100 times ULN. In cirrhosis, only moderate levels—approximately four times ULN—are detected (see Chapter 24). Skeletal muscle disorders, such as the muscular dystrophies, and inflammatory conditions also cause increases in AST levels (4 to 8× ULN).

AST exists as two isoenzyme fractions located in the cell cytoplasm and mitochondria. The intracellular concentration of AST may be 7,000 times higher than the extracellular concentration. The cytoplasmic isoenzyme is the predominant form occurring in serum. In disorders producing cellular necrosis, the mitochondrial form may be significantly increased. Isoenzyme analysis of AST is not routinely performed in the clinical laboratory.

Assay for Enzyme Activity

Assay methods for AST are generally based on the principle of the Karmen method, which incorporates a coupled enzymatic reaction using malate dehydrogenase (MD) as the indicator reaction and monitors the change in absorbance at 340 nm continuously as NADH is oxidized to NAD^+ (Eq. 13-11). The optimal pH is 7.3 to 7.8.

$$Aspartate + \alpha\text{-}ketoglutarate \underset{}{\overset{AST}{\rightleftharpoons}}$$
$$Oxaloacetate + glutamate$$
$$Oxaloacetate + NADH + H^+ \rightleftharpoons Malate + NAD^+$$

(Eq. 13-11)

Source of Error

Hemolysis should be avoided because it can dramatically increase serum AST concentration. AST activity is stable in serum for 3 to 4 days at refrigerated temperatures.

Reference Range

AST, 5–35 U/L (37°C)

Alanine Aminotransferase

Alanine aminotransferase (ALT) is a transferase with enzymatic activity similar to that of AST. Specifically, it catalyzes the transfer of an amino group from alanine to α-ketoglutarate with the formation of glutamate and pyruvate. The older terminology was serum *glutamic-pyruvic transaminase* (*SGPT*, or *GPT*). Equation 13-12 indicates the transferase reaction. Pyridoxal phosphate acts as the coenzyme.

$$\underset{\text{Alanine}}{\begin{array}{c}CH_3 \\ | \\ HC-NH_2 \\ | \\ COOH\end{array}} + \underset{\substack{\alpha\text{-Keto-}\\\text{glutarate}}}{\begin{array}{c}COOH \\ | \\ C=O \\ | \\ CH_2 \\ | \\ CH_2 \\ | \\ COOH\end{array}} \overset{ALT}{\rightleftharpoons} \underset{\text{Pyruvate}}{\begin{array}{c}CH_3 \\ | \\ C=O \\ | \\ COOH\end{array}} + \underset{\text{Glutamate}}{\begin{array}{c}COOH \\ | \\ HC-NH_2 \\ | \\ CH_2 \\ | \\ CH_2 \\ | \\ COOH\end{array}}$$

(Eq. 13-12)

CASE STUDY 13.2

While a 67-year-old female is shopping for groceries, she faints and falls. She is driven home by a friend. When home, she realizes that she is bleeding from her mouth and is slightly disoriented. She appears injured from the fall, but she does not remember tripping or falling. The woman is taken to a local emergency department. The examining physician determines that there was a loss of consciousness; to determine the reason, he orders a head CT and ECG and the following laboratory tests: CBC, PT, aPTT, CK, LDH, AST, and troponin T and troponin I. All tests are within normal limits. The woman is sutured for the mouth injuries and admitted to a 24-hour observation unit.

Questions

1. What possible diagnoses is the physician considering?
2. What laboratory tests would be elevated at 6, 12, and 24 hour if this patient had an AMI?
3. What isoenzyme tests would be useful with this patient?

Tissue Source

ALT is distributed in many tissues, with comparatively high concentrations in the liver. It is considered the more liver-specific enzyme of the transferases.

Diagnostic Significance

Clinical applications of ALT assays are confined mainly to evaluation of hepatic disorders. Higher elevations are found in hepatocellular disorders than in extrahepatic or intrahepatic obstructive disorders. In acute inflammatory conditions of the liver, ALT elevations are frequently higher than those of AST and tend to remain elevated longer as a result of the longer half-life of ALT in serum (16 and 24 hours, respectfully).

Cardiac tissue contains a small amount of ALT activity, but the serum level usually remains normal in AMI unless subsequent liver damage has occurred. ALT levels have historically been compared with levels of AST to help determine the source of an elevated AST level and to detect liver involvement concurrent with myocardial injury.

Assay for Enzyme Activity

The typical assay procedure for ALT consists of a coupled enzymatic reaction using LDH as the indicator enzyme, which catalyzes the reduction of pyruvate to lactate with the simultaneous oxidation of NADH. The change in absorbance at 340 nm measured continuously is directly proportional to ALT activity. The reaction proceeds according to Equation 13-13. The optimal pH is 7.3 to 7.8.

$$\text{Alanine} + \alpha\text{-ketoglutarate} \overset{ALT}{\rightleftharpoons} \text{Pyruvate} + \text{glutamate}$$
$$\text{Pyruvate} + NADH + H^+ \overset{LD}{\rightleftharpoons} \text{Lactate} + NAD^+$$

(Eq. 13-13)

Source of Error

ALT is stable for 3 to 4 days at 4°C. It is relatively unaffected by hemolysis.

Reference Range

ALT, 7–45 U/L (37°C)

Alkaline Phosphatase

ALP belongs to a group of enzymes that catalyze the hydrolysis of various phosphomonoesters at an alkaline pH. Consequently, ALP is a nonspecific enzyme capable of reacting with many different substrates. Specifically, ALP functions to liberate inorganic phosphate from an organic phosphate ester with the concomitant production of an alcohol. The reaction proceeds according to Equation 13-14:

$$\underset{\text{Phosophomonoester}}{\begin{array}{c}O \\ \| \\ R-P-O^- \\ | \\ O^-\end{array}} + H_2O \overset{ALP}{\underset{pH\ 9\text{-}10}{\rightleftharpoons}} \underset{\text{Alcohol}}{R-OH} + \underset{\text{Phosphate ion}}{\begin{array}{c}O \\ \| \\ HO-P-O^- \\ | \\ O^-\end{array}}$$

(Eq. 13-14)

The optimal pH for the reaction is 9.0 to 10.0, but optimal pH varies with the substrate used. The enzyme requires Mg^{2+} as an activator.

Tissue Source

ALP activity is present on cell surfaces in most human tissue. The highest concentrations are found in the intestine, liver, bone, spleen, placenta, and kidney. In the liver, the enzyme is located on both sinusoidal and bile canalicular membranes; activity in bone is confined to the osteoblasts, those cells involved in the production of bone matrix. The specific location of the enzyme within this tissue accounts for the more predominant elevations in certain disorders.

Diagnostic Significance

Elevations of ALP are of most diagnostic significance in the evaluation of hepatobiliary and bone disorders. In hepatobiliary disorders, elevations are more predominant in obstructive conditions than in hepatocellular disorders; in bone disorders, elevations are observed when there is involvement of osteoblasts.

In biliary tract obstruction, ALP levels range from 3 to 10 times ULN. Increases are primarily a result of increased synthesis of the enzyme induced by cholestasis. In contrast, hepatocellular disorders, such as hepatitis and cirrhosis, show only slight increases, usually less than three times ULN. Because of the degree of overlap of ALP elevations that occurs in the various liver disorders, a single elevated ALP level is difficult to interpret. It assumes more diagnostic significance when evaluated along with other tests of hepatic function (see Chapter 24).

Elevated ALP levels may be observed in various bone disorders. Perhaps the highest elevations of ALP activity occur in Paget's disease (osteitis deformans). Other bone disorders include osteomalacia, rickets, hyperparathyroidism, and osteogenic sarcoma. In addition, increased levels are observed in healing bone fractures and during periods of physiologic bone growth.

In normal pregnancy, increased ALP activity, averaging approximately 1½ times ULN, can be detected between weeks 16 and 20 and 2 to 3 time the ULN during the third trimester. ALP activity increases and persists until the onset of labor. Activity then returns to normal within 3 to 6 days.[24] Elevations also may be seen in complications of pregnancy such as hypertension, preeclampsia, and eclampsia, as well as in threatened abortion.

ALP levels are significantly decreased in the inherited condition of hypophosphatasia. Subnormal activity is a result of the absence of the bone isoenzyme and results in inadequate bone calcification.

ALP exists as a number of isoenzymes, which have been studied by a variety of techniques. The major isoenzymes, which are found in the serum and have been most extensively studied, are those derived from the liver, bone, intestine, and placenta.[25]

Electrophoresis is considered the most useful single technique for ALP isoenzyme analysis. However, because there may still be some degree of overlap between the fractions, electrophoresis in combination with another separation technique may provide the most reliable information. A direct immunochemical method for the measurement of bone-related ALP is now available; this has made ALP electrophoresis unnecessary in most cases.

The liver fraction migrates the fastest, followed by bone, placental, and intestinal fractions. Because of the similarity between liver and bone phosphatases, there often is not a clear separation between them. Quantitation with use of a densitometer is sometimes difficult because of the overlap between the two peaks. The liver isoenzyme can actually be divided into two fractions—the major liver band and a smaller fraction called *fast liver*, or α_1 liver, which migrates anodal to the major band and corresponds to the α_1 fraction of protein electrophoresis. When total ALP levels are increased, the major liver fraction is the most frequently

elevated. Many hepatobiliary conditions cause elevations of this fraction, usually early in the course of the disease. The fast-liver fraction has been reported in metastatic carcinoma of the liver, as well as in other hepatobiliary diseases. Its presence is regarded as a valuable indicator of obstructive liver disease. However, it is occasionally present in the absence of any detectable disease state.

The bone isoenzyme increases due to osteoblastic activity and is normally elevated in children during periods of growth and in adults older than age 50. In these cases, an elevated ALP level may be difficult to interpret.[26]

The presence of intestinal ALP isoenzyme in serum depends on the blood group and secretor status of the individual. Individuals who have B or O blood group and are secretors are more likely to have this fraction. Apparently, intestinal ALP is bound by erythrocytes of group A. Furthermore, in these individuals, increases in intestinal ALP occur after consumption of a fatty meal. Intestinal ALP may increase in several disorders, such as diseases of the digestive tract and cirrhosis. Increased levels are also found in patients undergoing chronic hemodialysis.

Difference in heat stability is the basis of a second approach used to identify the isoenzyme source of an elevated ALP. Typically, ALP activity is measured before and after heating the serum at 56°C for 10 minutes. If the residual activity after heating is less than 20% of the total activity before heating, then the ALP elevation is assumed to be a result of bone phosphatase. If greater than 20% of the activity remains, the elevation is probably a result of liver phosphatase. These results are based on the finding that placental ALP is the most heat stable of the four major fractions, followed by intestinal, liver, and bone fractions in decreasing order of heat stability. Placental ALP will resist heat denaturation at 65°C for 30 minutes.

Heat inactivation is an imprecise method for differentiation because inactivation depends on many factors, such as correct temperature control, timing, and analytic methods sensitive enough to detect small amounts of residual ALP activity. In addition, there is some degree of overlap between heat inactivation of liver and bone fractions in both liver and bone diseases.

A third approach to identification of ALP isoenzymes is based on selective chemical inhibition. Phenylalanine is one of several inhibitors that have been used. Phenylalanine inhibits intestinal and placental ALP to a much greater extent than liver and bone ALP. With phenylalanine use, however, it is impossible to differentiate placental from intestinal ALP or liver from bone ALP.

In addition to the four major ALP isoenzyme fractions, certain abnormal fractions are associated with neoplasms. The most frequently seen are the Regan and Nagao isoenzymes. They have been referred to as *carcinoplacental alkaline phosphatases* because of their similarities to the placental isoenzyme. The frequency of occurrence ranges from 3% to 15% in cancer patients. The Regan isoenzyme has been characterized as an example of an ectopic production of an enzyme by malignant tissue. It has been detected in various carcinomas, such as the lung, breast, ovarian, and colon, with the highest incidences in ovarian and gynecologic cancers. Because of its low incidence in cancer patients, diagnosis of malignancy is rarely based on its presence. It is, however, useful in monitoring the effects of therapy because it will disappear on successful treatment.

The Regan isoenzyme migrates to the same position as the bone fraction and is the most heat stable of all ALP isoenzymes, resisting denaturation at 65°C for 30 minutes. Its activity is inhibited by phenylalanine.

The Nagao isoenzyme may be considered a variant of the Regan isoenzyme. Its electrophoretic, heat stability, and phenylalanine inhibition properties are identical to those of the Regan fraction. However, Nagao also can be inhibited by L-leucine. Its presence has been detected in metastatic carcinoma of pleural surfaces and in adenocarcinoma of the pancreas and bile duct.

Assay for Enzyme Activity

Because of the relative nonspecificity of ALP with regard to substrates, a variety of methodologies for its analysis have been proposed and are still in use today. The major differences between these relate to the concentration and types of substrate and buffer used and the pH of the reaction. A continuous monitoring technique based on a method devised by Bowers and McComb allows calculation of ALP activity based on the molar absorptivity of *p*-nitrophenol. The reaction proceeds according to Equation 13-15:

(Eq. 13-15)

p-Nitrophenylphosphate (colorless) is hydrolyzed to *p*-nitrophenol (yellow), and the increase in absorbance at 405 nm, which is directly proportional to ALP activity, is measured.

Source of Error

Hemolysis may cause slight elevations because ALP is approximately six times more concentrated in erythrocytes than in serum. ALP assays should be run as soon as possible after collection. Activity in serum increases approximately

3% to 10% on standing at 25°C or 4°C for several hours. Diet may induce elevations in ALP activity of blood group B and O individuals who are secretors. Values may be 25% higher following ingestion of a high-fat meal.

Reference Range

ALP (total), (37°C)

Males–Females	4–15 y	54–369 U/L
Males	20–50 y	53–128 U/L
	≥60 y	56–119 U/L
Females	20–50 y	42–98 U/L
	≥60 y	53–141 U/L

Acid Phosphatase

Acid phosphatase (ACP) belongs to the same group of phosphatase enzymes as ALP and is a **hydrolase** that catalyzes the same type of reactions. The major difference between ACP and ALP is the pH of the reaction. ACP functions at an optimal pH of approximately 5.0. Equation 13-16 outlines the reaction sequence:

$$R-P-O^- + H_2O \xrightarrow[\text{pH 5}]{\text{ACP}} R-OH + HO-P-O^-$$

Phosphomonoester   Alcohol   Phosphate ion

(Eq. 13-16)

Tissue Source

ACP activity is found in the prostate, bone, liver, spleen, kidney, erythrocytes, and platelets. The prostate is the richest source, with many times the activity found in other tissue.

Diagnostic Significance

Historically, ACP measurement has been used as an aid in the detection of prostatic carcinoma, particularly metastatic carcinoma of the prostate. Total ACP determinations are relatively insensitive techniques, detecting elevated ACP levels resulting from prostatic carcinoma in the majority of cases only when the tumor has metastasized. Newer markers, such as prostate-specific antigen (PSA), are more useful screening and diagnostic tools (see Chapter 31).

One of the most specific substrates for prostatic ACP is thymolphthalein monophosphate. Chemical inhibition methods used to differentiate the prostatic portion most frequently use tartrate as the inhibitor. The prostatic fraction is inhibited by tartrate. Serum and substrate are incubated both with and without the addition of L-tartrate. ACP activity remaining after inhibition with L-tartrate is subtracted from total ACP activity determined without inhibition, and the difference represents the prostatic portion:

Total ACP – ACP after tartrate inhibition
= prostatic ACP   (Eq. 13-17)

The reaction is not entirely specific for prostatic ACP; lysosomal ACP are also inhibited by tartrate. However, other tissue sources are largely uninhibited.

Neither of these methods of ACP determination is sensitive to prostatic carcinoma that has not metastasized. Values are usually normal in the majority of cases and, in fact, may be elevated only in about 50% of cases of prostatic carcinoma that has metastasized.

One technique with much improved sensitivity over conventional ACP assays is the immunologic approach using antibodies that are specific for the prostatic portion. Immunochemical techniques, however, are not of value as screening tests for prostatic carcinoma.

PSA is more likely than ACP to be elevated at each stage of prostatic carcinoma, even though a normal PSA level may be found in stage D tumors. PSA is particularly useful to monitor the success of treatment; however, PSA is controversial as a screening test for prostatic malignancy because PSA elevation may occur in conditions other than prostatic carcinoma, such as benign prostatic hypertrophy and prostatitis.[27–29]

Other prostatic conditions in which ACP elevations have been reported include hyperplasia of the prostate and prostatic surgery. There are conflicting reports of elevations following rectal examination and prostate massage. Certain studies have reported ACP elevations; others have indicated no detectable change. When elevations are found, levels usually return to normal within 24 hours.[30]

ACP assays have proved useful in forensic clinical chemistry, particularly in the investigation of rape. Vaginal washings are examined for seminal fluid–ACP activity, which can persist for up to 4 days.[31] Elevated activity is presumptive evidence of rape in such cases.

Serum ACP activity may frequently be elevated in bone disease. Activity has been shown to be associated with the osteoclasts.[32] Elevations have been noted in Paget's disease, in breast cancer with bone metastases, and in Gaucher's disease, in which there is an infiltration of bone marrow and other tissue by Gaucher cells rich in ACP activity. Because of ACP activity in platelets, elevations are observed when platelet damage occurs, as in the thrombocytopenia resulting from excessive platelet destruction from idiopathic thrombocytopenic purpura.

Assay for Enzyme Activity

Assay procedures for total ACP use the same techniques as in ALP assays but are performed at an acid pH:

$$p\text{-Nitrophenolphosphate} \underset{\text{pH5}}{\overset{\text{ACP}}{\rightleftharpoons}} \quad \text{(Eq. 13-18)}$$
$$p\text{-Nitrophenol} + \text{phosphate ion}$$

The reaction products are colorless at the acid pH of the reaction, but the addition of alkali stops the reaction and transforms the products into chromogens, which can be measured spectrophotometrically.

Some substrate specificities and chemical inhibitors for prostatic ACP measurements have been discussed previously. Thymolphthalein monophosphate is the substrate of choice for quantitative end point reactions. For continuous monitoring methods, α-naphthyl phosphate is preferred.

Immunochemical techniques for prostatic ACP use several approaches, including RIA, counterimmunoelectrophoresis, and immunoprecipitation. Also, an immunoenzymatic assay (Tandem E) includes incubation with an antibody to prostatic ACP followed by washing and incubation with p-nitrophenylphosphate. The p-nitrophenol formed, measured photometrically, is proportional to the prostatic ACP in the sample.

Source of Error

Serum should be separated from the red cells as soon as the blood has clotted to prevent leakage of erythrocyte and platelet ACP. Serum activity decreases within 1 to 2 hours if the sample is left at room temperature without the addition of a preservative. Decreased activity is a result of a loss of carbon dioxide from the serum, with a resultant increase in pH. If not assayed immediately, serum should be frozen or acidified to a pH lower than 6.5. With acidification, ACP is stable for 2 days at room temperature. Hemolysis should be avoided because of contamination from erythrocyte ACP.

RIA procedures for measurement of prostatic ACP require nonacidified serum samples. Activity is stable for 2 days at 4°C.

Reference Range

Prostatic ACP, 0–3.5 ng/mL
Tartrate-resistant ACP, adults: 1.5–4.5 U/L (37°C); children: 3.5–9.0 U/L (37°C)

γ-Glutamyltransferase

γ-Glutamyltransferase (GGT) is an enzyme involved in the transfer of the γ-glutamyl residue from γ-glutamyl peptides to amino acids, H_2O, and other small peptides. In most biologic systems, glutathione serves as the γ-glutamyl donor. Equation 13-19 outlines the reaction sequence:

$$\text{Glutathione + amino acid} \overset{\text{AST}}{\rightleftharpoons} \text{Glutamyl peptide + L-cysteinylglycine} \quad \text{(Eq. 13-19)}$$

The specific physiologic function of GGT has not been clearly established, but it is suggested that GGT is involved in peptide and protein synthesis, regulation of tissue glutathione levels, and the transport of amino acids across cell membranes.[33]

Tissue Source

GGT activity is found primarily in tissue of the kidney, brain, prostate, pancreas, and liver. Clinical applications of assay, however, are confined mainly to evaluation of liver and biliary system disorders.

Diagnostic Significance

In the liver, GGT is located in the canaliculi of the hepatic cells and particularly in the epithelial cells lining the biliary ductules. Because of these locations, GGT is elevated in virtually all hepatobiliary disorders, making it one of the most sensitive of enzyme assays in these conditions (see Chapter 24). Higher elevations are generally observed in biliary tract obstruction.

Within the hepatic parenchyma, GGT exists to a large extent in the smooth endoplasmic reticulum and is, therefore, subject to hepatic microsomal induction. Therefore, GGT levels will be increased in patients receiving enzyme-inducing drugs such as warfarin, phenobarbital, and phenytoin. Enzyme elevations may reach levels four times ULN.

Because of the effects of alcohol on GGT activity, elevated GGT levels may indicate alcoholism, particularly chronic alcoholism. Generally, enzyme elevations in persons who are alcoholics or heavy drinkers range from two to three times ULN, although higher levels have been observed. GGT assays are useful in monitoring the effects of abstention from alcohol and are used as such by alcohol treatment centers. Levels usually return to normal within 2 to 3 weeks after cessation but can rise again if alcohol consumption is resumed. Because of the susceptibility to enzyme induction, any interpretation of GGT levels must be done with consideration of the consequent effects of drugs and alcohol.

GGT levels are also elevated in other conditions, such as acute pancreatitis, diabetes mellitus, and myocardial infarction. The source of elevation in pancreatitis and diabetes is probably the pancreas, but the source of GGT in MI is unknown. GGT assays are of limited value in the diagnosis of these conditions and are not routinely requested.

GGT activity is useful in differentiating the source of an elevated ALP level because GGT levels are normal in skeletal disorders and during pregnancy. It is particularly useful in evaluating hepatobiliary involvement in adolescents because ALP activity will invariably be elevated as a result of bone growth.

Assay for Enzyme Activity

The most widely accepted substrate for use in GGT analysis is γ-glutamyl-p-nitroanilide. The γ-glutamyl residue is transferred to glycylglycine, releasing p-nitroaniline, a chromogenic product with a strong absorbance at 405 to 420 nm. The reaction, which can be used as a continuous monitoring or fixed-point method, is outlined in Equation 13-20:

(Eq. 13-20)

Source of Error

GGT activity is stable, with no loss of activity for 1 week at 4°C. Hemolysis does not interfere with GGT levels because the enzyme is lacking in erythrocytes.

Reference Range

GGT: male, 6–55 U/L (37°C); female, 5–38 U/L (37°C)

Values are lower in females, presumably because of suppression of enzyme activity resulting from estrogenic or progestational hormones.

Amylase

Amylase (AMY) is an enzyme belonging to the class of hydrolases that catalyze the breakdown of starch and glycogen. Starch consists of both amylose and amylopectin. Amylose is a long, unbranched chain of glucose molecules, linked by α-1,4-glycosidic bonds; amylopectin is a branched chain polysaccharide with α, 1–6 linkages at the branch points. The structure of glycogen is similar to that of amylopectin but is more highly branched. α-AMY attacks only the α-1,4-glycosidic bonds to produce degradation products consisting of glucose, maltose, and intermediate chains, called *dextrins*, which contain α, 1–6 branching linkages. Cellulose and other structural polysaccharides consisting of linkages are not attacked by α-AMY. AMY is therefore an important enzyme in the physiologic digestion of starches. The reaction proceeds according to Equation 13-21:

(Eq. 13-21)

AMY requires calcium and chloride ions for its activation.

Tissue Source

The acinar cells of the pancreas and the salivary glands are the major tissue sources of serum AMY. Lesser concentrations are found in skeletal muscle and the small intestine and fallopian tubes. AMY is the smallest enzyme, with a molecular weight of 50,000 to 55,000. Because of its small size, it is readily filtered by the renal glomerulus and also appears in the urine.

Digestion of starches begins in the mouth with the hydrolytic action of salivary AMY. Salivary AMY activity, however, is of short duration because, on swallowing, it is inactivated by the acidity of the gastric contents. Pancreatic AMY then performs the major digestive action of starches once the polysaccharides reach the intestine.

Diagnostic Significance

The diagnostic significance of serum and urine AMY measurements is in the diagnosis of acute pancreatitis.[34] Disorders of tissue other than the pancreas can also produce elevations in AMY levels. Therefore, an elevated AMY level is a nonspecific finding. However, the degree of elevation of

AMY is helpful, to some extent, in the differential diagnosis of acute pancreatitis. In addition, other laboratory tests (e.g., measurements of urinary AMY levels, AMY clearance studies, AMY isoenzyme studies, and measurements of serum lipase [LPS] levels), when used in conjunction with serum AMY measurement, increase the specificity of AMY measurements in the diagnosis of acute pancreatitis.

In acute pancreatitis, serum AMY levels begin to rise 5 to 8 hours after the onset of an attack, peak at 24 hours, and return to normal levels within 3 to 5 days. Values generally range from 250 to 1,000 Somogyi units per dL (2.55 × ULN). Values can reach much higher levels.

Other disorders causing an elevated serum AMY level include salivary gland lesions, such as mumps and parotitis, and other intra-abdominal diseases, such as perforated peptic ulcer, intestinal obstruction, cholecystitis, ruptured ectopic pregnancy, mesenteric infarction, and acute appendicitis. In addition, elevations have been reported in renal insufficiency and diabetic ketoacidosis. Serum AMY levels in intra-abdominal conditions other than acute pancreatitis are usually less than 500 Somogyi units per dL.

An apparently asymptomatic condition of hyperamylasemia has been noted in approximately 1% to 2% of the population. Hyperamylasemia can occur in neoplastic diseases with elevated results as high as 50 times ULN. *Macroamylasemia* is a condition that results when the AMY molecule combines with immunoglobulins to form a complex that is too large to be filtered across the glomerulus. Serum AMY levels increase because of the reduction in normal renal clearance of the enzyme and, consequently, the urinary excretion of AMY is abnormally low. The diagnostic significance of macroamylasemia lies in the need to differentiate it from other causes of hyperamylasemia.

Much interest has been focused recently on the possible diagnostic use of AMY isoenzyme measurements.[34,35] Serum AMY is a mixture of a number of isoenzymes that can be separated on the basis of differences in physical properties, most notably electrophoresis, although chromatography and isoelectric focusing also have been applied. In normal human serum, two major bands and as many as four minor bands may be seen. The bands are designated as P-type and S-type isoamylase. P isoamylase is derived from pancreatic tissue; S isoamylase is derived from salivary gland tissue, as well as the fallopian tube and lung. The isoenzymes of salivary origin (S1, S2, S3) migrate most quickly, whereas those of pancreatic origin (P1, P2, P3) are slower. In normal human serum, the isoamylases migrate in regions corresponding to the β- to α-globulin regions of protein electrophoresis. The most commonly observed fractions are P2, S1, and S2.

In acute pancreatitis, there is typically an increase in P-type activity, with P3 being the most predominant isoenzyme. However, P3 also has been detected in cases of renal failure and, therefore, is not entirely specific for acute pancreatitis. S-type isoamylase represents approximately two-thirds of AMY activity of normal serum, whereas P-type predominates in normal urine.

TABLE 13.6	Amylase Methodologies
Amyloclastic	Measures the disappearance of starch substrate
Saccharogenic	Measures the appearance of the product
Chromogenic	Measures the increasing color from production of product coupled with a chromogenic dye
Continuous monitoring	Coupling of several enzyme systems to monitor amylase activity

Assay for Enzyme Activity

AMY can be assayed by a variety of different methods, which are summarized in Table 13.6. The four main approaches are categorized as amyloclast, saccharogenic, chromogenic, and continuous monitoring. Continuous monitoring has replaced previous methods for AMY activity.

In the amyloclastic method, AMY is allowed to act on a starch substrate to which iodine has been attached. As AMY hydrolyzes the starch molecule into smaller units, the iodine is released and a decrease occurs in the initial dark-blue color intensity of the starch–iodine complex. The decrease in color is proportional to the AMY concentration.

The saccharogenic method uses a starch substrate that is hydrolyzed by the action of AMY to its constituent carbohydrate molecules that have reducing properties. The amount of reducing sugars is then measured where the concentration is proportional to AMY activity. The saccharogenic method, the classic reference method for determining AMY activity, is reported in Somogyi units. Somogyi units are an expression of the number of milligrams of glucose released in 30 minutes at 37°C under specific assay conditions.

Chromogenic methods use a starch substrate to which a chromogenic dye has been attached, forming an insoluble dye–substrate complex. As AMY hydrolyzes the starch substrate, smaller dye–substrate fragments are produced, and these are water soluble. The increase in color intensity of the soluble dye–substrate solution is proportional to AMY activity.

Recently, coupled enzyme systems have been used to determine AMY activity by a continuous monitoring technique in which the change in absorbance of NAD^+ at 340 nm is measured. Equation 13-22 is an example of a continuous monitoring method. For AMY activity, the optimal pH is 6.9.

$$\text{Maltopentose} \xrightleftharpoons{\text{AMS}} \text{Maltrotriose} + \text{maltose}$$

$$\text{Maltrotriose} + \text{maltose} \xrightleftharpoons{\alpha\text{-glucosidase}} \text{5-Glucose}$$

$$\text{5-Glucose} + \text{5 ATP} \xrightleftharpoons{\text{Hexokinase}}$$

$$\text{5-Glucose-6-phosphate} + \text{5 ADP}$$

$$\text{5-Glucose-6-phosphate} + \text{5 NAD} + \xrightleftharpoons{\text{G-6-PD}}$$

$$\text{5,6-Phosphogluconolactone} + \text{5 NADH}$$

(Eq. 13-22)

Because salivary AMY is preferentially inhibited by wheat germ lectin, salivary and pancreatic AMY can be estimated by measuring total AMY in the presence and absence of lectin. Specific immunoassays are also available for measuring isoenzymes of AMY.

Source of Error

AMY in serum and urine is stable. Little loss of activity occurs at room temperature for 1 week or at 4°C for 2 months. Because plasma triglycerides suppress or inhibit serum AMY activity, AMY values may be normal in acute pancreatitis with hyperlipemia.

The administration of morphine and other opiates for pain relief before blood sampling will lead to falsely elevated serum AMY levels. The drugs presumably cause constriction of the sphincter of Oddi and of the pancreatic ducts, with consequent elevation of inarticulate pressure causing regurgitation of AMY into the serum.

Reference Range

AMY: serum, 28–100 (37°C) U/L; urine, 1–15 U/h

Because of the various AMY procedures currently in use, activity is expressed according to each procedure. There is no uniform expression of AMY activity, although Somogyi units are frequently used. The approximate conversion factor between Somogyi units and international units is 1.85.

Lipase

Lipase (LPS) is an enzyme that hydrolyzes the ester linkages of fats to produce alcohols and fatty acids. Specifically, LPS catalyzes the partial hydrolysis of dietary triglycerides in the intestine to the 2-monoglyceride intermediate, with the production of long-chain fatty acids. The reaction proceeds according to Equation 13-23:

(Eq. 13-23)

The enzymatic activity of pancreatic LPS is specific for the fatty acid residues at positions 1 and 3 of the triglyceride molecule, but substrate must be an emulsion for activity to occur. The reaction rate is accelerated by the presence of colipase and a bile salt.

Tissue Source

LPS concentration is found primarily in the pancreas, although it is also present in the stomach and small intestine.

Diagnostic Significance

Clinical assays of serum LPS measurements are confined almost exclusively to the diagnosis of acute pancreatitis.

Serum LPS activity increases 4 to 8 hours after an attack of acute pancreatitis, concentrations peak at 24 hours, and decrease within 8 to 14 days. LPS is similar in this respect to AMY measurements but is considered more specific for pancreatic disorders than AMY measurement. Both AMY and LPS levels rise quickly, but LPS elevations persist for approximately 8 days in acute pancreatitis, whereas AMY elevations persist for only 2 to 3 days. The extent of elevations does not correlate with severity of disease. Elevated LPS levels also may be found in other intra-abdominal conditions but with less frequency than elevations of serum AMY. Elevations have been reported in cases of penetrating duodenal ulcers and perforated peptic ulcers, intestinal obstruction, and acute cholecystitis. In contrast to AMY levels, LPS levels are normal in conditions of salivary gland involvement. Therefore, LPS levels are useful in differentiating serum AMY elevation as a result of pancreatic versus salivary involvement. Of the three lipase isoenzymes, L2 is thought to be the most clinically specific and sensitive.

Assay for Enzyme Activity

Procedures used to measure LPS activity include estimation of liberated fatty acids (titrimetric) and turbidimetric methods. The reaction is outlined in Equation 13-24:

$$\text{Triglyceride} + 2\,H_2O \underset{(pH = 8.6-9.0)}{\overset{LPS}{\rightleftharpoons}}$$
$$\text{2-Monoglyceride} + \text{2 fatty acids}$$

(Eq. 13-24)

Early methods for LPS were historically poor. The classic Cherry-Crandall method used an olive oil substrate and measured the liberated fatty acids by titration after a 24-hour incubation. Modifications of the Cherry-Crandall method have been complicated by the lack of stable and uniform substrates. However, triolein is one substrate now used as a more pure form of triglyceride.

Turbidimetric methods are simpler and more rapid than titrimetric assays. Fats in solution create a cloudy emulsion. As the fats are hydrolyzed by LPS, the particles disperse, and the rate of clearing can be measured as an estimation of LPS activity. Colorimetric methods are also available and are based on coupled reactions with enzymes such as peroxidase or glycerol kinase.

Source of Error

LPS is stable in serum, with negligible loss in activity at room temperature for 1 week or for 3 weeks at 4°C. Hemolysis should be avoided because hemoglobin inhibits the activity of serum LPS, causing falsely low values.

Reference Range

LPS, < 38 U/L (37°C)

Glucose-6-Phosphate Dehydrogenase

Glucose-6-phosphate dehydrogenase (G-6-PD) is an **oxidoreductase** that catalyzes the oxidation of glucose-6-phosphate to 6-phosphogluconate or the corresponding lactone. The reaction is important as the first step in the pentose-phosphate shunt of glucose metabolism with the ultimate production of NADPH. The reaction is outlined in Equation 13-25:

$$\text{Glucose-6-phosphate} + \text{NADP} + \xrightarrow{\text{G-6-PD}}$$

$$\text{6-Phosphogluconate}$$

(Eq. 13-25)

Tissue Source
Sources of G-6-PD include the adrenal cortex, spleen, thymus, lymph nodes, lactating mammary gland, and erythrocytes. Little activity is found in normal serum.

Diagnostic Significance
Most of the interest of G-6-PD focuses on its role in the erythrocyte. Here, it functions to maintain NADPH in reduced form. An adequate concentration of NADPH is required to regenerate sulfhydryl-containing proteins, such as glutathione, from the oxidized to the reduced state. Glutathione in the reduced form, in turn, protects hemoglobin from oxidation by agents that may be present in the cell. A deficiency of G-6-PD results in an inadequate supply of NADPH and, ultimately, in the inability to maintain reduced glutathione levels. When erythrocytes are exposed to oxidizing agents, hemolysis occurs because of oxidation of hemoglobin and damage of the cell membrane.

G-6-PD deficiency is an inherited sex-linked trait. The disorder can result in several different clinical manifestations, one of which is drug-induced hemolytic anemia. When exposed to an oxidant drug such as primaquine, an antimalarial drug, affected individuals experience a hemolytic episode. The severity of the hemolysis is related to the drug concentration. G-6-PD deficiency is most common in African Americans but has been reported in virtually every ethnic group.

Increased levels of G-6-PD in the serum have been reported in myocardial infarction and megaloblastic anemias. No elevations are seen in hepatic disorders. G-6-PD levels, however, are not routinely performed as diagnostic aids in these conditions.

CASE STUDY 13.3

A 32-year-old Hispanic female presents to the emergency department with abdominal pain, weakness, and loss of appetite. She had not traveled in recent months. She has not been well for several days.

Questions
1. What laboratory tests should be ordered to help diagnose this patient?
2. What enzyme tests will be useful in diagnosing this patient?
3. What two diagnoses are most likely for this patient?

Assay for Enzyme Activity
The assay procedure for G-6-PD activity is outlined in Equation 13-26:

$$\text{Glucose-6-phosphate} + \text{NADPH}^+ \xrightarrow{\text{G-6-PD}} \text{6-Phosphogluconate} + \text{NADPH} + \text{H}^+$$

(Eq. 13-26)

A red cell hemolysate is used to assay for deficiency of the enzyme; serum is used for evaluation of enzyme elevations.

Reference Range
G-6-PD, 7.9–16.3 U/g Hgb

Macroenzymes
Macroenzymes are high-molecular-mass forms of the serum enzymes (ACP, ALP, ALT, amylase, AST, CK, GGT, LDH, lipase) that can be bound to either an immunoglobulin (macroenzyme type 1) or a nonimmunoglobulin substance (macroenzyme type 2). Macroenzymes are usually found in patients who have an unexplained persistent increase of enzyme concentrations in serum.[36] The presence of macroenzymes can also increase with increasing age.[37] Enzymes can bind to immunoglobulins in a nonspecific manner, but there is also evidence that the enzyme–immunoglobulin complex can be formed by specific interactions between circulating autoantibodies and serum enzymes.[36] The reason for the formation of antienzyme antibodies is not known, but there are two theories to explain their formation. According to the "antigen-driven theory," the self-antigen becomes immunogenic by being altered or released from a sequestered site and reacts with an antibody that is initially formed against a foreign antigen.[38] The dysregulation of immune tolerance theory explains the formation of enzymes with autoantibodies in patients with autoimmune disorders.[38] To date, there has not been a strong correlation between the presence of

antienzyme antibodies and the pathogenesis of disease.[36] However, the presence of macroenzymes should be documented in the patient's medical records because macroenzymes can persist for long periods.[36]

Macroenzymes accumulate in the plasma because their high molecular masses prevent them from being filtered out of the plasma by the kidneys. The detection of macroenzymes is clinically significant because the presence of macroenzymes can cause difficulty in the interpretation of diagnostic enzyme results. The formation of high molecular weight enzyme complexes can cause false elevations in plasma enzymes, or they can falsely decrease the activity of the enzyme by blocking the activity of the bound enzyme.[36]

The principal method to identify enzymes that are bound to immunoglobulins and nonimmunoglobulins is protein electrophoresis. The binding of enzymes to high molecular weight complexes can alter the normal electrophoretic pattern of enzymes (see Fig. 13.5 for an example). Antienzyme antibodies can cause the formation of new enzyme bands on a gel, they can alter the intensity of enzyme bands, and they can cause band broadening on the gel.[36] Other test methods used to determine the presence of macroenzymes include gel filtration, immunoprecipitation, immunoelectrophoresis, counterimmunoelectrophoresis, and immunofixation. Last, the immunoinhibition test can also be used to determine the presence of macro-CK.

Drug-Metabolizing Enzymes

Drug-metabolizing enzymes function primarily to transform xenobiotics into inactive, water-soluble compounds for excretion through the kidneys. Metabolic enzymes can also transform inactive prodrugs into active drugs, convert xenobiotics into toxic compounds, or prolong the elimination half-life. Drug-metabolizing enzymes catalyze addition or removal of functional groups through hydroxylation, oxidation, dealkylation, dehydrogenation, reduction, deamination, and desulfuration reactions. These transformation reactions are referred to as phase I reactions and are often mediated by cytochrome P-450 (CYP 450) enzymes. Xenobiotics can also become transformed into more polar compounds through enzyme-mediated conjugation reactions, also known as phase II reactions, in which xenobiotics are conjugated with glucuronide (UDP-glucuronosyltransferase 1A1 [UGT1A1]), acetate (N-acetyltransferase [NAT]), glutathione (glutathione-S-transferase [GST]), sulfate (sulfotransferase), and methionine groups.[39]

CYP 450 enzymes are a superfamily of isoenzymes that are involved in the metabolism of more than 50% of all drugs. These enzymes contain heme molecules, and they are given the name CYP 450 because they absorb the maximum amount of light at 450 nm. More than 500 CYP 450 enzymes that have been identified, and they are classified into families according to their homology to other enzymes.[40] There are at least four CYP 450 (CYP 1, 2, 3, and 4) families that are expressed primarily in the liver, but some isoforms are also expressed in extrahepatic tissues such as the lung, kidney,

gastrointestinal tract, skin, and placenta.[39] The specific isozyme is classified by not only its family number but also by a subfamily letter, a number for an individual isozyme within the subfamily, and, if applicable, an asterisk followed by a number for each genetic (allelic) variant. Genetic variants have been identified that lead to complete enzyme deficiency (e.g., a frame shift, splice variant, stop codon, or a complete gene deletion), reduced enzyme function or expression, or enhanced enzyme function or expression. Recognition of genetic variants can explain interindividual differences in drug response and pharmacokinetics.[40–43] For example, four phenotypes are recognized for CYP 2D6: ultrametabolizers, extensive metabolizers, intermediate metabolizers, and poor metabolizers. Patients who are poor metabolizers for the CYP 2D6 enzyme are at risk for therapeutic failure when inactive prodrugs such as tamoxifen require CYP 2D6 for drug activation. Tricyclic antidepressants such as nortriptyline require CYP 2D6 for inactivation. Thus, CYP 2D6 poor metabolizers may require lower-dose requirements than will patients with extensive ("normal") metabolism and may be at high risk for adverse drug reactions.[39,42]

In addition to xenobiotic metabolism, CYP 450 enzymes are also involved in the biosynthesis of endogenous compounds. The CYP 5 family consists of thromboxane synthases that catalyze the reaction that leads to platelet aggregation. CYP 7 and CYP 27 families catalyze the hydroxylation of cholesterol for the biosynthesis of bile acids. The CYP 24 family catalyzes the hydroxylation and inactivation vitamin D_3. CYP 450 enzymes are also found in steroid-producing tissues and function to synthesize steroid hormones from cholesterol (CYP 11, 17, 19, and 21).[40]

Genetic variants that affect drug-metabolizing enzyme function and expression are recognized for other enzymes such as NAT, UGT1A1, GST, and TPMT. These variants are associated with distinct extensive (fast), intermediate, or poor (slow) metabolizer phenotypes, which could lead to adverse drug reactions or therapeutic failure. For example, two phenotypes—fast and slow acetylators—are recognized for N-acetyltransferase 2 (NAT2). NAT2 is the primary enzyme involved in the acetylation of isoniazid, a drug used to treat tuberculosis. Acetylation is the primary mechanism for the elimination of isoniazid, and therefore, patients with low NAT2 activity will not be able to inactivate isoniazid, putting those patients at increased risk for adverse drug reactions.[39] UGT1A1 has polymorphisms that can lead to a nonfunctioning enzyme. UGT1A1 is responsible for the metabolism of bilirubin; patients with nonfunctioning UGT1A1 are at risk for hyperbilirubinema.[43] Last, thiopurine methyltransferase (TPMT) is an enzyme that can be found in bone marrow and erythrocytes and functions to inactivate chemotherapeutic thiopurine drugs like azathioprine and 6-mercaptopurine. The TPMT enzyme has genetic polymorphisms, which causes variable responses (normal, intermediate, and low activity) to thiopurine metabolism. Patients with low TPMT activity are at risk of developing severe bone marrow toxicity when the standard dose therapy for thiopurine drugs is administered;

thus, genetic testing is essential for identifying patients with metabolizing enzyme polymorphisms.[43]

Pharmacogenetic testing is often used prior to drug therapy to assist clinicians in identifying patients with genetic polymorphisms, to guide drug and dose selection. Pharmacogenetic testing can be performed through phenotype tests that measure metabolic enzyme activity, through administration of a probe drug and subsequent evaluation of metabolic ratios, or through genotype testing that identifies clinically significant genetic variants.

The activity of drug-metabolizing enzymes can also be altered by food, nutritional supplements, or other drugs.

Compounds that stimulate an increase in the synthesis CYP 450 enzymes are called *inducers*. Inducers will increase the metabolism of drugs and reduce the bioavailability of the parent compound. Compounds that reduce the expression or activity of a drug-metabolizing enzyme are referred to as *inhibitors*. For example, inhibitors can compete with substrates for the active site of the CYP 450 and thereby decrease the metabolism of drugs and increase the bioavailability of the parent compound, or block activity or expression through noncompetitive means.[39] Table 13.7 lists the common families of CYP 450 enzymes along with some of their substrates and drugs that can induce or inhibit enzyme activity.

TABLE 13.7   Common Substrates for Drug-Metabolizing Enzymes

Enzyme	Substrates	Inducers	Inhibitors
CYP 1A1	(R)-Warfarin	Omeprazole TCDD Benzo[a]pyrene, 3MC	
CYP 1A2	Acetaminophen Caffeine (R)-Warfarin Estradiol Theophylline	Insulin Tobacco Polycyclic aromatic hydrocarbons	Ciprofloxacin Cimetidine Amiodarone Fluoroquinolones
CYP 2A6	Cyclophosphamide Halothane Zidovudine Coumarin	Dexamethasone	Pilocarpine Coumarin
CYP 2B6	Cyclophosphamide Diazepam Bupropion	Phenobarbital Rifampin	Ticlopidine
CYP 2C9	(S)-Warfarin Ibuprofen Tolbutamide Diclofenac Losartan Phenytoin	Rifampin Secobarbital	Fluconazole Amiodarone Isoniazid Probenecid Sertraline Sulfamethoxazole
CYP 2C19	Diazepam Omeprazole Clomipramine Indomethacin	Barbiturate Phenytoin	Omeprazole Chloramphenicol Cimetidine Ketoconazole Indomethacin
CYP 2D6	Carvedilol Amitriptyline Haloperidol Amphetamine Chlorpromazine Dextromethorphan Codeine	Dexamethasone Rifampin	Bupropion Fluoxetine Quinidine Amiodarone Sertraline Celecoxib Chlorpromazine
CYP 2E1	Acetaminophen Chlorzoxazone Halothane Ethanol	Ethanol Isoniazid	Disulfiram Diethyldithiocarbamate
CYP 3A4	Erythromycin Quinidine Diazepam	HIV antivirals Barbiturates Carbamazepine	HIV antivirals Ketoconazole Erythromycin

TABLE 13.7	Common Substrates for Drug-Metabolizing Enzymes (continued)		
Enzyme	**Substrates**	**Inducers**	**Inhibitors**
	Cortisol	Phenobarbital	Grapefruit juice
	Cyclosporine	Phenytoin	Cimetidine
	Indinavir	Rifampin	Chloramphenicol
	Chlorpheniramine	St. John's wort	
	Nifedipine	Troglitazone	
	Lovastatin		
	Testosterone		
	Cocaine		
	Fentanyl		
	Tamoxifen		
TPMT	Azathioprine		Naproxen
	6-Mercaptopurine		Furosemide

Source: Rendic S, Di Carlo FJ. Human cytochrome P450 enzymes: a status report summarizing their reactions, substrates, inducers, and inhibitors. *Drug Metab Rev.* 1997;29:413–580.

For additional student resources, please visit thePoint® at http://thepoint.lww.com

Questions

1. When a reaction is performed in zero-order kinetics
   a. The rate of the reaction is independent of the substrate concentration
   b. The substrate concentration is very low
   c. The rate of reaction is directly proportional to the substrate concentration
   d. The enzyme level is always high

2. Activation energy is
   a. Decreased by enzymes
   b. The energy needed for an enzyme reaction to stop
   c. Increased by enzymes
   d. Very high in catalyzed reactions

3. Enzyme reaction rates are increased by increasing temperatures until they reach the point of denaturation at
   a. 40–60°C
   b. 25–35°C
   c. 100°C
   d. 37°C

4. An example of using enzymes as reagents in the clinical laboratory is
   a. The hexokinase glucose method
   b. The diacetyl monoxime blood urea nitrogen (BUN) method
   c. The alkaline picrate creatinine method
   d. The biuret total protein method

5. Activity of enzymes in serum may be determined rather than concentration because
   a. The amount of enzyme is too low to measure
   b. The temperature is too high
   c. There is not enough substrate
   d. The amount of enzyme is too high to measure

6. The isoenzymes LD-4 and LD-5 are elevated in
   a. Liver disease
   b. Pulmonary embolism
   c. Renal disease
   d. Myocardial infarction

7. Which CK isoenzyme is elevated in muscle diseases?
   a. CK-MM
   b. CK-BB
   c. CK-MB
   d. CK-NN

8. Elevation of serum amylase and lipase is commonly seen in
   a. Acute pancreatitis
   b. Acute appendicitis
   c. Gallbladder disease
   d. Acid reflux disease

9. The saccharogenic method for amylase determinations measures
   a. The amount of product produced
   b. The amount of substrate consumed
   c. The amount of iodine present
   d. The amount of starch present

(continues on page 286)

review questions (continued)

10. Elevation of tissue enzymes in serum may be used to detect
  a. Tissue necrosis or damage
  b. Inflammation
  c. Infectious diseases
  d. Diabetes mellitus

11. Which of the following enzyme patterns is MOST diagnostic of Duchenne-type muscular dystrophy?
  a. Total CK level that is 5 to 10 times the ULN
  b. Total CK level that is 25 times the ULN
  c. Total CK level that is 50 to 100 times the ULN
  d. Total CK level that is 1,000 times the ULN

12. Which of the following preanalytical errors most commonly causes false increases in serum enzyme measurements?
  a. The patient was not fasting prior to blood draw.
  b. The blood sample was not maintained on ice upon collection and during transport to the laboratory.
  c. The serum was not separated from red blood cells within 1 hour.
  d. The patient smoked three cigarettes just prior to blood collection.
  e. The blood sample was not protected from light upon collection and during transport to the laboratory.

references

1. Enzyme Nomenclature 1978. *Recommendations of the Nomenclature Committee of the International Union of Biochemistry on the Nomenclature and Classification of Enzymes.* New York, NY: Academic Press; 1979.
2. Baron DN, Moss DW, Walker PG, et al. Abbreviations for names of enzymes of diagnostic importance. *J Clin Pathol.* 1971;24:656.
3. Baron DN, Moss DW, Walker PG, et al. Revised list of abbreviations for names of enzymes of diagnostic importance. *J Clin Pathol.* 1975;28:592.
4. Rej R. Accurate enzyme measurements. *Arch Pathol Lab Med.* 1998;117:352.
5. Spitzer M, Pinto A. Early diagnosis of ectopic pregnancy: can we do it accurately using a chemical profile? *J Womens Health Gend Based Med.* 2000;9:537.
6. Na Kafusa J, et al. The importance of serum creatine phosphokinase levels in the early diagnosis, and as a prognostic factor, of *Vibrio vulnificus* infection. *Br Med J.* 2001;145:2.
7. Galen RS. The enzyme diagnosis of myocardial infarction. *Hum Pathol.* 1975;6:141.
8. Wilkinson JH. *The Principles and Practice of Diagnostic Enzymology.* Chicago, IL: Year Book Medical Publishers; 1976:395.
9. Silverman LM, Dermer GB, Zweig MH, et al. Creatine kinase BB: a new tumor-associated marker. *Clin Chem.* 1979;25:1432.
10. Lang H, ed. *Creatine Kinase Isoenzymes: Pathophysiology and Clinical Application.* Berlin, Germany: Springer-Verlag; 1981.
11. Irvin RG, Cobb FR, Roe CR. Acute myocardial infarction and MB creatine phosphokinase: relationship between onset of symptoms of infarction and appearance and disappearance of enzyme. *Arch Intern Med.* 1980;140:329.
12. Bark CJ. Mitochondrial creatine kinase—a poor prognostic sign. *JAMA.* 1980;243:2058.
13. Batsakis J, Savory J, eds. Creatine kinase. *Crit Rev Clin Lab Sci.* 1982;16:291.
14. Lang H, Wurzburg U. Creatine kinase, an enzyme of many forms. *Clin Chem.* 1982;28:1439.
15. Lott JA. Electrophoretic CK and LDH isoenzyme assays in myocardial infarction. *Lab Mgmt.* 1983.
16. Pesce MA. The CK isoenzymes: findings and their meaning. *Lab Mgmt.* 1982.
17. Roche Diagnostics. *Isomune-CK Package Insert.* Nutley, NJ: Hoffman-La Roche; 1979.
18. Faulkner WR, Meites S, eds. *Selected Methods for the Small Clinical Chemistry Laboratory: Selected Methods of Clinical Chemistry.* Vol. 9. Washington, DC: American Association for Clinical Chemistry; 1982:475.
19. Lott JA, Stang JM. Serum enzymes and isoenzymes in the diagnosis and differential diagnosis of myocardial ischemia and necrosis. *Clin Chem.* 1980;26:1241.
20. Leung FY, Henderson AR. Influence of hemolysis on the serum lactate dehydrogenase-1/lactate dehydrogenase-2 ratio as determined by an accurate thin-layer agarose electrophoresis procedure. *Clin Chem.* 1981;27:1708.
21. Bhagavan NV, Darm JR, Scottolini AG. A sixth lactate dehydrogenase isoenzyme (LDH-6) and its significance. *Arch Pathol Lab Med.* 1982;106:521.
22. Cabello B, Lubin J, Rywlin AM, et al. Significance of a sixth lactate dehydrogenase isoenzyme (LDH$_6$). *Am J Clin Pathol.* 1980;73:253.
23. Goldberg DM, Werner M, eds. *LDH-6, A Sign of Impending Death From Heart Failure, Selected Topics in Clinical Enzymology.* New York, NY: Walter de Gruyter; 1983:347.
24. Posen S, Doherty E. The measurement of serum alkaline phosphatase in clinical medicine. *Adv Clin Chem.* 1981;22:165.
25. Warren BM. *The Isoenzymes of Alkaline Phosphatase.* Beaumont, TX: Helena Laboratories; 1981.
26. Fleisher GA, Eickelberg ES, Elveback LR. Alkaline phosphatase activity in the plasma of children and adolescents. *Clin Chem.* 1977;23:469.
27. Gittes RF. Carcinoma of the prostate. *N Engl J Med.* 1991;324:236.
28. Gittes RF. Prostate specific antigen. *N Engl J Med.* 1987;318:954.
29. Oesterling JE. Prostate specific antigen: a critical assessment of the most useful tumor marker for adenocarcinoma of the prostate. *J Urol.* 1991;145:907.

30. Griffiths JC. The laboratory diagnosis of prostatic adenocarcinoma. *Crit Rev Clin Lab Sci.* 1983;19:187.

31. Lantz RK, Berg MJ. From clinic to court: acid phosphatase testing. *Diagn Med.* 1981;Mar/Apr:55.

32. Yam LT. Clinical significance of the human acid phosphatases. A review. *Am J Med.* 1974;56:604.

33. Rosalki SB. Gamma-glutamyl transpeptidase. *Adv Clin Chem.* 1975;17:53.

34. Salt WB II, Schenker S. Amylase: its clinical significance. A review of the literature. *Medicine.* 1976;4:269.

35. Murthy U, et al. Hyperamylasemia in patients with acquired immunodeficiency syndrome. *Am J Gastroenterol.* 1992;87:332.

36. Remaley AT, Wilding P. Macroenzymes: biochemical characterization, clinical significance, and laboratory detection. *Clin Chem.* 1989;35:2261–2270.

37. Turecky L. Macroenzymes and their clinical significance. *Bratisl Lek Listy.* 2004;105:260–263.

38. Theofilopoulous AN. Autoimmunity. In: Stites DP, Stobo JD, Wells JV, eds. *Basic and Clinical Immunology.* 6th ed. Norwalk, CT: Appleton & Lange; 1987:128–158.

39. Hardman JG, Limbird LE, eds. *Goodman and Gilman's The Pharmacological Basis of Therapeutics.* 9th ed. New York, NY: McGraw-Hill; 1996:11–16.

40. Rendic S, Di Carlo FJ. Human cytochrome P450 enzymes: a status report summarizing their reactions, substrates, inducers, and inhibitors. *Drug Metab Rev.* 1997;29:413–580.

41. Wilkinson GR. Drug metabolism and variability among patients in drug response. *N Engl J Med.* 2005;352:2211–2221.

42. Nebert DW, Dieter MZ. The evolution of drug metabolism. *Pharmacology.* 2000;61:124–135.

43. McMillin GA. *Pharmacogenetics Fundamental of Molecular Diagnostics.* St Louis, MO: WB Saunders; 2007:197–215.

14

Carbohydrates

VICKI S. FREEMAN

chapter outline

key terms

Albuminuria
Carbohydrates
Diabetes mellitus
Disaccharides
Embden-Meyerhof pathway
Fisher projection
Glucagon
Gluconeogenesis
Glycogen
Glycogenolysis
Glycolysis
Glycosylated hemoglobin
Haworth projection
Hyperglycemic
Hypoglycemic
Insulin
Ketone
Monosaccharides
Oligosaccharides
Polysaccharides
Trioses

chapter objectives

Upon completion of this chapter, the clinical laboratorian should be able to do the following:

- Classify carbohydrates into their respective groups.
- Discuss the metabolism of carbohydrates in the body and the mode of action of hormones in carbohydrate metabolism.
- Differentiate the types of diabetes by clinical symptoms and laboratory findings according to the American Diabetes Association.
- Explain the clinical significance of the three ketone bodies.
- Relate expected laboratory results and clinical symptoms to the following metabolic complications of diabetes:
  - Ketoacidosis
  - Hyperosmolar coma
- Distinguish between reactive and spontaneous hypoglycemia.
- Describe the principle, specimen of choice, and the advantages and disadvantages of the glucose analysis methods.

> For additional student resources, please visit thePoint® at http://thepoint.lww.com

chapter objectives (continued)

- Describe the three commonly encountered methods of glycated hemoglobin, specimen of choice, and source of error.
- Describe the use of glycosylated hemoglobin in the long-term monitoring of diabetes.
- Discuss the methods of analysis and the advantages and disadvantages of ketone bodies.

Organisms rely on the oxidation of complex organic compounds to obtain energy. Three general types of such compounds are carbohydrates, amino acids, and lipids. Although all three are used as a source of energy, carbohydrates are the primary source for brain, erythrocytes, and retinal cells in humans. **Carbohydrates** are the major food source and energy supply for the body and are stored primarily as liver and muscle glycogen. Disease states involving carbohydrates are split into two groups—hyperglycemia and hypoglycemia. Early detection of diabetes mellitus is the aim of the American Diabetes Association (ADA) guidelines. Acute and chronic complications may be avoided with proper diagnosis, monitoring, and treatment. The laboratory plays an important role through periodic measurements of glycosylated hemoglobin and microalbumin.

GENERAL DESCRIPTION OF CARBOHYDRATES

Carbohydrates are compounds containing C, H, and O. The general formula for a carbohydrate is $C_x(H_2O)_y$. All carbohydrates contain C=O and –OH functional groups. There are some derivatives from this basic formula because carbohydrate derivatives can be formed by the addition of other chemical groups, such as phosphates, sulfates, and amines. The classification of carbohydrates is based on four different properties: (1) the size of the base carbon chain, (2) the location of the CO function group, (3) the number of sugar units, and (4) the stereochemistry of the compound.

Classification of Carbohydrates

Carbohydrates can be grouped into generic classifications based on the number of carbons in the molecule. For example, **trioses** contain three carbons, tetroses contain four, pentoses contain five, and hexoses contain six. In actual practice, the smallest carbohydrate is glyceraldehyde, a three-carbon compound.

Carbohydrates are hydrates of aldehyde or ketone derivatives based on the location of the CO functional group (Fig. 14.1). The two forms of carbohydrates are aldose and ketose (Fig. 14.2). The aldose form has a terminal carbonyl group (O=CH–) called an aldehyde group, whereas the ketose form has a carbonyl group (O=C) in the middle linked to two other carbon atoms (called a ketone group).

Several models are used to represent carbohydrates. The **Fisher projection** of a carbohydrate has the aldehyde or ketone at the top of the drawing. The carbons are numbered starting at the aldehyde or ketone end. The compound can be represented as a straight chain or might be linked to show a representation of the cyclic, hemiacetal form (Fig. 14.3). The **Haworth projection** represents the compound in the cyclic form that is more representative of the actual structure. This structure is formed when the functional (carbonyl) group (ketone or aldehyde) reacts with an alcohol group on the same sugar to form a ring called either a *hemiketal* or a *hemiacetal ring*, respectively (Fig. 14.4).

Stereoisomers

The central carbons of a carbohydrate are asymmetric (chiral)—four different groups are attached to the carbon atoms. This allows for various spatial arrangements around each asymmetric carbon (also called stereogenic centers) forming molecules called *stereoisomers*. Stereoisomers have the same order and types of bonds but different spatial arrangements and different properties. For each asymmetric carbon, there are 2^n possible isomers; therefore, there are 2^1, or two, forms of glyceraldehyde. Because an aldohexose contains four asymmetric carbons, there are 2^4, or 16, possible isomers. A monosaccharide is assigned to the D or the L series according to the configuration at the highest numbered asymmetric carbon. This asymmetrically substituted carbon atom is called the "configurational atom" or chiral center. Thus, if the hydroxyl group (or the oxygen bridge of the ring form) projects to the right in the Fisher projection, the sugar belongs to the D series and receives the prefix D-, and if it projects to the left, then it belongs to the L series and receives the prefix L-. These stereoisomers, called enantiomers, are images that cannot be overlapped and are nonsuperimposable. In Figure 14.5, D-glucose is represented in the Fisher projection with the hydroxyl group on carbon number 5 positioned on the right. L-glucose has

FIGURE 14.1 Pathways in glucose metabolism.

FIGURE 14.2 Two forms of carbohydrates.

FIGURE 14.3 Fisher projection of glucose. **Left:** Open-chain Fisher projections. **Right:** Cyclic Fisher projection.

FIGURE 14.5 Stereoisomers of glucose.

the hydroxyl group of carbon number 5 positioned on the left. Most sugars in humans are in the D-form.

Monosaccharides, Disaccharides, and Polysaccharides

Another classification of carbohydrates is based on the number of sugar units in the chain: monosaccharides, disaccharides, oligosaccharides, and polysaccharides. This chaining of sugars relies on the formation of glycoside bonds that are bridges of oxygen atoms. When two carbohydrate molecules join, a water molecule is produced. When they split, one molecule of water is used to form the individual compounds. This reaction is called *hydrolysis*. The glycoside linkages of carbohydrate can involve any number of carbons; however, certain carbons are favored, depending on the carbohydrate.

Monosaccharides are simple sugars that cannot be hydrolyzed to a simpler form. These sugars can contain three, four, five, and six or more carbon atoms (known as trioses, tetroses, pentoses, and hexoses, respectively). The most common include glucose, fructose, and galactose.

Disaccharides are formed when two monosaccharide units are joined by a glycosidic linkage. On hydrolysis, disaccharides will be split into two monosaccharides by disaccharide enzymes (e.g., lactase) located on the microvilli of the intestine. These monosaccharides are then actively absorbed. The most common disaccharides are maltose (comprising two D-glucose molecules in a 1 → 4 linkage), lactose, and sucrose.

Oligosaccharides are the chaining of 2 to 10 sugar units, whereas **polysaccharides** are formed by the linkage of many monosaccharide units. On hydrolysis, polysaccharides will yield more than 10 monosaccharides. Amylase hydrolyzes starch to disaccharides in the duodenum. The most common polysaccharides are starch (glucose molecules) and glycogen (Fig. 14.6).

Chemical Properties of Carbohydrates

Some carbohydrates are reducing substances; these carbohydrates can reduce other compounds. To be a reducing substance, the carbohydrate must contain a ketone or an aldehyde group. This property was used in many laboratory methods in the past in the determination of carbohydrates.

Carbohydrates can form glycosidic bonds with other carbohydrates and with noncarbohydrates. Two sugar molecules can be joined in tandem forming a glycosidic bond between the hemiacetal group of one molecule and the hydroxyl group on the other molecule. In forming the glycosidic bond, an acetal is generated on one sugar (at carbon 1) in place of the hemiacetal. If the bond forms with one of the other carbons on the carbohydrate other than the anomeric (reducing) carbon, the anomeric carbon is unaltered and the resulting compound remains a reducing substance. Examples of reducing substances include glucose, maltose, fructose, lactose, and galactose. If the bond is formed with the anomeric carbon on the other carbohydrate, the resulting compound is *no longer* a reducing substance. Nonreducing carbohydrates *do not* have an active ketone or aldehyde group. They *will not* reduce other compounds. The most common nonreducing sugar is sucrose—table sugar (Fig. 14.7).

All monosaccharides and many disaccharides are reducing agents. This is because a free aldehyde or ketone (the open-chain form) can be oxidized under the proper conditions. As disaccharide remains a reducing agent when the hemiacetal or ketal hydroxyl group is not linked to another molecule, both maltose and lactose are reducing agents, whereas sucrose is not.

Glucose Metabolism

Glucose is a primary source of energy for humans. The nervous system, including the brain, totally depends on glucose from the surrounding extracellular fluid (ECF) for energy. Nervous tissue cannot concentrate or store carbohydrates; therefore, it is critical to maintain a steady supply of glucose to the tissue. For this reason, the concentration of glucose in the ECF must be maintained in a narrow range. When the

FIGURE 14.4 Haworth projection of glucose.

FIGURE 14.6 Linkage of monosaccharides.

FIGURE 14.7 Haworth projection of sucrose.

concentration falls below a certain level, the nervous tissue loses the primary energy source and is incapable of maintaining normal function.

Fate of Glucose

Most of our ingested carbohydrates are polymers, such as starch and **glycogen**. Salivary amylase and pancreatic amylase are responsible for the digestion of these nonabsorbable polymers to dextrins and disaccharides, which are further hydrolyzed to monosaccharides by maltase, an enzyme released by the intestinal mucosa. Sucrase and lactase are two other important gut-derived enzymes that hydrolyze sucrose to glucose and fructose and lactose to glucose and galactose.

When disaccharides are converted to monosaccharides, they are absorbed by the gut and transported to the liver by the hepatic portal venous blood supply. Glucose is the only carbohydrate to be directly used for energy or stored as glycogen. Galactose and fructose must be converted to glucose before they can be used. After glucose enters the cell, it is quickly shunted into one of three possible metabolic pathways, depending on the availability of substrates or the nutritional status of the cell. The ultimate goal of the cell is to convert glucose to carbon dioxide and water. During this process, the cell obtains the high-energy molecule adenosine triphosphate (ATP) from inorganic phosphate and adenosine diphosphate. The cell requires oxygen for the final steps in the electron transport chain (ETC). Nicotinamide adenine dinucleotide (NAD) in its reduced form (NADH) will act as an intermediate to couple glucose oxidation to the ETC in the mitochondria where much of the ATP is gained.

The first step for all three pathways requires glucose to be converted to glucose-6-phosphate using the high-energy molecule, ATP. This reaction is catalyzed by the enzyme hexokinase (Fig. 14.8). Glucose-6-phosphate can enter the

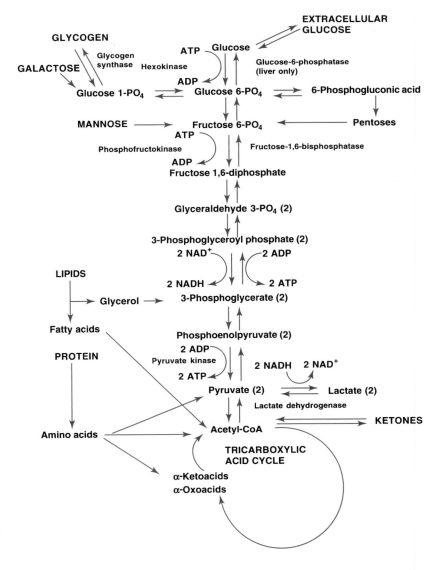

FIGURE 14.8 The Embden-Meyerhof pathway for anaerobic glycolysis.

Embden-Meyerhof pathway or the *hexose monophosphate pathway* (HMP) or can be converted to glycogen (Fig. 14.8). The first two pathways are important for the generation of energy from glucose; the conversion to glycogen pathway is important for the storage of glucose.

In the Embden-Meyerhof pathway, glucose is broken down into two- and three-carbon molecules of pyruvic acid that can enter the *tricarboxylic acid* (TCA) *cycle* on conversion to acetyl-coenzyme A (acetyl-CoA). This pathway requires oxygen and is called the *aerobic pathway* (Fig. 14.8). Other substrates have the opportunity to enter the pathway at several points. Glycerol released from the hydrolysis of triglycerides can enter at 3-phosphoglycerate, and fatty acids and ketones and some amino acids are converted or catabolized to acetyl-CoA, which is part of the TCA cycle. Other amino acids enter the pathway as pyruvate or as deaminated α-ketoacids and α-oxoacids. The conversion of amino acids by the liver and other specialized tissue, such as the kidney, to substrates that can be converted to glucose is called **gluconeogenesis**. Gluconeogenesis also encompasses the conversion of glycerol, lactate, and pyruvate to glucose.

Anaerobic **glycolysis** is important for tissue such as muscle, which often have important energy requirements without an adequate oxygen supply. These tissues can derive ATP from glucose in an oxygen-deficient environment by converting pyruvic acid into lactic acid. The lactic acid diffuses from the muscle cell, enters the systemic circulation, and is then taken up and used by the liver (Fig. 14.8). For anaerobic glycolysis to occur, 2 mol of ATP must be consumed for each mole of glucose; however, 4 mol of ATP are directly produced, resulting in a net gain of 2 mol of ATP. Further gains of ATP result from the introduction of pyruvate into the TCA cycle and NADH into the ETC.

The second energy pathway is the HMP *shunt*, which is actually a detour of glucose-6-phosphate from the glycolytic pathway to become 6-phosphogluconic acid. This oxidized product permits the formation of ribose-5-phosphate and NADP in its reduced form (NADPH). NADPH is important to erythrocytes that lack mitochondria and are therefore incapable of the TCA cycle. The reducing power of NADPH is required for the protection of the cell from oxidative and free radical damage. Without NADPH, the lipid bilayer membrane of the cell and critical enzymes would eventually be destroyed, resulting in cell death. The HMP shunt also permits pentoses, such as ribose, to enter the glycolytic pathway.

When the cell's energy requirements are being met, glucose can be stored as glycogen. This third pathway, which is called *glycogenesis*, is relatively straightforward. Glucose-6-phosphate is converted to glucose-1-phosphate, which is then converted to uridine diphosphoglucose and then to glycogen by glycogen synthase. Several tissues are capable of the synthesis of glycogen, especially the liver and muscles. Hepatocytes are capable of releasing glucose from glycogen or other sources to maintain the blood glucose concentration. This is because the liver synthesizes the

TABLE 14.1	**Pathways in Glucose Metabolism**
Glycolysis	Metabolism of glucose molecule to pyruvate or lactate for production of energy
Gluconeogenesis	Formation of glucose-6-phosphate from noncarbohydrate sources
Glycogenolysis	Breakdown of glycogen to glucose for use as energy
Glycogenesis	Conversion of glucose to glycogen for storage
Lipogenesis	Conversion of carbohydrates to fatty acids
Lipolysis	Decomposition of fat

enzyme glucose-6-phosphatase. Without this enzyme, glucose is trapped in the glycolytic pathway. Muscle cells do not synthesize glucose-6-phosphatase and, therefore, they are incapable of dephosphorylating glucose. Once glucose enters a muscle cell, it remains as glycogen unless it is catabolized. **Glycogenolysis** is the process by which glycogen is converted back to glucose-6-phosphate for entry into the glycolytic pathway. Table 14.1 outlines the major energy pathways involved either directly or indirectly with glucose metabolism.

Overall, dietary glucose and other carbohydrates either can be used by the liver and other cells for energy or can be stored as glycogen for later use. When the supply of glucose is low, the liver will use glycogen and other substrates to elevate the blood glucose concentration. These substrates include glycerol from triglycerides, lactic acid from skin and muscles, and amino acids. If the lipolysis of triglycerides is unregulated, it results in the formation of ketone bodies, which the brain can use as a source of energy through the TCA cycle. The synthesis of glucose from amino acids is gluconeogenesis. This process is used in conjunction with the formation of ketone bodies when glycogen stores are depleted—conditions normally associated with starvation. The principal pathway for glucose oxidation is through the Embden-Meyerhof pathway. NADPH can be synthesized through the HMP shunt, which is a side pathway from the anaerobic glycolytic pathway (Fig. 14.8).

Regulation of Carbohydrate Metabolism

The liver, pancreas, and other endocrine glands are all involved in controlling the blood glucose concentrations within a narrow range. During a brief fast, glucose is supplied to the ECF from the liver through glycogenolysis. When the fasting period is longer than 1 day, glucose is synthesized from other sources through gluconeogenesis. Control of blood glucose is under two major hormones: insulin and glucagon, both produced by the pancreas. Their actions oppose each other. Other hormones and neuroendocrine substances also exert some control over blood glucose concentrations, permitting the body to respond to increased demands for glucose or to survive prolonged

TABLE 14.2 **The Action of Hormones**

Action of Insulin
Increases glycogenesis and glycolysis: glucose → glycogen → pyruvate → acetyl-CoA
Increases lipogenesis
Decreases glycogenolysis

Action of Glucagon
Increases glycogenolysis: glycogen → glucose
Increases gluconeogenesis: fatty acids → acetyl-CoA → ketone, proteins → amino acids

fasts. It also permits the conservation of energy as lipids when excess substrates are ingested.

Insulin is the primary hormone responsible for the entry of glucose into the cell. It is synthesized by the β-cells of islets of Langerhans in the pancreas. When these cells detect an increase in body glucose, they release insulin. The release of insulin causes an increased movement of glucose into the cells and increased glucose metabolism. Insulin is normally released when glucose levels are high and is *not* released when glucose levels are decreased. It decreases plasma glucose levels by increasing the transport entry of glucose in muscle and adipose tissue by way of nonspecific receptors. It also regulates glucose by increasing glycogenesis, lipogenesis, and glycolysis and inhibiting glycogenolysis. Insulin is the only hormone that decreases glucose levels and can be referred to as a **hypoglycemic** agent (Table 14.2).

Glucagon is the primary hormone responsible for increasing glucose levels. It is synthesized by the α-cells of islets of Langerhans in the pancreas and released during stress and fasting states. When these cells detect a decrease in body glucose, they release glucagon. Glucagon acts by increasing plasma glucose levels by glycogenolysis in the liver and an increase in gluconeogenesis. It can be referred to as a **hyperglycemic** agent (Table 14.2).

Two hormones produced by the adrenal gland affect carbohydrate metabolism. *Epinephrine*, produced by the adrenal medulla, increases plasma glucose by inhibiting insulin secretion, increasing glycogenolysis, and promoting lipolysis. Epinephrine is released during times of stress. *Glucocorticoids*, primarily cortisol, are released from the adrenal cortex on stimulation by adrenocorticotropic hormone (ACTH). Cortisol increases plasma glucose by decreasing intestinal entry into the cell and increasing gluconeogenesis, liver glycogen, and lipolysis.

Two anterior pituitary hormones, growth hormone and ACTH, promote increased plasma glucose. *Growth hormone* increases plasma glucose by decreasing the entry of glucose into the cells and increasing glycolysis. Its release from the pituitary is stimulated by decreased glucose levels and inhibited by increased glucose. Decreased levels of cortisol stimulate the anterior pituitary to release ACTH. ACTH, in turn, stimulates the adrenal cortex to release cortisol and increases plasma glucose levels by converting liver glycogen to glucose and promoting gluconeogenesis.

Two other hormones affect glucose levels: thyroxine and somatostatin. The thyroid gland is stimulated by the production of thyroid-stimulating hormone to release *thyroxine* that increases plasma glucose levels by increasing glycogenolysis, gluconeogenesis, and intestinal absorption of glucose. *Somatostatin*, produced by the δ-cells of the islets of Langerhans of the pancreas, increases plasma glucose levels by the inhibition of insulin, glucagon, growth hormone, and other endocrine hormones.

HYPERGLYCEMIA

Hyperglycemia is an increase in plasma glucose levels. In healthy patients, during a hyperglycemia state, insulin is secreted by the β-cells of the pancreatic islets of Langerhans. Insulin enhances membrane permeability to cells in the liver, muscle, and adipose tissue. It also alters the glucose metabolic pathways. Hyperglycemia, or increased plasma glucose levels, is caused by an imbalance of hormones.

Diabetes Mellitus

Diabetes mellitus is actually a group of metabolic diseases characterized by hyperglycemia resulting from defects in insulin secretion, insulin action, or both. In 1979, the National Diabetes Data Group developed a classification and diagnosis scheme for diabetes mellitus.[1] This scheme included dividing diabetes into two broad categories: type 1, insulin-dependent diabetes mellitus (IDDM), and type 2, non–insulin-dependent diabetes mellitus (NIDDM).

Established in 1995, the International Expert Committee on the Diagnosis and Classification of Diabetes Mellitus, working under the sponsorship of the ADA, was given the task of updating the 1979 classification system. The proposed changes included eliminating the older terms of IDDM and NIDDM. The categories of type 1 and type 2 were retained, with the adoption of Arabic numerals instead of Roman numerals (Table 14.3).[2]

Therefore, the ADA/World Health Organization (WHO) guidelines recommend the following categories of diabetes:

• Type 1 diabetes
• Type 2 diabetes
• Other specific types of diabetes
• Gestational diabetes mellitus (GDM) (diagnosed in the second or third trimester of pregnancy that is not clearly overt diabetes)

TABLE 14.3 Classification of Diabetes Mellitus

Classification	Pathogenesis
Type 1	β-Cell destruction Absolute insulin deficiency Autoantibodies • Islet cell autoantibodies • Insulin autoantibodies • Glutamic acid decarboxylase autoantibodies • Tyrosine phosphatase IA-2 and IA-2B autoantibodies
Type 2	Insulin resistance with an insulin secretory defect Relative insulin deficiency
Other	Associated with secondary conditions • Genetic defects of β-cell function • Pancreatic disease • Endocrine disease • Drug or chemical induced • Insulin receptor abnormalities • Other genetic syndromes
Gestational	Glucose intolerance during pregnancy Due to metabolic and hormonal changes

CASE STUDY 14.1

An 18-year-old male high school student who had a 4-year history of diabetes mellitus was brought to the emergency department because of excessive drowsiness, vomiting, and diarrhea. His diabetes had been well controlled with 40 units of NPH insulin daily until several days ago when he developed excessive thirst and polyuria. For the past 3 days, he has also had headaches, myalgia, and a low-grade fever. Diarrhea and vomiting began 1 day ago.

Urinalysis Results		Chemistry Test Results	
Specific gravity	1.012	Sodium	126 mmol/L
pH	5.0	Potassium	6.1 mmol/L
Glucose	4+	Chloride	87 mmol/L
Ketone	Large	Bicarbonate	6 mmol/L
		Plasma glucose	600 mg/dL
		BUN	48 mg/dL
		Creatinine	2.0 mg/dL
		Serum ketones	4+

Questions

1. What is the probable diagnosis of this patient based on the data presented?
2. What laboratory test(s) should be performed to follow this patient and aid in adjusting insulin levels?
3. Why are the urine ketones positive?
4. What methods are used to quantitate urine ketones? Which ketone(s) do they detect?

Type 1 diabetes is characterized by inappropriate hyperglycemia primarily a result of pancreatic islet β-cell destruction and a tendency to ketoacidosis. Type 2 diabetes, in contrast, includes hyperglycemia cases that result from insulin resistance with an insulin secretory defect. An intermediate stage, in which the fasting glucose is increased above normal limits but not to the level of diabetes, has been named *impaired fasting glucose*. Use of the term *impaired glucose tolerance* to indicate glucose tolerance values above normal but below diabetes levels was retained. Also, the term GDM was retained for women who develop glucose intolerance during pregnancy.

Type 1 diabetes mellitus is a result of cellular-mediated autoimmune destruction of the β-cells of the pancreas, causing an absolute deficiency of insulin secretion. Upper limit of 110 mg/dL on the fasting plasma glucose is designated as the upper limit of normal blood glucose. Type 1 constitutes only 10% to 20% of all cases of diabetes and commonly occurs in childhood and adolescence. This disease is usually initiated by an environmental factor or infection (usually a virus) in individuals with a genetic predisposition and causes the immune destruction of the β-cells of the pancreas and, therefore, a decreased production of insulin. Characteristics of type 1 diabetes include abrupt onset, insulin dependence, and ketosis tendency. This diabetic type is genetically related. One or more of the following markers are found in 85% to 90% of individuals with fasting hyperglycemia: islet cell autoantibodies, insulin autoantibodies, glutamic acid decarboxylase autoantibodies, and tyrosine phosphatase IA-2 and IA-2B autoantibodies.

Signs and symptoms include polydipsia (excessive thirst), polyphagia (increased food intake), polyuria (excessive urine production), rapid weight loss, hyperventilation, mental confusion, and possible loss of consciousness (due to increased glucose to brain). Complications include microvascular problems such as nephropathy, neuropathy, and retinopathy. Increased heart disease is also found in patients with diabetes. Table 14.4 lists the laboratory findings in hyperglycemia. *Idiopathic type 1 diabetes* is a form of type 1 diabetes that has no known etiology, is strongly inherited, and does not have β-cell autoimmunity. Individuals with this form of diabetes have episodic requirements for insulin replacement.

TABLE 14.4	Laboratory Findings in Hyperglycemia

Increased glucose in plasma and urine
Increased urine-specific gravity
Increased serum and urine osmolality
Ketones in serum and urine (ketonemia and ketonuria)
Decreased blood and urine pH (acidosis)
Electrolyte imbalance

Type 2 diabetes mellitus is characterized by hyperglycemia as a result of an individual's resistance to insulin with an insulin secretory defect. This resistance results in a relative, not an absolute, insulin deficiency. Type 2 constitutes the majority of the diabetes cases. Most patients in this type are obese or have an increased percentage of body fat distribution in the abdominal region. This type of diabetes often goes undiagnosed for many years and is associated with a strong genetic predisposition, with patients at increased risk with an increase in age, obesity, and lack of physical exercise. Characteristics usually include adult onset of the disease and milder symptoms than in type 1, with ketoacidosis seldom occurring. However, these patients are more likely to go into a hyperosmolar coma and are at an increased risk of developing macrovascular and microvascular complications.

Other specific types of diabetes are associated with certain conditions (secondary), including genetic defects of β-cell function or insulin action, pancreatic disease, diseases of endocrine origin, drug- or chemical-induced insulin receptor abnormalities, and certain genetic syndromes. The characteristics and prognosis of this form of diabetes depend on the primary disorder. Maturity-onset diabetes of youth is a rare form of diabetes that is inherited in an autosomal dominant fashion.[3]

GDM has been defined as any degree of glucose intolerance with onset or first recognition during pregnancy. However, the latest recommendations suggest that "high-risk women found to have diabetes at their initial prenatal visit, using standard criteria (Table 14.5), receive a diagnosis

TABLE 14.5	Diagnostic Criteria for Diabetes Mellitus

1. HbA₁c ≥ 6.5% using a method that is NGSP certified and standardized to the DCCT assay[a]
2. Fasting plasma glucose ≥ 126 mg/dL (≥7.0 mmol/L)[a]
3. 2-h plasma glucose ≥ 200 mg/dL (≥11.1 mmol/L) during an OGTT[a]
4. Random plasma glucose ≥ 200 mg/dL (≥11.1 mmol/L) plus symptoms of diabetes[a]

HbA₁c, hemoglobin A₁c; NGSP, National Glycohemoglobin Standardization Program; OGTT, oral glucose tolerance test.
[a]In the absence of unequivocal hyperglycemia, these criteria should be confirmed by repeat testing on a different day. The fourth measure (OGTT) is not recommended for routine clinical use.

of overt, not gestational, diabetes."[4] Women identified through the oral glucose tolerance, listed in Table 14.8, should receive a diagnosis of GDM. Causes of GDM include metabolic and hormonal changes. Patients with GDM frequently return to normal postpartum. However, this disease is associated with increased perinatal complications and an increased risk for the development of diabetes in later years. Infants born to mothers with diabetes are at increased risk for respiratory distress syndrome, hypocalcemia, and hyperbilirubinemia. Fetal insulin secretion is stimulated in the neonate of a mother with diabetes. However, when the infant is born and the umbilical cord is severed, the infant's oversupply of glucose is abruptly terminated, causing severe hypoglycemia.

Pathophysiology of Diabetes Mellitus

In both type 1 and type 2 diabetes, the individual will be hyperglycemic, which can be severe. Glucosuria can also occur after the renal tubular transporter system for glucose becomes saturated. This happens when the glucose concentration of plasma exceeds roughly 180 mg/dL in an individual with normal renal function and urine output. As hepatic glucose overproduction continues, the plasma glucose concentration reaches a plateau around 300 to 500 mg/dL (17 to 28 mmol/L). Provided renal output is maintained, glucose excretion will match the overproduction, causing the plateau.

The individual with type 1 diabetes has a higher tendency to produce ketones. Patients with type 2 diabetes seldom generate ketones but instead have a greater tendency to develop hyperosmolar nonketotic states. The difference in glucagon and insulin concentrations in these two groups appears to be responsible for the generation of ketones through increased β-oxidation. In type 1, there is an absence of insulin with an excess of glucagon. This permits gluconeogenesis and lipolysis to occur. In type 2, insulin is not absent and may, in fact, present as hyperinsulinemia at times; therefore, glucagon is attenuated. Fatty acid oxidation is inhibited in type 2. This causes fatty acids to be incorporated into triglycerides for release as very low-density lipoproteins.

The laboratory findings of a patient with diabetes with ketoacidosis tend to reflect dehydration, electrolyte disturbances, and acidosis. Acetoacetate, β-hydroxybutyrate, and acetone are produced from the oxidation of fatty acids. The two former ketone bodies contribute to the acidosis. Lactate, fatty acids, and other organic acids can also contribute to a lesser degree. Bicarbonate and total carbon dioxide are usually decreased due to Kussmaul-Kien respiration (deep respirations). This is a compensatory mechanism to blow off carbon dioxide and remove hydrogen ions in the process. The anion gap in this acidosis can exceed 16 mmol/L. Serum osmolality is high as a result of hyperglycemia; sodium concentrations tend to be lower due in part to losses (polyuria) and in part to a shift of water from cells because of the hyperglycemia. The sodium value should not be falsely underestimated because of hypertriglyceridemia. Grossly elevated triglycerides will displace plasma volume and give the appearance of decreased electrolytes when flame photometry or prediluted, ion-specific electrodes are used for sodium determinations. Hyperkalemia is almost always present as a result of the displacement of potassium from cells in acidosis. This is somewhat misleading because the patient's total body potassium is usually decreased.

More typical of the untreated patient with type 2 diabetes is the nonketotic hyperosmolar state. The individual presenting with this syndrome has an overproduction of glucose; however, there appears to be an imbalance between production and elimination in urine. Often, this state is precipitated by heart disease, stroke, or pancreatitis. Glucose concentrations exceed 300 to 500 mg/dL (17 to 28 mmol/L) and severe dehydration is present. The severe dehydration contributes to the inability to excrete glucose in the urine. Mortality is high with this condition. Ketones are not observed because the severe hyperosmolar state inhibits the ability of glucagon to stimulate lipolysis. The laboratory findings of nonketotic hyperosmolar coma include plasma glucose values exceeding 1,000 mg/dL (55 mmol/L), normal or elevated plasma sodium and potassium, slightly decreased bicarbonate, elevated blood urea nitrogen (BUN) and creatinine, and an elevated osmolality (>320 mOsm/dL). The gross elevation in glucose and osmolality, the elevation in BUN, and the absence of ketones distinguish this condition from diabetic ketoacidosis.

Other forms of impaired glucose metabolism that do not meet the criteria for diabetes mellitus include impaired fasting glucose and impaired glucose tolerance. These forms are discussed in the following section.

CASE STUDY 14.2

A 58-year-old obese man with frequent urination was seen by his primary care physician. The following laboratory work was performed, and the following results were obtained:

Casual Plasma Glucose	225 mg/dL		
Urinalysis Results			
Color and appearance	Pale/clear	Blood	Negative
pH	6.0	Bilirubin	Negative
Specific	1.025	Urobilinogen	Negative
Glucose	2+	Nitrites	Negative
Ketones	Negative	Leukocyte esterase	Negative

Questions

1. What is the probable diagnosis of this patient?
2. What other test(s) should be performed to confirm this? Which is the preferred test?
3. What values from no. 2 would confirm the diagnosis of diabetes?
4. After diagnosis, what test(s) should be performed to monitor his condition?

Criteria for Testing for Prediabetes and Diabetes

The testing criteria for asymptomatic adults for type 2 diabetes mellitus were modified by the ADA Expert Committee to allow for earlier detection of the disease. According to the ADA recommendations, all adults beginning at the age of 45 years should be tested for diabetes every 3 years using the hemoglobin A_1c (HbA_1c), fasting plasma glucose, or a 2-hour 75 g oral glucose tolerance test (OGTT) unless the individual has otherwise been diagnosed with diabetes.[4] Testing should be carried out at an earlier age or more frequently in individuals who display overweight tendencies, that is, BMI greater than or equal to 25 kg/m² (at-risk BMI may be lower in some ethnic groups, i.e., Asian Americans ≥23 kg/m²), and have additional risk factors, as follows:

- Habitually physically inactive
- Family history of diabetes in a first-degree relative
- In a high-risk minority population (e.g., African American, Latino, Native American, Asian American, and Pacific Islander)
- History of GDM or delivering a baby weighing more than 9 lb (4.1 kg)
- Hypertension (blood pressure ≥ 140/90 mm Hg)
- Low high-density lipoprotein (HDL) cholesterol concentrations (<35 mg/dL [0.90 mmol/L])
- Elevated triglyceride concentrations > 250 mg/dL (2.82 mmol/L)
- A1C ≥ 5.7% (33 mmol/mol), IGT, or IFG on previous testing
- History of impaired fasting glucose/impaired glucose tolerance
- Women with polycystic ovarian syndrome (PCOS)
- Other clinical conditions associated with insulin resistance (e.g., severe obesity and acanthosis nigricans)
- History of cardiovascular disease

In the absence of the above criteria, testing for prediabetes and diabetes should begin at the age of 45 years. If results are normal, testing should be repeated at least at 3-year intervals, with consideration of more frequent testing depending on initial results and risk status.

As the incidence of adolescent type 2 diabetes has risen dramatically in the past few years, criteria for the testing for type 2 diabetes in asymptomatic children have been developed. These criteria include initiation of testing at the age

10 years or at the onset of puberty, if puberty occurs at a younger age, with follow-up testing every 2 years. Testing should be carried out on children who display the following characteristics: overweight (BMI >85th percentile for age and sex, weight for height >85th percentile, or weight >120% of ideal for height) plus any two of the following risk factors:

- Family history of type 2 diabetes in first- or second-degree relative
- Race/ethnicity (e.g., Native American, African American, Latino, Asian American, and Pacific Islander)
- Signs of insulin resistance or conditions associated with insulin resistance (e.g., acanthosis nigricans, hypertension, dyslipidemia, and PCOS)
- Maternal history of diabetes or GDM

CASE STUDY 14.3

A 14-year-old male student was seen by his physician. His chief complaints were fatigue, weight loss, and increases in appetite, thirst, and frequency of urination. For the past 3 to 4 weeks, he had been excessively thirsty and had to urinate every few hours. He began to get up three to four times a night to urinate. The patient has a family history of diabetes mellitus.

Laboratory Data		
Fasting plasma glucose	160 mg/dL	
Urinalysis	Specific gravity	1.040
	Glucose	4+
	Ketones	Moderate

Questions

1. Based on the preceding information, can this patient be diagnosed with diabetes?

2. What further tests might be performed to confirm the diagnosis?

3. According to the ADA, what criteria are required for the diagnosis of diabetes?

4. Assuming this patient has diabetes, which type would be diagnosed?

Criteria for the Diagnosis of Diabetes Mellitus

Four methods of diagnosis are suggested: (1) HbA$_1$c greater than or equal to 6.5% using a National Glycohemoglobin Standardization Program (NGSP)-certified method, (2) a

TABLE 14.6	Categories of Fasting Plasma Glucose
Normal fasting glucose	FPG 70–99 mg/dL (3.9–5.5 mmol/L)
Impaired fasting glucose	FPG 100–125 mg/dL (5.6–6.9 mmol/L)
Provisional diabetes diagnosis	FPG ≥126 mg/dL (≥7.0 mmol/l)[a]

FPG, fasting plasma glucose.
[a]Must be confirmed.

fasting plasma glucose greater than or equal to 126 mg/dL (7.0 mmol/L), or (3) an OGTT with a 2-hour postload (75 g glucose load) level greater than or equal to 200 mg/dL (11.1 mmol/L), and (4) symptoms of diabetes plus a random plasma glucose level greater than or equal to 200 mg/dL (11.1 mmol/L), each of which should be confirmed on a subsequent day by any one of the first three methods (Tables 14.5–14.7). Any of the first three methods are considered appropriate for the diagnosis of diabetes. The decision on which method to use is the decision of the health care provider depending on various patient factors. Point-of-care (POC) assay methods for either plasma glucose or HbA$_1$c are not recommended for diagnosis.

An intermediate group of individuals who did not meet the criteria of diabetes mellitus but who have glucose levels above normal be placed into three categories for the risk of developing diabetes. First, those individuals with fasting glucose levels greater than or equal to 100 mg/dL but less than 126 mg/dL are placed in the impaired fasting glucose category. Another set of individuals who have 2-hour OGTT levels greater than or equal to 140 mg/dL but less than 200 mg/dL are placed in the impaired glucose tolerance category. Additionally, individuals with a HbA$_1$c of 5.7% to 6.4% are placed in the third at-risk category. Individuals in these three categories are referred to as having "prediabetes" indicating the relatively high risk for the development of diabetes in these patients.

TABLE 14.7	Categories of Oral Glucose Tolerance
Normal glucose tolerance	2-h PG ≤ 140 mg/dL (≤7.8 mmol/L)
Impaired glucose tolerance	2-h PG140–199 mg/dL (7.8–11.1 mmol/l)
Provisional diabetes diagnosis	2-h PG ≥ 200 mg/dL (≥11.1 mmol/L)[a]

PG, plasma glucose.
[a]Must be confirmed.

Criteria for the Testing and Diagnosis of GDM

The diagnostic criteria for gestational diabetes were revised by the International Association of the Diabetes and Pregnancy Study Groups. The revised criteria recommend that all nondiabetic pregnant women should be screened for GDM at 24 to 28 weeks of gestation.

CASE STUDY 14.4

A 13-year-old girl collapsed on a playground at school. When her mother was contacted, she mentioned that her daughter had been losing weight and making frequent trips to the bathroom in the night. The emergency squad noticed a fruity breath. On entrance to the emergency department, her vital signs were as follows:

Blood pressure	98/50 mm Hg
Respirations	Rapid
Temperature	99 °F

Stat lab results included:

Random Urine		Serum Chemistries	
pH	5.5	Glucose	500 mg/dL
Protein	Negative	Ketones	Positive
Glucose	4+	BUN	6 mg/dL
Ketones	Moderate	Creatinine	0.4 mg/dL
Blood	Negative		

Questions

1. Identify this patient's most likely type of diabetes.
2. Based on your identification, circle the common characteristics associated with that type of diabetes in the case study above.
3. What is the cause of the fruity breath?

The approach for screening and diagnosis is either a one-step or two-step approach. The one-step approach is the performance of a 2-hour OGTT using a 75 g glucose load. Glucose measurements should be taken at fasting, 1 hour, and 2 hours. A fasting plasma glucose value greater than or equal to 92 mg/dL (5.1 mmol/L), a 1-hour value greater than or equal to 180 mg/dL (10 mmol/L), or a 2-hour glucose value greater than or equal to 153 mg/dL (8.5 mmol/L) is diagnostic of GDM if any one of the three criteria are met. This test should be performed in the morning after an overnight fast of at least 8 hours (Table 14.8).

TABLE 14.8	Diagnostic Criteria for Gestational Diabetes
One-Step Approach	
Fasting plasma glucose	≥92 mg/dL (5.1 mmol/L)
1-h plasma glucose	≥180 mg/dL (10 mmol/L)
2-h plasma glucose	≥153 mg/dL (8.5 mmol/L)
Two-Step Approach	
Fasting	≥95 mg/dL (5.3 mmo/L)
1-h plasma glucose	≥180 mg/dL (10.0 mmol/L)
2-h plasma glucose	≥155 mg/dL (8.6 mmol/L)
3-h plasma glucose	≥140 mg/dL (7.8 mmol/L)

In the two-step approach, an initial measurement of plasma glucose at 1-hour postload (50-g glucose load) is performed. A plasma glucose value 140 mg/dL (≥7.8 mmol/L) indicates the need to perform a 3-hour OGTT using a 100 g glucose load. GDM is diagnosed when any two of the following four values are met or exceeded: fasting, >95 mg/dL (5.3 mmol/L); 1 hour, greater than or equal to 180 mg/dL (10.0 mmol/L); 2 hours, greater than or equal to 155 mg/dL (8.6 mmol/L); or 3 hours, greater than or equal to 140 mg/dL (7.8 mmol/L). This test should be performed in the morning after an overnight fast of between 8 and 14 h, after at least 3 days of unrestricted diet (≥150 g carbohydrate per day) and unlimited physical activity. NOTE: The National Diabetes Data Group's levels are slightly higher than those listed above.

HYPOGLYCEMIA

Hypoglycemia involves decreased plasma glucose levels and can have many causes—some are transient and relatively insignificant, but others can be life threatening. Hypoglycemia causes brain fuel deprivation, which can result in impaired judgment and behavior, seizures, comas, functional brain failure, and death. Hypoglycemia is the result of an imbalance in the rate of glucose appearance and disappearance from the circulation. This imbalance may be caused by treatment, such as diabetic drugs or biological factors. The plasma glucose concentration at which glucagon and other glycemic factors are released is between 65 and 70 mg/dL (3.6 to 3.9 mmol/L); at about 50 to 55 mg/dL (2.8 to 3.1 mmol/L), observable symptoms of hypoglycemia appear. The warning signs and symptoms of hypoglycemia are all related to the central nervous system. The release of epinephrine into the systemic circulation and of norepinephrine at nerve endings of specific neurons acts in unison with glucagon to increase plasma glucose. Glucagon is released from the islet cells of the pancreas and inhibits insulin. Epinephrine is released from the adrenal gland and increases glucose metabolism and inhibits insulin. In addition, cortisol and growth hormone are released and increase glucose metabolism.

Historically, hypoglycemia was classified as postabsorptive (fasting) and postprandial (reactive) hypoglycemia.

TABLE 14.9	Classification of Hypoglycemia
Severe hypoglycemia	Requires assistance to actively administer carbohydrates and glucagon or take other corrective actions
Documented symptomatic hypoglycemia	Symptoms of hypoglycemia Measured plasma glucose concentration ≤70 mg/dL (≤3.9 mmol/L)
Asymptomatic hypoglycemia	No symptoms of hypoglycemia Measured plasma glucose concentration ≤70 mg/dL (≤3.9 mmol/L)
Probable symptomatic hypoglycemia	Symptoms typical of hypoglycemia No plasma glucose determination performed
Pseudohypoglycemia	Symptoms of hypoglycemia Measured plasma glucose concentration > 70 mg/dL (>3.9 mmol/L) but approaching that level

Source: Seaquist ER, Anderson J, Childs B, et al. Hypoglycemia and diabetes: a report of a workgroup of the American Diabetes Association and the Endocrine Society. *Diabetes Care.* 2013;36:1384–1395.

Postpranial hypoglycemia describes the timing of hypoglycemia (within 4 hours after meals). Current approaches suggest classifying postprandial hypoglycemia based on the severity of symptoms and measured plasma glucose levels. This approach is especially important for individuals with diabetes, who are a high risk for hypoglycemic episodes (Table 14.9).[5] The ADA and the Endocrine Society recommend that a plasma concentration of less than or equal to 70 mg/dL (□3.9 mmol/L) be used as cut-off as well as an alert value to prevent a clinical hypoglycemic episode. This value also allows for a margin of error for self-monitoring glucose devices. Patients with diabetes who present with iatrogenic hypoglycemia may potentially be harmed by the low glucose level.

Hypoglycemia is rare in individuals with normal glucose metabolism. In individuals without diabetes, a diagnosis of hypoglycemia should be made only in those who demonstrate the Whipple triad: (1) hypoglycemic symptoms; (2) plasma glucose concentration is low (<50 mg/dL) when the symptoms are present; and (3) symptoms are relieved by correction of the hypoglycemia when administered glucose or glucagon.[6] Symptoms of hypoglycemia include increased hunger, sweating, nausea and vomiting, dizziness, nervousness and shaking, blurring of speech and sight, and mental confusion. When hypoglycemia symptoms present in individuals in a postabsorptive (fasting) state, an insulinoma might be suspected. Laboratory findings include decreased plasma glucose levels during hypoglycemic episode and extremely elevated insulin levels in patients with pancreatic β-cell tumors (insulinoma). To investigate an insulinoma, the patient is required to fast under controlled conditions. Men and women have different metabolic patterns in prolonged fasts. The healthy male will maintain plasma glucose of 55 to 60 mg/dL (3.1 to 3.3 mmol/L) for several days. Healthy females will produce ketones more readily and permit plasma glucose to decrease to 40 mg/dL (2.2 mmol/L) or lower. Diagnostic criteria for an insulinoma include a change in glucose level greater than or equal to 25 mg/dL (1.4 mmol/L) coincident with an insulin level greater than or equal to 6 μU/mL (41.7 pmol/L), C-peptide levels greater than or equal to 0.2 nmol/L, proinsulin levels greater than or equal to 5 pmol/L, and/or β-hydroxybutyrate levels less than or equal to 2.7 mmol/L.[7]

Genetic Defects in Carbohydrate Metabolism

Glycogen storage diseases are the result of the deficiency of a specific enzyme that causes an alternation of glycogen metabolism. The most common congenital form of glycogen storage disease is glucose-6-phosphatase deficiency type 1, which is also called von Gierke disease, an autosomal recessive disease. This disease is characterized by severe hypoglycemia that coincides with metabolic acidosis, ketonemia, and elevated lactate and alanine. Hypoglycemia occurs because glycogen cannot be converted back to glucose by way of hepatic glycogenolysis. A glycogen buildup is found in the liver, causing hepatomegaly. The patients usually have severe hypoglycemia, hyperlipidemia, uricemia, and growth retardation. A liver biopsy will show a positive glycogen stain. Although the glycogen accumulation is irreversible, the disease can be kept under control by avoiding the development of hypoglycemia. Liver transplantation corrects the hypoglycemic condition. Other enzyme defects or deficiencies that cause hypoglycemia include glycogen synthase, fructose-1,6-bisphosphatase, phosphoenolpyruvate carboxykinase, and pyruvate carboxylase. Glycogen debrancher enzyme deficiency does not cause hypoglycemia but does cause hepatomegaly.

CASE STUDY 14.5

A 28-year-old woman delivered a 9.5-lb infant. The infant was above the 95th percentile for weight and length. The mother's history was incomplete; she claimed to have had no medical care through her pregnancy. Shortly after birth, the infant became lethargic and flaccid. A whole blood glucose and ionized calcium were performed in the nursery with the following results:

Whole blood glucose	25 mg/dL
Ionized calcium	4.9 mg/dL
Plasma glucose was drawn and analyzed in the main laboratory to confirm the whole blood findings.	
Plasma glucose	33 mg/dL
An intravenous glucose solution was started and whole blood glucose was measured hourly.	

Questions

1. Give the possible explanation for the infant's large birth weight and size.

2. If the mother was a gestational diabetic, why was her baby hypoglycemic?

3. Why was there a discrepancy between the whole blood glucose concentration and the plasma glucose concentration?

4. If the mother had been monitored during pregnancy, what laboratory tests should have been performed and what criteria would have indicated that she had gestational diabetes?

Galactosemia, a cause of failure to thrive syndrome in infants, is a congenital deficiency of one of three enzymes involved in galactose metabolism, resulting in increased levels of galactose in plasma. The most common enzyme deficiency is galactose-1-phosphate uridyltransferase. Galactosemia occurs because of the inhibition of glycogenolysis and is accompanied by diarrhea and vomiting. Galactose must be removed from the diet to prevent the development of irreversible complications. If left untreated, the patient will develop mental retardation and cataracts. The disorder can be identified by measuring erythrocyte galactose-1-phosphate uridyltransferase activity. Laboratory findings include hypoglycemia, hyperbilirubinemia, and galactose accumulation in the blood, tissue, and urine following milk ingestion. Another enzyme deficiency, fructose-1-phosphate aldolase deficiency, causes nausea and hypoglycemia after fructose ingestion.

Specific inborn errors of amino acid metabolism and long-chain fatty acid oxidation are also responsible for hypoglycemia. There are also alimentary and idiopathic hypoglycemias. Alimentary hypoglycemia appears to be caused by an increase in the release of insulin in response to rapid absorption of nutrients after a meal or the rapid secretion of insulin-releasing gastric factors.

ROLE OF LABORATORY IN DIFFERENTIAL DIAGNOSIS AND MANAGEMENT OF PATIENTS WITH GLUCOSE METABOLIC ALTERATIONS

The demonstration of hyperglycemia or hypoglycemia under specific conditions is used to diagnose diabetes mellitus and hypoglycemic conditions. Other laboratory tests have been developed to identify insulinomas and to monitor glycemic control and the development of renal complications.

CASE STUDY 14.6

Laboratory tests were performed on a 50-year-old lean white woman during an annual physical examination. She had no family history of diabetes or any history of elevated glucose levels during pregnancy.

Laboratory Results	
Fasting blood glucose (FBG)	90 mg/dL
Cholesterol	140 mg/dL
HDL	40 mg/dL
Triglycerides	90 mg/dL

Questions

1. What is the probable diagnosis of this patient?

2. Describe the proper follow-up for this patient?

3. What are the appropriate screening tests for diabetes in nonpregnant adults?

4. What are the risk factors that would indicate a potential of this patient's developing diabetes?

Methods of Glucose Measurement

Glucose can be measured from serum, plasma, or whole blood. Today, most glucose measurements are performed on serum or plasma. The glucose concentration in whole blood is approximately 11% lower than the glucose concentration in plasma. Serum or plasma must be refrigerated and separated from the cells within 1 hour to prevent substantial loss of glucose by the cellular fraction, particularly if the white blood cell count is elevated. Sodium fluoride ions (gray-top tubes) are often used as an anticoagulant and preservative of whole blood, particularly if analysis is delayed. The fluoride inhibits glycolytic enzymes. However, although fluoride maintains long-term glucose stability, the rates of decline of glucose in the 1st hour after sample collection in tubes with and without fluoride are virtually identical. Therefore, the plasma should be separated from the cells as soon as possible. FBG should be obtained in the morning after an approximately 8- to 10-hour fast (not longer than 16 h). Fasting plasma glucose values have a diurnal variation with the mean FBG higher in the morning than in the afternoon.[8] Diabetes in patients tested in the afternoon may be missed because of this variation. Cerebrospinal fluid and urine can also be analyzed. Urine glucose measurement is not used in diabetes diagnosis; however, some patients use this measurement for monitoring purposes.

CASE STUDY 14.7

For three consecutive quarters, a fasting glucose and glycosylated hemoglobin were performed on a patient. The results are as follows:

	Quarter 1	Quarter 2	Quarter 3
Plasma glucose, fasting	280 mg/dL	85 mg/dL	91 mg/dL
Glycosylated hemoglobin	7.8%	15.3%	8.5%

Questions

1. In which quarter was the patient's glucose best controlled? The least controlled?

2. Do the fasting plasma glucose and glycosylated hemoglobin match? Why or why not?

3. What methods are used to measure glycosylated hemoglobin?

4. What potential conditions might cause erroneous results?

The ability of glucose to function as a reducing agent has been useful in the detection and quantitation of carbohydrates in body fluids. Glucose and other carbohydrates are capable of converting cupric ions in alkaline solution to cuprous ions. The solution loses its deep-blue color and a red precipitate of cuprous oxide forms. Benedict's and Fehling's reagents, which contain an alkaline solution of cupric ions stabilized by citrate or tartrate, respectively, have been used to detect reducing agents in urine and other body fluids. Another chemical characteristic that used to be exploited to quantitate carbohydrates is the ability of these molecules to form Schiff bases with aromatic amines. *O*-toluidine in a hot acidic solution will yield a colored compound with an absorbance maximum at 630 nm. Galactose, an aldohexose, and mannose, an aldopentose, will also react with *O*-toluidine and produce a colored compound that can interfere with the reaction. The Schiff base reaction with *O*-toluidine is of historical interest only

and has been replaced by more specific enzymatic methods, which are discussed in the following section.

The most common methods of glucose analysis use the enzyme glucose oxidase or hexokinase (Table 14.10). Glucose oxidase is the most specific enzyme reacting with only β-D-glucose. Glucose oxidase converts β-D-glucose to gluconic acid. Mutarotase may be added to the reaction to facilitate the conversion of α-D-glucose to β-D-glucose. Oxygen is consumed and hydrogen peroxide (H_2O_2) is produced. The reaction can be monitored polarographically either by measuring the rate of disappearance of oxygen using an oxygen electrode or by consuming H_2O_2 in a side reaction. Horseradish peroxidase is used to catalyze the second reaction, and the H_2O_2 is used to oxidize a dye compound. Two commonly used chromogens are 3-methyl-2-benzothiazolinone hydrazone and *N,N*-dimethylaniline. The shift in absorbance can be monitored spectrophotometrically and is proportional to the amount of glucose present in the specimen. This coupled reaction is known as the Trinder reaction. However, the peroxidase coupling reaction used in the glucose oxidase method is subject to positive and negative interference. Increased levels of uric acid, bilirubin, and ascorbic acid can cause falsely decreased values as a result of these substances being oxidized by peroxidase, which then prevents the oxidation and detection of the chromogen. Strong oxidizing substances, such as bleach, can cause falsely increased values. An oxygen consumption electrode can be used to perform the direct measurement of oxygen by the polarographic technique, which avoids this interference. Oxygen depletion is measured and is proportional to the amount of glucose present. Polarographic glucose analyzers measure the rate of oxygen consumption because glucose is oxidized under first-order conditions using glucose oxidase reagent. The H_2O_2 formed must be eliminated in a side reaction to prevent the reaction from reversing. Molybdate can be used to catalyze the oxidation of iodide to iodine by H_2O_2 or catalase can be used to catalyze oxidation of ethanol by H_2O_2, forming acetaldehyde and H_2O.

The hexokinase method is considered more accurate than the glucose oxidase methods because the coupling reaction using glucose-6-phosphate dehydrogenase is highly specific; therefore, it has less interference than the coupled glucose oxidase procedure. Hexokinase in the presence of ATP converts glucose to glucose-6-phosphate. Glucose-6-phosphate and the cofactor NADP$^+$ are converted to 6-phosphogluconate and NADPH by glucose-6-phosphate dehydrogenase. NADPH has a strong absorbance maximum at 340 nm, and

TABLE 14.10 Methods of Glucose Measurement

Glucose oxidase	Glucose + O_2 + H_2O $\xrightarrow{\text{glucose oxidase}}$ gluconic acid + H_2O_2
	H_2O_2 + reduced chromogen $\xrightarrow{\text{peroxidase}}$ oxidized chromogen + H_2O
	Glucose + ATP $\xrightarrow{\text{hexokinase}}$ glucose-6-PO_4 + ADP
Hexokinase	Glucose-6-PO_4 + NADP$^+$ $\xrightarrow{\text{G-6-PD}}$ NADPH + 6-phosphogluconate
Clinitest	Cu^{2+} $\xrightarrow{\text{Reducing substance}}$ $Cu^{1+}O$

the rate of appearance of NADPH can be monitored spectrophotometrically and is proportional to the amount of glucose present in the sample. Generally accepted as the reference method, this method is not affected by ascorbic acid or uric acid. Gross hemolysis and extremely elevated bilirubin may cause a false decrease in results. The hexokinase method may be performed on serum or plasma collected using heparin, ethylenediaminetetraacetic acid (EDTA), fluoride, oxalate, or citrate. The method can also be used for urine, cerebrospinal fluid, and serous fluids.

Nonspecific methods of measuring glucose are still used in the urinalysis section of the laboratory primarily to detect reducing substances other than glucose. The method given next is the Benedict's modification, also called the Clinitest reaction.

Self-Monitoring of Blood Glucose

The ADA has recommended that individuals with diabetes monitor their blood glucose levels in an effort to maintain levels as close to normal as possible. For persons with type 1 diabetes, the recommendation is three to four times per day; for persons with type 2 diabetes, the optimal frequency is unknown. Recommended glycemic target for many nonpregnant adult is a preprandial capillary plasma glucose of 80 to 130 mg/dL (4.4 to 7.2 mmol/L). This recommendation has been determined to correlate with the achievement of an HbA_1c of less than 7%. Peak postprandial, 1 to 2 hours after the beginning of a meal, capillary plasma glucose of less than 180 mg/dL (<10.0 mmol/L) may be suggested for individuals who are not achieving the HbA_1c target. It is important that patients be taught how to use control solutions and calibrators to ensure the accuracy of their results.[9] Urine glucose testing should be replaced by self-monitoring of blood glucose; however, urine ketone testing will remain for type 1 and gestational diabetes.

Glucose Tolerance and 2-Hour Postprandial Tests

Guidelines for the performance and interpretation of the 2-hour postprandial test were set by the Expert Committee. A variation of this test is to use a standardized load of glucose. A solution containing 75 g of glucose is administered, and a specimen for plasma glucose measurement is drawn 2 hours later. Under this criterion, the patient drinks a standardized (75 g) glucose load and a glucose measurement is taken 2 hours later. If that level is greater than or equal to 200 mg/dL and is confirmed on a subsequent day by either an increased random or fasting glucose level, the patient is diagnosed with diabetes (see earlier discussion).

The OGTT is not recommended for routine use under the ADA guidelines. This procedure is inconvenient to patients and is not being used by physicians for diagnosing diabetes. However, if OGTT is used, the WHO recommends the criteria listed in Table 14.7. It is important that proper patient preparation be given before this test is performed. The patient should be ambulatory and on a normal-to-high carbohydrate intake for 3 days before the test. The patient

should be fasting for at least 10 hours and not longer than 16 hours, and the test should be performed in the morning because of the hormonal diurnal effect on glucose. Just before tolerance and while the test is in progress, patients should refrain from exercise, eating, drinking (except that the patient may drink water), and smoking. Factors that affect the tolerance results include medications such as large doses of salicylates, diuretics, anticonvulsants, oral contraceptives, and corticosteroids. Also, gastrointestinal problems, including malabsorption problems, gastrointestinal surgery, and vomiting and endocrine dysfunctions, can affect the OGTT results. The guidelines recommend that only the fasting and the 2-hour sample be measured, except when the patient is pregnant. The adult dose of glucose solution (Glucola) is 75 g; children receive 1.75 g/kg of glucose to a maximum dose of 75 g.

CASE STUDY 14.8

A 25-year-old healthy female patient complained of dizziness and shaking 1 hour after eating a large, heavy-carbohydrate meal. The result of a random glucose test performed via fingerstick was 60 mg/dL.

Questions

1. Identify the characteristics of hypoglycemia in this case study.
2. What test(s) should be performed next to determine this young woman's problem?
3. To which category of hypoglycemia would this individual belong?
4. What criteria would be used to diagnose a potential insulinoma?

Glycosylated Hemoglobin/HbA_1c

The aim of diabetic management is to maintain the blood glucose concentration within or near the nondiabetic range with a minimal number of fluctuations. Serum or plasma glucose concentrations can be measured by laboratories in addition to patient self-monitoring of whole blood glucose concentrations. Long-term blood glucose regulation can be followed by measurement of glycosylated hemoglobin.

Glycosylated hemoglobin is the term used to describe the formation of a hemoglobin compound produced when glucose (a reducing sugar) reacts with the amino group of hemoglobin (a protein). The glucose molecule attaches nonenzymatically to the hemoglobin molecule to form a ketoamine. The rate of formation is directly proportional to the plasma glucose concentrations. Because the average red blood cell lives approximately 120 days, the glycosylated hemoglobin level at any one time reflects the average blood glucose level over the previous 2 to 3 months. Therefore, measuring the glycosylated hemoglobin provides the clinician with a time-averaged picture of the patient's blood glucose concentration over the past 3 months.

HbA$_1$c, the most commonly detected glycosylated hemoglobin, is a glucose molecule attached to one or both N-terminal valines of the β-polypeptide chains of normal adult hemoglobin.[10] HbA$_1$c is a more reliable method of monitoring long-term diabetes control than random plasma glucose. Normal values range from 4.0% to 6.0%. Studies have shown that there is a strong linear relationship between average blood glucose and HbA$_1$c. Using a linear regression model, Nathan et al.[11] determined that an estimated average glucose (eAG) can be calculated from the HbA$_1$c reported value using the equation eAG (mg/dL) = 28.7 × HbA$_1$c − 46.7 (Table 14.11). However, this information needs to be used carefully, as another study has shown that the relationship between average plasma glucose and HbA$_1$c can differ substantially depending on the glycemic control of the population studied.[12] It is also important to remember that two factors determine the glycosylated hemoglobin levels: the average glucose concentration and the red blood cell life span. If the red blood cell life span is decreased because of another disease state such as hemoglobinopathies, the hemoglobin will have less time to become glycosylated and the glycosylated hemoglobin level will be lower. Other conditions associated with increased red cell turnover include pregnancy (second and third trimesters), recent blood loss or transfusion, erythropoietin therapy, or hemolysis.

Current ADA guidelines recommend that an HbA$_1$c test be performed at least two times a year with patients who are meeting treatment goals and who have stable glycemic control. For patients whose therapy has changed or who are not meeting glycemic goals, a quarterly HbA$_1$c test is recommended. The use of POC testing for HbA$_1$c allows for more timely decisions on therapy changes and has been shown to result in tighter glycemic control.[13] However, using POC assays for diagnostic purposes is not recommended since proficiency testing of personnel is not required.[1] Lowering HbA$_1$c to an average of less than 7% has clearly been shown to reduce the microvascular, retinopathic, and neuropathic complications of diabetes. Therefore, the HbA$_1$c goal for nonpregnant adults in general is less than 7%. Further studies have shown a small benefit to lowering HbA$_1$c to less than 6%, making this a goal for selected individual patients if possible without significant hypoglycemia. More (<6.5%) or less (<8%) stringent goals might be selected for individual patients based on their medical history. For pediatric populations, the recommended target A1C is less than 7.5%.

The specimen requirement for HbA$_1$c measurement is an EDTA whole blood sample. Before analysis, a hemolysate must be prepared. The methods of measurement are grouped into two major categories: (1) based on charge differences between glycosylated and nonglycosylated hemoglobin (cation-exchange chromatography, electrophoresis, and isoelectric focusing) and (2) structural characteristics of glycogroups on hemoglobin (affinity chromatography and immunoassay).

In the clinical laboratory, affinity chromatography is the preferred method of measurement. In this method, the glycosylated hemoglobin attaches to the boronate group of the resin and is selectively eluted from the resin bed using a buffer. This method is not temperature dependent and not affected by hemoglobin F, S, or C. Another method of measurement uses cation-exchange chromatography in which the negatively charged hemoglobins attach to the positively charged resin bed. The glycosylated hemoglobin is selectively eluted from the resin bed using a buffer of specific pH in which the glycohemoglobins are the most negatively charged and elute first from the column. However, this method is highly temperature dependent and affected by hemoglobinopathies. The presence of hemoglobin F yields false increased levels, and the presence of hemoglobins S and C yields false decreased levels. A common POC instrument HbA$_1$c assay is based on a latex immunoagglutination inhibition methodology. In this method, both the concentration of HbA$_1$c specifically and the concentration of total hemoglobin are measured, and the ratio reported as percent HbA$_1$c. In this method, glycated hemoglobin F is not measured, so at a very high level of hemoglobin F (>10%), the amount of HbA$_1$c will be lower than expected because a greater proportion of the glycated hemoglobin will be in the form of glycated hemoglobin F. High-performance liquid chromatography (HPLC) and electrophoresis methods are also used to separate the various forms of hemoglobin. With HPLC, all forms of glycosylated hemoglobin—A$_1$a, A$_1$b, and A$_1$c—can be separated.

Standardization of glycosylated hemoglobin has been a continuing problem; there was no consensus on the reference method and no single standard is available to be used in the assays. Because of this, HbA$_1$c values vary with the method and laboratory performing them (Table 14.12). The International Federation of Clinical Chemistry and Laboratory Medicine (IFCC) developed a common

TABLE 14.11 Translating the A$_1$c Assay into eAG Values and A$_1$c Levels

Estimated Average Glucose (eAG)	A$_1$C (%)
97 mg/dL (5.4 mmol/L)	5
126 mg/dL (7.0 mmol/L)	6
154 mg/dL (8.6 mmol/L)	7
183 mg/dL (10.2 mmol/L)	8
212 mg/dL (11.8 mmol/L)	9
240 mg/dL (13.4 mmol/L)	10
269 mg/dL (14.9 mmol/L)	11
298 mg/dL (16.5 mmol/L)	12

Source: Nathan DM, Kuenen J, Borg R, et al. Translating the A1C assay into estimated average glucose values. *Diabetes Care*. 2008;31: 1473–1478; Kilpatrick ES, Rigby AS, Atkin SL. Variability in the relationship between mean plasma glucose and HbA$_1$c: implications for the assessment of glycemic control. *Clin Chem*. 2007;53:897–901.

TABLE 14.12   Methods of Glycated Hemoglobin Measurement

Methods Based on Structural Differences

Immunoassays	Polyclonal or monoclonal antibodies toward the glycated N-terminal group of the β-chain of hemoglobin	
Affinity chromatography	Separates based on chemical structure using borate to bind glycosylated proteins	Not temperature dependent Not affected by other hemoglobins

Methods Based on Charge Differences

Ion-exchange chromatography	Positive-charge resin bed	Highly temperature dependent Affected by hemoglobinopathies
Electrophoresis	Separation is based on differences in charge	Hemoglobin F values > 7% interfere
Isoelectric focusing	Type of electrophoresis using isoelectric point to separate	Pre-HbA₁c interferes
High-pressure liquid chromatography	A form of ion-exchange chromatography	Separates all forms of glyco-Hb: A₁a, A₁b, and A₁c

definition for HbA₁c and a reference method that specifically measures the concentration of only one molecular species of glycated A₁c, the glycated N-terminal residue of the β-chain of hemoglobin. This method, using either HPLC/electrospray mass spectrometry or HPLC/capillary electrophoresis, is only used to standardize A₁c assays and cannot be used for the clinical measurement of HbA₁c.[14] International consensus groups have determined that HbA₁c results will be represented worldwide in IFCC units (mmol HbA1c/mol Hb) and derived NGSP units (%) using the IFCC–NGSP master equation.[15] The master equation for this conversion is NGSP = [0.09148 × IFCC] + 2.152. HbA₁c reagent and instrument manufacturers are required to document their traceability to the IFCC reference system with both the IFCC units (mmol/mol) and derived NGSP units (%). In the United States, the NGSP, with the Diabetes Control and Complications Trial (DCCT) HPLC method, is used as a primary reference method. An allowable error of 5 mmol HbA1c/mol Hb (0.46%) has been determined as acceptable.[16–18] With these developments, HbA₁c measurement has become a more reliable indicator of the long-term patient blood glucose regulation with more consistency in the results from laboratory to laboratory.

Ketones

Ketone bodies are produced by the liver through metabolism of fatty acids to provide a ready energy source from stored lipids at times of low carbohydrate availability. The three ketone bodies are acetone (2%), acetoacetic acid (20%), and 3-β-hydroxybutyric acid (78%). A low level of ketone bodies is present in the body at all times. However, in cases of carbohydrate deprivation or decreased carbohydrate use such as diabetes mellitus, starvation/fasting, high-fat diets, prolonged vomiting, and glycogen storage disease, blood levels increase to meet the energy needs. The term *ketonemia* refers to the accumulation of ketones in blood, and the term *ketonuria* refers to the accumulation of ketones in urine (Fig. 14.9). The measurement of ketones is recommended for patients with type 1 diabetes during acute illness, stress, pregnancy, or elevated blood glucose levels above 300 mg/dL or when the patient has signs of ketoacidosis.

The specimen requirement is *fresh* serum or urine; the sample should be tightly stoppered and analyzed immediately. No method used for the determination of ketones reacts with all three ketone bodies. The historical test (Gerhardt's) that used ferric chloride reacted with acetoacetic acid to produce a red color. The procedure had many interfering substances, including salicylates. A more common method using sodium nitroprusside ($NaFe[CN]_5NO$) reacts with acetoacetic acid in an alkaline pH to form a purple color. If the reagent contains glycerin, then acetone is also detected. This method is used with the urine reagent strip test and Acetest tablets. A newer enzymatic method adapted to some automated instruments uses the enzyme 3-hydroxybutyrate dehydrogenase to detect either 3-β-hydroxybutyric acid or acetoacetic acid, depending on the pH of the solution. A pH of 7.0 causes the reaction to proceed to the right (decreasing absorbance) and a pH of 8.5 to 9.5 causes the reaction to proceed to left (increasing absorbance; Table 14.13).

FIGURE 14.9 The three ketone bodies.

Acetone   **Acetoacetic acid**   **β-Hydroxybutyric acid**

TABLE 14.13 Methods of Ketone Measurement

Nitroprusside	Acetoacetic acid + nitroprusside $\xrightarrow{\text{alkaline pH}}$ purple color
Enzymatic	3-β-hydroxybutyrate + NAD$^+$ $\xrightarrow{\text{3-Hbd}}$ acetoacetate + H$^+$ + NADH

Albuminuria

Diabetes mellitus causes progressive changes to the kidneys and ultimately results in diabetic renal nephropathy, now referred to as diabetic kidney disease. This complication progresses over years and may be delayed by aggressive glycemic control. An early sign that diabetic kidney disease is occurring is an increase in urinary albumin. In the latest guidelines, the term microalbumin is no longer used "since albuminuria occurs on a continuum."[19] **Albuminuria** measurements are useful to assist in diagnosis at an early stage and before the development of proteinuria. An annual assessment of kidney function by the determination of urinary albumin excretion is recommended for diabetic patients. Persistent albuminuria, defined as an albumin–creatinine ratio of 30 to 299 mg/g creatinine in two out of three urine collections over a 3- to 6-month period, is an early indicator of diabetic kidney disease. Factors that may elevate the urinary excretion of albumin include exercise within 24 hours, infection, fever, congestive heart failure, marked hyperglycemia, and marked hypertension.[20]

The use of a random spot collection for the measurement of the albumin–creatinine ratio is the preferred method.[21] Using the spot method, without the simultaneous creatinine measurement, may result in false-positive and false-negative results because of variation in urine concentration. The two other alternatives, a 24-hour collection and a timed 4-hour overnight collection, which are more burdensome to the patient and add little to prediction or accuracy, are seldom required.

Islet Autoantibody and Insulin Testing

The presence of autoantibodies to the β-islet cells of the pancreas is characteristic of type 1 diabetes. However, islet autoantibody testing is not currently recommended for routine screening for diabetes diagnosis. In the future, this testing might identify at-risk, prediabetic patients. Insulin measurements are not required for the diagnosis of diabetes mellitus, but in certain hypoglycemic states, it is important to know the concentration of insulin in relation to the plasma glucose concentration.

CASE STUDY 14.9

A nurse caring for patients with diabetes performed a fingerstick glucose test on the Accu-Chek glucose monitor and obtained a value of 200 mg/dL. A plasma sample, collected at the same time by a phlebotomist and performed by the laboratory, resulted in a glucose value of 225 mg/dL.

Questions

1. Are these two results significantly different?
2. Explain.

key points

- **Carbohydrates** are the major food source and energy supply for the body and are stored primarily as liver and muscle glycogen.
- Disease states involving carbohydrates are split into two groups—hyperglycemia and hypoglycemia.
- Early detection of diabetes mellitus is the aim of the ADA guidelines.
- Hemoglobin A1c (HbA1c), fasting plasma glucose, or a 2-hour 75 g OGTT can be used for diagnosis of diabetes.

- Glycosylated hemoglobin level reflects the average blood glucose level over the previous 2 to 3 months.
- Albuminuria measurements are useful to assist in diagnosis at an early stage and before the development of proteinuria.

For additional student resources, please visit thePoint at http://thepoint.lww.com

questions

1. Which of the following hormones promotes gluconeogenesis?
   a. Growth hormone
   b. Hydrocortisone
   c. Insulin
   d. Thyroxine

2. Glucose oxidase oxidizes glucose to gluconic acid and
   a. H_2O_2
   b. CO_2
   c. HCO_3
   d. H_2O

3. From glucose and ATP, hexokinase catalyzes the formation of
   a. Acetyl-CoA
   b. Fructose-6-phosphate
   c. Glucose-6-phosphate
   d. Lactose

4. What is the preferred specimen for glucose analysis?
   a. EDTA plasma
   b. Fluoride oxalate plasma
   c. Heparinized plasma
   d. Serum

5. Hyperglycemic factor produced by the pancreas is
   a. Epinephrine
   b. Glucagon
   c. Insulin
   d. Growth hormone

6. Polarographic methods of glucose assay are based on which principle?
   a. Nonenzymatic oxidation of glucose
   b. Rate of oxygen depletion measured
   c. Chemiluminescence caused by the formation of ATP
   d. Change in electrical potential as glucose is oxidized

7. Select the enzyme that is most specific for β-D-glucose:
   a. Glucose oxidase
   b. Glucose-6-phosphate dehydrogenase
   c. Hexokinase
   d. Phosphohexose isomerase

8. Select the coupling enzyme used in the hexokinase method for glucose:
   a. Glucose dehydrogenase
   b. Glucose-6-phosphatase
   c. Glucose-6-phosphate dehydrogenase
   d. Peroxidase

9. All of the following are characteristic of von Gierke disease EXCEPT
   a. Hypoglycemia
   b. Hypolipidemia

   c. Increased plasma lactate
   d. Subnormal response to epinephrine

10. The preferred screening test for diabetes in nonpregnant adults is measurement of
    a. Fasting plasma glucose
    b. 2 hour postprandial
    c. Glycohemoglobin
    d. No one test is preferred over another for diagnosis

11. Following the 2015 ADA guidelines, the times of measurement for plasma glucose levels during an OGTT in nonpregnant patients are
    a. Fasting, 1 hour, and 2 hours
    b. Fasting and 60 minutes
    c. 30, 60, 90, and 120 minutes
    d. Fasting and 30, 60, 90, and 120 minutes.

12. Monitoring the levels of ketone bodies in the urine via nitroprusside reagents provides a semiquantitative measure of
    a. Acetoacetate
    b. 3-β-Hydroxybutyrate
    c. Acetone
    d. All three ketone bodies

13. A factor, other than average plasma glucose values, that can affect the HbA_1c level is
    a. Serum ketone bodies level
    b. Red blood cell life span
    c. Ascorbic acid intake
    d. Increased triglyceride levels

14. Monitoring the levels of ketone bodies in the urine is
    a. Considered essential on a daily basis for all diabetic patients
    b. A reliable method of assessing long-term glycemic control
    c. Recommended for patients with type 1 diabetes on sick days
    d. Not recommended by the ADA

15. A urinalysis identifies a positive result for reducing sugars, yet the test for glucose (glucose oxidase reaction) was negative on the dipstick. What do these results suggest?
    a. This is commonly observed with ascorbic acid interference.
    b. This may suggest the patient has a deficiency in galactose-1-phosphate uridyltransferase.
    c. This may suggest a pancreatic beta-cell tumor.
    d. This may suggest a deficiency in glycogen debrancher enzyme.
    e. It is not possible to obtain these results and there is an analytic error in testing.

review questions (continued)

16. Urinalysis of a diabetic patient identified the following:
Year 1: Urine albumin was 15 mg/g creatinine.
Year 2: Urine albumin was 25 mg/g creatinine.
Year 3: Urine albumin was 40 mg/g creatinine.
What do these clinical data suggest?
a. These levels of albumin in the urine are normal, and no follow-up is necessary.

b. These levels of albumin in the urine suggest that kidney function is compromised.

c. As these values of urinary albumin are not greater than 300 mg/g creatinine, the patient is not likely to have compromised kidney function.

d. An additional urinary albumin test is required in 3 to 6 months to verify diminishing kidney function.

references

1. National Diabetes Data Group. Classification and diagnosis of diabetes mellitus and other categories of glucose tolerance. *Diabetes.* 1979;28:1039–1057.
2. American Diabetes Association. Classification and diagnosis of diabetes. Sec. 2. In Standards of Medical Care in Diabetes. 2016. *Diabetes Care.* 2015;39(suppl 1):S13–S22.
3. Malchoff CD. Diagnosis and classification of diabetes mellitus. *Conn Med.* 1991;55(11):625.
4. American Diabetes Association. Diagnosis and classification of diabetes mellitus. *Diabetes Care.* 2012;35:S64–S71.
5. Seaquist ER, Anderson J, Childs B, et al. Hypoglycemia and diabetes: a report of a workgroup of the American Diabetes Association and the Endocrine Society. *Diabetes Care.* 2013;36:1384–1395.
6. Cryer PE, Axelrod L, Grossman AB, et al.; Endocrine Society. Evaluation and management of adult hypoglycemic disorders: an Endocrine Society Clinical Practice Guideline. *J Clin Endocrinol Metab.* 2009;94:709–728.
7. Service FJ. Medical progress: hypoglycemic disorders. *N Engl J Med.* 1995;332(17):1144–1152.
8. Troisi RJ, Cowie CC, Harris MI. Diurnal variation in fasting plasma glucose: implications for diagnosis of diabetes in patients examined in the afternoon. *JAMA.* 2000;284:3157–3159.
9. American Diabetes Association. Tests of glycemia in diabetes. *Diabetes Care.* 2004;27(suppl 1):S91–S93.
10. Eckfeldt JH, Bruns DE. Another step towards standardization of methods for measuring hemoglobin A_{1c}. *Clin Chem.* 1997;43(10):1811–1813.
11. Nathan DM, Kuenen J, Borg R, et al. Translating the A1C assay into estimated average glucose values. *Diabetes Care.* 2008;31:1473–1478.
12. Kilpatrick ES, Rigby AS, Atkin SL. Variability in the relationship between mean plasma glucose and HbA_1c:

implications for the assessment of glycemic control. *Clin Chem.* 2007;53:897–901.
13. American Diabetes Association. Standards of medical care in diabetes—2016. *Diabetes Care.* 2016;39(suppl 1):S1–S109.
14. Jeppsson JO, Kobold U, Barr J, et al. International Federation of Clinical Chemistry and Laboratory Medicine (IFCC): Approved IFCC reference method for the measurement of HbA1c in human blood. *Clin Chem Lab Med.* 2002;40:78–89.
15. Geistanger A, Arends S, Berding C, et al. Statistical methods for monitoring the relationship between the IFCC reference measurement procedure for hemoglobin A1c and the designated comparison methods in the United States, Japan, and Sweden. *Clin Chem.* 2008;54:1379–1385.
16. Weykamp CW, Mosca A, Gillery P, et al. The analytical goals for hemoglobin A1c measurement in IFCC units and National Glycohemoglobin Standardization Program units are different. *Clin Chem.* 2011;57:1204–1206.
17. Weykamp C, John G, Gillery P, et al. Investigation of 2 models to set and evaluate quality targets for Hb A1c: biological variation and sigmametrics. *Clin Chem.* 2015;61:752–759.
18. Braga F, Panteghini M. Standardization and analytical goals for glycated hemoglobin measurement. *Clin Chem Lab Med.* 2013;51(9):1719–1726.
19. American Diabetes Association. Microvascular complications and foot care. Sec. 9. In Standards of Medical Care in Diabetes-2016. *Diabetes Care.* 2016;39(suppl 1):S72–S66, S80.
20. Sacks DB, Arnold M, Bakris GL, et al. Guidelines and recommendations for laboratory analysis in the diagnosis and management of diabetes mellitus. *Clin Chem.* 2011;57:p.e1–p.e47. Published May 26, 2011.
21. National Kidney Foundation. KDOQI Clinical Practice Guideline for Diabetes and CKD: 2012 update. *Am J Kidney Dis.* 2012;60(5):850–886.

15

Lipids and Lipoproteins

RAFFICK A. R. BOWEN, AMAR A. SETHI,
G. RUSSELL WARNICK, and ALAN T. REMALEY

chapter outline

key terms

Arteriosclerosis
Cholesterol
Chylomicrons
Dyslipidemias
Endogenous pathway
Exogenous pathway
Fatty acids
Friedewald equation
HDL
LDL
Lipoprotein
Lp(a)
Phospholipids
Triglycerides
VLDL

chapter objectives

Upon completion of this chapter, the clinical laboratorian should be able to do the following:

• Explain lipoprotein physiology and metabolism.

For additional student resources, please visit thePoint®
at http://thepoint.lww.com

chapter objectives (continued)

- Describe the structure of fatty acids, phospholipids, triglycerides, cholesterol, and the various types of lipoprotein particles.
- Describe the laboratory tests used to assess lipids and lipoproteins, including principles and procedures.
- Identify common lipid disorders from clinical and laboratory data.
- Discuss the incidence and types of lipid and lipoprotein abnormalities.
- Identify the reference ranges for the major serum lipids.
- Relate the clinical significance of lipid and lipoprotein values in the assessment of coronary heart disease.
- Describe the role of standardization in the measurement of lipids and lipoproteins.

Lipoproteins constitute the body's "petroleum industry." Like the great oil tankers that travel the oceans of the world transporting petroleum for fuel needs, chylomicrons are large, lipid-rich transport vessels that ferry their cargo dietary triglycerides, the main oil in the body, throughout the circulatory system to peripheral tissues, finally docking when nearly empty at the liver as chylomicron remnants. The very-low-density lipoproteins (**VLDLs**) are like tanker trucks, redistributing dietary and hepatic synthesized triglycerides to peripheral cells mostly during fasting for energy needs or storage as fat. The low-density lipoproteins (**LDLs**), rich in cholesterol, which start out as VLDLs, are like nearly empty tankers that just deliver cholesterol to peripheral cells and return to the liver after their main cargo triglycerides have been off-loaded. The high-density lipoproteins (**HDLs**) are the cleanup crew, gathering up excess cholesterol for transport back to the liver. Cholesterol is used by the body for such useful functions as facilitating triglyceride transport by lipoproteins and maintaining the normal structure and integrity of cell membranes and as a precursor for steroid hormone synthesis, but when in excess, it can lead to cardiovascular disease.

Lipids and lipoproteins, which are central to the energy metabolism of the body, have become increasingly important in clinical practice, primarily because of their association with coronary heart disease (CHD). Numerous epidemiologic studies have demonstrated that, especially in affluent countries with high fat consumption, there is a clear association between the blood lipid levels and the development of atherosclerosis. Decades of basic research have also contributed to knowledge about the nature of the lipoproteins and their lipid and protein constituents, as well as their role in the pathogenesis of the atherosclerotic process.

The accurate measurement of the various lipid and lipoprotein parameters is critical in the diagnosis and treatment of patients with **dyslipidemia**. International efforts to reduce the impact of CHD on public health have focused attention on improving the reliability and convenience of the lipid and lipoprotein assays. Expert panels have developed guidelines for the detection and treatment of high cholesterol, as well as laboratory performance goals of accuracy and precision for the measurement of the lipid and lipoprotein analytes. This chapter begins with a review of lipid chemistry and

lipoprotein metabolism, followed by the diagnosis and treatment of dyslipidemia. Finally, the clinical laboratory measurement of lipids and lipoproteins will be discussed in the context of various national and international guidelines, such as from the National Cholesterol Education Program (NCEP).

LIPID CHEMISTRY

Lipids, commonly referred to as fats, are ubiquitous constituents of all living cells and have a dual role. First, because they are composed of mostly carbon–hydrogen (C–H) bonds, they are a rich source of energy and an efficient way for the body to store excess calories. Because of their unique physical properties, lipids are also an integral part of cell membranes and, therefore, also play an important structural role in cells. Lipids are also precursors for the steroid hormones, prostaglandins, leukotrienes, and lipoxins. The lipids transported by lipoproteins, namely, triglycerides, phospholipids, cholesterol, and cholesteryl esters, are also the principal lipids found in cell membranes and intracellular lipid droplets and the main focus of this section.

Fatty Acids

Fatty acids, as seen in the structure shown in Figure 15.1, are simply linear chains of C–H bonds that terminate with a carboxyl group (–COOH). In plasma, only a relatively small amount of fatty acids exists in the free or unesterified form, most of which are noncovalently bound to albumin. The majority of plasma fatty acids are instead found as a constituent of triglycerides or phospholipids (Fig. 15.1). Fatty acids are covalently attached to the glycerol backbone of triglycerides and phospholipids by an ester bond that forms between the carboxyl group on the fatty acid and the hydroxyl group (–OH) on glycerol (Fig. 15.1). Fatty acids are variable in length and can be classified as short-chain (4 to 6 carbon atoms), medium-chain (8 to 12 carbon atoms), long-chain (12 to 18 carbon atoms), or very-long-chain (>20 carbon atoms) fatty acids. Most fatty acids in our diet are of the long-chain variety and contain an even number of carbon atoms, such as palmitic acid (16 carbons) and stearic, oleic, linoleic, and linolenic acids (18 carbons). Not all of the carbon atoms in fatty acids are fully saturated or, in other words, bonded with hydrogen atoms; some of

Saturated fatty acid

cis Unsaturated fatty acid

Glycerol

Triglyceride

Phospholipid (phosphatidylcholine)

Cholesterol

Bile acid (cholic acid)

FIGURE 15.1 Chemical structures of lipids. Fatty acids are abbreviated as (R) for triglycerides and phospholipids.

them may instead form unsaturated carbon–carbon (C=C) double bonds. Depending on the number of C=C double bonds, fatty acids can be classified as being saturated (no double bonds) like palmitic acid, monounsaturated (one double bond) like oleic acid, or polyunsaturated (two or more double bonds) like linoleic and linolenic acids. The C=C double bonds of unsaturated fatty acids are typically arranged in the cis configuration, with both hydrogen atoms on the same side of the C=C double bond, which causes a bend in their molecular structure (Fig. 15.1). These bends increase the space that unsaturated fatty acids require when packed in a lipid layer, and as a result, these fatty acids are more fluid because they do not as readily self-associate and pack together tightly. Fatty acid C=C double bonds can also occur in the trans configuration, with both hydrogen atoms on opposite sides of the C=C double bond. Because of the spatial orientation of their double bonds, trans fatty acids do not bend and have physical properties more similar to saturated fatty acids. The trans fatty acids are not commonly found in nature; however, they are present in our diet because of the chemical hydrogenation treatment used in food processing to increase the viscosity of oils (harden fat) by converting polyunsaturated plant oils into solid margarine, which introduces trans double bonds. The major dietary trans fatty acid is elaidic acid, an 18-carbon fatty acid with one double bond. Both metabolic and

epidemiological studies have shown that the consumption of trans fatty acids increases the risk of CHD and hence the recent public health measures to reduce the content of trans fatty acids in our foods. The adverse effects of trans fatty acids are mostly attributed to an elevation of LDL and a decrease in HDL.[1] Most fatty acids are synthesized in the body from carbohydrate precursors, except linoleic and linolenic acids, which are referred to as essential fatty acids.[2] These two fatty acids are found in plants and must be ingested in the diet. Both of these essential fatty acids are important for growth, maintenance, and proper functioning of many physiological processes.

The polyunsaturated fatty acids are classified into omega-3, omega-6, and omega-9 families, depending on the position of the first double bond from the terminal (omega) methyl group of the fatty acid chain. Polyunsaturated fatty acids are precursors for the synthesis of eicosanoids that include prostaglandins, thromboxanes, prostacyclins, and leukotrienes. These fatty acids play a vital role in the structure and function of most biological membranes, and some fatty acids like omega-3 polyunsaturated fatty acids found in fish oils are beneficial in lowering the risk of cardiovascular disease.

Triglycerides

As can be inferred from the name, **triglycerides** contain three fatty acid molecules attached to one molecule of glycerol by ester bonds in one of three stereochemically distinct bonding positions, referred to as sn-1, sn-2, and sn-3 (Fig. 15.1). Each fatty acid in the triglyceride molecule can potentially be different in structure, thus producing many possible types of triglycerides. Triglycerides containing saturated fatty acids, which do not have bends in their structure (Fig. 15.1), pack together more closely and tend to be solid at room temperature. In contrast, triglycerides, containing cis unsaturated fatty acids (Fig. 15.1), typically form oils at room temperature. Most triglycerides from plant sources, such as corn, sunflower seeds, and safflower seeds, are rich in polyunsaturated fatty acids and are oils, whereas triglycerides from animal sources contain mostly saturated fatty acids and are usually solid at room temperature. As can be seen by inspecting the structure of triglycerides (Fig. 15.1), there are no charged or polar hydrophilic groups, making it very hydrophobic and virtually water insoluble. Because it is uncharged, triglyceride is classified as a neutral lipid.

Phospholipids

Phospholipids are similar in structure to triglycerides except that they only have two esterified fatty acids (Fig. 15.1). The third position on the glycerol backbone instead contains a phospholipid head group. There are several types of phospholipid head groups, such as choline, inositol, inositol phosphates, glycerol, serine, and ethanolamine, which are all hydrophilic in nature. The various types of phospholipids are named based on the type of phospholipid head group present. Phosphatidylcholine (often referred as lecithin) (Fig. 15.1) has a choline head group and is the most common phospholipid found on lipoproteins and in cell membranes. The two asymmetrically positioned fatty acids in phospholipids are typically 14 to 24 carbon atoms long, with one fatty acid commonly saturated and the other unsaturated most commonly in the sn-2 position.

Because phospholipids contain both hydrophobic fatty acid C–H chains and a hydrophilic head group, they are by definition amphipathic lipid molecules and, as such, are found on the surface of lipid layers or on the surface of lipoprotein particles. The polar hydrophilic head group faces outward toward the aqueous environment, whereas the fatty acid chains face inward away from the water in a perpendicular orientation with respect to the lipid surface. Phospholipids are synthesized in the cytosolic compartment of all organs of the body, especially in the liver, with phosphatidylcholine and phosphatidylethanolamine being the most abundant phospholipids in the body.

Cholesterol

Cholesterol is an unsaturated steroid alcohol containing four rings (A, B, C, and D), and it has a single C–H side chain tail similar to a fatty acid in its physical properties (Fig. 15.1). The only hydrophilic part of cholesterol is the hydroxyl group in the A-ring. Cholesterol is, therefore, also an amphipathic lipid and is found on the surface of lipid layers along with phospholipids. Cholesterol is oriented in lipid layers so that the four rings and the side chain tail are buried in the membrane in a parallel orientation to the fatty acid acyl chains on adjacent phospholipid molecules. The polar hydroxyl group on the cholesterol A-ring faces outward, away from the lipid layer, allowing it to interact with water by noncovalent hydrogen bonding or with the polar head groups of phospholipids.

Cholesterol can also exist in an esterified form called cholesteryl ester, with the hydroxyl group conjugated by an ester bond to a fatty acid, in the same way as in triglycerides. In contrast to free cholesterol, there are no polar groups on cholesteryl esters, making them very hydrophobic. Because it is not charged, cholesteryl esters are also classified as a neutral lipid and are not found on the surface of lipid layers but instead are located in the center of intracellular lipid droplets or in the hydrophobic core of lipoproteins, along with triglycerides.

Cholesterol is almost exclusively synthesized by animals, but plants do contain other sterols (called phytosterols) similar in structure to cholesterol. Dietary phytosterols are known to lower plasma total cholesterol and LDL cholesterol (LDL-C) and raise HDL cholesterol (HDL-C) levels most likely by competing with the intestinal absorption of cholesterol.

Cholesterol is synthesized in most tissues of the body from acetyl-CoA in the microsomal and cytosolic compartments of the cell. More than 25 enzymes are involved in the formation of cholesterol from acetyl-CoA. The principal steps include the conversion of acetyl-CoA derived from either the β-oxidation of fatty acids or the oxidative decarboxylation of pyruvate to β-hydroxy β-methyl glutaryl CoA (HMG-CoA).[3] HMG-CoA is then converted to mevalonic acid by the enzyme HMG-CoA reductase, the rate-limiting enzyme in cholesterol biosynthesis.[3] Mevalonic acid is phosphorylated, isomerized, and converted to geranyl- and farnesyl pyrophosphate, which, in turn, forms squalene.[3] Cyclization of squalene occurs with oxidation, methyl group transfer reactions, saturation of the side chain, and double bond shifting to produce cholesterol.[3]

Cholesterol is also unique in that, unlike other lipids, it is not readily catabolized by most cells and, therefore, does not serve as a source of fuel. Cholesterol can, however, be converted in the liver to primary bile acids, such as cholic acid (Fig. 15.1) and chenodeoxycholic acid, which promote fat absorption in the intestine by acting as detergents. A small amount of cholesterol can also be converted by some tissue, such as the adrenal gland, testis, and ovary, to steroid hormones, such as glucocorticoids, mineralocorticoids, and estrogens. Finally, a small amount of cholesterol, after first being converted to 7-dehydrocholesterol, can also be transformed to vitamin D_3 in the skin by irradiation from sunlight.

GENERAL LIPOPROTEIN STRUCTURE

The prototypical structure of a lipoprotein particle is shown in Figure 15.2. Lipoproteins are typically spherical in shape and range in size from as small as 10 nm to more than 1 μm (Table 15.1) As the name implies, lipoproteins are

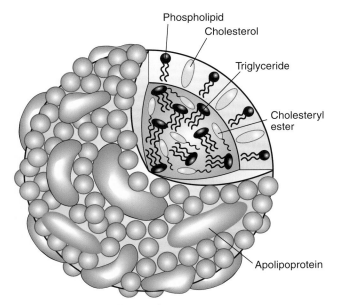

Phospholipid
Cholesterol
Triglyceride
Cholesteryl ester
Apolipoprotein

FIGURE 15.2 Model of lipoprotein structure.

composed of both lipids and proteins, called apolipoproteins. The amphipathic cholesterol and phospholipid molecules are primarily found on the surface of lipoproteins as a single monolayer, whereas the hydrophobic and neutral triglyceride and cholesteryl ester molecules are found in the central or core region and thus are micelles (Fig. 15.2). Because the main role of lipoproteins is the delivery of fuel to peripheral cells, the core of the lipoprotein particle essentially represents the cargo that is being transported by lipoproteins. The size of the lipoprotein particle correlates with its core neutral lipid content. The larger lipoprotein particles have correspondingly larger core regions and, therefore, contain relatively more triglyceride and cholesteryl ester. The larger lipoprotein particles also contain more lipid relative to protein and thus are lighter in density. The various lipoprotein particles were originally separated by ultracentrifugation into different density fractions (chylomicrons [chylos], VLDL, LDL, and HDL), which still form the basis for the most commonly used lipoprotein classification system (Table 15.1).

Apolipoproteins are primarily located on the surface of lipoprotein particles (Table 15.2). They help maintain the structural integrity of lipoproteins and also serve as ligands for cell receptors and as activators and inhibitors of the various enzymes that modify lipoprotein particles (Table 15.2). Apolipoproteins contain a structural motif called an amphipathic alpha helix, which accounts for the ability of these proteins to bind to lipids. Amphipathic helices are protein segments arranged in coils so that the hydrophobic amino acid residues interact with lipids, whereas the part of the helix containing hydrophilic amino acids faces away from the lipids and toward the aqueous environment.

Apolipoprotein (apo) A-I, the major protein of HDL, is frequently used as a measure of the amount of the antiatherogenic HDL present in plasma.[4] Apo B is a large protein with a molecular weight of approximately 500 kD and the principal protein of LDL, VLDL, and chylomicrons.[5] Apo B exists in two forms: apo B-100 and apo B-48. Apo B-100 is found in LDL and VLDL and is a ligand for the LDL receptor,[6] and it is, therefore, critical in the uptake of LDL by cells. Apo B-48, exclusively found in chylomicrons, is essentially the first 48% or half of the apo B molecule and is produced by posttranscriptional editing of the apo B-100 mRNA found in chromosome 2.[7] Apo B also contains amphipathic alpha helices but unlike other apolipoproteins also contain amphipathic beta sheets that avidly bind to lipids. Apo B-100 can also be found covalently linked to apo (a),[8] a plasminogen-like protein that is found in a proatherogenic lipoprotein particle called lipoprotein (a) [**Lp(a)**]. Apo E, another important apolipoprotein found in many types of lipoproteins (LDL, VLDL, and HDL), also serves as a ligand for the LDL receptor and the chylomicron remnant receptor. There are three major isoforms of apo E: apo E2, E3, and E4. The apo E isoforms affect lipoprotein metabolism because they differ in their ability to interact with the LDL receptor. For example, patients who are homozygous for the apo E2 isoform are at an increased risk for developing type III hyperlipoproteinemia and have low affinity for the LDL receptor. The connection with lipid metabolism is not completely understood, but individuals with the apo E4 isoform have higher affinity for the LDL receptor and have been shown to have an increased risk of developing Alzheimer's disease.[10,11]

Chylomicrons

Chylomicrons, which contain apo B-48, are the largest and the least dense of the lipoprotein particles, having diameters

Characteristics	CHYLOS	VLDL	LDL	HDL
Density (g/mL)	<0.93	0.93–1.006	1.019–1.063	1.063–1.21
Molecular weight (kD)	$(0.4–30) \times 10^9$	$(10–80) \times 10^6$	2.75×10^6	$(1.75–3.6) \times 10^5$
Diameter (nm)	80–1,200	30–80	18–30	5–12
Total lipid (% by weight)	98	89–96	77	50
Triglycerides (% by weight)	84	44–60	11	3
Total cholesterol (% by weight)	7	16–22	62	19

TABLE 15.1 Characteristics of the Major Human Lipoproteins

CHYLOS, chylomicrons; VLDL, very-low-density lipoprotein; LDL, low-density lipoprotein; HDL, high-density lipoprotein.

TABLE 15.2 Characteristics of the Major Human Apolipoproteins

Apolipoprotein	Molecular Weight (kD)	Plasma Concentration (mg/dL)	Major Lipoprotein Location	Function
Apo A-I	28,000	100–200	HDL	Structural, LCAT activator, ABCA1 lipid acceptor
Apo A-II	17,400	20–50	HDL	Structural
Apo A-IV	44,000	10–20	Chylos, VLDL, HDL	Structural
Apo B-100	5.4×10^5	70–125	LDL, VLDL	Structural, LDL receptor ligand
Apo B-48	2.6×10^5	<5	Chylos	Structural, remnant receptor ligand
Apo C-I	6,630	5–8	Chylos, VLDL, HDL	Structural
Apo C-II	8,900	3–7	Chylos, VLDL, HDL	Structural, LPL cofactor
Apo C-III	9,400	10–12	Chylos, VLDL, HDL	Structural, LPL inhibitor
Apo E	34,400	3–15	VLDL, HDL	Structural, LDL receptor ligand
Apo(a)	$(3–7) \times 10^5$	<30	Lp(a)	Structural, plasminogen inhibitor

HDL, high-density lipoprotein; Chylos, chylomicrons; LCAT, lecithin–cholesterol acyltransferase; VLDL, very-low-density lipoprotein; LDL, low-density lipoprotein; LPL, lipoprotein lipase.

as large as 1,200 nm[9] (Table 15.1). Because of their large size, they scatter light, which accounts for the turbidity or milky appearance of postprandial plasma. Because they are so light, they also readily float to the top of plasma when stored for hours or overnight at 4°C and form a creamy layer. Chylomicrons are produced by the intestine, where they are packaged with absorbed dietary lipids and apolipoproteins. Once they enter the circulation, triglycerides and cholesteryl esters in chylomicrons are rapidly hydrolyzed by lipases, such as lipoprotein lipase (LPL), and, within a few hours, are transformed into chylomicron remnant particles, which are recognized by proteoglycans and remnant receptors in the liver, facilitating their uptake.[9] The principal role of chylomicrons is the delivery of dietary lipids to hepatic and peripheral cells.

Very-Low-Density Lipoproteins

VLDL is produced primarily by the liver and contains apo B-100, the main apolipoprotein, apo E, and apo Cs; like chylomicrons, they are also rich in triglycerides. They are the major carriers of endogenous (hepatic-derived) triglycerides and transfer triglycerides from the liver to peripheral tissue mostly during the fasting state for energy utilization and storage. Like chylomicrons, they also reflect light and account for most of the turbidity observed in fasting hyperlipidemic plasma specimens, although they do not form a creamy top layer like chylomicrons, because they are smaller and less buoyant (Table 15.1). Excess dietary intake of carbohydrate, saturated fatty acids, and trans fatty acids enhances the hepatic synthesis of triglycerides, which in turn increases VLDL production. Free fatty acids released into the circulation by adipocytes are avidly taken up by the liver, which also stimulates VLDL secretion.

Intermediate-Density Lipoproteins

Intermediate-density lipoproteins (IDLs), also referred to as VLDL remnants, normally only exist transiently during the conversion of VLDL to LDL. The triglyceride and cholesterol contents of IDL are intermediate between those of VLDL and LDL. Normally, the conversion of VLDL to IDL proceeds so efficiently that appreciable quantities of IDL usually do not accumulate in the plasma after an overnight fast; thus, IDLs are not typically present in high quantities in normal plasma. In patients with type III hyperlipoproteinemia (dysbetalipoproteinemia or broad beta disease), a rare inborn error of metabolism, elevated levels of IDLs can be found in plasma. This defect is due to an abnormal form of apo E that delays the clearance of IDL. Individuals with this disorder are at a significant risk for peripheral vascular disease (PVD) and coronary artery disease (CAD), presumably because these lipoprotein particles like LDL are damaging to the vessel wall.

Low-Density Lipoproteins

LDL primarily contains apo B-100 and is more cholesterol rich than other apo B–containing lipoproteins (Table 15.1). They form as a consequence of the lipolysis of VLDL. LDL is readily taken up by cells via the LDL receptor in the liver and peripheral cells. In addition, because LDL particles are significantly smaller than VLDL particles and chylomicrons, they can infiltrate into the extracellular space of the vessel wall, where they can be oxidized and taken up by macrophages through various scavenger receptors.[12] Macrophages that take up too much lipid become filled with intracellular lipid drops and turn into foam cells, which is the predominant cell type of fatty streaks, an early precursor of atherosclerotic plaques.

LDL particles can exist in various sizes and compositions and have been separated into as many as eight subclasses through density ultracentrifugation or gradient gel electrophoresis.[13–15] The LDL subclasses differ largely in their content of core lipids; the smaller particles are denser and have relatively more triglyceride than cholesteryl esters. Recently, there has been great interest in measuring LDL subfractions, because small, dense, LDL particles have been shown to be more proatherogenic and may be a better marker for CHD risk.

Lipoprotein (a)

Lp(a) particles are LDL-like particles that contain one molecule of apo (a) linked to apo B-100 by a single disulfide bond. Lp(a) particles are heterogeneous in both size and density, as a result of a differing number of repeating peptide sequences, called kringles, in the apo (a) portion of the molecule. Lp(a) is larger than LDL and has a higher lipid content and a slightly lower density. The concentration of Lp(a) is inversely related to the size of the isoform; the larger size isoforms are not as efficiently secreted from the liver. Plasma levels of Lp(a) vary widely among individuals in the general population but remain relatively constant within an individual. Lp(a) appears to be poorly cleared by the LDL receptor, but the kidney has been postulated as the site of removal.[16]

Elevated levels of Lp(a) (>30 mg/dL) are now known to increase the risk of premature CHD and stroke. Because the kringle domains of Lp(a) have a high level of homology with plasminogen, a precursor of plasmin that promotes clot lysis via fibrin cleavage, it has been proposed that Lp(a) may compete with plasminogen for binding sites on endothelium and on fibrin, thereby promoting clotting. Clinical studies have demonstrated increasing risk of both myocardial infarction and stroke with increasing Lp(a) concentration; however, the measurement of Lp(a) is often underutilized in clinical practice. Part of the reason is due to the fact that the accurate measurement of Lp(a) is difficult and specific therapies for reducing its concentration in blood are limited but several are in development. Measuring Lp(a) is recommended for patients with a strong family history of CHD, particularly in the absence of other known risk factors, such as increased LDL-C, or for patients that develop CHD on statin therapy or for patients with premature aortic stenosis, which has been shown to be caused by high Lp(a) levels.

High-Density Lipoproteins

HDL, the smallest and most dense lipoprotein particle, is synthesized by both the liver and the intestine (Table 15.1). HDL can exist as either disk-shaped particles or, more commonly, spherical particles.[4] Discoidal HDL typically contains two molecules of apo A-I, which form a ring around a central lipid bilayer of phospholipid and cholesterol. Discoidal HDL is believed to represent nascent or newly secreted HDL and is the most active form in removing excess cholesterol from peripheral cells. The ability of HDL to remove cholesterol from cells, called reverse cholesterol transport, is one of the main mechanisms proposed to explain the antiatherogenic property of HDL. When discoidal HDL has acquired an additional lipid, cholesteryl esters and triglycerides form a core region between its phospholipid bilayer, which transforms discoidal HDL into spherical HDL. HDL is highly heterogeneous in size and lipid and protein composition and is separable into as many as 13 or 14 different subfractions. There are two major types of spherical HDL based on density differences: HDL_2 (1.063 to 1.125 g/mL) and HDL_3 (1.125 to 1.21 g/mL). HDL_2 particles are larger in size, less dense, and richer in lipid than HDL_3 and may be more efficient in the delivery of lipids to the liver.

Lipoprotein X

Lipoprotein X is an abnormal lipoprotein present in patients with biliary cirrhosis or cholestasis and in patients with mutations in lecithin–cholesterol acyltransferase (LCAT), the enzyme that esterifies cholesterol. Lipoprotein X is different from other lipoproteins in the endogenous pathway due to the lack of apo B-100. Phospholipids and nonesterified cholesterol are its main lipid components (~90% by weight) and albumin and apo C are the main protein components (<10% by weight). Lipoprotein X is mainly removed by the reticuloendothelial system of the liver and the spleen. Other organs, such as the kidney, also actively clear lipoprotein X from the plasma, which may account for renal disease in patients with genetic LCAT deficiency.[17] Lipoprotein X is typically included in the LDL-C value as calculated by the **Friedewald equation**, as well as in some direct methods for LDL-C but can be separated by LDL-C by ultracentrifugation.

LIPOPROTEIN PHYSIOLOGY AND METABOLISM

The four major pathways involved in lipoprotein metabolism are shown in Figure 15.3. The lipid absorption pathway, the **exogenous pathway**, and the **endogenous pathway** all depend on apo B–containing lipoprotein particles and can be viewed as the process to transport dietary lipid and hepatic-derived lipid to peripheral cells. In terms of energy metabolism, these three pathways are critical in the transport to peripheral cells of fatty acids, which are generated during the lipolysis of triglycerides and, to a lesser degree, cholesteryl esters on lipoproteins. In regard to the pathogenesis of atherosclerosis, the net result of these three pathways is the net delivery or forward transport of cholesterol to peripheral cells, which can lead to atherosclerosis when the cells in the vessel wall accumulate too much cholesterol. Peripheral cells are prone to accumulating cholesterol because they also synthesize their own cholesterol, and, unlike liver cells, they do not have the enzymatic pathways to catabolize cholesterol. Furthermore, cholesterol is relatively water insoluble and cannot readily diffuse away from its site of deposition or synthesis.

The principal way that peripheral cells maintain their cholesterol equilibrium is the reverse cholesterol transport pathway (Fig. 15.3), which is mediated by HDL. In this pathway, excess cholesterol from peripheral cells is

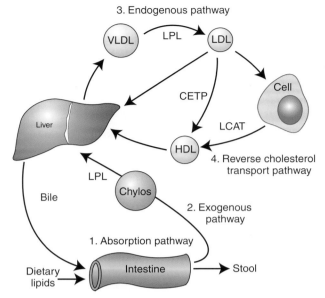

FIGURE 15.3 Diagram of major lipoprotein metabolism pathways.

transported back to the liver, where it can be excreted into the bile as free cholesterol or after being converted to bile acids. The liver is, therefore, involved in both forward and reverse cholesterol transport pathways and, in many ways, acts as a buffer in helping the body maintain its overall cholesterol homeostasis. There are several genetic defects in the genes that encode for proteins in the forward and reverse cholesterol transport pathways, which result in a predisposition for atherosclerosis. The majority of individuals with CAD, however, do not have a clear, single, genetic defect but instead have multiple genetic variations or gene polymorphisms that most likely interact with various lifestyle habits, such as exercise, diet, and smoking, leading to a predisposition for disease.

Lipid Absorption

Because fats are water insoluble, special mechanisms are required to facilitate the intestinal absorption of the 60 to 130 g of fat consumed per day in a typical Western diet. During the process of digestion, pancreatic lipase, by cleaving off fatty acids, first converts dietary lipids into more polar compounds with amphipathic properties. Thus, triglycerides are transformed into monoglycerides and diglycerides; cholesterol esters are transformed into free cholesterol; and phospholipids are transformed into lysophospholipids. These amphipathic lipids in the intestinal lumen form large aggregates with bile acids called micelles. Lipid absorption occurs when the micelles come in contact with the microvillus membranes of the intestinal mucosal cells. Absorption of some of these lipids may occur via a passive transfer process; however, recent evidence suggests that, in some cases, it might also be facilitated by specific transporters, such as the NPC1L-1 transporter for cholesterol. Short-chain free fatty acids, with 10 or fewer carbon atoms, can readily pass directly into the portal circulation and are

carried by albumin to the liver. The absorbed long-chain fatty acids, monoglycerides, and diglycerides are reesterified in intestinal cells to form triglycerides and cholesteryl esters. The newly formed triglycerides and cholesteryl esters are then packaged into chylomicrons by the microsomal transfer protein, along with apo B-48.

Triglyceride absorption is efficient; greater than 90% of dietary triglycerides are taken up by the intestine. In contrast, only about half of the 500 mg of cholesterol in the typical diet is absorbed each day. Even a smaller fraction of plant sterols is absorbed by the intestine. Recently, a specific transport system, involving the ABCG5 and ABCG8 transporters, has been described that prevents excess absorption of dietary cholesterol and plant sterols. Individuals with defective ABCG5 or ABCG8 transporters have a disease called sitosterolemia and have a predisposition for atherosclerosis and xanthomatosis because of increased cholesterol and plant sterol absorption.[18] ABCG5 and ABCG8 are also present in the liver and defects in these proteins also impair the elimination of plant sterols into bile for removal from the body.[19]

Exogenous Pathway

The newly synthesized chylomicrons in the intestine (Fig. 15.3) are initially secreted into the lacteals and then pass into the lymphatic ducts and eventually enter the circulation by way of the thoracic duct. After entering the circulation, chylomicrons interact with proteoglycans, such as heparin sulfate, on the luminal surface of capillaries in various tissues, such as skeletal muscle, heart, and adipose tissue. The proteoglycans along with a specific protein called GPIHBPI on capillaries also promote the binding of LPL,[20] which hydrolyzes triglycerides on chylomicrons. The free fatty acids and glycerol generated by the hydrolysis of triglycerides by LPL can then be taken up by cells and used as a source of energy. Excess fatty acids, particularly in fat cells (adipocytes), are reesterified into triglycerides for long-term energy storage in intracellular lipid drops. A key protein in triglyceride metabolism is apo C-II, which is found on VLDL and is critical in the activation of LPL. Hormone-sensitive lipase, another lipase that is found inside adipose cells, releases free fatty acids from triglycerides in stored fat, during fasting, when energy sources from carbohydrates are insufficient for the body's energy needs. The hormones epinephrine and cortisol play a key role in the mobilization and hydrolysis of triglycerides from adipocytes, whereas insulin right after a meal prevents lipolysis by adipocytes and promotes fat storage and glucose utilization.

During lipolysis of chylomicrons, there is a transfer of lipid (mainly triglyceride) and apolipoproteins (apo A-I and C-II) onto HDL, and chylomicrons are converted within a few hours after a meal into chylomicron remnant particles. Chylomicron remnants are rapidly taken up by the liver through interaction of apo E with the LDL receptor and another receptor on the surface of liver cells called LDL-related receptor protein.[21] Once in the liver, lysosomal enzymes break down the remnant particles to release free fatty acids, free cholesterol, and amino acids. Some cholesterol is converted to bile acids. Both bile acids and free cholesterol are directly excreted into the bile, but not all of the excreted cholesterol and bile salt exit the body. As previously described, approximately half of the excreted biliary cholesterol is reabsorbed by the intestine, with the remainder appearing in the stool, as fecal neutral steroids. In the case of bile acids, almost all of the bile acids are reabsorbed and reused by the liver for bile production.

Endogenous Pathway

Most triglycerides in the liver that are packaged into VLDL are derived from the diet after recirculation from adipose tissue. Normally, only a small fraction is synthesized de novo in the liver from dietary carbohydrate. VLDL particles, once secreted into the circulation, undergo a lipolytic process similar to that of chylomicrons (Fig. 15.3). VLDL loses core lipids, causing dissociation and transfer of apolipoproteins and phospholipids to other lipoprotein particles like HDL, primarily by the action of LPL, resulting in the conversion of VLDL to denser particles, called IDLs or VLDL remnants. IDL persists for short periods of time and receives cholesterol esters from HDL in exchange for triglycerides via cholesteryl ester transport protein. As with chylomicron remnants, IDL is taken up by the liver via apo E and the LDL receptor and the triglyceride in IDL are removed by hepatic triglyceride lipase, located on hepatic endothelial cells, producing LDL. About half of VLDL is eventually completely converted to LDL, and the remainder is taken up as VLDL remnants by the liver remnant receptors.

LDL particles are the major lipoproteins responsible for the delivery of exogenous cholesterol to peripheral cells due to the efficient uptake of LDL by the LDL receptors.[16] LDL can pass between capillary endothelial cells and bind to LDL receptors on cell membranes that recognize apo B-100. Once bound to LDL receptors, they are endocytosed by cells and transported to the lysosome, where they are degraded. The triglycerides in LDL are converted by acid lipase into free fatty acids and glycerol and further metabolized by the cell for energy or are reesterified and stored in lipid drops for later use. Free cholesterol derived from degraded LDL can be used for membrane biosynthesis, and excess cholesterol is converted by acyl-CoA–cholesterol acyltransferase (ACAT) into cholesteryl esters and stored in intracellular lipid drops. The regulation of cellular cholesterol biosynthesis is, in part, coordinated by the availability of cholesterol delivered by the LDL receptor. Many enzymes in the cholesterol biosynthetic pathway (e.g., HMG-CoA reductase, the main target for the cholesterol-lowering statin-type drugs) are down-regulated, along with the LDL receptor, when there is excess cellular cholesterol by a complex mechanism involving both gene regulation and posttranscriptional gene regulation.

Abnormalities in LDL receptor function result in elevation of LDL in the circulation and lead to hypercholesterolemia and premature atherosclerosis. Patients who are heterozygous for a disease called familial hypercholesterolemia (FH), with an incidence of approximately 1:500, have only approximately half the normal LDL receptors, which results in decreased hepatic uptake of LDL by the liver and increased hepatic cholesterol biosynthesis. The LDL that accumulates in the plasma of these individuals often leads to the development of CHD by midadulthood in heterozygotes and even earlier for homozygotes.

Individuals can be classified into two distinct phenotypes based on LDL, namely, types A and B. Type A individuals have large buoyant LDL particles, whereas in type B, LDL particles are smaller.[22] Elevated VLDL is associated with an exchange of VLDL triglycerides for cholesterol esters in HDL, resulting in triglyceride-rich HDL with decreased cholesterol content.[22] Cholesterol esters in LDL are also exchanged for VLDL triglycerides.[22] The triglycerides in LDL and HDL are subsequently removed by the action of lipases, producing smaller, more dense cholesterol-containing particles.[22] Small, dense LDL particles have been found to be an independent predictor of CHD and is also associated with increased risk of metabolic syndrome, which is a group of interrelated metabolic risk factors that appear to promote the development of atherosclerotic cardiovascular disease.[22] Small, dense LDL particles have a longer half-life in circulation than normal LDL and are more likely to be modified and taken up by scavenger receptors on macrophage, which will develop into foam cells, one of the critical steps in the development of atheroma.[22] It is difficult, however, to define the degree of increased risk with small, dense LDL particles quantitatively because of the common association between small LDLs with other risk factors of atherogenic dyslipidemia.

Reverse Cholesterol Transport Pathway

As previously described, one of the major roles of HDL is to maintain the equilibrium of cholesterol in peripheral cells by the reverse cholesterol transport pathway (Fig. 15.3). HDL is believed to remove excess cholesterol from cells by multiple pathways. In the aqueous diffusion pathway, HDL acts as a sink for the small amount of cholesterol that can diffuse away from the cells. Although cholesterol is relatively water insoluble, because it is an amphipathic lipid, it is soluble in plasma in micromolar amounts and can spontaneously dissociate from the surface of cell membranes and enter the extracellular fluid. Some free cholesterol will then bind to nascent HDL in the extracellular space, and once bound, it becomes trapped in lipoproteins after it is converted to cholesteryl ester by the enzyme LCAT, which resides on nascent HDL and is activated by its cofactor, apo A-I. The nascent HDL is first converted to HDL_3. The formation of cholesteryl ester via LCAT increases the capacity of the surface of HDL_3 particle to absorb more free cholesterol from cell membranes along with apo C-I, C-II, C-III, and E and phospholipids from VLDL and chylomicrons and is converted to HDL_2. HDL_2 can then directly deliver cholesterol to the liver by the scavenger receptor type B1 (SR-B1) and, possibly, other receptors. HDL particles can also transfer cholesteryl esters to chylomicrons and VLDL remnants to be transported to liver. Approximately half of the cholesterol on HDL is returned to the liver by the LDL receptor, after first being transferred from HDL to LDL by the cholesteryl ester transfer protein (CETP), which connects the forward and reverse cholesterol transport pathways (Fig. 15.3). Cholesterol that reaches the liver is then directly excreted into the bile or first converted to a bile acid before excretion.

Another pathway in which HDL mediates the removal of cholesterol from cells involves the ABCA1 transporter. The ABCA1 transporter is a member of the ATP-binding cassette transporter family,[23] which pumps various ligands across the plasma membrane. Defects in the gene for the ABCA1 transporter lead to Tangier disease, a disorder associated with low HDL and a predisposition to premature CHD.[24] The exact substrate for the ABCA1 transporter is not known, but it is believed that the transporter modifies the plasma membrane by transferring a lipid, which then enables apo A-I that has dissociated from HDL to bind to the cell membrane. In a detergent-like extraction mechanism, apo A-I then removes excess cholesterol and phospholipid from the plasma membrane of cells to form a discoidal-shaped HDL particle. The newly formed HDL is then competent to accept additional cholesterol by the aqueous diffusion pathway and is eventually converted into spherical HDL by the action of LCAT (Fig. 15.3). Recently, ABCG1, ABCG5 and ABCG8, which are other ABC transporters, have been described to facilitate the efflux of cholesterol to lipid-rich spherical HDL via a mechanism that appears to be different than the ABCA1 transporter.[25]

The ability of the body to remove excess cholesterol has for decades been measured in vitro using a cell-based assay, which tests the capacity of cholesterol-loaded macrophages to efflux cholesterol through the ABCA1 transporter.[26] This test provides additional knowledge about the function of the HDL particle beyond the HDL-C measurement. Recently, it was reported that efflux capacity, independent of HDL-C levels, was inversely correlated with intima–media thickness and the presence of CHD.[27] In fact, efflux capacity was a better predictor of disease status than conventional risk factors such as diabetes, smoking, LDL-C, and hypertension.[27] The importance of the efflux capacity was also reported in a population-based study where low levels were associated with incident atherosclerotic cardiovascular disease suggesting an impaired efflux capacity in the investigated subjects.[28]

LIPID AND LIPOPROTEIN POPULATION DISTRIBUTIONS

Serum lipoprotein concentrations differ between adult men and women, primarily as a result of differences in sex hormone levels, with women having, on average, higher

TABLE 15.3 **Adult Reference Ranges For Lipids**

Analyte	Reference Range
Total cholesterol	140–200 mg/dL (3.6–5.2 mmol/L)
HDL-C	40–75 mg/dL (1.0–2.0 mmol/L)
LDL-C	50–130 mg/dL (1.3–3.4 mmol/L)
Triglycerides	60–150 mg/dL (0.7–1.7 mmol/L)

HDL-C, high-density lipoprotein cholesterol; LDL-C, low-density lipoprotein cholesterol.

HDL-C levels and lower total cholesterol and triglyceride levels than men. The difference in total cholesterol, however, disappears after menopause as estrogen decreases. Men and women both show a tendency toward increased total cholesterol, LDL-C, and triglyceride concentrations with age. HDL-C concentrations generally remain stable after the onset of puberty and do not drop in women with the onset of menopause. General adult reference ranges are shown in Table 15.3.

Circulating levels of total cholesterol, LDL-C, and triglycerides in young children are generally much lower than those seen in adults.[29] In addition, concentrations do not significantly differ between boys and girls. HDL-C levels for both boys and girls are comparable to those of adult women. At the onset of puberty, however, HDL-C concentrations in boys fall to adult male levels, a drop of approximately 20%, whereas those of girls do not significantly change. It is the lower concentration of HDL-C in men, combined with their higher LDL-C and triglyceride levels, which accounts for much of the increased risk of premature heart disease in men.

The incidence of heart disease is strongly associated with serum cholesterol concentration, particularly LDL-C. Comparisons across different societies show that eating less animal fat and more grains, fruits, and vegetables, as is common in many Asian populations, is associated with lower LDL-C and lower rates of heart disease compared with societies that ingest more fat, particularly animal fat, and are more sedentary. These differences can be attributed to both genetic and lifestyle factors in the various countries and ethnic groups. The importance of diet was clearly shown in a study that compared the dietary patterns and heart disease rates in Japanese men living in Japan, Hawaii, and California.[30] In this study, as dietary intake became more Westernized, with increased consumption of fat and cholesterol, the LDL-C concentrations increased, as did the rates of heart disease. Japanese men living in California were found to have much higher rates of heart disease than Japanese men living in Japan; those in Hawaii were intermediate. Within societies in which diet tends to be more homogeneous, LDL-C levels become somewhat less discriminatory as a risk factor, and HDL-C levels become more important as a negative risk factor.

CASE STUDY 15.1

A 52-year-old man went to his physician for a physical examination. The patient had been a district manager for an automobile insurance company for the past 10 years and was a 24-lb overweight. He had missed his last two appointments with the physician because of business. The urinalysis dipstick finding was not remarkable. His blood pressure was elevated. The blood chemistry results are listed in Case Study Table 15.1.1.

Laboratory Results

Analyte	Patient Value	Reference Range
Na^+	151	135–143 mmol/L
K^+	4.5	3.0–5.0 mmol/L
Cl^-	106	98–103 mmol/L
CO_2 content	13	22–27 mmol/L
Total protein	5.7	6.5–8.0 g/dL
Albumin	1.6	3.5–5.0 g/dL
Ca^{2+}	7.9	9.0–10.5 mg/dL
Cholesterol	210	140–200 mg/dL
Uric acid	6.2	3.5–7.9 mg/dL
Creatinine	2.5	0.5–1.2 mg/dL
BUN	95	7–25 mg/dL
Glucose	88	75–105 mg/dL
Total bilirubin	1.2	0.2–1.0 mg/dL
Alkaline phosphatase	27	7–59 IU/L
Lactate dehydrogenase	202	90–190 IU/L
Aspartate transaminase	39	8–40 IU/L
Amylase	152	76–375 IU/L

Questions

1. Given the abnormal tests, what additional information would you like to have?

2. If this patient had triglycerides of 100 mg/dL (1.1 mmol/L) and an HDL-C of 23 mg/dL (0.6 mmol/L), what would be his calculated LDL-C value?

3. If, however, his triglycerides were 476 mg/dL (5.4 mmol/L), with an HDL-C of 23 mg/dL (0.6 mmol/L), what would be his calculated LDL-C value?

The NCEP was formed to alert the American population to the risk factors associated with heart disease. The NCEP has used panels of experts, including Adult Treatment Panels (ATPs), the Children and Adolescents Treatment Panel, and the Laboratory Standardization Panel, to produce various recommendations.[31] In 1988, the first NCEP ATP developed a list of heart disease risk factors. These guidelines were most recently updated by ATP IV in 2013.[32]

In general, the ATP guidelines and other similar guidelines are based on the central tenant that lifestyle changes, such as a low-fat diet, increased physical activity, and weight control, should be the first-line treatment for all patients at risk for cardiovascular disease (CVD) but that more aggressive drug therapy should also be considered for the highest risk individuals and/or for those that do not respond to lifestyle changes. According to the new ATP IV guidelines,[32,33] patients at high risk for CVD (diabetics and preexisting CVD) or those with an LDL-C greater than 190 mg/dL are advised to initiate simultaneous lifestyle changes along with drug therapy, defined as high-dose statin in order to reduce LDL-C by 50% from baseline.[32,33] Lower-risk patients between age 40 and 75 should have their 10-year CVD risk calculated and be treated with high- or moderate-dose statin if their risk score is greater than 7.5% and moderate-dose statin when their risk score is between 5% and 7.5%. For those patients with a 10-year risk less than 5% or if they fall outside the age range for the risk calculator (<40 years or >75 years), only lifestyle changes would typically be recommended, but statins could be considered if they have other extenuating circumstances, such as a strong family history or at risk based on other risk marker like CRP. Repeat laboratory testing is recommended to monitor compliance and to determine if at least a 50% reduction in LDL-C is achieved, but there are no longer any specific treatment target goals for LDL-C like in past guidelines. The current list of risk factors used in calculating the 10-year risk of CVD is shown in Table 15.4. It is recommended that all adults (20 years and older) have a fasting lipoprotein profile performed (total cholesterol, LDL-C, and HDL-C and triglycerides) once every 5 years. As described below, the Children and Adolescents Treatment Panel has developed similar guidelines for CVD risk assessment in the pediatric population.[29]

Dyslipidemia and Children

It is well recognized and documented that the atherosclerotic process begins in childhood, with dyslipidemia as one of the main risk factors for cardiovascular disease (CVD). A recent analysis of National Health and Nutrition Examination Survey data collected between 1998 and 2010 estimated that 24.6% of US children aged 9 to 11 had either abnormally low HDL cholesterol or elevated non–HDL cholesterol.[34] Elevated total cholesterol, LDL-C, VLDL-C, and decreased HDL-C concentrations are significantly associated with early atherosclerotic lesions in adolescent and young adults.[35] Thus, early identification and treatment of children with hyperlipidemia is likely to delay the atherosclerotic process and reduce CVD risk in adulthood. Guidelines for the assessment and treatment of CVD risk in children and adolescents have been published by the National Heart, Lung, and Blood Institute (NHLBI).[29]

TABLE 15.4 Coronary Heart Disease Risk Factors Determined by the NCEP Adult Treatment Panels

Positive Risk Factors
- Age: ≥45 y for men; ≥55 y or premature menopause for women
- Family history of premature CHD
- Current cigarette smoking
- Hypertension (blood pressure ≥ 140/90 mm Hg or taking antihypertensive medication)
- LDL-C concentration ≥ 160 mg/dL (≥4.1 mmol/L), with ≤1 risk factor
- LDL-C concentration ≥ 130 mg/dL (3.4 mmol/L), with ≥2 risk factors
- LDL-C concentration ≥ 100 mg/dL (2.6 mmol/L), with CHD or risk equivalent
- HDL-C concentration < 40 mg/dL (<1.0 mmol/L)
- Diabetes mellitus = CHD risk equivalent
- Metabolic syndrome (multiple metabolic risk factors)

Negative Risk Factors
- HDL-C concentration ≥ 60 mg/dL (≥1.6 mmol/L)
- LDL-C concentration < 100 mg/dL (<2.6 mmol/L)

CHD, coronary heart disease; LDL-C, low-density lipoprotein cholesterol; HDL-C, high-density lipoprotein cholesterol.

National Cholesterol Education Program

The goal of the NCEP (created in 1985 by NHLBI) is to educate the public and medical professionals about the benefits of lowering cholesterol levels to reduce the risk of CHD. The NCEP published the first set of pediatric guidelines for dyslipidemia in 1992.[29] These guidelines had two approaches: both diet and lifestyle changes for all children and a targeted lipid screening for individual children with a family history of heart disease, FH, or familial combined hyperlipidemia (FCH).[29] Some considered the reliance of these guidelines on family history to be too restrictive, and several studies demonstrated a significant number of children with elevated cholesterol levels would have been missed by these guidelines. For example, the Coronary Artery Risk Detection in Appalachian Communities (CARDIAC) Project, which utilized universal screening, found that 36% of children with severe dyslipidemia would have been overlooked.[36]

National Heart, Lung, and Blood Institute

With childhood obesity on the rise and almost half of obese children having at least one abnormal lipid level, the NHLBI Expert panel in 2011 published a comprehensive updated evidence-based guideline for the identification, management, and treatment of all major CV risk factors (including diabetes, hypertension, cigarette smoking, and obesity) in pediatric patients.[29] Universal lipid screening of all children from 9 to 11 years and again at 17 to 21 years with a nonfasting, non–HDL-C levels and targeted lipid screening are both supported by the NHLBI guidelines and endorsed by the American Academy of Pediatrics.[29]

The 9 to 11 age range is important because that is when then atherosclerotic process appears to accelerate but before the decline in LDL-C seen with puberty. Universal screening is not recommended for children before 9 years of age due to insufficient information on the safety and impact of lipid-lowering medications.[29] The NCEP guidelines also recommend selective screening to identify children at high dyslipidemia risk with two fasting lipid profiles between 2 and 8 years and again between 12 and 16 years. NHLBI guidelines provide algorithms to assist clinicians with the screening process, risk factor management, and treatment of dyslipidemia.[29] The NHLBI universal screening recommendations for lipid abnormalities in children and adolescents are controversial, and some health care providers have resisted.[37] Acceptable lipid levels for nonfasting blood specimens for youth and young adults are shown in Table 15.5.[29] If a nonfasting lipid profile reveals

TABLE 15.5 Lipid Cut Points (mg/dL)

	For Youth <17 y			For Young Adults 17–21 y		
Category	Acceptable	Borderline*	High**	Acceptable[a]	Borderline[a]	High[a]
TC	<170	170–199	≥200	>190	190–225	≥200
LDL-C	<110	110–129	≥130	<120	120–160	≥130
Non–HDL-C	<120	120–144	≥145	<150	150–190	≥145
Triglycerides						
0–9 y	<75	75–99	≥100			
10–19 y	<90	90–129	≥130	<115	115–150	≥150
Category	**Acceptable**	**Borderline**	**Low***	**Acceptable**	**Borderline**	**Low**
HDL-C	>45	45–40	<40	>45	45–40	<40

Values represent approximately the *75th and **95th percentiles and approximately the ***10th percentile for low HDL-C.
[a]The cut points for TC, HDL-C, and non–HDL-C represent the 95th percentile for 20- to 24-year-old subjects; acceptable values are at the <75th percentile. For HDL-C, low is <25th percentile and acceptable values are >50th percentile.
HDL-C, high-density lipoprotein cholesterol; LDL-C, low-density lipoprotein cholesterol; TC, total cholesterol.
From Expert Panel on Integrated Guidelines for Cardiovascular Health and Risk Reduction in Children and Adolescents, National Heart, Lung, and Blood Institute. Expert panel on integrated guidelines for cardiovascular health and risk reduction in children and adolescents: summary report. *Pediatrics.* 2011;128(suppl 5):S213–S256.

	Precision	Bias	Total Error
Total cholesterol	3% CV	±3%	±8.9%
HDL-C			
≥42 mg/dL	4% CV	±5%	±12.8%
<42 mg/dL	SD	<1.7 mg/dL	
LDL-C	4% CV	±4%	±11.8%
Triglycerides	5% CV	±5%	±14.8%

TABLE 15.6 NCEP Analytic Performance Goals

CV, coefficient of variation; HDL-C, high-density lipoprotein cholesterol; SD, standard deviation; LDL-C, low-density lipoprotein cholesterol.

a non–HDL-C greater than 145 mg/dL, then two separate fasting lipid profiles should be done at least 2 weeks apart but within 3 months of each other and the results averaged to confirm the abnormality. If an initial fasting lipid profile reveals an LDL-C ≥130 mg/dL, then another fasting lipid profile should be obtained at least 2 weeks later but within 3 months and the results averaged. The NHLBI recommends that children identified with dyslipidemia should begin with diet and lifestyle changes along with patient education and progress to more stringent diet and lifestyle changes.[29] If dyslipidemia persists, then pharmacological treatment and/or referral to a lipid specialist may be recommended for children aged ≥10 years.[29] Likewise, children with a genetic dyslipidemia, such as FH, should also be referred to a lipid specialist for more aggressive-type therapy.[29] Future studies are needed, however, to firmly establish if treatment of hyperlipidemia early in life prevents CHD in adulthood.

The NCEP Laboratory Standardization Panel and its successor, the Lipoprotein Measurement Working Group,[38–40] set laboratory guidelines for acceptable precision and accuracy when measuring total cholesterol, triglycerides, and lipoprotein cholesterol (HDL-C and LDL-C) (Table 15.6).

Obviously, the best way to reduce the prevalence of heart disease is through prevention. Learning and practicing good dietary and exercise patterns early in life, maintaining these patterns throughout life,[41] refraining from smoking, and controlling blood pressure are important means for reducing the incidence of CHD and stroke. Lipoprotein profile measurements provide a method of identifying individuals who may have levels that put them at risk so that they can receive appropriate treatment. Treatment of other diseases that may affect lipoproteins, such as diabetes mellitus, hypothyroidism, and renal disease, is also important. A prudent diet, low in fat, with a caloric intake adjusted to meet and maintain ideal body weight, along with regular exercise, can significantly reduce the risk of heart disease, stroke, diabetes, and cancer.[42] Additionally, saturated fat is more atherogenic than unsaturated fat.[41] The American Heart Association has recommended dietary guidelines for the intake of fat and cholesterol for most adult Americans (Table 15.7).

TABLE 15.7 Composition of the Therapeutic Lifestyle Changes Diet Recommended by the NCEP Adult Treatment Panel III (Compared with the Average American Diet)

Dietary Nutrient	TLC Diet	Average American Diet
Total fat	25%–35%	36% (% total calories)
Saturated	<7%	15%
Monounsaturated	≤20%	15%
Polyunsaturated	≤10%	6%
Cholesterol		>400 mg/d
Carbohydrate	50%–60%	
Fiber	20–30 g/d	
Protein	<15%	

TLC, therapeutic lifestyle changes.

DIAGNOSIS AND TREATMENT OF LIPID DISORDERS

Diseases associated with abnormal lipid concentrations are referred to as dyslipidemias. They can be caused directly by genetic abnormalities or through environmental/lifestyle imbalances, or they can develop secondarily, as a consequence of other diseases. Dyslipidemias are generally defined by the clinical characteristics of patients and the results of laboratory tests and are not necessarily defined by the specific genetic defect associated with the abnormality. Many, but not all, dyslipidemias, regardless of etiology, are associated with CHD or arteriosclerosis.

Arteriosclerosis

In the United States and many other developed countries, **arteriosclerosis** is the single leading cause of death and disability. The mortality rate has leveled off and started to decrease in the United States in the past three decades, partly as a result of advances in diagnosis and treatment but also because of changes in lifestyle in the American population. This increased awareness of the importance of diet and exercise in preventing CHD has resulted in an overall decrease in the average serum cholesterol concentration and in a lower prevalence of heart disease; however, it still exceeds all other causes of death combined. Although as many women as men now develop arteriosclerosis, they typically develop it 10 years later than men, and unfortunately, it sometimes goes unrecognized because of lack of awareness and because symptoms of myocardial infarction are sometimes subtler in women.

The relationship between heart disease and dyslipidemias stems from the deposition of lipids, mainly in the form of esterified cholesterol, in artery walls. This lipid deposition first results in fatty streaks, which are thin streaks of excess fat in macrophages in the subendothelial space. Autopsy studies have shown that fatty streaks occur in almost everyone older than age 15.[43] Fatty streaks can develop over time into plaques that contain increased number of smooth muscle cells, extracellular lipid, calcification, and fibrous tissue, which can partially block or occlude blood flow. Also, established plaque for unknown reasons can become vulnerable to rupture or erosion, triggering a thrombosis that can block circulation. When plaque develops in arteries of the arms or legs, it is called PVD; when it develops in the heart, it is referred to as CAD; and, when it develops in the vessels of the brain, it is called cerebrovascular disease. CAD is associated with angina and myocardial infarction, and CVD is associated with stroke. Many genetic and acquired dyslipidemias may also lead to lipid deposits in the liver and kidney, resulting in impaired function of these vital organs. Lipid deposits in skin form nodules called xanthomas, which are often a clue to the presence of an underlying genetic abnormality.

Plaque formation involves repeated cycles of cell injury, followed by infiltration and cell proliferation to repair the site. LDL is believed to play a central role in initiating and promoting plaque formation. It is deposited into the subendothelial space where it is taken up by various cells, including macrophages. This alters the gene and protein expression pattern of these cells and can promote an inflammatory response, particularly when LDL becomes oxidized.[44] Injury signals from the evolving plaque trigger the expression of adhesion proteins on endothelial cells and the production of soluble chemotactic proteins from resident macrophages, which promotes the attachment and infiltration of additional macrophages, lymphocytes, and platelets to the plaque. Continual injury and repair lead to additional narrowing of the vessel opening, or lumen, causing the blood to circulate in a nonlaminar manner under greater and greater pressure, which further aggravates plaque formation. The final event leading to complete occlusion of blood flow occurs when there is a hemorrhage into the plaque, which results in the formation of a thrombus that blocks blood flow and precipitates a myocardial infarction.

CASE STUDY 15.2

A 30-year-old man with chest pain was brought to the emergency department after a softball game. He was placed in the coronary care unit when his ECG showed erratic waves in the ST region. A family history revealed that his father died of a heart attack at the age of 45 years. The patient had always been athletic in high school and college, so he had not concerned himself with a routine physical. The laboratory tests listed in Case Study Table 15.2.1 were run.

Laboratory Results		
Patient Analyte	Values	Range
Na$^+$	139	135–143 mmol/L
K$^+$	4.1	3.0–5.0 mmol/L
Cl$^-$	101	98–103 mmol/L
CO_2 content	29	22–27 mmol/L
Total protein	6.9	6.5–8.0 g/dL
Albumin	3.2	3.5–5.0 g/dL
Ca^{2+}	9.3	9.0–10.5 mg/dL
Cholesterol	278	140–200 mg/dL
Uric acid	5.9	3.5–7.9 mg/dL
Creatinine	1.1	0.5–1.2 mg/dL
BUN	20	7–25 mg/dL
Glucose	97	75–105 mg/dL
Total bilirubin	0.8	0.2–1.0 mg/dL
Alkaline phosphatase	20	7–59 IU/L
Lactate dehydrogenase	175	90–190 IU/L
Aspartate transaminase	35	8–40 IU/L
Amylase	98	76–375 IU/L

Questions

1. Given the symptoms and the family history, what additional tests should be recommended?

2. If his follow-up total cholesterol remains in the same range after he is released from the hospital, and his triglycerides and HDL-C are within the normal range, what course of treatment should be recommended?

Because lipid deposits in the vessel walls are frequently associated with increased serum concentrations of LDL-C, lowering LDL is an important step in preventing and treating CHD.[45–47] It is estimated that for every 1% decrease in LDL-C concentration, there is a 2% decrease in the risk of developing arteriosclerosis.[48] For patients with established heart disease, studies have shown that aggressive treatment to reduce LDL-C levels below 100 mg/dL (2.6 mmol/L) or even lower is effective in the stabilization and sometimes regression of plaques.[49] Stabilization of plaque is thought to be at least as important as plaque regression in terms of rupture potential.

In some individuals, high levels of blood cholesterol or triglycerides are caused by genetic abnormalities in which either too much is synthesized or too little is removed. High levels of cholesterol and/or triglycerides in most people, however, are a result of increased consumption of foods rich in fat and cholesterol, smoking, and lack of exercise or a result of other disorders or disease states that affect lipid metabolism, such as diabetes, hypertension, hypothyroidism, obesity, liver and kidney diseases, and alcoholism. Low levels of HDL-C are also associated with increased risk of heart disease, but there are currently limited ways to pharmacologically raise HDL-C levels and it is unclear to what degree low HDL is causal in the pathogenesis of atherosclerosis. Existing drugs for increasing HDL-C are primarily fibric acid derivatives (fibrates) and niacin-containing compounds, but recent studies have failed to show a clear benefit from raising HDL with these drugs.[50] Newer drugs that raise HDL-C by inhibiting CETP may play a role in the future, but so far, these drugs have also failed to show a benefit. Other drugs using reconstituted HDL particles or administration of apo A-I mimetic peptides is also being actively investigated.[51]

Laboratory analyses are an important adjunct to managing patients with dyslipidemia, because accurate measurement of total cholesterol, HDL-C, and LDL-C and triglyceride levels is needed to determine the most appropriate diet or diet and drug therapy. As shown in Table 15.8 from the older ATP III guidelines, individuals on a low-fat diet, who continue to have LDL-C levels of 190 mg/dL (4.9

mmol/L) or higher on repeated measurement, will likely benefit from drug intervention. If they have two or more CAD risk factors and continue to have LDL-C levels of 160 mg/dL (4.1 mmol/L) or higher, they also would benefit from drug therapy. And if they have already been previously diagnosed with heart disease, drug therapy should be considered when the LDL-C level is 130 mg/dL (3.4 mmol/L) or higher. The average of at least two measurements, taken 1 to 8 weeks apart, should be used to determine the best treatment approach.[31]

Classic bile acid sequestrant drug treatments, such as cholestyramine, colesevelam, and colestipol, work by sequestering cholesterol in the gut so that it is not absorbed; this action enhances conversion of cholesterol into bile acids in the liver, reduces hepatic cholesterol content, and enhances the activity of LDL receptors, and until recently, these were considered to be the only safe drugs for use in children.[48] These bile acid sequestrants lower LDL-C concentrations by 15% to 30% but may increase triglycerides.[52] It is important to note that these agents interfere with the absorption of fat-soluble vitamins and some drugs like digoxin, warfarin, and thyroid supplements, resulting in altered blood concentrations of

 TABLE 15.8 **Treatment Guidelines Established by the NCEP Adult Treatment Panels (Initial Testing Should Consist of Fasting for ≥12 Hours)**

Risk Category and Action

TC, <200 mg/dL (<5.2 mmol/L); TG, <150 mg/dL (<1.7 mmol/L); LDL-C, <130 mg/dL (<3.4 mmol/L); HDL-C, ≥40 mg/dL (≥1.0 mmol/L)
Repeat within 5 y
Provide risk reduction information
TC, 200–239 mg/dL (5.2–6.2 mmol/L); TG, 150–199 mg/dL (1.7–2.2 mmol/L); LDL-C, 130–159 mg/dL (3.4–4.1 mmol/L); HDL-C, ≥40 mg/dL (≥1.0 mmol/L); and 0–1 risk factors
Provide therapeutic lifestyle changes diet and physical activity information and reevaluate in 1 y
Provide risk reduction information
TC, ≥200 mg/dL (≥5.2 mmol/L); TG, ≥200 mg/dL (≥2.2 mmol/L); LDL-C, 130–159 mg/dL (3.4–4.1 mmol/L); HDL-C, <40 mg/dL (<1.0 mmol/L); and ≥2 risk factors
Do clinical evaluation, including family history
Start dietary therapy (see below)
TC, ≥240 mg/dL (6.2 mmol/L)
Perform lipoprotein (LDL-C) analysis (see below)

Treatment Decisions

Risk Category	Action Level	Goal
Dietary Therapy		
No CHD; 0–1 risk factors	≥160 mg/dL (4.1 mmol/L)	<160 mg/dL (4.1 mmol/L)
No CHD; ≥2 risk factors (10-y risk, ≥ 20%)	≥130 mg/dL (3.4 mmol/L)	<130 mg/dL (3.4 mmol/L)
CHD; CHD risk equivalent (10-y risk, >20%)	>100 mg/dL (2.6 mmol/L)	<100 mg/dL (2.6 mmol/L)
Drug Therapy		
No CHD; 0–1 risk factors	≥190 mg/dL (4.9 mmol/L)	<160 mg/dL (4.1 mmol/L)
No CHD; 2 risk factors (10-y risk, ≤10%)	≥160 mg/dL (4.1 mmol/L)	<130 mg/dL (3.4 mmol/L)
No CHD; ≥2 risk factors (10-y risk, 10%–20%)	≥130 mg/dL (4.1 mmol/L)	<100 mg/dL (3.4 mmol/L)
CHD; CHD risk equivalent	≥130 mg/dL (3.4 mmol/L)	<100 mg/dL (2.6 mmol/L)

CHD, coronary heart disease; HDL-C, high-density lipoprotein cholesterol; LDL-C, low-density lipoprotein cholesterol; TC, total cholesterol; TG, triglycerides.

these drugs and prothrombin times. Bile acid sequestrants are contraindicated in individuals with triglyceride levels greater than 400 mg/dL (4.5 mmol/L). Bile acid sequestrants have uncomfortable adverse effects such as bloating and constipation and are poorly tolerated.

The most effective class of drugs for managing patients with dyslipidemia are the HMG-CoA reductase drug inhibitors, such as lovastatin, atorvastatin, and rosuvastatin. These drugs, commonly known as statins, block intracellular cholesterol synthesis by inhibiting HMG-CoA reductase, a rate-limiting enzyme in cholesterol biosynthesis. The reduced level of cholesterol in hepatocytes increases the expression of the LDL receptor, which removes LDL from the circulation, thus reducing the deposition of LDL into vessels and the formation of plaques. All statins are probably identical in their main mechanism but differ in dose–response curves. The major safety issues with statins are myositis and hepatotoxic effects; however, patient monitoring in clinical trials has shown that fewer than 2% of patients have sustained increases in liver enzymes. Routine monitoring of serum transaminases is recommended and creatine kinase for patients complaining of muscle-related symptoms. These drugs typically reduce LDL-C by as much as 20% to 40%, raise HDL-C by 5% to 10%, and can lower triglyceride by 7% to 43%, depending on the initial triglyceride level.[45,53] Statins are generally well tolerated, with maximum effects observed after 4 to 6 weeks.[45,53] Clinical trials have shown that statin is beneficial for both the primary and secondary prevention of CHD.[31]

Niacin or nicotinic acid at high doses (~2 to 6 g/d) is also a potent drug for reducing LDL-C levels (by 5% to 25%) and is the only effective drug at this time for significantly raising HDL-C levels (by 15% to 35%).[54] Niacin can also lower triglyceride levels by 20% to 50%[55]; however, it causes flushing, pruritus, hyperuricemia, and diarrhea in many patients and can be hepatotoxic.[56] The precise mechanism of action for niacin is not known, although it appears to act in the liver to reduce the formation of LDL and VLDL by inhibiting lipolysis of triglyceride in adipose tissue and triglyceride synthesis in the liver. This action is sufficient to control severe hypertriglyceridemia. Newer slow-release formulations of niacin and combination drugs reduce incidence of flushing.[57]

Fibric acid derivatives, such as clofibrate, gemfibrozil, fenofibrate, and etofibrate, are most often used to reduce triglyceride by 20% to 50% and increase HDL-C levels by 10% to 20%.[50,56] The effects of fibric acid derivatives on LDL-C concentrations are less predictable and depend on the individual's level of triglyceride. Individuals receiving fibric acid agents should have liver function tests monitored, because these drugs are associated with elevations in transaminases, as well as creatine kinase for patients complaining of muscle ache. Patients on fibrates and warfarin should also have their prothrombin time monitored, because fibrates can displace warfarin from their protein-binding sites.[52]

Ezetimibe is a new drug that inhibits the absorption of cholesterol by inhibiting the Niemann-Pick C1-like 1 (NPC1-L1) transporter in the intestine without impacting the absorption of fat-soluble nutrients. Ezetimibe therapy has been shown to decrease LDL-C concentrations by approximately 20%.[58] Ezetimibe in conjunction with statins results in greater reductions in LDL-C concentration than with statin alone. As with the use of statin drugs, liver function tests should be performed on individuals taking ezetimibe.[58]

Fish oil products that contain omega-3 fatty acids, eicosapentaenoic and docosahexaenoic acids, can be used to lower triglyceride levels (up to 45%) and raise HDL-C (up to 13%) in patients, although the mechanism of action is not fully understood; it has been shown that fish oils decrease hepatic triglyceride synthesis[59] via inhibition of diacylglycerol acyltransferase, fatty acid synthase, and acetyl-CoA carboxylase enzyme activities. Fish oils also enhance fatty acid β-oxidation by stimulating peroxisome proliferator–activated receptors. In addition, fish oils decrease the hepatic pool of triglycerides by suppressing transcription of the SREBP-1c gene, thereby inhibiting de novo synthesis of fatty acids and triglycerides.[60] However, elevations in LDL-C concentrations (up to 40%) have been observed in some patients receiving omega-3 fatty acids,[61] but LDL-C changes from small, dense atherogenic particles to larger, more buoyant and less atherogenic particles. Also, the rise in LDL-C is usually less than the decrease in VLDL cholesterol (VLDL-C). In addition, elevations in serum transaminases have been reported and these enzymes should be monitored periodically for those patients taking omega-3 fatty acids.

Hyperlipoproteinemia

Disease states associated with abnormal serum lipids are generally caused by malfunctions in the synthesis, transport, or catabolism of lipoproteins. Dyslipidemias can be subdivided into two major categories: hyperlipoproteinemias, which are diseases associated with elevated lipoprotein levels, and hypolipoproteinemias, which are associated with decreased lipoprotein levels. The hyperlipoproteinemias can be subdivided into hypercholesterolemia, hypertriglyceridemia, and combined hyperlipidemia, with elevations of both cholesterol and triglycerides.

Hypercholesterolemia

Hypercholesterolemia is the lipid abnormality most closely linked to heart disease.[62] One form of the disease, which is associated with genetic abnormalities that predispose affected individuals to elevated cholesterol levels, is called FH. Homozygotes for FH are fortunately rare (1:1 million in the population) and can have total cholesterol concentrations as high as 800 to 1,000 mg/dL (20 to 26 mmol/L). These patients can have their first heart attack when still in their teenage years.[63] Heterozygotes for the disease are seen much more frequently (1:500 in the population), because it is an autosomal codominant disorder; a defect in just one of the two copies of the LDL receptor can adversely affect lipid levels. Heterozygotes tend to have total cholesterol concentrations in the range of 300 to 600 mg/dL (8 to 15 mmol/L) and, if not treated, become symptomatic for heart disease in their twenties to fifties. Approximately 5% of patients younger than age 50 with CAD are FH heterozygotes. Other symptoms associated with FH include tendinous and tuberous xanthomas, which are cholesterol deposits under the skin, and arcus, which are cholesterol deposits in the cornea.[64]

In both homozygotes and heterozygotes, the cholesterol elevation is primarily associated with an increase in LDL-C. These individuals synthesize intracellular cholesterol normally but lack, or are deficient in, active LDL receptors. There are several classes of defects in the LDL receptor gene that are associated with FH. Class 1 mutations result in null allele where no LDL receptor protein is identified. Class 2 mutation, which accounts for the majority of clinical mutations in FH, creates a membrane protein that is synthesized but not transported to the Golgi efficiently and, thus, is degraded. Class 3 mutations result in an LDL receptor that cannot bind LDL. Class 4 mutations create an LDL receptor that cannot internalize the LDL and transport it to the Golgi, and class 5 mutations create LDL receptors that do not recyle.[65] Mutations in the LDL receptor gene promoter region have also been described. Consequently, LDL builds up in the circulation, because there are insufficient receptors to bind the LDL and transfer the cholesterol into the cells. Cells, however, which require cholesterol for use in cell membrane and hormone production, synthesize cholesterol intracellularly at an increased rate to compensate for the lack of cholesterol from the receptor-mediated mechanism.

CASE STUDY 15.3

A 43-year-old white man was diagnosed with hyperlipidemia at age 13 years, when his father died of a myocardial infarction at age 34 years. The man's grandfather had died at age 43 years, also of a myocardial infarction. Currently, the man is active and asymptomatic with regard to CHD. He is taking 40 mg of lovastatin (Mevacor), two times per day (maximum dose). He had previously taken niacin but could not tolerate it because of flushing and gastrointestinal distress, nor could he tolerate cholestyramine resin (Questran). His physical examination is remarkable for bilateral Achilles tendon thickening/xanthomas and a right carotid bruit (see Case Study Table 15.3.1).

Laboratory Results	
Triglycerides	91 mg/dL
Total cholesterol	269 mg/dL
HDL-C	47 mg/dL
LDL-C	204 mg/dL
Aspartate aminotransferase	34 U/L
Alanine aminotransferase	36 U/L
Alkaline phosphatase	53 U/L
Electrolytes and fasting glucose	Normal

Questions

1. What is his diagnosis?
2. Does he need further workup?
3. What other laboratory tests should be done?
4. Does he need further drug treatment? If so, what?

In FH heterozygotes and other forms of hypercholesterolemia, reduction in the rate of internal cholesterol synthesis, by inhibition of HMG-CoA reductase with statin drugs, stimulates the production of additional LDL receptors, particularly in the liver, which removes LDL from the circulation. Homozygotes, however, do not usually fully benefit as much from this type of therapy, because they do not have enough functional receptors to stimulate. Homozygotes can be treated by a technique called LDL apheresis, a method similar to the dialysis treatment, in which blood is periodically drawn from the patient, processed to remove LDL, and returned to the patient.[66]

Most individuals with elevated LDL-C levels do not have FH but are still at increased risk for premature CHD[31,48,62] and should be maintained on a low-fat diet and receive statin treatment when necessary (Table 15.8). Regular physical activity should also be incorporated, with drug therapy (Table 15.8).

PCSK9

The principal route of clearance of circulating LDL-C from the blood is hepatocyte endocytosis, a process mediated by binding of LDL-C to LDL-R on the hepatocyte cell membrane.[67] Proprotein convertase subtilisin/kexin type 9 (PCSK9) is a 72-kDa serine protease expressed in the liver, kidney, and intestine that plays an important role in LDL metabolism. PCSK9 binds to the extracellular epidermal growth factor–like repeat A (EGF-A) domain of LDL-R on the cell surface and is subsequently cointernalized with the LDL-R in clathrin-coated vesicles and escorted to lysosomes for degradation of the LDL-R. The binding of PCSK9 thus prevents the receptor from recycling to the plasma membrane, which can occur up to 150 times before it is normally inactivated or degraded. Thus, because of its role as major inhibitor of LDL-R, PCSK9 gene inactivation (with antisense oligonucleotides or small interfering RNA and immunological blockade of PCSK9 action and EGF-A to mimetic peptide) is an attractive target for lipid-lowering therapy. Several anti-PCSK9 monoclonal antibodies have recently been approved by the FDA for treatment of patients with severe dyslipidemias.[68] Gain-of-function mutations in PCSK9 gene account for 1% to 3% of individuals with FH and are associated with early-onset CVDs.[68] Gain-of-function mutations in PCSK9 enhance the interaction of PCSK9 for LDL-R and intracellular trafficking of LDLR for degradation by endosomal/lysosome, resulting in decreased LDL-R levels on plasma membrane and high plasma LDL-C levels. In contrast, loss-of-function mutation in the PCSK9 gene leads to an increase in the number of LDL-R on the surface of liver cells.[69] These can remove LDL-C from blood faster than usual, resulting in reduced plasma LDL-C concentration and lower-than-average risk of CVD.[69] The loss of PCSK9 appears to have no adverse consequences.

Hypertriglyceridemia

The NCEP ATP III has identified borderline high triglycerides as levels of 150 to 200 mg/dL (1.7 to 2.3 mmol/L), high as 200 to 500 mg/dL (2.3 to 5.6 mmol/L), and very high as greater than 500 mg/dL (>5.6 mmol/L).[31] Hypertriglyceridemia can be a consequence of genetic abnormalities, called FH, or the result of secondary causes, such as hormonal abnormalities associated with the pancreas, adrenal glands, and pituitary, or of diabetes mellitus or nephrosis. Diabetes mellitus leads to increased shunting of glucose into the pentose pathway, causing increased fatty acid synthesis. Renal failure depresses the removal of large-molecular-weight constituents like triglycerides, causing increased serum levels. Hypertriglyceridemia is generally a result of an imbalance between synthesis and clearance of VLDL in the circulation. In some studies, hypertriglyceridemia has not been shown as an independent risk factor for CHD, but many CHD patients have moderately elevated triglycerides in conjunction with decreased HDL-C levels.[70] It is often difficult to separate the risk associated with increased triglycerides from that of decreased HDL-C, but hypertriglyceridemia is now generally considered an important and potentially treatable risk factor for CHD by some guidelines but not others.

Triglycerides are influenced by a number of hormones, such as insulin, glucagon, pituitary growth hormone, adrenocorticotropic hormone (ACTH), thyrotropin, and adrenal medulla epinephrine and norepinephrine from the nervous system. Epinephrine and norepinephrine influence serum triglyceride levels by triggering production of hormone-sensitive lipase, which is located in adipose tissue.[71] Other body processes that trigger hormone-sensitive lipase activity are cell growth (growth hormone), adrenal stimulation (ACTH), thyroid stimulation (thyrotropin), and fasting (glucagon). Each process, through its action on hormone-sensitive lipase, results in an increase in serum triglyceride values.

Although severe hypertriglyceridemia (>500 mg/dL [>5.6 mmol/L]) is usually not associated with high risk of CHD, it is a potentially life-threatening abnormality because it can cause acute and recurrent pancreatitis.[56,72] It is, therefore, imperative that these patients be diagnosed and treated with low-fat diets and triglyceride-lowering medication. Severe hypertriglyceridemia is generally caused by a deficiency of LPL located on chromosome 8 or by a deficiency in apo C-II located on chromosome 19, which is a necessary cofactor for LPL activity.[73] Other rarer type of mutations in other proteins involved in triglyceride metabolism has also been described. Normally, LPL hydrolyzes triglycerides carried in chylomicrons and VLDL to provide cells with free fatty acids for energy from exogenous and endogenous triglyceride sources. A deficiency in LPL or apo C-II activity keeps chylomicrons from being cleared and serum triglycerides remain extremely elevated, even when the patient has fasted for longer than 12 to 14 hours.

Treatment of hypertriglyceridemia consists of dietary modifications, fish oil, and/or triglyceride-lowering drugs (primarily fibric acid derivatives) in cases of severe hypertriglyceridemia or when accompanied with low HDL-C.[74] It is possible that certain subspecies of chylomicrons and VLDL are atherogenic. Remnants of chylomicrons and VLDL represent subspecies that have been partially hydrolyzed by lipases and are thought to be potentially atherogenic.

Combined Hyperlipidemia

Combined hyperlipoproteinemia is generally defined as the presence of elevated levels of serum total cholesterol and triglycerides. Individuals presenting with this syndrome are considered at increased risk for CHD. In one genetic form of this condition, called familial combined hyperlipidemia (FCH), individuals from an affected kindred may only have elevated cholesterol, whereas others only have elevated triglycerides, and yet others, elevations of both. FCH is due in part to excessive hepatic synthesis of apoprotein B, leading to increased VLDL secretion and increased production of LDL from VLDL. These patients may have eruptive xanthomas and are at high risk for developing CHD. Another rare genetic form of combined hyperlipoproteinemia is called familial dysbetalipoproteinemia or type III hyperlipoproteinemia. The name type III hyperlipoproteinemia is a holdover from a lipoprotein typing system developed by Fredrickson et al.,[75] which otherwise is generally no longer used. The disease results from an accumulation of cholesterol-rich VLDL and chylomicron remnants as a result of defective catabolism of those particles. The disease is associated with the presence of a relatively rare form of apo E, called apo E2/2. The apo E2/2 cannot bind with hepatic E receptor, and therefore, VLDL and chylomicron remnant uptake is impaired.[75] Individuals with type III will frequently have total cholesterol values of 200 to 300 mg/dL (5 to 8 mmol/L) and triglycerides of 300 to 600 mg/dL (3 to 7 mmol/L). This disorder is associated with an increased risk of PVD and coronary disease.[76] Patients often have palmar xanthomas and tuberoeruptive xanthomas.[77] To distinguish them from other forms of combined hyperlipoproteinemias, it is first necessary to isolate the VLDL fraction with ultracentrifugation. A ratio derived from the cholesterol concentration in VLDL to total serum triglycerides will be greater than 0.30 in the presence of type III hyperlipoproteinemia. If the VLDL fraction is analyzed by agarose electrophoresis, the particles will migrate in a broad β region rather than in the normal pre-β region. Definitive diagnosis requires a determination of apo E isoforms by isoelectric focusing or DNA typing, resulting in either apo E2/2 homozygosity or, rarely, apo E mutation or deficiency. As with other dyslipidemias, these patients can be treated with a combination of drugs, such as niacin, gemfibrozil, HMG-CoA reductase inhibitors, and low-fat diets. Because of the cholesterol-enriched composition of these particles, use of the Friedewald equation[78] to calculate LDL-C levels will result in an underestimation of VLDL-C and, therefore, an overestimation of LDL-C, compared with beta-quantification ultracentrifugation procedure.[79]

CASE STUDY 15.4

A 60-year-old woman came to her physician because she was having problems with urination. Her previous history included hypertension and episodes of edema. The physician ordered various laboratory tests on blood drawn in his office. The results are shown in Case Study Table 15.4.1.

Laboratory Results

Patient Analyte	Values	Reference Range
Na⁺	149	135–143 mmol/L
K⁺	4.5	3.0–5.0 mmol/L
Cl⁻	120	98–103 mmol/L
CO₂ content	12	22–27 mmol/L
Total protein	5.7	6.5–8.0 g/dL
Albumin	2.3	3.5–5.0 g/dL
Ca²⁺	7.6	9.0–10.5 mg/dL
Cholesterol	201	140–200 mg/dL
Uric acid	15.4	3.5–7.9 mg/dL
Creatinine	4.5	0.5–1.2 mg/dL
BUN	87	7–25 mg/dL
Glucose	88	75–105 mg/dL
Total bilirubin	1.3	0.2–1.0 mg/dL
Triglycerides	327	65–157 mg/dL
Lactate dehydrogenase	200	90–190 IU/L
Aspartate transaminase	45	8–40 IU/L
Amylase	380	76–375 IU/L

Questions

1. What are the abnormal results in this case?
2. Why do you think the triglycerides are abnormal?
3. What is the primary disease exhibited by this patient's laboratory data?

Lp(a) Elevation

Elevations in the serum concentration of Lp(a), especially in conjunction with elevations of LDL, increase the risk of CHD and CVD.[80] Higher Lp(a) levels have been observed in most studies more frequently in patients with CHD than in normal control subjects. Lp(a) are variants of LDL with an extra apolipoprotein, called apo (a); the size and serum concentrations of Lp(a) are largely genetically determined. Because apo (a) has a high degree of homology with the coagulation factor plasminogen,[81] it has been proposed that it competes with plasminogen for fibrin binding sites, thus increasing plaque formation.[82] Most LDL-lowering drugs have no effect on Lp(a) concentration, even when LDL-C is significantly lowered. The two drugs shown to have some effect are niacin and estrogen replacement in postmenopausal women, but the value of specifically treating patients for high Lp(a) is still not clear, and instead, lowering LDL-C should probably be the first goal. New therapies for specifically lowering Lp(a) are currently being developed. Studies have shown that increased plasma concentrations of Lp(a) significantly correlate with increased risk of restenosis following percutaneous coronary intervention (PCI) for the treatment of CAD.[83] However, other studies have reported inconsistent data, which may be due to confounding factors and with problems with the assay.[84] Restenosis after PCI has been shown to be significantly reduced by decreasing Lp(a) concentrations with lipoprotein apheresis treatment.[85] Further studies are needed to clarify the precise mechanism by which Lp(a) causes restenosis following PCI.

Non–HDL Cholesterol

Although LDL-C is widely recognized as an established risk marker for CVD, many studies have demonstrated that LDL-C alone does not provide sufficient measure of atherogenesis, especially in hypertriglyceridemic patients. To address this issue, the calculation of non–HDL-C has been employed. Non–HDL-C reflects total cholesterol minus HDL-C and encompasses all cholesterol present in potentially atherogenic, apo B–containing lipoproteins [LDL, VLDL, IDL, and Lp(a)]. Unlike LDL-C, which can be incorrectly calculated using the Friedewald equation in the presence of postprandial hypertriglyceridemia, non–HDL-C is reliable when measured in the nonfasting state.[86] On average, non–HDL-C levels are approximately 30 mg/dL higher than LDL-C levels.[31,87] Recent studies have shown that elevated levels of non–HDL-C are associated with increased CVD risk, even if the LDL-C levels are normal.[88] In clinical studies, non–HDL-C has been found to be an independent predictor of CVD and for diabetes patients; it may be a stronger predictor than LDL-C and triglycerides.[88]

Hypobetalipoproteinemia

Hypobetalipoproteinemia is associated with isolated low levels of LDL-C as a result of a defect in the Apo B gene, but because it is not generally associated with CHD, it is not discussed further here. Abetalipoproteinemia, which is due to a defect in the microsomal transfer protein used in the synthesis and secretion of VLDL, can also present with low LDL and apo B–like hypobetalipoproteinemia. It is an autosomal recessive disorder and like hypobetalipoproteinemia patients, they are not at an increased risk of cardiovascular disease but can develop several neurologic and ophthalmologic problems from fat-soluble vitamin deficiencies.

Hypoalphalipoproteinemia

Hypoalphalipoproteinemia indicates an isolated decrease in circulating HDL, typically defined as an HDL-C concentration less than 40 mg/dL (1.0 mmol/L),[31] without the presence of hypertriglyceridemia. The term alpha denotes the region in which HDL migrates on agarose electrophoresis. There are several defects, often genetically determined, which are associated with hypoalphalipoproteinemia, such as LCAT, apo A-I, and ABCA1 transporter gene mutations.[89,90] Most of these defects are associated with a somewhat increased risk of premature CHD, but the association is not as strong as seen with genetic disorders that result in increased LDL-C. An extreme form of hypoalphalipoproteinemia, Tangier disease, is associated with HDL-C concentrations as low as 1 to 2 mg/dL (0.03 to 0.05 mmol/L) in homozygotes, accompanied by total cholesterol concentrations of 50 to 80 mg/dL (1.3 to 2.1 mmol/L).

Treatment options of individuals with isolated decreases of HDL-C are limited and the clinical utility is not clear. Niacin is somewhat effective in raising HDL-C but can have adverse effects, such as flushing or even hepatotoxicity, although newer, timed-release preparations may ameliorate those effects.[56,63,91] Lifestyle modifications, which can raise HDL-C, and treatment of any coexisting disorders that increase CHD risk are likely to be beneficial in these patients.

Acute, transitory hypoalphalipoproteinemia can also be seen in cases of severe physiologic stress, such as acute infections (primarily viral), other acute illnesses, and surgical procedures. HDL-C, as well as total cholesterol, concentrations can be significantly reduced under these conditions but will return to normal levels as recovery proceeds. For this reason, lipoprotein concentrations drawn during hospitalization or with a known disease state should be reassessed in the healthy, nonhospitalized state before intervention is considered.

LIPID AND LIPOPROTEIN ANALYSES

Lipid Measurement

Lipids and lipoproteins are important indicators of CHD risk, which is a major reason for their measurement in research, as well as in clinical practice. Decision cut points used to characterize CHD risk have been developed by various guidelines based on consideration of population distributions from large epidemiologic studies, intervention studies that demonstrated the efficacy of treatment regimens, and cost-effectiveness.[31] To improve the reliability of the analytic measurements, standardization programs have been implemented for the research laboratories performing the population and intervention studies, which helped to make results comparable among laboratories and over time.[92] More recently, standardization programs have been extended to diagnostic manufacturers and routine clinical

laboratories to facilitate reliable classification of patients using the national decision cut points. Thus, accuracy and standardization of results are especially important with the lipid and lipoprotein analytes.

Cholesterol Measurement

Serum or plasma specimens collected from patients in blood collection tubes who have fasted for at least 12 hours are usually preferred for total cholesterol testing but does not usually significantly change after a meal. If analysis is delayed, the serum/plasma specimen can be refrigerated at 4°C for several days. The lipid workup traditionally has begun with measurement of total serum cholesterol. Early analytic methods used strong acids (e.g., sulfuric and acetic) sometimes together with other chemicals (e.g., acetic anhydride or ferric chloride) to produce a measurable color with cholesterol.[93] Because the strong acid reactions are relatively nonspecific, partial or full extraction by organic solvents was sometimes used to improve specificity. In the past, the reference method for cholesterol involved hexane extraction after hydrolysis with alcoholic KOH followed by reaction with Liebermann-Burchard color reagent, which comprises sulfuric and acetic acids and acetic anhydride.[94,95] Recently, the reference method has changed to a gas chromatography–mass spectrometry (GC–MS) method that now specifically measures cholesterol and does not detect related sterols. This method shows good agreement with the gold standard method developed and applied at the U.S. National Institute of Standards and Technology, the so-called Definitive Method, using isotope dilution mass spectrometry.[96]

Enzymatic reagents have generally replaced strong acid chemistries in the routine laboratory. Enzymes, selected for specificity to the analyte of interest, provide reasonably accurate quantitation without the necessity for extraction or other pretreatment. Enzymatic reagents are mild compared with the earlier acid reagents and better suited for automated chemistry analyzers. The lipoproteins, HDL and LDL, are generally quantified based on their cholesterol content. Thus, the common lipid panel, including measurements of total cholesterol, LDL-C, and HDL-C, together with triglycerides, can be completed routinely using chemistry analyzers.

Although several enzymatic reaction sequences have been described, one sequence (Fig. 15.4) is most common for measuring cholesterol. The enzyme cholesteryl ester hydrolase cleaves the fatty acid residue from cholesteryl esters, which comprise about two-thirds of circulating cholesterol, converting them to unesterified or free cholesterol. The free cholesterol is reacted by the second enzyme, cholesterol oxidase, producing hydrogen peroxide (H_2O_2), a substrate for a common enzymatic color reaction using horseradish peroxidase to couple two colorless chemicals into a colored compound. The intensity of the resulting color, proportional to the amount of cholesterol, can be measured by a spectrophotometer, usually at a wavelength around 500 nm. Enzymes and reagents have improved so that most appropriately calibrated commercial reagents can be expected to give reliable results. This reaction sequence is generally

1. Cholesteryl ester + H_2O $\xrightarrow{\text{Cholesteryl esterase}}$ Cholesterol + Fatty acid

2. Cholesterol + O_2 $\xrightarrow{\text{Cholesterol oxidase}}$ Cholestenone + H_2O_2

3. H_2O_2 + Dye $\xrightarrow{\text{Peroxidase}}$ Color

FIGURE 15.4 Enzymatic assay sequence—cholesterol.

used on serum without an extraction step but can be subject to interference. For example, vitamin C and bilirubin are reducing agents that could interfere with the peroxidase-catalyzed color reaction, unless appropriate additional enzyme systems are added to eliminate the interference.

Triglyceride Measurement

Measurement of serum triglycerides in conjunction with cholesterol is useful in detecting certain genetic and other types of metabolic disorders, as well as in characterizing the risk of CVDs. The triglyceride value is also commonly used in the estimation of LDL-C by the Friedewald equation and is usually done on a fasting sample because triglycerides can sometimes significantly increase after a meal. Several enzymatic reaction sequences are available for triglyceride measurement, all including lipases to cleave fatty acids from the glycerol backbone.[97] The freed glycerol participates in any one of several enzymatic sequences. One of the more common earlier reactions, ending in a product measured in the ultraviolet (UV) region, used glycerol kinase and pyruvate kinase, culminating in the conversion of NADH to NAD+, with an associated decrease in absorbance.[98] This reaction is susceptible to interference and side reactions. The UV endpoint is also less convenient for modern analyzers, so this and other UV reaction sequences have been replaced by a second sequence (Fig. 15.5), involving glycerol kinase and glycerophosphate oxidase, coupled to the same peroxidase color reaction described for cholesterol.

The enzymatic triglyceride reaction sequences also react with any endogenous free glycerol, which is universally present in serum and can be a significant source of interference.[99] In most specimens, the endogenous free glycerol contributes a 10 to 20 mg/dL (0.11 to 0.023 mmol/L) overestimation of triglycerides. About 20% of specimens will have higher glycerol, with levels increased in certain conditions, such as diabetes and liver disease, or from glycerol-containing medications. Reagents are available that correct for endogenous free glycerol and are used by many research laboratories, but such methods are less efficient and hence uncommon in clinical laboratories. The most common

correction, designated "double-cuvette blank," is accomplished with a second parallel measurement using the triglyceride reagent without the lipase enzyme to quantify only the free glycerol blank. The glycerol blank measurement is subtracted from the total glycerol measurement obtained with the complete reagent to determine a net or blank-corrected triglyceride result. Another approach, designated "single-cuvette blank," begins with the lipase-free reagent. After a brief incubation, a blank reading is taken to measure only endogenous free glycerol. The lipase enzyme is then added as a second separate reagent and, after additional incubation, a final reading is taken that, after correcting for the blank by the instrument, gives a net or glycerol-blanked triglyceride value. A convenient and easily implemented alternative that does not increase cost—designated calibration blanking—can be done by simply adjusting the calibrator set points to net or blank-corrected values, compensating for the average free glycerol content of specimens. This approach, which is used by some diagnostic reagent companies, is usually reasonably accurate because free glycerol levels are generally relatively low and fairly consistent in most specimens. Most specimens will be blank corrected reasonably well and only a few specimens will be undercorrected but will still be better than without the calibration adjustment.

Until recently, the triglyceride reference method involved alkaline hydrolysis, solvent extraction, and a color reaction with chromotropic acid, an assay that is tedious and poorly characterized and was largely only done by the lipid standardization laboratory at the Centers for Disease Control and Prevention (CDC). Like the reference method for cholesterol, the CDC has recently switched to a GC–MS method that involves the hydrolysis of fatty acids on triglycerides and the measurement of glycerol. However, it must be noted that accuracy in triglyceride measurements for clinical purposes might be considered less relevant than that for cholesterol because the physiologic variation is so large, with the coefficient of variation (CV) in the range of 25% to 30%, making the contribution of analytic variation relatively insignificant.

1. Triglyceride + H_2O $\xrightarrow{\text{Bacterial lipase}}$ Fatty acid + Glycerol

2. Glycerol + ATP $\xrightarrow{\text{Glycerokinase}}$ Glycerophosphate + ADP

3. Glycerophosphate + O_2 $\xrightarrow{\text{Glycerophosphate oxidase}}$ Dihydroxyacetone + H_2O_2

4. H_2O_2 + Dye $\xrightarrow{\text{Peroxidase}}$ Color

FIGURE 15.5 Enzymatic assay sequence—triglycerides.

Lipoprotein Methods

Various methods have been used for the separation and quantitation of serum lipoproteins, taking advantage of physical properties, such as density, size, charge, and apolipoprotein content. The range in density observed among the lipoprotein classes is a function of the relative lipid and protein content and enables fractionation by density, using ultracentrifugation. Electrophoretic separations take advantage of differences in charge and size. Chemical precipitation methods, once common in clinical laboratories and now primarily used in research laboratories, depend on particle size, charge, and differences in the apolipoprotein content. Antibodies specific to apolipoproteins can be used to bind and separate lipoprotein classes. Chromatographic methods take advantage of size differences in molecular sieving methods or composition in affinity methods, using, for example, heparin sepharose. Most common in clinical laboratories are direct homogeneous reagents designed for fully automated use with chemistry analyzers, using combinations of detergents and, in some cases, antibodies to selectively assay cholesterol in lipoprotein classes.

Many ultracentrifugation methods have been used in the research laboratory, but ultracentrifugation is uncommon in the clinical laboratory. The most common approach, called preparative ultracentrifugation, uses sequential density adjustments of serum to fractionate major and minor lipoprotein classes. Density gradient methods, either nonequilibrium techniques in which separations are based on the rate of flotation or equilibrium techniques in which the lipoproteins separate based on their density, permit fractionation of several or all classes in a single run.[100] The available methods use different types of ultracentrifuge rotors: swinging bucket, fixed angle, vertical, and zonal. Newer methods have trended toward smaller-scale separations in small rotors, using tabletop ultracentrifuges. Ultracentrifugation, although tedious, expensive, and technically demanding, remains a workhorse for separation of lipoproteins for quantitative purposes and preparative isolations. Ultracentrifugation is also used in the reference methods for lipoprotein quantitation, because lipoproteins are classically defined in terms of hydrated density.

Electrophoretic methods allow separation and quantitation of major lipoprotein classes, as well as subclasses, and provide a visual display useful in detecting unusual or variant patterns.[101] Agarose gel has been the most common medium for separation of intact lipoproteins, providing a clear background and convenience in use.[102,103] Electrophoretic methods, in general, were considered useful for qualitative analysis but less than desirable for lipoprotein quantitation because of poor precision and large systematic biases, compared with other methods.[104] Using newer commercial automated electrophoretic systems, lipoprotein determinations can be precise and accurate but are no longer widely used.[105]

Electrophoresis in polyacrylamide gels is used for separation of lipoprotein classes, subclasses, and the apolipoproteins.[106] Of particular interest are methods that fractionate LDL subclasses to characterize the more atherogenic smaller, denser, lipid-depleted fractions versus the larger, lighter subclasses.

Chemical precipitation, usually with polyanions, such as heparin and dextran sulfate, together with divalent cations, such as manganese or magnesium, can be used to separate any of the lipoproteins but are most common for HDL.[107] Apo B in VLDL and LDL is rich in positively charged amino acids, which preferentially form complexes with polyanions. The addition of divalent cations neutralizes the charged groups on the lipoproteins, making them aggregate and become insoluble, resulting in their precipitation leaving HDL in solution. At appropriate concentrations of polyanion and divalent cation, the separation is reasonably specific.

Immunochemical methods, using antibodies specific to epitopes on the apolipoproteins, have been useful in both research and routine methods.[108] Antibodies have been immobilized on solid supports, such as a column matrix or latex beads. For example, the apo B–containing lipoproteins as a group can be bound by antibodies to apo B. Selectivity within the apo B–containing lipoproteins, such as removing VLDL while retaining LDL, can be obtained by including antibodies to minor apolipoproteins. HDL can be selectively bound using antibodies to apo A-I, the major protein of HDL. As another example, immobilized monoclonal antibodies have been used to separate a fraction of remnant lipoproteins designated RLP (remnant-like particles), shown to be particularly atherogenic.[109]

HDL Methods

For routine diagnostic purposes, HDL for many years was separated almost exclusively by chemical precipitation, involving a two-step procedure with manual pretreatment. A precipitation reagent added to serum or plasma aggregated non-HDLs, which were sedimented by centrifugation, at forces of approximately 1,500 g (gravity) with lengthy centrifugation times of 10 to 30 minutes or higher forces of 10,000 to 15,000 g, decreasing centrifugation times to 3 minutes. HDL is then quantified as cholesterol in the supernate, usually by one of the enzymatic assays modified for the lower HDL-C range.

CASE STUDY 15.5

A 49-year-old woman was referred for a lipid evaluation by her dermatologist after she developed a papular rash over her trunk and arms. The rash consisted of multiple, red, raised lesions with yellow centers. She had no previous history of such a rash and no family history of lipid disorders or CHD. She is postmenopausal, on standard estrogen replacement therapy, and otherwise healthy (see Case Study Table 15.5.1).

Laboratory Results	
Serum	Grossly Lipemic
Triglycerides	6,200 mg/dL
Total cholesterol	458 mg/dL
Fasting glucose	160 mg/dL
Liver function tests and electrolytes	Normal

Questions

1. What is the rash? What is the cause of her rash?
2. Is her oral estrogen contributing?
3. Is her glucose contributing?
4. What treatments are warranted, and what is her most acute risk?

The earliest common precipitation method used heparin in combination with manganese to precipitate the apo B–containing lipoproteins.[110] Because manganese interfered with enzymatic assays, alternative reagents were developed. Sodium phosphotungstate[111] with magnesium became commonly used, but because of its sensitivity to reaction conditions and greater variability, it was largely replaced by dextran sulfate (a synthetic heparin) with magnesium.[112] The earliest dextran sulfate methods used material of 500 kD, which was replaced by a 50 kD material, considered to be more specific.[113] Polyethylene glycol also precipitates lipoproteins, but it requires 100-fold higher reagent concentrations with highly viscous reagents, which are difficult to pipette precisely.[114] Numerous commercial versions of these precipitation reagents became available, which in earlier years often gave quite different results but gradually became more comparable as standardization programs were implemented.

A significant problem with HDL precipitation methods is interference from elevated triglyceride levels.[115] When triglyceride-rich VLDL and chylomicrons are present, the low density of the aggregated lipoproteins may prevent them from sedimenting or may even cause floating during centrifugation. This incomplete sedimentation, indicated by cloudiness, turbidity, or particulate matter floating in the supernate, results in overestimation of HDL-C. High-speed centrifugation reduces the proportion of turbid supernate. Predilution of the specimen promotes clearing but may lead to errors in the cholesterol analysis. Turbid supernates may also be cleared by ultrafiltration, a method that is reliable but tedious and inefficient. Because of these drawbacks and the fact that the laborious pretreatment step is not amenable to full automation, the precipitation methods became increasingly out of step with the modern automated clinical laboratory.

The result has been development of a new class of direct, sometimes termed homogeneous, methods, which automate the HDL quantification, making them better suited for the modern chemistry laboratory. Specific polymers, detergents, and even modified enzymes are used to suppress the enzymatic cholesterol reaction in lipoproteins other than HDL.[116] In general, a first reagent is added to "block" non-HDLs, followed by a second reagent with the enzymes to quantify the accessible (HDL) cholesterol. Homogeneous assays, which appear to be highly precise and reasonably accurate, have generally replaced pretreatment methods in the routine laboratory.[117] However, the methods have been shown to lack specificity for HDL in unusual specimens, for example, from patients with liver or kidney conditions. Also, the reagents have been subject to frequent modifications by the manufacturers in an effort to improve performance, which can affect results in long-term studies. For these reasons, precipitation-based methods are still used by some reference labs and often done by research laboratories.

The accepted reference method for HDL-C is a three-step procedure developed at the CDC. This method involves ultracentrifugation to remove VLDL, heparin manganese precipitation from the 1.006 g/mL infranate to remove LDL, and analysis of supernatant cholesterol by the Abell-Kendall assay.[95] Because this method is tedious and expensive, a simpler, direct precipitation method has been validated by the CDC Network Laboratory Group as a designated comparison method, using direct dextran sulfate (50 kD) precipitation of serum with Abell-Kendall cholesterol analysis.[92]

LDL Methods

LDL-C, well validated as a treatable risk factor for CHD, is the primary basis for treatment decisions in all guidelines. The most common research method for LDL-C quantitation and the basis for the reference method has been designated beta-quantification, in which beta designation refers to the electrophoretic term for LDL. Beta-quantification combines ultracentrifugation and chemical precipitation.[110,118] Ultracentrifugation of serum at the native density of 1.006 g/mL is used to float VLDL and any chylomicrons for separation. The fractions are recovered by pipetting after separating the fractions by slicing the tube. Ultracentrifugation has been preferred for VLDL separation because other methods, such as precipitation, are not as specific for VLDL and may be subject to interference from chylomicrons. In general, ultracentrifugation is a robust but tedious technique that can give reliable results, provided the technique is meticulous.

In a separate step, chemical precipitation is used to separate HDL from either the whole serum or the infranate obtained from ultracentrifugation. Cholesterol is quantified in serum, in the 1.006 g/mL infranate, and in the HDL supernate by enzymatic or other assay methods. LDL-C is calculated as the difference between cholesterol measured in the infranate and in the HDL fraction. VLDL-C is usually calculated as the difference between that in whole serum and the amount in the infranate fraction. The requirement for the need of an ultracentrifuge has generally limited beta-quantification to lipid specialty laboratories.

Beta-quantification is also the basis for the accepted reference method for LDL. The method is the same as that described for HDL above, with the measured HDL-C subtracted from that in the bottom fraction to obtain LDL-C.

A more common approach, bypassing ultracentrifugation and commonly used in routine and sometimes research laboratories, is calculating LDL-C by the Friedewald calculation.[78] HDL-C is quantified either after precipitation or using one of the direct methods, and total cholesterol and triglycerides are measured in the serum. VLDL-C is estimated as the triglyceride level divided by 5 (when using mg/dL units), an approximation that works reasonably well in most normolipemic specimens. The presence of elevated triglycerides (400 mg/dL [4.52 mmol/L] is the accepted limit), chylomicrons, and β-VLDL characteristic of the rare type III hyperlipoproteinemia precludes this estimation. The estimated VLDL-C and measured HDL-C are subtracted from total serum cholesterol to estimate or derive LDL-C. Thus, LDL-C = total cholesterol − HDL − Trig/5. This method, commonly performed as the lipid panel, is widely used in estimating LDL-C in routine clinical practice, having been recommended in the NCEP guidelines. Investigations in lipid specialty laboratories have suggested that the method is reasonably reliable for patient classification, provided the underlying measurements are made with appropriate accuracy and precision. There has been concern about the reliability in routine laboratories, however, because the error in calculating LDL-C combines the error in the underlying measurements: total cholesterol, triglycerides, and HDL-C. The NCEP Laboratory Expert Panel, considering performance as represented by proficiency surveys, concluded that the level of analytic performance required to derive LDL-C accurately enough to meet clinical needs was beyond the capability of most routine laboratories. To meet the NCEP precision goal of 4% CV for LDL-C (Table 15.6), a laboratory would be required to achieve half the NCEP goals for each of the underlying measurements. The NCEP panel concluded that better methods are needed for routine diagnostic use, preferably methods that directly separate LDL for cholesterol quantitation.[39]

Like for HDL, direct LDL-C methods have been developed or refined for general use, similar to the homogeneous assays for HDL-C.[119] Besides achieving full automation of the challenging LDL-C separation, these assays have the potential to streamline the measurement while improving precision. However, separating LDL with adequate specificity from other lipoproteins in this manner is more challenging even than that for HDL.[120] Because of the extra cost compared to Friedewald calculations and analytical concerns, direct LDL-C assays are not as widely used as direct HDL-C assays, although they have the advantage of being able to be used on nonfasting samples.

Compact Analyzers

The common lipids and lipoproteins can be measured with compact analysis systems designed for use in point-of-care testing at the patient's bedside, in the physician's office, in wellness centers, and even in the home. These compact devices that are used outside the clinical laboratory are considered waived from the Clinical Laboratory Improvement Amendments. The earliest systems, introduced in the 1980s, were relatively large and measured cholesterol and triglycerides as well as other common analytes, usually separately and sequentially. Newer systems have become smaller and more sophisticated, offering integrated separation of HDL and analysis of cholesterol and triglycerides simultaneously from fingerstick blood. Systems can measure cholesterol, triglycerides, HDL-C, and glucose simultaneously from a fingerstick sample. Noninstrumented systems are also available. These new technologies offer the capability of measuring lipids and lipoproteins with reasonable reliability outside the conventional laboratory.

Apolipoprotein Methods

Lipids by nature tend to be insoluble in the aqueous environment of the circulation; hence, the lipoproteins include various protein constituents, designated apolipoproteins, which enhance solubility, as well as playing other functional roles (Table 15.2). Apolipoproteins are commonly measured in research and some specialty laboratories supporting cardiovascular practices or clinical studies measure them routinely in addition to the lipoproteins. For clinical diagnostic purposes, three apolipoproteins in particular have been of interest. Apo B, the major protein of LDL and VLDL, is an indicator of combined LDL and VLDL concentration that can be measured directly in serum by immunoassay. Some studies suggest that apo B may be a better indicator of atherogenic particles than LDL-C.[121] Apo A-I, as the major protein of HDL, could be measured directly in serum in place of separation and analysis of HDL-C; however, because quantification in terms of cholesterol content is more common, the latter practice has prevailed. Lp(a), the variant of LDL, shown to be an independent indicator of CHD risk, is sometimes determined in managing patients. Measurement of these three apolipoproteins, considered to be emerging markers, can be useful in patient management by experienced practitioners.

Lp(a) has pre-β mobility on agarose electrophoresis and can be quantified by this technique. However, the apolipoproteins are commonly measured by immunoassays of various types, with several commercial kit methods available.[122] Most common in routine laboratories are turbidimetric assays for chemistry analyzers or nephelometric assays for dedicated nephelometers. Especially for apo B and Lp(a), these light-scattering assays may be subject to interference from the larger triglyceride-rich lipoproteins (chylomicrons) and VLDL. Enzyme-linked immunosorbent assay (ELISA), radial immunodiffusion (RID), and radioimmunoassay (RIA) methods have also been available, but the latter two methods are becoming less common. Antibodies used in the immunoassays may be polyclonal or monoclonal. International efforts to develop reference materials and standardization programs for the assays are in progress. Because Lp(a) is genetically heterogeneous and the levels and CHD risk correlate with the isoform size, qualitative assessment of isoform distribution may also be useful.[123]

Phospholipid Measurement

Quantitative measurements of phospholipids are primarily done for research but not as part of routine laboratory assessments of lipids and lipoproteins, because they have not been shown to add any value for cardiovascular risk prediction. The choline-containing phospholipids lecithin, lysolecithin, and sphingomyelin, which account for at least 95% of total phospholipids in serum, can be measured by an enzymatic reaction sequence using phospholipase D, choline oxidase, and horseradish peroxidase.[124]

Fatty Acid Measurement

Although studies suggest that fatty acids have potential in assessing CHD risk (e.g., the n-3 fatty acids), analysis is also primarily used in research laboratories for studies of diet. Less common is their measurement in the diagnosis of rare genetic conditions. Individual fatty acids can be analyzed by gas–liquid chromatography—after extraction, alkaline hydrolysis, and conversion to methyl esters of diazomethane[125] but enzymatic exist for measuring total plasma free fatty acids.[126]

STANDARDIZATION OF LIPID AND LIPOPROTEIN ASSAYS

Precision

Precision is a prerequisite for accuracy; a method may have no overall systematic error or bias, but if it is imprecise, it will still be inaccurate on some individual measurements. With the shift to modern automated analyzers, analytic variation has generally become less of a concern than biologic and other sources of preanalytic variation. Cholesterol levels are affected by many factors that can be categorized into biologic, clinical, and sampling sources.[127] Changes in lifestyle that affect diet, exercise, weight, and smoking patterns can result in fluctuations in the observed cholesterol and triglyceride values and the distribution of the lipoproteins. Similarly, the presence of clinical conditions, various diseases, or the medications used in their treatment can affect the circulating lipoproteins. Conditions present during blood collection, such as fasting status, posture, the choice of anticoagulant in the collection tube, and storage conditions, can alter the measurements. Typical observed biologic variation for more than 1 year for total cholesterol averages approximately 6.1% CV. In the average patient, measurements made over the course of a year would fall 66% of the time within ±6.1% of the mean cholesterol concentration and 95% of the time within twice this range. Some patients may exhibit substantially more biologic variation. Thus, preanalytic variation is generally relatively large in relation to the usual analytic variation, which is typically less than 3% CV, and must be considered in interpreting cholesterol results. Some factors, such as posture and blood collection, can be standardized to minimize the

variation. The NCEP guidelines recommend averaging at least two successive measurements to reduce the effects of both preanalytic and analytic sources.[31] The use of stepped cut points also reduces the practical effect of variation.

CASE STUDY 15.6

Three patients are seen in clinic:

- Patient 1 is a 40-year-old man with hypertension, who also smokes, but has not been previously diagnosed with CHD. His father developed CHD at age 53 years. He is fasting, and the results of his lipids include a total cholesterol concentration of 210 mg/dL, triglycerides of 150 mg/dL, and an HDL-C value of 45 mg/dL. He has a fasting glucose level of 98 mg/dL.
- Patient 2 is a 60-year-old woman with no family history of CHD and who is normotensive and does not smoke, with a total cholesterol concentration of 220 mg/dL, triglycerides of 85 mg/dL, and an HDL-C value of 80 mg/dL. Her fasting glucose level is 85 mg/dL.
- Patient 3 is a 49-year-old man with no personal or family history of CHD and who is not hypertensive and does not smoke. His fasting total cholesterol level is 260 mg/dL, his triglycerides are 505 mg/dL, his HDL-C is 25 mg/dL, and his glucose level is 134 mg/dL

Questions

For each patient seen in clinic:

1. What is the LDL-C level, as calculated using the Friedewald calculation?
2. Which patient, if any, should have his or her LDL-C measured, rather than calculated? Why?
3. How many known CHD risk factors does each patient have?
4. Based on what is known, are these patients recommended for lipid therapy (diet or drug) and, if so, on what basis?

Accuracy

Accuracy or trueness is ensured by demonstrating traceability or agreement through calibration to the respective "gold standard" reference system. With cholesterol, the reference system is advanced and complete, having served as a model for standardization of other laboratory analytes. The definitive method at the National Institute of Standards and Technology provides the ultimate accuracy target but is too expensive and complicated for frequent use.[96] The reference method developed and applied at the CDC, and calibrated by an approved primary reference standard to the definitive method, provides a transferable, practical reference link.[95] The reference method has been made conveniently accessible through a network of standardized laboratories, the Cholesterol Reference Method Laboratory Network. This network was established in the United States and other countries to extend standardization to manufacturers and clinical laboratories.[92] The network provides accuracy comparisons leading to certification of performance using fresh native serum specimens, necessary for reliable accuracy transfer because of analyte–matrix interaction problems on processed reference materials.[128,29]

Matrix Interactions

In the early stages of cholesterol standardization, which were directed toward diagnostic manufacturers and routine laboratories, commercial lyophilized or freeze-dried materials were used. These materials, made in large quantities, often with spiking or artificial addition of analytes, were assayed by the definitive and/or reference methods and distributed widely for accuracy transfer. Subsequently, biases were observed with some systems on fresh patient specimens even though they appeared to be accurate on the reference materials. Although such manufactured reference materials are convenient, stable, and amenable to shipment at ambient temperatures, the manufacturing process, especially spiking and lyophilization, altered the measurement properties in enzymatic assays such that results were not representative of those on patient specimens. To achieve reliable feedback on accuracy and facilitate transfer of the accuracy base, direct comparisons with the reference methods on actual patient specimens were determined to be necessary.[92] In response to these problems, the College of American Pathologists, a major provider of proficiency testing, now offers Accuracy-Based Lipid survey, which is made of fresh frozen serum and is commutable and without any matrix problems. Lipid and lipoprotein values are assigned to the material using reference methods.

CDC Cholesterol Reference Method Laboratory Network

The CDC cholesterol reference method laboratory network program was organized to improve the accuracy of lipid and lipoprotein testing. (Information is available at http://www.cdc.gov/labstandards/crmln.html.) The network offers formal certification programs for total cholesterol, HDL-C, and LDL-C and triglycerides whereby laboratories and manufacturers can document traceability to the national reference systems.[92] Through this program, clinical laboratories are able to identify certified commercial methods. Certification does not ensure all aspects of quality in a reagent system but primarily ensures that the accuracy is traceable to reference methods within accepted limits and that precision can meet the NCEP targets. The certification process is somewhat tedious and, thus, most efficient through manufacturers, but individual laboratories desiring to confirm the performance of their systems can complete a scaled-down certification protocol for cholesterol.

Analytic Performance Goals

The NCEP laboratory panels have established analytic performance goals based on clinical needs for routine measurements (Table 15.6).[38–40,130] For analysis of total cholesterol, the performance goal for total error is 8.9%. That is, the overall error should be such that each individual cholesterol measurement falls within ±8.9% of the reference method value. Actually, because the goals are based on 95% certainty, 95 of 100 measurements should fall within the total error limit. One can assay a specimen many times and calculate the mean to determine the usual value or the central tendency. The scatter or random variation around the mean is described by the standard deviation, an interval around the mean that includes, by definition, two-thirds of the observations. In the laboratory, because the scatter or imprecision is often proportional to the concentration, random variation is usually specified in relative terms as CV—the coefficient of variation or relative standard deviation, calculated as the standard deviation divided by the mean. Overall accuracy or systematic error is described as bias or trueness, the difference between the mean and the true value. Bias is primarily a function of the method's calibration and may vary by concentration. Of greatest concern in this context is bias at the NCEP decision cut points. The bias and CV targets presented in Table 15.6 are representative of performance that will meet the NCEP goals for total error.

Quality Control

Achieving acceptable analytic performance requires the use of reliable quality control materials, which should preferably closely emulate actual patient specimens. Commercial control materials have improved in recent years but may not approximate results with patients' specimens. Control materials can also be prepared in-house from freshly collected patient serum, aliquoted into securely sealed vials, quick frozen, and stored at −70°C. Such pools of fresh frozen serum are less subject to matrix interactions than the usual commercial materials, which is most important in monitoring accuracy in lipoprotein separation and analysis and preferable for monitoring cholesterol and other lipid measurements. At least two pools should be analyzed, preferably with levels at or near decision points for each analyte.

Specimen Collection

Serum, usually collected in serum separator vacuum tubes with clotting enhancers, has been the fluid of choice for lipoprotein measurement in the routine clinical laboratory. Ethylenediaminetetraacetic acid (EDTA) plasma was the traditional choice in lipid research laboratories, especially for lipoprotein separations, because the anticoagulant was thought to enhance stability by chelating metal ions. EDTA, however, has potential disadvantages that discourage routine use. Microclots, which can form in plasma during storage, could plug the sampling probes on the modern chemistry analyzers. EDTA also osmotically draws water from red cells, diluting the plasma constituents, and the dilution effect can vary depending on such factors as fill volume, the analyte being measured, and the extent of mixing. Because the NCEP cut points are based on serum values, cholesterol measurements made on EDTA plasma require correction by the factor of 1.03.

For additional student resources, please visit the**Point**® at http://thepoint.lww.com

q u e s t i o n s

1. Which of the following methods for lipoprotein electrophoresis depends on charge *and* molecular size?
   a. Polyacrylamide gel
   b. Paper
   c. Cellulose acetate
   d. Agarose

2. Which of the following statements concerning chylomicrons is FALSE?
   a. The major lipid transported by this lipoprotein is cholesterol.
   b. This lipoprotein is produced in the intestinal mucosa.
   c. The primary function is to carry dietary (exogenous) lipids to the liver.
   d. It remains at the origin (point of application) during lipoprotein electrophoresis.

3. The lipoprotein that contains the greatest amount of protein is called
   a. HDL
   b. Chylomicrons
   c. VLDL
   d. LDL

4. True or False? Pre–beta (VLDL)-lipoproteins migrate further toward the anode on polyacrylamide gel than they do on cellulose acetate or agarose.

5. Several enzymatic triglyceride methods measure the production or consumption of
   a. NADH
   b. Fatty acids
   c. Glycerol
   d. Diacetyl lutidine

6. The most likely cause for serum/plasma to appear "milky" is the presence of
   a. Chylomicrons
   b. VLDL
   c. LDL
   d. HDL

7. In the colorimetric determination of cholesterol using the enzyme cholesterol oxidase, the agent that oxidizes the colorless organic compound 4-aminoantipyrine to a pink complex is
   a. Hydrogen peroxide
   b. Cholest-4-ene-3-one
   c. NAD
   d. Phenol

8. Which lipoprotein is the major carrier of cholesterol *to* peripheral tissue?
   a. LDL
   b. Chylomicrons
   c. VLDL
   d. HDL

9. True or false? Increased levels of apo A-I are associated with increased risk of CAD.

10. A patient is admitted to the hospital with intense chest pains. The patient's primary care physician requests the emergency department doctor to order several tests, including a lipid profile with cholesterol fractionation. Given the patient's results provided below, what would be the LDL-C for this patient?
Total cholesterol = 400 mg/dL; triglycerides = 300 mg/dL; HDL-C = 100 mg/dL; LP electrophoresis, pending.
   a. 240 mg/dL
   b. 160 mg/dL
   c. 200 mg/dL
   d. 300 mg/dL

11. A patient is admitted to the hospital with intense chest pains. The patient's primary care physician requests the emergency department doctor to order several tests, including a lipid profile with cholesterol fractionation. Given the patient's results provided below, what would be this patient's LDL-C status?
Total cholesterol = 400 mg/dL; triglycerides = 300 mg/dL; HDL-C = 100 mg/dL; LP electrophoresis, pending
   a. High
   b. Optimal
   c. Desirable
   d. Borderline

review questions (continued)

12. As part of a lipoprotein phenotyping, it is necessary to perform total cholesterol and triglyceride determinations, as well as lipoprotein electrophoresis. The test results obtained from such studies were

- Triglyceride, 340 mg/dL (reference range, <150 mg/dL)
- Total cholesterol, 180 mg/dL (reference range, <200 mg/dL)
- Pre–beta-lipoprotein fraction increased
- Beta-lipoprotein fraction normal
- No chylomicrons present
- Serum appearance turbid

The best explanation for these results would be that the patient exhibits a phenotype indicative of

    a. Type IV hyperlipoproteinemia
    b. Type I hyperlipoproteinemia
    c. Type II hyperlipoproteinemia
    d. Type III hyperlipoproteinemia
    e. Type V hyperlipoproteinemia

13. Which of the following results is the most consistent with high risk of CHD?
    a. 20 mg/dL HDL-C and 250 mg/dL total cholesterol
    b. 35 mg/dL HDL-C and 200 mg/dL total cholesterol
    c. 50 mg/dL HDL-C and 190 mg/dL total cholesterol
    d. 55 mg/dL HDL-C and 180 mg/dL total cholesterol
    e. 60 mg/dL HDL-C and 170 mg/dL total cholesterol

14. What is the presumed defect in most cases of familial type IIa hyperlipoproteinemia?
    a. Defective receptors for LDL
    b. Deficiency of hydroxymethylglutaryl (HMG)-CoA reductase
    c. Deficiency of cholesterol esterase
    d. Deficiency of LPL
    e. Defective esterifying enzymes LCAT and ACAT

15. Hyperchylomicronemia (type I) in childhood has been associated with which of the following?
    a. A deficiency of apo C-II
    b. A deficiency of LCAT
    c. A deficiency of LPL
    d. A deficiency of apo A-I

references

1. Muller H, Kirkhus B, Pedersen JI. Serum cholesterol predictive equations with special emphasis on trans and saturated fatty acids. an analysis from designed controlled studies. *Lipids.* 2001;36(8):783–791.
2. Cunnane SC. Problems with essential fatty acids: time for a new paradigm? *Prog Lipid Res.* 2003;42(6):544–568.
3. Jones PJ. Regulation of cholesterol biosynthesis by diet in humans. *Am J Clin Nutr.* 1997;66(2):438–446.
4. Segrest JP, et al. Structure and function of apolipoprotein A-I and high-density lipoprotein. *Curr Opin Lipidol.* 2000;11(2):105–115.
5. Burnett JR, Barrett PH. Apolipoprotein B metabolism: tracer kinetics, models, and metabolic studies. *Crit Rev Clin Lab Sci.* 2002;39(2):89–137.
6. Javitt NB. Cholesterol homeostasis: role of the LDL receptor. *FASEB J.* 1995;9(13):1378–1381.
7. Law SW, et al. Human apolipoprotein B-100: cloning, analysis of liver mRNA, and assignment of the gene to chromosome 2. *Proc Natl Acad Sci U S A.* 1985;82(24):8340–8344.
8. Kostner KM, Kostner GM. Lipoprotein(a): still an enigma? *Curr Opin Lipidol.* 2002;13(4):391–396.
9. Cooper AD. Hepatic uptake of chylomicron remnants. *J Lipid Res.* 1997;38(11):2173–2192.
10. Lane RM, Farlow MR. Lipid homeostasis and apolipoprotein E in the development and progression of Alzheimer's disease. *J Lipid Res.* 2005;46(5):949–968.
11. Corder EH, et al. The role of APOE polymorphisms in late-onset dementias. *Cell Mol Life Sci.* 1998;54(9):928–934.
12. Kruth HS. Sequestration of aggregated low-density lipoproteins by macrophages. *Curr Opin Lipidol.* 2002;13(5):483–488.
13. Warnick GR, et al. Polyacrylamide gradient gel electrophoresis of lipoprotein subclasses. *Clin Lab Med.* 2006;26(4):803–846.
14. Kulkarni KR. Cholesterol profile measurement by vertical auto profile method. *Clin Lab Med.* 2006;26(4):787–802.
15. McNamara JR, et al. Differences in LDL subspecies involve alterations in lipid composition and conformational changes in apolipoprotein B. *J Lipid Res.* 1996;37(9):1924–1935.
16. Albers JJ, Koschinsky ML, Marcovina SM. Evidence mounts for a role of the kidney in lipoprotein(a) catabolism. *Kidney Int.* 2007;71(10):961–962.
17. Nishiwaki M, et al. Human lecithin:cholesterol acyl-transferase deficiency: in vivo kinetics of low-density

lipoprotein and lipoprotein-X. *Arterioscler Thromb Vasc Biol.* 2006;26(6):1370–1375.

18. Lee MH, Lu K, Patel SB. Genetic basis of sitosterolemia. *Curr Opin Lipidol.* 2001;12(2):141–149.

19. Graf GA, et al. ABCG5 and ABCG8 are obligate heterodimers for protein trafficking and biliary cholesterol excretion. *J Biol Chem.* 2003;278(48):48275–48282.

20. Mead JR, Irvine SA, Ramji DP. Lipoprotein lipase: structure, function, regulation, and role in disease. *J Mol Med (Berl).* 2002;80(12):753–769.

21. Vaziri ND. Causes of dysregulation of lipid metabolism in chronic renal failure. *Semin Dial.* 2009;22(6):644–651.

22. Rizzo M, Berneis K. Small, dense low-density-lipoproteins and the metabolic syndrome. *Diabetes Metab Res Rev.* 2007;23(1):14–20.

23. Dean M, Hamon Y, Chimini G. The human ATP-binding cassette (ABC) transporter superfamily. *J Lipid Res.* 2001;42(7):1007–1017.

24. Nofer JR, Remaley AT. Tangier disease: still more questions than answers. *Cell Mol Life Sci.* 2005;62(19–20):2150–2160.

25. Wang N, et al. ATP-binding cassette transporters G1 and G4 mediate cellular cholesterol efflux to high-density lipoproteins. *Proc Natl Acad Sci U S A.* 2004;101(26):9774–9779.

26. Kilsdonk EP, et al. Cellular cholesterol efflux mediated by cyclodextrins. *J Biol Chem.* 1995;270(29):17250–17256.

27. Khera AV, et al. Cholesterol efflux capacity, high-density lipoprotein function, and atherosclerosis. *N Engl J Med.* 2011;364(2):127–135.

28. Rohatgi A, et al. HDL cholesterol efflux capacity and incident cardiovascular events. *N Engl J Med.* 2014;371(25):2383–2393.

29. Expert Panel on Integrated Guidelines for Cardiovascular Health and Risk Reduction in Children and Adolescents; National Heart, Lung, and Blood Institute. Expert panel on integrated guidelines for cardiovascular health and risk reduction in children and adolescents: summary report. *Pediatrics.* 2011;128(suppl 5):S213–S256.

30. Kato H, et al. Epidemiologic studies of coronary heart disease and stroke in Japanese men living in Japan, Hawaii and California. *Am J Epidemiol.* 1973;97(6):372–385.

31. National Cholesterol Education Program (NCEP) Expert Panel on Detection, Evaluation, and Treatment of High Blood Cholesterol in Adults (Adult Treatment Panel III. Third Report of the National Cholesterol Education Program (NCEP) Expert Panel on Detection, Evaluation, and Treatment of High Blood Cholesterol in Adults (Adult Treatment Panel III) final report. *Circulation.* 2002;106(25):3143–3421.

32. Jensen MD, et al. 2013 AHA/ACC/TOS guideline for the management of overweight and obesity in adults: a report of the American College of Cardiology/American Heart Association Task Force on Practice Guidelines and The Obesity Society. *Circulation.* 2014;129(25 suppl 2):S102–S138.

33. Stone NJ, et al. 2013 ACC/AHA guideline on the treatment of blood cholesterol to reduce atherosclerotic cardiovascular risk in adults: a report of the American College of Cardiology/American Heart Association Task Force on Practice Guidelines. *Circulation.* 2014;129(25 suppl 2):S1–S45.

34. Kit BK, et al. Trends in serum lipids among US youths aged 6 to 19 years, 1988–2010. *JAMA.* 2012;308(6):591–600.

35. McMahan CA, et al. Pathobiological determinants of atherosclerosis in youth risk scores are associated with early and advanced atherosclerosis. *Pediatrics.* 2006;118(4):1447–1455.

36. Ritchie SK, et al. Universal versus targeted blood cholesterol screening among youth: the CARDIAC project. *Pediatrics.* 2010;126(2):260–265.

37. Newman TB, Pletcher MJ, Hulley SB. Overly aggressive new guidelines for lipid screening in children: evidence of a broken process. *Pediatrics.* 2012;130(2):349–352.

38. Warnick GR, Wood PD. National Cholesterol Education Program recommendations for measurement of high-density lipoprotein cholesterol: executive summary. The National Cholesterol Education Program Working Group on Lipoprotein Measurement. *Clin Chem.* 1995;41(10):1427–1433.

39. Bachorik PS, Ross JW. National Cholesterol Education Program recommendations for measurement of low-density lipoprotein cholesterol: executive summary. The National Cholesterol Education Program Working Group on Lipoprotein Measurement. *Clin Chem.* 1995;41(10):1414–1420.

40. Stein EA, Myers GL. National Cholesterol Education Program recommendations for triglyceride measurement: executive summary. The National Cholesterol Education Program Working Group on Lipoprotein Measurement. *Clin Chem.* 1995;41(10):1421–1426.

41. Schaefer EJ, et al. Lipoproteins, nutrition, aging, and atherosclerosis. *Am J Clin Nutr.* 1995;61(3 suppl):726S–740S.

42. Niebauer J, et al. Attenuated progression of coronary artery disease after 6 years of multifactorial risk intervention: role of physical exercise. *Circulation.* 1997;96(8):2534–2541.

43. Stary HC. Macrophages, macrophage foam cells, and eccentric intimal thickening in the coronary arteries of young children. *Atherosclerosis.* 1987;64(2–3):91–108.

44. Keaney JF Jr. Atherosclerosis: from lesion formation to plaque activation and endothelial dysfunction. *Mol Aspects Med.* 2000;21(4–5):99–166.

45. Scandinavian Simvastatin Survival Study Group. Randomised trial of cholesterol lowering in 4444 patients with coronary heart disease: the Scandinavian Simvastatin Survival Study (4S). *Lancet.* 1994;344(8934):1383–1389.

46. National Institutes of Health Consensus Conference. Triglyceride, HDL cholesterol and coronary heart disease. *JAMA.* 1993;269:505.

47. Shepherd J, et al. Prevention of coronary heart disease with pravastatin in men with hypercholesterolemia. 1995. *Atheroscler Suppl.* 2004;5(3):91–97.

48. The Lipid Research Clinics Coronary Program Primary Prevention Trial results. I. Reduction in incidence of coronary heart disease. *JAMA.* 1984;251(3):351–364.

49. Matthan NR, et al. Impact of simvastatin, niacin, and/or antioxidants on cholesterol metabolism in CAD patients with low HDL. *J Lipid Res.* 2003;44(4):800–806.

50. Rubins HB, Robins SJ, Collins D, et al. Gemfibrozil for the secondary prevention of coronary heart disease in men with low levels of high-density lipoprotein cholesterol. Veterans Affairs High-Density Lipoprotein Cholesterol Intervention Trial Study Group. *N Engl J Med.* 1999;341:410–418.

51. Sethi AA, et al. Apolipoprotein AI mimetic peptides: possible new agents for the treatment of atherosclerosis. *Curr Opin Investig Drugs.* 2007;8(3):201–212.

52. Gotto AM. Management of dyslipaemia. *Am J Med.* 2002;112:105–185; (supplement).

53. Shepherd J, et al. Prevention of coronary heart disease with pravastatin in men with hypercholesterolemia. West of Scotland Coronary Prevention Study Group. *N Engl J Med.* 1995;333(20):1301–1307.

54. Ganji SH. Niacin and cholesterol: role in cardiovascular disease (review). *J Nutr Biochem.* 2003;14:298–305.

55. Knopp RH. Drug treatment of lipid disorders. *N Engl J Med.* 1999;341(7):498–511.

56. Batiste MC, Schaefer EJ. Diagnosis and management of lipoprotein abnormalities. *Nutr Clin Care.* 2002;5(3):115–123.

57. Guyton JR. Niacin in cardiovascular prevention: mechanisms, efficacy, and safety. *Curr Opin Lipidol.* 2007;18(4):415–420.

58. Kosoglou T, et al. Ezetimibe: a review of its metabolism, pharmacokinetics and drug interactions. *Clin Pharmacokinet.* 2005;44(5):467–494.

59. Nestel PJ. Suppression by diets rich in fish oil of very low density lipoprotein production in man. *J Clin Invest.* 1984;74:82–89.

60. Price PT. Omega-3 polyunsaturated fatty acid regulation of gene expression. *Curr Opin Lipidol.* 2000;11:3–7.

61. McKenney JM, Sica D. Role of prescription omega-3 fatty acids in the treatment of hypertriglyceridemia. *Pharmacotherapy.* 2007;27(5):715–728.

62. Castelli WP, et al. Incidence of coronary heart disease and lipoprotein cholesterol levels. The Framingham Study. *JAMA.* 1986;256(20):2835–2838.

63. Marais AD, Firth JC, Blom DJ. Homozygous familial hypercholesterolemia and its management. *Semin Vasc Med.* 2004;4(1):43–50.

64. Schaefer EJ, McNamara JR. Overview of the diagnosis and treatment of lipid disorders. In: Rifai N, Warnick GR, eds. *Handbook of Lipoprotein Testing.* Washington, DC: AACC Press; 1997.

65. Chang JH, et al. Identification and characterization of LDL receptor gene mutations in hyperlipidemic Chinese. *J Lipid Res.* 2003;44(10):1850–1858.

66. Palcoux JB, et al. Comparison of different treatment regimens in a case of homozygous familial hypercholesterolemia. *Ther Apher.* 2002;6(2):136–139.

67. Ling H, Burns TL, Hilleman DE. An update on the clinical development of proprotein convertase subtilisin kexin 9 inhibitors, novel therapeutic agents for lowering low-density lipoprotein cholesterol. *Cardiovasc Ther.* 2014;32(2):82–88.

68. Giugliano RP, Sabatine MS. Are PCSK9 inhibitors the next breakthrough in the cardiovascular field? *J Am Coll Cardiol.* 2015;65(24):2638–2651.

69. Cohen JC. Emerging LDL therapies: using human genetics to discover new therapeutic targets for plasma lipids. *J Clin Lipidol.* 2013;7(3 suppl):S1–S5.

70. Genest J Jr, Cohn J. Plasma triglyceride-rich lipoprotein and high density lipoproteins disorders associated with atherosclerosis. *J Investig Med.* 1998;46(8):351–358.

71. Reynisdottir S, et al. Impaired activation of adipocyte lipolysis in familial combined hyperlipidemia. *J Clin Invest.* 1995;95(5):2161–2169.

72. Yadav D, Pitchumoni CS. Issues in hyperlipidemic pancreatitis. *J Clin Gastroenterol.* 2003;36(1):54–62.

73. Jackson RL, McLean LR, Demel RA. Mechanism of action of lipoprotein lipase and hepatic triglyceride lipase. *Am Heart J.* 1987;113(2 Pt 2):551–554.

74. Santamarina-Fojo S. The familial chylomicronemia syndrome. *Endocrinol Metab Clin North Am.* 1998;27(3):551–567, viii.

75. Fredrickson DS, Levy RI, Lees RS. Fat transport in lipoproteins—an integrated approach to mechanisms and disorders. *N Engl J Med.* 1967;276(5):273–281.

76. Civeira F, et al. Apo E variants in patients with type III hyperlipoproteinemia. *Atherosclerosis.* 1996;127(2):273–282.

77. Sijbrands EJ, et al. Severe hyperlipidemia in apolipoprotein E2 homozygotes due to a combined effect of hyperinsulinemia and an SstI polymorphism. *Arterioscler Thromb Vasc Biol.* 1999;19(11):2722–2729.

78. Friedewald WT, Levy RI, Fredrickson DS. Estimation of the concentration of low-density lipoprotein cholesterol in plasma, without use of the preparative ultracentrifuge. *Clin Chem.* 1972;18(6):499–502.

79. Jialal I, et al. Comparison of an immunoprecipitation method for direct measurement of LDL-cholesterol with beta-quantification (ultracentrifugation). *Am J Clin Pathol.* 1995;104(1):76–81.

80. Hopkins PN, et al. Lipoprotein(a) interactions with lipid and non-lipid risk factors in patients with early onset coronary artery disease: results from the NHLBI Family Heart Study. *Atherosclerosis.* 1998;141(2):333–345.

81. McLean JW, et al. cDNA sequence of human apolipoprotein(a) is homologous to plasminogen. *Nature.* 1987;330(6144):132–137.

82. Hajjar KA, et al. Lipoprotein(a) modulation of endothelial cell surface fibrinolysis and its potential role in atherosclerosis. *Nature.* 1989;339(6222):303–305.

83. Qin SY, et al. Association between baseline lipoprotein (a) levels and restenosis after coronary stenting: meta-analysis of 9 cohort studies. *Atherosclerosis.* 2013;227(2):360–366.

84. Schumacher M, et al. Lipoprotein (a) is not a risk factor for restenosis after percutaneous transluminal coronary angioplasty. *Am J Cardiol.* 1992;69(5):572.

85. Daida H, et al. Prevention of restenosis after percutaneous transluminal coronary angioplasty by reducing lipoprotein (a) levels with low-density lipoprotein apheresis. Low-Density Lipoprotein Apheresis Angioplasty Restenosis Trial (L-ART) Group. *Am J Cardiol.* 1994;73(15):1037–1040.

86. Bittner V. Non-high-density lipoprotein cholesterol and cardiovascular disease. *Curr Opin Lipidol.* 2003;14(4):367–371.

87. Mora S, et al. Fasting compared with nonfasting lipids and apolipoproteins for predicting incident cardiovascular events. *Circulation.* 2008;118(10):993–1001.

88. Charlton-Menys V, et al. Targets of statin therapy: LDL cholesterol, non-HDL cholesterol, and apolipoprotein B in type 2 diabetes in the Collaborative Atorvastatin Diabetes Study (CARDS). *Clin Chem.* 2009;55(3):473–480.

89. Mott S, et al. Decreased cellular cholesterol efflux is a common cause of familial hypoalphalipoproteinemia: role of the ABCA1 gene mutations. *Atherosclerosis.* 2000;152(2):457–468.

90. Baldassarre D, Amato M, Pustina L, et al. Increased carotid artery intima-media thickness in subjects with primary hypoalphalipoproteinemia. *Arterioscler Thromb Vasc Biol.* 2002;22:317–322.

91. McCormack PL, Keating GM. Prolonged-release nicotinic acid: a review of its use in the treatment of dyslipidaemia. *Drugs.* 2005;65(18):2719–2740.

92. Myers GL, Cooper GR, Greenberg N, et al. Standardization of lipid and lipoprotein measurements. In: Rifai N, Warnick GR, Dominczak MH, eds. *Handbook of Lipoprotein Testing.* 2nd ed. Washington, DC: AACC Press; 2000.

93. Zak B. Cholesterol methodologies: a review. *Clin Chem.* 1977;23(7):1201–1214.

94. Abel LL, et al. A simplified method for the estimation of total cholesterol in serum and demonstration of its specificity. *J Biol Chem.* 1952;195(1):357–366.

95. Duncan IW, Mather A, Cooper GR. *The procedure for the proposed cholesterol reference method.* Atlanta, GA: Division of Environmental Health Laboratory Sciences, Center for Environmental Health, Centers for Disease Control and Prevention; 1985.

96. Cohen A, et al. Total serum cholesterol by isotope dilution/mass spectrometry: a candidate definitive method. *Clin Chem.* 1980;26(7):854–860.

97. Klotzsch SG, McNamara JR. Triglyceride measurements: a review of methods and interferences. *Clin Chem.* 1990;36(9):1605–1613.

98. Bucolo G, Yabut J, Chang TY. Mechanized enzymatic determination of triglycerides in serum. *Clin Chem.* 1975;21(3):420–424.

99. Stinshoff K, et al. Relation between concentrations of free glycerol and triglycerides in human sera. *Clin Chem.* 1977;23(6):1029–1032.

100. Patsch JR, Patsch W. Zonal ultracentrifugation. *Methods Enzymol.* 1986;129:3–26.

101. Schmitz G, Boettcher A, Barlage S. New approaches to the use of lipoprotein electrophoresis in the clinical laboratory. In: Rifai N, Warnick GR, Dominczak MH, eds. *Handbook of Lipoprotein Testing.* 2nd ed. Washington, DC: AACC Press; 2000.

102. Warnick GR, et al. Lipoprotein quantification: an electrophoretic method compared with the Lipid Research Clinics method. *Clin Chem.* 1982;28(10):2116–2120.

103. Greenspan P, et al. Advances in agarose gel electrophoresis of serum lipoproteins. *J Chromatogr A.* 1995;698(1–2):333–339.

104. Rifai N, et al. Measurement of low-density-lipoprotein cholesterol in serum: a status report. *Clin Chem.* 1992;38(1):150–160.

105. Warnick GR, Leary ET, Goetsch J. Electrophoretic quantification of LDL-cholesterol using the Helena REP. *Clin Chem.* 1993;39:1122.

106. Li Z, et al. Analysis of high density lipoproteins by a modified gradient gel electrophoresis method. *J Lipid Res.* 1994;35(9):1698–1711.

107. Burstein M, Legmann P. Lipoprotein precipitation. *Monogr Atheroscler.* 1982;11:1–131.

108. Schumaker VN, et al. Anti-apoprotein B monoclonal antibodies detect human low density lipoprotein polymorphism. *J Biol Chem.* 1984;259(10):6423–6430.

109. Nakajima K, et al. Cholesterol in remnant-like lipoproteins in human serum using monoclonal anti apo B-100 and anti apo A-I immunoaffinity mixed gels. *Clin Chim Acta.* 1993;223(1–2):53–71.

110. National Institutes of Health. *Manual of Laboratory Operations, Lipid Research Clinics Program, Lipid and Lipoprotein Analysis.* Washington, DC: U.S. Department of Health and Human Services; 1983.

111. Lopes-Virella MF, et al. Cholesterol determination in high-density lipoproteins separated by three different methods. *Clin Chem.* 1977;23(5):882–884.

112. Warnick GR, Cheung MC, Albers JJ. Comparison of current methods for high-density lipoprotein cholesterol quantitation. *Clin Chem.* 1979;25(4):596–604.

113. Warnick GR, Benderson J, Albers JJ. Dextran sulfate-Mg^{2+} precipitation procedure for quantitation of high-density-lipoprotein cholesterol. *Clin Chem.* 1982;28(6):1379–1388.

114. Demacker PN, et al. Measurement of high-density lipoprotein cholesterol in serum: comparison of six isolation methods combined with enzymic cholesterol analysis. *Clin Chem.* 1980;26(13):1780–1786.

115. Warnick GR, et al. Multilaboratory evaluation of an ultrafiltration procedure for high density lipoprotein cholesterol quantification in turbid heparin-manganese supernates. *J Lipid Res.* 1981;22(6):1015–1020.

116. Sugiuchi H, et al. Direct measurement of high-density lipoprotein cholesterol in serum with polyethylene glycol-modified enzymes and sulfated alpha-cyclodextrin. *Clin Chem.* 1995;41(5):717–723.

117. Harris N, Galpchian V, Rifai N. Three routine methods for measuring high-density lipoprotein cholesterol compared with the Reference Method. *Clin Chem.* 1996;42(5):738–743.

118. Bachorik PS. Lipid and lipoprotein analysis with desktop analyzers. In: Rifai N, Warnick GR, Dominczak MH, eds. *Handbook of Lipoprotein Testing.* 2nd ed. Washington, DC: AACC Press; 2000.

119. Sugiuchi H, et al. Homogeneous assay for measuring low-density lipoprotein cholesterol in serum with triblock copolymer and alpha-cyclodextrin sulfate. *Clin Chem.* 1998;44(3):522–531.

120. Rifai N, et al. Analytical and clinical performance of a homogeneous enzymatic LDL-cholesterol assay compared with the ultracentrifugation-dextran sulfate-Mg^{2+} method. *Clin Chem.* 1998;44(6 Pt 1):1242–1250.

121. Barter PJ, et al. Apo B versus cholesterol in estimating cardiovascular risk and in guiding therapy: report of the thirty-person/ten-country panel. *J Intern Med.* 2006;259(3):247–258.

122. Bhatnager D, Durrington PN. Measurement and clinical significance of apolipoproteins A-1 and B. In: Rifai N, Warnick GR, Dominczak MH, eds. *Handbook of Lipoprotein Testing.* 2nd ed. Washington, DC: AACC Press; 2000.

123. Marcovina SM, Koschinsky ML. Lipoprotein (a): structure, measurement, and clinical significance. In: Rifai N, Warnick GR, Dominczak MH, eds. *Handbook of Lipoprotein Testing.* 2nd ed. Washington, DC: AACC Press; 2000.

124. McGowan MW, Artiss JD, Zak B. A procedure for the determination of high-density lipoprotein choline-containing phospholipids. *J Clin Chem Clin Biochem.* 1982;20(11):807–812.

125. Hellerstein MK. Methods for measurement of fatty acid and cholesterol metabolism. *Curr Opin Lipidol.* 1995;6(3):172–181.

126. Husek P, Simek P, Tvrzická E. Simple and rapid procedure for the determination of individual free fatty acids in serum. *Anal Chim Acta.* 2002;465:433–439.

127. Cooper GR, et al. Blood lipid measurements. Variations and practical utility. *JAMA.* 1992;267(12):1652–1660.

128. Bernert JT Jr, et al. Factors influencing the accuracy of the national reference system total cholesterol reference method. *Clin Chem.* 1991;37(12):2053–2061.

129. Eckfeldt JH, Copeland KR. Accuracy verification and identification of matrix effects. The College of American Pathologists' Protocol. *Arch Pathol Lab Med.* 1993;117(4):381–386.

130. Report from the Laboratory Standardization Panel of the National Cholesterol Education Program. *Recommendations for Improving Cholesterol Measurement.* Bethesda, MD: National Institutes of Health; 1990; (No. 902964).

16

Electrolytes

JAMES MARCH MISTLER

chapter outline

chapter objectives

Upon completion of this chapter, the clinical laboratorian should be able to do the following:

- Define electrolyte, osmolality, anion gap, anion, and cation.
- Discuss the physiology of each electrolyte described in the chapter.
- State the clinical significance of each of the electrolytes mentioned in the chapter.
- Calculate osmolality, osmolal gap, and anion gap and discuss the clinical usefulness of each.
- Discuss the analytic techniques used to assess electrolyte concentrations.
- Correlate the information with disease state, given patient data.
- Identify the reference ranges for sodium, potassium, chloride, bicarbonate, magnesium, and calcium.
- State the specimen of choice for the major electrolytes.
- Discuss the role of the kidney in electrolyte excretion and conservation in a healthy individual.
- Discuss the usefulness of urine electrolyte results: sodium, potassium, calcium, and osmolality.

key terms

Active Transport
Anion
Anion Gap (AG)
Cation
Diabetes Insipidus
Diffusion
Electrolyte
Extracellular Fluid (ECF)
Hypercalcemia
Hyperchloremia
Hyperkalemia
Hypermagnesemia
Hypernatremia
Hyperphosphatemia
Hypocalcemia
Hypochloremia
Hypokalemia
Hypomagnesemia
Hyponatremia
Hypophosphatemia
Hypovolemia
Intracellular Fluid (ICF)
Osmolal Gap
Osmolality
Osmolarity
Osmometer
Polydipsia
Tetany

For additional student resources, please visit thePoint® at http://thepoint.lww.com

Electrolytes are ions (minerals) capable of carrying an electric charge. They are classified as either anions or cations based on the type of charge they carry. Anion and cation classifications are based on how the ion migrates in an electric field; those electrolytes with a positive charge are **cations** that move toward the cathode, while those with a negative charge are **anions** that move toward the anode.

Electrolytes are an essential component in numerous processes, including volume and osmotic regulation (sodium [Na^+], chloride [Cl^-], potassium [K^+]); myocardial rhythm and contractility (K^+, magnesium [Mg^{2+}], calcium [Ca^{2+}]); cofactors in enzyme activation (e.g., Mg^{2+}, Ca^{2+}, zinc [Zn^{2+}]); regulation of adenosine triphosphatase (ATPase) ion pumps (Mg^{2+}); acid–base balance (bicarbonate [HCO_3^-], K^+, Cl^-); blood coagulation (Ca^{2+}, Mg^{2+}); neuromuscular excitability (K^+, Ca^{2+}, Mg^{2+}); and the production and use of ATP from glucose (e.g., Mg^{2+}, phosphate PO_4^-). Because many of these functions require electrolyte concentrations to be held within very narrow ranges, the body has complex systems for monitoring and maintaining electrolyte concentrations.

This chapter explores both the metabolic physiology and regulation of each electrolyte and relates these factors to the clinical significance of electrolyte measurements. In addition, methodologies used in determining concentrations of the individual analytes are discussed.

WATER

The average water content of the human body varies from 40% to 75% of total body weight, with values declining with age and especially with obesity. Women have lower average water content than do men as a result of a higher fat content. Water is the solvent for all processes in the human body as it is responsible for transporting nutrients to cells, determining cell volume by its transport into and out of cells, removal of waste products by way of urine, and acting as the body's coolant by way of sweating. Water is located in both intracellular and extracellular compartments. **Intracellular fluid (ICF)** is the fluid inside the cells and accounts for about two-thirds of total body water. **Extracellular fluid (ECF)** accounts for the other one-third of total body water and can be subdivided into the *intravascular ECF (plasma)* and the *interstitial cell fluid* that surrounds the cells in the tissue. Normal plasma is about 93% water, with the remaining volume occupied by lipids and proteins. The concentrations of ions within cells and in plasma are maintained both by energy-consuming active transport processes and by diffusion or passive transport processes.

Active transport is a mechanism that requires energy to move ions across cellular membranes. For example, maintaining a high intracellular concentration of K^+ and a high extracellular (plasma) concentration of Na^+ requires use of energy, which comes from the breakdown of ATP by ATPase-dependent ion pumps. **Diffusion** is the passive movement of ions (no energy consumed) across a membrane and depends on both the size and charge of the ion being transported, and on the nature of the membrane through which it is passing. The rate of diffusion of various ions also may be altered by physiologic and hormonal processes.

Distribution of water in the various body fluid compartments is controlled by maintaining the concentration of electrolytes and proteins in the individual compartments. Because most biologic membranes are freely permeable to water but not to ions or proteins, the concentration of ions and proteins on either side of the membrane will influence the flow of water across a membrane (known as an osmoregulator). In addition to the osmotic effects of Na^+, other ions, proteins, and blood pressure influence the flow of water across a membrane.

Osmolality

Osmolality is a physical property of a solution that is based on the concentration of solutes (expressed as millimoles) per kilogram of solvent (w/w). Osmolality is related to several changes in the properties of a solution relative to pure water, such as freezing point depression and vapor pressure decrease. These colligative properties (see Chapter 5) are the basis for routine measurements of osmolality in the laboratory. The term **osmolarity** is still occasionally used, with results reported in milliosmoles per liter (w/v), but it is inaccurate in cases of hyperlipidemia or hyperproteinemia; for urine specimens; or in the presence of certain osmotically active substances, such as alcohol or mannitol. Both the sensation of thirst and arginine vasopressin hormone (AVP), formerly called antidiuretic hormone (ADH), secretion are stimulated by the hypothalamus in response to an increased osmolality of blood. The natural response to the thirst sensation is to consume more fluids, increasing the water content of the ECF, therefore diluting the elevated solute (Na^+) levels and decreasing the osmolality of the plasma. Thirst, therefore, is important in mediating fluid intake. The other means of controlling osmolality is by secretion of AVP. This hormone is secreted by the posterior pituitary gland and acts on the cells of the collecting ducts in the kidneys to increase water reabsorption. This is an example of a negative feedback loop; as water is conserved, the osmolality decreases, which in turn shuts off AVP secretion (feedback loops are discussed more in Chapter 20).[1]

Clinical Significance of Osmolality

Osmolality in plasma is important because it is the parameter to which the hypothalamus responds. The regulation of osmolality also affects the Na^+ concentration in plasma, largely because Na^+ and its associated anions account for approximately 90% of the osmotic activity in plasma. Another important process affecting the Na^+ concentration in blood is the regulation of blood volume. As discussed later, although osmolality and volume are regulated by separate mechanisms (except for AVP and thirst), they are related because osmolality (Na^+) is regulated by changes in water balance, whereas volume is regulated by changes in Na^+ balance.[1]

To maintain a normal plasma osmolality (275 to 295 mOsm/kg of plasma H_2O), osmoreceptors in the hypothalamus respond quickly to small changes in osmolality. A 1% to 2% increase in osmolality causes a fourfold increase in the circulating concentration of AVP, and a 1% to 2% decrease in osmolality shuts off AVP production. AVP acts by increasing the reabsorption of water in the cortical and medullary collecting tubules but has a half-life in the circulation of only 15 to 20 minutes.

Renal water regulation by AVP and thirst play important roles in regulating plasma osmolality. Renal water excretion is more important in controlling water excess, whereas thirst is more important in preventing water deficit (dehydration). Consider what happens in several conditions.

Water Load

As excess intake of water (e.g., in polydipsia) begins to lower plasma osmolality, both AVP and thirst are suppressed. In the absence of AVP, water is not reabsorbed causing a large volume of dilute urine to be excreted; as much as 10 to 20 L of water daily can be excreted, well above any normal intake of water. Therefore, hypoosmolality and hyponatremia usually occur only in patients with impaired renal excretion of water.[1]

Water Deficit

As the deficit of water begins to increase plasma osmolality, both AVP secretion and thirst are activated. Although AVP contributes by minimizing renal water loss, thirst is the major defense against hyperosmolality and hypernatremia. Although hypernatremia rarely occurs in a person with a normal thirst mechanism and access to water, it becomes a concern in infants, unconscious patients, or anyone who is unable to either drink or ask for water. Osmotic stimulation of thirst progressively diminishes in people who are older than age 60. In the older patient with illness and diminished mental status, dehydration becomes increasingly likely. An example of the effectiveness of thirst in preventing dehydration can be seen in patients with **diabetes insipidus**, where there is either no AVP production or no ability to respond to the AVP in circulation. In these patients, excretion may increase to 10 L of urine per day; however, because thirst persists, water intake matches output and plasma Na^+, and therefore plasma osmolality, remain normal.[1]

Regulation of Blood Volume

Adequate blood volume is essential to maintain blood pressure and ensure good perfusion to all tissues and organs. Regulation of both Na^+ and water is interrelated in controlling blood volume. The renin–angiotensin–aldosterone hormone system responds primarily to a decreased blood volume. Renin is secreted near the renal glomeruli in response to decreased renal blood flow (decreased blood volume or blood pressure). Renin converts the hormone angiotensinogen to angiotensin I, which then becomes angiotensin II. Angiotensin II causes vasoconstriction, which quickly increases blood pressure, and secretion of aldosterone, which increases retention of Na^+ and the water that accompanies the Na^+. The effects of blood volume and osmolality on Na^+ and water metabolism are shown in Figure 16.1. Changes in blood volume (which is actually a change in pressure) are initially detected by a series of stretch receptors located in areas such as the cardiopulmonary circulation, carotid sinus, aortic arch, and glomerular arterioles. These receptors then activate a series of responses (effectors) that restore volume by appropriately varying vascular resistance, cardiac output, and renal Na^+ and water retention.[1]

Four other factors affect blood volume: (1) atrial natriuretic peptide (ANP), released from the myocardial atria in response to volume expansion, promotes Na^+ excretion in the kidney (B-type natriuretic peptide and ANP act together in regulating blood pressure and fluid balance);

FIGURE 16.1 Responses to changes in blood osmolality and blood volume. ANP, atrial natriuretic peptide; ADH, antidiuretic hormone; ACE, angiotensin-converting enzyme. The primary stimuli are shown in *boxes* (e.g., hypovolemia).

(2) volume receptors independent of osmolality stimulate the release of AVP, which conserves water by renal reabsorption; (3) glomerular filtration rate (GFR) increases with volume expansion and decreases with volume depletion; and (4) all other things equal, an increased plasma Na^+ will increase urinary Na^+ (and therefore water) excretion and vice versa. The normal reabsorption of 98% to 99% of filtered Na^+ by the tubules conserves nearly all of the 150 L of glomerular filtrate produced daily, while a 1% to 2% reduction in tubular reabsorption of Na^+ can increase water loss by several liters per day.

Urine osmolality values may vary widely depending on water intake and the circumstances of collection. However, it is generally decreased in diabetes insipidus and **polydipsia** (excessive H_2O intake) and increased in conditions such as the syndrome of inappropriate antidiuretic hormone (SIADH) secretion and **hypovolemia** (although urinary Na^+ is usually decreased).

Determination of Osmolality

Specimen
Osmolality may be measured in serum or urine. Major electrolyte concentrations, mainly sodium, chloride, and bicarbonate, provide the largest contribution to the osmolality value of serum. Plasma use is not recommended because osmotically active substances may be introduced into the specimen from the anticoagulant.

Discussion
The methods for determining osmolality are based on properties of a solution that are related to the number of molecules of solute per kilogram of solvent (colligative properties), such as changes in freezing point and vapor pressure. An increase in osmolality decreases both the freezing point temperature and the vapor pressure. Measurements of freezing point depression and vapor pressure decrease (actually, the dew point) are the two most frequently used methods of analysis. For detailed information on theory and methodology, consult Chapter 5 or the operator's manual of the instrument being used.

Samples must be free of particulate matter to obtain accurate results. Turbid serum and urine samples should be centrifuged before analysis to remove any extraneous particles. If reusable sample cups are used, they should be thoroughly cleaned, disinfected, and dried between each use to prevent contamination.

Osmometers that operate by freezing point depression are standardized using sodium chloride reference solutions. After calibration, the appropriate amount of sample is pipetted into the required cuvette or sample cup and placed in the analyzer. The sample is then supercooled to −7°C and seeded to initiate the freezing process. When temperature equilibrium has been reached, the freezing point is measured, with results for serum and urine osmolality reported as milliosmoles per kilogram.

Calculation of osmolality has some usefulness either as an estimate of the true osmolality or to determine the **osmolal gap**, which is the difference between the measured

TABLE 16.1 **Reference Ranges for Osmolality**

Serum	275–295 mOsm/kg
Urine (24 h)	300–900 mOsm/kg
Urine/serum ratio	1.0–3.0
Random urine	50–1,200 mOsm/kg
Osmolal gap	5–10 mOsm/kg

osmolality and the calculated osmolality. The osmolal gap indirectly indicates the presence of osmotically active substances other than Na^+, urea, or glucose, such as ethanol, methanol, ethylene glycol, isopropanol, lactate, or β-hydroxybutyrate.

Two formulas are presented, each having theoretic advantages and disadvantages. Both are adequate for the purpose previously described. For more discussion, the reader may consult other references.[2]

$$2\,Na + \frac{glucose\,(mg/dL)}{20} + \frac{BUN\,(mg/dL)}{3}$$
$$or \qquad\qquad (Eq.\ 16\text{-}1)$$
$$1.86\,Na + \frac{glucose}{18} + \frac{BUN}{2.8} + 9$$

Reference Ranges
See Table 16.1.[3]

THE ELECTROLYTES

Sodium
Na^+ is the most abundant cation in the ECF, representing 90% of all extracellular cations, and largely determines the osmolality of the plasma. A normal plasma osmolality is approximately 295 mmol/L, with Na^+ and associated anions accounting for 270 mmol/L.

Na^+ concentration in the ECF is much larger than inside the cells. Because a small amount of Na^+ can diffuse through the cell membrane, the two sides would eventually reach equilibrium. To prevent equilibrium and to ensure a concentration gradient, active transport systems, such as ATPase ion pumps, are present in all cells. K^+ (see section "Potassium") is the major intracellular cation. Like Na^+, K^+ would eventually diffuse across the cell membrane until equilibrium is reached. The Na^+/K^+-ATPase ion pump moves three Na^+ ions out of the cell in exchange for two K^+ ions moving into the cell as ATP is converted to ADP. Because water follows electrolytes across cell membranes, the continual removal of Na^+ from the cell prevents osmotic rupture of the cell by also drawing water from the cell.

Regulation
The plasma Na^+ concentration depends greatly on the intake and excretion of water and, to a somewhat lesser degree, on the renal regulation of Na^+. Three processes are of primary importance: (1) the intake of water in response to thirst, as stimulated or suppressed by plasma osmolality;

(2) the excretion of water, largely affected by AVP release in response to changes in either blood volume or osmolality; and (3) the blood volume status, which affects Na$^+$ excretion through aldosterone, angiotensin II, and ANP. The kidneys have the ability to conserve or excrete large amounts of Na$^+$, depending on the Na$^+$ content of the ECF and the blood volume. Normally, 60% to 75% of filtered Na$^+$ is reabsorbed in the proximal tubule; electroneutrality is maintained by either Cl$^-$ reabsorption or hydrogen ion (H$^+$) secretion. Some Na$^+$ is also reabsorbed in the loop and distal tubule and (controlled by aldosterone) exchanged for K$^+$ in the connecting segment and cortical collecting tubule. The regulation of osmolality and volume has been summarized in Figure 16.1.

TABLE 16.2	Causes of Hyponatremia

Increased Sodium Loss
Hypoadrenalism
Potassium deficiency
Diuretic use
Ketonuria
Salt-losing nephropathy
Prolonged vomiting or diarrhea
Severe burns

Increased Water Retention
Renal failure
Nephrotic syndrome
Hepatic cirrhosis
Congestive heart failure

Water Imbalance
Excess water intake
SIADH
Pseudohyponatremia

SIADH, syndrome of inappropriate arginine vasopressin hormone secretion.

CASE STUDY 16.1

A 32-year-old woman was admitted to the hospital following 2½ days of severe vomiting. Before this episode, she was reportedly well. Physical findings revealed decreased skin turgor and dry mucous membranes. Admission study results were as follows:

Serum
- Na$^+$: 129 mmol/L
- K$^+$: 5.0 mmol/L
- Cl$^-$: 77 mmol/L
- HCO$_3^-$: 9 mmol/L
- Osmolality: 265 mOsm/kg

Urine
- Na$^+$: 8 mmol/d
- Ketones: trace

Questions

1. What is the cause for each abnormal plasma electrolyte result?

2. What is the significance of the urine sodium and serum osmolality results?

Clinical Applications

Hyponatremia

Hyponatremia is defined as a serum/plasma level less than 135 mmol/L, and levels below 130 mmol/L are clinically significant.[4] Hyponatremia is one of the most common electrolyte disorders in hospitalized and nonhospitalized patients and can be assessed either by the cause of the decrease or with the osmolality level.[5,6]

Decreased levels may be caused by increased Na$^+$ loss, increased water retention, or water imbalance (Table 16.2). *Increased* Na$^+$ *loss* in the urine can occur with decreased aldosterone production, certain diuretics (thiazides), ketonuria (Na$^+$ lost with ketones), or a salt-losing nephropathy (with some renal tubular disorders). K$^+$ deficiency also causes Na$^+$ loss because of the inverse relationship of the two ions in the renal tubules; when serum K$^+$ levels are low, the renal tubules will conserve K$^+$ and excrete Na$^+$ in exchange for the loss of the monovalent cation. Each disorder results in an increased urine Na$^+$ level ($\geq$20 mmol/d), which exceeds the amount of water loss.[7]

Prolonged vomiting, diarrhea, or severe burns can result in Na$^+$ loss. Urine Na$^+$ levels are usually less than 20 mmol/d in these disorders, which can be used to differentiate among causes for urinary loss.

Increased water retention causes dilution of serum/plasma Na$^+$ as with acute or chronic renal failure. In nephrotic syndrome and hepatic cirrhosis, plasma proteins are decreased, resulting in a decreased colloid osmotic pressure in which intravascular fluid migrates to the tissue (edema results). The low plasma volume causes AVP to be produced, causing fluid retention and resulting in dilution of Na$^+$. This compensatory mechanism is also seen with congestive heart failure (CHF) as a result of increased venous pressure. Urine Na$^+$ levels can be used to differentiate the cause for increased water retention; when urine Na$^+$ is $\geq$20 mmol/d, acute or chronic renal failure is the likely cause, and when urine levels are less than 20 mmol/d, water retention may be a result of nephrotic syndrome, hepatic cirrhosis, or CHF.[7]

Water imbalance can occur as a result of excess water intake, as with polydipsia (increased thirst). The increased intake must be chronic before water imbalance occurs, which may cause mild or severe hyponatremia. In a normal individual, excess intake will not affect Na$^+$ levels. SIADH causes an increase in water retention because of increased AVP (ADH) production. A defect in AVP regulation has been associated with pulmonary disease, malignancies, central nervous system (CNS) disorders, infections (e.g., *Pneumocystis carinii* pneumonia), or trauma.[7] Pseudohyponatremia can occur

TABLE 16.3	Classification of Hyponatremia by Osmolality

With Low Osmolality
Increased sodium loss
Increased water retention

With Normal Osmolality
Increased nonsodium cations
Lithium excess
Increased γ-globulins—cationic (multiple myeloma)
Severe hyperkalemia
Severe hypermagnesemia
Severe hypercalcemia
Pseudohyponatremia
Hyperlipidemia
Hyperproteinemia
Pseudohyperkalemia as a result of in vitro hemolysis

With High Osmolality
Hyperglycemia
Mannitol infusion

when Na$^+$ is measured using indirect ion-selective electrodes (ISEs) in a patient who is hyperproteinemic or hyperlipidemic. An indirect ISE dilutes the sample prior to analysis, and as a result of serum/plasma water displacement, the ion levels are falsely decreased. (For detailed information on the theory of water displacement with indirect ISEs, consult Chapter 5.)

Hyponatremia can also be *classified according to serum/plasma osmolality* (Table 16.3). Because Na$^+$ is a major contributor to osmolality, both levels can assist in identifying the cause of hyponatremia. There are three categories of hyponatremia—low osmolality, normal osmolality, or high osmolality.[4] Most instances of **hyponatremia** occur *with decreased osmolality.* This may be a result of Na$^+$ loss or water retention, as previously mentioned.

Hyponatremia with a normal osmolality may be a result of a high increase in nonsodium cations as listed in Table 16.4. In multiple myeloma, the cationic γ-globulins replace some

TABLE 16.4	Causes of Hypernatremia

Excess Water Loss
Diabetes insipidus
Renal tubular disorder
Prolonged diarrhea
Profuse sweating
Severe burns

Decreased Water Intake
Older persons
Infants
Mental impairment

Increased Intake or Retention
Hyperaldosteronism
Sodium bicarbonate excess
Dialysis fluid excess

Na$^+$ to maintain the electroneutrality; however, because it is a multivalent cation, it has little effect on osmolality.

Pseudohyponatremia, as mentioned earlier, may also be seen with in vitro hemolysis, considered the most common cause for a false decrease.[4] When red blood cells (RBCs) lyse, Na$^+$, K$^+$, and water are released, and since Na$^+$ concentration is lower in RBCs, this results in a false decrease. *Hyponatremia with a high osmolality* is associated with hyperglycemia. The elevated levels of glucose increase the serum osmolality and cause a shift of water from the cells to the blood, resulting in a dilution of Na$^+$.

Symptoms of hyponatremia. Symptoms depend on the serum level. Between 125 and 130 mmol/L, symptoms are primarily gastrointestinal (GI). More severe neuropsychiatric symptoms are seen below 125 mmol/L, including nausea and vomiting, muscular weakness, headache, lethargy, and ataxia. More severe symptoms also include seizures, coma, and respiratory depression.[7] A level below 120 mmol/L for 48 hours or less (acute hyponatremia) is considered a medical emergency.[8] Serum and urine electrolytes are monitored as treatment to return Na$^+$ levels to normal occurs.[9]

Treatment of hyponatremia. Treatment is directed at correction of the condition that caused either water loss or Na$^+$ loss in excess of water loss. In addition, the onset of hyponatremia—acute or chronic (less than or more than 48 hours)—and the severity of hyponatremia are considered in treatment. Conventional treatment of hyponatremia involves fluid restriction and providing hypertonic saline and/or other pharmacologic agents that may take several days to reach the desired effect and may have deleterious side effects.[5] Correcting severe hyponatremia too rapidly can cause cerebral myelinolysis and too slowly can cause cerebral edema.[9] Appropriate management of fluid administration is critical. Fluid administration and monitoring are required during treatment of the underlying cause of the hyponatremia.

A newer type of pharmacologic agent, an AVP receptor antagonist, has been found to be an effective treatment for euvolemic or hypervolemic hyponatremia. Conivaptan has been approved by the U.S. Food and Drug Administration for use in the United States and blocks the action of AVP in the collecting ducts of the nephron, thus decreasing water reabsorption.[10] This AVP receptor antagonist tends to restore Na$^+$ levels within 24 hours.[5] Euvolemic hypernatremia is associated with SIADH, hypothyroidism, and adrenal insuffiency.[6] Hypervolemic hyponatremia is associated with liver cirrhosis with ascites, CHF, and overhydrated postoperative patients.[8] Conivaptan is not an effective treatment with hypovolemic hyponatremia because the increased water loss would accentuate the volume depletion problem.[10]

Hypernatremia

Hypernatremia (increased serum Na$^+$ concentration) results from excess loss of water relative to Na$^+$ loss, decreased water intake, or increased Na$^+$ intake or retention. Hypernatremia is less commonly seen in hospitalized patients than is hyponatremia.[7]

Loss of hypotonic fluid may occur either by the kidney or through profuse sweating, diarrhea, or severe burns.

Hypernatremia may result from loss of water in diabetes insipidus, either because the kidney cannot respond to AVP (nephrogenic diabetes insipidus) or because AVP secretion is impaired (central diabetes insipidus). Diabetes insipidus is characterized by copious production of dilute urine (3 to 20 L/d). Because people with diabetes insipidus drink large volumes of water, hypernatremia usually does not occur unless the thirst mechanism is also impaired. Partial defects of either AVP release or the response to AVP may also occur. In such cases, urine is concentrated to a lesser extent than appropriate to correct the hypernatremia. Excess water loss may also occur in renal tubular disease, such as acute tubular necrosis, in which the tubules become unable to fully concentrate the urine.

The measurement of urine osmolality is necessary to evaluate the cause of hypernatremia. With renal loss of water, the urine osmolality is low or normal. With extrarenal fluid losses, the urine osmolality is increased. Interpretation of the urine osmolality in hypernatremia is shown in Table 16.5.

Water loss through the skin and by breathing (insensible loss) accounts for about 1 L of water loss per day in adults. Any condition that increases water loss, such as fever, burns, diarrhea, or exposure to heat, will increase the likelihood of developing hypernatremia. Commonly, hypernatremia occurs in those persons who may be thirsty but who are unable to ask for or obtain water, such as adults with altered mental status and infants. When urine cannot be fully concentrated (e.g., in neonates, young children, older persons, and certain patients with renal insufficiency), a relatively lower urine osmolality may occur.

Chronic hypernatremia in an alert patient is indicative of hypothalamic disease, usually with a defect in the osmoreceptors rather than from a true resetting of the osmostat. A reset osmostat may occur in primary hyperaldosteronism, in which excess aldosterone induces mild hypervolemia that retards AVP release, shifting plasma Na^+ upward by approximately 3 to 5 mmol/L.[1]

Hypernatremia may be from excess ingestion of salt or administration of hypertonic solutions of Na^+, such as sodium bicarbonate or hypertonic dialysis solutions. Neonates are especially susceptible to hypernatremia from this cause. In these cases, AVP response is appropriate, resulting in urine osmolality of greater than 800 mOsm/kg (Table 16.5).

Symptoms of hypernatremia. Symptoms most commonly involve the CNS as a result of the hyperosmolar state. These symptoms include altered mental status, lethargy, irritability, restlessness, seizures, muscle twitching, hyperreflexes, fever, nausea or vomiting, difficult respiration, and increased thirst. Serum Na^+ of more than 160 mmol/L is associated with a mortality rate of 60% to 75%.[7]

Treatment of hypernatremia. Treatment is directed at correction of the underlying condition that caused the water depletion or Na^+ retention. The speed of correction depends on the rate with which the condition developed. Hypernatremia must be corrected gradually because too rapid a correction of serious hypernatremia ($\geq$160 mmol/L) can induce cerebral edema and death; the maximal rate should be 0.5 mmol/L/h.[1]

Determination of Sodium

Specimen

Serum, plasma, and urine are all acceptable for Na^+ measurements. When plasma is used, lithium heparin, ammonium heparin, and lithium oxalate are suitable anticoagulants. Hemolysis does not cause a significant change in serum or plasma values as a result of decreased levels of intracellular Na^+. However, with marked hemolysis, levels may be decreased as a result of a dilutional effect.

Whole blood samples may be used with some analyzers; however, consult the instrument operation manual for acceptability. The specimen of choice in urine Na^+ analyses is a 24-hour collection. Sweat is also suitable for analysis, and its collection and analysis are discussed in Chapter 29.

Methods

Through the years, Na^+ has been measured in various ways, including chemical methods, flame emission spectrophotometry, atomic absorption spectrophotometry (AAS), and ISEs. Chemical methods are outdated because of large sample volume requirements and lack of precision. ISEs are the most routinely used method in clinical laboratories.

The ISE method uses a semipermeable membrane to develop a potential produced by having different ion concentrations on either side of the membrane. In this type of system, two electrodes are used. One electrode has a constant potential, making it the reference electrode, and the difference in potential between the reference and measuring electrodes can be used to calculate the "concentration" of the ion in solution. However, it is the activity of the ion, not the concentration that is being measured (see Chapter 5). Most analyzers use a glass ion-exchange membrane in its ISE system for Na^+ measurement (Fig. 16.2). There are two types of ISE measurement, based on sample preparation: direct and indirect. Direct measurement provides an undiluted

TABLE 16.5	**Hypernatremia (150 mmol/L) Related to Urine Osmolality**

Urine Osmolality <300 mOsm/kg
Diabetes insipidus (impaired secretion of AVP or kidneys cannot respond to AVP)

Urine Osmolality 300–700 mOsm/kg
Partial defect in AVP release or response to AVP
Osmotic diuresis

Urine Osmolality >700 mOsm/kg
Loss of thirst
Insensible loss of water (breathing, skin)
GI loss of hypotonic fluid
Excess intake of sodium

AVP, arginine vasopressin hormone.

Na⁺ Electrode

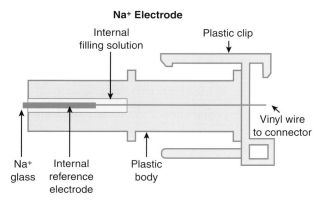

FIGURE 16.2 Diagram of sodium ISE with glass capillary membrane. (Courtesy of Nova Biomedical, Waltham, MA.)

TABLE 16.6	Reference Ranges for Sodium
Serum, plasma	135–145 mmol/L
Urine (24 h)	40–220 mmol/d, varies with diet
Cerebrospinal fluid	135–150 mmol/L

sample to interact with the ISE membrane. With the indirect method, a diluted sample is used for measurement. There is no significant difference in results, except when samples are hyperlipidemic or hyperproteinemic. In these samples, excess lipids or proteins displace plasma water, which leads to a falsely decreased measurement of ionic activity in millimoles per liter of plasma, whereas the direct method measures in plasma water only. In these cases, direct ISE is more accurate.

One source of error with ISEs is protein buildup on the membrane through continuous use. The protein-coated membranes cause poor selectivity, which results in poor reproducibility of results. A routine maintenance of these ISEs requires removal of this protein buildup to ensure quality results.

VITROS analyzers (Ortho-Clinical Diagnostics) use a single-use direct ISE potentiometric system. Each disposable slide contains a reference and measuring electrode (Fig. 16.3). A drop of sample fluid and a drop of reference fluid are simultaneously applied to the slide, and the potential difference between the two is measured, which is proportional to the Na⁺ concentration.[11]

Reference Ranges

See Table 16.6.[3]

Potassium

Potassium (K⁺) is the major intracellular cation in the body, with a concentration 20 times greater inside the cells than outside. Many cellular functions require that the body maintain a low ECF concentration of K⁺ ions. As a result, only 2% of the body's total K⁺ circulates in the plasma. Functions of K⁺ in the body include regulation of neuromuscular excitability, contraction of the heart, ICF volume, and H⁺ concentration.[1]

The K⁺ concentration has a major effect on the contraction of skeletal and cardiac muscles. An elevated plasma K⁺ decreases the resting membrane potential (RMP) of the cell (the RMP is closer to zero), which decreases the net difference between the cell's resting potential and threshold (action) potential. A lower than normal difference increases cell excitability, leading to muscle weakness. Severe **hyperkalemia** can ultimately cause a lack of muscle excitability (as a result of a higher RMP than action potential), which may lead to paralysis or a fatal cardiac arrhythmia.[1] Hypokalemia decreases cell excitability by increasing the RMP, often resulting in an arrhythmia or paralysis.[1] The heart may cease to contract in extreme cases of either hyperkalemia or hypokalemia.

K⁺ concentration also affects the H⁺ concentration in the blood. For example, in hypokalemia (low serum K⁺), as K⁺ is lost from the body, Na⁺ and H⁺ move into the cell. The H⁺ concentration is, therefore, decreased in the ECF, resulting in alkalosis.

1. **Upper slide mount**

2. **Paper bridge**

3. **Ion-selective membrane**
   • Methyl monensin

4. **Reference layer**
   • NaCl
   • Buffer at pH 5.6

5. **Silver, silver chloride layer**

6. **Support layer**

7. **Lower slide mount**

FIGURE 16.3 Schematic diagram of the ISE system for the potentiometric slide on the VITROS. (Courtesy of OCD, a Johnson & Johnson company, Rochester, NY.)

Regulation

Renal function related to tubular reabsorption and secretion is important in the regulation of potassium balance. Initially, the proximal tubules reabsorb nearly all the K^+. Then, under the influence of aldosterone, additional K^+ is secreted into the urine in exchange for Na^+ in both the distal tubules and the collecting ducts. Thus, the distal nephron is the principal determinant of urinary K^+ excretion. Most individuals consume far more K^+ than needed; the excess is excreted in the urine but may accumulate to toxic levels if renal failure occurs.

K^+ uptake from the ECF into the cells is important in normalizing an acute rise in plasma K^+ concentration due to an increased K^+ intake. Excess plasma K^+ rapidly enters the cells to normalize plasma K^+. As the cellular K^+ gradually returns to the plasma, it is removed by urinary excretion. Note that chronic loss of cellular K^+ may result in cellular depletion before there is an appreciable change in the plasma K^+ concentration because excess K^+ is normally excreted in the urine.

Three factors that influence the distribution of K^+ between cells and ECF are as follows: (1) K^+ loss frequently occurs whenever the Na^+, K^+-ATPase pump is inhibited by conditions such as hypoxia, hypomagnesemia, or digoxin overdose; (2) insulin promotes acute entry of K^+ into skeletal muscle and liver by increasing Na^+, K^+-ATPase activity; and (3) catecholamines, such as epinephrine (β_2-stimulator), promote cellular entry of K^+, whereas propanolol (β-blocker) impairs cellular entry of K^+. Dietary deficiency or excess is rarely a primary cause of hypokalemia or hyperkalemia. However, with a preexisting condition, dietary deficiency (or excess) can enhance the degree of hypokalemia (or hyperkalemia).

Exercise

K^+ is released from muscle cells during exercise, which may increase plasma K^+ by 0.3 to 1.2 mmol/L with mild to moderate exercise and by as much as 2 to 3 mmol/L with exhaustive exercise. These changes are usually reversed after several minutes of rest. Forearm exercise during venipuncture can cause erroneously high plasma K^+ concentrations.[12]

Hyperosmolality

Hyperosmolality, as with uncontrolled diabetes mellitus, causes water to diffuse from the cells, carrying K^+ with the water, which leads to gradual depletion of K^+ if kidney function is normal.

Cellular Breakdown

Cellular breakdown releases K^+ into the ECF. Examples are severe trauma, tumor lysis syndrome, and massive blood transfusions.

Clinical Applications

Hypokalemia

Hypokalemia is a plasma K^+ concentration below the lower limit of the reference range. Hypokalemia can occur with GI or urinary loss of K^+ or with increased cellular uptake of K^+. Common causes of hypokalemia are shown in Table 16.7. Of

TABLE 16.7	**Causes of Hypokalemia**

Gastrointestinal Loss
Vomiting
Diarrhea
Gastric suction
Intestinal tumor
Malabsorption
Cancer therapy—chemotherapy, radiation therapy
Large doses of laxatives

Renal Loss
Diuretics—thiazides, mineralocorticoids
Nephritis
Renal tubular acidosis
Hyperaldosteronism
Cushing's syndrome
Hypomagnesemia
Acute leukemia

Cellular Shift
Alkalosis
Insulin overdose

Decreased Intake

these, therapy with thiazide-type diuretics is the most common.[13] GI loss occurs when GI fluid is lost through vomiting, diarrhea, gastric suction, or discharge from an intestinal fistula. Increased K^+ loss in the stool also occurs with certain tumors, malabsorption, cancer therapy (chemotherapy or radiation therapy), and large doses of laxatives.

Renal loss of K^+ can result from kidney disorders such as K^+-losing nephritis and renal tubular acidosis (RTA). In RTA, as tubular excretion of H^+ decreases, K^+ excretion increases. Because aldosterone promotes Na^+ retention and K^+ loss, hyperaldosteronism can lead to hypokalemia and metabolic alkalosis.[1] Hypomagnesemia can lead to hypokalemia by promoting urinary loss of K^+. Mg^{2+} deficiency also diminishes the activity of Na^+, K^+-ATPase and enhances the secretion of aldosterone. Effective treatment requires supplementation with both Mg^{2+} and K^+.[1] Renal K^+ loss also occurs with acute myelogenous leukemia, acute myelomonocytic leukemia, and acute lymphocytic leukemia.[13] Although reduced dietary intake of K^+ rarely causes hypokalemia in healthy persons, decreased intake may intensify hypokalemia caused by use of diuretics, for example.

Increased cellular uptake of potassium is encountered in alkalemia and with elevated levels of insulin via therapeutic treatment of diabetes. Both alkalemia and insulin increase the cellular uptake of K^+. Because alkalemia promotes intracellular loss of H^+ to minimize elevation of intracellular pH, both K^+ and Na^+ enter cells to preserve electroneutrality. Plasma K^+ decreases by about 0.4 mmol/L per 0.1 unit rise in pH.[1]

Insulin promotes the entry of K^+ into skeletal muscle and liver cells. Because insulin therapy can sometimes uncover an underlying hypokalemic state, plasma K^+ should be monitored carefully whenever insulin is administered to susceptible patients.[1] A rare cause of hypokalemia is associated with a blood sample from a leukemic patient with a significantly elevated white blood cell count as the K$^+$ present in the sample is taken up by the white cells if the sample is left at room temperature for several hours.[13]

Symptoms of hypokalemia. Symptoms (e.g., weakness, fatigue, and constipation) often become apparent as plasma K$^+$ decreases below 3 mmol/L. Hypokalemia can lead to muscle weakness or paralysis, which can interfere with breathing. The dangers of hypokalemia concern all patients, but especially those with cardiovascular disorders because of an increased risk of arrhythmia, which may cause sudden death in certain patients. Mild hypokalemia (3.0 to 3.4 mmol/L) is usually asymptomatic.

Treatment of hypokalemia. Treatment typically includes oral KCl replacement of K$^+$ over several days. In some instances, intravenous (IV) replacement may be indicated. In some cases, chronic mild hypokalemia may be corrected simply by including food in the diet with high K$^+$ content, such as dried fruits, nuts, bran cereals, bananas, and orange juice. Plasma electrolytes are monitored as treatment to return K$^+$ levels to normal occurs.

Hyperkalemia
The most common causes of hyperkalemia are shown in Table 16.8. Patients with hyperkalemia often have an underlying disorder, such as renal insufficiency, diabetes mellitus, or metabolic acidosis, that contributes to hyperkalemia.[12] For example, during administration of KCl, a person with renal insufficiency is far more likely to develop hyperkalemia than is a person with normal renal function. The most common cause of hyperkalemia in hospitalized patients is due to therapeutic K$^+$ administration. The risk is greatest with IV K$^+$ replacement.[12]

In healthy persons, an acute oral load of K$^+$ will briefly increase plasma K$^+$ because most of the absorbed K$^+$ rapidly moves intracellularly. Normal cellular processes gradually release this excess K$^+$ back into the plasma, where it is normally removed by renal excretion. Impairment of urinary K$^+$ excretion is usually associated with chronic hyperkalemia.[1]

If a shift of K$^+$ from cells into plasma occurs too rapidly to be removed by renal excretion, acute hyperkalemia develops. In diabetes mellitus, insulin deficiency promotes cellular loss of K$^+$. Hyperglycemia also contributes by producing a hyperosmolar plasma that pulls water and K$^+$ from cells, promoting further loss of K$^+$ into the plasma.[1] In metabolic acidosis, as excess H$^+$ moves intracellularly to be buffered, K$^+$ leaves the cell to maintain electroneutrality. Plasma K$^+$ increases by 0.2 to 1.7 mmol/L for each 0.1 unit reduction of pH.[1] Because cellular K$^+$ often becomes depleted in cases of acidosis with hyperkalemia (including diabetic ketoacidosis), treatment with agents such as insulin and bicarbonate can cause a rapid intracellular movement of K$^+$, producing severe hypokalemia.

Various drugs may cause hyperkalemia, especially in patients with either renal insufficiency or diabetes mellitus. These drugs include captopril (inhibits angiotensin-converting enzyme), nonsteroidal anti-inflammatory agents (inhibit aldosterone), spironolactone (K$^+$-sparing diuretic), digoxin (inhibits Na$^+$–K$^+$ pump), cyclosporine (inhibits renal response to aldosterone), and heparin therapy (inhibits aldosterone secretion).

Hyperkalemia may result when K$^+$ is released into the ECF during enhanced tissue breakdown or catabolism, especially if renal insufficiency is present. Increased cellular breakdown may be caused by trauma, administration of cytotoxic agents, massive hemolysis, tumor lysis syndrome, and blood transfusions. In banked blood, K$^+$ is gradually released from erythrocytes during storage, often causing elevated K$^+$ concentration in plasma supernatant.

Patients on cardiac bypass may develop mild elevations in plasma K$^+$ during warming after surgery because warming causes cellular release of K$^+$, whereas hypothermia causes movement of K$^+$ into cells.

Symptoms of hyperkalemia. Hyperkalemia can cause muscle weakness, tingling, numbness, or mental confusion by altering neuromuscular conduction. Muscle weakness does not usually develop until plasma K$^+$ reaches 8 mmol/L.[1]

Hyperkalemia disturbs cardiac conduction, which can lead to cardiac arrhythmias and possible cardiac arrest. Plasma K$^+$ concentrations of 6 to 7 mmol/L may alter the electrocardiogram (ECG), and concentrations more than 10 mmol/L may cause fatal cardiac arrest.[1]

Treatment of hyperkalemia. Treatment should be immediately initiated when serum K$^+$ is 6.0 to 6.5 mmol/L or greater or if there are ECG changes.[12] To offset the effect of K$^+$, which lowers the resting potential of myocardial cells, Ca^{2+} may be given to reduce the threshold potential of myocardial cells. Therefore, Ca^{2+} provides immediate but short-lived protection to the myocardium against the effects of hyperkalemia. Substances that acutely shift K$^+$ back into cells, such as sodium bicarbonate, glucose, or insulin, may also be administered. K$^+$ may be quickly removed from the body by use

TABLE 16.8   Causes of Hyperkalemia

Decreased Renal Excretion
Acute or chronic renal failure (GFR < 20 mL/min)
Hypoaldosteronism
Addison's disease
Diuretics

Cellular Shift
Acidosis
Muscle/cellular injury
Chemotherapy
Leukemia
Hemolysis

Increased Intake
Oral or intravenous potassium replacement therapy

Artifactual
Sample hemolysis
Thrombocytosis
Prolonged tourniquet use or excessive fist clenching

GFR, glomerular filtration rate.

---

of diuretics (loop), if renal function is adequate, or sodium polystyrene sulfonate (Kayexalate) enemas, which bind to K^+ secreted in the colon. Hemodialysis can be used if other measures fail.[12] Patients treated with these agents must be monitored carefully to prevent hypokalemia as K^+ moves back into cells or is removed from the body.

Collection of Samples

Proper collection and handling of samples for K^+ analysis is extremely important because there are many causes of artifactual hyperkalemia. First, the coagulation process releases K^+ from platelets, so that serum K^+ may be 0.1 to 0.7 mmol/L higher than plasma K^+ concentrations.[2] If the patient's platelet count is elevated (thrombocytosis), serum K^+ may be further elevated. Second, if a tourniquet is left on the arm too long during blood collection or if patients excessively clench their fists or otherwise exercise their forearms before venipuncture, cells may release K^+ into the plasma. The first situation may be avoided by using a heparinized tube to prevent clotting of the specimen and the second by using proper care in the drawing of blood. Third, because storing blood on ice promotes the release of K^+ from cells, whole blood samples for K^+ determinations should be stored at room temperature (never iced) and analyzed promptly or centrifuged to remove the cells.[14] Fourth, if hemolysis occurs after the blood is drawn, K^+ may be falsely elevated—the most common cause of artifactual hyperkalemia. Slight hemolysis ($\approx$50 mg/dL of hemoglobin) can cause an increase of approximately 3%, while gross hemolysis (>500 mg/dL of hemoglobin) can cause an increase of up to 30%.[2]

Determination of Potassium

Specimen

Serum, plasma, and urine may be acceptable for analysis. Hemolysis must be avoided because of the high K^+ content of erythrocytes. Heparin is the anticoagulant of choice. Whereas serum and plasma generally give similar K^+ levels, serum reference intervals tend to be slightly higher. Significantly elevated platelet counts may result in the release of K^+ during clotting from rupture of these cells, causing a spurious hyperkalemia. In this case, plasma is preferred. Whole blood samples may be used with some analyzers; however, one should consult the instrument's operations manual for acceptability. Urine specimens should be collected over a 24-hour period to eliminate the influence of diurnal variation.

Methods

As with Na^+, the current method of choice is ISE. For ISE measurements, a valinomycin membrane is used to selectively bind K^+, causing an impedance change that can be correlated to K^+ concentration where KCl is the inner electrolyte solution.

Reference Ranges

See Table 16.9.[3]

Chloride

Chloride (Cl^-) is the major extracellular anion, and its precise function in the body is not well understood; however,

TABLE 16.9	Reference Ranges for Potassium
Serum	3.5–5.1 mmol/L
Plasma	Males: 3.5–4.5 mmol/L
	Females: 3.4–4.4 mmol/L
Urine (24 h)	25–125 mmol/d

it is involved in maintaining osmolality, blood volume, and electric neutrality. In most processes, Cl^- shifts secondarily to a movement of Na^+ or HCO_3^-.

Cl^- ingested in the diet is almost completely absorbed by the intestinal tract. Cl^- is then filtered out by the glomerulus and passively reabsorbed, in conjunction with Na^+, by the proximal tubules. Excess Cl^- is excreted in the urine and sweat. Excessive sweating stimulates aldosterone secretion, which acts on the sweat glands to conserve Na^+ and Cl^-.

Cl^- maintains electrical neutrality in two ways. First, Na^+ is reabsorbed along with Cl^- in the proximal tubules. In effect, Cl^- acts as the rate-limiting component, in that Na^+ reabsorption is limited by the amount of Cl^- available. Electroneutrality is also maintained by Cl^- through the *chloride shift*. In this process, CO_2 generated by cellular metabolism within the tissue diffuses out into both the plasma and the red cell. In the red cell, CO_2 forms carbonic acid (H_2CO_3), which splits into H^+ and HCO_3^- (bicarbonate). Deoxyhemoglobin buffers H^+, whereas the HCO_3^- diffuses out into the plasma and Cl^- diffuses into the red cell to maintain the electric balance of the cell (Fig. 16.4).

Clinical Applications

Cl^- disorders are often a result of the same causes that disturb Na^+ levels because Cl^- passively follows Na^+. There are a few exceptions. **Hyperchloremia** may also occur when there is an excess loss of HCO_3^- as a result of GI losses, RTA, or metabolic acidosis. **Hypochloremia** may also occur with excessive loss of Cl^- from prolonged vomiting, diabetic ketoacidosis, aldosterone deficiency, or salt-losing renal diseases such as pyelonephritis. A low serum level of Cl^- may also be encountered in conditions associated with high serum HCO_3^- concentrations, such as compensated respiratory acidosis or metabolic alkalosis.

Determination of Chloride

Specimen

Serum or plasma may be used, with lithium heparin being the anticoagulant of choice. Hemolysis does not cause a significant change in serum or plasma values as a result of decreased levels of intracellular Cl^-. However, with marked hemolysis, levels may be decreased as a result of a dilutional effect.

Whole blood samples may be used with some analyzers; however, one should consult the instrument's operation manual for acceptability. The specimen of choice in urine Cl^- analyses is 24-hour collection because of the large diurnal variation. Sweat is also suitable for analysis. Sweat collection and analysis are discussed in Chapter 29.

FIGURE 16.4 Chloride shift mechanism. See text for details. (Reprinted from Burtis CA, Ashwood ER, eds. *Tietz Textbook of Clinical Chemistry*. 2nd ed. Philadelphia, PA: WB Saunders; 1994, with permission.)

Methods

There are several methodologies available for measuring Cl⁻, including ISEs, amperometric-coulometric titration, mercurimetric titration, and colorimetry. The most commonly used is ISE. For ISE measurement, an ion-exchange membrane is used to selectively bind Cl⁻ ions.

Amperometric–coulometric titration is a method using coulometric generation of silver ions (Ag^+), which combine with Cl⁻ to quantitate the Cl⁻ concentration.

$$Ag^{2+} + 2Cl^- \rightarrow AgCl_2 \qquad \text{(Eq. 16-2)}$$

When all Cl⁻ in a patient is bound to Ag^+, excess or free Ag^+ is used to indicate the endpoint. As Ag^+ accumulates, the coulometric generator and timer are turned off. The elapsed time is used to calculate the concentration of Cl⁻ in the sample. The digital (Cotlove) chloridometer (Labconco Corporation) uses this principle in Cl⁻ analysis.

Reference Ranges

See Table 16.10.[3]

Bicarbonate

Bicarbonate is the second most abundant anion in the ECF. Total CO_2 comprises the bicarbonate ion (HCO_3^-), H_2CO_3, and dissolved CO_2, with HCO_3^- accounting for more than 90% of the total CO_2 at physiologic pH. Because HCO_3^- composes the largest fraction of total CO_2, total CO_2 measurement is indicative of HCO_3^- measurement.

TABLE 16.10	**Reference Ranges for Chloride**
Plasma, serum	98–107 mmol/L
Urine (24 h)	110–250 mmol/d, varies with diet

HCO_3^- is the major component of the buffering system in the blood. Carbonic anhydrase in RBCs converts CO_2 and H_2O to H_2CO_3, which dissociates into H^+ and HCO_3^-.

$$CO_2 + H_2O \xleftrightarrow{\text{CA}} H_2CO_3 \xleftrightarrow{\text{CA}} H^+ + HCO_3^- \qquad \text{(Eq. 16-3)}$$

where CA is carbonic anhydrase. HCO_3^- diffuses out of the cell in exchange for Cl⁻ to maintain ionic charge neutrality within the cell (chloride shift; see Fig. 16.4). This process converts potentially toxic CO_2 in the plasma to an effective buffer: HCO_3^-. HCO_3^- buffers excess H^+ by combining with acid, then eventually dissociating into H_2O and CO_2 in the lungs where the acidic gas CO_2 is eliminated.

Regulation

Most of the HCO_3^- in the kidneys (85%) is reabsorbed by the proximal tubules, with 15% being reabsorbed by the distal tubules. Because tubules are only slightly permeable to HCO_3^-, it is usually reabsorbed as CO_2. This happens as HCO_3^-, after filtering into the tubules, combines with H^+ to form H_2CO_3, which then dissociates into H_2O and CO_2. The CO_2 readily diffuses back into the ECF. Normally, nearly all the HCO_3^- is reabsorbed from the tubules, with little lost in the urine. When HCO_3^- is filtered in excess of H^+ available, almost all excess HCO_3^- flows into the urine.

In alkalosis, with a relative increase in HCO_3^- compared with CO_2, the kidneys increase excretion of HCO_3^- into the urine, carrying along a cation such as Na^+. This loss of HCO_3^- from the body helps correct pH.

Among the responses of the body to acidosis is an increased excretion of H^+ into the urine. In addition, HCO_3^- reabsorption is virtually complete, with 90% of the filtered HCO_3^- reabsorbed in the proximal tubule and the remainder in the distal tubule.[1]

Clinical Applications

Acid–base imbalances cause changes in HCO_3^- and CO_2 levels. A decreased HCO_3^- may occur from metabolic acidosis as HCO_3^- combines with H^+ to produce CO_2, which is exhaled by the lungs. The typical response to metabolic acidosis is compensation by hyperventilation, which lowers pco_2. Elevated total CO_2 concentrations occur in metabolic alkalosis as HCO_3^- is retained, often with increased pco_2 as a result of compensation by hypoventilation. Typical causes of metabolic alkalosis include severe vomiting, hypokalemia, and excessive alkali intake.

Determination of CO₂

Specimen

This chapter deals specifically with venous serum or plasma determinations. For discussion of arterial and whole blood pco_2 measurements, refer Chapter 17.

Serum or lithium heparin plasma is suitable for analysis. Although specimens should be anaerobic for the highest accuracy, many current analyzers (excluding blood gas analyzers) do not permit anaerobic sample handling. In most instances, the sample is capped until the serum or plasma is separated and the sample is analyzed immediately. If the sample is left uncapped before analysis, CO_2 escapes. Levels can decrease by 6 mmol/L/h.[2]

CO_2 measurements may be obtained in several ways; however, the actual portion of the total CO_2 being measured may vary with the method used. Two common methods are ISE and an enzymatic method.

One type of ISE for measuring total CO_2 uses an acid reagent to convert all the forms of CO_2 to CO_2 gas and is measured by a pco_2 electrode (see Chapter 5).

The enzyme method alkalinizes the sample to convert all forms of CO_2 to HCO_3^-. HCO_3^- is used to carboxylate phosphoenolpyruvate (PEP) in the presence of PEP carboxylase, which catalyzes the formation of oxaloacetate:

$$Phosphoenolpyruvate + HCO_3^- \xrightarrow{PEF carboxylate} Oxalocetate + H_2PO_4^- \quad \text{(Eq. 16-4)}$$

This is coupled to the following reaction, in which NADH is consumed as a result of the action of malate dehydrogenase:

$$Oxaloacetate + NADH + H^+ \xrightarrow{MDH} Malate + NAD^+ \quad \text{(Eq. 16-5)}$$

The rate of change in absorbance of NADH is proportional to the concentration of HCO_3^-.

Reference Ranges

CO_2, venous 23 to 29 mmol/L (plasma, serum).[3]

Magnesium
Magnesium Physiology

Magnesium (Mg^{2+}) is the fourth most abundant cation in the body and second most abundant intracellular ion. The average human body (70 kg) contains 1 mol (24 g) of Mg^{2+}. Approximately 53% of Mg^{2+} in the body is found in bone and 46% in muscle, other organs, and soft tissue, and less than 1% is present in serum and RBCs.[15] Of the Mg^{2+} present in serum, about one-third is bound to protein, primarily albumin. Of the remaining two-thirds, 61% exists in the free or ionized state, and about 5% is complexed with other ions, such as PO_4^- and citrate. Similar to Ca^{2+}, it is the free ion that is physiologically active in the body.[16]

The role of Mg^{2+} in the body is widespread. It is an essential cofactor of more than 300 enzymes, including those important in glycolysis; transcellular ion transport; neuromuscular transmission; synthesis of carbohydrates, proteins, lipids, and nucleic acids; and the release of and response to certain hormones.

The clinical usefulness of serum Mg^{2+} levels has greatly increased in the past 10 years as more information about the analyte has been discovered. The most significant findings are the relationship between abnormal serum Mg^{2+} levels and cardiovascular, metabolic, and neuromuscular disorders. Although serum levels may not reflect total body stores of Mg^{2+}, they are useful in determining acute changes in the ion.

Regulation

Rich sources of Mg^{2+} in the diet include raw nuts, dry cereal, and "hard" drinking water; other sources include vegetables, meats, fish, and fruit.[15] Processed foods, an ever-increasing part of the average US diet, have low levels of Mg^{2+} that may cause an inadequate intake. This in turn may increase the likelihood of Mg^{2+} deficiency. The small intestine may absorb 20% to 65% of the dietary Mg^{2+}, depending on the need and intake.

The overall regulation of body Mg^{2+} is controlled largely by the kidney, which can reabsorb Mg^{2+} in deficiency states or readily excrete excess Mg^{2+} in overload states. Of the nonprotein-bound Mg^{2+} that gets filtered by the glomerulus, only 25% to 30% is reabsorbed by the proximal convoluted tubule (PCT), unlike Na^+ in which 60% to 75% is absorbed in the PCT. Henle's loop is the major renal regulatory site, where 50% to 60% of filtered Mg^{2+} is reabsorbed in the ascending limb. In addition, 2% to 5% are reabsorbed in the distal convoluted tubule.[17] The renal threshold for Mg^{2+} is approximately 0.60 to 0.85 mmol/L ($\approx$1.46 to 2.07 mg/dL). Because this is close to normal serum concentration, slight excesses of Mg^{2+} in serum are rapidly excreted by the kidneys. Normally, only about 6% of filtered Mg^{2+} is excreted in the urine per day.[15]

Mg^{2+} regulation appears to be related to that of Ca^{2+} and Na^+. Parathyroid hormone (PTH) increases the renal reabsorption of Mg^{2+} and enhances the absorption of Mg^{2+} in the intestine. However, changes in ionized Ca^{2+} have a far greater effect on PTH secretion. Aldosterone and thyroxine apparently have the opposite effect of PTH in the kidney, increasing the renal excretion of Mg^{2+}.[16]

Clinical Applications

Hypomagnesemia

Hypomagnesemia is most frequently observed in hospitalized individuals in intensive care units (ICUs) or those receiving diuretic therapy or digitalis therapy (CHF, atrial fibrillation). These patients most likely have an overall tissue depletion of Mg^{2+} as a result of severe illness or loss, which leads to low serum levels. Hypomagnesemia is rare in nonhospitalized individuals.[16]

There are many causes of hypomagnesemia; however, it can be grouped into general categories (Table 16.11). Reduced intake is least likely to cause severe deficiencies in the United States. A Mg^{2+}-deficient diet as a result of starvation, chronic alcoholism, or Mg^{2+}-deficient IV therapy can cause a loss of the ion.

Various GI disorders may cause decreased absorption by the intestine, which can result in an excess loss of Mg^{2+} via the feces. Malabsorption syndromes; intestinal resection or bypass surgery; nasogastric suction; pancreatitis; and prolonged vomiting, diarrhea, or laxative use may lead to an Mg^{2+} deficiency. Neonatal hypomagnesemia has been reported as a result of various surgical procedures. A primary deficiency has also been reported in infants as a result of a selective malabsorption of the ion.[16]

A chronic congenital hypomagnesemia with secondary hypocalcemia (autosomal recessive disorder) has also been reported; molecular studies have revealed a specific transport protein defect in the intestine.[18]

Mg^{2+} loss due to increased excretion by way of urine can occur as a result of various renal and endocrine disorders or the effects of certain drugs on the kidneys. Renal tubular disorders and other select renal disorders may result in excess amounts of Mg^{2+} being lost through the urine because of decreased tubular reabsorption.

Several endocrine disorders can cause a loss of Mg^{2+}. Hyperparathyroidism and hypercalcemia may cause increased renal excretion of Mg^{2+} as a result of excess Ca^{2+} ions. Excess serum Na^+ levels caused by hyperaldosteronism may also cause increased renal excretion of Mg^{2+}. A pseudohypomagnesemia may also be the result of hyperaldosteronism caused by increased water reabsorption. Hyperthyroidism may result in an increased renal excretion of Mg^{2+} and may also cause an intracellular shift of the ion. In persons with diabetes, excess urinary loss of Mg^{2+} is associated with glycosuria; hypomagnesemia can aggravate the neuromuscular and vascular complications commonly found in this disease. Some studies have shown a relationship between Mg^{2+} deficiency and insulin resistance; however, Mg^{2+} is not thought to play a role in the pathophysiology of diabetes mellitus. The American Diabetes Association has issued a statement regarding dietary intake of Mg^{2+} and measurement of serum Mg^{2+} in patients with diabetes.[19]

Several drugs, including diuretics, gentamicin, cisplatin, and cyclosporine, increase renal loss of Mg^{2+} and frequently result in hypomagnesemia. The loop diuretics, such as furosemide, are especially effective in increasing renal loss of Mg^{2+}. Thiazide diuretics require a longer period of use to cause hypomagnesemia. Cisplatin has a nephrotoxic effect that inhibits the ability of the renal tubule to conserve Mg^{2+}. Cyclosporine, an immunosuppressant, severely inhibits the renal tubular reabsorption of Mg^{2+} and has many adverse effects, including nephrotoxicity, hypertension, hepatotoxicity, and neurologic symptoms such as seizures and tremors. Cardiac glycosides, such as digoxin and digitalis, can interfere with Mg^{2+} reabsorption; the resulting hypomagnesemia is a significant finding because the decreased level of Mg^{2+} can amplify the symptoms of digitalis toxicity.[16]

Excess lactation has been associated with hypomagnesemia as a result of increased use and loss through milk production. Mild deficiencies have been reported in pregnancy, which may cause a hyperexcitable uterus, anxiety, and insomnia.

Symptoms of hypomagnesemia. A patient who is hypomagnesemic may be asymptomatic until serum levels fall below 0.5 mmol/L.[16] A variety of symptoms can occur, and the most frequent involve cardiovascular, neuromuscular, psychiatric, and metabolic abnormalities (Table 16.12). The cardiovascular and neuromuscular symptoms result primarily from the ATPase enzyme's requirement for Mg^{2+}. Mg^{2+} loss leads to decreased intracellular K^+ levels because of a faulty Na^+/K^+ pump (ATPase). This change in cellular RMP causes increased excitability that may lead to cardiac arrhythmias. This condition may also lead to digitalis toxicity.

Muscle contraction also requires Mg^{2+} and ATPase for normal Ca^{2+} uptake following contraction. Normal nerve

---

TABLE 16.11 Causes of Hypomagnesemia

Reduced intake
Poor diet/starvation
Prolonged magnesium-deficient intravenous therapy
Chronic alcoholism

Decreased absorption
Malabsorption syndrome
Surgical resection of small intestine
Nasogastric suction
Pancreatitis
Vomiting
Diarrhea
Laxative abuse
Neonatal
Primary
Congenital

Increased Excretion—Renal
Tubular disorder
Glomerulonephritis
Pyelonephritis

Increased Excretion—Endocrine
Hyperparathyroidism
Hyperaldosteronism
Hyperthyroidism
Hypercalcemia
Diabetic ketoacidosis

Increased Excretion—Drug Induced
Diuretics
Antibiotics
Cyclosporine
Digitalis

Miscellaneous
Excess lactation
Pregnancy

Adapted from Polancic JE. Magnesium: metabolism, clinical importance, and analysis. *Clin Lab Sci.* 1991;4(2):105–109.

TABLE 16.12	Symptoms of Hypomagnesemia

Cardiovascular	*Psychiatric*
Arrhythmia	Depression
Hypertension	Agitation
Digitalis toxicity	Psychosis
Neuromuscular	*Metabolic*
Weakness	Hypokalemia
Cramps	Hypocalcemia
Ataxia	Hypophosphatemia
Tremor	Hyponatremia
Seizure	
Tetany	
Paralysis	
Coma	

Adapted from Polancic JE. Magnesium: metabolism, clinical importance, and analysis. *Clin Lab Sci.* 1991;4(2):105–109.

and muscle cell stimulation requires Mg^{2+} to assist with the regulation of acetylcholine, a potent neurotransmitter. Hypomagnesemia can cause a variety of symptoms from weakness to tremors, **tetany** (irregular muscle spasms), paralysis, or coma. The CNS can also be affected, resulting in psychiatric disorders that range from subtle changes to depression or psychosis.

Metabolic disorders are also associated with hypomagnesemia. Studies have indicated that approximately 40% of hospitalized patients with hypokalemia are also hypomagnesemic.[17] In addition, 20% to 30% of patients with hyponatremia, hypocalcemia, or hypophosphatemia are also hypomagnesemic.[17] Mg^{2+} deficiency can impair PTH release and target tissue response, resulting in hypocalcemia. Replenishing any of these deficient ions alone often does not remedy the disorder unless Mg^{2+} therapy is provided. Mg^{2+} therapy alone may restore both ion levels to normal; serum levels of the ions must be monitored during treatment.

Treatment of hypomagnesemia. The preferred form of treatment is by oral intake using magnesium lactate, magnesium oxide, or magnesium chloride or an antacid that contains Mg^{2+}. In severely ill patients, an $MgSO_4$ solution is given parenterally. Before initiation of therapy, renal function must be evaluated to avoid inducing hypermagnesemia during treatment.[17]

Hypermagnesemia
Hypermagnesemia is observed less frequently than is hypomagnesemia.[16] Causes for elevated serum Mg^{2+} levels are summarized in Table 16.13; the most common is renal failure

CASE STUDY 16.2

A 60-year-old man entered the emergency department after 2 days of "not feeling so well." History revealed a myocardial infarction 5 years ago, when he was prescribed digoxin. Two years ago, he was prescribed a diuretic after

periodic bouts of edema. An ECG at time of admission indicated a cardiac arrhythmia. Admitting lab results are shown in Case Study Table 16.2.1.

CASE STUDY TABLE 16.2.1	Laboratory Results
Venous Blood	
Digoxin: 1.4 ng/mL, therapeutic 0.5–2.2 (1.8 nmol/L, therapeutic 0.6–2.8)	
Na^+: 137 mmol/L	
K^+: 2.5 mmol/L	
Cl^-: 100 mmol/L	
HCO_3^-: 25 mmol/L	
Mg^{2+}: 0.4 mmol/L	
Ion/free Ca^{2+}: 1.0 mmol/L	

Questions

1. Because the digoxin level is within the therapeutic range, what may be the cause for the arrhythmia?
2. What is the most likely cause for the hypomagnesemia?
3. What is the most likely cause for the decreased potassium and ionized calcium levels?
4. What type of treatment would be helpful?

(GFR < 15 mL/min). The most severe elevations are usually a result of the combined effects of decreased renal function and increased intake of commonly prescribed Mg^{2+}-containing medications, such as antacids, enemas, or cathartics. Nursing home patients are at greatest risk for this occurrence.[16]

TABLE 16.13	Causes of Hypermagnesemia

Decreased Excretion
Acute or chronic renal failure
Hypothyroidism
Hypoaldosteronism
Hypopituitarism (↓growth hormone)

Increased Intake
Antacids
Enemas
Cathartics
Therapeutic—eclampsia, cardiac arrhythmia

Miscellaneous
Dehydration
Bone carcinoma
Bone metastases

Adapted from Polancic JE. Magnesium: metabolism, clinical importance, and analysis. *Clin Lab Sci.* 1991;4(2):105–109.

Hypermagnesemia has been associated with several endocrine disorders. Thyroxine and growth hormone cause a decrease in tubular reabsorption of Mg^{2+}, and a deficiency of either hormone may cause a moderate elevation in serum Mg^{2+}. Adrenal insufficiency may cause a mild elevation as a result of decreased renal excretion of Mg^{2+}.[16]

$MgSO_4$ may be used therapeutically with preeclampsia, cardiac arrhythmia, or myocardial infarction; Mg^{2+} is a vasodilator and can decrease uterine hyperactivity in eclamptic states and increase uterine blood flow. This therapy can lead to maternal hypermagnesemia, as well as neonatal hypermagnesemia due to the immature kidney of the newborn. Premature infants are at greater risk to develop actual symptoms.[16] Studies have shown that IV Mg^{2+} therapy in myocardial infarction patients may reduce early mortality.[15]

Dehydration can cause a pseudohypermagnesemia, which can be corrected with rehydration. Because of increased bone loss, mild serum Mg^{2+} elevations can occur in individuals with multiple myeloma or bone metastases.

Symptoms of hypermagnesemia. Symptoms of hypermagnesemia typically do not occur until the serum level exceeds 1.5 mmol/L.[16] The most frequent symptoms involve cardiovascular, dermatologic, GI, neurologic, neuromuscular, metabolic, and hemostatic abnormalities (Table 16.14). Mild to moderate symptoms, such as hypotension, bradycardia, skin flushing, increased skin temperature, nausea, vomiting, and lethargy, may occur when serum levels are 1.5 to 2.5 mmol/L.[16] Life-threatening symptoms, such as ECG changes, heart block, asystole, sedation, coma, respiratory depression or arrest, and paralysis, can occur when serum levels reach 5.0 mmol/L.[16]

Elevated Mg^{2+} levels may inhibit PTH release and target tissue response. This may lead to hypocalcemia and hypercalciuria.[16] Normal hemostasis is a Ca^{2+}-dependent process that may be inhibited as a result of competition between increased levels of Mg^{2+} and Ca^{2+} ions. Thrombin generation and platelet adhesion are two processes in which interference may occur.[16]

Treatment of hypermagnesemia. Treatment of Mg^{2+} excess associated with increased intake is to discontinue the source of Mg^{2+}. Severe symptomatic hypermagnesemia requires immediate supportive therapy for cardiac, neuromuscular, respiratory, or neurologic abnormalities. Patients with renal failure require hemodialysis. Patients with normal renal function may be treated with a diuretic and IV fluid.

Determination of Magnesium
Specimen
Nonhemolyzed serum or lithium heparin plasma may be analyzed. Because the Mg^{2+} concentration inside erythrocytes is 10 times greater than that in the ECF, hemolysis must be avoided, and the serum should be separated from the cells as soon as possible. Oxalate, citrate, and ethylenediaminetetraacetic acid (EDTA) anticoagulants are unacceptable because they will bind with Mg^{2+}. A 24-hour urine sample is preferred for analysis because of a diurnal variation in excretion. The urine must be acidified with HCl to avoid precipitation.

Methods
The three most common methods for measuring total serum Mg^{2+} are colorimetric: calmagite, formazan dye, and methylthymol blue. In the calmagite method, Mg^{2+} binds with calmagite to form a reddish-violet complex that may be read at 532 nm. In the formazan dye method, Mg^{2+} binds with the dye to form a colored complex that may be read at 660 nm. In the methylthymol blue method, Mg^{2+} binds with the chromogen to form a colored complex. Most methods use a Ca^{2+} shelter to prohibit interference from this divalent cation. The reference method for measuring Mg^{2+} is AAS.

Although the measurement of total Mg^{2+} concentrations in serum remains the usual diagnostic test for detection of Mg^{2+} abnormalities, it has limitations. First, because approximately 25% of Mg^{2+} is protein bound, total Mg^{2+} may not reflect the physiologically active, free ionized Mg^{2+}. Second, because Mg^{2+} is primarily an intracellular ion, serum concentrations will not necessarily reflect the status of intracellular Mg^{2+}; even when tissue and cellular Mg^{2+} is depleted by as much as 20%, serum Mg^{2+} concentrations may remain normal.

Reference Ranges
See Table 16.15.[3]

Calcium
Calcium Physiology
In 1883, Ringer[20] showed that Ca^{2+} was essential for myocardial contraction. While attempting to study how bound and free forms of Ca^{2+} affected frog heart contraction, McLean and Hastings[21] showed that the ionized/free Ca^{2+} concentration was proportional to the amplitude of frog heart

TABLE 16.14	Symptoms of Hypermagnesemia	
Cardiovascular	**Neuromuscular**
Hypotension	*Decreased reflexes*
Bradycardia	Dysarthria
Heart block	Respiratory depression
	Paralysis
Dermatologic	*Metabolic*
Flushing	Hypocalcemia
Warm skin	
Gastrointestinal	*Hemostatic*
Nausea	Decreased thrombin generation
Vomiting	Decreased platelet adhesion
Neurologic	
Lethargy	
Coma	

Adapted from Polancic JE. Magnesium: metabolism, clinical importance, and analysis. *Clin Lab Sci.* 1991;4(2):105–109.

TABLE 16.15	Reference Range for Magnesium
Serum, colorimetric	0.63–1.0 mmol/L (1.26–2.10 mg/dL)

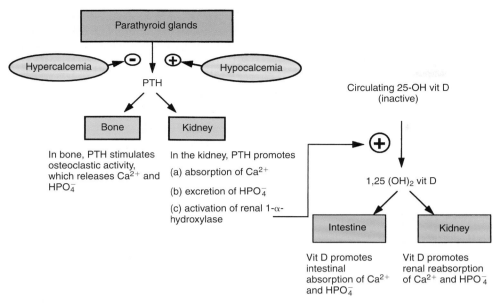

FIGURE 16.5 Hormonal response to hypercalcemia and hypocalcemia. PTH, parathyroid hormone; 25-OH vit D, 25-hydroxyvitamin D; 1,25(OH)₂ vit D, dihydroxyvitamin D.

contraction, whereas protein-bound and citrate-bound Ca^{2+} had no effect. From this observation, they developed the first assay for ionized/free Ca^{2+} using isolated frog hearts. Although the method had poor precision by today's standards, the investigators were able to show that blood-ionized Ca^{2+} was closely regulated and had a mean concentration in humans of about 1.18 mmol/L. Because decreased ionized Ca^{2+} impairs myocardial function, it is important to maintain ionized Ca^{2+} at a near-normal concentration during surgery and in critically ill patients. Decreased ionized Ca^{2+} concentrations in blood can cause neuromuscular irritability, which may become clinically apparent as tetany.

Regulation

Three hormones, PTH, vitamin D, and calcitonin, are known to regulate serum Ca^{2+} by altering their secretion rate in response to changes in ionized Ca^{2+}. The actions of these hormones are shown in Figure 16.5.

PTH secretion in blood is stimulated by a decrease in ionized Ca^{2+}, and conversely, PTH secretion is stopped by an increase in ionized Ca^{2+}. PTH exerts three major effects on both bone and kidney. In the bone, PTH activates a process known as *bone resorption*, in which activated osteoclasts break down bone and subsequently release Ca^{2+} into the ECF. In the kidneys, PTH conserves Ca^{2+} by increasing tubular reabsorption of Ca^{2+} ions. PTH also stimulates renal production of active vitamin D.

Vitamin D_3, a cholecalciferol, is obtained from the diet (seafood, dairy, egg yolks) or exposure of skin to sunlight. Vitamin D_3 is then converted in the liver to 25-hydroxycholecalciferol (25-OH-D_3), still an inactive form of vitamin D. In the kidney, 25-OH-D_3 is specifically hydroxylated to form 1,25-dihydroxycholecalciferol (1,25-[OH]₂-D_3), the biologically active form. This active form of vitamin D increases Ca^{2+} absorption in the intestine and enhances the effect of PTH on bone resorption.

Calcitonin, which originates in the medullary cells of the thyroid gland, is secreted when the concentration of Ca^{2+} in blood increases. Calcitonin exerts its Ca^{2+}-lowering effect by inhibiting the actions of both PTH and vitamin D. Although calcitonin is apparently not secreted during normal regulation of the ionized Ca^{2+} concentration in blood, it is secreted in response to a hypercalcemic stimulus.

Distribution

About 99% of Ca^{2+} in the body is part of bone, and the remaining 1% is mostly in the blood and other ECF, as little is in the cytosol of most cells. In fact, the concentration of ionized Ca^{2+} in blood is 5,000 to 10,000 times higher than in the cytosol of cardiac or smooth muscle cells. Maintenance of this large gradient is vital to maintain the essential rapid inward flux of Ca^{2+}.

Ca^{2+} in blood is distributed among several forms. About 45% circulates as free Ca^{2+} ions (referred to as ionized Ca^{2+}); 40% is bound to protein, mostly albumin; and 15% is bound to anions, such as HCO_3^-, citrate, and lactate. Clearly, this distribution can change in disease. It is noteworthy that concentrations of citrate, HCO_3^-, lactate, and albumin can change dramatically during surgery or critical care. This is why ionized Ca^{2+} cannot be reliably calculated from total Ca^{2+} measurements, especially in acutely ill individuals.

Clinical Applications

Tables 16.16 and 16.17 summarize causes of hypocalcemic and hypercalcemic disorders. Although both total Ca^{2+} and ionized Ca^{2+} measurements are available in many laboratories, ionized Ca^{2+} is usually a more sensitive and specific marker for Ca^{2+} disorders.

Hypocalcemia

When PTH is not present, as with *primary hypoparathyroidism*, serum Ca^{2+} levels are not properly regulated. Bone tends to "hang on" to its storage pool, and the kidney increases

TABLE 16.16 **Causes of Hypocalcemia**

Primary hypoparathyroidism—glandular aplasia, destruction, or removal
Hypomagnesemia
Hypermagnesemia
Hypoalbuminemia (total only, ionized calcium not affected by)—chronic liver disease, nephrotic syndrome, malnutrition
Acute pancreatitis
Vitamin D deficiency
Renal disease
Rhabdomyolysis
Pseudohypoparathyroidism

TABLE 16.17 **Causes of Hypercalcemia**

Primary hyperparathyroidism—adenoma or glandular hyperplasia
Hyperthyroidism
Benign familial hypocalciuria
Malignancy
Multiple myeloma
Increased vitamin D
Thiazide diuretics
Prolonged immobilization

excretion of Ca^{2+}. Because PTH is also required for normal vitamin D metabolism, the lack of vitamin D's effects also leads to a decreased level of Ca^{2+}. Parathyroid gland aplasia, destruction, and removal are obvious reasons for primary hypoparathyroidism.

Case Study 16.3

An 84-year-old nursing home resident was seen in the emergency department with the following symptoms: nausea, vomiting, decreased respiration, hypotension, and low pulse rate (46 bpm). Physical examination showed the skin was warm to the touch and flushed. Admission laboratory data are found in Case Study Table 16.3.1.

CASE STUDY TABLE 16.3.1 Laboratory Results

		Result	Reference Range
Serum	Total protein	5.6 g/dL	6.0–8.0 g/dL
	Albumin	3.0 g/dL	3.5–5.0 g/dL
	Total Ca^{2+}	8.2 mg/dL	8.6–10.0 mg/dL
	BUN	45 mg/dL	5–20 mg/dL
	Creatinine	2.3 mg/dL	0.7–1.5 mg/dL
	Mg^{2+}	4.0 mmol/L	0.63–1.0 mmol/L
Plasma	Na^+	129 mmol/L	136–145 mmol/L
	K^+	5.3 mmol/L	3.4–5.0 mmol/L
	Cl^-	96 mmol/L	98–107 mmol/L
	HCO_3^-	16 mmol/L	22–29 mmol/L

Questions

1. What is the most likely cause for the patient's symptoms?
2. What is the most likely cause for the hypermagnesemia?
3. What could be the cause for the hypocalcemia?

Because hypomagnesemia has become more frequent in hospitalized patients, chronic hypomagnesemia has also become recognized as a frequent cause of **hypocalcemia**. Hypomagnesemia may cause hypocalcemia by three mechanisms: (1) it inhibits the glandular secretion of PTH across the parathyroid gland membrane, (2) it impairs PTH action at its receptor site on bone, and (3) it causes vitamin D resistance.[15] Elevated Mg^{2+} levels may inhibit PTH release and target tissue response, perhaps leading to hypocalcemia and hypercalciuria.[16]

When total Ca^{2+} is the only result reported, hypocalcemia can appear with hypoalbuminemia. Common causes are associated with chronic liver disease, nephrotic syndrome, and malnutrition. In general, for each 1 g/dL decrease in serum albumin, there is a 0.2 mmol/L (0.8 mg/dL) decrease in total Ca^{2+} levels.[22]

About one-half of the patients with acute pancreatitis develop hypocalcemia. The most consistent cause appears to be a result of increased intestinal binding of Ca^{2+} as increased intestinal lipase activity occurs.[22] Vitamin D deficiency and malabsorption can cause decreased absorption, which leads to increased PTH production or secondary hyperparathyroidism.

Patients with renal disease caused by glomerular failure often have altered concentrations of Ca^{2+}, PO_4^-, albumin, Mg^{2+}, and H^+ (pH). In chronic renal disease, secondary hyperparathyroidism frequently develops as the body tries to compensate for hypocalcemia caused either by hyperphosphatemia (PO_4^- binds and lowers ionized Ca^{2+}) or altered vitamin D metabolism. Monitoring and controlling ionized Ca^{2+} concentrations may avoid problems due to hypocalcemia, such as osteodystrophy, unstable cardiac output or blood pressure, or problems arising from hypercalcemia, such as renal stones and other calcifications. Rhabdomyolysis, as with major crush injury and muscle damage, may cause hypocalcemia as a result of increased PO_4^- release from cells, which bind to Ca^{2+} ions.[22]

Pseudohypoparathyroidism is a rare hereditary disorder in which PTH target tissue response is decreased (end organ resistance). PTH production responds normally to loss of Ca^{2+}; however, without normal response (decreased cAMP [cyclic adenosine 3′,5′-phosphate] production), Ca^{2+} is lost in the urine or remains in the bone storage pool. Patients often have common physical features, including short stature, obesity, shortened metacarpals and metatarsals, and abnormal calcification.

Surgery and intensive care. Because appropriate Ca^{2+} concentrations promote good cardiac output and maintain adequate blood pressure, the maintenance of a normal ionized Ca^{2+} concentration in blood is beneficial to patients in either surgery or intensive care. Controlling Ca^{2+} concentrations may be critical in open heart surgery when the heart is restarted and during liver transplantation because large volumes of citrated blood are given.

Because these patients may receive large amounts of citrate, HCO_3^-, Ca^{2+} salts, or fluids, the greatest discrepancies between total Ca^{2+} and ionized Ca^{2+} concentrations may be seen during major surgical operations. Consequently, ionized Ca^{2+} measurements are the Ca^{2+} measurement of greatest clinical value.

Hypocalcemia occurs commonly in critically ill patients, that is, those with sepsis, thermal burns, renal failure, or cardiopulmonary insufficiency. These patients frequently have abnormalities of acid–base regulation and losses of protein and albumin, which are best suited to monitoring Ca^{2+} status by ionized Ca^{2+} measurements. Normalization of ionized Ca^{2+} may have beneficial effects on cardiac output and blood pressure.

Neonatal monitoring. Typically, blood-ionized Ca^{2+} concentrations in neonates are high at birth and then rapidly decline by 10% to 20% after 1 to 3 days. After about 1 week, ionized Ca^{2+} concentrations in the neonate stabilize at levels slightly higher than in adults.[23]

The concentration of ionized Ca^{2+} may decrease rapidly in the early neonatal period because the infant may lose Ca^{2+} rapidly and not readily reabsorb it. Several possible etiologies have been suggested: abnormal PTH and vitamin D metabolism, hypercholesterolemia, hyperphosphatemia, and hypomagnesemia.

Symptoms of hypocalcemia. Neuromuscular irritability and cardiac irregularities are the primary groups of symptoms that occur with hypocalcemia. Neuromuscular symptoms include paresthesia, muscle cramps, tetany, and seizures. Cardiac symptoms may include arrhythmia or heart block. Symptoms usually occur with severe hypocalcemia, in which total Ca^{2+} levels are below 1.88 mmol/L (7.5 mg/dL).[22]

Treatment of hypocalcemia. Oral or parenteral Ca^{2+} therapy may occur, depending on the severity of the decreased level and the cause. Vitamin D may sometimes be administered in addition to oral Ca^{2+} to increase absorption. If hypomagnesemia is a concurrent disorder, Mg^{2+} therapy should also be provided.

Hypercalcemia
Primary hyperparathyroidism is the main cause of **hypercalcemia**.[22] Hyperparathyroidism, or excess secretion of PTH, may show obvious clinical signs or may be asymptomatic. The patient population seen most frequently with primary hyperparathyroidism is older women.[22] Although either total or ionized Ca^{2+} measurements are elevated in serious cases, ionized Ca^{2+} is more frequently elevated in subtle or asymptomatic hyperparathyroidism. In general,

ionized Ca^{2+} measurements are elevated in 90% to 95% of cases of hyperparathyroidism, whereas total Ca^{2+} is elevated in 80% to 85% of cases.

The second leading cause of hypercalcemia is associated with various types of malignancy, with hypercalcemia sometimes being the sole biochemical marker for disease.[22] Many tumors produce PTH-related peptide (PTH-rP), which binds to normal PTH receptors and causes increased Ca^{2+} levels. Specific assays to measure PTH-rP are available because this abnormal protein is not detected by most PTH assays.

Because of the proximity of the parathyroid gland to the thyroid gland, hyperthyroidism can sometimes cause hyperparathyroidism. A rare, benign, familial hypocalciuria has also been reported. Thiazide diuretics increase Ca^{2+} reabsorption, leading to hypercalcemia. Prolonged immobilization may cause increased bone resorption. Hypercalcemia associated with immobilization is further compounded by renal insufficiency.

Symptoms of hypercalcemia. A mild hypercalcemia (2.62 to 3.00 mmol/L [10.5 to 12 mg/dL]) is often asymptomatic.[22] Moderate or severe Ca^{2+} elevations include neurologic, GI, and renal symptoms. Neurologic symptoms may include mild drowsiness or weakness, depression, lethargy, and coma. GI symptoms may include constipation, nausea, vomiting, anorexia, and peptic ulcer disease. Hypercalcemia may cause renal symptoms of nephrolithiasis and nephrocalcinosis. Hypercalciuria can result in nephrogenic diabetes insipidus, which causes polyuria that results in hypovolemia, which further aggravates the hypercalcemia.[22] Hypercalcemia can also cause symptoms of digitalis toxicity.

Treatment of hypercalcemia. Treatment of hypercalcemia depends on the level of hypercalcemia and the cause. Often people with primary hyperparathyroidism are asymptomatic. Estrogen deficiency in postmenopausal women has been implicated in primary hyperparathyroidism in older women.[22] Often, estrogen replacement therapy reduces Ca^{2+} levels. Parathyroidectomy may be necessary in some hyperparathyroid patients. Patients with moderate to severe hypercalcemia are treated to reduce Ca^{2+} levels. Salt and water intake is encouraged to increase Ca^{2+} excretion and avoid dehydration, which can compound the hypercalcemia. Thiazide diuretics should be discontinued. Bisphosphonates (a derivative of pyrophosphate) are the main drug class used to lower Ca^{2+} levels, achieved by its binding action to bone, which prevents bone resorption.[22]

Determination of Calcium
Specimen
The preferred specimen for total Ca^{2+} determinations is either serum or lithium heparin plasma collected without venous stasis. Because anticoagulants such as EDTA or oxalate bind Ca^{2+} tightly and interfere with measurement, they are unacceptable for use.

The proper collection of samples for ionized Ca^{2+} measurements requires greater care. Because loss of CO_2 will increase pH, samples must be collected anaerobically. Although heparinized whole blood is the preferred sample, serum from sealed evacuated blood collection tubes may be used if clotting and centrifugation are done quickly (<30 minutes) and at room temperature. No liquid heparin products should be used. Most heparin anticoagulants (Na^+ and lithium) partially bind to Ca^{2+} and lower ionized Ca^{2+} concentrations. A heparin concentration of 25 IU/mL, for example, decreases ionized Ca^{2+} by about 3%. Dry heparin products are available titrated with small amounts of Ca^{2+} or Zn^{2+} or with small amounts of heparin dispersed in an inert "puff" that essentially eliminates the interference by heparin.

For analysis of Ca^{2+} in urine, an accurately timed urine collection is preferred. The urine should be acidified with 6 mol/L HCl, with approximately 1 mL of the acid added for each 100 mL of urine.

Methods

The two commonly used methods for total Ca^{2+} analysis use either orthocresolphthalein complexone (CPC) or arsenazo III dye to form a complex with Ca^{2+}. Prior to the dye-binding reaction, Ca^{2+} is released from its protein carrier and complexes by acidification of the sample. The CPC method uses 8-hydroxyquinoline to prevent Mg^{2+} interference. AAS remains the reference method for total Ca^{2+}, although it is rarely used in the clinical setting.

Current commercial analyzers that measure ionized/free Ca^{2+} use ISEs for this measurement. These systems may use membranes impregnated with special molecules that selectively, but reversibly, bind Ca^{2+} ions. As Ca^{2+} binds to these membranes, an electric potential develops across the membrane that is proportional to the ionized Ca^{2+} concentration. A diagram of one such electrode is shown in Figure 16.6.

Reference Ranges

For total Ca^{2+}, the reference range varies slightly with age.[3] In general, Ca^{2+} concentrations are higher through adolescence when bone growth is most active. Ionized/free Ca^{2+} concentrations can change rapidly from day 1 to day 3 of life. Following this, they stabilize at relatively high levels, with a gradual decline through adolescence; see Table 16.18.

TABLE 16.18	Reference Ranges for Calcium
Total Calcium—Serum, Plasma	
Child, <12 y	2.20–2.70 mmol/L (8.8–10.8 mg/dL)
Adult	2.15–2.50 mmol/L (8.6–10.0 mg/dL)
Ionized Calcium—Serum	
Child	1.20–1.38 mmol/L (4.8–5.5 mg/dL)
Adult	1.16–1.32 mmol/L (4.6–5.3 mg/dL)
Ionized Calcium—Plasma	
Adult	1.03–1.23 mmol/L (4.1–4.9 mg/dL)
Ionized Calcium—Whole Blood	
Adult	1.15–1.27 mmol/L (4.6–5.1 mg/dL)
Total Calcium— Urine (24 H)	2.50–7.50 mmol/d (100–300 mg/d), varies with diet

Phosphate
Phosphate Physiology

Found everywhere in living cells, phosphate compounds participate in many of the most important biochemical processes. The genetic materials deoxyribonucleic acid and ribonucleic acid are complex phosphodiesters. Most coenzymes are esters of phosphoric or pyrophosphoric acid. The most important reservoirs of biochemical energy are ATP, creatine phosphate, and PEP. Phosphate deficiency can lead to ATP depletion, which is ultimately responsible for many of the clinical symptoms observed in hypophosphatemia.

Alterations in the concentration of 2,3-bisphosphoglycerate (2,3-BPG) in RBCs affect the affinity of hemoglobin for oxygen, with an increase facilitating the release of oxygen in tissue and a decrease making oxygen bound to hemoglobin less available. By affecting the formation of 2,3-BPG, the concentration of inorganic phosphate indirectly affects the release of oxygen from hemoglobin.

Understanding the cause of an altered phosphate concentration in the blood is often difficult because transcellular shifts of phosphate are a major cause of hypophosphatemia in blood. That is, an increased shift of phosphate into cells

FIGURE 16.6 Diagram of ionized calcium electrode for the ionized calcium analyzer. (Courtesy of Radiometer America, Westlake, OH.)

can deplete phosphate in the blood. Once phosphate is taken up by the cell, it remains there to be used in the synthesis of phosphorylated compounds. As these phosphate compounds are metabolized, inorganic phosphate slowly leaks out of the cell into the blood, where it is regulated principally by the kidney.

Regulation

Phosphate in blood may be absorbed in the intestine from dietary sources, released from cells into blood, and lost from bone. In healthy individuals, all these processes are relatively constant and easily regulated by renal excretion or reabsorption of phosphate.

Disturbances to any of these processes can alter phosphate concentrations in the blood; however, the loss of regulation by the kidneys will have the most profound effect. Although other factors, such as vitamin D, calcitonin, growth hormone, and acid–base status, can affect renal regulation of phosphate, the most important factor is PTH, which overall lowers blood concentrations by increasing renal excretion.

Vitamin D acts to increase phosphate in the blood. Vitamin D increases both phosphate absorption in the intestine and phosphate reabsorption in the kidney.

Growth hormone, which helps regulate skeletal growth, can affect circulating concentrations of phosphate. In cases of excessive secretion or administration of growth hormone, phosphate concentrations in the blood may increase because of decreased renal excretion of phosphate.

Distribution

Although the concentration of all phosphate compounds in blood is about 12 mg/dL (3.9 mmol/L), most of that is organic phosphate, and only about 3 to 4 mg/dL is inorganic phosphate. Phosphate is the predominant intracellular anion, with intracellular concentrations varying, depending on the type of cell. About 80% of the total body pool of phosphate is contained in bone, 20% in soft tissues, and less than 1% is active in the serum/plasma.

Clinical Applications
Hypophosphatemia

Hypophosphatemia occurs in about 1% to 5% of hospitalized patients.[24] The incidence of hypophosphatemia increases to 20% to 40% in patients with the following disorders: diabetic ketoacidosis, chronic obstructive pulmonary disease, asthma, malignancy, long-term treatment with total parenteral nutrition, inflammatory bowel disease, anorexia nervosa, and alcoholism. The incidence increases to 60% to 80% in ICU patients with sepsis. In addition, hypophosphatemia can also be caused by increased renal excretion, as with hyperparathyroidism, and decreased intestinal absorption, as with vitamin D deficiency or antacid use.[24] Although most cases are moderate and seldom cause problems, severe hypophosphatemia (<1.0 g/dL or 0.3 mmol/L) requires monitoring and possible replacement therapy. There is a 30% mortality rate in those who are severely hypophosphatemic versus a 15% rate in those with normal or mild hypophosphatemia.[24]

Hyperphosphatemia

Patients at greatest risk for **hyperphosphatemia** are those with acute or chronic renal failure.[24] An increased intake of phosphate or increased release of cellular phosphate may also cause hyperphosphatemia. Because they may not yet have developed mature PTH and vitamin D metabolism, neonates are especially susceptible to hyperphosphatemia caused by increased intake, such as from cow's milk or laxatives. Increased breakdown of cells can sometimes lead to hyperphosphatemia, as with severe infections, intensive exercise, neoplastic disorders, or intravascular hemolysis. Because immature lymphoblasts have about four times the phosphate content of mature lymphocytes, patients with lymphoblastic leukemia are especially susceptible to hyperphosphatemia. Hypoparathyroidism may also cause hyperphosphatemia.

Determination of Inorganic Phosphorus
Specimen

Serum or lithium heparin plasma is acceptable for analysis. Oxalate, citrate, or EDTA anticoagulants should not be used because they interfere with the analytic method. Hemolysis should be avoided because of the higher concentrations inside RBCs. Circulating phosphate levels are subject to circadian rhythm, with highest levels in late morning and lowest in the evening. Urine analysis for phosphate requires a 24-hour sample collection because of significant diurnal variations.

Methods

Most of the current methods for phosphorus determination involve the formation of an ammonium phosphomolybdate complex. This colorless complex can be measured by ultraviolet absorption at 340 nm or can be reduced to form molybdenum blue, a stable blue chromophore, which is read between 600 and 700 nm.

Reference Ranges

Phosphate values vary with age. Divided into age groups, the ranges are shown in Table 16.19.

Lactate
Lactate Biochemistry and Physiology

Lactate is a by-product of an emergency mechanism that produces a small amount of ATP when oxygen delivery is severely diminished. Pyruvate is the normal end product of glucose metabolism (glycolysis). The conversion of pyruvate to lactate is activated when a deficiency of oxygen leads to an accumulation of excess NADH (Fig. 16.7). Normally, sufficient oxygen maintains a favorably high ratio of NAD to NADH. Under these conditions, pyruvate is converted

TABLE 16.19 Reference Ranges for Inorganic Phosphorus

Serum	
Neonate	1.45–2.91 mmol/L (4.5–9.0 mg/dL)
Child ≤15 y	1.07–1.74 mmol/L (3.3–5.4 mg/dL)
Adult	0.78–1.42 mmol/L (2.4 – 4.4 mg/dL)
Urine (24 h)	13–42 mmol/d (0.4–1.3 g/d)

Aerobic Metabolism

Anaerobic Metabolism

FIGURE 16.7 Aerobic versus anaerobic metabolism of glucose.

to acetyl-coenzyme A (CoA), which enters the citric acid cycle and produces 38 mol of ATP for each mole of glucose oxidized. However, under hypoxic conditions, acetyl-CoA formation does not occur, and NADH accumulates, favoring the conversion of pyruvate to lactate through anaerobic metabolism. As a result, only 2 mol of ATP are produced for each mole of glucose metabolized to lactate, with the excess lactate released into the blood. This release of lactate into blood has clinical importance because the accumulation of

excess lactate in blood is an early, sensitive, and quantitative indicator of the severity of oxygen deprivation (Fig. 16.8).

Regulation

Because lactate is a by-product of anaerobic metabolism, it is not specifically regulated, as with K^+ or Ca^{2+}, for example. As oxygen delivery decreases below a critical level, blood lactate concentrations rise rapidly and indicate tissue hypoxia earlier than does pH. The liver is the major organ

FIGURE 16.8 Metabolic effects of hypoxia, leading to cell death.

for removing lactate by converting lactate back to glucose by a process called *gluconeogenesis*.

Clinical Applications

Measurements of blood lactate are useful for metabolic monitoring in critically ill patients, for indicating the severity of the illness, and for objectively determining patient prognosis.

There are two types of lactic acidosis. Type A is associated with hypoxic conditions, such as shock, myocardial infarction, severe CHF, pulmonary edema, or severe blood loss. Type B is of metabolic origin, such as with diabetes mellitus, severe infection, leukemia, liver or renal disease, and toxins (ethanol, methanol, or salicylate poisoning).

Determination of Lactate

Specimen Handling

Special care should be practiced when collecting and handling specimens for lactate analysis. Ideally, a tourniquet should not be used because venous stasis will increase lactate levels. If a tourniquet is used, blood should be collected immediately and the patient should not exercise the hand before or during collection.[14] After sample collection, glucose is converted to lactose by way of anaerobic glycolysis and should be prevented. Heparinized blood may be used but must be delivered on ice, and the plasma must be quickly separated. Iodoacetate and fluoride, which inhibit glycolysis without affecting coagulation, are usually satisfactory additives, but the specific method directions must be consulted.

Methods

Although lactate is a sensitive indicator of inadequate tissue oxygenation, the use of blood lactate measurements has been hindered because older methods were slow and laborious.

TABLE 16.20 **Reference Ranges for Lactate**

	Enzymatic Method, Plasma	Colorimetric, Whole Blood
Venous	0.5–2.2 mmol/L (4.5–19.8 mg/dL)	0.9–1.7 mmol/L (8.1–15.3 mg/dL)
Arterial	0.5–1.6 mmol/L (4.5–14.4 mg/dL)	<1.3 mmol/L (<11.7 mg/dL)
Cerebrospinal fluid	1.0–2.9 mmol/L (9–26 mg/dL)	

Other means of following perfusion or oxygenation have been used, such as indwelling catheters that measure blood flow, pulse oximeters, base-excess determinations, and measurements of oxygen consumption (Vo_2). Current enzymatic methods make lactate determination readily available.

The most commonly used enzymatic method uses lactate oxidase to produce pyruvate and H_2O_2:

$$\text{Lactate} + O_2 \xrightarrow{\text{Lactate oxidase}} \text{pyruvate} + H_2O_2 \quad \text{(Eq. 16-6)}$$

One of two couple reactions may then be used. Peroxidase may be used to produce a colored chromogen from H_2O_2:

$$H_2O_2 + \text{H donar} + \text{chromogen} \xrightarrow{\text{Peroxidase}} \text{colored dye} + 2H_2O \quad \text{(Eq. 16-7)}$$

Reference Ranges

See Table 16.20.[3]

Case Study 16.4

Consider the following laboratory results from three adult patients (Case Study Table 16.4.1):

CASE STUDY TABLE 16.4.1 **Laboratory Results**

	Reference Ranges				
Case	Ion CA^{2+} 1.16–1.32 mmol/L	Total MG^{2+} 0.63–1.0 mmol/L	PO_4^- 0.87–1.45 mmol/L	Hematocrit 35%–45%	Intact Parathyroid Hormone 13–64 ng/L
A	1.44	0.90	0.85	42	100
B	1.08	0.50	0.90	40	25
C	1.70	0.98	1.43	30	12

Questions

1. Which set of laboratory results (Case A, B, or C) is most likely associated with each of the following diagnoses?

- Primary hyperparathyroidism
- Malignancy
- Hypomagnesemic hypocalcemia

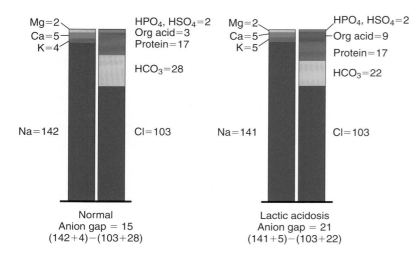

Normal
Anion gap = 15
(142+4)−(103+28)

Lactic acidosis
Anion gap = 21
(141+5)−(103+22)

FIGURE 16.9 Demonstration of anion gap from concentrations of anions and cations in normal state and in lactic acidosis.

ANION GAP

Routine measurement of electrolytes usually involves only Na^+, K^+, Cl^-, and HCO_3^- (as total CO_2). These values may be used to approximate the **anion gap (AG)**, which is the difference between unmeasured anions and unmeasured cations; however, there is never an actual "gap" between total cationic charges and anionic charges. The AG is calculated by the concentration difference between commonly measured cations (Na+K) and commonly measured anions (Cl+HCO₃), as shown in Figure 16.9. AG is useful in indicating an increase in one or more of the unmeasured anions in the serum and also as a form of quality control for the analyzer used to measure these electrolytes. Consistently abnormal AGs in serum from healthy persons may indicate an instrument problem.

There are two commonly used methods for calculating the AG. The first equation is

$$AG = Na^+ - (Cl^- + HCO_3^-) \qquad \text{(Eq. 16-8)}$$

It is equivalent to unmeasured anions minus the unmeasured cations in this way:

$$(PO_4^- + 2SO_4^{2-}) - (K^+ + 2Ca^{2+} + Mg^{2+}) \qquad \text{(Eq. 16-9)}$$

The reference range for the Ag^{2+} using this calculation is 7 to 16 mmol/L.[3] The second calculation method is

$$AG = (Na^+ + K^+) - (Cl^- + HCO_3^-) \qquad \text{(Eq. 16-10)}$$

It has a reference range of 10 to 20 mmol/L.[3]

An *elevated AG* may be caused by uremia/renal failure, which leads to PO4- and SO4² retention; ketoacidosis, as seen in cases of starvation or diabetes; methanol, ethanol, ethylene glycol, or salicylate poisoning; lactic acidosis; hypernatremia; and instrument error. *Low AG* values are rare but may be seen with hypoalbuminemia (decrease in unmeasured anions) or severe hypercalcemia (increase in unmeasured cations).

ELECTROLYTES AND RENAL FUNCTION

The kidney is central to the regulation and conservation of electrolytes in the body. For a review of kidney structure,

refer Figure 16.10 and Chapter 27. The following is a summary of electrolyte excretion and conservation in a healthy individual:

1. Glomerulus: This portion of the nephron acts as a filter, retaining large proteins and protein-bound constituents while most other plasma constituents pass into the filtrate. The concentrations in the filtered plasma should be approximately equal to ECF without protein.
2. Renal tubules:
   a. Phosphate reabsorption is inhibited by PTH and increased by 1,25-[OH]₂-D₃. Excretion of PO_4^- is stimulated by calcitonin.

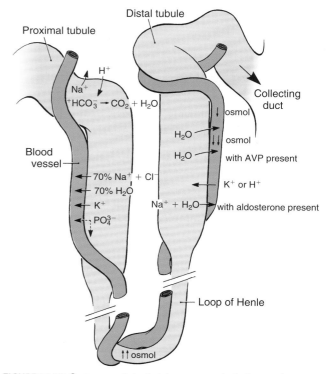

FIGURE 16.10 Summary of electrolyte movements in the renal tubules. AVP, arginine vasopressin hormone.

b. Ca^{2+} is reabsorbed under the influence of PTH and 1,25-$[OH]_2$-D_3. Calcitonin stimulates excretion of Ca^{2+}.

c. Mg^{2+} reabsorption occurs largely in the thick ascending limb of Henle's loop.

d. Sodium reabsorption can occur through three mechanisms:
   - Approximately 70% of the Na^+ in the filtrate is reabsorbed in the proximal tubules by isoosmotic reabsorption. It is limited, however, by the availability of Cl^- to maintain electrical neutrality.
   - Na^+ is reabsorbed in exchange for H^+. This reaction is linked with HCO_3^- and depends on carbonic anhydrase.
   - Stimulated by aldosterone, Na^+ is reabsorbed in exchange for K^+ in the distal tubules. (H^+ competes with K^+ for this exchange.)

e. Cl^- is reabsorbed, in part, by passive transport in the proximal tubule along the concentration gradient created by Na^+.

f. K^+ is reabsorbed by two mechanisms:
   - Active reabsorption in the proximal tubule almost completely conserves K^+.
   - Exchange with Na^+ is stimulated by aldosterone. H^+ competes with K^+ for this exchange.

g. Bicarbonate is recovered from the glomerular filtrate and converted to CO_2 when H^+ is excreted in the urine.
   - Henle's loop: With normal AVP function, it creates an osmotic gradient that enables water reabsorption to be increased or decreased in response to body fluid changes in osmolality.
   - Collecting ducts: Also under AVP influence, this is where final adjustment of water excretion is made.

CASE STUDY 16.5

A 15-year-old girl in a coma was brought to the emergency department by her parents. She has diabetes and has been insulin dependent for 7 years. Her parents stated that there have been several episodes of hypoglycemia and ketoacidosis in the past and that their daughter has often been "too busy" to take her insulin injections. The laboratory results obtained on admission are shown in Case Study Table 16.5.1.

Questions

1. What is the diagnosis?

2. Calculate the AG. What is the cause of the AG result in this patient?

3. Why are chloride and bicarbonate decreased? What is the significance of the elevated potassium value?

4. What is the significance of the plasma osmolality?

CASE STUDY TABLE 16.5.1   Laboratory Results

		Result	Reference Range
Venous blood	Na^+	145 mmol/L	136–145 mmol/L
	K^+	5.8 mmol/L	3.4–5.0 mmol/L
	Cl^-	87 mmol/L	98–107 mmol/L
	HCO_3^-	8 mmol/L	22–29 mmol/L
	Glucose	1,050 mg/dL	70–110 mg/dL
	Urea nitrogen	35 mg/dL	7–18 mg/dL
	Creatinine	1.3 mg/dL	0.5–1.3 mg/dL
	Lactate	5 mmol/L	0.5–2.2 mmol/L
	Osmolality	385 mOsm/kg	275–295 mOsm/kg
Arterial blood	pH	7.11	7.35–7.45
	po_2	98 mm Hg	83–100 mm Hg
	pco_2	20 mm Hg	35–45 mm Hg
Urine		Normal	
	Glucose	4+	Negative
	Ketones	4+	Negative

For additional student resources, please visit the Point® at http://thepoint.lww.com

questions

1. What is the major intracellular cation?
   a. Potassium
   b. Calcium
   c. Magnesium
   d. Sodium

2. What is the major extracellular cation?
   a. Sodium
   b. Chloride
   c. Magnesium
   d. Calcium

3. Osmolality can be defined as a measure of the concentration of a solution based on the
   a. Number of dissolved particles
   b. Number of ionic particles present
   c. Number and size of the dissolved particles
   d. Density of the dissolved particles

4. Hyponatremia may be caused by each of the following EXCEPT
   a. Hypomagnesemia
   b. Aldosterone deficiency
   c. Prolonged vomiting or diarrhea
   d. Acute or chronic renal failure

5. Hypokalemia may be caused by each of the following EXCEPT
   a. Acidosis
   b. Prolonged vomiting or diarrhea
   c. Hypomagnesemia
   d. Hyperaldosteronism

6. Hyperkalemia may be caused by each of the following EXCEPT
   a. Alkalosis
   b. Acute or chronic renal failure
   c. Hypoaldosteronism
   d. Sample hemolysis

7. The main difference between a direct and indirect ISE is
   a. Sample is diluted in the indirect method, not in the direct method
   b. The type of membrane that is used
   c. Direct ISEs use a reference electrode, whereas indirect ISEs do not
   d. Whole blood samples can be measured with the direct method and not with the indirect method

8. Which method of analysis will provide the most accurate electrolyte results if a grossly lipemic sample is used?
   a. Direct ISE
   b. Indirect ISE
   c. Flame emission photometry
   d. Atomic absorption

9. The most frequent cause of hypermagnesemia is due to
   a. Renal failure
   b. Increased intake of magnesium
   c. Hypoaldosteronism
   d. Acidosis

10. A hemolyzed sample will cause falsely increased levels of each of the following EXCEPT
    a. Sodium
    b. Potassium
    c. Phosphate
    d. Magnesium

11. The largest portion of total body water is found in which tissue?
    a. Intracellular fluid
    b. Extracellular fluid
    c. Intravascular extracellular fluid
    d. Interstitial cell fluid
    e. Plasma

12. Osmoreceptors in the hypothalamus are key to regulating blood osmolality. Typically, a 1% to 2% shift in osmolality causes a _____ change in circulating concentration of AVP.
    a. Twofold
    b. Fourfold
    c. Eightfold
    d. Tenfold

13. The quantitative relationship between changes in blood osmolality and the normal expected response by AVP is best described as a(n):
    a. Indirect relationship
    b. Direct relationship
    c. Logarithmic relationship
    d. There is no quantitative relationship

review questions (continued)

14. The sample of choice for measuring blood osmolality is:
 a. Serum
 b. Plasma
 c. Whole blood
 d. Serum or plasma may both be used

15. With increased water loss, burn patients are most likely to also experience:
 a. Hypernatremia
 b. Hyponatremia
 c. Hypomagnesemia
 d. Hypoosmolality

16. Which plasma electrolyte has the most narrow reference range and is MOST strictly regulated by the body?
 a. Sodium
 b. Magnesium
 c. Calcium
 d. Chloride
 e. Potassium

17. True or False? RBCs are key for oxygen transport, carbon dioxide transport, and maintaining electroneutrality in the blood.

references

1. Rose BD, ed. *Clinical Physiology of Acid–base and Electrolyte Disorders*. 5th ed. New York, NY: McGraw-Hill; 2001: 163–228, 241–257, 372–402, 696–793, 836–930.
2. Burtis CA, Ashwood ER, Bruns DE, eds. *Tietz Textbook of Clinical Chemistry and Molecular Diagnostics*. 4th ed. St. Louis, MO: Elsevier Saunders; 2006:49, 985, 991–992.
3. Wu HB, ed. *Tietz Clinical Guide to Laboratory Tests*. 4th ed. St. Louis, MO: Elsevier Saunders; 2006:118, 214, 198–200, 234–237, 650–653, 706–707, 786–789, 852–855, 880–883, 992–996.
4. Oh MS. Pathogenesis and diagnosis of hyponatremia. *Nephron*. 2002;92(suppl 1):2–8.
5. Munger MA. New agents for managing hyponatremia in hospitalized patients. *Am J Health Syst Pharm*. 2007;64:253–265.
6. Oh MS. Management of hyponatremia and clinical use of vasopressin antagonists. *Am J Med Sci*. 2007;333:101–105.
7. Kumar S, Tomas B. Sodium. *Lancet*. 1998;352:220–228.
8. Patel GP, Balk RA. Recognition and treatment of hyponatremia in acutely ill hospitalized patients. *Clin Ther*. 2007;29:211–229.
9. Crook M. The investigation and management of severe hyponatremia. *J Clin Pathol*. 2002;55:883.
10. Verbalis JG, Goldsmith SR, Greenberg A, et al. Hyponatremia treatment guidelines 2007: expert panel recommendations. *Am J Med*. 2007;120:S1–S21.
11. Ortho Clinical Diagnostics. *Vitros Na+ Package Insert, Version 5.0*. Rochester, NY: Ortho Clinical Diagnostics; 2015.
12. Gennari FJ. Disorders of potassium homeostasis: hypokalemia and hyperkalemia. *Crit Care Clin*. 2002;18:273–288.
13. Gennari FJ. Hypokalemia. *N Engl J Med*. 1998;339:451–458.
14. Burtis CA, Ashwood ER, Bruns DE, eds. *Tietz Fundamentals of Clinical Chemistry*. 6th ed. St. Louis, MO: Elsevier Saunders; 2008:394, 433.
15. Elin RJ. Magnesium: the fifth but forgotten electrolyte. *Am J Clin Pathol*. 1994;102:616–622.
16. Polancic JE. Magnesium: metabolism, clinical importance, and analysis. *Clin Lab Sci*. 1991;4:105–109.
17. Whang R. Clinical disorders of magnesium metabolism. *Comp Ther*. 1997;23:168–173.
18. Schlingmann KP, Weber S, Peters M, et al. Hypomagnesemia with secondary hypocalcemia is caused by mutations in TRPM6, a new member of the TRPM gene family. *Nat Genet*. 2002;31:166–170.
19. Whang R, Sims G. Magnesium and potassium supplementation in the prevention of diabetic vascular disease. *Med Hypotheses*. 2000;55:263–265.
20. Ringer S. A further contribution regarding the influence of different constituents of blood on contractions of the heart. *J Physiol*. 1883;4:29.
21. McLean FC, Hastings AB. A biological method for estimation of calcium ion concentration. *J Biol Chem*. 1934;107:337.
22. Bushinsky DA, Monk RD. Calcium. *Lancet*. 1998;352:23.
23. Wandrup J. Critical analytical and clinical aspects of ionized calcium in neonates. *Clin Chem*. 1989;35:2027.
24. Shiber JR, Mattu A. Serum phosphate abnormalities in the emergency department. *J Emerg Med*. 2002;23: 395–400.

17

Blood Gases, pH, and Buffer Systems

YACHANA KATARIA and MARK D. KELLOGG

chapter objectives

Upon completion of this chapter, the clinical laboratorian should be able to do the following:

- Describe the principles involved in the measurement of pH, pCO_2, pO_2, and the various hemoglobin species.
- Outline the interrelationship of the buffering mechanisms of bicarbonate, carbonic acid, and hemoglobin.
- Explain the clinical significance of the following pH and blood gas parameters: pH, pCO_2, pO_2, actual bicarbonate, carbonic acid, base excess, oxygen saturation, fractional oxyhemoglobin, hemoglobin oxygen (binding) capacity, oxygen content, and total CO_2.

For additional student resources, please visit thePoint® at http://thepoint.lww.com

chapter objectives (continued)

- Determine whether data are normal or represent metabolic or respiratory acidosis or metabolic or respiratory alkalosis using the Henderson-Hasselbalch equation and blood gas data. Identify whether the data represent uncompensated or compensated conditions.
- Identify some common causes of nonrespiratory acidosis and alkalosis, respiratory acidosis and alkalosis, and mixed abnormalities. State how the body attempts to compensate (kidney and lungs) for the various conditions.
- Describe the significance of the hemoglobin–oxygen dissociation curve and the impact of pH, 2,3-diphosphoglycerate (2,3-DPG), temperature, pH, and pCO_2 on its shape and release of O_2 to the tissues.
- Discuss problems and precautions in collecting and handling samples for pH and blood gas analysis. Include syringes, anticoagulants, mixing, icing, and capillary and venous samples as well as arterial samples in the discussion.
- Describe instrumental approaches to measuring various hemoglobin species and pH and blood gas parameters.
- Describe approaches to quality assurance, including quality control, proficiency testing, and delta checks to assess analytic quality.
- Discuss the reasons for possible discrepancies, given oxygen saturation data calculated by the blood gas analyzer and measured by the CO-oximeter.
- Calculate partial pressures of pCO_2 and pO_2 for various percentages of carbon dioxide and oxygen. In doing these calculations, account for the barometric pressure and vapor pressure of water.

An important aspect of clinical biochemistry is information on a patient's acid–base balance and blood gas homeostasis. These data often are used to assess patients in life-threatening situations. These test parameters are interrelated, focusing on only one test result can be misleading.

This chapter discusses exchange of gases, carbon dioxide and oxygen, together with the body's mechanisms to maintain an acid–base balance. The interpretation of data, from measurement of pH and other blood gas parameters, and the techniques and instrumentation used in these measurements are also described. In addition, preanalytical considerations and quality assurance of blood gas analysis are reviewed.

ACID–BASE BALANCE

Maintenance of H⁺

An *acid* is a substance that can donate hydrogen ions (H^+) when dissolved in water. A *base* is a substance that can accept hydrogen ions. pH of a solution is defined as the negative log of the hydrogen ion concentration. Accordingly, a decrease in one pH unit represents a 10-fold increase in H^+ concentration.

The logarithmic pH scale expresses H^+ concentration (c is concentration):

$$pH = \log \frac{1}{cH^+} = -\log cH^+ \qquad \text{(Eq. 17-1)}$$

Through metabolism, the body produces approximately 150 g of H^+ each day. Yet the concentration of H^+ in the extracellular body fluids is maintained within a narrow range from 36 to 44 nmol/L (pH 7.35 to 7.45). Through mechanisms that involve the lungs and kidneys, the body controls and excretes H^+ in order to maintain pH homeostasis. Imbalances between the rate of acid formation and excretion can occur and can lead to alterations in consciousness, neuromuscular irritability, tetany, coma, and death.

The relative strengths of acids and bases, their ability to dissociate in water, are described by their dissociation constant (K_a). Tables of dissociation constants can be found online and in most biochemistry texts. The pK_a is defined as the negative log of the dissociation constant. The dissociation constant is also known as the ionization constant. If the pH equals pK_a, then the solution in equilibrium and protonated and unprotonated species are present in equal concentrations. If the pH of the solution is less than pK_a then majority of the components will largely be protonated. Many species have more than one pK_a meaning they can accept or donate more than one H^+.

Buffer Systems: Regulation of H⁺ and the Henderson-Hasselbalch Equation

A *buffer* consists of a weak acid and a salt of its conjugate base, and it resists the change in pH upon adding acid or base. The effectiveness of a buffer depends on the pK_a of the buffering system and the pH of the environment in which it is placed. In plasma, the bicarbonate–carbonic acid system, is one of the principal buffers:

$$H_2CO_3 \leftrightarrow HCO_3^- + H^+ \qquad \text{(Eq. 17-2)}$$
$$\underset{\text{Carbonic acid}}{} \qquad \underset{\text{Bicarbonate}}{}$$

Buffers consist of a weak acid, such as carbonic acid (H_2CO_3), and a salt of its conjugate base, such as bicarbonate (HCO_3^-), which forms the bicarbonate–carbonic acid buffer system. H_2CO_3 is a weak acid because it does not completely dissociate into H^+ and HCO_3^-, whereas a strong acid, such as HCl, completely dissociates into H^+ and Cl^- in solution. When hydrogen ions are added to the bicarbonate–carbonic acid system, the HCO_3^- will combine with the H^+ to form H_2CO_3 (Eq. 17-2). Therefore, bicarbonate–carbonic acid reaction is driven to the right, increasing the amount of carbonic acid and consuming bicarbonate ion. Conversely when a strong base is added, H_2CO_3 will combine with the OH^- ions to form H_2O and the weaker conjugate base HCO_3^-.

Although the bicarbonate–carbonic acid system has low buffering capacity, it is still the most important buffer system in extracellular fluids for three reasons: (1) H_2CO_3 dissociates into CO_2 and H_2O, allowing CO_2 to be eliminated by the lungs and H^+ as water; (2) changes in CO_2 modify the ventilation (respiratory) rate; and (3) HCO_3^- concentration can be changed by the kidneys.

Proteins and phosphates are also involved in buffering, primarily in the intracellular fluids and to a minor extent in the extracellular spaces. Most circulating proteins have a net negative charge and are capable of binding H^+. The phosphate buffer system ($HPO_4^{2-} - H_2PO_4^-$) is the primary buffer in urine and is involved in the exchange of sodium ion in the urine filtrate. Hemoglobin plays a role in buffering the CO_2 as it is transported to the lungs for excretion.

The lungs and kidneys play important roles in extracellular fluid pH homeostasis. The interrelationship of the lungs and kidneys in maintaining pH is depicted by the Henderson-Hasselbalch equation (Eq. 17-3). The *Henderson-Hasselbalch equation* expresses acid–base relationships in a mathematical formula:

$$pH = pK_a' + \log \frac{cA^-}{cHA} \qquad \text{(Eq. 17-3)}$$

where A^- is the proton acceptor or base (e.g., HCO_3^-), HA is the proton donor or weak acid (e.g., H_2CO_3), and pK_a' is the pH at which there is an equal concentration of protonated and unprotonated species. Knowing any of the three variables allows for the calculation of the fourth.

Regulation of Acid–Base Balance: Lungs and Kidneys (Transport of Carbon Dioxide)

Carbon dioxide, the end product of most aerobic metabolic processes, easily diffuses out of the tissue where it is produced and into the plasma and red cells in the surrounding capillaries. In plasma, a small amount of CO_2

is physically dissolved or combined with amino groups of proteins to form carbamino compounds. However, most of the CO_2 freely diffuses into the red blood cells and catalysed by carbonic anhydrase, combines with H_2O to form H_2CO_3, that dissociates into H^+ and HCO_3^- (Fig. 17.1).

The dissociation of H_2CO_3 causes development of a concentration gradient due to the increase in HCO_3^- concentration; accordingly, biocarbonate ions diffuse from the red cells and diffuse into the plasma. To maintain electroneutrality (the same number of positively and negatively charged ions on each side of the red cell membrane), chloride diffuses into the cell. This is known as the *chloride shift* (also known as the Hamburger shift). The H^+ generated is buffered by binding with the recently deoxygenated hemoglobin molecules. This is why the abbreviation HHb is used to designate deoxygenated hemoglobin, because it has hydrogen bound instead of oxygen.

In the lungs, this process is reversed. Inspired O_2 diffuses from the alveoli into the blood and is bound to hemoglobin, forming oxyhemoglobin (O_2Hb). The H^+ that was carried on the (reduced) hemoglobin in the venous blood is released to recombine with HCO_3^- to form H_2CO_3, which dissociates into H_2O and CO_2. The CO_2 diffuses into the alveoli and is eliminated through ventilation. The net effect of these systems is a minimal change in H^+ concentration between the venous and arterial circulation. When the lungs do not remove CO_2 at the rate of its production, it accumulates in the blood, causing an increase in H^+ concentration. However, if CO_2 removal is faster than its production (hyperventilation), the H^+ concentration will be decreased. Therefore, the pH of the blood will increase. A change in the H^+ concentration of blood that results from nonrespiratory disturbances causes the respiratory center to respond by altering the rate of ventilation in an effort to restore the blood pH to normal. The lungs together with the buffer systems provide the first line of defense to change the acid–base status.

FIGURE 17.1 Interrelationship of the bicarbonate and hemoglobin buffering systems.

The kidneys regulate the excretion of both acid and base, making them an important player in the regulation of acid–base balance. Specifically, the kidney's main role is to reabsorb bicarbonate ion, HCO_3^-, from the glomerular filtrate in the proximal tubules (Fig. 17.2A). If bicarbonate ions were not reabsorbed and excreted in the urine, this would impact the bicarbonate–carbonic acid buffer system resulting causing a markedly increased levels of H^+ ions. Because the glomerular filtrate contains the same HCO_3^- concentration as plasma, passive reabsorption of HCO_3^- across the tubule membrane into the blood cannot occur. Instead, sodium (Na^+) in the glomerular filtrate is exchanged for H^+ in the tubular cell. The H^+ combines with HCO_3^- in the filtrate to form H_2CO_3, that is subsequently converted into H_2O and CO_2 by carbonic anhydrase. The CO_2 diffuses into the tubular cells and reacts with H_2O to reform H_2CO_3, which then largely disassociates into hydrogen and bicarbonate ions. The bicarbonate ion is reabsorbed into the blood along with sodium. The hydrogen ion provides a vehicle to reabsorb bicarbonate ion. In a healthy individual, virtually all of the filtered bicarbonate ion is reabsorbed.

During alkalosis, the kidney excretes HCO_3^- to compensate for the elevated blood pH. The exchange between H^+ and Na^+ suggests, in part, why clinicians order pH and blood gases together, along with electrolytes (Na^+, K^+, and Cl^-) to assess the acid–base status of a patient.

Under normal conditions, the body produces a net excess (50 to 100 mmol/L) of acid (H^+) each day that must be

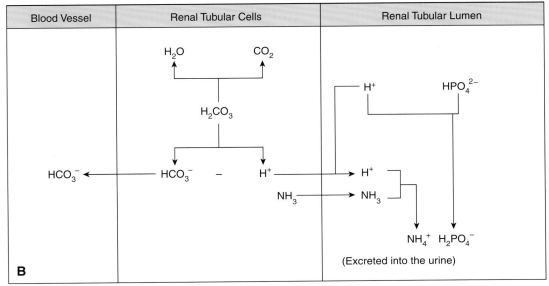

FIGURE 17.2 Bicarbonate reabsorption by the proximal tubule cell. C–A, carbonic anhydrase.

excreted by the kidney. The minimum urine pH that can be generated is 4.6, which limits the amount of free hydrogen ion excretion. The phosphate buffering system (Fig. 17.2B) allows for greater hydrogen ion excretion. Most of the H^+ ions in the glomerular filtrate combine with monohydrogen phosphate (HPO_4^{2-}) and ammonia (NH_3) and is excreted in the urine as dihydrogen phosphate ($H_2PO_4^-$) and ammonium ions (NH_4^+). Ammonia is produced by the deamination of glutamine and other amino acids. During acidosis ammonia production is increased to help buffer the excess hydrogen ions.

ASSESSMENT OF ACID–BASE HOMEOSTASIS

The Bicarbonate Buffering System

In assessing acid–base homeostasis, components of the bicarbonate buffering system are measured and calculated. Inferences can be made from these results about the systems produce, retain, and excrete the acids and bases. For the bicarbonate–carbonic acid buffer system, the dissolved CO_2 (dCO_2) is in equilibrium with CO_2 gas, which can be expelled by the lungs. Because the CO_2 can be removed, the bicarbonate buffering system is referred to as an *open* system, and the dCO_2, expelled by the lungs, is the *respiratory component*. The lungs participate rapidly in the regulation of blood pH through hypoventilation or hyperventilation. The kidneys, the nonrespiratory or also known as the metabolic component, control the bicarbonate concentration.

In plasma and at body temperature (37°C), the pK_a' of the bicarbonate–carbonic acid buffer system is 6.1. The concentration of H_2CO_3 is proportional to the partial pressure exerted by the dCO_2. In plasma at 37°C, the value for the combination of the solubility constant for pCO_2 and the factor to convert mm Hg to mmol/L is 0.0307 mmol/L/mm Hg. The solubility constant is dependent on temperature and the solvent. Both pH and pCO_2 are measured in blood gas analysis, and the pK_a' is a constant; therefore, HCO_3^- can be calculated:

$$pH = pK_a' + \log \frac{cHCO_3^-}{0.0307 \times pCO_2} \qquad \text{(Eq. 17-4)}$$

When the kidneys and lungs are functioning properly, the ratio of HCO_3^- to H_2CO_3 is 20:1, corresponding to a pH of 7.40. This can be calculated by substituting normal values (Table 17.1) for HCO_3^- and pCO_2 from the preceding equation:

$$\frac{24\,mmol/L}{(0.0307\,mmol/L-mm\,Hg) \times 40\,mm\,Hg}$$

$$= \frac{24}{1.2} = \frac{20}{1} \qquad \text{(Eq. 17-5)}$$

The normal pH of 7.4 can be derived by adding the log of 20 (1.3) to the pK_a' of the bicarbonate system ($7.40 = 6.1 + 1.3$).

TABLE 17.1	Arterial Blood Gas Reference Range at 37°C
pH	7.35–7.45
pCO_2 (mm Hg)	35–45
HCO_3^- (mmol/L)	22–29
Total CO_2 content (mmol/L)	23–27
pO_2 (mmol/L)	85–105
SO_2 (%)	>95
O_2Hb (%)	>95

The numerator (HCO_3^-) denotes the kidney function, whereas the denominator (pCO_2, which represents H_2CO_3) denotes the lung function. The lungs will impact pH through retention or elimination of CO_2 by changing the rate and volume of ventilation. The kidneys regulate pH by excreting acid, primarily in the ammonium ion, and by reclaiming HCO_3^- from the glomerular filtrate.

CASE STUDY 17.1

A 50-year-old man came to the emergency department after returning from foreign travel. His symptoms included persistent diarrhea over the past 3 days and rapid respirations (tachypnea). Blood sample for blood gas analysis was drawn with the following results:

pH	7.21
pCO_2	19 mm Hg
pO_2	96 mm Hg
HCO_3^-	7 mmol/L
SO_2	96% (calculated) (reference range, >95%)

Question

1. What is the patient's acid–base status?
2. Why is the HCO_3^- level low?
3. Why does the patient have rapid respirations?

Acid–Base Disorders: Acidosis and Alkalosis

Acid–base disorders result from imbalances in the acid base equilibrium. When blood pH is less than the reference range (7.35 to 7.45), it is termed **acidemia**. Similarly, a pH greater than the reference range is termed **alkalemia**. Acidemia will result if the hydrogen ion concentration increases through increased pCO_2 concentrations or decreases in the bicarbonate concentration. Alkalemia will result with hydrogen ion concentrations that are decreased, either from decreased pCO_2 or increased concentrations of bicarbonate. Technically, the suffix *-osis* refers to a process in the body; the suffix *-emia* refers to the corresponding state in blood (*-osis* is the cause of the *-emia*).

A disorder caused by ventilatory dysfunction (a change in the pCO_2, the respiratory component) is termed *primary respiratory acidosis* or *alkalosis*. A disorder resulting from a change in the bicarbonate level (a renal or metabolic function) is termed a *nonrespiratory or metabolic disorder*.

The response to maintain acid–base homeostasis is termed **compensation** and is accomplished by altering the factor not associated with the primary process. Mixed acid–base disorders arise from the presence of more than one process or compensatory mechanism in response to the primary disorder. For example, if the imbalance is of metabolic (nonrespiratory) origin, the body compensates by altering ventilation. Conversely, for disturbances of the respiratory component, the kidneys will compensate by selectively excreting or reabsorbing specific ions.

The lungs can immediately compensate by retaining or expelling carbon dioxide; however, this response is short term and often incomplete, whereas the kidneys are slower to respond (2 to 4 days), but the response is long term and sustained. *Fully compensated status* implies that the pH has returned to the normal range (the ratio of HCO_3^- to H_2CO_3 of 20:1 has been restored); *partially compensated* implies that the pH is approaching normal.

Acidosis may be caused by a primary metabolic or respiratory imbalance. In primary metabolic acidosis, the amount of acid exceeds the capacity of the buffer systems, and there is a decrease in bicarbonate to less than 24 mmol/L. The resulting decrease in pH is due to the decreased ratio of the metabolic to respiratory component in the Henderson-Hasselbalch equation:

$$pH \propto \frac{\downarrow cHCO_3^-}{N(0.0307 \times pCO_2)} < \frac{20}{1} \quad \text{(Eq. 17-6)}$$

where N is a normal value and $\propto$ indicates proportional.

The body compensates for metabolic acidosis through *hyperventilation*, which is an increase in the rate or depth of breathing. By expelling (i.e., "blowing off") CO_2, the base-to-acid ratio will normalize by reducing the pCO_2 and thereby elevating the pH. Secondary compensation occurs when the kidneys begin to correct the ratio by excreting hydrogen ions and reabsorbing bicarbonate ions.

Metabolic acidosis may be caused by the following reasons:

- Direct administration or ingestion of acid-producing substances (i.e., ammonium chloride, calcium chloride, salicylates, ethanol).
- Production of organic acids as seen with diabetic ketoacidosis (increased levels of acetoacetic acid and β-hydroxybutyric acid and lactic acid in lactic acidosis).
- Reduced excretion of acids as seen in renal tubular acidosis.
- Excessive loss of bicarbonate from diarrhea or drainage from a biliary, pancreatic, or intestinal fistula.

CASE STUDY 17.2

An 80-year-old woman fell on the ice and fractured her femur. After several hours, upon arrival to the emergency department, she was anxious, panting, and complaining of severe chest pain along with not being able to breathe. Her pulse was rapid (tachycardia) as was her respiration rate (tachypnea). A sample for blood gases was drawn and yielded the following results:

pH	7.31
pCO_2	27 mm Hg
pO_2	62 mm Hg
HCO_3^-	12 mmol/L
SO_2	78% (calculated) (reference range, >95%)

Question

1. What is the patient's acid–base status?
2. Why is the HCO_3^- level low?

Primary *respiratory acidosis* results from a decrease in alveolar ventilation (*hypoventilation*), causing a decreased elimination of CO_2 by the lungs:

$$pH \propto \frac{NcHCO_3^-}{\uparrow(0.0307 \times pCO_2)} < \frac{20}{1} \quad \text{(Eq. 17-7)}$$

Respiration is regulated in the medulla of the brain. Chemoreceptors present in the aortic arch and the carotid sinus respond to the levels of H^+ (pH), O_2, and CO_2 in the blood and cerebrospinal fluid.

Respiratory acidosis may be caused by the following reasons:

- Ineffective removal of CO_2 from the blood as seen in lung disease.
- Airway obstruction as seen in chronic obstructive pulmonary disease (COPD). Destructive changes in the airways and alveolar walls increase the size of the alveolar air spaces, resulting in a reduction of the lung surface area available for gas exchange. As a result, CO_2 is retained in the blood, causing chronic **hypercarbia** (elevated pCO_2).
- Drugs such as barbiturates, morphine, and alcohol will cause hypoventilation which subsequently increase blood pCO_2 levels.
- Decreased cardiac output, as observed with congestive heart failure, will result in less blood being presented to the lungs for gas exchange and, therefore, an elevated pCO_2.

In primary respiratory acidosis, the compensation occurs through metabolic processes. However, as previously mentioned, the metabolic processes, unlike the respiratory, require hours to days to affect the pH. Therefore, it takes days to weeks for full compensation to occur. The kidneys respond to respiratory acidosis by increasing the excretion of H^+ and reclamation of HCO_3^-. As a result of this, HCO_3^- in the blood increases causing the pH to return to normal.

As with acidosis, alkalosis can result from metabolic and respiratory causes. Primary *metabolic alkalosis* results from a gain in HCO_3^-, causing an increase in the pH:

$$pH \propto \frac{NcHCO_3^-}{\uparrow(0.0307 \times pCO_2)} > \frac{20}{1} \quad \text{(Eq. 17-8)}$$

Metabolic alkalosis maybe caused by the following reasons:

- Excess administration of sodium bicarbonate or through ingestion of bicarbonate-producing salts, such as sodium lactate, citrate, and acetate.
- Excessive loss of acid through vomiting, nasogastric suctioning, or prolonged use of diuretics that augment renal excretion of H^+ can produce an apparent increase in HCO_3^-.
- Hypokalemia and chloride deficit stimulate the reabsorption of HCO_3^- in the distal tubules.

The hydrogen ion sensors in the brain signal the respiratory center to depress respiration, which results in hypoventilation and increases the retention of CO_2 thereby increasing pCO_2 and lowering the pH. However, this response is erratic, and increases in pCO_2 is a stimulus itself to increase respiration. Ultimately, the primary cause of metabolic alkalosis needs to be corrected.

Primary *respiratory alkalosis* from an increased rate of alveolar ventilation causes excessive elimination of CO_2 by the lungs:

$$pH \propto \frac{NcHCO_3^-}{\downarrow(0.0307 \times pCO_2)} > \frac{20}{1} \quad \text{(Eq. 17-9)}$$

The causes of respiratory alkalosis include:

- Hypoxemia- and hysteria-induced hyperventilation.
- Chemical stimulation of the respiratory center by drugs, such as salicylates and nicotine that cause hyperventilation.
- Pulmonary emboli or pulmonary fibrosis in which pulmonary oxygen exchange is impaired.

The kidneys compensate by excreting HCO_3^- in the urine and reclaiming H^+ to the blood.

CASE STUDY 17.3

A 24-year-old graduate student was brought to the emergency department in a comatose state after being found unconscious in his room. A bottle of secobarbital (sedative) was found on his bed stand. He did not respond to painful stimuli, his respiration was barely perceptible, and his pulse was weak. A sample for blood gases was drawn and yielded the following results:

pH	7.10
pCO_2	70 mm Hg
pO_2	58 mm Hg
HCO_3^-	20 mmol/L
O_2Hb	80% (reference range, >95%)

Question

1. What is the patient's acid–base status?
2. What caused the profound hypoventilation?
3. Once the respiratory component returns to normal, what will be the patient's expected acid–base status?

CASE STUDY 17.4

A 24-year-old Himalayan man was accepted to graduate school in the United States. Before leaving home, he had an extensive physical exam that included various blood tests. When the medical staff at the US university reviewed his medical records, it was noted that all test results were normal except the HCO_3^-, which was 15 mmol/L (reference range, 22 to 26 mmol/L). The HCO_3^- was done separately on a serum sample. It was not part of a blood gas panel. To rule out nonrespiratory acidosis, the university physician wanted to check current status of the HCO_3^-. The value was 24 mmol/L.

Question

1. How would his blood gases results (pH, pCO_2, HCO_3^-) differ between home and the US?
2. Which direction does the oxygen dissociation curve shift at altitude?

OXYGEN AND GAS EXCHANGE

Oxygen and Carbon Dioxide

The role of oxygen in metabolism is crucial to life. In the mitochondria, electrons from the oxidation of NADH and $FADH_2$ are transferred through the electron transport chain to reduce molecular oxygen to water. pO_2 is measured to evaluate a patient's oxygen status and is typically measured along with pH and pCO_2 in routine blood gas analysis.

For adequate tissue oxygenation, the following seven conditions are necessary: (1) available atmospheric oxygen, (2) adequate ventilation, (3) gas exchange between the lungs and arterial blood, (4) binding of O_2 onto hemoglobin, (5) adequate hemoglobin, (6) adequate blood flow to tissues, and (7) release of O_2 to the tissue. Any disturbances in these conditions can result in hypoxia, poor tissue oxygenation.

The amount of O_2 available in atmospheric air depends on the barometric pressure (BP) and altitude. At sea level, the BP is 760 mm Hg. (In the International System of Units, 1 mm Hg = 0.133 kPa, where 1 Pa = 1 N/m^2.) Dalton's law states that total atmospheric pressure is the sum of the partial pressures of each of the gases in the atmosphere. One atmosphere exerts 760 mm Hg of pressure and is made up of O_2 (20.93%), CO_2 (0.03%), nitrogen (78.1%), and inert gases (~1%). The percentage for each gas is the same at all altitudes; the *partial pressure* for each gas in the atmosphere is equal to the BP at a particular altitude times the appropriate percentage for each gas. The vapor pressure of water (47 mm Hg) at 37°C must be accounted for in calculating the partial pressure for the individual gases (Fig. 17.3). In the body, these gases are always fully saturated with water. For example:

$$\text{Partial pressure of } O_2 \text{ at sea level (in the body)}$$
$$= (760 \text{ mm Hg} - 47 \text{ mm Hg}) \times 20.93\%$$
$$= 149 \text{ mm Hg (at 37°C)}$$

$$\text{Partial pressure of } CO_2 \text{ at sea level (in the body)}$$
$$= (760 \text{ mm Hg} - 47 \text{ mm Hg}) \times 0.03\%$$
$$= 2 \text{ mm Hg (at 37°C)}$$

Air is moved into the lungs through expansion of the thoracic cavity, which creates a temporary negative pressure gradient, causing air to move into the numer-

ous tracheal branches that terminate at the alveoli. Gas exchange between alveolar air and pulmonary blood occurs in the alveoli. At the beginning of inspiration, these airways are still filled with air (gas) retained from the previously expired breath. This air, termed *dead space air*, dilutes the air being inspired. The inspired air is warmed to 37°C and becomes saturated with water vapor and mixes with air in the alveoli. The resulting pO_2 in the alveoli averages about 110 mm Hg instead of the anticipated 149 mm Hg. There are many factors that can influence the amount of O_2 that moves to the alveoli, and some of the factors are as follows:

- *Destruction of the alveoli.* The normal surface area of the alveoli is as big as a tennis court. Diminished surface area in diseases such as emphysema will cause an inadequate amount of O_2 to move into the blood.
- *Pulmonary edema.* Gas diffuses from the alveoli into the capillary through a small space. With pulmonary edema, fluid "leaks" into this space and inhibits diffusion of gases.
- *Airway blockage.* In patients with asthma or bronchitis, airways are blocked, which prevents air from the atmosphere from reaching the alveoli.

There are factors that can influence the amount of O_2 to the tissue, and some common causes of inadequate perfusion are as follows:

- *Inadequate blood supply.* When the blood supply to the lung is inadequate, O_2 enters the blood in the lungs, but not enough blood is being carried away to the tissue where it is needed. This may be the consequence of a blockage in a pulmonary blood vessel (pulmonary embolism), pulmonary hypertension, or heart failure.
- *Diffusion of CO_2 and O_2.* O_2 diffuses 20 times slower than CO_2, it is more sensitive to problems with diffusion. In instances such as pulmonary edema, hypoxemia will develop but with minimal alteration to pCO_2. This type of hypoxemia is generally treated with supplemental O_2. The percentage of O_2 can be increased temporarily when needed; however, 60% or higher O_2 concentrations must be used with caution because it can be toxic to the lungs.
- *Intrapulmonary shunting.* Nonfunctional alveoli prohibits venous blood from being oxygenated that results in decreased oxygen content.
- Anemia. Blood with less hemoblogin will carry proportionally less oxygen.

Oxygen Transport

Most O_2 in arterial blood is transported to the tissue by hemoglobin. In the adult, hemoglobin (A_1) molecule can combine reversibly with four molecules of O_2. The actual amount of O_2 loaded onto hemoglobin depends on the availability of O_2; concentration and type(s) of hemoglobin present; presence of competing molecules, such as carbon monoxide (CO); pH; temperature of the blood; and levels of pCO_2 and 2,3-diphosphoglycerate (2,3-DPG). With adequate atmospheric and alveolar O_2 available and normal

FIGURE 17.3 Gas content in lungs and pulmonary and systemic circulation.

diffusion of O_2 to the arterial blood, more than 95% of "functional" hemoglobin (hemoglobin capable of *reversibly* binding O_2) will bind O_2. The percentage of O_2 in inspired air, or fraction of inspired oxygen (**FiO_2**), can be increased by breathing gas mixtures up to 100% O_2. Increasing FiO_2 further saturates hemoglobin. However, once the hemoglobin is 100% saturated, an increase in O_2 to the alveoli serves only to increase the concentration of dO_2 in the arterial blood. Prolonged administration of high concentrations of O_2 may cause oxygen toxicity and, in some cases, decreased ventilation that leads to hypercarbia.

Hemoglobin exists in one of four conditions:

1. O_2Hb is the erythrocyte hemoglobin. Ferrous iron (Fe^{2+}) in the heme group reversibly binds to O_2.
2. Deoxyhemoglobin (HHb), also known as reduced hemoglobin, is hemoglobin not bound to O_2 but capable of forming a bond when O_2 is available. Notably, hemoglobin increases its affinity to hydrogen ions as it loses O_2.
3. Carboxyhemoglobin (COHb) is hemoglobin bound to carbon monoxide (CO) and is not available for O_2 transport. This is because the bond between CO and Hb is 200 times stronger than the bond between O_2 and Hb.
4. Methemoglobin (MetHb) is hemoglobin unable to bind O_2 because iron (Fe) is in an oxidized (Fe^{3+}) rather than reduced state. The Fe^{3+} can be reduced by the enzyme methemoglobin reductase, which is found in red blood cells.

Dedicated spectrophotometers (CO-oximeters), discussed later in this chapter, are used to determine the relative concentrations (relative to total hemoglobin) of these hemoglobin species.

Assessment of a Patient's Oxygen Status

Four parameters are commonly used to assess a patient's oxygen status:

1. Oxygen saturation (SO_2);
2. Fractional (percent) oxyhemoglobin (FO_2Hb)
3. Trends in oxygen saturation assessed by transcutaneous (TC) and pulse oximetry (SpO_2)
4. Amount of O_2 dissolved in plasma (pO_2).

Oxygen saturation, SO_2, represents the percentage of the functional hemoglobin that is saturated with O_2 compared with the total amount of hemoglobin capable of binding O_2[1]:

$$SO_2 = \frac{cO_2Hb}{(cO_2Hb + cHHb)} \times 100 \quad \text{(Eq. 17-10)}$$

SO_2 is frequently measured by pulse oximetry (discussed later). These calculated results, however, can differ significantly from those determined by direct CO-oximeter measurement due to the assumption that normal, healthy subjects have fully functional hemoglobin and the oxyhemoglobin dissociation curve has a specific shape and location. These algorithms do not account for the presence

of other hemoglobin species, such as COHb and MetHb, that are incapable of reversibly binding O_2. These shortcomings can generate erroneous results; therefore, SO_2 should not be used to assess oxygenation status.[1,2]

Fractional (or percent) oxyhemoglobin (FO_2Hb) is calculated from the ratio of the concentration of oxyhemoglobin to the concentration of total hemoglobin ($ctHb$):

$$FO_2Hb = \frac{cO_2Hb}{ctHb} = \frac{cO_2Hb}{cO_2Hb + cHHb + cdysHb} \quad \text{(Eq. 17-11)}$$

where the $cdysHb$ represents hemoglobin derivatives, such as COHb and MetHb, that cannot reversibly bind with O_2 but still contribute to the "total" hemoglobin measurement.

These two terms, SO_2 and FO_2Hb, can be confused easily since in most healthy individuals (and even those individuals with some disease states), the numeric values for SO_2 to FO_2Hb. However, in the presence of dyshemoglobins, the values for FO_2Hb and SO_2 will deviate. They will also deviate when the patient is a smoker since CO preferentially binds to hemoglobin as opposed to O_2.

Partial pressure of oxygen dissolved in plasma (pO_2) accounts for little of the body's O_2 stores. A healthy adult breathing room air will have a pO_2 of 90 to 95 mm Hg. In an adult with a blood volume of 5 L, only 13.5 mL of O_2 will be available as dissolved oxygen (pO_2) in plasma, compared with more than 1,000 mL of O_2 carried as O_2Hb.

Noninvasive measurements for following trends in oxygenation status can be attained with *pulse oximetry* (SpO_2). These devices pass light of two or more wavelengths through the tissue in the capillary bed of the toe, finger, or earlobes. Pulse oximeters that calculate oxyhemoglobin saturation based only on oxyhemoglobin and deoxyhemoglobin will overestimate the oxyhemoglobin saturation in the presence of dyshemoglobins. In addition, the accuracy of pulse oximetry can be compromised by many factors, including poor perfusion and severe anemia. Recent technological advances in pulse oximetry have allowed for measurement of COHb and MetHb.

The maximum amount of O_2 that can be carried by hemoglobin in a given quantity of blood is the *hemoglobin oxygen (binding) capacity*. The molecular weight of tetramer hemoglobin is 64,458 g/mol. One mole of a perfect gas occupies 22,414 mL. Therefore, each gram of hemoglobin carries 1.39 mL of O_2:

$$\frac{22,414 \, mL/mol_4}{64,458 \, g/mol} = 1.39 \, mL/g \quad \text{(Eq. 17-12)}$$

When the total hemoglobin (tHb) is 15 g/dL, and the hemoglobin is 100% saturated with O_2, the O_2 capacity is

$$15 g/100 mL \times 1.39 mL/g = 20.8 mL \, O_2/100 mL \text{ of blood} \quad \text{(Eq. 17-13)}$$

Oxygen content is the total O_2 in blood and determined from the sum of the O_2 bound to hemoglobin (O_2Hb) and the amount dissolved in the plasma (pO_2). Normally, 97% to 99% of the available hemoglobin is saturated with O_2. Assuming a tHb of 15 g/dL, the O_2 content for every 100 mL of blood plasma becomes 20.5 mL.

$$0.3 mL + (20.8 mL \times 0.97) = 20.5 mL \quad \text{(Eq. 17-14)}$$

pO_2 and pCO_2 are only indices of gas exchange efficiency in the lungs, they do not reveal the *content* of either gas in the blood. For every 1 mm Hg pO_2, 0.00314 mL of O_2 will be dissolved in 100 mL of plasma at 37°C. For example, if the pO_2 is 100 mm Hg, 0.3 mL of O_2 will be dissolved in every 100 mL of blood plasma. The amount of dissolved O_2 is usually not clinically significant. However, it is of clinical significance when a patient is put in hyperbaric chamber to assess if hemoglobin delivery is impaired. This is accomplished by increasing the pressure of inspired air to force more O_2 in solution and changes can be subsequently evaluated.

Hemoglobin–Oxygen Dissociation

While adequate ventilation and gas exchange with the pulmonary circulation are important for tissue oxygenation, hemoglobin must also be able to release oxygen to prevent hypoxia. Hemoglobin has four heme molecules that transport and release oxygen to the tissues and subsequently transport H^+ and CO_2 from the tissue to the lungs. Increases in pO_2 will saturate hemoglobin with oxygen, whereas increased H^+ concentration and pCO_2 levels in the tissue change the molecular configuration of O_2Hb, facilitating O_2 release.

Oxygen dissociates from adult hemoglobin (A_1) in a characteristic sigmoidal fashion. This relationship is graphed (Fig. 17.4) with pO_2 on the *x*-axis and percent SO_2 on the *y*-axis. Once one oxygen molecule is bound, it becomes easier

for additional oxygen molecules to bind. A significant decrease in pO_2 can occur before changing the affinity of hemoglobin to oxygen, and this equates to approximately around 60 mm Hg. However, below this threshold, oxygen will readily be released. The position of the oxygen dissociation curve reflects the *affinity* of hemoglobin to O_2 that reflects rate of this dissociation.

The affinity of hemoglobin for O_2 depends on hydrogen ion activity (pH), pCO_2 and CO levels, body temperature, and 2,3-diphosphoglycerate (2,3-DPG) concentration. Changes in these variables will affect the affinity of hemoglobin for O_2 and therefore the position and shape of the oxygen dissociation curve. In actively metabolizing tissue, the conditions in the microenvironment promote the release of oxygen. Oxidative metabolism increases the temperature, H^+, CO_2, and 2,3-DPG concentrations, which results in a right shift of the dissociation curve. This decreased affinity of hemoglobin to O_2 facilitates oxygen uptake for the tissue. In the lungs, temperature, H^+, pCO_2, and 2,3-DPG decrease relative to tissue levels, shifting the oxygen dissociation curve slightly to the left. This enhances O_2 binding to hemoglobin and improve O_2 uptake.

The metabolic by-product, 2,3-DPG, is also involved in two seemingly unrelated adaptations to potentially hypoxic conditions. When the β-chains of the hemoglobin molecule bind 2,3-DPG, oxyhemoglobin dissociation curve shifts to the right, this results in release of oxygen for oxygen uptake by the tissue. Anemic patients have elevated levels of 2,3-DPG as a compensatory mechanism. In addition, as an adaptation mechanism, 2,3-DPG levels increase at high altitudes that results in the release of oxygen from hemoglobin. Dyshemoglobins, such as COHb or MetHb, can also affect the hemoglobin–oxygen dissociation curve. An elevation in CO from cigarette smoking causes the curve to shift to the left. As a consequence, increased affinity to hemoglobin makes release of O_2 inefficient. The preceding discussion refers to normal adult (A_1) hemoglobin. In newborns or patients with hemoglobinopathies, the pattern of dissociation differs. For example, fetal hemoglobin, a form of hemoglobin present while intrauterine and in the first few months of life, has a stronger affinity to oxygen compared to adult hemoglobin. Therefore, the fetal dissociation curve will be shifted to the left.

In summary, the unique structure of hemoglobin allows it to act as both an acid–base buffer and O_2 buffer. As hemoglobin moves through the body, exposure to the various microenvironments promotes association and dissociation of O_2, CO_2, and H^+. In tissue, exposure to elevated CO_2 and H^+ results in enhanced O_2 release (oxygen buffering). This release of oxygen from hemoglobin accelerates the uptake of CO_2 and H^+ by hemoglobin (acid–base buffering). In the lungs, the microenvironment promotes uptake of O_2 and release of CO_2.

MEASUREMENT

Spectrophotometric Determination of Oxygen Saturation (CO-Oximetry)

The *actual percent oxyhemoglobin* (O_2Hb) can be determined spectrophotometrically using a CO-oximeter designed to directly measure the various hemoglobin

FIGURE 17.4 Oxygen dissociation curves. *Curve B* is the normal human curve. *Curves A* and *C* are from blood with increased affinity and decreased affinity, respectively. 2,3-DPG, 2,3-diphosphoglycerate.

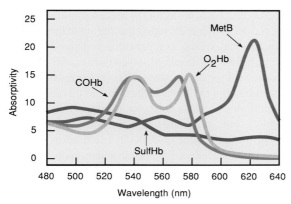

FIGURE 17.5 Optical absorption of hemoglobin fractions. (Reproduced from Clin Chem News 1990 [January], with permission.)

species. Each species of hemoglobin has a characteristic absorbance curve (Fig. 17.5). The number of hemoglobin species measured will depend on the number and specific wavelengths incorporated into the instrumentation. For example, two-wavelength instrument systems can measure only two hemoglobin species (i.e., O_2Hb and HHb), which are expressed as a fraction or percentage of the total hemoglobin.

At a minimum, instruments should have four wavelengths for measurements of HHb, O_2Hb, and the two most common dyshemoglobins, COHb and MetHb. Instruments with more than four wavelengths can recognize dyes and pigments, turbidity, other hemoglobin species, and abnormal proteins. Some CO-oximeters employ hundreds of wavelengths, which has reduced measurement interferences. Microprocessors control the sequencing of multiple wavelengths of light through the sample and apply the necessary matrix equations after absorbance readings are made to calculate the percentage of the individual hemoglobin species:

$$\begin{aligned} O_2HB &= a_1A_1 + a_2A_2 + \ldots + a_nA_n \\ HHb &= b_1A_1 + \ldots + b_nA_n \\ COHB &= c_1A_1 + c_2A_2 + \ldots + c_nA_n \\ MetHb &= d_1A_1 + d_2A_2 + d_nA_n \end{aligned} \quad \text{(Eq. 17-15)}$$

where a_1, a_n, b_n, etc., are coefficients that are analogues of the absorption constant (a) that are derived from established methods and A_1, A_2, and so on are the absorbances of the sample. The matrix equations will change depending on the number of wavelengths of light (which is manufacturer specific) passed through the sample.

The results from these instruments should not be confused with a calculated SO_2 from a blood gas analyzer, which *estimates* the SO_2 value from a measured pO_2 and an empirical equation based on the oxygen–hemoglobin dissociation curve. Only measured O_2Hb values reflect the patient's true status because calculated SO_2 and O_2Hb

values will be different in the presence of dyshemoglobins. For example, in CO poisoning, SO_2 will likely be normal with a significantly decreased O_2Hb level.

As with any spectrophotometric measurement, potential sources of error exist, including faulty calibration of the instrument and spectral-interfering substances. The presence of any substances absorbing light at the same wavelengths used in the measurement is a potential source of error. Product claims for specific instruments must be consulted for specific interferences.

The primary purpose of determining O_2Hb is to assess oxygen transport from the lungs. So before blood sample collection, it is best to stabilize the patient's ventilation status. An appropriate waiting period before the sample is drawn should follow changes in supplemental O_2 or mechanical ventilation. All blood samples should be collected under anaerobic conditions and mixed immediately with heparin or other appropriate anticoagulant. All samples should be analyzed promptly to avoid changes in saturation resulting from the consumption of oxygen by metabolizing cells.

Blood Gas Analyzers: pH, *p*CO₂, and *p*O₂

Blood gas analyzers use *electrodes* (macroelectrochemical or microelectrochemical sensors) as sensing devices to measure pO_2, pCO_2, and pH. The pO_2 measurement is amperometric, the reduction of oxygen produces a current that is proportional to the amount of oxygen present in the sample, whereas the pCO_2 and pH measurements are potentiometric, in which a change in voltage indicates the activity of each analyte. Advances in microsensor technology have greatly expanded the analytic menu of whole blood analyzers. In addition to pH and blood gas measurements, many manufacturers include hemoglobin and/or hematocrit, sodium, potassium, chloride, metabolites such as glucose, lactate, creatinine, and blood urea nitrogen, and CO-oximetry with their instrumentation. The blood gas analyzer can also calculate several additional parameters: bicarbonate, total CO_2, base excess, and SO_2.

Measurement of *p*O₂

The pO_2 electrode is an amperometric electrode, often referred to as a Clarke electrode. An oxygen permeable membrane covers the tip of the electrode to selectively allow O_2 to diffuse into the electrolyte solution. A small, constant polarizing potential (approximately –0.65 V) is applied between the anode and cathode. As a result, the electrons are drawn from the anode to the cathode. The oxygen diffuses from the sample to the cathode, where it is subsequently reduced. The current produced in this circuit is proportional to the amount of O_2 reduced at the cathode. A *microammeter* placed in the circuit between the anode and cathode measures the movement of electrons (current). The semipermeable membrane will also allow other gases to pass, such as CO_2 and N_2, but these gases will not be reduced at the cathode if the polarizing voltage is tightly controlled.

CASE STUDY 17.5

A 37-year-old man was admitted to the emergency department. He presented with the following symptoms: shortness of breath, dizzy, flushed (hyperemic), sweating (diaphoretic), and nauseous. Shortly after being admitted, blood gases were drawn:

pH	7.48
pCO_2	32 mm Hg
pO_2	96 mm Hg
HCO_3^-	24 mmol/L
SO_2	98% (calculated)
SpO_2	99% (pulse oximetry oxygen saturation)

After a few hours, the patient's symptoms diminished, and he was released from the hospital. Two weeks later, he was admitted again to the emergency department with the same symptoms. This time, arterial blood was drawn for both blood gases and CO-oximetry measurements. The results were as follows:

pH	7.49
pCO_2	33 mm Hg
pO_2	95 mm Hg
HCO_3^-	23 mmol/L
SO_2	98% (calculated) (reference range, >95%)
SpO_2	99% (pulse oximetry oxygen saturation) (reference range, >95%)

Spectrophotometric (CO-oximeter) measurement of hemoglobin species:

Hb	13.5 g/L
O_2Hb	73% (reference range, >95%)
COHb	22% (reference range, <2%; higher with smokers)
MetHb	1% (reference range, <1.5%)

Question

1. Is the patient hypoxic on the first admission to the ED?
2. Considering the new laboratory data, is this patient hypoxic on the second admission to the ED?
3. Why is there discrepancy between calculated SO_2, SpO_2, and O_2Hb?

The primary source of error for pO_2 measurement is associated with the buildup of protein material on the surface of the membrane. This buildup attenuates oxygen diffusion and slows the electrode response.

It is of utmost importance to not to expose the sample to room air when collecting, transporting, and making O_2 measurements. Contamination of the sample with room air ($pO_2 > 150$ mm Hg) can result in significant error because leukocytes continue to metabolize O_2. Additionally, when the white blood cell count is elevated markedly, low pO_2 values may be observed if not analyzed immediately after the blood draw.

CASE STUDY 17.6

A 48-year-old man with diabetes with a history of alcohol abuse was admitted to the emergency department. He had an elevated heart rate (tachycardia) and was experiencing extreme shortness of breath. Blood was drawn for glucose and blood gases and urine collected for the assessment of ketones:

Glucose	570 mg/dL
Urinary ketones	Large (reference range, negative)
pH	7.00
pCO_2	48 mm Hg
pO_2	68 mm Hg
HCO_3^-	12 mmol/L
SO_2	81% (calculated)
tHb	10 g/dL

Question

1. Is the patient's acidemia a result of respiratory or metabolic disturbances or a combination of both?
2. If the patient was not having respiratory problems, how would you classify the acid–base disturbance?
3. What is the significance of the urinary ketones that result in terms of identifying the type of diabetes?

Measurement of pH and pCO_2

To measure pH, a glass membrane sensitive to H^+ is placed around an internal Ag–AgCl electrode to form a measuring electrode. Potential develops at the glass membrane as a result of H^+ diffusion from the unknown solution into the membrane's surface. Hydrogen ions are proportional to the difference in cH^+ between the unknown sample and the buffer solution inside the electrode. The developed potential at the glass membrane is measured by placing a reference electrode in the solution and both electrodes must be connected to a pH (volt) meter. The indicator voltage is compared to the reference electrode that (commonly either a calomel [Hg–HgCl] or an Ag–AgCl half-cell) provides a steady reference voltage. The pH meter reflects the potential difference between the two electrodes. For the cell described, the Nernst equation predicts that a change of +59.16 mV, at 25°C, results in a 10-fold increase in H^+ activity, equivalent to a decrease of one pH unit (e.g., pH 7.0 to 6.0). However, this response is temperature specific. For example, at 37°C, a change of one pH unit elicits a 61.5 mV change.

pCO_2 method is based on the pH electrode. It has an outer semipermeable membrane that allows CO_2 to diffuse and dissolve into an internal layer of electrolyte, usually a bicarbonate buffer. The CO_2 that diffuses across the membrane reacts with the buffer, forming *carbonic acid*. Carbonic acid then dissociates into bicarbonate and hydrogen ions. The change in H^+ activity is measured by the pH electrode and is related to the amount of CO_2 present in the sample.

As with any electrode, the buildup of protein material on the membrane will affect diffusion and cause errors. pCO_2 electrodes are slower to respond because of the chemical reaction that must be completed. As previously mentioned, electrodes are also sensitive to temperatures and barometric pressure. Other sources of error include erroneous calibration caused by incorrect or contaminated calibration materials.

Types of Electrochemical Sensors

Macroelectrode sensors have been used in blood gas instruments since the beginning of the clinical measurement of blood gases. These have been modified over time in an effort to simplify their use and minimize the required sample volume and maintenance. *Microelectrodes* basically are miniaturized macroelectrodes. Miniaturization became possible with better manufacturing capabilities and with the development of the sophisticated electronics required to handle minute changes in signal.

Thick and thin film technology is a further modification of electrochemical sensors. Although the measurement principle is identical, the sensors are reduced to tiny wires embedded in a printed circuit card. The special card has etched grooves to separate components. A special paste material containing the required components (similar in function to the electrolytes of macroelectrodes) is spread over the sensors. To reduce the required sample volume, several sensors can be placed on a single small card. These sensors are disposable and less expensive to manufacture, which reduces maintenance.

Optical Sensors

Optical sensors is another form of technology that is utilized for blood gas measurements. Optical sensors (optodes) measure fluorescence or phosphorescence of organic dyes with O_2, CO_2, and H^+. The dye is separated from the sample by a membrane, as with electrodes, and the analyte diffuses into the dye, causing either an increase in or a quenching of fluorescence proportional to the amount of analyte. Calibration is used to establish the relationship between concentration and fluorescence. Normally, a single calibration will suffice for long periods because this technology is not subject to the drifts seen in electrochemical technology.

Optical technology has been applied to indwelling blood gas systems.[3] Fiberoptic bundles carry light to sensors positioned at the tip of catheters, and other bundles carry light back, allowing changes in fluorescence to be measured in a catheter within the patient's arterial system. The commercial development of indwelling systems has been limited by the increased probability of thrombogenesis and protein buildup on the membrane, separating the sample from the fluorescing dyes. This buildup impedes free sample diffusion into the measuring chamber.

Calibration

Calibration of a blood gas analyzer will vary among manufacturers. Normally, two different gas mixtures with known pCO_2 and pO_2 levels are used. One of the mixtures is used to calibrate the lower end, and the composition of this mixture is 0% O_2 and 5% CO_2, whereas the second mixture is used to calibrate the gases on the upper end, and the composition of the mixture is 20% O_2 and 10% CO_2.

Most blood gas instruments will calibrate automatically at specified time intervals since electrodes are drifted over time. Most electrodes will require calibration every 30 to 60 minutes. Instruments are programmed to prompt the operator if the values deviate from the expected value. For example, if the value(s) obtained during calibration exceed(s) a programmed tolerance limit, flagging of a *drift* error will occur at the time of calibration, and corrective action will need to be taken before patient samples can be analyzed.

The pH electrode is calibrated against two primary traceable buffer solutions traceable to standards that meet specifications set by the National Institute of Standards and Technology (NIST). Typically, there are two calibrators, a low and high calibrators, with pH values of 6.8 and 7.38, respectively. The calibrators must be stored at the stated temperature and not exposed to room air since pH changes with the absorption of CO_2.

pH and blood gas measurements are extremely sensitive to temperature. It is critical that the electrode sample chamber be maintained at constant temperature for all measurements. All blood gas analyzers have electrode chambers thermostatically controlled to 37°C ± 0.1°C as small temperature variations can drastically change the pH and blood gas values. Accordingly, the Nernst equation is temperature specific; if the temperature of the measurement system changes, the output (voltage) will change. The solubility of gases in a liquid medium also depends on the temperature; as the temperature goes down, the solubility of the gas increases.

CASE STUDY 17.7

A 64-year-old woman with COPD was admitted to the emergency department with extreme shortness of breath. She had a bluish color that was particularly pronounced on her lips and nail beds and she displayed a weak and persistent cough with diminished but rattling breath sounds. Home medications included bronchodilators, steroids, Lasix (a loop diuretic that does not conserve plasma potassium), and digitalis. Vital signs: heart rate, 148 bpm; blood pressure, 100/88 mm Hg; temperature, 37°C; and respiratory rate, 38/min. Initial blood gas results on room air were the following:

pH	7.289
pCO_2	91 mm Hg
pO_2	53 mm Hg
HCO_3^-	43 mmol/L

Questions

1. What is the patient's acid–base status?
2. Would the pH be normal if the patient was able to decrease her pCO_2 to 50 mm Hg?

Correction for Temperature

Values for pH, pCO_2, and pO_2 are temperature dependent. By convention, these aforementioned measurements are made at 37°C. But what happens when a patient's body temperature differs from 37°C, should the blood gas values be 'corrected' to the actual temperature of the patient? The blood gas instrument software can easily perform these corrections. However, the data are difficult to interpret because appropriate reference ranges *for the patient's temperature* must be used, but these are not available. When temperature-corrected results are reported, it is critical that results also be reported with the 37°C (noncorrected) results.

Calculated Parameters

Several acid–base parameters can be calculated from measured pH and pCO_2 values. Manufacturers of blood gas instruments include algorithms to perform these calculations. No calculated parameter is universally used; many physicians have preferred parameters for identifying various pathologies.

HCO_3^- measurement is based on the Henderson-Hasselbalch equation. This can be calculated when pH and pCO_2 are known. The Henderson-Hasselbach equation makes the assumption that the pK_a of the bicarbonate buffer system in plasma at 37°C is 6.1.

Carbonic acid (H_2CO_3) concentration can be calculated using the solubility coefficient of CO_2 in plasma at 37°C. The solubility constant to convert pCO_2 to mmol/L of H_2CO_3 is 0.0307. If the temperature or the composition of plasma changes (e.g., an increase in lipids, in which gases are more soluble), the constant will also change.

Total carbon dioxide content ($ctCO_2$) is the bicarbonate plus the dCO_2 (carbonic acid) plus the associated CO_2 with proteins (carbamates). A blood gas analyzer approximates $ctCO_2$ by adding the bicarbonate and carbonic acid values ($ctCO_2 = cHCO_3^- + [0.0307\ pCO_2]$).

Some clinicians use **base excess** to assess the metabolic component. Base excess is calculated from an algorithm that uses the patient's pH, pCO_2, and hemoglobin. A positive base excess value indicates an excess of bicarbonate or relative deficit of noncarbonic acid and suggests *metabolic alkalosis*, whereas a negative value (base deficit) indicates a deficit of bicarbonate or relative excess of noncarbonic acids and suggests *metabolic acidosis*. Because the indicated nonrespiratory alkalosis or acidosis may be a result of primary disturbances or compensatory mechanisms, base excess values should not be used alone in assessing a patient's acid–base status.

QUALITY ASSURANCE

Preanalytic Considerations

Blood gas measurements, like all laboratory measurements, are subject to preanalytic, analytic, and postanalytic errors. Blood gas measurements are particularly affected by **preanalytic errors**—those introduced during sample collection and transportation of samples before analysis.[1,4]

The quality assurance cycle is shown in Figure 17.6. The steps included in the analytic phase are under the direct control of the laboratory. Notably, most of the quality assurance cycle lies outside the laboratory; therefore, the laboratorian must take an active role in educating *all* individuals involved to ensure quality. The preanalytic considerations start with proper patient identification, which is absolutely essential before any blood specimen is collected. Once collected, the specimen must be correctly labeled with accurate information.

Only trained personnel who have the knowledge about possible sources of error and the experience with the blood drawing equipment and technique should draw samples for blood gas analyses. Because arterial blood collection may be painful and results in patient hyperventilation, which lowers the pCO_2 and increases the pH, the ability to reassure the patient is essential. The choice of site—radial, brachial, femoral, or temporal artery—depends on the predominant patient population (e.g., pediatric patients, burn patients, and outpatients) within an institution. The Clinical and Laboratory Standards Institute (CLSI) publication *Procedures for the Collection of Arterial Blood Specimens* is an excellent reference.[4]

Although arterial samples for pH and blood gas studies are recommended, peripheral venous samples can be

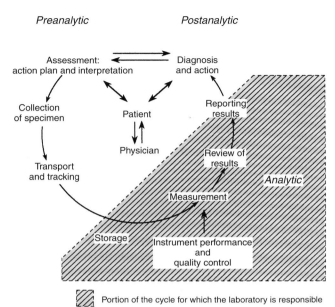

Blood Gas Analysis Quality
Assurance Cycle

Preanalytic   *Postanalytic*

Portion of the cycle for which the laboratory is responsible

FIGURE 17.6 Blood gas analysis quality assurance cycle. (Courtesy of Robert F. Moran.)

O_2) and body temperature—at the time of sample collection must also be documented.

In most instances, the ideal collection device for arterial blood sampling is a 1- to 3-mL self-filling, plastic, disposable syringe, containing the appropriate type and amount of anticoagulant. Evacuated collection tubes are not appropriate for blood gases. While both dry (lyophilized) and liquid lithium heparin are acceptable anticoagulants, the liquid form is not recommended because liquid heparin can dilute the sample and possibly alter the sample due to equilibration with room air.[1,4] Once drawn, the blood in the syringe must be mixed thoroughly with the heparin to prevent microclots from forming. Adequate mixing is also important immediately before analysis to resuspend the settled cells. Although sodium and lithium salts of heparin are recommended for pH and blood gas analysis, other forms are available: ammonium, zinc, electrolyte balanced, and calcium titrated. Selection of the proper type of heparin is particularly important with instruments combining blood gas, electrolyte, and metabolite measurements. It is important to consult the manufacturer's product insert.

used if pulmonary function or O_2 transport is not being assessed. For venous samples, the source of the specimen must be clearly identified and the appropriate (venous) reference ranges included with the results for data interpretation. Depending on the patient, capillary blood may need to be collected to assess pH and pCO_2. The correlation with arterial blood is good for pH and pCO_2. However, capillary pO_2 values do not correlate well with arterial pO_2 values as a result of exposure to room air. Central venous (pulmonary artery) blood samples are obtained to assess O_2 consumption, which is calculated from the O_2 content of arterial and pulmonary artery blood and the cardiac output. For sample collection from an indwelling arterial line, an appropriate blood volume must initially be withdrawn and discarded from the line to assure that the actual collected sample contains only arterial blood. Proper flushing procedure minimizes the chance of specimen contamination with solutions (i.e., liquid heparin, medication, or electrolyte fluids) that may be in the line.[1]

Sources of error in the collection and handling of blood gas specimens include the following:

• Collection device
• Form and concentration of heparin used for anticoagulation
• Speed of syringe filling
• Maintenance of the anaerobic environment
• Mixing of the sample to ensure dissolution and distribution of the heparin and transport and storage time before analysis

For proper interpretation of blood gas results, the patient's status—ventilation (on room air or supplemental

CASE STUDY 17.8

A 23-year-old woman with a history of asthma was brought to the emergency department by ambulance. She was extremely short of breath. Her level of consciousness was diminished greatly, and she was only able to respond to questions with nods or one-word responses. She had a weak cough, with nearly inaudible breath sounds. After drawing blood gases, she was placed on supplemental oxygen. Vital signs: heart rate, 160 bpm; blood pressure, 120/84 mm Hg; temperature, 37°C; and respiratory rate, 36/min. Her initial blood gas and total hemoglobin results were as follows:

pH	7.330
pCO_2	25 mm Hg
pO_2	58 mm Hg
HCO_3^-	13 mmol/L
tHb	12.4 g/L

Questions

1. What is the patient's acid–base and oxygenation status?
2. What is the cause of the acid–base disturbance?
3. Estimate how long it may take for the patient to partially and then fully compensate for the acid–base dysregulation

Slow filling of the syringe may be caused by a mismatch of syringe and needle sizes. While a too small of a needle reduces patient's pain and therefore the likelihood of arteriospasm and hematoma, it may produce bubbles that affect pCO_2 and pO_2 measurement. It may also cause hemolysis of the blood, which significantly alters potassium levels, an electrolyte frequently ordered along with pH and blood gases. Maintenance of an anaerobic environment is critical to correct results. Any air trapped in the syringe during the draw should be immediately expelled at the completion of the draw.

Transport time and analysis should be minimal to reduce cellular metabolism. Anaerobic condition results in oxygen and glucose consumption and carbon dioxide and lactate production. Placing the filled syringe in an ice water slurry promptly after the draw minimizes cell metabolism. There is potential for pO_2 to increase due to oxygen diffusing from the water through the pores of the plastic syringe. In addition, lower temperatures cause increased oxygen solubility in blood and a left shift in the oxyhemoglobin dissociation curve resulting in more oxygen combining with hemoglobin. As a consequence, when the sample is heated by the blood gas analyzer, the measured pO_2 is falsely elevated.[5] The best practice in avoiding many of these aforementioned preanalytic errors is to analyse the sample as quickly as possible. Oxygen and carbon dioxide levels in blood kept at cool room temperatures for up to 20 to 30 minutes are minimally affected except in the presence of an elevated leukocyte or platelet count. In the presence of elevated leukocytes, glycolysis will also be elevated, which has a pronounced effect on pH, pO_2, and pCO_2. The CLSI guidelines advocate samples be kept at room temperature and analyzed in less than 30 minutes.[1] Preanalytical errors of samples that will be utilized on multianalyte instruments should also be considered. For example, prolonged ice water slurry storage can result in falsely elevated potassium in whole blood samples.

Seeing as sample procurement and handling are the source of most errors in blood gas analysis, it is necessary that procedures and policies are carefully constructed, and adherence is monitored to ensure quality. At this time, no quality assessment approach can detect all preanalytic problems associated with blood gas analysis.

Analytic Assessments: Quality Control and Proficiency Testing

Quality control (QC) assesses the process in the three components of analytic phase—preanalytic, analytic, and postanalytic—testing process. Ideally, to evaluate the performance of a test method, a control should reflect an actual patient sample matrix; however, this is not possible for blood gases. Nonetheless, there are several approaches to asses quality control for blood gases.[1]

Surrogate liquid control materials are the basis of most of the traditional QC practices.[6] Usually, these are sold in sealed glass containers with solutions equilibrated with gases of known concentration. The containers can be snapped open and then analyzed by an analyst similar to a patient's sample. Alternatively, the instrument can automatically assess the liquid at programmed intervals for analysis. Surrogate

liquid controls are typically available in at least three levels, corresponding to values observed with low, expected (i.e., "normal"), and elevated values for each of the measured analytes. The QC materials vary in stability and are susceptible to temperature variation in storage and handling. Furthermore, liquid control materials have significantly different matrices than fresh whole blood; therefore, the laboratorian must be aware that they may not detect problems that can affect patient samples or they may detect errors induced by improper handling of the commercial controls.

Aqueous-based controls consist of buffered medium sealed in vials with gas mixtures. These have low O_2 solubility, making them sensitive to factors that affect pO_2. Aqueous controls must be at room temperature for analysis, and manufacturer recommendations must be followed closely or pO_2 results may be unreliable. Hemoglobin-containing and emulsion-based controls have increased O_2 solubility to better resist O_2 changes. *Tonometry* is the equilibration of a fluid with gases of known concentration and under controlled conditions, such as constant temperature, BP, and humidification.[1] When whole blood is used, it is considered the reference procedure to establish the accuracy for pCO_2 and pO_2. However, tonometry is rarely used today because the technique is considered to be cumbersome and time consuming.

Duplicate assays using two or more instruments for simultaneous analysis of a patient sample is another quality control approach. The delta checks, or the difference in values obtained on the two instruments, often identify problems that might be missed by routine QC. The allowable difference in duplicates should be tighter than those observed with surrogate liquid controls. Further investigation is usually needed as discrepancies between results provide no clue regarding which data point is wrong or which instrument is malfunctioning. Consequently, the duplicate assay approach cannot be used as the sole method of QC. It can be a useful approach for detection of errors and for troubleshooting instruments.

Nonsurrogate QC is becoming particularly popular for testing devices used in point of care. This category includes a variety of quality assurance mechanisms that are integrated into the design of the device, such as electronic QC (which simulates sensor signals to test electronic components), automated procedural controls (which ensures that certain steps of the method occur appropriately), and automated internal checks (which may, e.g., ensure the quality of a raw electronic signal). Such controls may check all, but usually just a portion, of the test system's analytic components each time the test is performed.

Whatever the QC approach may be, the QC needs of the blood gas laboratory contrast sharply with those of the general laboratory, which can analyze many patient samples as a group and includes multiple control specimens with each run. In blood gas instruments, the critical nature of the measurements and the limited patient sample volume do not always allow for repeat analyses, if problems exist. Consequently, the blood gas laboratory must perform *prospective* QC because instruments must be *prequalified* to ensure proper performance before the patient sample arrives for analysis.

Several manufacturers have devised onboard QC systems that greatly reduce operator handling errors. Advances in computer technology and software monitoring algorithms now can automatically analyze QC products, continuously monitor instrument performance, and detect some preanalytical problems (i.e., microclots and hemolysis) for improved reliability and error detection in blood gas and multianalyte instruments.

Participating in external, interlaboratory surveys or proficiency testing programs is another essential component of ensuring the quality of blood gas measurements.[7] Ongoing comparisons of results through proficiency testing help ensure that systematic (accuracy) errors do not slowly increase and go undetected by internal QC procedures. A rigorous internal QC program ensures internal consistency. Good performance in a proficiency testing program ensures the absence of significant bias relative to other laboratories and further confirms the validity of a laboratory's patient results. If an individual analyzer does not produce proficiency testing results consistent with its peer laboratories (those using the same method/instrument) or if the differences between values change over time, suspicion of the instrument's performance is warranted.

For additional student resources, please visit the**Point** at http://thepoint.lww.com

questions

1. The presence of dyshemoglobins will cause a calculated % SO_2 result to be falsely (elevated, decreased) and a pulse oximeter % SpO_2 result to be falsely (elevated, decreased).
   a. Elevated, elevated
   b. Decreased, decreased
   c. Elevated, decreased
   d. Decreased, elevated

2. The preferred anticoagulant for arterial blood gas measurements is _____ in the _____ state.
   a. Lithium heparin; dry
   b. EDTA; dry
   c. Potassium oxalate; liquid
   d. Sodium citrate; dry

3. At a pH of 7.10, the H^+ concentration is equivalent to
   a. 80 nmol/L
   b. 20 nmol/L
   c. 40 nmol/L
   d. 60 nmol/L

4. In respiratory alkalosis, the kidneys compensate by (excretion, retention) of bicarbonate and (increased, decreased) excretion of NaH_2PO_4.
   a. Excretion, decreased
   b. Excretion, increased
   c. Retention, increased
   d. Retention, decreased

5. The normal ratio of carbonic acid to bicarbonate in arterial blood is
   a. 1:20
   b. 7.4:6.1
   c. 0.003:1.39
   d. 20:1

6. When arterial blood from a normal patient is exposed to room air
   a. pCO_2 increases; pO_2 decreases
   b. pCO_2 decreases; pO_2 increases
   c. pCO_2 decreases; pO_2 decreases
   d. pCO_2 increases; pO_2 increases

7. A patient's arterial blood gas results are as follows: pH 7.37; pCO_2, 75 mm Hg; HCO_3^-, 37 mmol/L. These values are consistent with
   a. Compensated respiratory acidosis
   b. Compensated nonrespiratory acidosis
   c. Uncompensated respiratory alkalosis
   d. Uncompensated nonrespiratory alkalosis

8. A patient's arterial blood gas results are as follows: pH 7.48; pCO_2 54 mm Hg; HCO_3^- 38 mmol/L. These values are consistent with
   a. Compensated nonrespiratory alkalosis
   b. Compensated respiratory alkalosis
   c. Uncompensated respiratory alkalosis
   d. Uncompensated nonrespiratory alkalosis

9. In the circulatory system, bicarbonate leaves the red blood cells and enters the plasma through an exchange mechanism with _____ to maintain electroneutrality.
   a. Chloride
   b. Carbonic acid
   c. Lactate
   d. Sodium

10. Hypoventilation can compensate for which of the following acid–base disorders:
    a. Nonrespiratory acidosis
    b. Mixed alkalosis
    c. Mixed acidosis
    d. Nonrespiratory alkalosis

review questions (continued)

11. What is the oxygen binding capacity of hemoglobin in a blood sample that is 100% saturated with O_2 and has a total hemoglobin value of 12 g/dL
  a. 17 mL O_2/dL
  b. 4 mL O_2/dL
  c. 8 mL O_2/dL
  d. 34 mL O_2/dL

12. Carbonic acid concentration in blood plasma is equivalent to
  a. 0.0307 mmol/L/mm Hg times the pCO_2 value in mm Hg
  b. Apparent pK_a of carbonic acid, 6.1, plus the pCO_2 value in mm Hg
  c. pCO_2 value in mm Hg plus HCO_3^- value in mm Hg
  d. Bicarbonate concentration divided by the pCO_2 value in mm Hg

13. Oxygen content in blood reflects
  a. pO_2 value
  b. O_2Hb only
  c. O_2 dissolved in blood plasma only
  d. The patient's total hemoglobin value
  e. All of these

references

1. D'Orazio P, et al. *Blood Gas and pH Analysis and Related Measurements; Approved Guideline.* Wayne, PA: Clinical and Laboratory Standards Institute; 2009.
2. Ehrmeyer S, Ancy J, Laessig R. Oxygenation: measure the right thing. *J Respir Care Pract.* 1998;11:25–30.
3. Roupie EE. Continuous assessment of arterial blood gases. *Crit Care.* 1997;1(1):11–14.
4. Blonshine S, et al. *Procedures for the Collection of Arterial Blood Specimens; Approved Standard.* 4th ed. Wayne, PA: Clinical and Laboratory Standards Institute (formerly NCCLS); 2012.
5. Ancy J. Blood gases and preanalytic error prevention. *RT Magazine.* 2012:7–10.
6. Westgard JO, et al. *Statistical Quality Control for Quantitative Measurement Procedures: Principles and Definitions; Approved Guideline.* Wayne, PA: CLSI; 2006.
7. Ehrmeyer S, Laessig R. Benefits for voluntary proficiency testing. *Adv Lab Admin.* 2006;15(8):3.

18

Trace and Toxic Elements

FREDERICK G. STRATHMANN and CARRIE J. HAGLOCK-ADLER

chapter outline

key terms

Atomic absorption spectroscopy
Atomic emission spectroscopy
Emission spectrum
Essential
Inductively coupled plasma
Mass spectrometry
Mass-to-charge ratio
Metalloenzyme
Metalloprotein
Nonessential

For additional student resources, please visit the Point
at http://thepoint.lww.com

Zinc
Introduction
Absorption, Transport, and Excretion
Health Effects, Deficiency, and
Toxicity

Laboratory Evaluation of Zinc
Status
Questions
Bibliography
References

chapter objectives

Upon completion of this chapter, the clinical laboratorian should be able to do the following:

- Define metalloprotein, metalloenzyme, cofactor, trace element, ultratrace element, essential trace element, and nonessential trace element.
- State the biological functions of trace and toxic elements included in the chapter.
- Discuss the absorption, transport, and excretion of trace and toxic elements included in the chapter.
- Distinguish between essential and nonessential trace elements.
- Discuss the clinical significance of deficiency and toxicity of trace elements included in the chapter.
- Discuss specimen collection considerations and common laboratory methods for measuring trace and toxic elements.
- Determine the optimal specimen type for the assessment of trace and toxic elements.

OVERVIEW AND OBJECTIVES

Almost half of the elements listed in the periodic table have been found in the human body.[1] An element is considered **essential** if a deficiency impairs a biochemical or functional process and replacement of the element corrects this impairment. Decreased intake, impaired absorption, increased excretion, and genetic abnormalities are all examples of conditions that could result in deficiency of one or several trace elements. The World Health Organization has established the dietary requirement for nutrients as the smallest amount of the nutrient needed to maintain optimal function and health. Any element that is not considered essential is classified as **nonessential**. Nonessential trace elements are of medical interest primarily because many of them are toxic.

The trace and toxic elements included in this chapter all have biochemical importance, whether minor or major. The essential trace elements are often associated with an enzyme (**metalloenzyme**) or another protein (**metalloprotein**) as a cofactor. Deficiencies typically impair one or more biochemical functions, and excess concentrations are associated with at least some degree of toxicity. Although trace elements, such as iron, copper, and zinc, are found in mg/L or part per million (ppm) concentrations, ultratrace elements, such as selenium, chromium, and manganese, are found in µg/L or part per billion (ppb) concentrations.

This chapter provides an overview of the trace and toxic elements frequently encountered in the clinical laboratory. The absorption, transport, distribution, metabolism (if relevant), and elimination will be described and related to the clinical significance of disease states or toxicity. In addition, an introduction to the most common testing methodologies is provided. No reference intervals have been included in the chapter text; however, several

excellent sources for toxic element thresholds and trace element reference intervals are included in the bibliography. As always, the use of published thresholds and reference intervals as more than general guidelines must be done with caution, as variations in geographical location, testing methodologies, and population differences can often compromise their validity.

INSTRUMENTATION AND METHODS

For many years, the most commonly used instrumentation for trace and toxic metal analysis has been the atomic absorption spectrometer, either with flame (FAAS) or flameless (i.e., graphite furnace, GFAAS) atomization. Atomic emission spectrometry is also useful for some elements, particularly if used in the form of inductively coupled plasma atomic emission spectroscopy (ICP-AES) for atomization and excitation. Recently, **inductively coupled plasma** mass spectrometry (ICP-MS) is becoming more widely used because of its sensitivity, wide range of elements covered, and relative freedom from interferences. There is no single technique that is best for all purposes. A summary of the relative advantages and disadvantages of the main techniques is given in Table 18.1.

Sample Collection and Processing

Specimens for analysis of trace elements must be collected with scrupulous attention to details such as anticoagulant, collection apparatus, and specimen type (urine, serum, plasma, or blood). Because of the low concentration in biologic specimens and the ubiquitous presence in the environment, extraordinary measures are required to prevent contamination of the specimen. This includes using special sampling and collection devices, specially cleaned glassware, and water and reagents of high purity. The selection

TABLE 18.1 Relative Advantages and Disadvantages of Main Techniques for Elemental Analysis				
	Flame AA	**GFAA**	**ICP-AES**	**ICP-MS**
Sensitivity	Moderate	Excellent	Moderate	Excellent
Selectivity	Excellent	Good	Poor	Good
Elemental coverage	Moderate	Good	Good	Excellent
Speed for one analyte	Fast	Slow	Fast	Fast
Multielement capabilities	No	No	Yes	Yes
Initial cost of instrument	Low	Moderate	Moderate	High
Cost of consumables	Very low	Very high	Low	Moderate
Ease of operation	Excellent	Poor	Moderate	Moderate

of needles, evacuated blood collection tubes, anticoagulants and other additives, water and other reagents, pipettes, and sample cups must be carefully evaluated for use in trace and ultratrace analyses. In addition, the laboratory environment must be carefully controlled. Recommended measures include placing the trace elements laboratory in a separate room incorporating rigorous contamination control features, such as sticky mats at doors, nonshedding ceiling tiles, carefully controlled airflow to minimize particulate contamination, disposable booties worn over shoes, particle monitoring equipment, etc. Many useful measures are borrowed from those employed in semiconductor clean rooms.

Atomic Emission Spectroscopy

The simplified principle of the **atomic emission spectroscopy** (AES) instruments is presented in Figure 18.1.

The three most important components of AE spectrophotometer are as follows:

1. A source, in which the sample is atomized at a sufficient temperature to produce an excited-state species. Those species will emit radiation upon relaxation back to the ground state.
2. A wavelength selecting device (monochromator), for the spectral dispersion of the radiation and separation of the analytical line from other radiation.
3. A detector permitting measurement of radiation intensity.

A liquid sample, containing element(s) of interest, is converted into an aerosol and delivered into the source, where it receives energy sufficient to emit radiation. The intensity of the emitted radiation is correlated to the concentration of an analyte and is the basis for quantitation. The most

commonly used sources in AES are flame and inductively coupled plasma. Flames are capable of producing temperatures up to 3,000 K. Typical fuel gases include hydrogen and acetylene, while oxidant gases include air, oxygen, or nitrous oxide. The gases are combined in a specially designed mixing chamber. A sample is also introduced into the mixing chamber using a nebulizer that converts liquid into a fine spray. The mixing chamber and burner assembly are shown in Figure 18.2. The same assembly can be used for atomic absorption instrumentation.

In AES, both atomic and ionic excited states can be produced (depending on the element and the source), which leads to the production of complicated emission spectra. The "**emission spectrum**" of an element is composed of a series of very narrow peaks (sometimes known as "lines"), with each line at a different wavelength and each line matched to a specific transition. Each element has its own characteristic emission spectrum. For example, sodium can be detected by tuning the monochromator to a wavelength of 589 nm. Ideally, each emission line of a given element would be distinct from all other emission lines of other elements. However, there are many cases where emission lines from distinct elements overlap resulting in interferences. The choice of interference-free wavelength (atomic or ionic line) may be challenging. While there are several possible wavelengths for a given element, wavelengths producing suitable

FIGURE 18.2 Mixing chamber burner for flame AA. (Courtesy of Perkin-Elmer, Waltham, MA.)

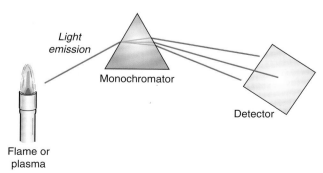

FIGURE 18.1 Simplified schematic of AES.

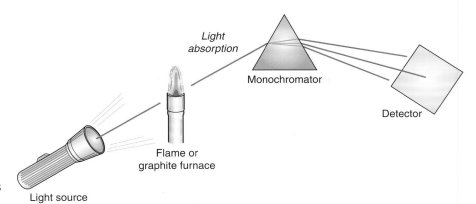

Light absorption

Monochromator

Detector

Flame or graphite furnace

FIGURE 18.3 Simplified schematic of AAS instrumentation.

Light source

analytical performance, such as limit of quantitation, freedom from interferences, robustness, etc., are selected.

The first detectors in AES used photographic film. Contemporary AES instruments feature photomultiplier tubes or array-based detector systems.

Atomic Absorption Spectroscopy

Atomic absorption spectroscopy (AAS) is an analytical procedure for the quantitative determination of elements through the absorption of optical radiation by free atoms in the gas phase. The spectra of the atoms are line spectra that are specific for the absorbing elements.

Absorption is governed by the Beer-Lambert law:

$$A = -\log_{10}\left(\frac{I_1}{I_0}\right) \varepsilon L C_g \quad \text{(Eq. 18-1)}$$

where A is the absorbance of the sample, I_0 is the incident light intensity, I_1 is the transmitted light intensity, ε is the molar absorptivity of the target analyte for the wavelength being used, L is the path length, and C_g is the gas-phase concentration of the target analyte. Under some simplifying assumptions, this equation takes the form:

$$A = KC \quad \text{(Eq. 18-2)}$$

where K is a constant determined by calibration, and C is the solution phase concentration of the analyte.

The simplified principle of the AAS instruments is presented in Figure 18.3.

The four most important components of AA spectrophotometer are:

1. Radiation (light) source, which emits the spectrum of the analyte element
2. Atomizer, in which the atoms of the element of interest in the sample are formed
3. Monochromator, for the spectral dispersion of the radiation and separation of the analytical line from other radiation
4. Detector permitting measurement of radiation intensity

Typical radiation sources for AAS are hollow cathode lamps (HCLs) and electrodeless discharge lamps (EDLs). The HCL contains a quantity of the target element in the form of

a hollow cylinder. During operation, a small quantity of the target element is vaporized, and some of the gas-phase atoms of the target element become electronically excited and emit photons with the right wavelength to be absorbed by atoms of the target element in the atomizer. While HCLs are an ideal source for determining most elements by atomic absorption, for volatile elements, the use of EDLs is recommended.

The most common sources in AAS are flame (FAAS) and graphite furnace (GFAAS, also called flameless or electrothermal AAS). The mixing chamber burner, which produces laminar flames of high optical transparency, was already described in the section on AES in this chapter. Copper, iron, and zinc are often measured by FAAS.

The graphite tubes are the most commonly used atomizers in flameless AAS. Tubes are made of high-purity polycrystalline electrographite and coated with pyrolytic graphite and can be heated to a high temperature by an electrical current. A small aliquot (usually 20 µL) of liquid sample is placed in the tube at the ambient temperature. The heating program (specifying the temperatures and times) is designed to first dry the sample, then pyrolyze, vaporize, and atomize the sample, followed by a cleaning step.

Selenium, cadmium, and lead are often measured by GFAAS. GFAAS allows for measurements of both liquid and solid samples. A common problem in GFAAS is that analyte volatility depends on the molecular form of the analyte and the sample matrix. To overcome this limitation, chemical modifiers (palladium nitrate, magnesium nitrate, or a mixture of both) are frequently added to samples, calibrators, and controls.

Inductively Coupled Plasma Mass Spectrometry

Inductively coupled plasma **mass spectrometry** (ICP-MS) is a state-of-the-art analytical technique for elemental analysis. The term *plasma* in ICP refers to an ionized gas (typically argon), in which a certain proportion of electrons are free.

Like other mass spectrometers, the ICP-MS measures the **mass-to-charge ratio** (molecular mass divided by ionic charge [m/z]) of selected analyte ions) and includes the following components: (1) an ion source, (2) a mass analyzer, and (3) an ion detector. A simplified schematic of an ICP-MS is given in Figure 18.4.

FIGURE 18.4 Simplified schematic of ICP-MS instrumentation.

The argon plasma induced by commercial ICP instruments (both ICP-AES and ICP-MS) generates temperatures ranging from 6,000 K to 10,000 K and serves several purposes. First, it dries and then vaporizes the droplets produced by the nebulizer. This step is followed by atomization of any molecular species. Finally, atoms are thermally ionized, at which point they are ready for introduction into the mass spectrometer

Nearly all ICP torches consist of three concentric quartz tubes surrounded by a coil carrying radiofrequency (RF) power. The middle tube of the torch carries the argon (Ar) that forms the plasma.

Quantitative analysis for clinical samples is best performed with the use of an internal standard. All patient samples, calibrators, and controls are diluted with an internal standard, usually a solution of an uncommon element such as yttrium. Rather than using the raw signal level of the target elements as the basis for quantitation, the signal for each of the target elements is divided by the signal of the internal standard to give signal ratios (i.e., normalized intensities).

Quadrupole Mass Spectrometers
The typical mass spectrometer used for ICP-MS is a quadrupole mass spectrometer. The analyzer consists of four parallel conducting rods arranged in a square array. Applying RF and constant (DC) voltages to the rods, the instrument can be tuned so that only ions of a specific m/z ratio can pass through the device to reach the detector. This type of instrument tends to be relatively simple to use and maintain, but the resolution (the ability to discriminate between closely spaced m/z values) is limited, being able to well resolve peaks separated by one m/z unit but not able to resolve peaks separated by a small fraction of an m/z unit.

High-Resolution Mass Spectrometers
Other ICP-MS instruments incorporate high-resolution mass spectrometers. These are usually "double focusing sector field" instruments. Such instruments separate ions of different m/z values via deflection in a magnetic field, with ions of greater m/z being deflected to a lesser degree than those of lower m/z. The magnetic field is adjusted so as to allow only ions of a selected m/z to reach the detection

system at any given point in time. A second device known as an electrostatic analyzer corrects for certain nonideal effects, allowing the instrument to achieve high resolution. Commercially available high-resolution ICP-MS instruments are capable of a resolution of 10,000 (10% valley). This is enough to resolve, for example, $^{75}As^+$ from $^{75}ArCl^+$, both nominally 75 m/z units, but which differ by 1×10^3 units when viewed at high resolution. However, magnetic sector instruments are not able to resolve elemental isobaric interferences such as $^{115}Sn/^{115}In$ or $^{40}Ca/^{40}Ar$, which would require resolution much higher than 10,000.

Interferences
In general, the interferences in elemental analysis are classified as spectroscopic or nonspectroscopic.

Spectroscopic
Spectral interferences generally result from a spectral overlap with the spectrum of the target analyte. For example, in AA, certain molecular species may have broad absorption spectra that may overlap the line spectra of the elements of interest, leading to false elevations of the target element concentrations. A much less common occurrence would be for the absorption spectrum of one element to overlap with that of another.

Various strategies are used to deal with spectral interferences in AAS. A continuum source background corrector may be included in the instrument design at the cost of some instrument complication. Another alternative is Zeeman background correction, which relies on shifting the atomic spectral lines by the application of a magnetic field.

In ICP-MS, spectral interferences include polyatomic species whose m/z may overlap m/z of the target analyte. For example, $^{56}(ArO^+)$ has the same nominal m/z as $^{56}Fe^+$. The argon oxide ion, which can be a significant component of plasma generated by an ICP torch, can potentially interfere with iron analysis by ICP-MS. Another well-known polyatomic interference is argon chloride ion $^{75}(ArCl)^+$ on determination of $^{75}As^+$. An extensive table of polyatomic interferences in ICP-MS has been published.[2]

Several approaches are used to deal with polyatomic interferences in ICP-MS. One applies algebraic equations, together with relative isotopic abundance information, to mathematically correct for interferences.[3] Another approach interposes a reaction cell or collision cell between the main ion lenses and the mass analyzer.[4] A small amount of a gas such as helium or ammonia introduced into the cell removes interferences, either by chemical reaction or by an energy-filtering process, using the fact that polyatomic species, with their larger collisional cross sections, lose energy faster than atomic ions. Recently, a tandem mass spectrometer has been introduced to the market. Similar to conventional tandem mass spectrometers, the design includes two mass filtering quadrupoles separated by an octopole collision/reaction cell. High-resolution mass spectrometers provide a third way to remove interferences as discussed in an earlier section.

A second source of spectral interferences in ICP-MS arises from nearby elements in the periodic table. For example, tin (Sn) and cadmium (Cd) both have isotopes at 114 Da (amu), so they could potentially interfere with each other if the instrument is set to measure 114 m/z. This can usually be handled by using a different isotope for the analysis. For example, cadmium also has an isotope at 111 Da that is free from isobaric elemental interferences.

A third source of spectral interferences in ICP-MS comes from doubly charged ions. For example, $^{136}Ba^{2+}$ appears at the same m/z as $^{68}Zn^+$ (136/2 equals 68/1). These are relatively uncommon and can usually be avoided, such as by choosing a different isotope for analysis or tuning the torch to reduce multiply charged ions.

Nonspectroscopic

Matrix interferences involve the bulk physical properties of the sample to be analyzed. The aqueous samples may behave differently than organic and biological specimens, depending upon the technology used and the analyte of interest. The properties of significance are viscosity, presence of easily ionized elements, and presence of carbon. Matrix matching of the calibrators, controls, and specimens helps to overcome matrix interferences. Dilution of the specimens helps to minimize matrix effect, but it is only applicable to certain analytical techniques and to the determination of analytes with higher concentrations.

Anything that could interfere with atomization of the sample could be classified as a nonspectral interference. For example, in AA, a flame may not be hot enough for efficient atomization. Difference in sample viscosity between standards and unknown samples, resulting in differing rates of sample introduction, is another example of a nonspectral interference. In AES, anything that would prevent the efficient excitation or emission of spectral lines used for the analysis would constitute a nonspectral interference.

Elemental Speciation

The toxicity of elements may depend on their chemical forms. For example, arsenobetaine is a relatively nontoxic form of arsenic. Methylated forms of arsenic are intermediate in toxicity, and inorganic arsenic, such as As(V) and As(III), is highly toxic. In the medical evaluation of patients, it can be important to know whether an elevated arsenic level is due to relatively innocuous forms, such as arsenobetaine, perhaps from a seafood meal ingested up to 3 days before the specimen collection or by dangerous forms such as inorganic arsenic. In addition, the concentrations of methylated forms may be useful information for monitoring recovery from toxic exposure. The methodologies for elemental analysis discussed in previous sections are generally not capable of specifying the chemical form of the target elements.

So-called hyphenated techniques allow for speciation determinations. In a hyphenated analysis, the combination of two or more complementary analytical techniques is used to measure the specific form of an analyte. A classic example of this approach is liquid chromatography-ICP-MS (LC-ICP-MS). The sample is injected into a liquid chromatograph, which separates the different chemical forms of the analyte producing a characteristic retention time. Concurrently, the eluting sample is continuously analyzed by a mass spectrometer. The retention time partially identifies the analytes, and the mass spectrometer further identifies the element. In some cases, AA may substitute for MS in elemental speciation schemes. Methods for elemental speciation are becoming more common, especially in Europe. Despite clinical matrices being among the most difficult for speciation, several applications are reported; among them are the following:

Arsenic speciation in urine by LC-ICP-MS and HG-GFAAS
Copper in urine by size exclusion chromatography (SEC)-ICP-MS
Copper in red blood cells (RBCs) by SEC-ICP-MS
Lead in blood by gas chromatography (GC)-GFAAS
Selenium in serum by SEC-GFAAS
Zinc in urine by anion exchange chromatography (AEC)-ICP-MS

Alternative Analytical Techniques

Voltametric methods, such as anodic stripping voltammetry (ASV) and adsorptive stripping voltammetry (ADSV) can be used in determination of selected metals and are the basis for some point-of-care devices.[5] Ion chromatography (IC) can be used for the determination of copper, iron, and zinc in blood, serum, and plasma and for the determination of zinc in urine.

Gas chromatography–mass spectrometry (GC-MS) is capable of determination of cadmium, chromium, cobalt, copper, lead, and selenium in urine, copper in serum, and lead in blood.

The methods accommodating direct analysis of solid samples, for instance, laser ablation ICP-MS (LA-ICP-MS), are gaining recognition for selected clinical applications.

ALUMINUM

Introduction

Aluminum (Al) is a crystalline silver-white ductile metal. Aluminum is the most abundant metal in the earth's crust (~8%). It is always found combined with other elements such as oxygen, silicon, and fluorine. Aluminum as the metal is obtained from aluminum-containing minerals.

Due to its good conductivity of heat and electricity, ease of welding, tensile strength, light weight, and corrosion-resistant oxide coat, aluminum is applicable to a wide variety of industrial and household uses. Aluminum is used for beverage cans, pots and pans, airplanes, siding and roofing, and foil. Aluminum is often mixed with small amounts of other metals to form aluminum alloys, which are stronger and harder than aluminum alone.

Aluminum compounds have many different uses, for example, as alums in water treatment and alumina in abrasives and furnace linings. They are also found in consumer products such as antacids, astringents, buffered aspirin, food additives, cosmetics, and antiperspirants.

Absorption, Transport, and Excretion

The average adult in the United States ingests about 7 to 9 mg aluminum per day in food.[6] The human organism can absorb aluminum and its compounds orally, by inhaling and parenterally. There is no indication of dermal absorption. Approximately 1.5% to 2% of inhaled and 0.01% to 5% of ingested aluminum are absorbed. The absorption efficiency is dependent on chemical form, particle size (inhalation), and concurrent dietary exposure to chelators such as citric acid or lactic acid.[6,7]

After a relatively quick uptake of aluminum into the intestinal walls, its passage into the blood is much slower. In plasma, aluminum is bound to carrier proteins such as transferrin.[8] Aluminum binds to various ligands in the blood and distributes to every organ, with highest concentrations ultimately found in bone (~50% of the body burden) and lung tissues (~25% of the body burden). Aluminum levels in lungs increase with age.[6]

Urine accounts for 95% of aluminum excretion with 2% eliminated in the bile.

Health Effects and Toxicity

The mechanisms by which aluminum applies its toxicity are not well understood, though aluminum has been shown to interfere with a variety of enzymatic processes[9] and administration of aluminum to experimental animals is known to produce encephalopathy similar to that seen in Alzheimer's disease in man.[10] Although aluminum-containing over-the-counter oral products are considered safe in healthy individuals at recommended doses, some adverse effects have been observed following long-term use in some individuals. Workers who breathe large amounts of aluminum dusts can have lung problems, such as coughing or changes that show up in chest x-rays.

Signs and symptoms of aluminum toxicity include encephalopathy (stuttering, gait disturbance, myoclonic jerks, seizures, coma, abnormal EEG), osteomalacia or aplastic bone disease (painful spontaneous fractures, hypercalcemia, and tumorous calcinosis), proximal myopathy, increased risk of infection, microcytic anemia, increased left ventricular mass, and decreased myocardial function.[7]

Aluminum toxicity occurs in people with renal insufficiencies who are treated by dialysis with aluminum-contaminated solutions or oral agents that contain aluminum. The clinical manifestations of aluminum toxicity include anemia, bone disease, and progressive dementia with increased concentrations of aluminum in the brain. Prolonged intravenous feeding of preterm infants with solutions containing aluminum is associated with impaired neurologic development.

Laboratory Evaluation of Aluminum Status

Aluminum is primarily measured using ICP-MS or GFAAS. Accurate measurements are often complicated by the increased risk for environmental contamination of specimens. Urine and serum levels are useful in determining toxic exposures, monitoring exposure over time, and monitoring chelation therapy.[11]

ARSENIC

Introduction

Arsenic (As) is a ubiquitous element displaying both metallic and nonmetallic properties. Its content in the earth's crust is estimated at 1.5 to 2.0 mg/kg. For most people, food is the largest source of arsenic exposure (about 25 to 50 micrograms per day [µg/d]), with lower amounts coming from drinking water and air.[12] Anthropogenic sources of arsenic (production of metals, burning of coil, fossil fuels, timber and its use in agriculture) release three times more of arsenic than natural sources. The main current use of arsenic is as a wood preservative. Other current and past uses of arsenic include pesticides, pigments, poison gases, ammunition manufacturing, semiconductor processing, and medicines.[13]

Health Effects and Toxicity

The relation of clinical signs and symptoms to arsenic exposure depends on the duration and extent of the exposure to inorganic and methylated species of arsenic, as well as the underlying clinical status of the patient. For acute arsenic exposure, the symptoms may include gastrointestinal (nausea, emesis, abdominal pain, rice water diarrhea), bone marrow (pancytopenia, anemia, basophilic stippling), cardiovascular (EKG changes), central nervous system (encephalopathy, polyneuropathy), renal (renal insufficiency, renal failure), and hepatic (hepatitis) systems. For chronic arsenic exposure, systems and symptoms may include dermatologic (Mees lines, hyperkeratosis, hyperpigmentation, alopecia), hepatic (cirrhosis, hepatomegaly), cardiovascular (hypertension, peripheral vascular disease), central nervous system ("socks and glove" neuropathy, tremor), and malignancies (squamous cell skin, hepatocellular, bladder, lung, renal). Chronic arsenic exposure has been shown to cause blackfoot disease (BFD), a severe form of peripheral vascular disease (PVD) that leads to gangrenous changes.

The white powder of arsenic trioxide is odorless, tasteless, and one of the most common poisons in human history. Doses of 0.01 to 0.05 g produce toxic symptoms. The lethal dose is reported to be between 0.12 and 0.3 g; however, recoveries from higher doses have been reported.[13] Immediate treatment of expected exposure consists of lavage and use of activated charcoal to reduce arsenic absorption. The most effective antidotes for arsenic poisoning are the following chelating agents: dimercaprol (a.k.a British anti-Lewisite, BAL), penicillamine, and succimer.[14]

In the year 2000, the U.S. FDA approved the use of arsenic trioxide for the treatment of acute promyelocytic leukemia (APL),[15] which is diagnosed in approximately 1,500 people in United States every year.

Absorption, Transport, and Excretion

The main routes of exposure are ingestion of arsenic-containing foods, water and beverages, or inhalation of contaminated air; however, arsenic toxicity is a complex topic. Organic forms of arsenic such as arsenocholine and arsenobetaine are commonly found in fish and seafood, are considered relatively nontoxic, and are cleared rapidly (1 to 2 days).[16] Inorganic species of arsenic are highly toxic and occur naturally in rocks, soil, and groundwater. They are also found in many synthetic products, poisons, and industrial processes. Methylated species are intermediate in toxicity and arise primarily from metabolism of inorganic species, but small amounts may arise directly from food. Organic methylated arsenic compounds such as MMA and DMA are formed by hepatic metabolism of As(+3) and As(+5). The methylated inorganic forms are considered less toxic than As(+3) and As(+5); however, they are eliminated slowly (1 to 3 weeks). The Biological Exposure Index established by the American Conference of Governmental Industrial Hygienists (ACGIH) for the sum of inorganic and methylated metabolites of arsenic in urine is 35 µg/L. However, clinical symptoms may not be evident at 35 µg/L.[14]

CASE STUDY 18.1

A 27-year-old male has been seen regularly by his physician for skin lesions and increasing peripheral neuropathy over a period of several months coinciding with a home project using reclaimed wood treated with chromated copper arsenate. The initial total arsenic urine level was found to be 47 µg/L. Reflexive arsenic speciation indicated 13 µg/L As, total inorganic, 33 µg/L As, total methylated, and less than 10 µg/L of As, organic.

Questions

1. Discuss the metabolism of arsenic after inorganic arsenic ingestion.
2. What is a likely cause of the elevated total arsenic result?
3. Would blood arsenic levels have helped in the diagnosis?

Laboratory Evaluation of Arsenic Status

Arsenic is primarily measured using ICP-MS, GFAAS, or HG-AAS. In most cases, arsenic is best detected by urine due to the short half-life of arsenic in blood. When arsenic speciation is desired (typically following a high total urine arsenic value reported by ICP-MS or AA), a separation method is employed either online or off-line prior to elemental analysis.

CADMIUM

Introduction

Cadmium (Cd) is a soft, bluish-white metal, which is easily cut with a knife. Principal industrial uses of cadmium include manufacture of pigments and batteries, as well as in the metal-plating and plastics industries. In the United States, the burning of fossil fuels such as coal or oil and the incineration of municipal waste materials constitute the largest sources of airborne cadmium exposure, along with zinc, lead, or copper smelters in some locations. Cadmium-containing waste products and soil contamination, primarily as a result of human activity, are becoming of concern, and the U.S. Environmental Protection Agency (EPA) has established loading rates of 20 kg/ha for high cation exchange capacity soils with a pH of 6.5 and a lower rate of 5 kg/ha for acid soils.[17]

Absorption, Transport, and Excretion

Based on renal function (development of proteinuria), the reference dose for cadmium in drinking water is 0.0005 mg per kg per day (mg/kg/d), and the dose for dietary exposure to cadmium is 0.001 mg/kg/d.[18] Absorption of cadmium is higher in females than in males due to differences in iron stores. The absorption of inhaled cadmium in air is 10% to 50% with gastrointestinal absorption of cadmium estimated to be 5%. The absorption of cadmium in cigarette smoke is 10% to 50%, and smokers of tobacco products have about twice the cadmium abundance in their bodies as nonsmokers. For nonsmokers, the primary exposure to cadmium is through ingested food.[19] Ninety percent of ingested cadmium is excreted in the feces due to the low absorbance of cadmium from the gut.[20]

Health Effects and Toxicity

Cadmium has no known role in normal human physiology. Toxicity is believed to be a result of protein-Cd adducts causing denaturation of the associated proteins, resulting in a loss of function.[20] Ingestion of high amounts of cadmium may lead to a rapid onset with severe nausea, vomiting, and abdominal pain.[20] Renal dysfunction is a common presentation for chronic cadmium exposure, often resulting in slow-onset proteinuria. Acute effects of inhalation of fumes containing cadmium include respiratory distress due to chemical pneumonitis and edema and can cause death. Breathing of cadmium vapors can also result in nasal epithelial damage and lung damage similar to emphysema.[20] Cadmium exposure can affect the liver, bone, immune, blood, and nervous systems.[19,21]

EDTA (ethylenediaminetetraacetic acid) can be used as a chelating agent in cadmium poisoning.

Laboratory Evaluation of Cadmium Status

Cadmium is usually quantified by GFAAS and ICP-MS; ICP-AES is also used. In blood, cadmium is found mostly (70%) in the red blood cells. Cadmium in blood reflects the average uptake during the past few months and can be used for monitoring purposes but does not accurately reflect a recent exposure. Urinary excretion is about 0.001% and 0.01% of the body burden per 24 hours. At low exposure, urine cadmium reflects the total accumulation.[22]

CHROMIUM

Introduction

Chromium (Cr), from the Greek word *chroma* ("color"), makes rubies red and emeralds green. Chromium is the 21st most abundant element in the earth's crust and is used in the manufacturing of stainless steel. Occupational exposure to chromium occurs in wood treatment, stainless steel welding, chrome plating, the leather tanning industry, and the use of lead chromate or strontium chromate paints. Chromium exists in two main valency states: trivalent and hexavalent.

Absorption, Transport, and Excretion

Cr(+6) is better absorbed and much more toxic than Cr(+3).[22] Both transferrin and albumin are involved in chromium absorption and transport.[23] Transferrin binds the newly absorbed chromium at site B, while albumin acts as an acceptor and transporter of chromium if the transferrin sites are saturated.[24] Other plasma proteins, including β- and γ-globulins and lipoproteins, bind chromium.

Health Effects, Deficiency, and Toxicity

Cr(+3) is an essential dietary element and plays a role in maintaining normal metabolism of glucose, fat, and cholesterol. The estimated safe and adequate daily intake of chromium for adults is in the range of 50 to 200 µg/d, although data are insufficient to establish a recommended daily allowance.[25]

Dietary chromium deficiency is relatively uncommon, and most cases occur in persons with specific clinical situations such as total parenteral nutrition, diabetes, or malnutrition. Chromium deficiency is characterized by glucose intolerance, glycosuria, hypercholesterolemia, decreased longevity, decreased sperm counts, and impaired fertility.[25]

Cr(+6) compounds are powerful oxidizing agents and are more toxic systemically than Cr(+3) compounds, given similar amounts and solubilities. At physiological pH, Cr(+6) forms CrO_4^{-2} and readily passes through cell membranes due to its similarity to essential phosphate and sulfate oxyanions. Intracellularly, Cr(+6) is reduced to reactive intermediates, producing free radicals and oxidizing DNA, both potentially inducing cell death.[26] Severe dermatitis and skin ulcers can result from contact with Cr(+6) salts. Up to 20% of chromium workers develop contact dermatitis.

Allergic dermatitis with eczema has been reported in printers, cement workers, metal workers, painters, and leather tanners. Data suggest that a Cr(+3)–protein complex is responsible for the allergic reaction.[25]

When inhaled, Cr(+6) is a respiratory tract irritant, resulting in airway irritation, airway obstruction, and possibly lung cancer. The target organ of inhaled chromium is the lung; the kidneys, liver, skin, and immune system may also be affected.

Low-dose, chronic chromium exposure typically results only in transient renal effects. Elevated urinary β2-microglobulin levels (an indicator of renal tubular damage) have been found in chrome platers, and higher levels have generally been observed in younger persons exposed to higher Cr(+6) concentrations.[25]

In May 2011, the FDA issued orders for postmarket surveillance studies to manufacturers of metal-on-metal (MoM) hip replacement systems in response to an increasing concern over failed implant devices reported in Europe.[27] In the United States, no guidelines have been established for the assessment of metal ions in asymptomatic patients due to a lack of knowledge regarding the prevalence of adverse events in the US population and no clear threshold levels associated with an adverse event.

Laboratory Evaluation of Chromium Status

Chromium may be determined by GFAAS, NAA, or ICP-MS. Plasma, serum, and urine do not indicate the total body status of the individual, whereas urine levels may be useful for metabolic studies.[23] In the setting of suspected failure of MoM hip implants that use a cobalt–chrome alloy femoral head, serum is the preferred specimen type for both chromium and cobalt analysis.[28]

COPPER

Introduction

Copper (Cu) is a relatively soft yet tough metal with excellent electrical and heat conducting properties. Copper is widely distributed in nature both in its elemental form and in compounds. Copper forms alloys with zinc (brass), tin (bronze), and nickel (cupronickel, widely used in coins). Copper is an essential trace element found in four oxidation states, Cu(0), Cu(+1), Cu(+2), and Cu(+3), with Cu(+2) the most stable of all oxidation states.[29] Copper is an important cofactor for several metalloenzymes and is critical for the reduction of iron in heme synthesis.

Absorption, Transport, and Excretion

The copper content in the normal human adult is 50 to 120 mg. Copper is distributed through the body with the highest concentrations found in the liver, brain, heart, and kidneys. Hepatic copper accounts for about 10% of the total copper in the body.[30] Copper is also found in the cornea, spleen, intestine, and lung. The amount of copper absorbed from the intestine is 50% to 80% of ingested copper.[25] The average daily intake is approximately 10 mg or more of copper.[30] The exact mechanisms by which copper is absorbed and transported by the intestine are unknown, but an active transport mechanism at low concentrations and passive diffusion at high concentrations have been proposed. Copper is transported to the liver bound to albumin, transcuprein, and low-molecular-weight components in the portal system. In the liver, copper is incorporated into ceruloplasmin for distribution throughout the body.[29] Ceruloplasmin is an α_2-globulin, and each 132,000-molecular-weight molecule contains six atoms of copper.[30]

In a normal physiological state, 98% of copper excretion is through the bile, with copper losses in the urine and sweat constituting approximately 2% of dietary intake.[25] Menstrual losses of copper are minor.

Health Effects, Deficiency, and Toxicity

Copper is a component of several metalloenzymes, including ceruloplasmin, cytochrome C oxidase, superoxide dismutase, tyrosinase, metallothionein, dopamine hydroxylase, lysyl oxidase, clotting factor V, and an unknown enzyme that cross-links keratin in hair.

Copper deficiency is observed in premature infants, and copper absorption is impaired in severe diffuse diseases of small bowel, lymph sarcoma, and scleroderma.[30] Copper deficiency is related to malnutrition, malabsorption, chronic diarrhea, hyperalimentation, and prolonged feeding with low-copper, total-milk diets. Signs of copper deficiency include (1) neutropenia and hypochromic anemia in the early stages, (2) osteoporosis and various bone and joint abnormalities that reflect deficient copper-dependent cross-linking of bone collagen and connective tissue, (3) decreased pigmentation of the skin and general pallor, and (4) in the later stages, possible neurologic abnormalities (hypotonia, apnea, psychomotor retardation).[25]

Subclinical copper depletion contributes to an increased risk of coronary heart disease. An extreme form of copper deficiency is seen in Menkes' disease, with symptoms usually appearing at the age of 3 months and death usually occurring by the age of 5. This invariably fatal, progressive brain disease is characterized by peculiar hair, called kinky or steely, and retardation of growth. Clinical signs include progressive mental deterioration, coarse feces, disturbance of muscle tone, seizures, and episodes of severe hypothermia.

Copper toxicity has been associated with living near copper-producing facilities, using water from copper pipes or cooking with copper-lined vessels or exposure to algaecides, herbicides, pyrotechnics, ceramic glazes, electrical wiring, or welding supplies. Because of its redox potential, copper is an irritant to epithelia and mucous membranes and can cause hepatic and renal damage with hemolysis.[31] Copper-induced emesis has a characteristic blue-green color.

Wilson's disease is a genetically determined copper accumulation disease that usually presents between the ages of 6 and 40 years. Clinical findings include neurologic disorders, liver dysfunction, and Kayser-Fleischer rings (green-brown discoloration) in the cornea caused by copper deposition. Early diagnosis of Wilson's disease is important because complications can be effectively prevented, and in some cases, the disease can be halted with use of zinc acetate or chelation therapy.[25] Serum ceruloplasmin levels and the direct measurement of free copper are key diagnostic steps in the diagnosis of Wilson's disease.[32]

Laboratory Evaluation of Copper Status

Copper is measured by flame AAS, ICP-MS, ICP-AES, and ASV. Serum copper and urine copper are used to monitor for nutritional adequacy and subacute management of copper toxicity. Direct measurement of free copper and ceruloplasmin in serum is used to screen for Wilson's disease. Common trends in laboratory testing seen in various diseases states are summarized in Table 18.2.

IRON

Introduction

Iron (Fe) is fourth most abundant element in the earth's crust and the most abundant transition metal. Methods of extracting iron from ore have been known for centuries. The physical properties of iron alloys can be varied over an enormous range by appropriate alloying and heat-treating methods, giving a range of strength, hardness, toughness, corrosion resistance (in the form of stainless steels), and

TABLE 18.2 Interpretation of Copper Testing Results

	Serum Copper	Urine Copper
Nutritional deficiency	↓	↓
Menkes' syndrome	↓	↑
Acute copper toxicity	↑ or ↑↑	↑
Chronic copper toxicity	↑	↑
Wilson's disease	N or ↓	↑ or ↑↑
Smoking, inflammatory conditions	↑ or ↑↑	N
Estrogen, pregnancy	↑ or ↑↑	N

N, normal; ↓, decreased; ↑, increased; ↑↑, significantly increased.
Source: Jacobs DS, DeMott WR, Oxley DK. *Jacobs & DeMott Laboratory Test Handbook*. 5th ed. Hudson, OH: Lexi-Comp.; 2001:1031.

magnetic properties and ability to take and hold a sharp edge.

Although highly abundant in the earth's crust, iron is classified as a trace element in the body. Iron ions are able to participate in redox chemistry in both the ferrous [Fe(+2)] and ferric [Fe(+3)] states, allowing iron to fill numerous biochemical roles as a carrier of other biochemically active substances (e.g., oxygen) and as an agent in redox and electron transfer reactions (e.g., via various cytochromes). Iron's high activity is a double-edged sword, and free iron ions in the body also participate in destructive chemistry, primarily in catalyzing the formation of toxic free radicals. As a result, very little free iron is normally found in the body.

Absorption, Transport, and Excretion

Absorption of iron from the intestine is the primary means of regulating the amount of iron within the body. Typically, only about 10% of the 1 g/d of dietary iron is absorbed. To be absorbed by intestinal cells, iron must be in the ferrous oxidation state and bound to protein. Because Fe(+3) is the predominant form of iron in foods, it must first be reduced to Fe(+2) by agents such as vitamin C or ferric reductases present in the intestinal epithelium before it can be absorbed. In the intestinal mucosal cell, Fe(+2) can be bound by ferritin for storage and eliminated after sloughing off or be exported to the basolateral side. From there, iron is oxidized to Fe(+3) and bound by apotransferrin for transport throughout the body. The peptide hormone hepcidin regulates iron absorption in the upper gastrointestinal tract by modulating the export of iron from cells by ferroportin.[33] After about 120 days in circulation, red cells are degraded by the spleen, liver, and macrophages, which return Fe to the circulation for reuse. Absorption and transport capacity can be increased in conditions such as iron deficiency, anemia, or hypoxia. Iron is lost primarily by desquamation and red cell loss to urine and feces. With each menstrual cycle, women lose approximately 20 to 40 mg of iron.

Health Effects, Deficiency, and Toxicity

Of the 3 to 5 g of iron in the body, approximately 2 to 2.5 g of iron is in hemoglobin, mostly in RBCs and red cell precursors. A moderate amount of iron (~130 mg) is in myoglobin, the oxygen-carrying protein of muscle. A small (8 mg), but extremely important pool is bound in tissue to enzymes that require iron for full activity. These include peroxidases, cytochromes, and many of the Krebs cycle enzymes. Iron is also stored as ferritin and hemosiderin, primarily in the bone marrow, spleen, and liver. Only 3 to 5 mg of iron is found in plasma, almost all of it associated with transferrin, albumin, and free hemoglobin.[34]

Iron deficiency affects about 15% of the worldwide population. Those with a higher than average risk of iron deficiency anemia include pregnant women, young children, adolescents, and women of reproductive age.[35] Increased blood loss, decreased dietary iron intake, or decreased release from ferritin may result in iron deficiency. Reduction in iron stores usually precedes both a reduction in circulating iron and anemia, as demonstrated by a decreased red blood cell count, mean corpuscular hemoglobin concentration, and microcytic RBCs.

Iron overload states are collectively referred to as hemochromatosis (HH), whether or not tissue damage is present. Primary Fe overload is most frequently associated with hereditary HH. HH is a single-gene homozygous recessive disorder leading to abnormally high Fe absorption, culminating in Fe overload. HH causes tissue accumulation of iron, affects liver function, and often leads to hyperpigmentation of the skin. Some conditions associated with severe HH include diabetes mellitus, arthritis, cardiac arrhythmia or failure, cirrhosis, hypothyroidism, impotence, and liver cancer. Treatment may include therapeutic phlebotomy or administration of *chelators*, such as deferoxamine. Transferrin can be administered in the case of atransferrinemia.[33]

Secondary Fe overload may result from excessive dietary, medicinal, or transfusional Fe intake or be due to metabolic dysfunction. Hemosiderosis has been used to specifically designate a condition of iron overload as demonstrated by an increased serum iron and total iron-binding capacity (TIBC) or transferrin, in the absence of demonstrable tissue damage.

Iron may play a role as a *pro-oxidant*, contributing to lipid peroxidation,[36,37] atherosclerosis,[37,38] deoxyribonucleic acid (DNA) damage,[36–38] carcinogenesis,[39,40] and neurodegenerative diseases.[41,42] Fe(+3), released from binding proteins, can enhance production of free radicals to cause oxidative damage. In iron-loaded individuals with thalassemia who are treated with chelators to bind and mobilize iron, intake of ascorbic acid may actually promote the generation of free radicals.[43]

Laboratory Evaluation of Iron Status

Disorders of iron metabolism are evaluated primarily by packed cell volume, hemoglobin, red cell count and indices, total iron and TIBC, percent saturation, transferrin, and ferritin.[44] Common trends in laboratory testing seen in various diseases states are summarized in Table 18.3.

Total Iron Content (Serum Iron)

Measurement of serum iron concentration refers specifically to the Fe^{+3} bound to transferrin and not to the iron circulating as free hemoglobin in serum. The specimen may be collected as serum without anticoagulant or as plasma with heparin. Oxalate, citrate, or ethylenediaminetetraacetic acid binds Fe ions, and all are unacceptable anticoagulants. Early morning sampling is preferred because of the diurnal variation in iron concentration. Specimens with visible hemolysis should be rejected.

Total Iron-Binding Capacity

TIBC refers to the theoretical amount of iron that could be bound if transferrin and other minor iron-binding proteins present in the serum or plasma sample were saturated.

TABLE 18.3 **Laboratory Markers of Iron Status in Several Disease States[7]**

Condition	Serum Iron	Transferrin	Ferritin	Percent Saturation	TIBC
Iron deficiency	↓	↑	↓	↓	↑
Iron overdose	↑	↓	↑	↑	↓
Hemochromatosis	↑	Slightly ↓	↑	↑	↓
Malnutrition	↓	↓	↓	Variable	↓
Chronic infection	↓	↓	↑	↓	↓
Acute liver disease	↑	Variable	↑	↑	Variable
Chronic anemia	↓	N or ↓	N or ↑	↓	N or ↓

N, normal; ↓, decreased; ↑, increased.

Typically, only one-third of the iron-binding sites on transferrin are saturated.

Percent Saturation

The percent saturation, also called the transferrin saturation, is the ratio of serum iron to TIBC. The normal range for this is approximately 20% to 50%, but it varies with age and sex.

Transferrin and Ferritin

Transferrin is measured by immunochemical methods such as nephelometry. Transferrin is increased in iron deficiency and decreased in iron overload and HH. Transferrin may also be decreased in chronic infections and malignancies.

Ferritin is measured in serum by various immunochemical methods. Ferritin is decreased in iron deficiency anemia and increased in iron overload and HH. Ferritin is often increased in several other conditions including chronic infections, malignancy, and viral hepatitis.

A liver biopsy sample can be digested and analyzed for iron by AAS or ICP-MS as a follow-up to abnormal blood tests consistent with a HH diagnosis.[45] Iron quantification in liver is not used for evaluation of acute iron toxicity. Hepcidin testing has not yet been shown to be clinically useful.

CASE STUDY 18.2

An asymptomatic 1-year-old African American male had a BLL of 39 µg/dL during a follow-up visit scheduled after a 44 µg/dL routine capillary blood test 5 days prior. The child shows no signs of developmental delay and has been staying with relatives since the initial BLL result.

Questions

1. What is a common source of lead exposure for children?

2. Discuss the various methods for chelation after toxic lead exposure.

3. Is chelation therapy indicated in this case?

LEAD

Introduction

Metallic lead (Pb) is soft, bluish white, highly malleable, and ductile. It is a poor conductor of electricity and heat and is resistant to corrosion. Lead is widely distributed in the earth's crust, and the main lead ores are galena, cerrusite, and anglesite.[46] Lead is used in production of storage batteries, ammunition, solder, and foils. Tetraethyl lead was once used extensively as an additive in gasoline (petrol) for its ability to increase the fuel's octane rating and is present in many paints manufactured before 1970. The manufacture of lead-based household paints was banned in the United States in 1972, but is still used in paints intended for nondomestic use. Toxic concentrations of lead can be found in areas adjacent to homes painted with lead-based paints and around highways where it has accumulated from the past use of leaded gasoline. In recent years, there have been massive recalls of toys and costume jewelry produced in China, due to concerns over elevated lead content. Lead plays no known role in normal human physiology.

Absorption, Transport, and Excretion

Exposure to lead is primarily respiratory or gastrointestinal. Inhalation results in 30% to 40% absorption efficiency. Gut absorption depends on a variety of factors, including age and nutritional status, with enhanced gastrointestinal absorption occurring in children younger than 6 years of age. Certain substances, such as iron, calcium, magnesium, alcohol, and fat, may weaken lead absorption, while low dietary zinc, ascorbic acid, and citric acid can enhance the absorption of lead.[46] Ninety-nine percent of absorbed lead is taken up by erythrocytes where it interferes with heme synthesis. Lead distributes to soft tissues, such as the liver, kidneys, and brain, with the skeletal lead concentrations containing greater than 90% of the body burden of lead.[47] Absorbed lead is excreted primarily in urine (76%) and feces (16%), and the remaining 8% is excreted in hair, sweat, nails, and others.[46]

Health Effects and Toxicity

The clinical presentation of lead toxicity is variable. In children, obvious symptoms are usually seen at blood levels of 60 µg/dL or higher with 45 µg/dL the typical threshold for acute, clinical intervention. IQ declines are seen in children with blood lead levels of 10 µg/dL or higher. Other CNS symptoms of lead toxicity in children may include clumsiness, gait abnormalities, headache, behavioral changes, seizures, and severe cognitive and behavioral problems. Gastrointestinal symptoms include abdominal pain, constipation, and colic. Other conditions may include acute nephropathy and anemia. The U.S. Centers for Disease Control and Prevention (CDC) estimates an incidence of more than 450,000 for children with blood lead levels higher than 10 µg/dL. In adults, the following symptoms may be observed: peripheral neuropathies, motor weakness, chronic renal insufficiency, systolic hypertension, and anemia.

Lead exposure primarily arises in two settings: childhood exposure, usually through paint chips, and adult occupational exposure in the smelting, mining, ammunitions, soldering, plumbing, ceramic glazing, and construction industries. Other sources include lead-glazed ceramics and certain Asian herbal remedies. US government Web sites contain extensive information on the health and environmental impacts of lead.[48]

Laboratory Evaluation of Lead Status

The most common specimen type is whole venous blood, the result of which is commonly referred to as the blood lead level or BLL. This is preferred over plasma and serum as circulating lead is predominantly associated with red blood cells. Elevated lead levels in capillary blood specimens should be confirmed with a venous specimen to avoid the potential contribution of external contamination.

Urine lead may be useful for detecting recent exposures to lead or to monitor chelation therapy. Other testing, such as plasma aminolevulinic acid, whole blood zinc protoporphyrin, or free erythrocyte protoporphyrins, may be useful for screening in occupational exposures. Noninvasive measurements of lead in bone may be available radiographically. Removal of further lead exposure and parental education are essential parts to management for patients with elevated blood lead levels.[31]

ICP-MS is a preferred method of analysis, although ICP-AES and GFAAS are also used.

CASE STUDY 18.3

A 42-year-old woman with a history of diabetes was seen by her physician for weight loss, anorexia, and general fatigue. As part of the physical examination, both "bronze" skin pigmentation and an enlarged liver were noted. Her initial chemistry panel showed the following relevant results (Reference intervals provided in parentheses):

Albumin	3.7 g/dL (3.8–5.0)
AST	180 U/L (14–50)
ALT	200 U/L (10–60)
Total bilirubin	2.5 mg/dL (0.2–1.2)
Serum iron	180 µg/dL (45–150)

Further testing for the elevated iron showed the following:

Serum iron	170 µg/dL (45–150)
Transferrin	210 mg/dL (200–380)
Ferritin	300 µg/L (10–250)
% Transferrin saturation	80 (20–50)

Genetic testing confirmed the patient had an *HFE* 3 mutation and was diagnosed with HH.

Questions

1. Are the test results consistent with iron deficiency or toxicity?

2. Are this patient's conditions and symptoms typical of hemochromatosis?

3. What is a treatment plan for iron overload, and what is the main goal?

MERCURY

Introduction

Mercury (Hg), also called quicksilver, is a heavy, silvery metal. Along with bromine, mercury is one of only two elements that are liquid at room temperature and pressure. There are three naturally occurring oxidation states of mercury: Hg(0), Hg(+1), and Hg(+2). Organic mercury refers to various forms of mercury bound to a carbon atom, with mercury usually in the +2 oxidation state.

Mercury is released to the atmosphere as a product of the natural degassing of rock (30,000 tons per year) and through various human activities (20,000 tons per year). Mercury is used in dental amalgams, electronic switches, germicides, fungicides, and fluorescent light bulbs.[49] The use of mercury in medicine has greatly declined in all respects; however, mercury compounds are found in some over-the-counter drugs, including topical antiseptics, stimulant laxatives, diaper rash ointment, eye drops, and nasal sprays. Mercury is widely used in the production of eye cosmetics, especially mascara.

Absorption, Transport, and Excretion

Routes of exposure include (1) inhalation, primarily as elemental mercury vapor but occasionally as dimethyl mercury; (2) ingestion of $HgCl_2$ and mercury-containing foods such as predatory fish species; (3) cutaneous absorption of methyl mercury through the skin and even through latex gloves; (4) injection of relatively inert liquid mercury and mercury-containing tattoo pigments; and (5) dental amalgams. Inhaled mercury vapor is retained in the lungs to about 80%, whereas liquid metallic mercury passes through the gastrointestinal tract largely unabsorbed.[50]

Mercury enters the food chain primarily by volcanic activity and manmade sources such as coal combustion and smelting.

Most of the dietary intake comes from consumption of meat and fish products, with estimates of dietary intake varying based upon geographical location and dietary sources.[49] The kidney is the major storage organ after elemental or inorganic mercury exposure. Methyl mercury is efficiently absorbed from the gastrointestinal tract, and distribution to tissues, including the brain, appears complete in 48 hours. Movement of MeHg across the blood–brain barrier appears to be dependent on coupling with the amino acid cysteine.[51]

There is relatively little bioaccumulation of inorganic and elemental mercury. Half-lives vary according to the route of exposure and form of mercury, from 5 days in blood for phenylmercury to 90 days in urine for chronic exposure to inorganic mercury. Normally, the highest accumulation of mercury is in the kidney, liver, spleen, and brain. Mercury can accumulate in the pituitary and thyroid glands, the pancreas, and the reproductive organs. The bulk of mercury accumulated in the body is eliminated in approximately 60 days; however, organic forms of mercury can accumulate in the brain and may take up to several years to be eliminated.

Fecal and urinary excretions are the main elimination routes for inorganic and organic mercury. A special form of elimination is the transfer of mercury from mother to fetus through the placenta.

Health Effects and Toxicity

Mercury has no known function in normal human physiology. Toxicities have been observed following inhalation, ingestion, and dermal absorption of mercury compounds. Mercurial salts were historically used as diuretics, topical disinfectants, and laxatives before mercury toxicity was well understood. Since the 1930s, some vaccines have contained the preservative thimerosal, a mercury-containing compound metabolized into ethylmercury. Although it was widely speculated that this mercury-based preservative can cause or trigger autism in children, scientific studies showed no evidence supporting any such link. Nevertheless, thimerosal has been removed from or reduced to trace amounts in all US vaccines recommended for children 6 years of age and younger, with the exception of the inactivated influenza vaccine.

Organic mercury and elemental mercury vapor are toxic to both the central and peripheral nervous systems. Mercury attacks the CNS well before a victim shows symptoms. Professor Karen Wetterhahn, the founding director of Dartmouth College's Toxic Metals Research Program and an expert in the mechanisms of metal toxicity, died in 1997, at the age of 48, as a result of a tragic laboratory accident involving the use of dimethylmercury.

Elemental mercury readily vaporizes, and its inhalation can produce harmful effects on the nervous, digestive, and immune systems and the lungs and kidneys. The inorganic salts of mercury can affect the skin, eyes, gastrointestinal tract, and kidneys.

The toxicity of mercury is primarily through reaction with protein sulfhydryl groups (MSH), resulting in dysfunction and inactivation. Liquid elemental mercury is poorly absorbed and relatively nontoxic, but elemental mercury vapor is highly absorbed and is highly toxic. Inorganic, ionized forms of mercury are toxic. Further bioconversion to an alkyl mercury, such as methyl mercury, yields a very toxic species of mercury that is highly selective for lipid-rich mediums such as the brain.[52]

Mercury intoxication can manifest in many signs and symptoms that affect several organ systems, including headache, tremor, impaired coordination, abdominal cramps, diarrhea, dermatitis, polyneuropathy, proteinuria, and hepatic dysfunction.[53] Because many of these are relatively nonspecific signs and symptoms, laboratory testing provides a key role in assessing mercury intoxication.

Laboratory Evaluation of Mercury Status

Mercury is usually determined as total mercury levels in blood and urine without regard to chemical form. Analytical methods include ICP-MS and cold vapor atomic absorption spectroscopy.

MANGANESE

Introduction

As the twelfth most abundant element in the earth's crust, manganese (Mn) is found in over 250 minerals, of which 15 have commercial importance. Nearly all the elemental manganese is used in the production of the alloy ferromanganese widely used in steel production. Other uses of elemental manganese include a scavenger role in copper and aluminum alloys and in a production of dry cell batteries. Various manganese compounds are widely used in fertilizers, animal feeds, pharmaceutical products, dyes, paint dryers, catalysts, and wood preservatives and in production of glass and ceramics. The manganese-based compound methylcyclopentadienyl manganese tricarbonyl is a fuel supplement used to increase the octane level of gasoline and though banned in 1977 is currently approved for use in the United States.[54]

Absorption, Transport, and Excretion

Roughly 2% to 15% of dietary manganese is absorbed in the small intestine. Dietary factors that affect manganese absorption include iron, calcium, phosphates, and fiber.[25] Manganese absorption is age dependent, with infants retaining higher levels of manganese than adults. Manganese is a normal component in tissue with the highest levels found in fat and bone. Though accumulation of manganese in the healthy population has not been observed, chronic liver disease or other types of liver dysfunction can reduce manganese elimination and promote accumulation in various regions of the brain.[54] Manganese elimination occurs predominately through the bile.

Health Effects, Deficiency, and Toxicity

Manganese is biochemically essential as a constituent of metalloenzymes and as an enzyme activator. Manganese-containing enzymes include arginase, pyruvate carboxylase, and manganese superoxide dismutase in the mitochondria. Manganese-activated enzymes include hydrolases, kinases, decarboxylases, and transferases. Many of these activations are not specific to manganese, and other metal ions (magnesium, iron, or copper) can replace manganese as an activator and mask the effects of manganese deficiency.[25]

Blood clotting defects, hypocholesterolemia, dermatitis, and elevated serum calcium, phosphorus, and alkaline phosphatase activity have been observed in some subjects who underwent experimental manganese depletion.[25] Low levels of manganese have been associated with epilepsy,[7] hip abnormalities, joint disease, congenital malformation,[25] heart and bone problems, and stunted growth in children.[55]

Manganese toxicity causes nausea, vomiting, headache, disorientation, memory loss, anxiety, and compulsive laughing or crying. Chronic manganese toxicity resembles Parkinson's disease with akinesia, rigidity, tremors, and masklike faces.[7] A clinical condition named *locura manganica* (manganese madness) was described in Chilean manganese miners with acute manganese aerosol intoxication.[56]

Laboratory Evaluation of Manganese Status

Manganese is measured by ICP-MS and GFAAS. Urine manganese is used in conjunction with serum manganese to evaluate possible toxicity or deficiency.

MOLYBDENUM

Introduction

Molybdenum (Mo) is a hard, silvery white metal occurring naturally as molybdenite, wulfenite, and powelite. Most molybdenum is used for the production of alloys, as well as catalysts, corrosion inhibitors, flame retardants, smoke depressants, lubricants, and molybdenum blue pigments. Molybdenum is an essential trace element with the importance of molybdenum-containing organic compounds in biological systems identified over 80 years ago.[57]

Absorption, Transport, and Excretion

Between 25% and 80% of ingested molybdenum is absorbed predominately in the stomach and small intestine,[25] with the majority of absorbed molybdenum retained in the liver, skeleton, and kidney. In blood, molybdenum is extensively bound to α_2-macroglobulin and to red blood cell membranes.[57] Molybdenum can cross the placental barrier, and high levels of molybdenum in the diet of the mother can increase the molybdenum in the liver of the neonate.[58]

Health Effects, Deficiency, and Toxicity

Molybdenum is vital to human health through its inclusion in at least three enzymes: xanthine oxidase, aldehyde oxidase, and sulfite oxidase. The active site of these enzymes binds molybdenum in the form of a cofactor "molybdopterin."[7]

Dietary molybdenum deficiency is rare with a single case reported as a result of total parenteral nutrition in a man

with Crohn's disease.[57] Molybdenum cofactor deficiency is a recessively inherited error of metabolism due to a lack of functional molybdopterin. The symptoms include seizures, anterior lens dislocation, decreased brain weight, and usually death prior to 1 year of age.[7]

Molybdenum toxicity is rarely reported as there are few known cases of human exposure to excess molybdenum. High dietary and occupational exposures to molybdenum have been linked to elevated uric acid in blood and an increased incidence of gout.[25]

Molybdenum is rapidly eliminated in both urine and bile, with urine excretion predominating when intake is high.[57]

Laboratory Evaluation of Molybdenum Status

Molybdenum levels are measured by ICP-MS and GFAAS. Blood levels are less than 60 µg/L.[57]

SELENIUM

Introduction

Selenium (Se) is a naturally occurring metalloid with many chemical and physical properties similar to those of sulfur. Selenium is an essential trace element and a major constituent of 40 minerals and a minor constituent of 37 others.[59] Most processed selenium is used in the electronics industry; however, other uses include nutritional supplements, pigments, pesticides, rubber production, antidandruff shampoos, and fungicides.

Absorption, Transport, and Excretion

Selenium is well absorbed from the gastrointestinal tract (~50%). Selenium exposure occurs primarily from food but can be found in drinking water, usually in the form of inorganic sodium selenate or sodium selenite. Selenium homeostasis is largely achieved by excretion via urine and feces. Other routes or elimination include sweat and, at very high intakes, exhalation of volatile forms of selenium.[60]

Health Effects, Deficiency, and Toxicity

In the 1930s, selenium was considered a toxic element; in the 1940s, a carcinogen; in the 1950s, it was declared an essential element; and since the 1960s and especially the 1970s, it has been viewed as an anticarcinogen. Glutathione peroxidase (in the form of selenocysteine) is part of the cellular antioxidant defense system against free radicals,[25] and selenium is also involved in the metabolism of thyroid hormones[61] (e.g., deiodinase enzymes and thioredoxin reductase).[60]

Selenium deficiency has been associated with cardiomyopathy, skeletal muscle weakness, and osteoarthritis. A significant negative correlation was observed between selenium intakes and the rate of cancer of the large intestine, rectum, prostate, breast, ovary, and lungs and leukemia.[59]

Keshan disease, an endemic cardiomyopathy that affects mostly children and women in childbearing age in certain areas in China, has been associated with selenium deficiency. Symptoms include dizziness, malaise, loss of appetite, nausea, chills, abnormal electrocardiograms, cardiogenic shock, cardiac enlargements, and congestive heart failure. Selenium supplementation has been shown to effectively control Keshan disease.[25] Kashin-Beck disease, an endemic osteoarthritis that occurs during adolescent and preadolescent years, is another disease linked to low selenium status in northern China, North Korea, and eastern Siberia.[62]

Acute oral exposure to extremely high levels of selenium may produce gastrointestinal symptoms (nausea, vomiting, and diarrhea) and cardiovascular symptoms such as tachycardia. Chronic exposure to very high levels can cause dermal effects, including diseased nails and skin and hair loss, as well as neurologic problems such as unsteady gait or paralysis.[60] In 1984, 12 cases of selenium toxicity were reported to the FDA and CDC, because of the ingestion of selenium supplements, containing levels almost 200 times higher than stated on the label. The most common symptoms reported in these cases were nausea and vomiting, nail changes, hair loss, fatigue, abdominal cramps, watery diarrhea, and garlicky breath. No abnormalities of blood chemistry were seen in 67% of the victims, and renal and liver functions were normal.[63]

The EPA has determined that one specific form of selenium, selenium sulfide, is a probable human carcinogen. Selenium sulfide is a very different chemical from the organic and inorganic selenium compounds found in foods and in the environment.[62] In Hubei Province (China) during 1961 through 1964, almost half of the population of many villages died from chronic selenosis. The most common signs of selenium poisoning were loss of hair and nails, skin lesions, tooth decay, and abnormalities of the nervous system.[59]

Laboratory Evaluation of Selenium Status

Selenium is most often determined by ICP-MS or GFAAS. The determination of urinary and blood selenium is a useful measure of selenium status.

ZINC

Introduction

Zinc (Zn) is a bluish-white, lustrous metal that is stable in dry air and becomes covered with a white coating when exposed to moisture. Zinc is used in a production of alloys, especially brass (with copper), in galvanizing steel, in die casting, in paints, in skin lotions, as treatment for Wilson's disease, and in many over-the-counter medications. Zinc is an essential trace element, and deficiency is common throughout life, especially in individuals who do not ingest meat.

Absorption, Transport, and Excretion

The body content in a normal individual varies substantially with age and is predominantly distributed in muscle (60%) and the skeleton (30%). The remaining 10% is distributed in various other tissues with highest concentrations found in the eyes, prostate, and hair. Zinc absorption mainly occurs in the small intestine and especially in the jejunum.[64] Factors increasing zinc absorption include the presence of animal proteins[65]

and amino acids in a meal,[66] intake of calcium,[67] and unsaturated fatty acids.[68] Conversely, factors decreasing zinc absorption include the intake of iron,[69,70] taking zinc on an empty stomach,[68] presence of copper at high levels,[71] and age.[72] In blood, the absorbed zinc is distributed between red blood cells (80%), plasma (17%), and white blood cells (3%).[73] In normal dietary circumstances, about 90% of zinc is excreted in feces.[74]

Health Effects, Deficiency, and Toxicity

Zinc is second only to iron in importance as an essential trace element. The main biochemical role of zinc is seen in its influence on the activity of more than 300 enzymes in classes such as oxidoreductases, transferases, hydrolases, leases, isomerases, and lipases. As a result of the importance of zinc for the structure, regulation, and catalytic action of various enzymes, zinc is indirectly involved in the synthesis and metabolism of DNA and RNA, the synthesis and metabolism of proteins, the metabolism of glucose and cholesterol, membrane structure maintenance, insulin function, and growth factor effects.[64] Chronic oral zinc supplementation interferes with copper absorption and may cause copper deficiency forming the basis for using zinc to treat Wilson's disease.

Zinc deficiency causes growth retardation, slows skeletal maturation, causes testicular atrophy, and reduces taste perception. Old age, pregnancy, lactation, and alcoholism are also associated with poor zinc nutrition.[25] Infants with acrodermatitis enteropathica (zinc malabsorption) first develop a characteristic facial and diaper rash. Untreated, symptoms progress and include growth retardation, diarrhea, impaired T-cell immunity, insufficient wound healing, infections, delayed testicular development in adolescence, and early death.[7] Zn deficiency in adolescents is manifested by slow growth or weight loss, altered taste, delayed puberty, dwarfism, impaired dark adaptation, alopecia, emotional instability, and tremors. In severe cases, lymphopenia and death can result from an overwhelming infection.[7]

Zinc is relatively nontoxic. Nevertheless, high doses (1 g) or repetitive doses of 100 mg/d for several months may lead to gastrointestinal tract symptoms, decrease in heme synthesis due to an induced copper deficiency, and hyperglycemia.[64] Exposure to ZnO fumes and dust may cause "zinc fume fever," with symptoms including chemically induced pneumonia, severe pulmonary inflammation, fever, hyperpnea, coughing, pains in legs and chest, and vomiting.[64]

Laboratory Evaluation of Zinc Status

Zinc is measured by flame AAS, ICP-AES, and ICP-MS. Low urine zinc levels in the presence of low serum zinc levels usually confirm zinc deficiency.[7] Low serum zinc in an apparently healthy (nonstressed, nonseptic) patient who has normal serum albumin levels can be used as evidence of zinc deficiency, especially if urine zinc levels are also low. Normal serum zinc cannot be interpreted as evidence of normal zinc stores. Zinc concentration in red blood cells is approximately ten times that in serum.[25] Copper status should be monitored in patients on long-term zinc therapy.[7,72]

For additional student resources, please visit the Point® at http://thepoint.lww.com

questions

1. Extreme copper deficiency is seen in what fatal condition?
   a. Menkes' disease
   b. Klinefelter's syndrome
   c. Meese disease
   d. Kayser-Fleischer rings

2. Suppose the controller on a GFAAS is defective and the furnace is running cold. What effect will this likely have on the number of photons absorbed in the measurements?
   a. It will decrease the number of photons absorbed.
   b. It will increase the number of photons absorbed.
   c. It will have little effect.
   d. It is not a relevant question because AAS relies on emission of light from electronically excited atoms.

3. Why would a clinical chemist develop an arsenic method that combines liquid chromatography with ICP-MS?
   a. To separate and quantitate several different arsenic-containing species in the same sample
   b. To eliminate interference by sodium from the analysis
   c. To shorten the run time of the measurement
   d. To lower the coefficient of variation for total arsenic measurements

4. Select the answer that designates three techniques widely used for elemental analysis, identified according to the initials for the techniques.
   a. AAS, ICP-MS, AES
   b. NMR, ICP-MS, AES
   c. GC-MS, ICP-MS, AES
   d. HPLC-ICP-MS, AAS, FTIR

5. One of the calcium isotopes (^{40}Ca) has an atomic weight of 40. At what positions in a mass spectrum would singly and doubly charged ions of this isotope of calcium appear? Assume that singly charged Ca is listed first.
   a. 40 and 20
   b. 40 and 60
   c. 40 and 80
   d. 40 and 40

6. What primary purposes does the torch serve in ICP-MS?
   a. Vaporization, atomization, and ionization
   b. Vaporization, atomization, and electronic excitation
   c. Nebulization, atomization, and photon absorption
   d. Droplet transport, vaporization, and ion detection

7. Manganese toxicity resembles the following disease:
   a. Parkinson's disease
   b. Wilson's disease
   c. Alzheimer's disease
   d. Menkes' disease

8. Iron is physiologically active only in the ferrous form in
   a. Hemoglobin
   b. Cytochromes
   c. Ferritin
   d. Transferrin

9. A metal ion required for optimal enzyme activity is best termed a(an)
   a. Cofactor
   b. Accelerator
   c. Coenzyme
   d. Catalyst

10. Which trace metal is contained in glucose tolerance factor?
   a. Chromium
   b. Copper
   c. Selenium
   d. Zinc

11. What metal may be used as a treatment for Wilson's disease?
   a. Zinc
   b. Copper
   c. Molybdenum
   d. Fluorine

12. The metal ion essential for the activity of xanthine oxidase and xanthine dehydrogenase is
   a. Molybdenum
   b. Iron
   c. Zinc
   d. Manganese

bibliography

Holstege CP. Heavy metals. In: Holstege CP, Borloz MP, Benner JP, eds. *Toxicology Recall*. Baltimore, MD: Lippincott Williams & Wilkins; 2009:256–310.

Jacobs DS, DeMott WR, Oxley DK. *Jacobs & DeMott Laboratory Test Handbook*. 5th ed. Lexi-Comp's Clinical Reference Library. Hudson, OH: Lexi-Comp.; 2001:1031.

Nordberg G, Fowler B, Nordberg M, et al. *Handbook on the Toxicology of Metals*. 3rd ed. Amsterdam; Boston, MA: Academic Press; 2007:xlvii, 975.

Pais I, Jones JB. *The Handbook of Trace Elements*. Boca Raton, FL: St. Lucie Press; 1997:xv, 223.

Seiler HG, Sigel A, Sigel H. *Handbook on Metals in Clinical and Analytical Chemistry*. New York, NY: Marcel Dekker; 1994:xx, 753.

Thomas R. *Practical Guide to ICP-MS: a Tutorial for Beginners*. 2nd ed. Practical spectroscopy. Boca Raton, FL: CRC Press; 2008:xxv, 347.

references

1. Rodushkin I, Odman F, Branth S. Multielemental analysis of whole blood by high resolution inductively coupled plasma mass spectrometry. *Fresenius J Anal Chem*. 1999;364:338–346.
2. May T, Wiedmeyer R. A table of polyatomic interferences in ICP-MS. *Atom Spectrosc*. 1998:19.
3. Vaughan M, Horlick G. Correction procedures for rare earth analysis in inductively coupled plasma-mass spectrometry. *Appl Spectrosc*. 1990;44:587–593.
4. Thomas R. *Practical Guide to ICP-MS: a Tutorial for Beginners*. 2nd ed. Boca Raton, FL: CRC Press; 2008:xxv, 347.
5. Sobin C, Parisi N, Schaub T, et al. A bland–altman comparison of the lead care® system and inductively coupled plasma mass spectrometry for detecting low-level lead in child whole blood samples. *J Med Toxicol*. 2011;7:24–32.
6. Agency for Toxic Substances & Disease Registry. Aluminum. http://www.atsdr.cdc.gov/toxfaqs/tf.asp?id=190&tid=34 (Accessed January 2012).
7. Jacobs DS, DeMott WR, Oxley DK. *Jacobs & Demott Laboratory Test Handbook*. 5th ed. Hudson, OH: Lexi-Comp.; 2001:1031.
8. Schaller K, Letzel S, Angerer J. Aluminum. In: Seiler H, Sigel A, Sigel H, eds. *Handbook on Metals in Clinical and Analytical Chemistry*. New York, NY: Marcel Dekker; 1994:217–226.
9. Alfrey A. Aluminum. In: Mertz W, Underwood EJ, eds. *Trace Elements in Human and Animal Nutrition*. Vol. 1. 5th ed. St. Louis, MO: Academic Press; 1986:399–413.
10. Baselt R. Disposition of toxic drugs and chemicals in man. In: Baselt R, ed. *Disposition of Toxic Drugs and Chemicals in Man*. 8th ed. Seal Beach, CA: Biomedical Publications; 2004:39–41.
11. Sjögren B, Iregren A, Elinder C, et al. Aluminum. In: Nordberg G, Fowler B, Nordberg M, et al., eds. *Handbook on the Toxicology of Metals*. 3rd ed. Amsterdam; Boston, MA: Academic Press; 2007:339–352.
12. U.S. Environmental Protection Agency. Arsenic compounds. www.epa.gov/ttn/atw/hlthef/arsenic.html (Accessed January 2012).
13. Iffland R. Arsenic. In: Seiler H, Sigel A, Sigel H, eds. *Handbook on Metals in Clinical and Analytical Chemistry*. New York, NY: Marcel Dekker; 1994:237–253.
14. Fowler B, Chou C-HS, Jones R, et al. Arsenic. In: Nordberg G, Fowler B, Nordberg M, et al., eds. *Handbook on the Toxicology of Metals*. 3rd ed. Amsterdam; Boston, MA: Academic Press; 2007:367–406.
15. Kamimura T, Miyamoto T, Harada M, et al. Advances in therapies for acute promyelocytic leukemia. *Cancer Sci*. 2011;102:1929–1937.
16. Anke M. Arsenic. In: Mertz W, Underwood EJ, eds. *Trace Elements in Human and Animal Nutrition*. Vol. 2. 5th ed. St. Louis, MO: Academic Press; 1986:347–372.
17. Pais I, Jones JB. *The Handbook of Trace Elements*. Boca Raton, FL: St. Lucie Press; 1997:xv, 223.
18. U.S. Environmental Protection Agency. Cadmium. http://www.epa.gov/iris/subst/0141.htm (Accessed January 2012).
19. Agency for Toxic Substances & Disease Registry. Cadmium. http://www.atsdr.cdc.gov/substances/toxsubstance.asp?toxid=15 (Accessed January 2012).
20. Moyer T, Burritt M, Butz J. Toxic metals. In: Burtis CA, Ashwood ER, Bruns DE, eds. *Tietz Textbook of Clinical Chemistry and Molecular Diagnostics*. 4th ed. Philadelphia, PA: WB Saunders; 2006:1377–1378.
21. Herber RFM. Cadmium. In: Seiler HG, Sigel A, Sigel H, et al., eds. *Handbook on Metals in Clinical and Analytical Chemistry*. New York, NY: Marcel Dekker; 1994:283–297.
22. Nordberg G, Nogawa K, Nordberg M, et al. Cadmium. In: Nordberg G, Fowler B, Nordberg M, et al., eds. *Handbook on the Toxicology of Metals*. 3rd ed. Amsterdam; Boston, MA: Academic Press; 2007:445–486.
23. Herold DA, Fitzgerald RL. Chromium. In: Seiler H, Sigel A, Sigel H, eds. *Handbook on Metals in Clinical and Analytical Chemistry*. New York, NY: Marcel Dekker; 1994:321–332.
24. Offenbacher EG, Pi-Sunyer FX. Chromium in human nutrition. *Annu Rev Nutr*. 1988;8:543–563.
25. Shenkin A, Baines M, Lyon T. Vitamins and trace elements. In: Burtis CA, Ashwood ER, Bruns DE, eds. *Tietz Textbook of Clinical Chemistry and Molecular Diagnostics*. 4th ed. Philadelphia, PA: WB Saunders; 2006:1075–1164.
26. Langård S, Costa M. Chromium. In: Nordberg G, Fowler B, Nordberg M, et al., eds. *Handbook on the Toxicology of Metals*. 3rd ed. Amsterdam; Boston, MA: Academic Press; 2007:487–510.
27. U.S. Food and Drug Administration. Information for all health care professionals who provide treatment to patients with a metal-on-metal hip implant system. http://www.fda.gov/MedicalDevices/ProductsandMedicalProcedures/ImplantsandProsthetics/MetalonMetalHipImplants/ucm241744.htm (Accessed January 2012).
28. Walter LR, Marel E, Harbury R, et al. Distribution of chromium and cobalt ions in various blood fractions after resurfacing hip arthroplasty. *J Arthroplasty*. 2008;23:814–821.
29. Ellingsen D, Horn N, Aaseth J. Copper. In: Nordberg G, Fowler B, Nordberg M, et al., eds. *Handbook on the Toxicology of Metals*. 3rd ed. Amsterdam; Boston, MA: Academic Press; 2007:529–546.
30. Sarkar B. Copper. In: Seiler HG, Sigel A, Sigel H, eds. *Handbook on Metals in Clinical and Analytical Chemistry*. New York, NY: Marcel Dekker; 1994:339–347.
31. Holstege CP. Heavy metals. In: Holstege CP, Borloz MP, Benner JP, eds. *Toxicology Recall*. Baltimore, MD: Lippincott Williams & Wilkins; 2009:256–310.
32. McMillin GA, Travis JJ, Hunt JW. Direct measurement of free copper in serum or plasma ultrafiltrate. *Am J Clin Pathol*. 2009;131:160–165.

33. Higgins T, Beutler E, Doumas B. Hemoglobin, iron, and bilirubin. In: Burtis CA, Ashwood ER, Bruns DE, eds. *Tietz Textbook of Clinical Chemistry and Molecular Diagnostics.* 4th ed. Philadelphia, PA: WB Saunders; 2006:1165–1208.
34. Rossi E. Hepcidin—the iron regulatory hormone. *Clin Biochem Rev.* 2005;26:47–49.
35. Beard JL, Dawson H, Piñero DJ. Iron metabolism: a comprehensive review. *Nutr Rev.* 1996;54:295–317.
36. Meneghini R. Iron homeostasis, oxidative stress, and DNA damage. *Free Radic Biol Med.* 1997;23:783–792.
37. Smith C, Mitchinson MJ, Aruoma OI, et al. Stimulation of lipid peroxidation and hydroxyl-radical generation by the contents of human atherosclerotic lesions. *Biochem J.* 1992;286(Pt 3):901–905.
38. Schwartz CJ, Valente AJ, Sprague EA, et al. The pathogenesis of atherosclerosis: an overview. *Clin Cardiol.* 1991;14:I1–I16.
39. Anghileri LJ. Iron, intracellular calcium ion, lipid peroxidation and carcino-genesis. *Anticancer Res.* 1995;15:1395–400.
40. Weinberg ED. Cellular iron metabolism in health and disease. *Drug Metab Rev.* 1990;22:531–579.
41. McCord JM. Iron, free radicals, and oxidative injury. *Semin Hematol.* 1998;35:5–12.
42. Smith MA, Perry G. Free radical damage, iron, and alzheimer's disease. *J Neurol Sci.* 1995;134(suppl):92–94.
43. Herbert V, Shaw S, Jayatilleke E. Vitamin c-driven free radical generation from iron. *J Nutr.* 1996;126:1213S–1220S.
44. Tofaletti JG. Trace elements. In: Bishop ML, Fody EP, Schoeff LE, eds. *Clinical Chemistry: Principles, Procedures, Correlations.* 5th ed. Philadelphia, PA: Lippincott Williams & Wilkins; 2004.
45. ARUP Laboratories. I. Hemochromatosis. http://www.arupconsult.com/Topics/Hemochromatosis.html (Accessed January 2012).
46. Christensen J, Kristiansen J. Lead. In: Seiler H, Sigel A, Sigel H, eds. *Handbook on Metals in Clinical and Analytical Chemistry.* New York, NY: Marcel Dekker; 1994:425–440.
47. Skerfving S, Bergdahl I. Lead. In: Nordberg G, Fowler B, Nordberg M, et al., eds. *Handbook on the Toxicology of Metals.* 3rd ed. Amsterdam; Boston, MA: Academic Press; 2007:599–643.
48. Boffetta P, Nyberg F. Contribution of environmental factors to cancer risk. *Br Med Bull.* 2003;68:71–94.
49. Berlin M, Zalups R, Fowler B. Mercury. In: Nordberg G, Fowler B, Nordberg M, et al., eds. *Handbook on the Toxicology of Metals.* 3rd ed. Amsterdam; Boston, MA: Academic Press; 2007:675–729.
50. Drash G. Mercury. In: Seiler H, Sigel A, Sigel H, eds. *Handbook on Metals in Clinical and Analytical Chemistry.* New York, NY: Marcel Dekker; 1994:479–493.
51. Goyer R, Klaassen CD, Waalkes MP. Nervous system. In: Goyer RA, Klaassen CD, Waalkes MP, eds. *Metal Toxicology.* San Diego, CA: Academic Press; 1995:199–235.
52. Porter W, Moyer T. Clinical toxicology. In: Burtis CA, Ashwood ER, eds. *Tietz Fundamentals of Clinical Chemistry.* 4th ed. Philadelphia, PA: WB Saunders; 2006:427–456.
53. Ashwood E. *Clinical Testing.* New York, NY: ARUP Laboratories; 2004:101–102.
54. Šaric´ M, Lucchini R. Manganese. In: Nordberg G, Fowler B, Nordberg M, et al., eds. *Handbook on the Toxicology of Metals.* 3rd ed. Amsterdam; Boston, MA: Academic Press; 2007:645–674.
55. Kaiser J. State court to rule on manganese fume claims. *Science (New York, NY).* 2003;300:927.
56. Donaldson J. The physiopathologic significance of manganese in brain: its relation to schizophrenia and neurodegenerative disorders. *Neurotoxicology.* 1987;8:451–462.
57. Turnlund J, Friberg L. Molybdenum. In: Nordberg G, Fowler B, Nordberg M, et al., eds. *Handbook on the Toxicology of Metals.* 3rd ed. Amsterdam; Boston, MA: Academic Press; 2007:731–741.
58. Anke M, Giel M. Molybdenum. In: Seiler H, Sigel A, Sigel H, eds. *Handbook on Metals in Clinical and Analytical Chemistry.* New York, NY: Marcel Dekker; 1994:495–501.
59. Magee R, James B. Selenium. In: Seiler H, Sigel A, Sigel H, eds. *Handbook on Metals in Clinical and Analytical Chemistry.* New York, NY: Marcel Dekker; 1994:551–562.
60. Högberg J, Alexander J. Selenium. In: Nordberg G, Fowler B, Nordberg M, et al., eds. *Handbook on the Toxicology of Metals.* 3rd ed. Amsterdam; Boston, MA: Academic Press; 2007:783–807.
61. Gladyshev VN, Jeang KT, Stadtman TC. Selenocysteine, identified as the penultimate c-terminal residue in human t-cell thioredoxin reductase, corresponds to TGA in the human placental gene. *Proc Natl Acad Sci U S A.* 1996;93:6146–6151.
62. Agency for Toxic Substances & Disease Registry. Selenium. http://www.atsdr.cdc.gov/substances/toxsubstance.asp?toxid=28 (Accessed January 2012).
63. Levander O. Selenium. In: Mertz W, Underwood EJ, eds. *Trace Elements in Human and Animal Nutrition.* Vol. 1. 5th ed. St. Louis, MO: Academic Press; 1986:209–279.
64. Thunus L, Lejeune R. Zinc. In: Seiler H, Sigel A, Sigel H, eds. *Handbook on Metals in Clinical and Analytical Chemistry.* New York, NY: Marcel Dekker; 1994:667–674.
65. Solomons NW. Biological availability of zinc in humans. *Am J Clin Nutr.* 1982;35:1048–1075.
66. Sandstrom B, Cederblad A. Zinc absorption from composite meals. II. Influence of the main protein source. *Am J Clin Nutr.* 1980;33:1778–1783.
67. Sandstrom B, Arvidsson B, Cederblad A, et al. Zinc absorption from composite meals. I. The significance of whest extraction rate, zinc, calcium, and protein content in meals based on bread. *Am J Clin Nutr.* 1980;33:739–745.
68. Cunnane SC. Maternal essential fatty acid supplementation increases zinc absorption in neonatal rats: relevance to the defect in zinc absorption in acrodermatitis enteropathica. *Pediatr Res.* 1982;16:599–603.
69. Solomons NW. Competitive interaction of iron and zinc in the diet: consequences for human nutrition. *J Nutr.* 1986;116:927–935.
70. Sandström B, Davidsson L, Cederblad A, et al. Oral iron, dietary ligands and zinc absorption. *J Nutr.* 1985;115:411–414.
71. Lönnderdal B. Iron-zinc-copper interactions. In: *Micronutrient Interactions Impact on Child Health and Nutrition.* Washington, DC: International Life Sciences Institute; 1996:3–10.
72. Bales CW, Steinman LC, Freeland-Graves JH, et al. The effect of age on plasma zinc uptake and taste acuity. *Am J Clin Nutr.* 1986;44:664–669.
73. Fisher GL. Function and homeostasis of copper and zinc in mammals. *Sci Total Environ.* 1975;4:373–412.
74. Hambridge K, Casey C, Krebs N. Zinc. In: Mertz W, Underwood EJ, eds. *Trace Elements in Human and Animal Nutrition.* Vol. 1. 5th ed. St. Louis, MO: Academic Press; 1986:1–137.

19

Porphyrins and Hemoglobin

ELIZABETH L. FRANK and SARA A. TAYLOR

chapter outline

key terms

Cytochromes
Heme
Hemoglobin
Hemoglobinopathies
Myoglobin
Porphyrias
Porphyrin
Porphyrin precursors
Porphyrinogens
Porphyrinurias
Pyrrole
Thalassemias

chapter objectives

Upon completion of this chapter, the clinical laboratorian should be able to do the following:

- Describe the chemical structure and biological function of porphyrins and hemoglobin.
- Outline the biochemical pathway for the synthesis of heme.
- Define the role of porphyrins as intermediates in the heme biosynthetic pathway.
- Identify the properties of porphyrins and porphyrin precursor compounds that produce disease symptoms, facilitate detection, and differentiate the acute and cutaneous porphyrias.
- Describe the major pathological conditions associated with increased concentration and excretion of porphyrins and porphyrin precursors.
- State the specimen collection, transport, and storage requirements necessary for determinations of porphyrins and porphyrin precursors in the clinical laboratory.
- Discuss commonly used methods for the measurement of porphyrins and precursor compounds in blood, plasma, urine, and feces.
- Suggest possible clinical conditions associated with test results, given patient values for porphyrins and precursor compounds, and supporting clinical information.
- Describe the degradation of hemoglobin.
- Discuss the clinical significance and laboratory data associated with the hemoglobinopathies and thalassemias.
- Identify the laboratory tests used in the diagnosis of hemoglobinopathies and thalassemias.
- Discuss the structure and clinical significance of myoglobin in the body.

For additional student resources, please visit the Point®
at http://thepoint.lww.com

Hemoglobin and **myoglobin** are chemically similar molecules that contain **porphyrin** groups. Porphyrins are cyclic structures comprised of four **pyrrole** rings joined by methine bridges. The arrangement of the pyrrole nitrogen atoms in the porphyrin ring allows chelation of a metal ion to form functional groups that participate in oxidative metabolism. The chelation of ferrous iron to protoporphyrin produces **heme**, the prosthetic group of hemoglobin responsible for binding oxygen. The analysis of porphyrins in the laboratory aids in the diagnosis of a group of rare disorders called **porphyrias** that result from disturbances in heme synthesis.

Hemoglobin molecules are designed to bind, deliver, and release oxygen. Qualitative defects in the hemoglobin molecule result in a group of disorders called **hemoglobinopathies**. Quantitative defects in the production of hemoglobin molecules lead to another group of disorders, called **thalassemias**. Myoglobin is a simple heme protein found in cardiac and skeletal muscles. Damage to the heart or muscle releases myoglobin into the blood. Increased serum myoglobin is seen following acute myocardial infarction (AMI), muscle injury, and intense exercise.

PORPHYRINS

Porphyrins are chemical intermediates in the synthesis of hemoglobin, myoglobin, and other respiratory pigments called **cytochromes**. Iron is chelated to the porphyrin ring to form heme, which is incorporated into proteins to produce biologically functional hemoproteins, such as hemoglobin, myoglobin, cytochrome P450, and the peroxidase and catalase enzymes.[1] Porphyrins are analyzed in clinical chemistry to aid in the diagnosis of porphyrias, diseases that result from disturbances in heme synthesis. Excess amounts of these intermediate compounds in blood, urine, or feces indicate a metabolic block in heme synthesis.

Porphyrin Properties

There are many naturally occurring porphyrins. The pigment chlorophyll is a magnesium porphyrin that enables plants to use light energy to synthesize carbohydrates. Most porphyrins in the human body exist as **porphyrinogens**, reduced compounds that are intermediates in the biosynthesis of heme, the nonprotein, iron-containing prosthetic group of hemoglobin. Porphyrinogens are oxidized on exposure to air to porphyrins. Substitution of the pyrrole rings that make up the porphyrinogen macrocycle generates four isomers for every porphyrin compound; however, only type I and type III isomers occur naturally. These isomers differ in the spatial arrangement of the pyrrole substituents.[2] Only type III isomers form heme; however, in some disorders, the nonfunctional type I isomers may be found in excess in body fluids and tissue.

Porphyrins are photoactive due to extensive conjugation of the tetrapyrrole ring. Their dark red color is due to a strong absorbance in the visible region of the spectrum. The conjugated tetrapyrrole ring is highlighted in the diagram of protoporphyrin shown in Figure 19.1. The compounds

FIGURE 19.1 Structure of porphyrins: protoporphyrin.

absorb light of 400-nm wavelength and emit a characteristic orange-red fluorescence between 600 and 650 nm.[3] This property produces some of the manifestations of disease and provides a means for detection of the compounds in body fluids tested in the laboratory. Aqueous solubility of porphyrins varies with the number of carboxylic acid substituents present in the particular porphyrin compound. Uroporphyrin (Uro) has eight carboxylic acid groups, is the most soluble in water, and is excreted renally. Porphyrins with only two carboxyl groups are the least soluble. These compounds are present in blood and excreted in the feces. Coproporphyrin (Copro) has four carboxylic acid substituents and intermediate solubility. Coproporphyrins are found in blood, urine, and feces. Solubility influences the type of specimen selected for the measurement of particular porphyrin intermediates.

CASE STUDY 19.1

A 58-year-old man with a history of alcoholism complained of increased skin fragility and skin lesion formation on his hands, forehead, neck, and ears on exposure to the sun. On physical examination, hyperpigmentation and hypertrichosis were observed. Laboratory testing of a 24-hour urine specimen showed increased uroporphyrin, heptacarboxyl porphyrin, and a slight increase in coproporphyrin; testing for ALA and PBG was negative. Isocoproporphyrin was elevated in the feces. Serum ferritin and serum transaminase were increased.

Questions

1. What is the most probable disorder?
2. Which confirmatory test should be ordered?
3. What is the most probable precipitating factor?
4. What are other causes of acquired cases of this type of porphyria?
5. How is this type of porphyria differentiated from other porphyrias causing cutaneous symptoms?

CASE STUDY 19.2

A few days after a laparotomy for "intestinal obstruction," a young nurse from South Africa became emotionally disturbed and appeared to be hysterical. For more than 1 week before the surgery, she had taken barbiturate capsules as a sleep aid. She complained of severe abdominal and muscle pain and general weakness. Her tendon reflexes were absent, and she was vomiting and constipated. Her urine was dark in color on standing and gave a brilliant pink fluorescence when viewed in ultraviolet light. Within 24 hours, she was completely paralyzed, and after 2 days she expired.

Questions

1. What possible condition did this young woman have, and why did it manifest at this time?

2. Would members of her family be at risk for a similar disease?

3. Which enzyme defect should be suspected?

4. What other confirmatory tests, if any, could be performed?

Biochemistry: Synthesis of Heme

Although all cells contain hemoproteins and can synthesize heme, the bone marrow and liver are the primary sites for heme production.[2] Biosynthesis is accomplished in a sequence of reactions catalyzed by eight different enzymes in which one molecule of heme is produced from eight molecules of δ-aminolevulinic acid (ALA). The first and last three synthetic reactions require a significant amount of energy and take place in the mitochondrion. Other reactions, which do not require as much energy, occur in the cytosol. Each reaction in the pathway is catalyzed by a particular enzyme. Heme biosynthesis is diagrammed in Figure 19.2.

In the first step in the pathway, glycine and succinyl coenzyme A are condensed to form δ-aminolevulinic acid. In the next reaction, the enzyme porphobilinogen synthase catalyzes condensation of two molecules of ALA to form the monopyrrole porphobilinogen (PBG). Polymerization of four molecules of PBG creates a linear tetrapyrrole, hydroxymethylbilane. This process is catalyzed by the enzyme hydroxymethylbilane synthase (also called PBG deaminase). The enzyme uroporphyrinogen III synthase catalyzes an intramolecular rearrangement and ring closure. The product of this reaction is the cyclic isomer, uroporphyrinogen III. Sequential removal of one carboxyl group from each pyrrole ring in the cyclic tetrapyrrole is catalyzed by uroporphyrinogen decarboxylase. The hepta-, hexa-, penta-, and tetra-carboxyl intermediates are formed in succession. In subsequent reactions, coproporphyrinogen oxidase catalyzes the oxidation of two additional carboxylic acid substituents to form protoporphyrinogen IX, which is oxidized to protoporphyrin (Proto) in a reaction catalyzed by protoporphyrinogen oxidase. In the final step of biosynthesis, ferrochelatase catalyzes the insertion of ferrous iron into the porphyrin ring to form heme.

Heme formation is regulated by negative feedback. Control of the rate of heme synthesis in cells in the liver is achieved largely through regulation of the enzyme δ-aminolevulinic acid synthase (ALAS). Heme inhibits synthesis of the constitutive gene ALAS1 at transcription and translation and also controls transfer from the cytosol to mitochondria.[4] Increases in the pool of hepatic heme diminish the production of ALAS (a negative feedback mechanism). Conversely, ALAS production is increased with a depletion of heme. The size of the regulatory heme pool is influenced by the requirement for hemoproteins in the liver. Drugs and other compounds appear to induce ALAS synthesis by several different mechanisms, but all result in depletion of the regulatory heme pool. Therefore, the rate of heme synthesis can change rapidly in response to a variety of external stimuli. In bone marrow erythrocytes, other enzymes in the pathway and the rate of cellular iron uptake seem to control the rate of heme synthesis.[5]

FIGURE 19.2 Heme biosynthesis.

Spontaneous Formation of Porphyrin Isomers

When the intracellular concentration of PBG is sufficiently high, polymerization occurs without enzymatic catalysis. If the enzyme hydroxymethylbilane synthase is deficient, PBG accumulates and PBG monomers polymerize to the linear tetrapyrrole, hydroxymethylbilane, which spontaneously cyclizes. There is no intramolecular rearrangement and a different isomer, uroporphyrinogen I is formed.[2,4] Uroporphyrinogen I is a substrate for uroporphyrinogen decarboxylase and four carboxyl groups can be removed to produce coproporphyrinogen isomer I. Coproporphyrinogen oxidase cannot oxidize coproporphyrinogen I, which accumulates and is excreted. Deficiency of uroporphyrinogen III synthase allows hydroxymethylbilane to accumulate and cyclize to uroporphyrinogen I, which is decarboxylated to Copro I. In this case, too, coproporphyrinogen I accumulates and is excreted. The porphyrin isomers Uro I and Copro I are found in biological fluids from patients with particular porphyrias.

Pathophysiology: Disorders of Heme Biosynthesis

The porphyrias are a group of rare inherited or acquired metabolic disorders caused by loss or gain of function mutations in the enzymes responsible for heme biosynthesis.[6] The defective enzyme results in overproduction, accumulation, and excretion of toxic precursor compounds and porphyrins. Conditions corresponding to enzyme abnormalities have been identified in every step of heme synthesis. Most of the diseases have an autosomal dominant inheritance pattern (mutation of one gene causes disease), and there is a 50% reduction in activity of the affected enzyme. Some patients demonstrate an enzyme deficiency but do not experience clinical or biochemical manifestations of porphyria, indicating that other factors, such as demand for increased heme biosynthesis, operate to cause disease expression.

Deficient activity of the first enzyme in the pathway, ALA synthase, is associated with an X-linked recessive disorder and sideroblastic anemia—not a porphyria. An X-linked dominant gain-of-function mutation in the erythroid-specific ALAS enzyme results in increased enzyme activity and production of excess protoporphyrin.[7] Deficient activities of any of the other enzymes in the pathway cause a porphyria characterized by excessive accumulation and excretion of intermediate compounds that produce particular symptoms. In most cases, residual enzyme activity produces sufficient heme to prevent anemia. Autosomal recessive diseases also occur; these conditions are associated with more severe symptoms. Late-onset porphyria has been reported as a rare complication of hematologic disorders.[8,9]

Porphyrias can be grouped according to the clinical manifestations of disease.[6,10] An excess of the early precursors in the pathway of heme synthesis (ALA, PBG) causes neuropsychiatric symptoms, including abdominal pain, nausea, constipation, hypertension, psychiatric symptoms, fever, and paresthesia. Porphyrias in this category include ALA dehydratase deficiency porphyria (ADP) and acute intermittent porphyria (AIP). Excesses of porphyrin intermediates produce cutaneous symptoms of photosensitivity, blisters, excess facial hair, and hyperpigmentation. Congenital erythropoietic porphyria (CEP), porphyria cutanea tarda (PCT), erythropoietic protoporphyria (EPP), and X-linked protoporphyria (XLPP) are associated with cutaneous symptoms. Porphyrin-induced photosensitivity manifests through increased fragility of light-exposed skin, in CEP and PCT, or by burning of light-exposed skin, in EPP and XLPP. The photosensitizing effects of the porphyrins are attributed to absorption of light. Excesses of both precursor compounds and porphyrin intermediates cause neurocutaneous symptoms that are found in hereditary coproporphyria (HCP) and variegate porphyria (VP).

Conditions associated with neurological symptoms and serious acute attacks are termed acute porphyrias. The acute porphyrias are ADP, AIP, HCP, and VP. AIP is the most common acute porphyria, although most (~80%) individuals with a genetic defect are asymptomatic. Attacks usually begin in early adulthood, occur more often in women, and may be precipitated by a variety of factors. Severe neurological attacks can be life threatening. In HCP and VP, ineffective catalysis by coproporphyrinogen oxidase or protoporphyrinogen oxidase results in inhibition of hydroxymethylbilane synthase and consequent increase in PBG concentrations. For this reason, HCP and VP are classified as acute porphyrias. In these diseases, porphyrin intermediates accumulate also and symptoms associated with photosensitivity may occur.

The cutaneous (nonacute) porphyrias present as chronic conditions. Exposure to sunlight results in photosensitization of the skin due to accumulation of excess porphyrins in tissues. The porphyrins absorb light and react, producing blistering skin lesions on sun-exposed areas that characterize the disease. CEP, PCT, EPP, and XLPP are cutaneous porphyrias. PCT is the most common cutaneous porphyria and occurs more often as a sporadic condition. Exogenous factors including alcohol consumption, estrogen use, hepatitis C or HIV infection, and increased hepatic iron content, as occurs in hemochromatosis, may precipitate development of PCT. The autosomal recessive disease, CEP, is associated with extreme photosensitivity. Exposure to sunlight destroys the skin and may cause disfiguring changes to facial features, fingers, and toes, and corneal scarring. Hepatoerythropoietic porphyria (HEP) is a homozygous form of PCT characterized by severe clinical symptoms, which are similar to CEP. In EPP, deficiency of ferrochelatase causes accumulation of protoporphyrin in red blood cells, plasma, and feces. Redness, edema, and painful burning sensations occur when skin is exposed to sunlight. Disease onset happens early in life, and porphyria may be overlooked as the cause of these symptoms in a young child. XLPP manifests as increased activity of the erythroid-specific ALAS enzyme and massive production of protoporphyrin with consequent cutaneous symptoms similar to those found in EPP.

Treatment of porphyria is directed at modifying the biochemical abnormalities causing clinical symptoms. Intravenous hematin is used to counteract acute attacks of neurologic dysfunction. Hematin inhibits the enzyme ALAS1 and reduces porphyrin synthesis. Drugs and medications known to precipitate acute attacks must not be used. Cutaneous symptoms are managed by minimizing sun exposure, use of protective clothing and topical sun-blocking agents, and oral administration of β-carotene, which acts as a singlet oxygen trap, to prevent skin damage. Application of the synthetic α-melanocyte-stimulating hormone analogue, afamelanotide, provides photoprotection by increasing melanin in the skin.[11] Phlebotomy, to reduce iron stores, and low-dose chloroquine, to increase porphyrin excretion, are used to treat PCT. Precipitating factors, such as ingestion of alcohol or estrogens, should be avoided. Blood transfusion may be necessary in CEP and HEP. Severe cases of porphyria have been treated effectively with bone marrow or liver transplantation.[6]

Secondary Porphyrinurias

Secondary **porphyrinurias** are acquired conditions associated with increased excretion of urinary porphyrins.[3] The disorders are not the result of an inherited biochemical defect in heme synthesis but are due to another disorder or toxin interfering with heme formation or metabolism. Liver disease and heavy metal poisoning can cause excess urinary porphyrin excretion in the absence of porphyria. Impaired heme synthesis may result from functional changes due to liver diseases such as hepatitis, cirrhosis, and obstructive jaundice.[12] The toxic metal lead inhibits enzymatic formation of PBG, increasing concentrations of ALA, and coproporphyrinogen oxidase function, which causes Copro III to accumulate. Lead interferes with insertion of ferrous iron into heme, and an alternate product, zinc protoporphyrin, is formed by incorporation of zinc ions into the protoporphyrin ring. Some symptoms of lead intoxication are similar to those found in acute porphyria.

Biliary excretion of coproporphyrin isomers is altered in the inherited disorders of bilirubin metabolism (Dubin Johnson, Rotor, and Gilbert syndromes).[13] In Dubin Johnson syndrome, excretion of Copro I is increased and Copro III excretion is decreased. Total urinary coproporphyrin may be slightly elevated, and the ratio of Copro I to Copro III is greater than 80%. In Rotor syndrome, there is a shift from biliary to urinary porphyrin excretion, and total urinary Copro is increased. Copro I accounts for about 70% of the total amount. In Gilbert's syndrome, 50% of urinary coproporphyrin is the Copro I isomer. These ratios are the opposite of the expected coproporphyrin ratio. In unaffected individuals, more Copro III than Copro I is excreted in the urine; the Copro I: Copro III isomer ratio is approximately 30%:70%.[14,15]

Clinical Application

Testing for porphyrins and **porphyrin precursors** is used to diagnose and monitor porphyrias and other disorders of porphyrin metabolism. Methods available for identification of porphyrias include genetic assays to detect DNA mutations, functional and quantitative assays for the enzymes responsible for heme biosynthesis, and biochemical assays to identify and quantify porphyrins and precursor compounds. Only a few specialized laboratories perform molecular genetic testing and enzyme assays.[16] Clinical diagnostic tests for porphyrin disorders are based most often on identification of characteristic patterns of excess porphyrin precursor and intermediate compounds in body fluids (Table 19.1). The specimen tested (urine, blood, or feces) depends on solubility and excretion of the metabolic intermediates associated with particular disease symptoms.

TABLE 19.1 Heme Biosynthesis: Metabolites and Diseases

Pathway Step	Synthetic Reaction	Associated Enzyme	Accumulated Substrates Precursors	Porphyrins	Affected Body Fluids	Porphyria
1	Condensation	ALA synthase	—	Proto	Blood, feces	X-linked protoporphyria
2	Condensation	PBG synthase	ALA	Copro III	Urine	ALA dehydratase deficiency porphyria
3	Polymerization	Hydroxymethylbilane synthase	PBG	Uro	Urine	Acute intermittent porphyria
4	Ring inversion and cyclization	Uroporphyrinogen III synthase	—	Uro I, Copro I	Urine, blood, plasma, feces	Congenital erythropoietic porphyria
5	Decarboxylation	Uroporphyrinogen decarboxylase	—	Uro, Hepta, Hexa, Penta	Urine, plasma, feces	Porphyria cutanea tarda
6	Oxidation	Coproporphyrinogen oxidase	PBG	Copro III	Urine, plasma, feces	Hereditary coproporphyria
7	Oxidation	Protoporphyrinogen oxidase	PBG	Proto, Copro III	Blood, plasma, feces	Variegate porphyria
8	Chelation	Ferrochelatase	—	Proto	Blood, plasma, feces	Erythropoietic protoporphyria

ADP, ALA dehydratase deficiency porphyria; AIP, acute intermittent porphyria; ALA, δ-aminolevulinic acid; CEP, congenital erythropoietic porphyria; Copro, coproporphyrin(ogen); EPP, erythropoietic protoporphyria; HCP, hereditary coproporphyria; Hepta, heptacarboxyl porphyrin(ogen); Hexa, hexacarboxyl porphyrin(ogen); PBG, porphobilinogen; PCT, porphyria cutanea tarda; Penta, pentacarboxyl porphyrin(ogen); Proto, protoporphyrin(ogen); Uro, uroporphyrin(ogen); VP, variegate porphyria; XLPP, X-linked protoporphyria.

Acute symptoms indicate testing for the porphyrin precursors PBG and ALA in urine. Patients with cutaneous photosensitivity are evaluated by examination of blood, urine, and feces for excess porphyrin intermediates.

Testing for Porphyrin Disorders

When an acute porphyria is suspected, initial testing is determination of PBG in a urine specimen. If symptoms are present and due to porphyria, increased concentrations of PBG will be detected in a random urine specimen.[6] A positive test can be followed by measurement of the deficient enzyme, hydroxymethylbilane synthase (PBG deaminase) to identify AIP, and analysis of fecal porphyrins to differentiate among the acute porphyrias (AIP, VP, and HCP). PBG may not be increased in asymptomatic individuals and negative results do not exclude porphyria completely. Testing can be repeated on a specimen collected over 24 hours or when acute symptoms recur.

Initial testing for cutaneous disease requires measurement of porphyrins in a random or timed urine collection.[3] Increased excretion of porphyrins in a characteristic pattern particular for each disease is diagnostic for PCT and CEP. Testing for PBG is negative in these conditions. Suspected EPP or XLPP is evaluated by assessing porphyrins in plasma or whole blood. Plasma testing can be used to monitor PCT, but this specimen is not adequate for diagnosis.

Approach to Testing

Logical testing to investigate symptoms and exclude porphyria is based on the separation of disease symptoms into acute (neurological) and cutaneous categories and allows rapid diagnosis of the more common porphyrias—AIP and PCT—associated with each type.[17] Detection of increased concentrations of PBG in a urine specimen indicates an acute porphyria, and PCT symptoms are associated with a characteristic pattern of urinary porphyrin isomer excretion. Negative test results allow exclusion of porphyria as a cause of symptoms, while positive test results may provoke additional testing to enumerate the particular porphyria or condition.

In some areas, urine or plasma is screened to detect total porphyrin concentration, and additional (reflex) testing is performed on specimens determined to contain elevated amounts of porphyrins. Since this practice may delay diagnosis, it is not recommended if specimens must be submitted to a remote reference laboratory for testing. Genetic analysis to determine the causative mutation should be limited to individuals with positive biochemical test results that establish the diagnosis of a particular porphyria and family members at risk for disease.[10,18]

Analytical Methods

Testing for the precursor compounds, PBG and ALA, utilizes ion exchange chromatography to remove interferences and isolate each compound. Detection is accomplished by the addition of 4-dimethylaminobenzaldehyde (Ehrlich's

reagent) to produce a characteristic rose red color that is detected spectrophotometrically. The principle is that of the Watson-Schwartz assay.[19] The spectrum has an absorbance maximum at approximately 555 nm and a shoulder at 525 nm. Current assays allow quantitative measurement of analyte concentrations.

Porphyrin intermediates may be evaluated using liquid chromatography (HPLC) with fluorescent detection.[3] Urine is acidified to enhance the natural fluorescence of the porphyrins, and an aliquot is injected onto the HPLC system. Separation of the carboxylated porphyrin isomers helps to characterize the particular porphyria. The porphyrin isomers Uro I, Uro III, heptacarboxyl (Hepta), hexacarboxyl, pentacarboxyl, Copro I, and Copro III can be separated within 10 to 12 minutes using a reverse phase analytical column and gradient elution. A dicarboxylated porphyrin (deuteroporphyrin) is used as an internal standard for the assay since these compounds are not found naturally in urine. Measured porphyrin concentrations can be normalized (expressed as a ratio) to creatinine concentration for random urine collections. Results for 24-hour collections are expressed as excretion per day.

Chromatographic analysis of a negative urine specimen shows small amounts of uroporphyrin I and III, little heptacarboxyl porphyrin, more Copro than Uro, and more Copro III than Copro I. Chromatography for a urine specimen positive for PCT reveals large peaks of Uro I, Uro III and Hepta, and Hexa and Penta peaks. Isocoproporphyrin, an alternate metabolic product that is produced when uroporphyrinogen decarboxylase is deficient, is identified in specimens when excretion is high. Massive peaks corresponding to Uro I and Copro I, the isomers that are formed when Uro III synthase is deficient, will be found in a chromatogram characteristic of CEP.

Fecal porphyrin analysis using HPLC with fluorescent detection allows separation and quantification of coproporphyrin isomers and protoporphyrin to differentiate the acute porphyrias AIP, HCP, and VP. An aliquot of the fecal specimen is lyophilized and reconstituted in acidic solution to enhance the natural porphyrin fluorescence before it is subjected to chromatographic analysis. Copro is significantly increased in HCP, and both Proto and Copro may be elevated in VP. Fecal porphyrin excretion is within normal limits (negative) or only slightly increased in AIP. Testing for protoporphyrin to determine presence of EPP or XLPP is performed by scanning fluorescence of a plasma specimen and by analysis of whole blood.

Specimen Requirements

Specimens must be protected from light. Porphyrins and precursor compounds are stable in unpreserved urine at 4°C for up to 48 hours and can be frozen (−20°C) for several weeks. Dilute urine (creatinine <25 mg/dL) is not adequate for analysis. Porphyrins in fecal specimens can be stored frozen (−20°C) for several months. Whole blood collected for protoporphyrin measurement should be anticoagulated with EDTA and stored in the dark at 4°C.[3]

FIGURE 19.3 Hemoglobin A: structure of the hemoglobin molecule.

The amino acid sequences of the globin proteins vary and are the basis of fetal/adult chain nomenclature: α, β, δ, and γ.

The majority of hemoglobin in normal adults is designated as hemoglobin A, or A_1, which contains two α and two β chains (Fig. 19.3). Hemoglobin A_2, which comprises two α and two δ chains, makes up less than 3% of normal adult hemoglobin. The remainder is composed of hemoglobin F, which contains two α and two γ chains. Two types of γ chains may be present in hemoglobin F, $γ^G$ and $γ^A$. These two types of chains are functionally identical but differ in the amino acid present at the 136th position, glycine or alanine, respectively. Hemoglobin F is the main hemoglobin during fetal life and is about 60% of normal hemoglobin at birth. There is a gradual switch from production of γ chains to β chains, and by about age 9 months, hemoglobin F usually constitutes less than 1% of total hemoglobin. Hemoglobin F has a greater affinity for oxygen than hemoglobin A; therefore, it is a more efficient oxygen carrier for the fetus. Hemoglobin F is more resistant to alkali than hemoglobin A, and this is the basis of one laboratory test to differentiate these two types of hemoglobin.

Two other hemoglobin chains, designated ζ and ε, are present only in embryonic life. Production of these chains stops by week 8 of gestation, and γ chain production takes over. The three embryonic hemoglobins are identified as Gower I, two ζ chains and two ε chains; Gower II, two α chains and two ε chains; and Portland I, two ζ chains and two γ chains.

Genetic control of hemoglobin synthesis occurs in two areas: control of structure and control of rate and quantity of production. Defects in structure produce a group of diseases called the *hemoglobinopathies*. Defects in rate and quantity of production lead to disorders called the *thalassemias*. Structurally, each globin chain has its own genetic locus; therefore, it is the individual chains, not the whole hemoglobin molecule, that are under genetic control. The genes for the globin chains can be divided into two major groups: the α genes, located on chromosome 16, and the non–α genes, located on chromosome 11 (Fig. 19.4). In most persons, the α gene locus is duplicated—there are two α chain genes per haploid set of chromosomes, designated $α_1$ and $α_2$. The α gene and, hence, its polypeptide chains are identical in hemoglobins A, A_2, and F. The non–α genes for the β, δ, and γ chains are sufficiently close in genetic terms to be subjected to nonhomologous crossover, with the resulting production of fused or hybrid globin chains,

Since porphyrin analysis typically is offered by large reference laboratories or "porphyrin centers," the most important considerations may be appropriate selection of the test to perform and careful collection, storage, and transport of the specimen.

HEMOGLOBIN

Role in the Body

Hemoglobin has many important functions in the body. Its major role is oxygen transport to the tissue and CO_2 transport back to the lungs. The hemoglobin molecule is designed to take up oxygen in areas of high oxygen tension and release oxygen in areas of low oxygen tension. Hemoglobin is carried to all tissues of the body by erythrocytes. Hemoglobin is also one of the major buffering systems of the body.

Structure of Hemoglobin

The hemoglobin protein is a large, complex molecule that is roughly spherical in shape and is comprised of two major parts: a central oxygen binding, nonprotein heme molecule, and two pairs of identical globin chains (Fig. 19.3).

FIGURE 19.4 Chromosomal structure of the α- and β-globin gene clusters on chromosomes 16 and 11, respectively. Genes with a Ψ (psi) designation represent pseudo-genes. (Used with permission from themedicalbiochemistrypage.org, LLC.)

such as hemoglobin Lepore (δβ-globin chain) and Kenya (γβ-globin chain).

Based on the genetics of the globin chain production, the structural abnormalities, or *hemoglobinopathies*, can be divided into four groups:

1. Amino acid substitutions (e.g., hemoglobins S, C, D, E, O, and G)
2. Amino acid deletion—deletions of three or multiples of three nucleotides in deoxyribonucleic acid (DNA; e.g., hemoglobin Gun Hill)
3. Elongated globin chains resulting from chain termination, frame shift, or other mutations (e.g., hemoglobin Constant Spring)
4. Fused or hybrid chains resulting from nonhomologous crossover (e.g., hemoglobins Lepore and Kenya)

The amino acid substitutions are the most common abnormalities, with several hundred described so far. Approximately two-thirds of the hemoglobinopathies have an affected β chain. They may be clinically silent or they may cause severe damage, as with hemoglobin S. Amino acid substitutions, for the majority of defects, result from a single-base nucleotide substitution in DNA.

Absent or diminished synthesis of one of the polypeptide chains of human hemoglobin characterizes the *thalassemias*, a heterogeneous group of inherited disorders. In α-thalassemia, α-globin chain synthesis is absent or reduced; in β-thalassemia, β-globin chain synthesis is absent (β⁰-thal) or partially reduced (β⁺-thal).

Synthesis and Degradation of Hemoglobin

Hemoglobin synthesis occurs in the immature red blood cells (RBCs) located in the bone marrow. Normal synthesis depends on heme synthesis in the cell mitochondria, globin synthesis in the cytoplasm, and on an adequate iron supply. Newly synthesized heme exits the mitochondria and complexes with four globin molecules in the cell cytoplasm. Iron is transported from stores to the developing RBCs where it is inserted into heme and is available to bind oxygen.

Hemoglobin is degraded either in the blood vessels (intravascular hemolysis) or outside of the circulatory system within the phagocytic cells of the spleen, liver, and bone marrow (extravascular hemolysis). Laboratory measurement of hemoglobin degradation products can help to determine increased RBC destruction, such as in a hemolytic anemia (Chapters 11 and 27).

Clinical Significance and Disease Correlation
Hemoglobin Qualitative Defects: The Hemoglobinopathies
Hemoglobin S
The amino acid defect in hemoglobin S is at the sixth position on the β chain, where glutamic acid is substituted by valine, giving the hemoglobin a less negative charge than hemoglobin A. This is the most common hemoglobinopathy in the United States.

CASE STUDY 19.3

A 32-year-old African American woman came to the obstetrics and gynecology clinic of her local hospital because she was feeling a little weak. A CBC showed hemoglobin of 9.9 g/dL (reference range 11.7 to 15.7 g/dL), with an MCV of 87 fL (reference range 80 to 100 fL). The physician ordered a hemoglobin electrophoresis as a follow-up. The cellulose acetate pattern showed a peak of 58% at the hemoglobin A position, a peak of 35% at the hemoglobin S position, and a peak of 5% at the A₂ position. Further studies indicated a positive dithionite solubility test result and a hemoglobin F value of 1%.

Questions

1. What is the best possible diagnosis for this woman?
2. Does this condition require further follow-up and treatment?
3. What implications does this disease have for her unborn child?
4. Are the values for hemoglobins A₂ and F normal for this condition?

Individuals have either sickle cell trait (HbAS, the heterozygous state) or sickle cell disease (HbSS, the homozygous state). Black Africans and African Americans have the highest incidence: 1 of 500 infants has sickle cell anemia and 8% to 10% carry the HbAS trait. It is also found in Mediterranean countries, such as Greece, Italy, and Israel, as well as in Saudi Arabia and India.

Because of the high morbidity and mortality associated with homozygous expression of the gene, the frequency of the mutant gene would be expected to decline in the gene pool. However, a phenomenon known as balanced polymorphism exists, which indicates that the heterozygous state (HbAS) has a selective advantage over either of the homozygous states (HbAA or HbSS). It appears that the heterozygous condition offers protection from parasites, particularly *Plasmodium falciparum*, especially in children. When infected with *P. falciparum*, children with sickle cell trait have a lower parasite count, the infection is shorter in duration, and the incidence of death is low. It is thought that the infected RBCs are preferentially sickled and, therefore, efficiently destroyed by phagocytic cells.[20]

When hemoglobin S is deoxygenated in vitro under near-physiologic conditions, it becomes relatively insoluble as compared with hemoglobin A and aggregates into long, rigid polymers called *tactoids*. These cells appear as sickle- or crescent-shaped forms on stained blood films. Sickled cells may return to their original shape when oxygenated; however, after several sickling episodes, irreversible membrane damage occurs and cells are phagocytized by macrophages in the spleen, liver, or bone marrow, causing anemia. The severity of the hemolytic process is directly related to the number of damaged cells in circulation. The rigid sickled cells are unable to deform and circulate through small capillaries, resulting in blockage. Tissue hypoxia results, causing extreme pain and leading to tissue death. Infarctions in the spleen are common, causing excessive necrosis and scarring, leading to a nonfunctional spleen in most adults with sickle cell anemia. This is referred to as *autosplenectomy*. The amount of sickling is related to the amount of hemoglobin S in the cells. The reported inhibitory effect of hemoglobins A and F is due to a dilutional effect. There is also a lower tendency for hemoglobin F to copolymerize with hemoglobin S than with hemoglobin A. This is considered responsible for the observed protective effect of elevated hemoglobin F levels in individuals with sickle cell anemia.

Laboratory findings in the homozygous disease include a normocytic, normochromic anemia, increased reticulocyte count, and variation in size and shape of RBCs with target cells and sickle cells present. Polychromatophilia and nucleated RBCs are common. The heterozygous disease is clinically asymptomatic and usually has a normal blood film. The solubility test for hemoglobin S will be positive in both homozygous and heterozygous forms but should always be confirmed with hemoglobin electrophoresis. On cellulose acetate electrophoresis at an alkaline pH, hemoglobin S moves in a position between hemoglobin A and A_2. Of total hemoglobin, 85% to 100% will be hemoglobin S in the homozygous state and usually less than 50% in the heterozygous state. Hemoglobins D and G migrate in the same position as hemoglobin S, but both would be negative with the solubility test. Electrophoresis on citrate agar at an acid pH is necessary to separate these hemoglobins from hemoglobin S (see Fig. 19.4.1).

Hemoglobin C

The glutamic acid in the sixth position of the β chain is replaced by lysine, resulting in a net positive charge. Hemoglobin C is found in West Africa in the vicinity of North Ghana in 17% to 28% of the population and in 2% to 3% of African Americans.

The heterozygous form, hemoglobin AC, is asymptomatic. The homozygous form usually causes a mild, well-compensated anemia characterized by abdominal pain and splenomegaly. The most prominent laboratory feature is the presence of target cells. There is a tendency to form large, oblong, hexagonal crystalloid structures within the red cell. These structures are most prominent in patients who have undergone splenectomy.

A differential diagnosis is obtained by cellulose acetate electrophoresis. Hemoglobin C moves with hemoglobin A_2 and is negative with the solubility test. In the heterozygous form, hemoglobin C falls in the range of 35% to 48%. Hemoglobins E, O, and C_{Harlem} migrate with hemoglobin C. These hemoglobin variants can be readily distinguished from hemoglobin C by citrate agar electrophoresis at an acid pH.

Hemoglobin SC

Hemoglobin SC disease is the most common *mixed hemoglobinopathy*. One β gene codes for β-S chains and the other β gene codes for β-C chains, leaving no normal β chains to produce hemoglobin A. Clinically, this disease is less severe than homozygous sickle cell anemia but has similar clinical symptoms. The blood film characteristically shows many target cells and occasional abnormal shapes resembling the sickle cell, the hexagonal hemoglobin C crystal, and a combination of the two. The solubility test is positive, and electrophoresis on cellulose acetate shows about equal amounts of hemoglobin S and hemoglobin C.

Hemoglobin E

Hemoglobin E is an amino acid substitution of lysine for glutamic acid in the 26th position of the β chain, resulting in a net positive charge. Hemoglobin E is somewhat unstable when subjected to oxidizing agents.

Found in Asia, it is estimated to occur in about 20 million individuals, 80% of whom live in Southeast Asia. In the homozygous form, there is a mild anemia with microcytosis and target cells. In the heterozygous form, the patient is asymptomatic. The differential diagnosis is obtained by electrophoresis. On cellulose acetate, hemoglobin E moves with A_2, C, and O. It is present in the heterozygous form in amounts varying from 30% to 45%, which is somewhat lower than the percentage for hemoglobin C. This is probably a result of the somewhat unstable nature of hemoglobin E. On citrate agar, hemoglobin E migrates with A. It is more common to find this defect in association with both α- and β-thalassemia. E-β-thalassemia is a more severe disorder, with moderate anemia and splenomegaly.

Hemoglobin D

The letter D is given to any hemoglobin variant with an electrophoretic mobility on cellulose acetate similar to that of hemoglobin S but that has a negative solubility test. Hemoglobin $D_{Los\ Angeles}$ and its identical variant, hemoglobin D_{Punjab}, are the most common, with glycine substituted for glutamic acid at the 121st position of the β chain. Hemoglobin D_{Punjab} is found in Northwest India but occasionally can be seen in English, Portuguese, and French individuals because of the close historical connection of these countries with East India. Hemoglobin $D_{Los\ Angeles}$ is found in 0.02% of African Americans.

The homozygous state is rare. There is a mild anemia and/or splenomegaly and only a slight anisocytosis. The oxygen affinity is higher than in normal blood. Heterozygous individuals are asymptomatic. Differential diagnosis is accomplished with electrophoresis. On cellulose acetate, hemoglobin D migrates with hemoglobin S in proportions of 35% to 50%. On citrate agar, hemoglobin D migrates with A.

Hemoglobin Quantitative Defects: The Thalassemias

The thalassemias are a group of diseases in which a defect causes reduced synthesis of one or more of the hemoglobin chains, but the chains are structurally normal. Interaction among a large number of different molecular defects is the

CASE STUDY 19.4

A 54-year-old African American woman was admitted to the hospital with the chief complaint of left hip pain and lethargy. She had a long history of multiple emergency department visits for hip pain requiring medication. She previously had been found to have a positive solubility test for hemoglobin S but denied a history of sickle cell disease. There was family history of sickle cell trait. She had a mastectomy for breast cancer 10 years before. Admission laboratory values were as follows:

		Reference Range
Hemoglobin	5.3 g/dL	11.7–15.7 g/dL
Hematocrit	17%	35%–47%
MCV	82 fL	80–100 fL
MCHC	31%	32%–36%
WBC	12.0 × 10⁹/L	3.5–11.0 × 10⁹/L
Platelet count	53.0 × 10⁹/L	150–440 × 10⁹/L
Differential	Normal	
Reticulocyte count	6.4% (corrected, 2.4%)	0.5%–1.5%
RBC morphology	Target cells; spherocytes; schistocytes; basophilic stippling; and bizarre forms, including elongated, block-shaped, and more densely stained cells	

A hemoglobin electrophoresis was ordered. Patterns from the cellulose acetate and citrate agar electrophoresis are shown in Case Study Figure 19.4.1. Chest x-ray showed a right lower lobe infiltrate with pulmonary vascular congestion and an enlarged spleen. Fluid aspirated from the nasogastric tube was positive for blood.

The patient was given medication for an aspiration pneumonia, gastrointestinal bleeding, and congestive heart failure. She was given packed RBCs; fresh, frozen plasma; and platelets, but her condition continued to worsen. Six hours later, laboratory tests confirmed disseminated intravascular coagulation. A bone marrow biopsy was performed and revealed extensive necrosis of marrow elements. Three hours later, the patient died of cardiac arrest.

Questions

1. What hemoglobinopathy is indicated by the hemoglobin electrophoresis patterns?

2. What clinical feature of this disease differs from the typical picture in sickle cell anemia?

3. What other hemoglobins interact with hemoglobin S, and how can these be differentiated from hemoglobin C?

4. Was this patient's death due to the hemoglobinopathy? Is it unusual for hemoglobin SC to be life shortening?

FIGURE 19.4.1 Hemoglobin electrophoretic patterns. **A.** Cellulose acetate at pH 8.4. **B.** Citrate agar at pH 6.2. ● = origin. (Case study data courtesy of Margaret Uthman, MD, University of Texas Medical School at Houston.)

cause for decreased or absent globin chain synthesis.[21] The two most common types are α-thalassemia, resulting from defective production of α chains, and β-thalassemia, resulting from a defect in the production of β chains. Defects in the production of the δ and γ chains have been described, but these are not involved in the production of hemoglobin A and are, therefore, not clinically significant. Rarely, combinations of gene deletions, such as δ and β, may lead to clinical disease. Any form of unbalanced production of globin chains causes the erythrocytes to be small, hypochromic, and sometimes deformed. Intracellular accumulation of unmatched chains in the developing erythrocytes causes precipitation of the proteins, which leads to cell destruction in the bone marrow. Although erythropoiesis is occurring, it is ineffective because mature cells do not reach the peripheral blood to carry oxygen.

Thalassemia is inherited as an autosomal dominant disorder with heterogeneous expression of the disease. One of the most common hereditary disorders, it is distributed worldwide. The prevalence of the thalassemia gene has been attributed to the protection it offers against falciparum malaria. The heterozygous state produces a disorder called *thalassemia minor*, which is clinically asymptomatic and resembles iron deficiency. The homozygous state, *thalassemia major*, is usually lethal before birth or in childhood. Early and continuous treatment of some forms of the disease allows survival to young adulthood, but complications are many.

α-*Thalassemias*

Two α genes are located on each chromosome 16, one inherited from the mother and one from the father, yielding a total of four α genes. There are four principal clinical types of different severity known to occur in the population, and these four types can be explained, respectively, by deletions of four, three, two, or one of the α-globin gene loci (Fig. 19.5). α-Thalassemia occurs with high frequency in Asian populations but is also seen in the Black African, African American, Indian, and Middle Eastern populations. The type of α-thalassemia found in Black Africans and African Americans is also associated with deletion of the α-globin genes but in a different pattern than is found in the Asian population (Fig. 19.5). The four clinical types of α-thalassemia in order of most deletions to least deletions are the following:

1. Hydrops fetalis is the most clinically severe form of α-thalassemia because of the total absence of α chain synthesis. Hemoglobin Bart's, which is a tetramer of γ chains, is the main hemoglobin found in the red cells of affected infants. Hemoglobin Bart's has an extremely high O₂ affinity and allows almost no oxygen transport to the tissue. These infants are either stillborn or die of hypoxia shortly after birth.
2. Hemoglobin H disease has α chain synthesis at about one-third of the amount of β chain synthesis. As a result, β chains accumulate and form tetramers, which are called *hemoglobin H*. β chain precipitates (hemoglobin H inclusions) alter the shape and ability of the cell to deform, significantly shortening the life span of the cells. These

Thalassemias

α = Normal a gene locus   α⁰ = Deleted a gene locus

FIGURE 19.5 Deletions of α-globin gene loci on chromosome 16 in α-thalassemia.

individuals have a moderate hemolytic anemia, with 5% to 30% hemoglobin H, 1% hemoglobin A₂, and the remainder hemoglobin A. Hemoglobin H inclusions can be seen in the red cells with a supravital stain. Cord blood contains 10% to 20% hemoglobin Bart's.

3. α-Thalassemia trait results from two gene deletions, either on the same (—/αα) or on different chromosomes (–α/–α). The deletion on two separate chromosomes is more common in Black Africans and African Americans (Fig. 19.5). These individuals have a mild, microcytic, hypochromic anemia. Occasionally, excess β chains may form hemoglobin H inclusions. Cord blood contains 2% to 10% hemoglobin Bart's; however, after age 3 months, electrophoresis is normal.
4. Silent carriers are missing only one α gene, and the remaining genes direct production of sufficient α chains for normal hemoglobin production. This state is often characterized by expression of 1% to 2% of hemoglobin Bart's in a neonate. If hemoglobin Bart's is not detected in a neonate or prior to 3 months of age by standard testing, it can only be detected by more specialized testing, such as gene mapping, α:β-globin messenger ribonucleic acid (mRNA) ratio, or other polymerase chain reaction (PCR)–based methods.[21,22] It has been estimated that the frequency of this genetic disorder may be as high as 27% in the African American population.[21]

β-*Thalassemias*

In contrast to α-thalassemia, gene deletions usually do not cause β-thalassemia. More than 200 different mutations have been described resulting in failure to produce normal amounts of β-globin chains. A large majority of the defects result from point mutations.[22] The β-thalassemias are classically divided into homozygous disease, called thalassemia major or Cooley's anemia, and heterozygous disease, called thalassemia minor. However, the clinical expression of the disease is heterogeneous, depending on the type of genetic defect and involvement with other gene loci. The disease may be broadly divided into two major subtypes according to genetic expression: β+, in which β chains are produced in reduced amounts, and β0, which is complete absence of β chains.

β+-Thalassemia is the most common type. There is some synthesis of β-globin chains but in significantly reduced amounts (5% to 30%) of normal. The biochemical defect shows a quantitative deficiency of β-globin mRNA. The hemoglobin electrophoresis pattern and hemoglobin F and A_2 quantitation show about 2% to 8% hemoglobin A_2, an elevated but varying amount of hemoglobin F, and the remainder hemoglobin A. The mean cell volume (MCV) is low, with severe anemia, reticulocytes, nucleated RBCs, basophilic stippling, target cells, extreme poikilocytosis, and anisocytosis.

β0-Thalassemia accounts for 10% of homozygous β-thalassemia, with a total absence of β chain synthesis but intact synthesis of γ chains. In the homozygous form, there is 1% to 6% hemoglobin A_2 and 95% hemoglobin F. The hemoglobin concentration is low, with a severe anemia. The heterozygous form appears clinically the same as homozygous β+-thalassemia.

Homozygous β-thalassemia—β-thalassemia major—either β+ or β0, is a crippling disease of childhood. This is unlike α-thalassemia, in which the child either dies shortly after birth or leads a normal life. The hypochromic, microcytic anemia is a result of both the defect of functional hemoglobin tetramer synthesis and the premature destruction of RBCs, both intramedullary and extramedullary, due to increased α chains. The bone marrow compensates by enormously expanding in size, sometimes causing structural bone abnormalities. Treatment of severe forms of the disease includes regular transfusion therapy, iron chelation drugs to remove excess iron, and folic acid supplements.[23] Bone marrow transplantation has been successful if an HLA-identical donor is available.[21] Gene therapy is being studied as an alternative treatment of the future.[24–26]

Heterozygous β-thalassemia—thalassemia minor—may be caused by inheritance of one thalassemia gene, either β+ or β0. The other gene directing β chain production is normal, and RBC survival is not shortened. About 1% of African Americans are affected, and it also commonly occurs in individuals of Mediterranean and Arabic descent. Clinically, the condition is usually asymptomatic but may sometimes cause a mild microcytic anemia. The hematologic laboratory values resemble those of iron deficiency anemia, and it is important to distinguish the two because quite different treatments are required. The RBC count in thalassemia minor is usually higher than would be expected with the accompanying hemoglobin concentration, and a few target cells or occasional basophilic stippling may be seen on a stained smear. The red cell distribution width (RDW) parameter on automated instruments, which is a quantitative measure of RBC variation in size, may be helpful to distinguish the two disorders. It is typically normal in thalassemia and increased in iron deficiency as a result of the heterogeneity of the RBCs. Hemoglobin electrophoresis of thalassemia minor characteristically shows an increase in hemoglobin A_2. Quantitation of hemoglobin A_2 by column chromatography usually reveals values between 3.5% and 7%.

δ-β-Thalassemia is a rare type characterized by total absence of both β chain synthesis of hemoglobin A and δ chain synthesis of hemoglobin A_2. Homozygous patients have 100% hemoglobin F. Heterozygous individuals usually have less than 90% hemoglobin A, 2% to 3% hemoglobin A_2, and 5% to 20% hemoglobin F.

Patients are anemic and show a thalassemic phenotype because the γ chain synthesis of hemoglobin F is not equal to α chain synthesis. There is approximately one-third as much γ chain produced as α chain. Hemoglobin F is heterogeneously distributed among the erythrocytes, as revealed by the acid elution stain procedure.

Hereditary persistence of fetal hemoglobin (HPFH) is genetically and hematologically heterogeneous. In African Blacks and African Americans, there is a total absence of β as well as δ chain synthesis because of deletions in chromosome 11. γ Chain synthesis is present in the adult at a high level and, in contrast to synthesis of hemoglobin F in β-thalassemia or δ-β-thalassemia, is uniformly distributed. In heterozygotes, there is no imbalance of globin chain synthesis. There is 17% to 33% hemoglobin F. The patients are clinically normal. In homozygotes, there is 100% hemoglobin F, with no synthesis of hemoglobin A or A_2. There are no significant hematologic abnormalities, other than erythrocytosis, and these patients are also asymptomatic.

Analytical Methods

Most hemoglobinopathies and thalassemias can be diagnosed by the use of the complete blood count (CBC), blood film evaluation, solubility test, and cellulose acetate electrophoresis. Citrate agar electrophoresis may be necessary for confirmation of some abnormal hemoglobins. Thalassemias may require quantitation of hemoglobin A_2 or F by more definitive methods. A serum ferritin may be helpful to distinguish thalassemia minor from iron deficiency anemia. Hemoglobinopathies may also be diagnosed rapidly and accurately using newer automated techniques such as HPLC and isoelectric focusing (IEF).[27] The more complicated cases may require more specialized procedures, such as α/β-globin chain analysis,[28] cation-exchange HPLC,[28,29] or DNA technology testing.[30–34]

Solubility Test (Screening Test for Sickling Hemoglobins)

The solubility test is based on the principle that sickling hemoglobin, in the deoxygenated state, is relatively insoluble and forms a precipitate when placed in a high-molarity phosphate buffer solution.[35,36] The precipitate appears because the deoxygenated hemoglobin molecules form tactoids that refract and deflect light rays, producing a turbid solution. A small amount of packed RBCs is placed in a buffered solution of sodium dithionite with saponin to lyse the RBCs in a 12 × 75 mm glass tube. After mixing well and incubating at room temperature for 5 minutes, the tube containing the solution is placed approximately 1 in. in front of a heavy, black-lined index card. If there is no sickling hemoglobin present, the lines on the card will be easily seen. If sickling hemoglobin is present, the lines will be indistinct or impossible to read. The test is reported as positive or negative for sickling hemoglobin. A positive and a negative control should be run with each test batch.

CASE STUDY 19.5

A 5-year-old white boy was seen by a physician for an upper respiratory tract infection and splenomegaly was noted. A CBC was ordered and, subsequently, a hemoglobin electrophoresis. The following were the results:

		Reference Range
Hemoglobin	8.5 g/dL	11.7–15.7 g/dL
Hematocrit	27%	35%–47%
RBC	4.3×10^{12}/L	$3.8–5.2 \times 10^{12}$/L
MCV	62.3 fL	80–100 fL
MCHC	32.0%	32%–36%
RDW	18.5%	11.5%–14.5%
Platelet	538×10^9/L	$150–440 \times 10^9$/L
WBC	10.7×10^9/L	$3.5–11.0 \times 10^9$/L
Reticulocyte count	5.6%	0.5%–1.5%
WBC differential	Normal except for 1 nucleated RBC/100 WBCs	
RBC morphology	Moderate aniso-cytosis, moderate microcytosis, slight polychromasia, slight target cells, slight schistocytes	
Hemoglobin electrophoresis (cellulose acetate)		
Hemoglobin C	89%	
Hemoglobin F	11%	

A hemoglobin electrophoresis by citrate agar method confirmed hemoglobins C and F. Hemoglobin F was determined by the alkali denaturation method to be 7.5%. Hemoglobin A_2 could not be quantitated due to the presence of hemoglobin

C. The patient's father had been previously told that he was slightly anemic due to a blood disorder called thalassemia. The patient's mother and four older siblings were healthy and unaware of any abnormal hemoglobin.

Questions

1. What combination of disorders did the patient most probably inherit?
2. Why were the mother and the other siblings unaware of an abnormality?
3. Why was the patient unable to produce hemoglobin A?
4. What caused the discrepancy in values for hemoglobin F from electrophoresis and the alkali denaturation test?
5. Why was it unusual to find hemoglobin C in a white family?

Outdated reagents and reagents not at room temperature interfere with the test. False-negative tests may be due to anemia or recent transfusions or may occur in infants younger than age 6 months because of high concentrations of hemoglobin F. If whole blood is used instead of packed RBCs, false-positive results may occur due to erythrocytosis, hyperglobulinemia, extreme leukocytosis, or hyperlipidemia and false-negative results may occur in anemia. This test does not differentiate between the homozygous and heterozygous presence of hemoglobin S, and other rare sickling variants, such as hemoglobin C_{Harlem}, may give a positive test. Commonly used as a screening test for sickling hemoglobin in adults, this test may also be used as a confirmatory test for sickling hemoglobin after initial evaluation with cellulose acetate electrophoresis.

Cellulose Acetate Hemoglobin Electrophoresis

A fresh hemolysate made from a packed RBC sample is applied to a cellulose acetate plate using a buffer of alkaline pH (8.4 to 8.6), and electrophoresis is performed.[36–38] After electrophoresis, the membrane is stained and cleared. The patient's hemoglobin migration is compared with that of a control for test interpretation. A rough estimate of proportions of different hemoglobins may be made using a densitometer.

The order of electrophoretic mobility, from slowest to fastest, is hemoglobins C, S, F, and A (Fig. 19.6). (There are several mnemonic devices for remembering the migration pattern, such as Accelerated, Fast, Slow, and Crawl.) Hemoglobin that migrates beyond hemoglobin A is termed *fast hemoglobin*. Hemoglobin Bart's and hemoglobin H both migrate here. Any abnormal hemoglobin or any normal hemoglobin present in increased amounts, such as hemoglobin A_2 and F, should be confirmed. If there is abnormal hemoglobin, confirm with citrate agar electrophoresis and solubility test if hemoglobin S is suspected. If an increased amount of A_2 or

Cellulose Acetate Electrophoresis (pH 8.4–8.6)						
(−) po						(+)
	A2 C E	S D G	F	A	Bart's	HGB H
Normal adult	+/−	−	−	++++	−	−
Sickle cell disease	+	+++	++	−	−	−
Sickle cell trait	−	++	−	+++	−	−
Hemoglobin CC disease	+++	−	+	−	−	−
Hemoglobin AC disease	++	−	−	+++	−	−
Hemoglobin DD disease	−	+++	+	−	−	−
Hemoglobin AD disease	−	++	−	+++	−	−
Hemoglobin SC disease	++	++	+	−	−	−
β Thalassemia major	+	−	+++	−	−	−
β Thalassemia minor	+	−	+/−	+++	−	−
α Thalassemia major	−	−	−	−	++	++
α Thalassemia minor	−	−	−	+++	+	−

FIGURE 19.6 Hemoglobin migration patterns in several hemoglobinopathies and thalassemias. po = sample point of origin. The number of + signs denotes the relative amounts of hemoglobin detected; − denotes no or virtually no hemoglobin detected.

F occurs, then quantify the amount. Hemoglobin D and G comigrate with hemoglobin S in this method.

Universal newborn screening for hemoglobinopathies has become the norm since it was shown that early diagnosis and comprehensive care can reduce morbidity and mortality in infants with sickle cell disease. For mass screening, IEF and HPLC have replaced cellulose acetate electrophoresis in most cases due to their automation and high throughput.[20]

Citrate Agar Electrophoresis

Citrate agar electrophoresis is performed at an acid pH (6.0 to 6.2) after abnormal hemoglobin is detected on cellulose acetate electrophoresis.[36,39] In this method, an important factor in determining the mobility of hemoglobin is solubility. Hemoglobin F, with the fastest cathodal mobility, is also the most soluble, probably because it is most resistant to denaturation at pH 6.0. Adult hemoglobins with solubility similar to that of hemoglobin A, such as D, E, G, O, and I, move with hemoglobin A. The relatively insoluble hemoglobin S moves behind hemoglobin A, and the even more insoluble hemoglobin C moves behind hemoglobin S (Fig. 19.4.1).

Hemoglobin A₂ Quantitation

The quantity of hemoglobin A_2 may be estimated by hemoglobin electrophoresis; however, this yields only a rough estimate. Quantitation is best accomplished by microcolumn chromatography[36,40] or HPLC.[28,29,40]

Acid Elution Stain for Hemoglobin F

Erythrocytes containing an increased amount of hemoglobin F can be distinguished from normal adult cells by the acid elution technique.[36,41] This method may be helpful in the diagnosis of HPFH or to detect fetal cells in maternal circulation during problem pregnancies. In the microscopic method, adult hemoglobin, hemoglobin A, is eluted from the erythrocytes by incubation in an acid buffer. Hemoglobin F remains behind and is stained with eosin. Adult cells are negative and have no staining because they contain no hemoglobin F. Fetal RBCs may also be detected by flow cytometric assay methods.[42]

Hemoglobin F Quantitation

Fetal hemoglobin may be quantitated based on the principle that it is resistant to alkali denaturation in 1.25 mol/L NaOH for 2 minutes. Denatured hemoglobin A is precipitated out with ammonium sulfate and removed by filtration. The optical density of the clear supernatant solution is read at 540 nm, and the percentage of fetal hemoglobin is calculated against the optical density of the total hemoglobin solutions.[36] HPLC has been recommended as the method of choice for quantitation of fetal hemoglobin.[29]

The average adult has less than 1.5% fetal hemoglobin. However, elevated levels may be found in several inherited and acquired diseases. The HPFH should be suspected in individuals who possess 10% or more fetal hemoglobin with no other apparent clinical abnormalities.

The importance of accurate quantitation of hemoglobin F may increase in the future due to its use in experimental methods as a cure for hemoglobinopathies and thalassemia syndromes.[27,43] The protective effect of hemoglobin F in sickle cell disease is a main focus of current research for effective therapy. Investigation of the cellular and molecular mechanisms of the fetal to adult (γ to β) switch during the perinatal period and search for anti-switching drugs to maintain high levels of hemoglobin F is promising.[27]

DNA Technology

The definitive diagnosis of some hemoglobinopathies and thalassemias that involve combinations of genetic defects may require DNA analysis. The robust sensitivity and specificity of molecular techniques allows for precise analysis of hemoglobin abnormalities. Disadvantages of molecular methods include higher cost and lack of availability in most routine laboratories. The advantages are that it provides definitive information about the genotype of individuals tested, and in some cases, direct detection of the molecular lesions is possible. Whereas biochemical methods such as HPLC, denaturing HPLC (dHPLC), capillary electrophoresis

(CE), denaturing gradient gel electrophoresis (DGGE), and IEF are useful to screen for hemoglobinopathies and thalassemias, specific molecular techniques that facilitate diagnosis of complex cases include reverse oligonucleotide probe hybridization PCR (gap-PCR), high resolution melting (HRM), multiplex ligation–dependent probe amplification (MLPA), allele-specific oligonucleotide (ASO) hybridization, single strand conformation polymorphism (SSCP), and next generation sequencing (NGS). The mechanics of these techniques will be outlined here very briefly.

PCR utilizes short oligonucleotide sequences (primers) to amplify specific DNA sequences of interest. Gap-PCR is a variation of this method that is based upon the inability of PCR primers complementary to DNA sequences located far apart to produce amplification unless a deletion brings them closer together. Gap-PCR is utilized to detect α thalassemia deletions/duplications.[30]

CASE STUDY 19.6

A 22-year-old white woman of Italian heritage had been told that she was slightly anemic and had been treated with iron periodically throughout her life. She was a student in a clinical laboratory science program and had a CBC performed as a part of a hematology class.

Laboratory values were as follows:

		Reference Range
Hemoglobin	11.0 g/dL	11.7–15.7 g/dL
Hematocrit	34%	35%–47%
RBC	5.8×10^{12}/L	3.8–5.2×10^{12}/L
MCV	59.4 fL	80–100 fL
MCHC	31.9%	32%–36%
RDW	14.2%	11.5%–14.5%

From these values, the hematology instructor suspected an inherited disorder instead of iron deficiency and suggested that the student contact her physician for further testing. A hemoglobin electrophoresis revealed slightly increased amounts of hemoglobins F and A_2, which were subsequently quantitated to reveal hemoglobin F of 3.2% and hemoglobin A_2 of 4.2%. Iron studies were normal.

Questions

1. What is the most probable disorder?
2. What CBC values caused the instructor to suggest further testing?
3. Why is it important for this disorder to be correctly diagnosed?

HRM is a technique that can be used post PCR amplification as long as the probe utilized during the amplification process is complexed with a fluorescent detection dye that recognizes double-stranded DNA (such as SyB green). The PCR amplicon is heated incrementally until it denatures. Mutated DNA does not perfectly match its complementary probe and will denature at lower temperatures than does a perfectly matched DNA/probe hybrid. As long as the amplicon remains double stranded, fluorescence persists. Loss of fluorescence indicates that the amplicon has denatured, indicating that a mutation is present.

Multiplex PCR uses multiple primers to amplify several DNA targets simultaneously. MLPA is a related PCR technique that allows multiple DNA targets to be amplified with only a single primer pair. This is possible since MLPA relies on probe amplification to characterize DNA. The probe is split into two parts, one part is complementary to the forward primer and the other part is complementary to the reverse primer. When both parts of the probe hybridize to their adjacent targets, which is only possible in the presence of complete and correct DNA, ligation and subsequent amplification of the probe is possible. A single set of primers is possible since all the probes that are utilized carry tails for the binding of amplification primers with universal recognition sequences.[31]

ASO is also known as the reverse dot blot technique. To test for the presence of a mutation in a DNA sample, a DNA amplicon is applied to duplicate support membranes (dot blots). An ASO probe is synthesized so that it is complementary to the altered sequence, and a control probe recognizes the normal sequence. Each ASO probe is fully complementary to its target sequence (either mutated or wild type) and will bind strongly. A single mismatch against its nontarget allele leads to a weaker interaction which is visualized with a weaker signal. The two ASO probes are applied to both dot blots, and discrimination is possible between the fully complementary and the mismatched hybrids.[32]

The principle of SSCP relies on the fact that single-stranded DNA has a characteristic conformation, and single base changes in the sequence can cause DNA to migrate differently under nondenaturing electrophoresis conditions. Amplified DNA is first heated to denature it and then cooled to promote self-annealing. Wild-type and mutant DNA exhibit different banding patterns during electrophoretic separation that is reflective of their different nucleotide bases.[33]

Finally gene sequencing has been a powerful means for identifying the order of DNA nucleotides in a genome since its development by Frederick Sanger in 1977. The principle involves in vitro DNA replication employing DNA polymerase and a mix of uncorrupted nucleotides in addition to chain-terminating nucleotides. As long as the unadulterated nucleotides are incorporated into the DNA molecule, the polynucleotide extends in length. When a chain terminating nucleotide is randomly incorporated into the growing chain, polymerization ends. The resulting DNA chains of variable lengths are separated by gel electrophoresis. Shorter fragments migrate more quickly than longer fragments, which allow determination of base sequence. Sanger sequencing has largely been replaced by large-scale NGS. NGS yields thousands of sequences simultaneously, minimizing the effort and the cost of sequencing. The methodology differs between systems, but many systems employ genomic DNA which is first fragmented into libraries of short lengths. The libraries are ligated to synthetic adapter sequences that allow the DNA to be immobilized on a platform. The next step is to clonally amplify the library in order to generate millions of DNA clusters, each cluster containing multiple copies of the DNA template. Amplified DNA is exposed to fluorescently tagged nucleotides—each nucleotide (A, T, C, and G) receives a uniquely colored fluor (fluorophore?). Recording the color of each fluor as its vehicle nucleotide attaches to complementary DNA allows sequence determination. The instrument records the sequences of bases in each molecular cluster, and the groups of bases are assembled against themselves (de novo sequencing) or aligned to a reference genome (resequencing).[34]

A special strength of the DNA technology is in the prenatal diagnosis of thalassemia major. Because the globin genes are represented in all tissue, including those in which they are not active, prenatal diagnosis of thalassemic states may be made by sampling tissue that is relatively easy to obtain, such as chorionic villi or amniotic fluid cells, rather than fetal blood, which is obtained with much greater difficulty and at a much greater risk to the fetus.[35] Two new techniques for analysis of fetal DNA with even lower risk are the isolation of fetal cells from maternal blood by flow cytometry and the use of cell-free fetal DNA from the maternal serum. Maternal DNA molecules are longer than fetal-derived ones, allowing for accurate separation.[21,44] DNA technology also has been used in the prenatal diagnosis of sickle cell anemia. Fetal cells obtained by amniocentesis or chorionic villus sampling may be analyzed using similar techniques as in the thalassemias. PCR is the method of choice for prenatal diagnosis, if available.[27] Hemoglobin electrophoresis on a hemolysate of fetal blood cells can also be used in cases in which DNA technology is unavailable or when rapid results are needed, owing to a patient's advanced gestational age. Prenatal diagnosis is a major factor in controlling these severe genetic diseases because there is no effective cure at this time, other than HLA-matched allogeneic bone marrow transplant.[44]

MYOGLOBIN
Structure and Role in the Body

Myoglobin is a heme protein found in the skeletal and cardiac muscle. It can reversibly bind oxygen in a manner similar to the hemoglobin molecule; however, myoglobin is unable to release oxygen, except under low oxygen tension. Myoglobin is a simple heme protein containing one polypeptide chain and one heme group per molecule. The polypeptide chain contains 153 amino acids, making it slightly larger than one chain in the hemoglobin molecule. Therefore, its size is slightly larger than one-fourth that of a hemoglobin molecule, with a molecular weight of approximately 17,000.

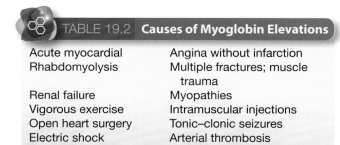

TABLE 19.2	Causes of Myoglobin Elevations
Acute myocardial	Angina without infarction
Rhabdomyolysis	Multiple fractures; muscle trauma
Renal failure	Myopathies
Vigorous exercise	Intramuscular injections
Open heart surgery	Tonic–clonic seizures
Electric shock	Arterial thrombosis
Certain toxins	Malignant hyperthermia
Muscular dystrophy	Systemic lupus erythematosus

The iron atom in the center of the heme group is the site of reversible oxygen binding, identical to the hemoglobin molecule. In the body, myoglobin acts as an oxygen carrier in the cytoplasm of the muscle cell. Transport of oxygen from the muscle cell membrane to the mitochondria is its main role. Myoglobin serves as an extra reserve of oxygen to help exercising muscle maintain activity longer.

Clinical Significance

Damage to muscles often results in elevated concentrations of serum and urine myoglobin (Table 19.2). Renal clearance is rapid, and myoglobinemia following a single injury tends to be transient. High concentrations of myoglobin may cause acute renal failure (ARF). Measurement of myoglobin in serum and urine can be used to calculate a myoglobin clearance rate. The combination of a high serum myoglobin (≥400 ng/mL) and a low clearance rate (≤4 mL/min) indicates a high risk of ARF.[45] Myoglobin in urine will cross-react with the hemoglobin test on the dipstick and cause a positive reaction. Confirmation of myoglobinuria by a more specific assay, such as an immunoassay, allows differentiation from hemoglobinuria. Myoglobin measurement in urine or serum may be performed when rhabdomyolysis or any disease/injury resulting in muscle damage is suspected.

Currently, the primary use of serum myoglobin testing is in the investigation of chest pain to diagnose or rule out AMI. The combined use of myoglobin and troponin or the MB isoenzyme of creatine kinase (CK-MB) is useful for the early exclusion of AMI.[46] Damaged heart muscle cells release myoglobin within the 1st few hours of onset of myocardial infarction, and peak values are reached within 2 to 3 hours and as early as 30 minutes. Myoglobin, therefore, is the first cardiac marker to rise, sooner than CK-MB or troponin (T or I). Although an increase of myoglobin in the circulation provides an early indicator of myocardial infarction, false-positive results may occur from any injury to skeletal muscle that also contains myoglobin. The use of myoglobin as an early marker should be followed by use of a definitive marker, such as troponin (T or I), that is more cardiac specific but does not appear in the blood as early. In cases in which thrombolytic therapy is used in the treatment of myocardial infarction, myoglobin levels combined with CK-MB and clinical indications may be used as monitors of reperfusion of the occluded artery.[47] Myoglobin also has been investigated to aid in the diagnosis and differentiation of the different types of hereditary progressive muscular dystrophy.[48] Myoglobin levels in urine are normally not detected or very low. Elevated levels of urine myoglobin indicate an increased risk of renal damage and failure. Myoglobin is discussed in greater detail in Chapter 11.

Analytical Methods

There are several immunoassay methods for measurement and identification of myoglobin. These procedures incorporate the binding of specific antibodies to myoglobin,

with a resulting chemical or physical change (e.g., fluorescence, chemiluminescence, and immunochromatic) that can be measured and correlated to myoglobin concentration. These methods have been adapted to point-of-care devices for rapid assessment of chest pain, as well as conventional methods for multianalyte analyzer platforms.[49,50] Although plasma is the specimen of choice for cardiac marker analysis, there is evidence that different anticoagulants have different effects on particular commercial assays for myoglobin.[49] It has also been shown that there are precision and reference range differences between the different myoglobin assays.[49]

For additional student resources, please visit **thePoint** at http://thepoint.lww.com

questions

1. The primary purpose of porphyrins in the human body is to
   a. Chelate free hemoglobin
   b. Contribute to the synthesis of heme
   c. Transport ferrous iron
   d. Transport oxygen to tissues

2. The chemical structure of porphyrin is described as a(n)
   a. Cyclic tetrapyrrole
   b. Heterocyclic pyrrole
   c. Linear tetrapyrrole
   d. Oxygen-binding prosthetic group

3. Which statement correctly describes a porphyrin property?
   a. Porphyrins absorb light in the visible region of the spectrum and fluoresce.
   b. Porphyrins are not soluble in aqueous solution.
   c. Porphyrins are oxidized to porphyrinogens when exposed to air.
   d. Porphyrins produced spontaneously are functional compounds.

4. The porphyrias can be classified according to disease symptoms as
   a. Congenital or acquired
   b. Erythropoietic or hepatic
   c. Hematologic or muscular
   d. Neurologic or cutaneous

5. Elevated urinary PBG concentration with negative fecal porphyrin results indicates
   a. Acute intermittent porphyria (AIP)
   b. Erythropoietic protoporphyria (EPP)
   c. Hereditary coproporphyria (HCP)
   d. Porphyria cutanea tarda (PCT)

6. Porphyria cutanea tarda (PCT) is identified by
   a. Chromatographic analysis of a 24-h urine collection
   b. Scanning fluorescence of plasma
   c. Screening for PBG in a random urine specimen
   d. Separation of fecal porphyrins in a 24-h specimen

7. Suspected erythropoietic protoporphyria (EPP) is evaluated by
   a. Assessing plasma or whole blood for protoporphyrin
   b. Enzymatic measurement of hydroxymethylbilane synthase
   c. HPLC analysis of a urine specimen
   d. Molecular testing for ferrochelatase

8. Porphobilinogen often is measured in the urine using
   a. Chromatography
   b. Electrophoresis
   c. Spectrophotometry
   d. The Watson-Schwartz method

9. In the clinical laboratory, testing to identify specific porphyrins is performed using
   a. Chemical derivatization and spectrophotometry
   b. Fluorometric emission scanning
   c. Liquid chromatography with fluorescent detection
   d. Thin layer chromatography

10. Specimens collected for evaluation of porphyria should be
    a. Allowed to clot at room temperature for an hour
    b. Diluted to less than 25 mg/dL creatinine
    c. Exposed to light and air to oxidize the analytes
    d. Protected from light and stored cold

(continues on page 420)

review questions (continued)

11. Inherited disorders in which a genetic defect causes abnormalities in rate and quantity of synthesis of structurally normal polypeptide chains of the hemoglobin molecule are called
  a. Hemoglobinopathies
  b. Molecular dyscrasias
  c. Porphyrias
  d. Thalassemias

12. Molecular diagnostic techniques that can help diagnose hemoglobin disorders such as hemoglobinopathies and thalassemias include
  a. Biochemical separation, identification, and quantification of mixture components
  b. Separation of macromolecules and their fragments, based on their size and charge
  c. DNA amplification, hybridization, and nucleotide sequencing
  d. The use of specific monoclonal antibodies

13. Which of the following abnormal hemoglobins, found frequently in individuals from Southeast Asia, migrates with hemoglobin A_2 on cellulose acetate electrophoresis?
  a. Hemoglobin C
  b. Hemoglobin D
  c. Hemoglobin E
  d. Hemoglobin Lepore

14. Which type of alpha-thalassemia results from deletion of three genes and produces a moderate hemolytic anemia?
  a. Hemoglobin Bart's
  b. Hemoglobin H disease
  c. Hydrops fetalis
  d. Thalassemia trait

15. The most effective way to quantitate hemoglobin A_2 is by
  a. Alkali denaturation test
  b. Citrate agar electrophoresis
  c. Column chromatography
  d. Densitometry

16. Serum or plasma myoglobin concentrations are used as
  a. An early marker of acute myocardial infarction
  b. An indicator of congestive heart failure
  c. Lead poisoning indicator
  d. Liver function tests

17. Which of the following is the best test to differentiate beta-thalassemia minor from iron deficiency anemia?
  a. Complete blood count
  b. Hemoglobin A_2 quantitation
  c. Hemoglobin electrophoresis (cellulose acetate, alkaline pH)
  d. Solubility test

18. Which is the correct sequence of electrophoretic migration of hemoglobins from slowest to fastest on cellulose acetate at an alkaline pH?
  a. A, F, S, C
  b. C, A, S, F
  c. C, S, A, F
  d. C, S, F, A

19. High-resolution melting (HRM) is a technique that can be used post PCR amplification as long as the probe utilized during the amplification process is complexed with a fluorescent detection dye that recognizes
  a. Single-stranded DNA
  b. Double-stranded DNA
  c. cDNA
  d. Specific primers

20. The two main sites of production of heme are
  a. Heart and lung
  b. Liver and bone marrow
  c. Liver and spleen
  d. Muscle and blood

21. Which hemoglobin is resistant to alkali denaturation in NaOH?
  a. Hb A
  b. Hb C
  c. Hb F
  d. Hb S

22. A patient has an abnormal hemoglobin band that migrates with Hb S on cellulose acetate (pH 8.4) hemoglobin electrophoresis. The solubility test is negative. Which test should be performed next?
  a. Citrate agar (pH 6.2) electrophoresis
  b. HbA_2 quantitation
  c. Acid elution stain
  d. Blood film evaluation

review questions (continued)

23. Silent carriers of alpha-thalassemia are missing how many alpha genes?
a. 1
b. 2
c. 3
d. 4

24. Which hemoglobin contains four gamma chains and has an extremely high affinity for oxygen?
a. Hb Bart's
b. Hb F
c. Hb Gower I
d. Hb Portland I

25. A patient with Southeast Asian heritage is found to have a mild microcytic anemia and a few target cells. Hemoglobin electrophoresis on cellulose acetate at pH 8.4 reveals a major band that migrates with Hb A_2 and no Hb A. On citrate agar electrophoresis, the band travels in the position of Hb A. What is the most probable abnormal hemoglobin present?
a. Hb A
b. Hb C
c. Hb D
d. Hb E

references

1. Bottomley SS, Muller-Eberhard U. Pathophysiology of heme synthesis. *Semin Hematol.* 1988;25:282–302.

2. Awad WM. Iron and heme metabolism. In: Devlin TM, ed. *Textbook of Biochemistry with Clinical Correlations.* 6th ed. Hoboken, NJ: Wiley-Liss; 2006:823–847.

3. Badminton MN, Whatley SD, Deacon AC, et al. The Porphyrias and other disorders of porphyrin metabolism. In: Burtis CA, Ashwood ER, Bruns DE, eds. *Tietz Textbook of Clinical Chemistry and Molecular Diagnostics.* 5th ed. St. Louis, MO: Elsevier Saunders; 2012:1031–1055.

4. Anderson KE, Sassa S, Bishop DF, et al. Disorders of heme biosynthesis: X-linked sideroblastic anemia and the porphyrias. In: Scriver CR, Beaudet AL, Sly WS, et al., eds. *The Metabolic and Molecular Bases of Inherited Disease.* 8th ed. New York: McGraw-Hill; 2001:2991–3062.

5. Desnick RJ, Balwani M. The Porphyrias. In: Kasper D, Fauci A, Hauser S, et al., eds. *Harrison's Principles of Internal Medicine.* 19th ed. New York: McGraw-Hill Medical; 2015. http://accessmedicine.mhmedical.com. Accessed February 2016.

6. Puy H, Gouya L, Deybach J-C. Porphyrias. *Lancet.* 2010;375:924–937.

7. Whatley SD, Ducamp S, Gouya L, et al. C-Terminal deletions in the ALAS2 gene lead to gain of function and cause X-linked dominant protoporphyria without anemia or iron overload. *Am J Hum Genet.* 2008;83:408–414.

8. Kontos AP, Ozog D, Bichakjian C, Lim HW. Congenital erythropoietic porphyria associated with myelodysplasia presenting in a 72-year-old man: report of a case and review of the literature. *Brit J Dermatol.* 2003;148:160–164.

9. Goodwin RG, Kell WJ, Laidler P, et al. Photosensitivity and acute liver injury in myeloproliferative disorder secondary to late-onset protoporphyria caused by deletion of a ferrochelatase gene in hematopoietic cells. *Blood.* 2006;107:60–62.

10. Balwani M, Desnick RJ. The porphyrias: advances in diagnosis and treatment. *Blood.* 2012;120:4496–4504.

11. Clinuvel SCENESSE®. http://www.clinuvel.com/en/scenesse/scenesse-afamelanotide. Accessed March 2016.

12. Kaczynski J, Hansson G, Wallerstedt S. Increased porphyrins in primary liver cancer mainly reflect a parallel liver disease. *Gastroenterol Res Pract.* 2009;2009:1–6.

13. Chowdhury JR, Wolkoff AW, Chowdhury NR, Arias IM. Hereditary jaundice and disorders of bilirubin metabolism. In: Valle D, Beaudet AL, Vogelstein B, et al., eds. *The Online Metabolic and Molecular Bases of Inherited Disease.* New York: McGraw-Hill Medical. 2001. http://ommbid.mhmedical.com/. Accessed February 2016.

14. Berthelot P, Dhumeaux D. New insights into the classification and mechanisms of hereditary, chronic, non-haemolytic hyperbilirubinaemias. *Gut.* 1978;19:474–480.

15. Frank M, Doss MO. Relevance of urinary coproporphyrin isomers in hereditary hyperbilirubinemias. *Clin Biochem.* 1989;22:221–222.

16. Molecular tests. https://www.genetests.org/tests/. Accessed March 2016.

17. Mathur SC, Schexneider KI, Hutchison RE. Hematopoiesis. In: McPherson RA, Pincus MR, eds. *Henry's Clinical Diagnosis and Management by Laboratory Methods.* 22nd ed. Philadelphia, PA: Saunders Elsevier; 2011:536–556.

18. Whatley SD, Badminton MN. Role of genetic testing in the management of patients with inherited porphyria and their families. *Ann Clin Biochem.* 2013;50:204–216.

19. Watson CJ, Schwartz S. A simple test for urinary porphobilinogen. *Exp Biol Med (Maywood).* 1941;47:393–394.

20. Wang WC. Sickle cell anemia and other sickling syndromes. In: Greer JP, Foerster J, Rodgers GM, et al., eds. *Wintrobe's Clinical Hematology.* 12th ed. Philadelphia, PA: Wolters Kluwer Health/Lippincott Williams & Wilkins; 2009:1038, 1062–1063.

21. Borgna-Pignatti C, Galanello R. The thalassemias and related disorders: quantitative disorders of hemoglobin synthesis. In: Greer JP, Foerster J, Rodgers GM, et al., eds. *Wintrobe's Clinical Hematology.* 12th ed. Philadelphia, PA: Wolters Kluwer Health/Lippincott Williams & Wilkins; 2009:1083, 1093.

22. Galanello R, Sollaine C, Paglietti E, et al. α-Thalassemia carrier identification by DNA analysis in the screening for thalassemia. *Am J Hematol.* 1998;59:273.

23. Harrison CR. Hemolytic anemias: intracorpuscular defects, IV. Thalassemia. In: Harmening DM, ed. *Clinical Hematology and Fundamentals of Hemostasis.* 4th ed. Philadelphia, PA: FA Davis; 2002:194.

24. Herzog RW, Hagstrom JN. Gene therapy for hereditary hematological disorders. *Am J Pharmacogenomics.* 2001;1:137.

25. Tisdale J, Sadelain M. Toward gene therapy for disorders of globin synthesis. *Semin Hematol.* 2001;38:382.

26. Quek L, Thein SL. Molecular therapies in beta-thalassemia. *Br J Haematol.* 2007:136:353–365.

27. Natarajan K, Townes TM, Kutlar A. Disorders of hemoglobin structure: sickle cell anemia and related abnormalities. In: Prchal JT, Kaushansky K, Lichtman MA, et al., eds. *Williams Hematology.* 8th ed. New York: McGraw-Hill; 2010; Chapter 48. http://0-www.accessmedicine.com.innopac.lsuhsc.edu/content.aspx?aID=6130552. Accessed January 30, 2012.

28. Tuzmen S, Schecter AN. Genetic diseases of hemoglobin: diagnostic methods for elucidating β-thalassemia mutations. *Blood Rev.* 2001;15:19.

29. Clarke GM, Higgins TN. Laboratory investigation of hemoglobinopathies and thalassemias: review and update. *Clin Chem.* 2000;46:1284.

30. Kho SL, Chua KH, George E, et al. A novel gap-PCR with high resolution melting analysis for the detection of α-thalassaemia Southeast Asian and Filipino β°-thalassaemia deletion. *Sci Rep.* 2015;5:13937.

31. Lee ST, Yoo EH, Kim JY, et al. Multiplex ligation-dependent probe amplification screening of isolated increased HbF levels revealed three cases of novel rearrangements/deletions in the beta-globin gene cluster. *Br J Haematol.* 2010;148(1):154–160.

32. Maggio A, Giambona A, Cai SP, et al. Rapid and simultaneous typing of hemoglobin S, hemoglobin C, and seven Mediterranean beta-thalassemia mutations by covalent reverse dot-blot analysis: application to prenatal diagnosis in Sicily. *Blood.* 1993;81(1):239–242.

33. Vallian S, Nassiri I. Development of a sensitive deaminated single-strand conformation polymorphism (DSSCP). *Appl Biochem Biotechnol.* 2010;160(3):927–931.

34. Xiong L, Barrett AN, Hua R, et al. Non-invasive prenatal diagnostic testing for β-thalassaemia using cell-free fetal DNA and next generation sequencing. *Prenat Diagn.* 2015;35(3):258–265.

35. Arcasoy MO, Gallagher PG. Molecular diagnosis of hemoglobinopathies and other red blood cell disorders. *Semin Hematol.* 1999;36:328.

36. Elghetany MT, Davey FR. Erythrocytic disorders. In: Henry JB, ed. *Clinical Diagnosis and Management by Laboratory Methods.* 20th ed. Philadelphia, PA: WB Saunders; 2001:562–563.

37. Briere RO, Golias T; Gatsakis JG. Rapid qualitative and quantitative hemoglobin fractionation. *Am J Clin Pathol.* 1965;44:695.

38. Graham JL, Grunbaum BW. A rapid method for microelectrophoresis and quantitation of hemoglobins on cellulose acetate. *Am J Clin Pathol.* 1963;39:567.

39. Milner PF, Gooden H. Rapid citrate-agar electrophoresis in routine screening for hemoglobinopathies using a simple hemolysate. *Am J Clin Pathol.* 1975;64:58.

40. Huisman THJ, Schroeder WA, Brodie AN, et al. Microchromatography of hemoglobins: II. A simplified procedure for the determination of hemoglobin A₂. *J Lab Clin Med.* 1975;86:700.

41. Clayton E, Foster BE, Clayton EP. New stain for fetal erythrocytes in peripheral blood smears. *Obstet Gynecol.* 1970;35:642.

42. Clinical and Laboratory Standards Institute (CLSI). *Fetal Red Cell Detection: Approved Guideline.* Wayne, PA: CLSI; 2001. (Document H52-A)

43. Mosca A, Paleari R, Ivaldi G. The relevance of hemoglobin F measurement in the diagnosis of thalassemias and related hemoglobinopathies. *Clin Biochem.* 2009;42:1798.

44. Harteveld CL, Kleanthous M, Traeger-Synodinos J. Prenatal diagnosis of hemoglobin disorders: present and future strategies. *Clin Biochem.* 2009;42:1768.

45. Wu AH, Laios I, Green S, et al. Immunoassays for serum and urine myoglobin: myoglobin clearance assessed as a risk factor for acute renal failure. *Clin Chem.* 1994;40(5):796–802.

46. Morrow DA, Cannon CP, Jesse RL, et al. National Academy of Clinical Biochemistry laboratory medicine practice guidelines: clinical characteristics and utilization of biochemical markers in acute coronary syndromes. *Clin Chem.* 2007;53:552.

47. Christenson RH, Azzazy HME. Biochemical markers of the acute coronary syndromes. *Clin Chem.* 1998;44:1855.

48. Poche H, Kattner E, Beckmann R, et al. Hereditary progressive muscular dystrophies: serum myoglobin pattern in patients with different types of muscular dystrophies. *Clin Physiol Biochem.* 1989;7:40.

49. Zaninotto M, Pagani F, Altinier S, et al. Multicenter evaluation of five assays for myoglobin determination. *Clin Chem.* 2000;46(10):1631–1637.

50. Apple FS, Christenson RH, Valdes R Jr, et al. Simultaneous rapid measurement of whole blood myoglobin, creatine kinase MB, and cardiac troponin I by the triage cardiac panel for detection of myocardial infarction. *Clin Chem.* 1999;45(2):199–205.

PART three

Assessment of Organ System Functions

20

Hypothalamic and Pituitary Function

ROBERT E. JONES and HEATHER CORN

chapter outline

key terms

Adenohypophysis
Adrenocorticotropin hormone (ACTH)
Anterior pituitary
Corticotropin-releasing hormone
Direct effector
Diurnal rhythms
Dopamine
Feedback loops
Follicle-stimulating hormone (FSH)
Gonadotropin-releasing hormone (GnRH)
Growth hormone
Growth hormone–releasing hormone (GHRH)
Hypothalamic–hypophyseal portal system
Hypothalamus
Infundibulum
Insulin-like growth factor (IGF)
Luteinizing hormone (LH)
Median eminence
Neurohypophysis
Oxytocin
Pituitary stalk
Posterior pituitary
Prolactin
Prolactin inhibitory factor (PIF)
Pulsatile secretion
Sella turcica
Somatostatin (SS)
Thyroid-stimulating hormone (TSH)
Thyrotropin-releasing hormone (TRH)
Tropic hormone
Vasopressin (ADH)

chapter objectives

Upon completion of this chapter, the clinical laboratorian should be able to do the following:

- Describe the functions of the anterior and posterior pituitary.
- Define the anatomic relationship between the pituitary and hypothalamus.
- Discuss the concept of open-loop negative feedback and relate this to the function of the various hypothalamic–pituitary–endocrine target gland loops.
- Describe the effects of pulsatility and cyclicity on the results of hormone measurements.
- Differentiate between tropic and direct effector in relationship to pituitary hormones.
- Discuss the regulation of prolactin secretion.
- State the nonneoplastic causes of prolactin elevation.
- Explain the difference between primary and secondary endocrine deficiency states.
- Describe the clinical features of the excess and deficiency states for growth hormone, prolactin, and vasopressin.
- Relate the physiology underlying the strategies used for screening and definitive testing for suspected disorders of growth hormone.

For additional student resources, please visit thePoint® at http://thepoint.lww.com

The term *pituitary* (derived from both Latin and Greek) literally means to "spit mucus," reflecting the primitive notion of pituitary function. In one way, the ancient physiologists were correct—they believed that the brain was responsible for signaling the pituitary to secrete; however, instead of mucus, it was later discovered that the brain directs the pituitary to secrete hormones that regulate other endocrine glands. When this was recognized, the pituitary was designated the "master gland" because, without the pituitary, there was a cessation of growth, together with profound alterations in intermediary metabolism and failure of gonadal, thyroidal, and adrenal function. The pituitary is also referred to as the *hypophysis*, from Greek meaning "undergrowth," attesting to its unique position under the hypothalamus.

Our concept of pituitary function and its role in regulating other endocrine glands has changed. Rather than viewed as the master gland, it is more appropriately recognized as a transponder that translates neural input into a hormonal product. Features that distinguish the function of the pituitary include **feedback loops, pulsatile secretions, diurnal rhythms**, and environmental or external modification of its performance. These characteristics of pituitary operation can vex the clinical evaluation of suspected endocrine disease or, alternatively, lend incredible insight into subtle defects in endocrinologic function.

EMBRYOLOGY AND ANATOMY

The three distinct parts of the pituitary are the **anterior pituitary**, or **adenohypophysis**; the intermediate lobe, or pars intermedialis; and the **posterior pituitary**, or **neurohypophysis**. The intermediate lobe is poorly developed in humans and has little functional capacity other than to confuse radiologists by forming nonfunctional, benign, cystic enlargements of the pituitary. The posterior pituitary, which arises from the diencephalon, is responsible for the storage and release of **oxytocin** and **vasopressin** (also called *antidiuretic hormone* [ADH]). The anterior pituitary, the largest portion of the gland, originates from Rathke pouch, an evagination of buccal ectoderm that progressively extends upward and is eventually enveloped by the sphenoid bone. The creation of the **median eminence**, the inferior portion of the hypothalamus, and the **pituitary stalk** is the other critical event in the formation of the hypothalamic–hypophyseal unit. Pituitary function can be detected between the seventh and ninth weeks of gestation. The ultimate determination of anterior pituitary cell types is dependent on the spatial relationships of progenitor cell types and an integrated flow of transcription factors that ultimately form lactotrophs (prolactin-secreting cells), somatotrophs (growth hormone [GH]-secreting cells), thyrotrophs (thyroid-stimulating hormone [TSH]-secreting cells), corticotrophs (adrenocorticotropin hormone [ACTH]-secreting cells), and gonadotrophs (luteinizing hormone [LH]- and follicle-stimulating hormone [FSH]-secreting cells).[1]

The pituitary resides in a pocket of the sphenoid (the **sella turcica**, meaning "Turkish saddle") and is surrounded by dura mater. The reflection of dura that separates the superior portion of the pituitary from the hypothalamus, the diaphragma sella, is penetrated by the **infundibulum**, or pituitary stalk, that connects the adenohypophysis to the *median eminence* and **hypothalamus**. The pituitary stalk contains both neural and vascular structures that terminate in the hypophysis. The posterior pituitary is connected to the supraoptic and paraventricular hypothalamic nuclei (where vasopressin and oxytocin are produced) by way of two, distinct neurosecretory tracts, the supraopticohypophyseal and tuberohypophyseal tracts, which pass through the stalk. The anterior pituitary receives 80% to 90% of its blood supply and many hypothalamic factors via the **hypothalamic–hypophyseal portal system**, also contained in the stalk. The primary plexus of this portal system is located in the median eminence and is composed of capillaries lacking a blood–brain barrier (fenestrated capillaries), where the hypothalamic nuclei that modulate pituitary function terminate their axons. In turn, the long portal vessels connect the primary plexus to the anterior pituitary and serve as a conduit for these hypothalamic–hypophysiotropic hormones. These anatomic relationships are illustrated in Figure 20.1.

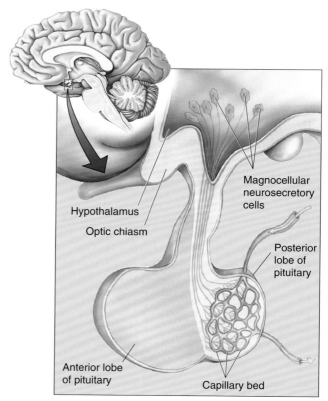

FIGURE 20.1 Relational anatomy of the pituitary and hypothalamus. (Reproduced with permission from Bear MF, Connors BW, Paradiso MA. *Neuroscience: Exploring the Brain*. 2nd ed. Baltimore, MD: Lippincott Williams & Wilkins; 2001:501.)

FUNCTIONAL ASPECTS OF THE HYPOTHALAMIC–HYPOPHYSEAL UNIT

Afferent pathways (inputs) to the hypothalamus are integrated in various specialized nuclei, processed, and then resolved into specific patterned responses. Because the hypothalamus has many efferent neural connections (outputs) to higher brain centers (the limbic system, the autonomic nervous system, and the pituitary), these responses appear to be rather diffuse but are actually stereotypical. The hypothalamic response patterns are similar for each specific pituitary hormone and characterized by open-loop negative feedback mechanisms, pulsatility, and cyclicity. Negative feedback resembles a typical servomechanism and forms the basis of our understanding of hypothalamic–pituitary function. An example of negative feedback is the relationship between a thermostat and a home heating unit. The thermostat is set to a given temperature. As the temperature in the home falls below this set point, the thermostat sends an electrical impulse to the furnace and turns the furnace on. Heat is restored to the room, and, when the temperature in the room exceeds the predetermined set point, the thermostat turns off the furnace. Because the thermostat set point can be adjusted for the comfort of the occupants, the furnace–thermostat functional relationship is termed an *open-loop negative feedback system*. Most endocrine feedback loops are of the open-loop variety, meaning that they are subject to external modulation and generally influenced or modified by higher neural input or other hormones.

A simple example of an endocrine feedback loop is the hypothalamic–pituitary–thyroidal axis. The hypothalamus produces the hypophysiotropic hormone, **thyrotropin-releasing hormone (TRH)**, and releases it into the portal system where it directs the thyrotrophs (or TSH-producing cells) in the anterior pituitary to secrete **TSH**. TSH circulates to the thyroid and stimulates several steps in the thyroid that are critical in the production and release of thyroid hormone (thyroxine). Thyroxine is released in the blood and circulates to the hypothalamus and pituitary to suppress further TRH and TSH production. This axis can be partially inhibited by adrenal steroids (glucocorticoids) and by cytokines; as a result, thyroid hormone production may decline during periods of severe physiologic stress.[2] The feedback of thyroxine at the level of the pituitary is called a *short feedback loop*, and feedback at the level of the hypothalamus is called a *long feedback loop*. Feedback between the pituitary and hypothalamus (when present) is called an *ultrashort feedback loop*. Figure 20.2 illustrates this simple feedback loop.

All anterior pituitary hormones are secreted in a pulsatile fashion. The pulse frequency of secretion is generally regulated by neural modulation and is specific for each hypothalamic–pituitary–end-organ unit. Perhaps the best example of pituitary pulsatility is the secretion of the hormones that regulate gonadal function (**LH and FSH**). In normal male subjects, the median interpulse interval for LH is 55 minutes, and the average LH peak duration is 40 minutes.[3]

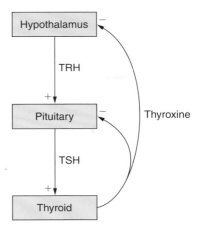

FIGURE 20.2 Simple feedback loop. TRH, thyrotropin-releasing hormone; TSH, thyroid-stimulating hormone.

The pulse frequency of the regulatory hypothalamic hormone, **gonadotropin-releasing hormone (GnRH)**, has profound effects on LH secretion profiles—increasing the frequency of GnRH pulses reduces the gonadotrope secretory response, and decreasing the GnRH pulse frequency increases the amplitude of the subsequent LH pulse.[4]

Another feature of the hypothalamic–pituitary unit is the cyclic nature of hormone secretion. The nervous system usually regulates this function through external signals, such as light–dark changes or the ratio of daylight to darkness. The term *zeitgeber* ("time giver") refers to the process of entraining or synchronizing these external cues into the function of internal biologic clocks. As a result, many pituitary hormones are secreted in different amounts, depending on the time of day. These circadian, or diurnal, rhythms are typified by **ACTH**, or TSH secretion. With ACTH, the nadir of secretion is between 11:00 PM and 3:00 AM, and the peak occurs on awakening or around 6:00 to 9:00 AM.[5] The circadian rhythm of ACTH is a result of variations in pulse amplitude and not alterations in pulse frequency.[6] The nocturnal levels of TSH are approximately twice the daytime levels; the nocturnal rise in TSH is a result of increased pulse amplitude.[7]

HYPOPHYSIOTROPIC OR HYPOTHALAMIC HORMONES

The hypothalamus produces many different products; however, only those that have a direct effect on classic pituitary function will be discussed in this chapter. Most products are peptides; however, bioactive amines are also synthesized and transported from the hypothalamus. Hypothalamic hormones may have multiple actions. For example, TRH stimulates the secretion of both TSH and **prolactin**; GnRH stimulates both LH and FSH production; and **somatostatin (SS)** inhibits GH and TSH release from the pituitary. In addition to its effects on water metabolism, vasopressin (ADH) can also stimulate *ACTH* secretion. The main stimulus for ACTH secretion is **corticotropin-releasing hormone**. These hypophysiotropic hormones are found

Hormone	Structure	Action
TRH	3 amino acids	Releases TSH and prolactin
GnRH	10 amino acids	Releases LH and FSH
CRH	41 amino acids	Releases ACTH
GHRH	44 amino acids	Releases GH
Somatostatin	14 and 28 amino acids	Inhibits GH and TSH release (additional effects on gut and pancreatic function)
Dopamine (prolactin inhibitory factor)	1 amino acid	Inhibits prolactin release

TRH, thyrotropin-releasing hormone; TSH, thyroid-stimulating hormone; GnRH, gonadotropin-releasing hormone; LH, luteinizing hormone; FSH, follicle-stimulating hormone; CRH, corticotropin-releasing hormone; ACTH, adrenocorticotropin hormone; GHRH, growth hormone–releasing hormone.

throughout the central nervous system and various other tissues, including the gut, pancreas, and other endocrine glands. Their function outside the hypothalamus and pituitary is poorly understood. The action of hypophysiotropic hormones on anterior pituitary function is summarized in Table 20.1.

ANTERIOR PITUITARY HORMONES

The hormones secreted from the anterior pituitary are larger and more complex than those synthesized in the hypothalamus. These pituitary hormones are either *tropic*, meaning their actions are specific for another endocrine gland, or they are **direct effectors**, because they act directly on peripheral tissue. TSH and its unique role in regulating thyroid function provide an example of tropic; an example of a direct effector is GH. GH has direct effects on substrate metabolism in numerous tissues and also stimulates the liver to produce growth factors that are critical in enhancing linear growth. The **tropic hormones** are LH, which directs testosterone production from Leydig cells in men and ovulation in women; FSH, which is responsible for ovarian recruitment and early folliculogenesis in women and spermatogenesis in men; TSH, which directs thyroid hormone production from the thyroid; and ACTH, which regulates adrenal steroidogenesis. Both GH and prolactin are direct effectors. A general summary of relationships among anterior pituitary hormones and their target organs and feedback effectors is provided in Table 20.2.

The actions of the tropic hormones are discussed in other chapters devoted to the specific target gland.

PITUITARY TUMORS

According to autopsy studies, up to 20% of people harbor clinically silent pituitary adenomas, and findings consistent with pituitary tumors are observed in 10% to 30% of normal individuals undergoing MRI examinations. In addition, pituitary tumors account for 91% of the lesions removed from carefully selected patients who have undergone transsphenoidal surgery.[8,9] Close medical follow-up is recommended if the incidentally discovered lesion is hormonally silent and is less than 1 cm in diameter. Prolactin-secreting pituitary tumors are the most common, followed by nonfunctioning or null cell tumors, and tumors that secrete GH, gonadotropins, ACTH, or TSH account for the remainder. The WHO defined "atypical pituitary tumors" as tumors that have an MIB-1 proliferative index greater than 3%, excessive p53 immunoreactivity, and increased mitotic activity.[10] Most of these "atypical" tumors are macroadenomas (i.e., >1 cm in diameter) and show invasion into surrounding structures like the cavernous sinuses. They may or may not be hormonally active and, interestingly, tend to stain commonly for GH or ACTH even though they may not produce clinically evident syndromes.[10] MIB-1 is a monoclonal antibody that is used to detect the Ki-67 antigen, a marker of cell proliferation, and a high "proliferation index" suggests higher degree of atypia.[11]

Physiologic enlargement of the pituitary can be seen during puberty and pregnancy. The enlargement seen during pregnancy is due to lactotroph hyperplasia. Thyrotroph and lactotroph or gonadotroph hyperplasia can also be seen in long-standing primary thyroidal or gonadal failure, respectively.

Pituitary Hormone	Target Gland	Structure	Feedback Hormone
LH	Gonad (tropic)	Dimeric glycoprotein	Sex steroids (E_2/T)
FSH	Gonad (tropic)	Dimeric glycoprotein	Inhibin
TSH	Thyroid (tropic)	Dimeric glycoprotein	Thyroid hormones (T_4/T_3)
ACTH	Adrenal (tropic)	Single peptide derived from POMC	Cortisol
Growth hormone	Multiple (direct effector)	Single peptide	IGF-I
Prolactin	Breast (direct effector)	Single peptide	Unknown

LH, luteinizing hormone; FSH, follicle-stimulating hormone; TSH, thyroid-stimulating hormone; ACTH, adrenocorticotropin hormone; T_4, thyroxine; T_3, triiodothyronine; E_2, estradiol; T, testosterone; POMC, pro-opiomelanocortin; IGF-I, insulin-like growth factor.

GROWTH HORMONE

The pituitary is vital for normal growth. Growth ceases if the pituitary is removed, and if the hormonal products from other endocrine glands that are acted on by the pituitary are replaced (thyroxine, adrenal steroids, and gonadal steroids), growth is not restored until GH is administered. However, if GH is given in isolation without the other hormones, growth is not promoted. Therefore, it takes complete functioning of the pituitary to establish conditions ripe for growth of the individual. It also takes adequate nutrition, normal levels of insulin, and overall good health to achieve a person's genetic growth potential.

GH, also called *somatotropin*, is structurally related to prolactin and human placental lactogen. A single peptide with two intramolecular disulfide bridges, it belongs to the direct effector class of anterior pituitary hormones. The somatotrophs, pituitary cells that produce GH, constitute over one-third of normal pituitary weight. Release of somatotropin from the pituitary is stimulated by the hypothalamic peptide **growth hormone–releasing hormone (GHRH)**; somatotropin's secretion is inhibited by SS.[12] GH is secreted in pulses, with an average interpulse interval of 2 to 3 hours, with the most reproducible peak occurring at the onset of sleep.[13] Between these pulses, the level of GH may fall below the detectable limit, resulting in the clinical evaluation of GH deficiency being based on a single, challenging measurement. Ghrelin, an enteric hormone that plays important roles in nutrient sensing, appetite and in glucose regulation, is also a potent stimulator of GH secretion.[14]

No other hypothalamic–hypophyseal system more vividly illustrates the concept of an open-loop paradigm than that seen with GH. The on-and-off functions of GHRH/SS and the basic pattern of secretory pulses of GH are heavily modulated by other factors (Table 20.3).

Actions of GH

GH has many diverse effects on metabolism; it is considered an amphibolic hormone because it directly influences both anabolic and catabolic processes. One major effect of GH is that it allows an individual to effectively transition from a fed state to a fasting state without experiencing a shortage of substrates required for normal intracellular oxidation. GH directly antagonizes the effect of insulin on glucose metabolism, promotes hepatic gluconeogenesis, and stimulates lipolysis.[15,16] From a teleologic viewpoint, this makes perfect sense—enhanced lipolysis provides oxidative substrate for peripheral tissue, such as skeletal muscle, and yet conserves glucose for the central nervous system by stimulating the hepatic delivery of glucose and opposing insulin-mediated glucose disposal. Indeed, isolated GH deficiency in children may be accompanied by hypoglycemia; however, hypoglycemia is more likely to occur if both GH and ACTH are deficient.[17]

The anabolic effects of GH are reflected by enhanced protein synthesis in skeletal muscle and other tissues. This is translated into a positive nitrogen balance and phosphate retention.

Although GH has direct effects on many tissues, it also has indirect effects that are mediated by factors that were initially called *somatomedins*. In early experiments, it became apparent that GH supplementation in hypophysectomized animals induced the production of an additional factor that stimulated the incorporation of sulfate into cartilage.[18,19] As this "protein" was purified, it was evident that there was more than one somatomedin, and because of their structural homology to proinsulin, the nomenclature shifted to **insulin-like growth factor (IGF)**.[20,21] For example, somatomedin C, the major growth factor induced by GH, is now IGF-I.[22] IGFs also have cell surface receptors that are distinct from insulin; however, supraphysiologic levels of IGF-II can "bleed" over on the insulin receptor and cause hypoglycemia,[23] and hyperinsulinemia can partially activate IGF-I receptors.[24] GH stimulates the production of IGF-I from the liver, and as a result, IGF-I becomes a biologic amplifier of GH levels. IGFs are complexed to specific serum *binding proteins* that have been shown to affect the actions of IGFs in multifaceted ways.[25] IGF-binding protein 3 (IGFBP-3) is perhaps the best studied member of the IGFBP family. Recently, IGFBPs and specifically IGFBP-3 have been shown to directly play a role in the pathophysiology of several human cancers (this may be independent of IGF-1 and IGF-1 receptor–mediated pathways).[26] The tumor suppressor gene, P53, has been shown to upregulate active IGFBP-3 secretion, which in turn inhibits IGF-1 signaled mutagenesis, and, thus, inhibits neoplastic cell proliferation.[27] Low levels of IGFBP-3 were positively correlated

TABLE 20.3 Other Modifiers of Growth Hormone Secretion

Stimulate Growth Hormone Secretion	Inhibit Growth Hormone Secretion
Sleep	Glucose loading
Exercise	β-Agonists (e.g., epinephrine)
Physiologic stress	α-Blockers (e.g., phentolamine)
Amino acids (e.g., arginine)	Emotional/psychogenic stress
Hypoglycemia	Nutritional deficiencies
Sex steroids (e.g., estradiol)	Insulin deficiency
α-Agonists (e.g., norepinephrine)	Thyroxine deficiency
β-Blockers (e.g., propranolol)	

with higher rates of colorectal cancer risk (in men) in a nested case–control study from the Physicians Health Study cohort.[28]

Testing

As noted above, a single, random measurement of GH is rarely diagnostic. The current testing paradigms for GH are soundly based on the dynamic physiology of the GH axis. For example, circulating levels of IGF-I and, perhaps, IGFBP-3 reasonably integrate the peaks of GH secretion, and elevated levels of both are consistent with, but may not be diagnostic of, a sustained excess of GH. Other conditions such as hepatoma can be associated with high levels of IGF-I, and levels of IGFBP-3 may be inappropriately normal in some people with active acromegaly. Conversely, low IGF-I levels may reflect inadequate production of GH; however, low IGF levels are also seen in patients with poorly controlled diabetes, malnutrition, or other chronic illnesses.[29] The inherent high biologic variability and assay performance issues further confound the use of IGF-I measurements in the clinical setting.[30] Recently, new recommendations to improve the assay performance for both IGF-I and GH have been published.[31]

Definitive testing for determining the autonomous production of GH relies upon the normal suppressibility of GH by oral glucose loading.[22,32,33] This test is performed after an overnight fast, and the patient is given a 100 g oral glucose load. GH is measured at time zero and at 60 and 120 minutes after glucose ingestion. Following oral glucose loading, GH levels are undetectable in normal individuals; however, in patients with acromegaly, GH levels fail to suppress and may even paradoxically rise.

Testing patients for suspected GH deficiency is more complicated. There are several strategies to stimulate GH, and new protocols are currently evolving. Once considered the gold standard, insulin-induced hypoglycemia is being replaced by less uncomfortable testing schemes.[34] Combination infusions of GHRH and the amino acid L-arginine or an infusion of L-arginine coupled with oral L-DOPA are the most widely used although acquiring some of the medications can be problematic.[35] If GH levels rise above 3 to 5 ng/mL, it is unlikely that the patient is GH deficient[34]; however, a lower threshold may be adopted because of improved sensitivity of the newer two-site GH assays.[35] On the other hand, several studies have shown that provocative GH testing may not be necessary in patients with low IGF-1 levels and otherwise documented panhypopituitarism.[29]

Acromegaly

Acromegaly results from pathologic or autonomous GH excess and, in the vast majority of patients, is a result of a pituitary tumor. There have been isolated case reports of tumors causing acromegaly as a result of the ectopic production of GHRH,[36–38] and although exceedingly interesting or instructive, the ectopic production of GHRH or GH remains rare.[37] Recent reports have documented mutations in the aryl hydrocarbon–interacting protein gene (AIP)[39] in cases of familial acromegaly and polymorphisms in the SS receptor type 5 gene in sporadic cases.[40] If a GH-producing tumor occurs before epiphyseal

closure, the patient develops gigantism[41] and may grow to an impressive height; otherwise, the patient develops classical, but insidious, features of bony and soft tissue overgrowth.[42] These features include progressive enlargement of the hands and feet as well as growth of facial bones, including the mandible and bones of the skull. In advanced cases, the patient may develop significant gaps between their teeth. Diffuse (not longitudinal if the condition occurred following puberty) overgrowth of the ends of long bones or the spine can produce a debilitating form of arthritis.[43] Because GH is an insulin antagonist, glucose intolerance or overt diabetes can occur. Hypertension; accelerated atherosclerosis; and proximal muscle weakness, resulting from acquired myopathy,[44] may be seen late in the illness. Sleep apnea is common. Organomegaly, especially thyromegaly, is common, but hyperthyroidism is exceedingly rare unless the tumor cosecretes TSH. GH excess is also a hypermetabolic condition, and as a result, acromegalic patients may complain of excessive sweating or heat intolerance. The features of acromegaly develop slowly over time, and the patient (or even their family) may be oblivious that changes in physiognomy have occurred. In these cases, the patient's complaints may center on the local effects of the tumor (headache or visual complaints) or symptoms related to the loss of other anterior pituitary hormones (hypopituitarism). A careful, retrospective review of older photographs may be crucial in differentiating coarse features due to inheritance from the classical consequences of acromegaly. If left untreated, acromegaly shortens life expectancy because of increased risk of heart disease, resulting from the combination of hypertension, coronary artery disease, and diabetes/insulin resistance. Because patients with acromegaly also have a greater lifetime risk of developing cancer, cancer surveillance programs (especially regular colonoscopy) are recommended.[22]

CASE STUDY 20.1

A 48-year-old man seeks care for evaluation of muscle weakness, headaches, and excessive sweating. He has poorly controlled hypertension and, on questioning, admits to noticing a gradual increase in both glove and shoe size, as well as a reduction in libido. A review of older photographs of the man documents coarsening of facial features, progressive prognathism, and broadening of the nose. Acromegaly is suspected.

Questions

1. What screening tests are available?
2. What is the definitive test for autonomous growth hormone production?
3. Because the patient complains of reduced libido, hypogonadism is suspected. What evaluation is appropriate?
4. How would your thinking change if she had galactorrhea but normal levels of prolactin?

Cosecretion of prolactin can be seen in up to 40% of patients with acromegaly.[45] Only a few TSH/GH-secreting tumors have also been reported.[46]

Confirming the diagnosis of acromegaly is relatively easy; however, some patients with acromegaly have normal random levels of GH. An elevated level of GH that does not suppress normally with glucose loading equates to an easy diagnosis. In those patients with normal, but inappropriately sustained, random levels of GH, elevated levels of IGF-I are helpful; however, nonsuppressibility of GH to glucose loading is the definitive test.[32,33]

Treatment of acromegaly can be challenging. The goal of treatment is tumor ablation, with continued function of the remainder of the pituitary. Transsphenoidal adenomectomy is the procedure of choice.[22] If normal GH levels and kinetics (normal suppressibility to glucose) are restored following surgery, the patient is likely cured. Unfortunately, GH-producing tumors may be too large or may invade into local structures that preclude complete surgical extirpation, and the patient is left with a smaller, but hormonally active, tumor. External beam or focused irradiation is frequently used at this point, but it may take several years before GH levels decline.[47,48] In the interim, efforts are made to suppress GH. Three different classes of agents, SS analogs (octreotide, pasireotide, and lanreotide), dopaminergic agonists (cabergoline and bromocriptine), and GH receptor antagonists (pegvisomant) may be employed for GH suppression.[49,50]

GH Deficiency

GH deficiency occurs in both children and adults. In children, it may be genetic or it may be due to tumors, such as craniopharyngiomas. In adults, it is a result of structural or functional abnormalities of the pituitary (see the section on *hypopituitarism* in this chapter); however, a decline in GH production is an inevitable consequence of aging, and the significance of this phenomenon is poorly understood.[51,52]

Although GH deficiency in children is manifest by growth failure, not all patients with short stature have GH deficiency[53] (see above). There have been several genetic defects identified in the GH axis. The most common type is a recessive mutation in the GHRH gene that causes a failure of GH secretion. A rarer mutation, loss of the GH gene itself, has also been observed. Mutations that result in GH insensitivity have also been reported. These mutations may involve the GH receptor, IGF-I biosynthesis, IGF-I receptors, or defects in GH signal transduction. As a result, patients with GH insensitivity do not respond normally to exogenously administered GH. Finally, structural lesions of the pituitary or hypothalamus may also cause GH deficiency and may be associated with other anterior pituitary hormone deficiencies.

An adult GH deficiency syndrome has been described in patients who have complete or even partial failure of the anterior pituitary. The symptoms of this syndrome are extremely vague and include social withdrawal, fatigue, loss of motivation, and a diminished feeling of well-being,[54] but

several studies have documented increased mortality in children who are GH deficient although this relationship is less clear in adults.[55] Osteoporosis and alterations in body composition (i.e., reduced lean body mass) are frequent concomitants of adult GH deficiency.[56]

GH replacement therapy has become relatively simple with the advent of recombinant human GH.[57] Currently, the cost of GH is the major limiting factor for replacement. GH has been employed by athletes as a performance-enhancing substance and as an aid in injury recovery; however, the effectiveness of GH for these purposes is controversial.[58]

PROLACTIN

Prolactin is structurally related to GH and human placental lactogen. Considered a stress hormone, it has vital functions in relationship to reproduction. Prolactin is classified as a direct effector hormone (as opposed to a tropic hormone) because it has diffuse target tissue and lacks a single endocrine end organ.

Prolactin is unique among the anterior pituitary hormones because its major mode of hypothalamic regulation is tonic inhibition rather than intermittent stimulation. **Prolactin inhibitory factor (PIF)** was once considered a polypeptide hormone capable of inhibiting prolactin secretion; **dopamine**, however, is the only neuroendocrine signal that inhibits prolactin and is now considered to be the elusive PIF. Any compound that affects dopaminergic activity in the median eminence of the hypothalamus will also alter prolactin secretion. Examples of medications that cause hyperprolactinemia include phenothiazines, butyrophenones, metoclopramide, reserpine, tricyclic antidepressants, α-methyldopa, and antipsychotics that antagonize the dopamine D2 receptor. Any disruption of the pituitary stalk (e.g., tumors, trauma, or inflammation) causes an elevation in prolactin as a result of interruption of the flow of dopamine from the hypothalamus to the lactotrophs, the pituitary prolactin-secreting cells. TRH directly stimulates prolactin secretion and increases in TRH (as seen in primary hypothyroidism) elevate prolactin levels.[59] Estrogens also directly stimulate lactotrophs to synthesize prolactin. Pathologic stimulation of the neural suckling reflex is the likely explanation of hyperprolactinemia associated with chest wall injuries. Hyperprolactinemia may also be seen in renal failure and polycystic ovary syndrome. Physiologic stressors, such as exercise and seizures, also elevate prolactin. The feedback effector for prolactin is unknown. Although the primary regulation of prolactin secretions is tonic inhibition (e.g., dopamine), it is also regulated by several hormones, including GnRH, TRH, and vasoactive intestinal polypeptide. Stimulation of breasts, as in nursing, causes the release of prolactin-secreting hormones from the hypothalamus through a spinal reflex arc.

As mentioned, the physiologic effect of prolactin is lactation. The usual consequence of prolactin excess is hypogonadism, either by suppression of gonadotropin secretion from the pituitary or by inhibition of gonadotropin action at the gonad.[60] The suppression of ovulation seen in lactating postpartum mothers is related to this phenomenon.

Prolactinoma

A prolactinoma is a pituitary tumor that directly secretes prolactin, and it represents the most common type of functional pituitary tumor. The clinical presentation of a patient with a prolactinoma depends on the age and gender of the patient and the size of the tumor. Premenopausal women most frequently complain of menstrual irregularity/amenorrhea, infertility, or galactorrhea; men or postmenopausal women generally present with symptoms of a pituitary mass, such as headaches or visual complaints. Occasionally, a man may present with reduced libido or complaints of erectile dysfunction. The reason(s) for the varied presentations of a prolactinoma are somewhat obscure but likely relate to the dramatic, noticeable alteration in menses or the abrupt onset of a breast discharge in younger women. By contrast, the decline in reproductive function in older patients may be overlooked as an inexorable consequence of "aging." One recently recognized complication of prolactin-induced hypogonadism is osteoporosis.[61]

CASE STUDY 20.2

A 23-year-old woman has experienced recent onset of a spontaneous, bilateral breast discharge and gradual cessation of menses. She reports normal growth and development and has never been pregnant.

Questions

1. What conditions could be causing her symptoms?
2. What medical conditions (other than a prolactinoma) are associated with hyperprolactinemia?
3. Which medications raise prolactin?

Other Causes of Hyperprolactinemia

There are many physiologic, pharmacologic, and pathologic causes of hyperprolactinemia, and a common error by clinicians is to ascribe any elevation in prolactin to a "prolactinoma." Generally, substantial elevations in prolactin (>150 ng/mL) indicate prolactinoma, and the degree of elevation in prolactin is correlated with tumor size.[62] Modest elevations in prolactin (25 to 100 ng/mL) may be seen with pituitary stalk interruption, use of dopaminergic antagonist medications, or other medical conditions such as primary thyroidal failure, renal failure, or polycystic ovary syndrome. Breast or genital stimulation may also modestly elevate prolactin. Significant hyperprolactinemia is also encountered during pregnancy. Under most circumstances, the principal form of prolactin is a 23-kD peptide; however, a 150-kD form may also be secreted. This larger prolactin

molecule has a markedly reduced biologic potency and does not share the reproductive consequences of the 23-kD variety. If the 150-kD form of prolactin predominates, this is called macroprolactinemia, and the clinical consequences are unclear, but most patients are relatively asymptomatic.[62] The prevalence of macroprolactinemia has been estimated at 10% to 22% of hyperprolactinemic samples[63] and can be excluded by precipitating serum samples with polyethylene glycol prior to measuring prolactin.

Clinical Evaluation of Hyperprolactinemia

A careful history and physical examination are usually sufficient to exclude most common, nonendocrine causes of hyperprolactinemia. It is essential to obtain TSH and free T_4 to eliminate primary hypothyroidism as a cause for the elevated prolactin. If a pituitary tumor is suspected, a careful assessment of other anterior pituitary function (basal cortisol, LH, FSH, and gender-specific gonadal steroid [either estradiol or testosterone]) and an evaluation of sellar anatomy with a high-resolution MRI should be obtained.

Management of Prolactinoma

The therapeutic goals are correction of symptoms that result from local invasion or extension of the tumor by reducing tumor mass, restoration of normal gonadal function and fertility, prevention of osteoporosis, and preservation of normal anterior and posterior pituitary function. The different therapeutic options include simple observation, surgery, radiotherapy, or medical management with dopamine agonists.[64] However, the management of prolactinoma also depends on the size of the tumor (macroadenomas [tumor size >10 mm] are less likely to be "cured" than are microadenomas [tumor size < 10 mm])[65] and the preferences of the patient.

Dopamine agonists are the most commonly used therapy for microprolactinomas. Tumor shrinkage is noted in more than 90% of patients treated with either bromocriptine mesylate (Parlodel) or cabergoline (Dostinex), dopamine receptor agonists. Both drugs also shrink prolactin-secreting macroadenomas.[64] A resumption of menses and restoration of fertility is also frequently seen during medical therapy. The adverse effects of bromocriptine include orthostatic hypotension, dizziness, and nausea. The gastrointestinal adverse effects of bromocriptine can be ameliorated through intravaginal administration, and its efficacy is otherwise uncompromised. Cabergoline has fewer adverse effects and may be administered biweekly because of its longer duration of action. By virtue of its ability to interact with the 5-hydroxytryptamine (5-HT)$_{2B}$ serotonergic receptor, cabergoline has been linked to the development of valvular heart disease,[66] although the doses of cabergoline required to elicit the risk of valvular damage are in vast excess to the doses used in the management of prolactinomas. Either agent should be discontinued during pregnancy unless tumor regrowth has been documented.

Neurosurgery is not a primary mode of prolactinoma management. The indications for neurosurgical intervention include pituitary tumor apoplexy (hemorrhage), acute visual loss due to macroadenoma, cystic prolactinoma, intolerance to medical therapy, or tumor resistance to dopaminergic agonists. Surgical cure rates are inversely proportional to tumor size and the degree of prolactin elevation. Radiotherapy is generally reserved for high surgical risk patients with locally aggressive macroadenomas who are unable to tolerate dopamine agonists.

Idiopathic Galactorrhea

Lactation occurring in women with normal prolactin levels is defined as *idiopathic galactorrhea*. This condition is usually seen in women who have been pregnant several times and has no pathologic implication, but may be a manifestation of a localized increased sensitivity to prolactin in breast tissue. It is to be remembered that this is a diagnosis of exclusion.

HYPOPITUITARISM

The failure of either the pituitary or the hypothalamus results in the loss of anterior pituitary function. Complete loss of function is termed *panhypopituitarism*; however, there may be a loss of only a single pituitary hormone, which is referred to as a *monotropic hormone deficiency*. The loss of a tropic hormone (ACTH, TSH, LH, and FSH) is reflected in function cessation of the affected endocrine gland. Loss of the direct effectors (GH and prolactin) may not be readily apparent. This section concentrates on the causes of hypopituitarism and certain subtleties involved in the therapy of panhypopituitarism; more detailed descriptions of various hormone deficiency states are covered in other chapters.

CASE STUDY 20.3

A 60-year-old man presented with intractable headaches. MRI was requested to evaluate this complaint, and a 2.5-cm pituitary tumor was discovered. In retrospect, he noted an unexplained 20-kg weight loss, cold intolerance, fatigue, and loss of sexual desire.

Questions

1. How would you approach the evaluation of his anterior pituitary function?

2. What additional testing may be required to confirm a loss in anterior pituitary function?

The laboratory diagnosis of hypopituitarism is relatively straightforward. In contrast to the primary failure of an endocrine gland that is accompanied by dramatic increases in circulating levels of the corresponding pituitary tropic hormone, secondary failure (hypopituitarism) is associated with low or normal levels of tropic hormone. In primary hypothyroidism, for example, the circulating levels of thyroxine are low and TSH levels may exceed 200 μU/mL (normal, 0.4 to 5.0 μU/mL). As a result of pituitary failure in hypothyroidism, TSH levels are inappropriately low and typically less than 1.0 μU/mL in association with low free thyroxine levels.

There are several important issues in distinguishing between primary and secondary hormone deficiency states. To differentiate between primary and secondary deficiencies, both tropic and target hormone levels should be measured when there is any suspicion of pituitary failure or as part of the routine evaluation of gonadal or adrenal function. If one secondary deficiency is documented, it is essential to search for other deficiency states and the cause for pituitary failure. For example, failure to recognize secondary hypoadrenalism may have catastrophic consequences if the patient is treated with thyroxine. Similarly, initially overlooking a pituitary or hypothalamic lesion could preclude early diagnosis and treatment of a potentially aggressive tumor.

Etiology of Hypopituitarism

The many causes of hypopituitarism are listed in Table 20.4. Direct effects of pituitary tumors, or the sequelae of treatment of tumors, are the most common causes of pituitary failure. Pituitary tumors may cause panhypopituitarism by compressing or replacing normal tissue or interrupting the flow of hypothalamic hormones by destroying the pituitary stalk. Large, nonsecretory pituitary tumors (chromophobe adenomas or null cell tumors) or macroprolactinomas are most commonly associated with this phenomenon. Parasellar tumors (meningiomas and gliomas), metastatic tumors (breast and lung), and hypothalamic tumors (craniopharyngiomas or dysgerminomas) can also cause hypopituitarism through similar mechanisms. Hemorrhage into a pituitary tumor (pituitary tumor apoplexy) is rare; however, when it occurs, it frequently causes complete pituitary failure.[67] Postpartum ischemic necrosis of the pituitary following a complicated delivery (Sheehan's syndrome) typically presents as profound, unresponsive shock or as

 TABLE 20.4 **Causes of Hypopituitarism**

1. Pituitary tumors
2. Parapituitary/hypothalamic tumors
3. Trauma
4. Radiation therapy/surgery
5. Infarction
6. Infection
7. Infiltrative disease
8. Immunologic
9. Familial
10. Idiopathic

failure to lactate in the puerperium. Infiltrative diseases, such as hemochromatosis, sarcoidosis, or histiocytosis, can also affect pituitary function. Fungal infections, tuberculosis, and syphilis can involve the pituitary or hypothalamus and may cause impairment of function. Lymphocytic hypophysitis,[68] an autoimmune disease of the pituitary, may only affect a single cell type in the pituitary, resulting in a monotropic hormone deficiency, or can involve all cell types, yielding total loss of function. Ipilimumab, a monoclonal antibody that blocks cytotoxic T-lymphocyte–associated antigen 4 (CTLA-4) and proven to increase survival in melanoma patients, has been associated with lymphocytic hypophysitis in up to 5% of treated patients.[69] Severe head trauma may shear the pituitary stalk or may interrupt the portal circulation. Similarly, surgery involving the pituitary may compromise the stalk and/or blood supply to the pituitary or may iatrogenically diminish the mass of functioning pituitary tissue. Panhypopituitarism can result from radiotherapy used to treat a primary pituitary tumor or a pituitary that was inadvertently included in the radiation port; loss of function, however, may be gradual and may occur over several years. There have been rare instances of familial panhypopituitarism[70] or monotropic hormone deficiencies. In Kallmann's syndrome, for example, GnRH is deficient, and the patient presents with secondary hypogonadism. Last, there may not be an apparent identified cause for the loss of pituitary function, and the patient is classified as having idiopathic hypopituitarism, although it is always prudent to continue the search for an underlying cause.

CASE STUDY 20.4

An 18-year-old woman was admitted to the neurologic intensive care unit following a severe closed head injury. Her course stabilized after 24 hours, but the nursing staff noticed a dramatic increase in the patient's urine output, which exceeded 1,000 mL/h.

Questions

1. What caused her increased urine production?
2. How could you prove your suspicions?
3. Could she have other possible endocrinologic problems?

Treatment of Panhypopituitarism

In the average patient, replacement therapy for panhypopituitarism is the same as for primary target organ failure. Patients are treated with thyroxine, glucocorticoids, and gender-specific sex steroids. It is less clear about GH replacement in adults, and additional studies are needed to clarify this issue. Replacement becomes more complicated in panhypopituitary patients who desire fertility. Pulsatile

GnRH infusions have induced puberty and restored fertility in patients with Kallmann's syndrome,[71] and gonadotropin preparations have restored ovulation/spermatogenesis in people with gonadotropin deficiency.[72]

POSTERIOR PITUITARY HORMONES

The posterior pituitary is an extension of the forebrain and represents the storage region for vasopressin (also called ADH) and oxytocin. Both of these small peptide hormones are synthesized in the supraoptic and paraventricular nuclei of the hypothalamus and transported to the neurohypophysis via their axons in the hypothalamoneurohypophyseal tract. This tract transits the median eminence of the hypothalamus and continues into the posterior pituitary through the pituitary stalk. The synthesis of each of these hormones is tightly linked to the production of neurophysin,[73] a larger protein whose function is poorly understood. Both hormones are synthesized outside of the hypothalamus in various tissues, and it is plausible they have an autocrine or a paracrine function.

Oxytocin

Oxytocin is a cyclic nonapeptide, with a disulfide bridge connecting amino acid residues 1 and 6. As a posttranslational modification, the C-terminus is amidated. Oxytocin has a critical role in lactation[74] and plays a major role in labor and parturition.[75] Oxytocin is also unique because its secretion responds to a positive feedback loop, meaning that circulating levels of oxytocin actually perpetuate further hormone secretion, instead of suppressing further hormone secretion as is the case with most anterior pituitary hormones. In this way, uterine contractions propagate oxytocin release, which causes further uterine contractions, which cause further oxytocin release until parturition occurs. Synthetic oxytocin, Pitocin, is used in obstetrics to induce labor. Recent studies have linked oxytocin to a variety of biosocial behaviors to include maternal nurturing and mother–infant bonding.[76] In addition to its reproductive and prosocial effects, oxytocin has been shown to have effects on pituitary, renal, cardiac, metabolic, and immune function.

Vasopressin

Structurally similar to oxytocin, vasopressin is a cyclic nonapeptide with an identical disulfide bridge; it differs from oxytocin by only two amino acids. Vasopressin's major action is to regulate renal free water excretion and, therefore, has a central role in water balance. The vasopressin receptors in the kidney (V_2) are concentrated in the renal collecting tubules and the ascending limb of the loop of Henle. They are coupled to adenylate cyclase, and once activated, they induce insertion of aquaporin-2, a water channel protein, into the tubular luminal membrane.[77] Vasopressin is also a potent pressor agent and effects blood clotting[78] by promoting factor VII release from hepatocytes and von Willebrand factor release from the endothelium. These vasopressin receptors (V_{1a} and V_{1b}) are coupled to phospholipase C.

Hypothalamic osmoreceptors and vascular baroreceptors regulate the release of vasopressin from the posterior pituitary. The osmoreceptors are extremely sensitive to even small changes in plasma osmolality, with an average osmotic threshold for vasopressin release in humans of 284 mOsm/kg. As plasma osmolality increases, vasopressin secretion increases. The consequence is a reduction in renal free water clearance, a lowering of plasma osmolality, and a return to homeostasis. The vascular baroreceptors (located in the left atrium, aortic arch, and carotid arteries) initiate vasopressin release in response to a fall in blood volume or blood pressure. A 5% to 10% fall in arterial blood pressure in normal humans will trigger vasopressin release; however, in contrast to an osmotic stimulus, the vasopressin response to a baroreceptor-induced stimulus is exponential. In fact, baroreceptor-induced vasopressin secretion will override the normal osmotic suppression of vasopressin secretion.

Diabetes insipidus (DI), characterized by copious production of urine (polyuria) and intense thirst (polydipsia), is a consequence of vasopressin deficiency. However, total vasopressin deficiency is unusual, and the typical patient presents with a partial deficiency. The causes of hypothalamic DI include apparent autoimmunity to vasopressin-secreting neurons, trauma, diseases affecting pituitary stalk function, and various central nervous system or pituitary tumors. A sizable percentage of patients (up to 30%) will have idiopathic DI.[79]

Depending on the degree of vasopressin deficiency, diagnosis of DI can be readily apparent or may require extensive investigation. Documenting an inappropriately low vasopressin level with an elevated plasma osmolality would yield a reasonably secure diagnosis of DI. In less obvious cases, the patient may require a water deprivation test in which fluids are withheld from the patient and serial determinations of serum and urine osmolality are performed in an attempt to document the patient's ability to conserve water. Under selected circumstances, a health care provider may simply offer a therapeutic trial of vasopressin or a synthetic analog such as desmopressin (dDAVP) and assess the patient's response. In this circumstance, amelioration of both polyuria and polydipsia would be considered a positive response, and a presumptive diagnosis of DI is made. However, if the patient has primary polydipsia (also known as compulsive water drinking), a profound hypo-osmolar state (water intoxication) can ensue due to the continued ingestion of copious amounts of fluids and a reduced renal excretion of free water. This scenario illustrates the importance of carefully evaluating each patient prior to therapy.

Vasopressin excess may also occur and is much more difficult to treat. Since excess vasopressin leads to the pathologic retention of free water, restricting free water intake to small amounts each day has been a historical cornerstone of treatment. Recently, conivaptan and tolvaptan,[80] vasopressin V_2 receptor antagonists, have been approved for the management of euvolemic hyponatremia due to vasopressin excess.

> **For additional student resources, please visit** thePoint® at http://thepoint.lww.com

questions

1. Open-loop negative feedback refers to the phenomenon of
  a. Negative feedback with a modifiable set point
  b. Blood flow in the hypothalamic–hypophyseal portal system
  c. Blood flow to the pituitary via dural-penetrating vessels
  d. Negative feedback involving an unvarying, fixed set point

2. The specific feedback effector for FSH is
  a. Inhibin
  b. Activin
  c. Progesterone
  d. Estradiol

3. Which anterior pituitary hormone lacks a stimulatory hypophysiotropic hormone?
  a. Prolactin
  b. Growth hormone
  c. Vasopressin
  d. ACTH

4. The definitive suppression test to prove autonomous production of growth hormone is
  a. Oral glucose loading
  b. Somatostatin infusion
  c. Estrogen priming
  d. Dexamethasone suppression

5. Which of the following is influenced by growth hormone?
  a. All of these
  b. IGF-I
  c. IGFBP-III
  d. Lipolysis

6. What statement concerning vasopressin secretion is NOT true?
  a. All of these.
  b. Vasopressin secretion is closely tied to plasma osmolality.
  c. Changes in blood volume also alter vasopressin secretion.
  d. A reduction in effective blood volume overrides the effects of plasma osmolality in regulating vasopressin secretion.

(continues on page 436)

review questions (continued)

7. What are the long-term sequelae of untreated or partially treated acromegaly?
   a. An increased risk of colon and lung cancer
   b. A reduced risk of heart disease
   c. Enhanced longevity
   d. Increased muscle strength

8. TRH stimulates the secretion of
   a. Prolactin and TSH
   b. Prolactin
   c. Growth hormone
   d. TSH

9. Estrogen influences the secretion of which of the following hormones?
   a. All of these
   b. Growth hormone
   c. Prolactin
   d. Luteinizing hormone

10. What is the difference between a tropic hormone and a direct effector hormone?
    a. Tropic and direct effector hormones are both similar in that both act directly on peripheral tissue.
    b. Tropic and direct effector hormones are both similar in that both act directly on another endocrine gland.
    c. Tropic hormones act on peripheral tissue, while direct effector hormones act on endocrine glands.
    d. Tropic hormones act on endocrine glands, while direct effector hormones act on peripheral tissues.

11. A deficiency in vasopressin can lead to which of the following?
    a. Euvolemic hypokalemia
    b. Euvolemic hyponatremia
    c. Diabetes insipidus
    d. Primary hypothyroidism

12. Which of the following hormones stimulate prolactin secretion?
    a. Dopamine
    b. GnRH
    c. TRH
    d. TSH

13. Which hormone most directly stimulates testosterone secretion?
    a. LH
    b. FSH
    c. GnRH
    d. TRH

14. Which of the following is NOT likely to be present in an "atypical pituitary tumor" as defined by the World Health Organization (WHO)?
    a. Invasion into surrounding structures such as the cavernous sinus
    b. MIB-1 proliferative index greater than 3%
    c. Excessive p53 immunoreactivity
    d. Decreased mitotic activity

15. Concerning secretion of growth hormone, which of the following is NOT true?
    a. Secretion is stimulated by GHRH.
    b. Secretion is pulsatile, occurring usually 2 to 3 times daily.
    c. The most reproducible surge is at the onset of sleep.
    d. It is secreted from somatotrophs that constitute over one-third of normal pituitary weight

16. Familial acromegaly is most likely caused by a mutation in which gene?
    a. GNAS
    b. AIP
    c. SS receptor type 5
    d. GHRH gene

17. Cosecretion of which hormone is most commonly seen with acromegaly?
    a. Prolactin
    b. TSH
    c. ACTH
    d. FSH

18. Which hormone is not secreted from the anterior pituitary?
    a. Prolactin
    b. Oxytocin
    c. FSH
    d. TSH

19. Which of the following is most suggestive of a diagnosis of diabetes insipidus?
    a. Low sodium in a patient who reports polydipsia and polyuria
    b. Persistent complaint of polydipsia and polyuria in a patient without diabetes mellitus
    c. Elevated serum osmolarity in the setting of decreased urine osmolarity, in the presence of hypernatremia
    d. Hyponatremia after a therapeutic trial of dDAVP

review questions (continued)

20. Vasopressin release is regulated by which of the following?
a. Hypothalamic osmoreceptors
b. Vascular baroreceptors
c. V2 receptors in the kidney
d. a and b

21. Replacement of thyroxine is potentially dangerous in the setting of which other hormonal abnormality?
a. GH deficiency
b. Hyperprolactinemia
c. Perimenopausal state
d. ACTH deficiency

22. Which of the following is NOT generally considered to be a function of oxytocin?
a. Uterine contraction during labor
b. Milk "letdown" for breast-feeding
c. Enhancement of insulin sensitivity in smooth muscle
d. Enhancement of mother–infant bonding

23. Which clinical presentation is consistent with Kallmann's syndrome?
a. Hypothyroidism and intermittent severe weakness or paralysis
b. ACTH deficiency together with GH excess
c. Hyperprolactinemia in the setting of pregnancy
d. Hypogonadism with the absence of smell

24. Which drug may cause panhypopituitarism?
a. Ipilimumab
b. Risperdal
c. Pitocin
d. Cabergoline

25. Which of the following is unlikely to be a cause of hyperprolactinemia?
a. Metoclopramide
b. Primary hypothyroidism
c. Primary hypogonadism
d. Pituitary stalk interruption

references

1. Kelberman D, Rizzoti K, Lovell-Badge R, et al. Genetic regulation of pituitary gland development in human and mouse. *Endocr Rev.* 2009;30(7):790–829.
2. Adler SM, Wartofsky L. The nonthyroidal illness syndrome. *Endocrinol Metab Clin North Am.* 2007;36(3):657–672.
3. Veldhuis JD, Keenan DM, Pincus SM. Regulation of complex pulsatile and rhythmic neuroendocrine systems: the male gonadal axis as a prototype. *Prog Brain Res.* 2010;181:79–110.
4. Nunemaker CS, Satin LS. Episodic hormone secretion: a comparison of the basis of pulsatile secretion of insulin and GnRH. *Endocrine.* 2014;47:49–63.
5. Dijk DJ, Duffy JF, Silva EJ, et al. Amplitude reduction and phase shifts of melatonin, cortisol and other circadian rhythms after a gradual advance of sleep and light exposure in humans. *PLoS One.* 2012;7(2):e30037.
6. Spiga F, Waite EJ, Liu Y, et al. ACTH-dependent ultradian rhythm of corticosterone secretion. *Endocrinology.* 2011;152:1448–1457.
7. Tonsfeldt KJ, Chappell PE. Clocks on top: the role of the circadian clock in the hypothalamic and pituitary regulation of endocrine physiology. *Mol Cell Endocrinol.* 2012;349:3–12.
8. Valassi E, Biller BM, Klibanski A, et al. Clinical features of non-pituitary sellar lesions in a large surgical series. *Clin Endocrinol (Oxf).* 2010;73:798–807.
9. Couldwell WT, Altay T, Krisht K, et al. Sellar and paracellar metastatic tumors. *Int J Surg Oncol.* 2012;2012:647256.
10. Zada G, Woodmansee WW, Ramkissoon S, et al. Atypical pituitary adenomas: incidence, clinical characteristics, and implications. *J Neurosurg.* 2011;114:336–344.
11. Marrelli D, Pinto E, Nari A, et al. Mib-1 proliferation index is an independent predictor of lymph node metastasis in invasive breast cancer: a prospective study on 675 patients. *Oncol Rep.* 2006;15(2):425–429.
12. Córdoba-Chacón J, Gahete MD, Castaño JP, et al. Somatostatin and its receptors contribute in a tissue specific manner to the sex-dependent metabolic (fed/fasting) control of growth hormone axis in mice. *Am J Physiol Endocrinol Metab.* 2011;300:E46–E54.
13. Ribeiro-Oliveira A, Barkan AL. Growth hormone pulsatility and its impact on growth and metabolism in humans. *Growth Hormone Relat Dis Ther Contemp Endocrinol.* 2011;(pt 1):33–56.
14. Pradhan G, Samson SL, Sun X. Ghrelin: much more than a hunger hormone. *Curr Opin Clin Nutr Metab Care.* 2013;16:619–624.
15. Chia DJ. Minireview: mechanisms of growth hormone-mediated gene regulation. *Mol Endocrinol.* 2014;28:1012–1025.
16. Møller N, Jørgensen JO. Effects of growth hormone on glucose, lipid, and protein metabolism in human subjects. *Endocr Rev.* 2009;30(2):152–177.
17. Cambiaso P, Schiaffini R, Pontrelli G, et al. Nocturnal hypoglycemia in ACTH and GH deficient children: role of continuous glucose monitoring. *Clin Endocrinol (Oxf).* 2013;79:232–237.
18. Salmon WD, Daughaday WH. A hormonally controlled serum factor which stimulates sulfate incorporation by cartilage in vitro. *J Lab Clin Med.* 1957;49:825–826.
19. Daughaday WH, Hall K, Raben MS, et al. Somatomedin: proposed designation for sulphation factor. *Nature.* 1972;235:107.
20. Klapper DG, Svoboda ME, Van Wyk JJ. Sequence analysis of somatomedin-C: confirmation of identity with insulin-like growth factor I. *Endocrinology.* 1983;112:2215–2217.
21. Rinderknecht E, Humbel RE. The amino acid sequence of human insulin-like growth factor I and its structural homology with proinsulin. *J Biol Chem.* 1978;253:2769–2776.

22. Melmed S, Colao A, Barkan A, et al. Guidelines for acromegaly management: an update. *J Clin Endocrinol Metab.* 2009;94(5):1509–1517.

23. Khowaja A, Johnson-Rabbett B, Bantle J, et al. Hypoglycemia mediated by paraneoplastic production of insulin-like growth factor-2 from a malignant renal solitary fibrous tumor—clinical case and literature review. *BMC Endocr Disord.* 2014;14:49.

24. Li G, Barrett EJ, Ko S-H, et al. Insulin and insulin-like growth factor-I receptors differentially mediate insulin-stimulated adhesion molecule production by endothelial cells. *Endocrinology.* 2009;150:3475–3482.

25. Forbes BE, McCarthy P, Norton RS. Insulin-like growth factor binding proteins: a structural perspective. *Front Endocrinol (Lausanne).* 2012;3:38.

26. Jogie-Brahim S, Feldman D, Oh Y. Unraveling insulin-like growth factor binding protein-3 actions in human disease. *Endocr Rev.* 2009;30(5):417–437.

27. Torng, P-L, Lin C-W, Chan MWY, et al. Promoter methylation of IGFBP-3 and p53 expression in ovarian endometrioid carcinoma. *Mol Cancer.* 2009;8:120.

28. Jing M, Pollack MN, Giovannucci E, et al. Prospective study of colorectal cancer risk in men and plasma levels of insulin-like growth factor (IGF)-I and IGF-binding protein-3. *J Natl Cancer Inst.* 1999;91(7):620–625.

29. Kwan AYM, Hartman ML. IGF-I measurements in the diagnosis of adult growth hormone deficiency. *Pituitary.* 2007;10(2):151–157.

30. Bancos I, Algeciras-Schimnich A, Grebe S, et al. Evaluation of variables influencing the measurement of insulin-like growth factor-I. *Endocr Pract.* 2014;20:421–426.

31. Clemmons, D.R..Consensus statement on the standardization and evaluation of growth hormone and insulin-like growth factor assays. *Clin Chem.* 2011;57:555–559.

32. Ben-Shlomo A, Melmed S. Acromegaly. *Endocrinol Metab Clin North Am.* 2008;37(1):101–122.

33. Melmed S. Medical progress: acromegaly. *N Engl J Med.* 2006;355(24):2558–2573.

34. Molitch ME, Clemmons DR, Malozowski S, et al. Evaluation and treatment of adult growth hormone deficiency: an Endocrine Society clinical practice guideline. *J Clin Endocrinol Metab.* 2011;96(6):1587–1609.

35. Bidlingmaier M, Freda PU. Measurement of human growth hormone by immunoassays: current status, unsolved problems and clinical consequences. *Growth Horm IGF Res.* 2010;20(1):19–25.

36. Faglia G, Arosio M, Bazzoni N. Ectopic acromegaly. *Endocrinol Metab Clin North Am.* 1992;21:575–596.

37. Ezzat S, Ezrin C, Yamashita S, et al. Recurrent acromegaly resulting from ectopic growth hormone gene expression by a metastatic pancreatic tumor. *Cancer.* 1993;71:66–70.

38. Gola M, Doga M, Bonadonna S, et al. Neuroendocrine tumors secreting growth hormone-releasing hormone: pathophysiological and clinical aspects. *Pituitary.* 2006;9(3):221–229.

39. Chahal HS, Stals K, Unterländer M, et al. AIP mutation in pituitary adenomas in the 18th century and today. *N Engl J Med.* 2011;364:43–50.

40. Ciganoka D, Balcere I, Kapa I, et al. Identification of somatostatin receptor type 5 gene polymorphisms associated with acromegaly. *Eur J Endocrinol.* 2011;165:517–525.

41. de Herder WW. Acromegaly and gigantism in the medical literature. Case descriptions in the era before and the early years after the initial publication of Pierre Marie (1886). *Pituitary.* 2009;12(3):236–244.

42. Reddy R, Hope S, Wass J. Acromegaly. *BMJ.* 2010;341:c4189.

43. Killinger Z, Rovenský J. Arthropathy in acromegaly. *Rheum Dis Clin North Am.* 2010;36(4):713–720.

44. McNab TL, Khandwala HM. Acromegaly as an endocrine form of myopathy: case report and review of literature. *Endocr Pract.* 2005;11(1):18–22.

45. Lopes MB. Growth hormone-secreting adenomas: pathology and cell biology. *Neurosurg Focus.* 2010;29(4):E2.

46. Johnston PC, Hamrahian AH, Prayson RA, et al. Thyrotoxicosis with the absence of clinical features of acromegaly in a TSH- and GH-secreting, invasive pituitary macroadenoma. *Endocrinol Diabetes Metab Case Rep.* 2015;2015:140070.

47. Del Porto LA, Liubinas SV, Kaye AH. Treatment of persistent and recurrent acromegaly. *J Clin Neurosci.* 2011;18(2):181–190.

48. Rowland NC, Aghi MK. Radiation treatment strategies for acromegaly. *Neurosurg Focus.* 2010;29(4):E12.

49. Sherlock M, Woods C, Sheppard MC. Medical therapy in acromegaly. *Nat Rev Endocrinol.* 2011;7(5):291–300.

50. Brue T, Castinetti F, Lundgren F, et al. Which patients with acromegaly are treated with pegvisomant? An overview of methodology and baseline data in ACROSTUDY. *Eur J Endocrinol.* 2009;161(suppl 1):S11–S17.

51. Mullis PE. Genetics of isolated growth hormone deficiency. *J Clin Res Pediatr Endocrinol.* 2010;2:52–62.

52. Bartke A. Growth hormone and aging: a challenging controversy. *Clin Interv Aging.* 2008;3(4):659–665.

53. Allen DB, Cuttler L. Clinical practice. Short stature in childhood—challenges and choices. *N Engl J Med.* 2013;368:1220–1228.

54. Reed ML, Merriam GR, Kargi AY. Adult growth hormone deficiency—benefits, side effects, and risks of growth hormone replacement. *Front Endocrinol (Lausanne)* 2013;4:64.

55. Friedrich N, Schneider H, Dörr M, et al. All-cause mortality and serum insulin-like growth factor I in primary care patients. *Growth Horm IGF Res.* 2011;21(2):102–106.

56. Woodhouse LJ, Mukerjee A, Shalet SM, et al. The influence of growth hormone status on physical impairments, functional limitations, and health-related quality of life in adults. *Endocr Rev.* 2006;27(3):287–317.

57. Svensson J, Bengtsson BA. Safety aspects of GH replacement. *Eur J Endocrinol.* 2009;161(suppl 1):S65-S74.

58. Erotokritou-Mulligan I, Holt RIG, Sönksen PH. Growth hormone doping: a review. *J Sports Med.* 2011;2:99–111.

59. Hekimsoy Z, Kafesçiler S, Güçlü F, et al. The prevalence of hyperprolactinemia in overt and subclinical hypothyroidism. *Endocr J.* 2010;57(12):1011–1015.

60. Shibli-Rahhal A, Schlechte J. Hyperprolactinemia and infertility. *Endocrinol Metab Clin North Am.* 2011;40(4):837–846.

61. Shibli-Rahhal A, Schlechte J. The effects of hyperprolactinemia on bone and fat. *Pituitary.* 2009;12(2):96–104.

62. Chahal J, Schlechte J. Hyperprolactinemia. *Pituitary.* 2008;11(2):141–146.

63. Gibney J, Smith TP, McKenna TJ. The impact on clinical practice of routine screening for macroprolactin. *J Clin Endocrinol Metab.* 2005;90:3927–3932.

64. Melmed S, Montori VM, Schlechte JA, et al.; Endocrine Society. Diagnosis and treatment of hyperprolactinemia: an Endocrine Society clinical practice guideline. *J Clin Endocrinol Metab.* 2011;96(2):273–288.

65. Dekkers OM, Lagro J, Burman P, et al. Recurrence of hyperprolactinemia after withdrawal of dopamine agonists: systematic review and meta-analysis. *J Clin Endocrinol Metab.* 2010;95(1):43–51.

66. Delgado V, Biermasz NR, van Thiel SW, et al. Changes in heart valve structure and function in patients treated with dopamine agonists for prolactinomas, a 2-year follow-up study. *Clin Endocrinol (Oxf).* 2012;77(1):99–105.

67. Nawar RN, Abdelmannan D, Selman WR, et al. Pituitary tumor apoplexy: a review. *J Intensive Care Med.* 2008;23:75–90.

68. Caturegli P, Lupi I, Landek-Salgado M, et al. Pituitary autoimmunity: 30 years later. *Autoimmun Rev.* 2008;7:631–637.

69. Hodi FS, O'Day SJ, McDermott DF, et al. Improved survival with ipilimumab in patients with metastatic melanoma. *N Engl J Med.* 2010;363:711–723.

70. Romero CJ, Nesi-Franca S, Radovick S. Molecular basis of hypopituitarism. *Trends Endocrinol Metab.* 2009;20:506–516.

71. Fechner A, Fong S, McGovern P. A review of Kallmann syndrome: genetics, pathophysiology, and clinical management. *Obstet Gynecol Surv.* 2008;63(3):189–194.

72. Du X, Yuan Q, Yao Y, et al. Hypopituitarism and successful pregnancy. *Int J Clin Exp Med.* 2014;7:4660–4665.

73. Elphick MR. NG peptides: a novel family of neurophysin-associated neuropeptides. *Gene.* 2010;458(1–2):20–26.

74. Lee H-J, Macbeth AH, Pagani J, et al. Oxytocin: the great facilitator OF LIFE. *Prog Neurobiol.* 2009;88:127–151.

75. Vrachnis N, Iliodromiti Z. The oxytocin-oxytocin receptor system and its antagonists as tocolytic agents. *Int J Endocrinol.* 2011;2011:350546.

76. Ross HE, Young LJ. Oxytocin and neural mechanisms regulating social cognition and affiliative behavior. *Front Neuroendocrinol.* 2009;30:534–547.

77. Wilson JLL, Miranda CA, Knepper MA. Vasopressin and the regulation of aquaporin-2. *Clin Exp Nephrol.* 2013;17:751–764.

78. Ozier Y, Bellamy L. Pharmacological agents: antifibrinolytics and desmopressin. *Best Pract Res Clin Anaesthesiol.* 2010;24(1):107–119.

79. Jane JA Jr, Vance ML, Laws ER. Neurogenic diabetes insipidus. *Pituitary.* 2006;9(4):327–329.

80. Cassagnol M, Shogbon AO, Saad M. The therapeutic use of vaptans for the treatment of dilutional hyponatremia. *J Pharm Pract.* 2011;24(4):391–399.

81. Clemmons DR. Value of insulin-like growth factor system markers in the assessment of growth hormone status. *Endocrinol Metab Clin North Am.* 2007;36(1):109–129.

82. Murad MH, Elamin MB, Malaga G, et al. The accuracy of diagnostic tests for GH deficiency in adults: a systematic review and meta-analysis. *Eur J Endocrinol.* 2011;165:841–849.

21

Adrenal Function

VISHNU SUNDARESH and DEEPIKA S. REDDY

chapter outline

key terms

chapter objectives

Upon completion of this chapter, the clinical laboratorian should be able to do the following:

- Explain how the adrenal gland functions to maintain blood pressure, potassium, and glucose homeostasis.
- Describe steroid biosynthesis, regulation, and actions according to anatomic location within the adrenal gland.
- Discuss the pathophysiology of adrenal cortex disorders, namely, Cushing's syndrome and Addison's disease.

For additional student resources, please visit thePoint® at http://thepoint.lww.com

chapter objectives (continued)

- List the appropriate laboratory tests to differentially diagnose primary and secondary Cushing's syndrome and Addison's disease.
- Differentiate the adrenal enzyme deficiencies and their blocking pathways in establishing a diagnosis.
- Describe the synthesis, storage, and metabolism of catecholamines.
- State the most useful measurements in supporting the diagnosis of pheochromocytoma.
- List the clinical findings associated with hypertension that suggest an underlying adrenal etiology is causing high blood pressure.

THE ADRENAL GLAND: AN OVERVIEW

The adrenal gland is a multifunctional organ that produces steroid hormones and neuropeptides essential for life. Despite the complex actions of adrenal hormones, most pathological conditions of the adrenal gland are manifested by their impact on blood pressure, electrolyte balance, and androgen excess.[1] An adrenal etiology should be considered in the differential diagnosis when patients presents with (i) **hypertension**, hypokalemia, and metabolic alkalosis (suspect hyperaldosteronism); (ii) hypertension, spells of anxiety, palpitations, dizziness, and diaphoresis (pheochromocytoma); (iii) hypertension, rapid unexplained weight gain, red/purple stretch marks, and proximal muscle weakness (Cushing's syndrome); (iv) inappropriate hirsutism/virilization and inability to conceive (congenital adrenal hyperplasia); and (v) loss of appetite, unintentional weight loss, and pigmented skin (primary adrenal insufficiency).

In clinical practice, patients often present with underproduction or overproduction of one or more adrenal hormones. Adrenal nodules are also discovered incidentally on abdominal imaging performed for other reasons. Hypofunction is treated with hormone replacement, and hyperfunction is treated with pharmacologic suppression and/or surgery.

EMBRYOLOGY AND ANATOMY

The adrenal gland is composed of two embryologically distinct tissue—the outer adrenal cortex and inner adrenal medulla. The cortex is derived from mesenchymal cells located near the urogenital ridge that differentiate into three structurally and functionally distinct zones (Fig. 21.1). The medulla arises from neural crest cells that invade the cortex during the 2nd month of fetal development. By adulthood, the medulla contributes 10% of total adrenal weight.

Adult adrenal glands are shaped like pyramids, located superior and medial to the upper pole of the kidneys in the retroperitoneal space (hence, also known as suprarenal glands). On cross section, both regions remain distinct; the cortex appears yellow, while the medulla is dark mahogany.[2]

Adrenal arterial supply is symmetric. Small arterioles branch to form a dense subcapsular plexus that drains into the sinusoidal plexus of the cortex. There is no direct arterial blood supply to middle and inner zones. In contrast, venous drainage from the central vein displays laterality. After crossing the medulla, the right adrenal vein empties into the inferior vena cava, and the left adrenal vein drains into the left renal vein. There is a separate capillary sinusoidal network from the medullary arterioles that also drains into the central vein and limits the exposure of cortical cells to medullary venous blood. Glucocorticoids from the cortex are carried directly to the adrenal medulla via the portal system, where they stimulate enzyme production of **epinephrine (EPI)** (Fig. 21.15).

Sympathetic and parasympathetic axons reach the medulla through the cortex. En route, these axons release neurotransmitters (e.g., catecholamines and neuropeptide Y) that modulate cortex blood flow, cell growth, and function. Medullary projections into the cortex have been found to contain cells that also synthesize and release neuropeptides, such as **vasoactive inhibitory peptide (VIP)**, adrenomedullin, and **atrial natriuretic peptide (ANP)**, and potentially influence cortex function.

THE ADRENAL CORTEX BY ZONE

The major adrenal cortical hormones, **aldosterone**, *cortisol*, and **dehydroepiandrosterone sulfate (DHEA-S)**, are uniquely synthesized from a common precursor cholesterol by cells located in one of three functionally distinct zonal layers of the adrenal cortex. These zonal layers are *zona glomerulosa*, **zona fasciculata**, and *zona reticularis*, respectively (Fig. 21.1).

Zona glomerulosa (G-zone) cells (outer 10%) synthesize aldosterone, a mineralocorticoid critical for sodium retention, potassium excretion, acid–base homeostasis, and regulation of blood pressure. They have low cytoplasmic-to-nuclear ratios and small nuclei with dense chromatin with intermediate lipid inclusions.

Zona fasciculata (F-zone) cells (middle 75%) synthesize glucocorticoids, such as cortisol and cortisone, critical for glucose homeostasis and blood pressure. Fasciculata cells are cords of clear cells, with a high cytoplasmic-to-nuclear ratio and lipids laden with "foamy" cytoplasm. The fasciculata cells also generate androgen precursors such as **dehydroepiandrosterone (DHEA)**, which is sulfated in the

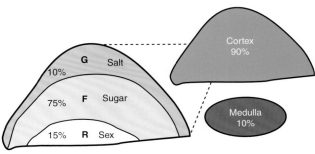

FIGURE 21.1 Adrenal gland by layer.

FIGURE 21.2 Conversion of cholesterol to pregnenolone. ACTH, adrenocorticotropic hormone; CRH, corticotropin-releasing hormone.

innermost **zona reticularis (R-zone)**. Subcapsular adrenal cortex remnants can regenerate into fasciculate adrenals, metastasize, and survive in ectopic locations such as the liver, gallbladder wall, broad ligaments, celiac plexus, ovaries, scrotum, and cranium.

Zona reticularis cells (inner 15%) sulfate DHEA to DHEA-S, which is the main adrenal androgen. The zone is sharply demarcated with lipid-deficient cords of irregular, dense cells with lipofuscin deposits.

Adrenal cell types are presumed to arise from stem cells. A proposed tissue layer between the zona glomerulosa and fasciculata may serve as a site for progenitor cells to regenerate zonal cells.[3]

Cortex Steroidogenesis

Control of steroid hormone biosynthesis is complex, including **adrenocorticotropic hormone (ACTH)** and **angiotensin II (AT II)**. It occurs via substrate availability, enzyme activity, and inhibitory feedback loops that are layer specific.

All adrenal steroids are derived by sequential enzymatic conversion of a common substrate, cholesterol. Adrenal parenchymal cells accumulate and store circulating low-density lipoproteins (LDLs). The adrenal gland can also synthesize additional cholesterol using the enzyme acetyl-CoA, ensuring that adrenal steroidogenesis remains normal in patients with variable lipid disorders and in patients on lipid-lowering agents.

Only free cholesterol can enter steroidogenic pathways in response to ACTH. The availability of free intracellular cholesterol is metabolically regulated by ACTH (stimulatory) and LDL (inhibitory) through multiple mechanisms. **Corticotropin-releasing hormone (CRH)** is secreted from the hypothalamus in response to circadian signals, low serum cortisol levels, and stress. CRH stimulates release of stored ACTH from the anterior pituitary gland, which stimulates transport of free cholesterol into adrenal mitochondria, initiating steroid production.

Conversion of cholesterol to pregnenolone is a rate-limiting step in steroid biosynthesis: six carbon atoms are removed from cholesterol by enzyme cytochrome P450 (CYP450) present in the mitochondrial membrane (Fig. 21.2). Newly synthesized pregnenolone is then returned to the cytosol for subsequent zonal conversion by microsomal enzymes in each layer by F-zone enzymes and/or androgens by enzymes in the R-zone (Fig. 21.3).

High serum glucocorticoids suppress release of CRH and ACTH via a negative feedback mechanism. Cortisol is the primary feedback regulator of ACTH-stimulated hormone production in the adrenal cortex. ACTH generally does not

FIGURE 21.3 Adrenocortical hormone synthesis by zone.

Enzyme Defect	New Classification	HTN	Virilization	High Lab Value
◻ 3β-Hydroxysteroid dehydrogenase	3β-HSD II	N	Slight	DHEA
◼ 17α-Hydroxylase	CYP17	Y	No	Aldosterone
◼ 11β-Hydroxylase	CYP11B1GF	Y	Marked	11-DOC
◼ 21β-Hydroxylase	CYP21A2	N	Marked	17-OH-progesterone

FIGURE 21.4 Congenital adrenal hyperplasia syndromes.

impact G-zone aldosterone synthesis, although cortisol has mineralocorticoid action.

Decreased activity of any enzyme required for biosynthesis can occur as an acquired or inherited (autosomal recessive) trait. Defects that decrease the production of cortisol cause increases in ACTH and CRH secretion in an attempt to stimulate cortisol levels and lead to adrenal hyperplasia or overproduction of androgens, depending on the affected enzyme.

Evaluation of adrenal function requires measuring relevant adrenal hormones, metabolites, and regulatory secretagogues. Diagnosis is based on the correlation of clinical and laboratory findings.[4]

Congenital Adrenal Hyperplasia

Congenital adrenal hyperplasia refers to a group of clinical entities that arise from absent or diminished activity of enzymes involved in steroidogenesis. The mineralocorticoid, glucocorticoid, and androgen production pathways can be affected to varying degrees based on the enzyme affected. Blocks in one pathway result in upstream substrate buildup and potential upregulation of another pathway. The most common enzyme affected is 21-hydroxylase. Deficiency in this enzyme results in decreased glucocorticoid, in some cases mineralocorticoid and increased adrenal androgen production.[5] A very high serum concentration of 17-hydroxyprogesterone, the normal substrate for 21-hydroxylase, is diagnostic of classic 21-hydroxylase deficiency. The "classic" presentation is seen in infants. It presents with features such as failure to thrive and low blood pressure. These infants need both glucocorticoid and mineralocorticoid replacement. A second "nonclassic" form is seen in adults. Woman with this form present in their reproductive years with complaints of hirsutism, menstrual irregularities, and infertility. They may need steroids during pregnancy. The different enzyme defects along with clinical and biochemcial abnormalities have been summarized in Figure 21.4.

PRIMARY ALDOSTERONISM

Overview

The clinical entity in which excessive secretion of aldosterone cannot be suppressed with salt or volume replacement is termed **primary aldosteronism (PA)**. PA results in hypertension, hypokalemia, metabolic alkalosis, and increased risk of vascular disease such as stroke as depicted in Figure 21.5. It is estimated that 5% to 10% of patients with hypertension have PA.[6] Endocrine Society guidelines on PA suggest that hypokalemia is found only in 37% of patients with PA.[7] The guidelines recommend more aggressive screening may be appropriate in those with SBP greater than 160/DBP greater than 100, drug-resistant hypertension, hypokalemia associated with hypertension, presence of adrenal mass, family history of early hypertension or stroke, and first-degree relatives of patients with PA.

Etiology

The most common causes of PA are:

- Aldosterone-producing adrenal adenoma
- Unilateral or bilateral adrenal hyperplasia

Other causes are as follows:

- Familial hyperaldosteronism such as glucocorticoid remediable aldosteronism (GRA)
- Adrenocortical carcinomas that secrete aldosterone
- Ectopic aldosterone secretion

Diagnosis

Plasma aldosterone concentration (PAC) and plasma renin activity (PRA) are used in the diagnosis of PA.[8] Presence of both PAC of greater than 15 ng/dL and PAC/PRA (plasma renin activity) of 30 or greater is suggestive of PA. The 2008 Endocrine Society guidelines recommend the labs be checked in AM after the patient has been up for at least

High Potassium
Angiotensin II

G-ZONE

Aldosterone

Main steroid: Aldosterone
Main regulator: Renin-angiotensin system (RAS)
Major function: Blood pressure and K$^+$ homeostasis

Syndrome:

Hypoaldosteronism (Distal RTA type IV)
Hyperaldosteronism (Aldosteronism)

Clinical Findings:

Hyperkalemia, renal salt wasting
HTN, hypokalemia, metabolic alkalosis

FIGURE 21.5 G-zone function and pathology. HTN, hypertension.

2 hours. The patient should be seated for 5 to 15 minutes before the draw and sodium intake should be unrestricted. Most antihypertensive medications do not need to be stopped prior to testing except mineralocorticoid antagonist. If clinical suspicion is high in a patient on ACE-I and testing is negative, the ACE-I should be discontinued and testing repeated. If the initial screening is suggestive of PA, confirmatory tests include aldosterone measurement following either oral salt loading or IV saline infusion.

Oral salt loading requires oral consumption of about 5,000 mg NaCl per day. On day 3, urine sodium, creatinine, and aldosterone are measured in a 24-hour urine collection. Presence of urine sodium greater than 200 mEq and urine aldosterone greater than 12 μg/24 hours is suggestive of PA. The saline infusion test involves IV infusion of 2 L NaCl in 2 hours. Following this, PAC normally will be less than 5 ng/dL, and in those with PA, the value is often greater than 10 ng/dL.

Biochemical evaluation is followed by adrenal imaging (CT, MRI). Presence of an adrenal mass should still prompt further testing before surgical intervention since adrenal adenomas are often nonfunctional. Aldosterone secretion may be due to bilateral hyperplasia. Adrenal venous sampling (AVS) is recommended to distinguish between hyperplasia and aldosterone-secreting adenoma.[9] Some authors do suggest that in persons less than 35 years, one may be able to proceed to surgery without AVS. The study requires technical expertise and should be performed by experienced practitioners. Adrenal vein to IVC cortisol ratios and aldosterone levels corrected for cortisol are used to determine appropriate placement of sampling catheters. If there is asymmetry in aldosterone release between adrenal glands (greater than 4:1), it is likely to be unilateral excess aldosterone production and the patient would benefit from surgical intervention. If less than 3:1 ratio exists, it is likely to be secondary to adrenal hyperplasia and the patient should be treated medically.

Treatment

Surgery is the treatment of choice for aldosterone-producing adenoma. Hypertension is controlled in 30% to 60% of the patients treated surgically.[10] Mineralocorticoid antagonists such as spironolactone or eplerenone should be used for adrenal hyperplasia. If GRA is suspected in patients with multiple family members with early onset of hypertension, steroids such as prednisone are the treatment of choice.

Isolated Hypoaldosteronism

Insufficient aldosterone secretion is seen with adrenal gland destruction, with chronic heparin therapy, following unilateral adrenalectomy (transient), and with G-zone enzyme deficiencies. Most hypoaldosteronism occurs in patients with mild renal insufficiency such as persons with diabetes who present with mild metabolic acidosis, high serum potassium$^+$, low urinary potassium$^+$ excretion (urine K^+ < urine Na^+), and low renin. Treatment is with dietary changes and Fludrocortisone (a synthetic mineralocorticoid), which enhances salt retention and the secretion of potassium$^+$ and hydrogen$^+$.

Types of aldosteronism are diagrammed in Figure 21.6 according to their PA (*y*-axis) and PRA (*x*-axis) values.

ADRENAL CORTICAL PHYSIOLOGY

Cortisol synthesis (8 to 15 mg/d) is critical to hemodynamics and glucose homeostasis. F-zone disorders manifest

FIGURE 21.6 Types of aldosteronism according to plasma aldosterone:plasma renin activity (PRA) ratio. HTN, hypertension.

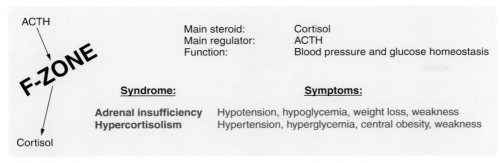

FIGURE 21.7 F-zone function and pathology. ACTH, adrenocorticotropic hormone.

with blood pressure and glucose abnormalities (Fig. 21.7). Glucocorticoids maintain blood glucose by inducing lipolysis and causing amino acid release from muscle for conversion into glucose (gluconeogenesis) and storage as liver glycogen.

ADRENAL INSUFFICIENCY

Overview

Adrenal insufficiency is a term that describes inadequate hormone secretion from the adrenal cortex. This may be a primary adrenal problem in which case there is inadequate release of glucocorticoids (such as cortisol), mineralocorticoids (such as aldosterone), and adrenal androgens. In primary adrenal insufficiency, there is reduced production of adrenal hormones despite adequate stimulation. In secondary adrenal insufficiency, adrenal gland function is preserved but the stimulus for hormone release is insufficient or absent. This would occur if the pituitary gland failed to release adequate adrenocorticotropic hormone (ACTH). The most common cause of adrenal insufficiency is autoimmune destruction of the adrenal gland.[11] Other causes of adrenal insufficiency include infections (tuberculosis and histoplasmosis), tumors, bilateral adrenal hemorrhage, etc.

Symptoms

Clinical symptoms of chronic adrenal insufficiency can be nonspecific with most patients complaining of fatigue, decreased appetite, weight loss, and nausea. Patients may also present with more severe findings such as low blood pressure, low blood sugar, low serum sodium, and high potassium levels as depicted in Figure 21.8.

Diagnosis

The diagnosis of adrenal insufficiency can be suspected if the 8 AM serum cortisol is low with concomitant elevation in ACTH levels. A cortisol level less than 3 µg/dL in the morning is highly suggestive of adrenal insufficiency. The diagnosis of primary adrenal insufficiency is made by performing an ACTH stimulation test. The test is performed at 8 AM in the fasting state.[12] Baseline cortisol and ACTH levels are obtained. The patient is then given 250 µg of cosyntropin (synthetic ACTH) intravenously and cortisol level is checked at 30 and 60 minutes post ACTH administration. A cortisol of 18 or greater at either 30 or 60 minutes post ACTH time point suggests normal adrenal function. In secondary adrenal insufficiency, the ACTH stimulation test may be normal or abnormal based on the duration of the disease. If secondary adrenal insufficiency is suspected, metyrapone suppression testing can be done.[13] Metyrapone blocks certain enzymes in the steroidogenesis pathway. When metyrapone is administered orally at midnight, in normal individuals, it will block 11β-hydroxylase increasing 11-deoxycortisol (>7 µg/dL) while cortisol decreases (<5 µg/dL). Secondary adrenal insufficiency is suggested in patients with a near-normal response to a 250-µg cosyntropin test but with an abnormal response to metyrapone. An alternative is to do an insulin tolerance test (ITT). Hypoglycemia is induced with insulin administration and ACTH, cortisol, and growth hormone response to hypoglycemia is measured. The ITT should be avoided in those with **cardiovascular disease** and seizure disorder. Figure 21.9 provides a summary of primary and secondary adrenal insufficiency.

Frequency	Symptoms	Signs
100%	Weakness Fatigue Anorexia	Weight loss
90%		Hyperpigmentation (primary adrenal insufficiency)
50%	Nausea Diarrhea	
10%	Pain	Adrenal calcification

FIGURE 21.8 Signs and symptoms of adrenal insufficiency.

FIGURE 21.9 Differential diagnosis of low cortisol states. ACTH, adrenocorticotropic hormone.

Stress

Infection

Severe obesity (visceral)

Polycystic ovary syndrome (up to 40% have slightly elevated urine cortisol)

Chronic alcoholism (cortisol normalizes with abstinence)

Depression (up to 80% have abnormal cortisol levels, disappears with remission)

Iatrogenic Cushing's (<1% inhaled, topical, oral glucocorticoid use)

Cushing's Syndrome	Symptoms of Cushing's Syndrome	
	HTN	(85%–90%)
	Central obesity	(90%)
	Glucose intolerance	(80%)
	Plethoric faces	(80%)
	Purple striae	(65%)
	Hirsutism	(65%)
	Abnormal menses	(60%)
	Muscle weakness	(60%)

FIGURE 21.10 Conditions associated with hypercortisolism. HTN, hypertension.

Treatment

The treatment of primary adrenal insufficiency includes both glucocorticoid replacement (prednisone or hydrocortisone) and mineralocorticoid replacement (fludrocortisone). In secondary adrenal insufficiency, only glucocorticoid replacement is required since aldosterone production remains normal.

HYPERCORTISOLISM (CUSHING'S SYNDROME)

Overview

Excess cortisol production presents with a constellation of clinical manifestations. Each is not unique to cortisol excess but when present together may suggest hypercortisolism. The common findings are as follows: There is progressive central obesity with sparing of extremities. Dorsocervical fat pad deposition and fat accumulation in the cheeks result in the "buffalo hump" and "moon face," respectively. A number of dermatologic manifestations can be seen such as atrophy of skin, easy bruising, wide purple striae, and hyperpigmentation based on the etiology of cortisol excess. In women, menstrual irregularity, signs of androgen excess such as acne, and hirsutism can be seen. Proximal muscle weakness and decreased bone mineral density may be present. Patients with cortisol excess also have increased risk of cardiovascular disease, thromboembolic events such as DVT, increased anxiety, and risk of infection including atypical fungal infections.[14]

Etiology

Cortisol excess may be due to adrenal tumors that make excess cortisol in which case pituitary release of ACTH levels is low. Alternatively, cortisol production could be due to elevated ACTH levels either from a pituitary tumor or from nonpituitary or ectopic sources often associated with malignancy such as lung cancer. The term Cushing's disease is used when the source of elevated ACTH is the pituitary gland, while other forms of cortisol excess are labelled as Cushing's syndrome. Cushing's disease is the most common reason for cortisol excess accounting for about 70% of cases (Figs. 21.10 and 21.11).

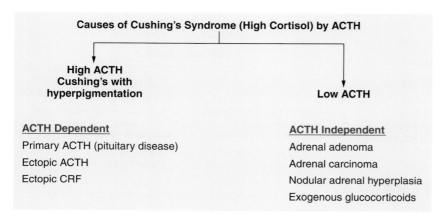

FIGURE 21.11 Differentiating source of adrenocorticotropic hormone (ACTH) secretion.

Diagnosis

Once exogenous cortisol use (oral, topical, injected, inhaled) is ruled out, initial screen tests for cortisol excess include (a) urine free cortisol collected over 24 hours (on two occasions to be considered positive), (b) midnight salivary cortisol (two occasions), and (c) dexamethasone suppression testing (1 mg overnight or 2 mg over 48 hours). A systematic review during the development of Endocrine Society guidelines in 2008 suggested that the three tests were similar in diagnostic accuracy.[15] The guidelines recommend demonstrating at least two positive tests for the diagnosis as this increases the diagnostic accuracy over any one test.

Urine free cortisol (UFC) measurement requires accurate collection and measurement of urine volume. Fluid intake greater than 5 L a day and urine volume greater than 3 L can lead to a false-positive test.[16] Depression and alcohol intake may also influence UFC resulting in so-called pseudo-Cushing's.[17] A cortisol level three times above normal is suggestive of cortisol excess but would have to be confirmed with another test. When liquid chromatography–tandem mass spectrometry is used, sensitivity of UFC was 97% and specificity was 91%.

Overnight 1 mg dexamethasone suppression test (DST) involves administration of 1 mg dexamethasone between 11 PM and midnight followed by an 8 AM serum cortisol level.[18] The test is considered negative if the AM cortisol level is less than 1.8 µg/dL. This is a stringent criterion and may have greater sensitivity and lower specificity. It is the test of choice when an adrenal nodule/mass is an incidental finding on abdominal imaging.

Late night salivary cortisol level (LNSC) is an alternate screening test. It takes advantage of the fact that patients with true excess endogenous production of cortisol lose diurnal variability in cortisol production. On the other hand, those with pseudo-Cushing's maintain that variability. A pooled analysis of seven studies suggested sensitivity of 93% and specificity of 96% of LNSC.[19] These numbers may be lower in mild hypercortisolism and in pregnancy.

Once hypercortisolism is established, a reliable two-site IRMA (immunoradiometric) assay for ACTH is used to determine the reason for high cortisol levels. If the 8 AM ACTH level is greater than 15 µg/dL, cortisol secretion is considered ACTH dependent. On the other hand, with ACTH less than 5 µg/dL, cortisol secretion is thought to be ACTH independent. While levels between 5 and 15 µg/dL are deemed indeterminate, there are little data to support these cutoffs, and the recommendations come from clinical guidelines. In ACTH-independent Cushing's syndrome, the next step is to obtain CT or MRI imaging of the adrenal glands.

In ACTH-dependent hypercortisolism, the source of ACTH is most often the pituitary gland. The source can also be "ectopic" such as lung cancers, pancreatic tumors, etc. Pituitary adenomas secreting ACTH are somewhat resistant to negative feedback regulation by glucocorticoids while most nonpituitary ACTH-secreting malignant tumors are highly resistant to feedback suppression. Therefore, dynamic testing employing high-dose steroids is used to distinguish between ectopic and pituitary source of ACTH.

The high-dose dexamethasone suppression test can be performed in two ways: overnight[18,20] or over 48 hours.

In the overnight test, a baseline AM serum cortisol level is determined and 8 mg of dexamethasone is administered at 11:00 PM followed by an 8:00 AM plasma ACTH and serum cortisol measurement. A cortisol level less than 5 µg/dL is considered significant suppression. Alternatively, if the cortisol post dexamethasone is suppressed by 50% or more compared to the baseline value, the source of ACTH is thought to be pituitary.

In the 2-day high-dose dexamethasone suppression test, baseline UFC from a 24-hour urine collection is obtained. Following this, 2 mg of dexamethasone is administered every 6 hours for 48 hours. At the end of the study, urine free cortisol (24 hours) or serum cortisol is measured. Low urinary cortisol and suppressed serum cortisol UFC less than 5 µg/dL would suggest pituitary ACTH production.

The gold standard for determining source of ACTH production is inferior petrosal sinus sampling (IPSS). This is an invasive procedure in which ACTH level in inferior petrosal sinus and peripheral vein is determined simultaneously. This study can also be done following stimulation with CRH. An inferior petrosal sinus to peripheral ACTH ratio of 2:1 or greater without CRH and 3:1 or greater with use of CRH is suggestive that ACTH hypersecretion is from the pituitary.[21] Laterality (left vs. right side of pituitary) can also be determined with IPSS. Imaging with MRI can then be used for localization of pituitary ACTH-secreting tumors. If it is ectopic, CT, MRI, or scintigraphy may be required for localization. Figure 21.12 summarizes the diagnostic testing algorithm.

Treatment

Cushing's Disease
Transsphenoidal resection of pituitary tumor is the treatment of choice.[22,23] Cure rates 80% to 90% can be achieved with microadenomas (<1 cm). Cure rates are around 60% or less when the pituitary tumor is greater than 1 cm (macroadenoma).

Cushing's Syndrome
Surgical resection (adrenal or ectopic) would be the first step in management.

If hypercortisolism persists after surgical intervention, medical therapy can be used. Adrenal enzyme inhibitors such as ketoconazole, adrenolytic agents such as mitotane, pituitary ACTH secretion suppressors such as pasireotide or cabergoline, and finally glucocorticoid receptor blockers are all available for use. Bilateral adrenalectomy is occasionally necessary if medical therapy is unable to suppress cortisol levels and the patient has infectious/thrombotic complications from cortisol excess.

FIGURE 21.12 Cushing's syndrome workup. Note that dexamethasone serum levels (for standard test, 2 ng/mL; suppression test, 6.5 ng/mL) can be drawn at 8:00 AM (or 6 hours after the last dose) to help clarify or determine compliance. Normal dexamethasone saliva levels have not been determined. ACTH, adrenocorticotropic hormone.

ADRENAL ANDROGENS

Androgens are produced as by-products of cortisol synthesis that are regulated by ACTH. Although prolactin, pro-opiomelanocortin peptides, and T lymphocytes are known stimulators of androgens, regulatory mechanisms of R-zone biosynthesis remain uncertain (Fig. 21.13). R-cells primarily produce DHEA and multiple 19-carbon steroids (androgens and estrogens) from 17α-hydroxylated pregnenolone and progesterone. DHEA is sulfated to DHEA-S by sulfotransferase, an adrenal enzyme, and secreted daily.

Both DHEA and DHEA-S are precursors to more active androgens (e.g., androstenedione, testosterone, and **5-dihydrotestosterone**) and estrogens (e.g., estradiol and estrone). Although DHEA and DHEA-S have minimal androgenic activity, adverse effects are caused by conversion to active androgens in the adrenal and peripheral tissue (e.g., hair follicles, sebaceous glands, genitalia, adipose, and prostate tissue). Although men derive less than 5% of their testosterone from adrenal or peripheral sources, women rely on the adrenals for 40% to 65% of their daily testosterone production from precursor.

Although observational data demonstrate adrenal androgen production increases in both genders in late childhood and correlates with the onset of pubic hair (adrenarche), it peaks in young adults and progressively declines with age.

Androgen Excess

Androgen excess causes ambiguous genitalia in female infants and precocious puberty in children of both sexes. Androgens stimulate organ development, linear growth, and epiphyseal fusion. Virilization in boys includes penile enlargement, androgen-dependent hair growth, and other secondary sexual characteristics. Girls develop hirsutism, acne, deepening of voice, and clitorimegaly. Excess

FIGURE 21.13 R-zone function and pathology. Manifestations of adrenal hyperandrogenism vary with age, onset, and gender. DHEA, dehydroepiandrosterone; DHEA-S, dehydroepiandrosterone sulfate.

FIGURE 21.14 Effects of DHEA supplementation. DHEA, dehydroepiandrosterone; IGF-1, insulin growth factor 1; HDL, high-density lipoprotein.

androgens can cause short stature by leading to early epiphyseal fusion.

In women, androgen overproduction can cause infertility, with masculinizing effects (e.g., hirsutism, acne, male pattern baldness, menstrual irregularities, and, in severe cases, virilization).

In men, excess adrenal androgens converted to estrogen can also cause infertility with feminizing effects and inhibition of pituitary gonadotropins, which lowers testicular testosterone production. Despite overall adrenal androgen excess, males can experience hypogonadal symptoms including loss of muscle mass and decreased hair growth, decrease in testes size, low testicular testosterone production, and suboptimal spermatogenesis.

Diagnosis

Gonads produce less than 10% of DHEA-S and DHEA; therefore, high DHEA-S and DHEA production strongly suggests adrenal hyperandrogenism, whereas elevated testosterone values are seen with either adrenal or gonadal hyperandrogenism.

Plasma DHEA-S, DHEA, or urinary 17-ketosteroids can identify patients with adrenal causes of pathologic masculinization (females) and feminization (males).

Treatment

Similar to the previously described disorders of overproduction, differentiation between ACTH-dependent and ACTH-independent secretion is assessed by dexamethasone suppression tests followed by imaging studies (CT, MRI). Adenomas and carcinomas are surgically removed. Glucocorticoid-suppressible causes are treated accordingly. Exogenous sources are discontinued and other nonadrenal conditions are treated. Drugs with antiandrogenic properties (e.g., minoxidil, spironolactone, birth control pills) are occasionally used.

Exogenous DHEA is a popular nutritional supplement with numerous purported properties (only a few studied), including vasodilatory, anti-inflammatory, antiaging, and antiatherosclerosis.

The clinical relevance of DHEA(S) interactions with nonandrogen/estrogen receptors remains unknown. DHEA (4 mg/d) and DHEA-S (7 to 15 mg/d) are secreted as the major components of adrenal androgens. There is no evidence that this molecule is required for health or that it contributes to disease. Steroid receptors for DHEA have not been clearly identified. DHEA actions are attributed to its downstream products, testosterone and estrogen.

In normal and compromised patients (e.g., adrenal insufficiency, glucocorticoid therapy, depression, older persons, and trained athletes), DHEA can increase the sense of well-being and raises or lowers a variety of serum markers (Fig. 21.14), although the changes are small. Supplementation (50 to 100 mg/d) in some androgen-deficient patients (e.g., those with adrenal insufficiency, ACTH deficiency, and glucocorticoid therapy) may help ameliorate adverse effects of deficiency and may inhibit glucocorticoid-induced bone loss. However, DHEA can cause adverse androgenic effects in women, and the long-term consequences of supplementation remain unknown.

THE ADRENAL MEDULLA

The adrenal medulla produces catecholamines from the amino acid tyrosine. The secreted catecholamines regulate the body's sympathetic response to stress. Catecholamine products serve as first responders to stress by acting within seconds (cortisol takes 20 minutes) to promote the fight-or-flight response, which increases cardiac output and blood pressure, diverts blood toward muscle and brain, and mobilizes fuel from storage.

Embryology

Sympathetic nervous system arises in the fetus from primordial neural crest stem cells. At about 5th week of gestation, they migrate from the spinal ganglia in the thoracic region. Initially, they form the sympathetic chain posterior to the dorsal aorta and later on migrate anteriorly. At the 6th week of gestation, these primitive cell groups migrate to the adrenal cortex to form the adrenal medulla. These cells are referred to as sympathogonia and pheochromoblasts, which later differentiate into pheochromocytes. The paraganglia are formed by migration of pheochromoblasts and pheochromocytes on either sides of the aorta.

Tumors that arise from either cell line share similar histologic and biochemical properties. Malignant

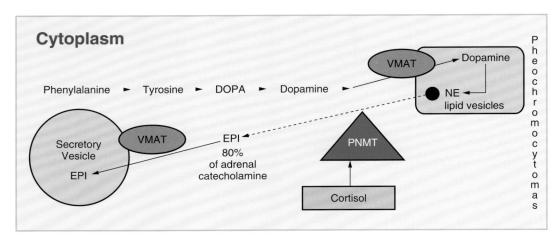

FIGURE 21.15 Biosynthesis and storage of catecholamines. VMAT, vesicular monoamine transporter; NE, norepinephrine; EPI, epinephrine; PNMT, phenylethanolamine *N*-methyltransferase.

neuroblastomas and benign ganglioneuromas arise from sympathoblasts, secrete **homovanillic acid**, and are rarely seen after adolescence. In contrast, tumors of chromaffin cells (pheochromocytomas) maintain the capacity to synthesize and store catecholamines (**norepinephrine [NE]** and EPI) throughout life.[24]

Biosynthesis, Storage, and Secretion of Catecholamines

Catecholamines have a benzene ring with a catechol nucleus and two hydroxyl side groups linked to a side-chain amine, hence the name "catecholamine," and include dopamine (DA), NE, and epinephrine (EPI). Biosynthesis begins with the sequential conversion of phenylalanine substrates in a tightly regulated, compartmentalized manner. All reactions take place in the cytoplasm, except for the production of NE, which occurs within lipid vesicles or outer mitochondrial membranes, as illustrated in Figure 21.15.

In the cytosol, NE is converted into EPI by a cortisol-dependent enzyme called **phenylethanolamine *N*-methyltransferase (PNMT)**. Any form of stress that increases cortisol levels stimulates EPI production.

In the adrenal medulla, EPI and NE are stored in neurosecretory vesicles but are in dynamic equilibrium with the surrounding cytoplasm. They diffuse into the cytoplasm and actively re-enter the vesicles via **vesicular monoamine transporters (VMATs)**. They enter the circulation via exocytosis of the vesicles. The cytoplasmic catecholamines may also be metabolized by enzyme catecholamine-*O*-methyltransferase (COMT) into metanephrines and normetanephrines, which enter circulation via diffusion.

EPI is the main catecholamine secreted by a normal adrenal medulla, which contains 80% of EPI. The ratio of NE to EPI in the serum is normally 9:1 (98% from postganglionic neurons, 2% from the medulla). In adrenal insufficiency (low cortisol), that ratio increases to 45:1 in females and 24:1 in males.

In sympathetic neurons, cytoplasmic dopamine is sequestered into vesicles, converted into NE, and stored until nerve stimulation causes its release into a synapse by exocytosis.

Metabolism and Excretion of Catecholamines

All catecholamines are rapidly eliminated from target cells and the circulation by three mechanisms:

1. Reuptake into secretory vesicles
2. Uptake in nonneuronal cells (mostly liver)
3. Degradation

Degradation relies on two enzymes—COMT (in nonneuronal tissues) and **monoamine oxidase (MAO)** (within neurons)—to produce metabolites (metanephrines and vanillylmandelic acid [VMA]) from free catecholamines. Metabolites and free catecholamines are eliminated by direct filtration into the urine and excreted as free NE (5%), conjugated NE (8%), metanephrines (20%), and VMA (30%) (Fig. 21.16).

PHEOCHROMOCYTOMA AND PARAGANGLIOMA

Overview

Pheochromocytomas are rare catecholamine-secreting tumors arising from the chromaffin cells. The name was coined based on the dusky color of the tumor after staining with chromium salts (in Greek phios=dusky, chromo=color, and cytoma=tumor). Those which arise from the adrenal medulla are referred to as **pheochromocytoma** and those from the sympathetic ganglia are referred to as paraganglioma (extra-adrenal pheochromocytoma). It is important to distinguish between them because of implications related to neoplastic associations, risk of malignancy, and genetic testing. In this chapter, **pheochromocytoma–paraganglioma (PPGL)** will be used to refer to both adrenal and extra-adrenal tumors.

Catecholamine elimination, degradation pathways, and metabolites

FIGURE 21.16 Catecholamine degradation. Free catecholamines (EPI and NE) are either sequestered into VMAT-containing vesicles or converted into metabolites, DOMA by neuronal MAOs and metanephrines by nonneuronal COMTs. These metabolites are ultimately degraded to VMA (DOMA by COMTs and metanephrines by MAOs) and excreted. EPI, epinephrine; NE, norepinephrine; VMAT, vesicular monoamine transporter; DOMA, 3,4-dihydroxymandelic acid; MAO, monoamine oxidase; COMT, catechol methyltransferases; VMA, vanillylmandelic acid.

Epidemiology

PPGLs occur in 0.2% to 0.6% of patients with hypertension and their annual incidence is approximately estimated to be 0.8 per 100,000 patient-years. PPGLs most commonly present between fourth and fifth decade of life and do not have a sex predilection.[25]

About 98% of tumors are located within the abdomen, 85% originating from the adrenal gland. 70% of the tumors are sporadic while 30% have a syndromic presentation. Associated syndromes are von Hippel-Lindau (VHL) syndrome, multiple endocrine neoplasia type 2 (MEN 2), and neurofibromatosis type 1 (NF1). Malignancy, defined by the occurrence of metastases, occurs in 10% among pheochromocytoma with a higher rate of 35% from the paraganglioma. Paragangliomas are located in multiple sites, which include skull base (glomus jugulare tumor), neck (carotid body tumor), thorax (heart and mediastinum), abdomen (organ of Zuckerkandl near the origin of inferior mesenteric artery), and pelvis (bladder wall).

Clinical Presentation

PPGLs are diagnosed in four different clinical situations: (i) patient presents with symptoms, (ii) during evaluation of an adrenal mass, (iii) screening of patients with related syndromes, and (iv) screening of family members diagnosed with PPGLs.[26]

The symptoms of PPGLs are due to paroxysmal secretion of catecholamines and occur in only 50% of patients. The classic triad includes spells of palpitations, headaches, and sweating. Half of them have paroxysmal hypertension while the remaining have sustained hypertension or normal blood pressure. Other symptoms include pallor, hand tremors, shortness of breath, and generalized weakness/fatigue. Patients may also present with symptoms of panic attack, especially tumors that produce EPI. Less common presentations include weight loss, dizziness, orthostatic hypotension, papilledema, cardiomyopathy, erythrosis, hyperglycemia, or psychiatric diagnoses. PPGLs should also be suspected if there is symptom of a spell during diagnostic procedures like endoscopy, during induction of anesthesia or surgical procedures, and during exposure to foods rich in tyramine or drugs like MAO inhibitors or metoclopramide. In a retrospective study, 40% of patients evaluated for pheochromocytoma met the criteria for panic disorder, compared with 5% of control patients with HTN (Fig. 21.17).

10%	90%
Incidentally discovered (imaging, surgery, autopsy)	**Intra-adrenal**
Multiple	**Intra-abdominal** (95%)
Extra-adrenal (chest, neck, abdomen, bladder)	**Single**
Malignant (invasion, distant metastases)	**Benign**
Familial (von Hippel-Lindau, MEN-II, parathyroid hyperplasia, medullary thyroid carcinoma, neurofibromatosis, paraganglioma)	

FIGURE 21.17 Pheochromocytomas.

Diagnosis

Evaluation for PPGLs should be based on clinical suspicion and testing should be performed in the following scenarios:

1. Symptoms and signs of PPGL, especially paroxysmal
2. Early- or late-onset HTN, resistant HTN, or atypical presentation of diabetes mellitus
3. Symptoms of PPGL provoked by drugs
4. Incidentally discovered adrenal nodules (irrespective of hypertension status)
5. Syndromic presentation
6. Idiopathic cardiomyopathy
7. History of gastric stromal tumor or pulmonay chondromas (Carney triad)
8. Personal or family history of PPGL

Interfering Medications

Certain medications may lead to false-positive testing due to (a) direct interference with the measurement method and/or (b) interference with disposition of catecholamines. These medications are acetaminophen, labetalol, sotalol, α-methyldopa, tricyclic antidepressants, buspirone, phenoxybenzamine, MAO inhibitors, sympathomimetics, cocaine, sulfasalazine, and levodopa. A review of the medications taken by patients should be performed prior to testing in order to avoid false-positive results.

Biochemical Testing

A high diagnostic sensitivity is of utmost importance to avoid missing a diagnosis of PPGL. Plasma-free metanephrines or 24-hour urine fractionated metanephrines and catecholamines may be used for initial testing. Some experts recommend to use plasma levels for patients suspected to have a high risk of PPGL and a 24-hour urine collection for those with low risk of PPGL.

Plasma-Free Metanephrines

The guidelines on PPGL by the endocrine society recommend blood draw for plasma-fractionated metanephrines to be measured with the patient in supine position for at least 30 minutes prior to blood sampling. This is based on the evidence that upright posture activates the sympathetic nervous system and stimulates the release of NE and metabolism to normetanephrines leading to false-positive results. Most laboratories use high-performance liquid chromatography or radioimmunoassays. This yields a high sensitivity of 96% to 100% but a poor specificity of 85% to 89%, which is even lower in patients older than 60 years at 77%.[27,28]

24-Hour Urine Fractionated Metanephrines and Catecholamines

The collection of 24-hour urine should be performed appropriately and patients should be counseled the proper method of collection. Urine volume should be quantified and creatinine tested to verify adequacy of collection. Most laboratories use high-performance liquid chromatography (HPLC) with electrochemical detection or tandem mass spectroscopy (MS/MS). This yields a high sensitivity of 98% and specificity of 98%.

24-hour VMA and plasma chromogranin A are not routinely measured since they have poor sensitivity and specificity.

Normal Results

If testing yields normal results, no further testing is indicated. Exception is for patients who present with spells, and repeat testing using a 24-hour urine collection should be performed during a spell. If one test is equivocal (less than threefold elevation above the upper limit of normal), a different test should be performed if clinical suspicion remains high.

If results of the preceding tests are equivocal, a clonidine suppression test (92% accurate) should be performed to separate patients with pheochromocytoma from those without pheochromocytoma who are experiencing similar symptoms secondary to increased sympathetic outflow.[29] Clonidine, an antihypertensive agent, acts as an α2-adrenoceptor agonist and inhibits release of neuronal NE in patients without PPGL alone.

Sympatholytic drugs should be stopped at least 48 hours prior to testing. Baseline plasma normetanephrine is measured and oral clonidine is given at 300 μg/70 kg body weight and plasma normetanephrines is measured 3 hours later. If the 3-hour plasma normetanephrine is elevated and decreases by less than 40% compared to baseline level, test is abnormal indicating a PPGL.

Case Detection

In general, the metanephrines and catecholamines should be elevated to above threefold upper limit of normal for the particular lab value to proceed with radiological investigation. A retrospective review of 1,896 patients reported a false-positive rate of 19% to 21% for both plasma-free and 24-hour urine fractionated metanephrines.[30] Below are the cutoff lab values for a positive case detection.

24-Hour Urine Fractionated Metanephrines and Catecholamines

Normetanephrine greater than 900 μg/24 hours or metanephrine greater than 400 μg/24 hours

Norepinephrine greater than 170 μg/24 hours
Epinephrine greater than 35 μg/24 hours
Dopamine greater than 700 μg/24 hours

Plasma-Fractionated Metanephrines

The normal ranges for plasma metanephrines and normetanephrines depend upon the method used to obtain the blood sample:

Sample obtained via an indwelling cannula placed for 20 minutes before the blood draw following an overnight fast:

Metanephrine less than 0.3 nmol/L

Normetanephrine less than 0.66 nmol/L

Sample obtained via venipuncture in a seated ambulant nonfasting patient:

Metanephrine less than 0.5 nmol/L

Normetanephrine less than 0.9 nmol/L

Radiographic Localization

Biochemical confirmation of pheochromocytoma should be followed by imaging for tumor localization.[31] Ninety five percent of the PPGLs are in the abdomen/pelvis. The most common sites for paragangliomas are the superior and inferior para-aortic areas (75%), bladder (10%), thorax (10%), and head, neck, and pelvis (5%).

Either a computed tomograph (CT) or magnetic resonance imaging (MRI) of the abdomen/adrenals is a reasonable option. They have a high sensitivity of 98% to 100% to detect sporadic pheochromocytoma but a low specificity of 70% due to presence of adrenal incidentalomas. Although the choice of imaging depends upon multiple factors such as radiation exposure, contrast agents, availability, and cost, CT is favored due to its excellent spatial resolution. CT is also the first choice for imaging the thorax and pelvis, while MRI is preferred for skull base and neck paraganglioma. ^{123}I-labeled metaiodobenzylguanidine scintigraphy (MIBG) is used for metastatic PPGLs, recurrent disease, and prior to radiotherapy with ^{131}I-MIBG. It has a low sensitivity and high specificity and should not be used for routine screening. Fluorodeoxyglucose–positron emission tomography (FDG–PET) is widely available and is an option for detection of metastatic disease with a higher sensitivity compared to 123-I MIBG and CT/MRI.

Treatment

Management of PPGL involves surgical removal of the tumor after appropriate medication therapy. It is extremely important to control blood pressure, heart rate, and volume status prior to therapy. Alpha-blockers, beta-blockers, and calcium channel blockers are the most commonly used drugs along with a high sodium diet in the preoperative period.

Surgical excision is a high-risk procedure and should be performed by experienced surgeons at tertiary-level care institutions. Patients with severe preoperative hypertension and highly secretory tumors or those undergoing repeat intervention are at highest risk for complications. After a successful surgery, plasma catecholamines usually normalize within a week.

Outcome, Prognosis, and Follow-up

Surgical removal of a pheochromocytoma is the primary therapy; nevertheless, excision does not necessarily lead to long-term cure of pheochromocytoma or hypertension (even in patients with benign tumors). Patients with familial pheochromocytomas, right adrenal tumors, and extra-adrenal tumors are more likely to have recurrence. In one retrospective series of 176 patients, pheochromocytoma recurred in 16% (52% of those were malignant). Hence, long-term monitoring is indicated in all patients, even those who are apparently cured.

Genetic Testing

Although most PPGLs are sporadic, up to 40% of them are familial and associated with a syndrome.[32] All the syndromes have autosomal dominant inheritance with frequencies (in parenthesis) and mutations as described below:

- Multiple endocrine neoplasia 2 (50%): mutations in the *RET* proto-oncogene
- von Hippel-Lindau syndrome (10% to 20%): mutations in the *VHL* tumor suppressor gene
- Neurofibromatosis type 1 (0.1% to 5.7%): mutations in the *NF1* gene

It is recommended to proceed with genetic testing in the following scenarios:

- Paraganglioma
- Bilateral pheochromocytoma
- Unilateral pheochromocytoma and a family history of PPGL
- Unilateral pheochromocytoma onset at age less than 45 years
- Clinical findings suggestive of one of the syndromes

Genetics is a rapidly changing field, and hence for the latest information, please refer to www.genetests.org.

ADRENAL INCIDENTALOMA

An adrenal incidentaloma is defined as an adrenal mass greater than 1 cm, which is discovered on imaging performed to evaluate nonadrenal pathology.[33] This is the result of advancement in medical imaging technology and the widespread use of imaging studies. The prevalence on CT abdomen is 4.4% and increases to 10% in the elderly, with 10% to 15% being bilateral nodules. Autopsies report a prevalence of 1% to 9%, with higher prevalence among people who have obesity, diabetes mellitus, and HTN. Workup requires biochemical testing to evaluate for hyperfunction, hypofunction, and imaging to define tumor characteristics (benign or malignant).

An adrenal protocol CT abdomen or MRI abdomen is the imaging of choice to determine tumor characteristics, while the FDG–PET scan is used selectively. Size of the nodule is important since 90% of the adrenocortical carcinomas are greater than 4 cm and smaller size at diagnosis correlates to better prognosis. Fine needle aspiration cytology, if performed, should be done after ruling out a pheochromocytoma. It will help distinguish between adrenal and extra-adrenal malignancy but cannot distinguish an adrenal adenoma from a carcinoma. It can also help diagnose infiltrative disorders (amyloidosis, sarcoidosis) and infectious diseases (histoplasmosis, tuberculosis).

In case of bilateral lesions, in addition to routine workup, appropriate biochemical testing should be performed to evaluate for adrenal insufficiency. Figure 21.18 illustrates a

Incidentaloma Function Evaluation		
	Clinical Features	**Screening Tests** **Negative Results**
Pheochromocytoma	**HTN** (paroxysmal) with spells (sweating, HA, or palpitations)	24-hour urine metanephrines <1 μg or 5.5 μmol/mg creatine
Cushing's syndrome	**HTN**, obesity (truncal) weakness	1 mg bedtime dexamethasone 8 AM cortisol < 3.6 μg/dL, or 24-hour urine free cortisol normal
Primary aldosteronism	**HTN**, hypokalemia, weakness	Serum potassium, *if low* urine K⁺ excretion (<30 mmol)
Adrenocarcinoma	Virilization (+ above)	Plasma renin:aldosterone ratio < 30 Plasma DHEAS (<9.2 μmol/L) Urine 17-ketosteroid < 20 mg

FIGURE 21.18 Brief functional screen for adrenal masses. HTN, hypertension; HA, hyperaldosteronism; DHEA-S, dehydroepiandrosterone sulfate.

brief functional screen for adrenal masses, which assesses the function of all adrenal layers and serves as a clinical summary.

CASE STUDIES

Hypertension is common and most often presents as an independent medical condition. Occasionally, hypertension is a result of an underlying illness and requires different treatment. Because adrenal function is critical for (1) blood pressure, (2) potassium, and (3) glucose homeostasis, an adrenal etiology should be considered in all patients with blood pressure problems accompanied by electrolyte abnormalities, unexplained change in weight, failure to thrive, inappropriate virilization, and anxiety periods.

Eight different clinical scenarios are presented below. Each presentation is associated with a different diagnosis and treatment. A discussion of adrenal causes, diagnoses, and treatments for each is found within the chapter. Each numbered case study completes the following opening statement: a 22-year-old woman (previously adopted, not currently taking medications, negative medical history) presents with …

CASE STUDY 21.2

… hypertension, with weakness and rapid onset of obesity. This patient also exhibits central fat pads, buffalo hump, plethora, thin skin, purple striae, easy bruising, osteoporosis, hyperglycemia/insulin resistance, and recurrent infections.

Question

1. What is the diagnosis?

CASE STUDY 21.3

… hypertension, with weakness, irregular menses, and hypokalemia. Her young age, borderline low cortisol, and low androgens also are significant.

Question

1. What is the diagnosis?

CASE STUDY 21.1

… hypertension, with weakness and hypokalemia. The patient also has a high urine potassium excretion without diuretics.

Question

1. What is the diagnosis?

CASE STUDY 21.4

… hypertension, with periods of panic attacks and hot flashes. She also presents with headache, hyperglycemia, hyperthyroidism, and gastrointestinal complaints.

Question

1. What is the diagnosis?

CASE STUDY 21.5

. . . hypertension, with virilization. This young woman presents with irregular menses diagnosed with polycystic ovary syndrome. She has a borderline low cortisol and elevated 17-OH progesterone.

Question

1. What is the diagnosis?

CASE STUDY 21.6

. . . hypertension and hyperkalemia. She has normal renal function (low urine potassium⁺) and metabolic acidosis.

Question

1. What is the diagnosis?

CASE STUDY 21.7

. . . hypotension, failure to thrive, weight loss, and weakness. Her laboratory results reveal hyperkalemia, fasting hypoglycemia, and metabolic acidosis.

Question

1. What is the diagnosis?

CASE STUDY 21.8

. . . new virilization and hirsutism. Laboratory results show increased IGF-1 (insulin growth factor 1), DHEA(S), and testosterone levels. She is a healthy food enthusiast who experiments with nutritional supplements.

Question

1. What is the diagnosis?

For additional student resources, please visit thePoint® at http://thepoint.lww.com

questions

1. When considering an endocrine cause for a patient's hypertension, the _____ _____ is the usual suspect.

2. When hypertension results from an endocrine disorder, what hormonal state is usually found: hormone underproduction or overproduction?

3. True or false? Major warning signs of adrenal disease include abnormal blood pressure, abnormal electrolytes (potassium, acid–base status, urine dilution), and unexplained weight change.

4. _____ is the common substrate from which all adrenal steroids are produced.

5. True or false? When produced, free catecholamines (NE and EPI) are short-lived. They are best measured in the urine, though catecholamine metabolites are best measured in the serum.

6. _____ is responsible for epinephrine production.

7. A primary hyperaldosteronemic state is characterized by:
   a. A urine potassium of 35 mmol/d
   b. A urine potassium of 21 mmol/d
   c. A spot urine test where the sodium levels are greater than potassium levels
   d. Within 3 hours of taking 50 mg of captopril, plasma aldosterone was low
   e. All of the above are characteristic of hypoaldosteronism

8. During a low-dose (1 mg) dexamethasone suppression test, total cortisol levels measured in a patient at 8:35 AM was 2.8 μg/dL. How is this interpreted?
   a. The patient is normal.
   b. The patient has Cushing's syndrome.
   c. The patient has a nonpituitary tumor causing ectopic ACTH syndrome.
   d. The patient has an ACTH-secreting pituitary adenoma.

(continues on page 456)

review questions (continued)

9. The most biologically active androgen in this list is:
  a. DHEA
  b. DHEA-S
  c. LH
  d. FSH
  e. Estrone

10. Which amino acid is needed for the biosynthesis of norepinephrine and epinephrine?
  a. Alanine
  b. Phenylalanine
  c. Isoleucine
  d. Leucine
  e. Serine

11. Which of the following describes catecholamines?
  a. Hydrophobic
  b. Degraded rapidly in nonneuronal cells by mono-amine reductase
  c. Have long half-lives
  d. Circulating blood catecholamines are 99% bound to albumin.
  e. None of the above accurately describes catecholamines.

12. The collection of a 24-hour urine is used for measuring:
  a. Creatinine clearance
  b. Norepinephrine
  c. Dopamine
  d. All of the above may be measured in a 24-hour urine
  e. All but one of the above may be measured in a 24-hour urine

references

1. Kacsoh D. In: Dolan J, ed. *Endocrine Physiology*. New York, NY: McGraw-Hill; 2000:360–448.
2. Clark O, Kebebew E, Clark OH. *Textbook of Endocrine Surgery*. Philadelphia, PA: Elsevier Saunders; 2005:557.
3. Miller W. In: Felig P, ed. *Endocrinology and Metabolism*. New York, NY: McGraw-Hill; 2001:387–493.
4. Lacroix A. In: Pinchera A, ed. *Endocrinology and Metabolism*. London, UK: McGraw-Hill; 2001:285–297.
5. Speiser PW, Azziz R, Baskin LS, et al. Congenital adrenal hyperplasia due to steroid 21 hydroxylase deficiency: an Endocrine Society clinical practice guideline. *J Clin Endocrinol Metab*. 2010;95(9):4133–4160. doi:10.1210/jc.2009-2631
6. Mulatero P, Stowasser M, Loh KC, et al. Increased diagnosis of primary aldosteronism, including surgically correctable forms, in centers from five continents. *J Clin Endocrinol Metab*. 2004;89(3):1045–1050. doi:10.1210/jc.2003-031337
7. Funder JW, Carey RM, Mantero F, et al. The management of primary aldosteronism: case detection, diagnosis, and treatment: an endocrine society clinical practice guideline. *J Clin Endocrinol Metab*. 2016;105(5):1889–1916. doi:10.1210/jc.2015-4061
8. Weinberger MH, Fineberg NS. The diagnosis of primary aldosteronism and separation of two major subtypes. *Arch Intern Med*. 1993;153(18):2125–2129.
9. Young WF, Stanson AW, Thompson GB, et al. Role for adrenal venous sampling in primary aldosteronism. *Surgery*. 2004;136(6):1227–1235. doi:10.1016/j.surg.2004.06.051
10. Meyer A, Brabant G, Behrend M. Long-term follow-up after adrenalectomy for primary aldosteronism. *World J Surg*. 2005;29(2):155–159. doi:10.1007/s00268-004-7496-z
11. Erichsen MM, Løvås K, Skinningsrud B, et al. Clinical, immunological, and genetic features of autoimmune primary adrenal insufficiency: observations from a Norwegian registry. *J Clin Endocrinol Metab*. 2009;94(12):4882–4890. doi:10.1210/jc.2009-1368
12. Dickstein G, Shechner C, Nicholson WE, et al. Adrenocorticotropin stimulation test: effects of basal cortisol level, time of day, and suggested new sensitive low dose test. *J Clin Endocrinol Metab*. 1991;72(4):773–778. doi:10.1210/jcem-72-4-773
13. Staub JJ, Noelpp B, Girard J, et al. The short metyrapone test: comparison of the plasma ACTH response to metyrapone and insulin-induced hypoglycaemia. *Clin Endocrinol (Oxf)*. 1979;10(6):595–601.
14. Nieman LK, Biller BM, Findling JW, et al. The diagnosis of Cushing's syndrome: an Endocrine Society clinical practice guideline. *J Clin Endocrinol Metab*. 2008;93(5):1526–1540. doi:10.1210/jc.2008-0125
15. Elamin MB, Murad MH, Mullan R, et al. Accuracy of diagnostic tests for Cushing's syndrome: a systematic review and metaanalyses. *J Clin Endocrinol Metab*. 2008;93(5):1553–1562. doi:10.1210/jc.2008-0139
16. Mericq MV, Cutler GB. High fluid intake increases urine free cortisol excretion in normal subjects. *J Clin Endocrinol Metab*. 1998;83(2):682–684. doi:10.1210/jcem.83.2.4555
17. Carroll BJ, Curtis GC, Davies BM, et al. Urinary free cortisol excretion in depression. *Psychol Med*. 1976;6(1):43–50.
18. Tyrrell JB, Findling JW, Aron DC, et al. An overnight high-dose dexamethasone suppression test for rapid differential diagnosis of Cushing's syndrome. *Ann Intern Med*. 1986;104(2):180–186.
19. Carroll T, Raff H, Findling JW. Late-night salivary cortisol for the diagnosis of Cushing syndrome: a meta-analysis. *Endocr Pract*. 2009;15(4):335–342. doi:10.4158/EP09023OR
20. Bruno OD, Rossi MA, Contreras LN, et al. Nocturnal high-dose dexamethasone suppression test in the aetiological diagnosis of Cushing's syndrome. *Acta Endocrinol*. 1985;109(2):158–162.
21. Oldfield EH, Doppman JL, Nieman LK, et al. Petrosal sinus sampling with and without corticotropin-releasing hormone for the differential diagnosis of Cushing's syndrome. *N Engl J Med*. 1991;325(13):897–905. doi:10.1056/NEJM199109263251301
22. Bigos ST, Somma M, Rasio E, et al. Cushing's disease: management by transsphenoidal pituitary microsurgery. *J Clin Endocrinol Metab*. 1980;50(2):348–354. doi:10.1210/jcem-50-2-348

23. Nieman LK, Biller BM, Findling JW, et al. Treatment of Cushing's syndrome: an Endocrine Society clinical practice guideline. *J Clin Endocrinol Metab.* 2015;100(8):2807–2831. doi:10.1210/jc.2015-1818

24. Fitzgerald PA. In: *Gardner D*, Shoback D, eds. *Greenspan's Basic & Clinical Endocrinology.* 9th ed. China: McGraw-Hill; 2011:345–356.

25. Martucci VL, Pacak K. Pheochromocytoma and paraganglioma: diagnosis, genetics, management, and treatment. *Curr Probl Cancer.* 2014;38(1):7–41. doi:10.1016/j.currproblcancer.2014.01.001

26. Lenders JW, Duh QY, Eisenhofer G, et al. Pheochromocytoma and paraganglioma: an endocrine society clinical practice guideline. *J Clin Endocrinol Metab.* 2014;99(6):1915–1942. doi:10.1210/jc.2014-1498

27. Lenders JW, Pacak K, Walther MM, et al. Biochemical diagnosis of pheochromocytoma: which test is best? *JAMA.* 2002;287(11):1427–1434.

28. Sawka AM, Jaeschke R, Singh RJ, et al. A comparison of biochemical tests for pheochromocytoma: measurement of fractionated plasma metanephrines compared with the combination of 24-hour urinary metanephrines and catecholamines. *J Clin Endocrinol Metab.* 2003;88(2):553–558. doi:10.1210/jc.2002-021251

29. Eisenhofer G, Goldstein DS, Walther MM, et al. Biochemical diagnosis of pheochromocytoma: how to distinguish true- from false-positive test results. *J Clin Endocrinol Metab.* 2003;88(6):2656–2666. doi:10.1210/jc.2002-030005

30. Yu R, Wei M. False positive test results for pheochromocytoma from 2000 to 2008. *Exp Clin Endocrinol Diabetes.* 2010;118(9):577–585. doi:10.1055/s-0029-1237699

31. Allen BC, Francis IR. Adrenal imaging and intervention. *Radiol Clin North Am.* 2015;53(5):1021–1035. doi:10.1016/j.rcl.2015.05.004

32. Rana HQ, Rainville IR, Vaidya A. Genetic testing in the clinical care of patients with pheochromocytoma and paraganglioma. *Curr Opin Endocrinol Diabetes Obes.* 2014;21(3):166–176. doi:10.1097/MED.0000000000000059

33. Ioachimescu AG, Remer EM, Hamrahian AH. Adrenal incidentalomas: a disease of modern technology offering opportunities for improved patient care. *Endocrinol Metab Clin North Am.* 2015;44(2):335–354. doi:10.1016/j.ecl.2015.02.005

22

Gonadal Function

MAHIMA GULATI

chapter outline

key terms

Amenorrhea
Androgen
Corpus luteum
Follicle-stimulating hormone
Follicular phase
Graafian follicle
Gynecomastia
Hirsutism
Hypogonadism
Inhibin
Leydig cells
Luteal phase
Luteinizing hormone
Ovulation
Sertoli cells
Virilization

chapter objectives

Upon completion of this chapter, the clinical laboratorian should be able to do the following:

- Discuss the biosynthesis, secretion, transport, and action of the sex steroids and gonadotropins.
- Identify the location of the pituitary, ovaries, and testes.
- Describe the hypothalamic–pituitary–ovarian and hypothalamic–pituitary–testicular axes and how they regulate sex steroid and gonadotropin hormone production.
- Explain the principles of each diagnostic test for pituitary–gonadal axes dysfunction.
- Correlate laboratory information with regard to suspected gonadal disorders, given a patient's clinical data.
- Describe the appropriate laboratory testing protocol to effectively evaluate or monitor patients with suspected gonadal disease.

For additional student resources, please visit thePoint®
at http://thepoint.lww.com

THE TESTES

By the 6th week of development in both sexes, the primordial germ cells have migrated from their extraembryonic location to the gonadal ridges, where they are surrounded by the sex cords to form a pair of primitive gonads. Whether chromosomally 46 XX or 46 XY, the developing gonad at this stage of development is bipotential.

The ovarian pathway is followed unless a gene on the short arm of the Y chromosome, designated TDF (testis-determined factor) also known as sex-determining region Y (SRY) gene, makes a DNA-binding protein that acts as a switch, diverting development into the male pathway. In the presence of the Y chromosome (and due to the SRY protein), the medullary tissue starts forming typical testes with seminiferous tubules and Leydig cells by 7 weeks of gestation. Leydig cells under the stimulation of human chorionic gonadotropin (hCG) from the placenta become capable of androgen secretion by week 10. The spermatogonia, derived from the primordial germ cells by 200 or more successive mitoses, form the walls of the seminiferous tubules together with supporting Sertoli cells.

While the primordial germ cells are migrating to the genital ridges, thickenings in the ridges indicate the developing genital ducts and the mesonephric (formerly called wolffian) and paramesonephric (formerly called müllerian) ducts. In the male, the Leydig cells of the fetal testes produce androgen, which stimulates the mesonephric ducts to form the male genital ducts (ductus deferens, epididymis, seminal vesicles, and ejaculatory ducts), and the Sertoli cells produce a hormone that suppresses formation of the paramesonephric ducts (antimüllerian hormone [AMH]). In the female (or in an embryo with no gonads), the mesonephric ducts regress, and the paramesonephric ducts develop into the female duct system. In the early embryo, the external genitalia consist of a genital tubercle, paired labioscrotal swellings, and paired urethral folds. From this undifferentiated state, male external genitalia develop under the influence of androgens or, in the absence of a testis, female external genitalia are formed regardless of whether an ovary is present.

There are three important steps in sexual differentiation and the development of the normal male phenotype. The first is the differentiation of bipotential gonad primordia (identical in both XX and XY fetuses) into the testes that secrete testosterone, which is under the control of the SRY protein coded by that Y chromosome gene. The second is the development of the internal reproductive tract, initiated by fetal testicular androgen production. In male fetuses, this requires the presence of AMH that causes involution of the müllerian ducts, the anlage for the female type reproductive tract. The third is the development of the external genitalia that requires testosterone and, in some target tissues, its more potent metabolite 5α-dihydrotestosterone (DHT).

Several genes are important for normal gonadal differentiation (and their mutations may lead to disorders of sexual differentiation). Steroidogenic factor 1 (SF-1)[1] is important for differentiation and maintenance of both gonadal and adrenal tissue, increasing the synthesis of testosterone and reducing its conversion to estradiol via the transcriptional regulation of the hydroxylases and P450 aromatase, respectively. It may also regulate transcription of the AMH[2] gene in synergy with WT1.[3] Testicular descent is regulated by the protein product of gene Insl3, which is a member of the insulin-like family and is secreted by Leydig cells. Insl3 seems to be important in gubernaculum formation, and mutations in its gene have been shown to be linked with bilateral cryptorchidism in male mice,[4] and in addition, Insl3 protein may also be a biomarker for Leydig cell function. Insl3 also seems to play a role in female fertility (see below).

Functional Anatomy of the Male Reproductive Tract

Adult testes are paired, ovoid organs that hang from the inguinal canal by the spermatic cord, which comprises a neurovascular pedicle, vas deferens, and cremasteric muscle. The testes are located outside the body, encased by a muscular sac. Blood flow is governed by an intricate plexus of arterial and venous blood flow that, together with contraction of the dartos muscle in the scrotal sac, regulates the temperature of the testicles to 2°C below core body temperature. This important function is vital to uninterrupted sperm production. Also encased in the muscular sheath is the spermatic cord, which has the ability to retract the testicles into the inguinal canal in instances of threatened injury. The testes themselves are comprised of two anatomical units: a network of tubules, known as the seminiferous tubules, and an interstitium. The tubules contain germ cells and Sertoli cells and are responsible for sperm production. The testes serve dual functions, which include (1) production of sperm and (2) production of reproductive steroid hormones.[5] In the embryonic stage, the dominant male sex hormone, testosterone (T), aids in development and differentiation of the primordial gonads.

Puberty marks the transition from a nonreproductive state into a reproductive state and is associated with adrenarche with increase in adrenal androgen and gonadarche. Tanner staging of the pubertal and axillary hair changes and genitalia is used in children to mark pubertal changes, which are characterized by growth spurt, increased muscle mass, psychological changes, and male pattern hair growth. The earliest sign of puberty in boys is testicular enlargement that results from rising **luteinizing hormone** (LH) and **follicle-stimulating hormone** (FSH). After puberty, throughout adulthood, and until late in old age, testosterone helps with sperm production and maintains secondary sexual characteristics.

The sperm move sequentially through the tubuli recti; rete testes; ductuli efferentes testes; the head, body, and tail of the epididymis; and, finally, into the vas deferens. Various secretory products of the seminal vesicles and prostate mix with sperm to form the final product: semen. Seminal vesicle secretions are rich in vitamin C and fructose, important for the preservation of motility of the sperm.

Physiology of the Testicles
Spermatogenesis

Sperm are formed from stem cells called *spermatogonia*. The spermatogonia undergo mitosis and meiosis; finally, the haploid cells transform to form mature sperm. The mature sperm has a head, body, and tail, which enables it to swim for the purpose of forming a zygote with the haploid ovum. Certain spermatogonia stagger division so that sperm production is uninterrupted and continuous. The Sertoli cells are polyfunctional cells that aid in the development and maturation of sperm.[6]

Hormonogenesis

Testosterone, the predominant hormone secreted by the testes, is controlled primarily by two pituitary hormones: FSH and LH.[7] Because these hormones were first described in women, they are named in reference to the menstrual cycle. Both hormones are produced by a single group of cells in the pituitary called *gonadotrophs*. FSH acts primarily on germinal stem cells[8] and LH acts primarily on the **Leydig cells**[7]—located in the testicular interstitium—that synthesize testosterone. Gonadotropins (LH and FSH) are glycoproteins and share an alpha subunit with thyroid-stimulating hormone (TSH) and hCG. The beta subunit confers biological specificity for them.

Hormonal Control of Testicular Function

The hypothalamus, located in the brain, generates a hormone called gonadotropin-releasing hormone (GnRH) in a pulsatile fashion. GnRH is synthesized in neurons situated in the arcuate nucleus and other nuclei of the hypothalamus and is released into the portal hypophyseal system that, in turn, determines the production of LH and FSH from the pituitary gland. Impaired pulse generation of GnRH leads to inadequate production of LH and FSH, resulting in **hypogonadism**.[9] The first, and rate-limiting, step in the testicular steroidogenesis is the conversion of cholesterol to pregnenolone. This cholesterol is either trapped by endocytosis from the blood lipoproteins or synthesized within the Leydig cells. The LH binds to the glycoprotein receptor in the cell wall and induces intracellular cyclic AMP production that, in turn, activates protein kinase A, which catalyzes protein phosphorylation. This latter step induces testosterone synthesis. The testicular steroidogenesis pathway is similar to the pathway in the adrenal cortex and they share the same enzymatic systems. Testosterone is the principal **androgen** hormone in the blood, and after puberty, the testes secrete 4 to 10 mg daily and less than 5% is derived from adrenal precursors such as dehydroepiandrosterone (DHEA) and androstenedione. It is largely bound, with 2% to 3% free. About 50% of testosterone is bound to albumin and about 45% is bound to sex hormone–binding globulin (SHBG). The concentration of binding protein determines the level of total testosterone but not the free testosterone levels during laboratory estimation. Testosterone and **inhibin** are the two hormones secreted by the testes that provide feedback control to the hypothalamus and pituitary. Leydig cell steroidogenesis of testosterone is primarily controlled by LH secretion, with negative feedback of testosterone and estradiol on the hypothalamic–pituitary axis. FSH acts on Sertoli cells to stimulate protein synthesis, inhibin, and androgen-binding protein. The actions of both testosterone and FSH on Sertoli cells are synergistic, permitting completion of spermatogenesis. FSH stimulates production of an androgen receptor that makes the Sertoli cell responsive to androgen and, in turn, androgens stimulate synthesis of FSH receptors. Feedback on FSH is attributed to inhibin.[10]

Testosterone concentration fluctuates in a circadian fashion, reflecting the parallel rhythms of LH and FSH levels. This fact should be considered when interpreting serum levels of testosterone: the highest level is found at about 6 AM and correlates with most laboratory normal ranges, and the lowest level is found at about 12 AM (in a male with a normal sleep–wake cycle).

Cellular Mechanism of Testosterone Action

Testosterone enters the cell and converts to DHT in cells rich in 5α-reductase, such as some hair follicles and prostate. DHT and testosterone complex with an intracellular receptor protein and this complex bind to the nuclear receptor, effecting protein synthesis and cell growth.

Physiologic Actions of Testosterone
Prenatal Development

Early in development, embryos have primordial components of the genital tracts of both sexes. The primitive gonads become distinguishable at about the 7th week of embryonic stage. Both chorionic gonadotropins and fetal LH stimulate production of testosterone by the fetal Leydig cells. In the fetus, the hypothalamo-hypophyseal vascular connections are responsible for LH release by hypothalamic GnRH and are established between 11 and 12 weeks after conception, which is 3 weeks after testosterone production by the Leydig cells of the testis. hCG, which has LH-like action, made by the placenta, accounts for this gap in stimulation of testosterone production by the fetal testes. Exposure of testosterone to the Wolffian duct leads to differentiation of the various components of the male genital tract. **Sertoli cells** produce AMH, which aids in regression of the female primordial genital tract. The scrotal skin is rich in 5α-reductase, which converts testosterone to DHT. Fetal exposure to drugs that block this enzyme and DHT formation leads to feminization of the genitalia of the male fetus.

Postnatal Development

Testicular function is reactivated during puberty after a period of quiescence to produce testosterone that results in development of secondary sex hair (face, chest, axilla, and pubis), enhanced linear skeletal growth, development of internal and external genitalia, increased upper body musculature, and development of larynx and vocal cords with deepening of the voice.[11–13] Possible mood changes and aggression are undesired effects that may occur during puberty. The linear growth effects of testosterone are finite, with epiphyseal closure when genetically determined height is achieved. Hypogonadism during puberty leads to imprecise closure of growth plates, leading to excessive height, long limbs, and disproportionate upper and lower body segments. Male secondary sexual characteristics can be staged by a system of development devised by Marshall and Tanner (Table 22.1).

Effect on Spermatogenesis
Stimulation of Leydig cells induces production of testosterone. Testosterone, acting with FSH, has paracrine effects on the seminiferous and Sertoli cells, inducing spermatogenesis. Exogenous overuse or abuse of testosterone, such as occurs with some athletes, will reduce the high intratesticular concentration of testosterone, leading to reduction of sperm production.

Effect on Secondary Sexual Effects
Testosterone has growth-promoting effects on various target tissues. The secondary sex characteristics that develop during puberty are maintained into late adulthood by testosterone.[13] The prostate enlarges progressively during adulthood, while exposure of scalp hair results in regression of the hair follicles (temporal hairline recession). Failure to develop secondary sexual characteristics should prompt evaluation for hypogonadism or constitutional delay in boys. Loss of secondary sexual characteristics might occur gradually and should prompt evaluation for hypogonadism because, among other effects, low testosterone levels lead to loss of bone mass and development of osteoporosis in males at any age.

TABLE 22.1 **Tanner Staging of Genital and Pubic Hair Development in Males**

Stages of Genital Development
1. Prepubertal
2. Enlargement of the scrotum and testes
3. Increased length of the penis, further enlargement of the testes
4. Enlargement of the testes, scrotum, and penis with growth of glans; darkening of scrotal skin
5. Mature genitalia

Stages of Pubic Hair Development
1. Lanugo-type hair (prepubertal)
2. Dark terminal hair at the base of the penis
3. Darker terminal hair spreading over junction of pubes
4. Terminal hair covering pubic region, no spread to medial thighs
5. Mature stage with horizontal distribution of terminal hair to inner thighs

Disorders of Sexual Development and Testicular Hypofunction
Pubertal development could be premature (precocious) or delayed, even if development is normal at birth.[14,15] Precocious sexual development results from the premature exposure of sex steroids, which might arise from early gonadotropin secretion or production by the adrenal glands or testes. Detailed descriptions of the sequence of hormonal pubertal abnormalities of hair, genitals, and breasts are beyond the scope of this text. The differential diagnosis of hypogonadism includes a diverse group of disorders affecting the testicles and the hypothalamic–pituitary regulation of the testes outlined in Box 22.1. Certain important disorders are explained in the following section.

Hypergonadotropic Hypogonadism
Hypergonadotropic hypogonadism incorporates a group of disorders characterized by low testosterone, elevated FSH or LH, and impaired sperm production.

BOX 22.1 Causes of Delayed Puberty

- Delayed puberty or hypogonadism, with increased gonadotropins (FSH and/or LH)
- Klinefelter's syndrome
- Bilateral gonadal failure
- Primary testicular failure
- Anorchia
- Vanishing testicles
- Chemotherapeutic agents
- Irradiation
- Trauma
- Infection (mumps orchitis)
- Delayed puberty with normal or low FSH and/or LH
- Constitutional delayed puberty[16]
- Hypothalamic dysfunction
- Malnutrition
- Chronic systemic illness
- Severe obesity
- Central nervous system tumors
- Hypopituitarism
- Panhypopituitarism
- Kallmann's syndrome (anosmia, cleft palate, and reduced FSH and LH levels)
- Isolated GH deficiency
- Hyperprolactinemia (prolactinoma or drug induced)
- Hypothyroidism
- Miscellaneous
- Prader-Willi syndrome
- Laurence-Moon syndrome
- LEOPARD syndrome
- Bloom syndrome
- Germ cell neoplasia
- Male pseudohermaphroditism
- Ataxia–telangiectasia
- Steroidogenic enzyme defects

Klinefelter's Syndrome

Klinefelter's syndrome occurs in about 1 of 400 to 600 men and is caused by the presence of an extra chromosome; in fact, it is the most common human sex chromosome abnormality. The most common karyotype is 47, XXY.11. Men with this disorder have small (<2.5 cm), firm testicles. **Gynecomastia** (enlargement of the male breast) is commonly present at the time of diagnosis. Due to reduced production of testosterone, LH levels are elevated. Due to deficient seminiferous tubule mass, FSH is elevated from underproduction of inhibin.[17] These men also have azoospermia and resultant sterility. Men with *mosaicism* may produce some sperm and pregnancies have been reported with such men. Elevated levels of FSH and LH induce increased aromatase activity, resulting in elevated estrogen levels. Men with Klinefelter's syndrome may have reduced bone density and breast cancer risk comparable to women.

Testicular Feminization Syndrome

Testicular feminization syndrome is the most severe form of androgen resistance syndrome, resulting from mutations of the androgen receptor and impaired androgen actions in target tissues. As a result of the lack of androgen and unopposed estrogen effects, the physical development pursues the female phenotype, with fully developed breast and female distribution of fat and hair. Most present for evaluation of primary amenorrhea, at which time the lack of female internal genitalia becomes apparent. The testicles are often undescended, and failure to promptly remove these organs is essential to abort malignant transformation. Biochemical evaluation reveals normal or elevated serum concentrations of testosterone with elevated FSH and LH levels. There is no utility or response to administration of exogenous testosterone. They are reared as girls. There is a wide variation in androgen insensitivity and in corresponding clinical deficits in male sexual development.

5α-Reductase Deficiency

Deficiency of 5α-reductase is a rare cause of androgen insensitivity and results in a mutation encoding the type 2 isoenzyme, maps to chromosome 2p23, and is expressed in XY males. A reduction in levels of the enzyme 5α-reductase results in decreased DHT concentrations. Physical development is similar to the female phenotype until puberty when the wolffian ducts virilize in response to testosterone. The female internal genitalia are absent and the male internal genitalia are well developed (epididymis, vas deferens, and seminal vesicle) in response to testosterone. DHT is essential for the development of the prostate and external genitalia during embryonic virilization.

Myotonic Dystrophy

Myotonic dystrophy (type 1 caused by DMPK gene mutation and type 2 caused by CNBP gene mutation) is inherited in an autosomal dominant fashion (almost always, an affected person has one parent with the condition) and presents with primary hypogonadism, frontal balding, diabetes, and muscle weakness, atrophy, and dystonia (an inability of the muscle to relax adequately after contraction). The incidence of DM is 1 in 8,000 worldwide. Testicular failure typically presents in the twenties and thirties; however, puberty progresses normally and male secondary sexual characteristics, height, bone growth, etc., are attained normally during pubertal course of development. Primary hypogonadism occurs with primarily germ cell compartment failure (i.e., oligozoospermia and infertility), with elevated serum FSH. In later stages, failure of Leydig cell compartment resulting in low serum testosterone, elevated LH concentrations, and testicular atrophy occurs. Testicular failure happens more commonly in DM1 (type 1 myotonic dystrophy) than in DM2.

Testicular Injury and Infection

Mumps orchitis develops in a third of postpubertal males with mumps and is the most frequent extrasalivary manifestation of this highly contagious infection. Mumps epididymo-orchitis is usually unilateral (85% of the times); therefore, permanent sterility is rare (contrary to popular belief). Most cases of orchitis occur within 4 to 6 days of parotitis, but it may precede parotitis or be the only manifestation of mumps. Intermittently, mumps outbreaks have been reported in secondary schools, colleges, universities, and military groups; however, the absolute numbers are still quite low at a few hundred cases reported in a year in the United States. Other infectious causes of orchitis like TB, Chlamydia, gonorrhea, etc., are fortunately rare in the United States. Radiation and chemotherapy for cancer can result in long-term testicular damage.

Sertoli Cell–Only Syndrome

Sertoli cell–only syndrome (SCO syndrome or germ cell aplasia) is characterized by a lack of germ cells. Men present with small testes, high FSH levels, azoospermia, and normal testosterone levels. Testicular biopsy, which is necessary for diagnosis, shows lack (or complete absence) of spermatozoa. This disorder may arise from Y chromosome microdeletions on Yq11 locus (AZF region: Azoospermia Factor). It is relatively rare, affecting 5% to 10% of all infertile men in the country.

Hypogonadotropic Hypogonadism

The hallmark of disorders of hypogonadotropic hypogonadism is the occurrence of low testosterone levels together with low or inappropriately normal FSH or LH levels.

Kallmann's Syndrome

The impaired secretion of GnRH has been elucidated in the X-linked form of congenital GnRH deficiency, which results from impaired migration of GnRH neurons and olfactory nerves to the ventral hypothalamus during embryogenesis. Proper migration of these neurons is dependent on the correct expression of anosmin, a 680–amino acid neural cell adhesion molecule–like protein, which is the product of the KAL1 gene.

Mutations in the KAL1 gene (a gene found on the X chromosome) occur less often in sporadic cases (<10%). In general, the clinical phenotypes of idiopathic hypogonadotropic hypogonadism (IHH) subjects with KAL1 mutations are characterized with a high incidence of microphallus, cryptorchidism, and small testes. X-linked KAL mutations have never been observed in families with normosmic IHH (nIHH) or in families with both anosmic and nonanosmic individuals.[18,19]

Kallmann's syndrome is a result of an inherited, X-linked recessive trait that manifests as hypogonadism during puberty. The frequency of this syndrome is 1 of 10,000 males. Certain men also have red-green color blindness, congenital deafness, or cerebellar dysfunction.

Hyperprolactinemia
Prolactin elevation resulting from any cause (drug-induced or prolactin-producing tumors of the pituitary) can result in hypogonadotropic hypogonadism[20,21] due to impairment of both frequency and amplitude of FSH and LH pulses, because of hypothalamic kisspeptin neuron–mediated disruption of GnRH pulsatile secretion.[22,23]

Type 2 Diabetes
Type 2 diabetes is also associated with hypogonadotropic hypogonadism in at least 25% to 50% of men.[24] It is characterized by low free or total serum concentrations of testosterone and inappropriately low LH.[25] This may stem from insulin resistance (insulin action seems to be important for LH release by gonadotropes), low SHBG levels, inflammation (hypogonadism in type 2 diabetic males was seen to be associated with high C-reactive protein levels, an inflammatory marker),[24] and even elevated estradiol levels (due to testosterone aromatization in adipose tissue). Of note, type 1 diabetes does not seem to be associated with hypogonadism, provided glycemic control has remained good and BMI is within normal limits.[26]

Age
There is a gradual reduction in testosterone after age 30, with an average decline of about 110 ng/dL every decade. The Baltimore Longitudinal Study of Aging revealed "hypogonadism" (reduced total testosterone concentrations) of 19% at age 60, 28% at age 70, and 49% at age 80,[27] with free testosterone concentrations much lower in these men. Age is also associated with elevation of SHBG by about 1%/year. Similar findings emerged from the Massachusetts Male Aging Study, which showed 1.6%/year decline in total testosterone levels and 2% to 3%/year decline in bioavailable testosterone (free and albumin-bound testosterone) levels.[28] Recently, the results of the Testosterone Trials were published that showed significant improvement in sexual function in older men greater than 65 years, given testosterone replacement for 1 year, but no significant improvement in physical function or vitality.[29]

Pituitary Disease
Acquired hypogonadism can follow injury to the pituitary as a result of tumors, surgical- or radiation-induced trauma, vascular injury, autoimmune hypophysitis, or granulomatous or metastatic disease. Hemochromatosis is a rare cause of pituitary dysfunction.

Opioid Use
Long-term or continuous use of narcotics has been linked to severe hypogonadotropic hypogonadism (due to μ-opioid receptor–mediated decreased GnRH pulsatile production) and even decrease in male fertility (decreased sperm motility, decreased sperm counts, and abnormal sperm morphology).[30]

Obstructive Sleep Apnea
It is unclear if sleep apnea leads to hypogonadotropic hypogonadism (due to hypoxemia and sleep deprivation),[31] or if the obesity (which is often present in men with sleep apnea) leads to decreased testosterone levels. It is to be noted that testosterone replacement therapy (especially high-dose testosterone) may worsen preexisting sleep apnea, possibly due to increased oxygen consumption; and therefore, the Endocrine Society guidelines[32] recommend not starting testosterone replacement therapy in men with untreated severe OSA, until first starting them on CPAP.

Diagnosis of Hypogonadism
Both clinical and biochemical features must be met (Fig. 22.1) to make the diagnosis of hypogonadism. Testosterone concentrations have a circadian rhythm and the time of sampling must be considered. Morning samples between 8 and 10 AM are recommended to match values from reference interval studies. Multiple estimation of free and bound testosterone levels should be done on different days before a diagnosis of testosterone deficiency is confirmed.[32] The distinction between primary (disease or destruction of the testes) versus secondary (disease or destruction of the pituitary) or tertiary (hypothalamic) is relatively easy to make. FSH and/or LH[33] values are elevated in primary hypogonadism and are inappropriately normal or low with secondary or tertiary etiologies. Pituitary MRI should be done in secondary hypogonadism in young individuals. Older individuals often have secondary or tertiary (hypothalamic) dysfunction as a result of reduced hypothalamic pulse generator frequency, resulting in low or inappropriately normal FSH and/or LH levels.[34] Clinical signs and symptoms of hypogonadism (e.g., loss of secondary sexual characteristics, decreased muscle mass, osteoporosis, etc.) should be corroborated with low testosterone levels, particularly when testosterone replacement therapy is considered.[32]

Testosterone Replacement Therapy
The following principles should guide testosterone therapy: testosterone should be administered only to a man who is hypogonadal, as evidenced by clinical symptoms and signs consistent with androgen deficiency and a distinctly subnormal serum testosterone concentration. Treating symptoms of hypogonadism without corroborating biochemical evidence of testosterone deficiency is not recommended. Restoring testosterone to midnormal concentrations can be achieved satisfactorily whether the testosterone deficiency is due to primary or secondary hypogonadism.

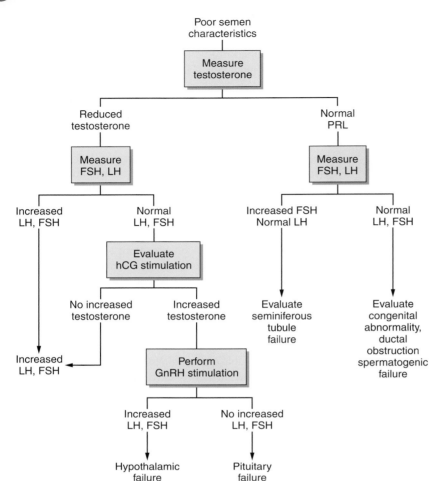

FIGURE 22.1 Clinical diagnostic evaluation of male hypogonadism. PRL, prolactin; FSH, follicle-stimulating hormone; LH, luteinizing hormone; hCG, human chorionic gonadotropin; GnRH, gonadotropin-releasing hormone.

The currently available modes[35] of testosterone administration in the United States are as follows:

1. **Parenteral testosterone.** This is the most widely available and cost-effective mode of administration. The cypionate and enanthate esters of testosterone are available for intramuscular injection. The peak level is achieved in 72 hours and the effect lasts for a period of 1 to 2 weeks. Weekly administration provides for a lower peak and less fluctuation within the normal range of testosterone levels. Usual dosing is 50 to 100 mg weekly or 150 to 250 mg once every 2 weeks. Testosterone dose should be based on lean body mass, not on body weight, and is best reached by administering a standard dose of testosterone, with minor dose escalations based on serum testosterone levels measured midpoint between two injections. The goal is to maintain this middose level at midpoint of the normal ranges. Recently, FDA has approved extra-long-acting testosterone undecanoate injection, which can be injected every 10 weeks (after the first 2 doses, which need to be injected in a 4-week interval), but this injection is available only under AVEED REMS program,[36] due to possible risk of serious adverse effects of pulmonary oil microembolism (POME) and anaphylaxis.

2. **Transdermal testosterone patch therapy.** This mode of administration provides more physiologic levels of testosterone. The patch is permeability enhanced to aid in the absorption of testosterone through normal skin. Local skin irritation can occur and often limits the patch use.

3. **Testosterone gel.** This hydroalcoholic gel preparation is applied to nongenital skin once daily. The absorption is gradual and provides blood levels of testosterone in the normal range for 24 hours. The main concern with this preparation is potential transmission to female partners or children on close skin contact.

4. **Testosterone buccal pellet.** This plastic tablet is placed along the gum line twice daily. Local discomfort (irritated gums) and the need for twice-daily dosing sometimes limit use.

5. **Subcutaneous testosterone pellet** (Testopel) involves implantation of three to six 75 mg testosterone pellets every 3 to 6 months, into the subdermal fat of the buttocks, lower abdominal wall, or thigh with a trocar under sterile conditions using a local anesthetic. This is not a very frequently used mode of testosterone replacement due to pellet extrusion, fibrosis, infection, and the need for an incision to implant the Testopel.

6. **Nasal testosterone gel (Natesto).** Natesto is administered into each nostril by a metered-dose pump applicator three times daily. The risk of testosterone transfer from a patient to his partner or children is mitigated, but the complications of testosterone replacement are acne, polycythemia, prostate enlargement, possible growth-promoting effect on undiagnosed prostate cancer, worsening of obstructive sleep apnea (OSA), peripheral edema, and gynecomastia.

Oral alkylated androgens are not recommended due to adverse effects of decreased high-density lipoprotein,[37] increase in low-density lipoprotein (LDL), and also incidence of cholestatic jaundice and peliosis hepatitis.

Monitoring Testosterone Replacement Therapy

Prostate-specific antigen (PSA), blood counts (for hematocrit), and lipid levels should be checked 3 to 6 months after initiation of testosterone replacement and at least yearly thereafter. Routine clinical evaluation for leg edema, worsening of sleep apnea, and prostate enlargement is also recommended. Pharmacologic use of testosterone may also reduce sperm count by reducing the intratesticular testosterone concentration that is manyfold higher than serum concentrations. If PSA elevation is noted after testosterone replacement, prostate evaluation with possible biopsy is recommended. Prostatic carcinoma is a contraindication to testosterone replacement.

THE OVARIES

Early Ovarian Development

If no Y chromosome or TDF is present, the gonad, by default, forms an ovary; the cortex develops, the medulla regresses, and oogonia begin to develop within follicles. The oogonia are derived from the primitive germ cells by a series of about 30 mitoses, far fewer than the number required for spermatogenesis. Beginning at about the end of the 3rd month, the oogonia enter meiosis I, but this process is arrested at a stage called dictyotene, in which the cell remains until ovulation occurs many years later (this cell is called primary oocyte). Many of the oogonia degenerate before birth, and only about 400 mature into ova during the 30 years or so of sexual maturity of the female. It is evident that the gonads are paired bilateral structures; in very rare circumstances, the developmental processes may be different on either side. Estrogen formation in the fetal ovary begins in early development despite primordial follicles not having begun forming until the second trimester of pregnancy (at 16 weeks of gestation). The gonadotropins from the pituitary gradually take over the role of maternal placental hCG, and fetal pituitary LH and FSH peak near midgestation and then fall to low concentrations at birth. Postpartum, a smaller peak of LH and FSH occur, which stimulates steroid secretion leading to neonatal milk production from the breast.

Pubertal Changes of Ovarian Function

The onset of puberty is characterized by increasing secretion of LH and FSH that stimulates gonadal activity and is driven by increased activity of the hypothalamic GnRH neurons. In the ovary, both LH and FSH are involved in the control of steroidogenesis, and there are numerous isoforms of circulating LH and FSH and their biological potency depends on the degree of glycosylation, which is associated with differences in assays for LH and FSH. The genes coding LH and FSH receptors are on chromosome 2p21. Inactivating mutations of the β-chain of the LH receptor have been described. Before the onset of puberty, both LH and FSH are secreted in small amounts, but as puberty approaches, the amplitude of LH and FSH pulsatile secretions increases and the nocturnal rise in LH secretion increases. The nocturnal rise disappears with adulthood.

The ovaries are paired organs that, like the male gonads, perform the dual functions of gamete (ovum) and steroid hormone production.[38–40] Unlike in the male, the primordial reproductive cells in the female typically produce a solitary gamete. Ovarian and menstrual events are carefully synchronized by a complex interplay of hormones among the hypothalamus, pituitary, and ovaries to prepare the uterus for implantation of an embryo. In the absence of implantation, the uterine lining is shed, resulting in menses.[41,42]

The length of the menstrual cycle is the time between any two consecutive cycles. The typical duration is 25 to 35 days, with average menstrual flow about 3 to 6 days.[42]

Functional Anatomy of the Ovaries

The ovaries are oval organs that lie in the pelvic fossa, formed by the posterior and lateral pelvic wall, and attach to the posterior surface of the broad ligament by the peritoneal fold, otherwise known as the mesovarium. They are positioned near the fimbrial end of the fallopian tubes, which are connected to the uterine cavity. An adult ovary averages 2 to 5 cm in length, weighs an average of 14 g, and typically contains 2 to 4 million primordial follicles.[43] These primordial follicles are present at birth; however, maturation is blocked until puberty. Following the onset of puberty, each ovarian cycle is marked by recruitment of a few primordial follicles for maturation. Typically, all but one of these follicles will then atrophy, in a process termed the **follicular phase**.

The single remaining follicle—known as the **graafian follicle**—is composed of an outer and inner layer (the theca externa and theca interna, respectively) encasing a central fluid-filled cavity and a layer of cells known as the granulosa layer.[44–46] The maturing ovum attaches to the inside of the follicle via cells derived from granulosa cells, called *cumulus cells*. During the **luteal phase** of the ovarian cycle, the graafian follicle releases its ovum in response to ovarian stimulation by LH. When the ovum is extruded, the graafian follicle undergoes a morphologic change with hypertrophy of the theca and granulosa cells to become the **corpus luteum**.

This process is called *luteinization*. The corpus luteum is rich in cholesterol and acts as a substrate for continued production of progesterone and estrogen, maintaining the endometrium for conception. If conception or implantation fails to occur, the endometrium is shed and the corpus luteum atrophies to an atretic follicle.

Hormonal Production by the Ovaries

As in the adrenal glands and the testes, the steroidogenic pathway and synthetic enzymes are present in the ovaries. Cholesterol is either synthesized from acetate or actively transported from the LDL particle in blood and then used as a substrate for hormonal production.[47]

Estrogen

Naturally synthesized estrogens are carbon-18 compounds. The principal estrogen produced in the ovary is estradiol. Estrone and estriol are primarily metabolites of intraovarian and extraglandular conversion. Estrogens promote breast, uterine, and vaginal development and also affect the skin, vascular smooth muscles, bone cells, and the central nervous system.[48] The lack of estrogen that naturally occurs with the onset of menopause leads to atrophic changes in these organs.[49] During the reproductive period, it is estrogen that is responsible for follicular phase changes in the uterus, with deficiency resulting in irregular and incomplete development of the endometrium.

Progesterone

Progesterone is a carbon-21 compound within the steroid family and is produced by the corpus luteum. Progesterone induces the secretory activity of those endometrial glands that have been primed by estrogen, readying the endometrium for embryo implantation. Other effects include thickening of the cervical mucus, reduction of uterine contractions, and thermogenic effect, in which basal body temperature rises after **ovulation**. This effect is of clinical use in marking the occurrence of ovulation. Progesterone is the dominant hormone responsible for the luteal phase, and deficiency results in failure of implantation of the embryo.[50]

Androgens

Ovaries produce the androgens androstenedione, dehydroandrostenedione, testosterone, and DHT, all of which are carbon-19 compounds. Excess production of ovarian androgens in women leads to excess hair growth (**hirsutism**), loss of female characteristics, and—in severe cases—development of overt male secondary sexual features (masculinization or **virilization**).[50–52] Unlike estrogen, which is not produced in the ovary after menopause, ovarian androgen synthesis continues well into advanced age.[53]

Others

Inhibins A and B, which are produced by the ovaries, are hormones that inhibit FSH production.[54] Activin is a hormone that enhances FSH secretion and induces steroidogenesis.[54]

Folliculostatin, relaxin,[55] follicle regulatory protein, oocyte maturation factor, and meiosis-inducing substance are hormones that appear to have important, yet not clearly characterized, functions.

The Menstrual Cycle

By convention, the menstrual cycle is considered to start on the 1st day of menses (day 1). The menstrual cycle consists of two phases of parallel events occurring at the ovaries and endometrium. Within the ovaries, these events are known as the follicular and luteal phases, while the concurrent endometrial events are known as the proliferative and secretory phases.[56]

The Follicular Phase

The follicular phase begins with the onset of menses and ends on the day of LH surge. Early in the follicular phase, the ovary secretes very little estrogen or progesterone. A rise in FSH, however, stimulates estrogen production. The estrogen secreted by the developing follicle within the ovary stimulates uterine epithelial cells, blood vessel growth, and endometrial gland development to increase the thickness of the endometrium.

The Luteal Phase

Estrogen levels peak 1 day before ovulation, at which point a positive feedback system results in an LH surge. The start of the luteal phase is marked by the extrusion of the ovum approximately 36 hours after this LH surge, with subsequent luteinization of the graafian follicle to form the corpus luteum. The corpus luteum secretes progesterone to aid in the implantation of the embryo. The intense secretory capacity of the uterine glands aids the implantation of the embryo. In the absence of fertilization, with a gradual decline in the production of progesterone and estrogen by the corpus luteum, there is a loss of endometrial blood supply; this results in shedding of the endometrium approximately 14 days after ovulation occurred. The typical duration of menstrual bleeding is 3 to 5 days, with blood loss averaging 50 mL. Onset of menses marks the end of the luteal phase.

Hormonal Control of Ovulation

The central control of FSH and LH secretion resides in the GnRH pulse generator of the arcuate nuclei and medial preoptic nuclei of the hypothalamus.[56] Positive and negative feedback responses exist among estrogen, progesterone, LH, and FSH production. It is because of the lack of estrogen after menopause that both FSH and LH levels rise.[57] During reproductive years, FSH levels are elevated early in the follicular phase. A midcycle surge in LH production stimulates a series of events that culminate in ovulation, with FSH levels falling after this event. Any injury to the hypothalamus or the presence of either psychosocial or physical stressors leads to changes in these hormonal cues and results in anovulation and amenorrhea.[58]

CASE STUDY 22.1

A 39-year-old woman presented with hot flashes and irregular menstrual cycles for 6 months. Clinical examination did not reveal abnormality. Laboratory evaluation reveals the following: CBC, normal; blood glucose, 89 mg/dL; TSH, 1.5 mIU/L; FSH, 128 IU/L; and LH, 30 IU/L.

This clinical situation is consistent with one of the following:

1. PCOS
2. Prolactinoma
3. Pituitary tumor
4. Menopause
5. Hypothalamic hormone deficiency

Pubertal Development in the Female

As with males, puberty in females consists of a sequence of hormonally mediated events resulting in the development of secondary sexual characteristics and attainment of final adult height. Thelarche (development of breast tissue) is typically the earliest sign of sexual development, followed by development of pubic hair. Menarche, or initiation of menses, occurs an average of 2 to 3 years after the onset of puberty.

Precocious Sexual Development

Precocious sexual development occurs in response to premature exposure of tissues to sex steroids from any source and is distinguished from precious puberty, which can be arrested by suppression of GnRH with analogs of GnRH that will suppress LH. If untreated, precious puberty or sexual development can lead to short stature. Premature breast development is characterized by isolated breast development and occurs in response to earlier estrogen secretion, albeit at low circulating concentrations. Premature adrenarche may occur between 4 and 8 years of age and is characterized by pubic hair growth, and most commonly, precious puberty does not ensue. Gonadotropins and gonadal steroid secretion help differentiate between them. DHEA and dehydroepiandrosterone sulfate (DHEAS) are elevated for age but match the child's bone age.

In girls with delayed puberty, sex steroids and gonadotropins are low, but they continue growing and may be tall because growth hormone (GH) and other pituitary hormones are unaffected unless pituitary or hypothalamic dysfunction is present.

Devised by Marshall and Tanner as a way to determine pubertal staging, the Tanner staging system, outlined in Table 22.2, is used to monitor and assess the growth stages of breast and pubic hair.[59]

| TABLE 22.2 | Tanner Staging of Breast and Pubic Hair Development in Females |

Stages of Breast Development
1. Prepubertal
2. Elevation of breast bud and papilla, areolar enlargement
3. Elevation of breast tissue and papilla
4. Elevation of areola and papilla in secondary mound above the level of the breast
5. Mature stage: recession of areola into the breast with projection of papilla only

Stages of Pubic Hair Development
1. Lanugo-type hair (prepubertal)
2. Dark terminal hair on labia majora
3. Terminal hair covering labia majora and spreading to the mons pubis
4. Terminal hair fully covering the labia majora and mons pubis
5. Terminal hair covering the labia majora, mons pubis, and inner thighs

Menstrual Cycle Abnormalities

The menstrual cycle ranges from 25 to 35 days, with an average of 28-day duration. The average age of menopause in the United States is between 45 and 55 years, with the median at 53 years.[57]

Amenorrhea is defined as the absence of menses. *Primary amenorrhea* is used to describe a woman who has never menstruated by age 16 years, while *secondary amenorrhea* is used to describe a woman who has had at least one menstrual cycle followed by absence of menses for a minimum of 3 to 6 months.[58] Frequency of the different etiologies for amenorrhea, both primary and secondary, is listed in Table 22.3.

Oligomenorrhea refers to infrequent irregular menstrual bleeding, with cycle lengths in excess of 35 to 40 days. Uterine bleeding in excess of 7 days is dysfunctional and is termed *menorrhagia*. In a patient with infertility, the diagnosis of inadequate luteal phase is made when the luteal phase is less than 10 days or when an endometrial biopsy indicates the progression of endometrial changes is delayed or out of phase, resulting in implantation failure.[60] The

TABLE 22.3	Etiologies of Amenorrhea	
	Primary (%)	Secondary (%)
Hypothalamus	27	38
Pituitary	2	15
Polycystic ovarian syndrome	7	30
Ovary	43	12
Uterus/outflow	19	7

Target	Result	Cause
Female		
Hypothalamus	Decreased GnRH	Drugs
		Increased stress
		Diet
Pituitary	Decreased FSH and LH	Destructive tumor or vesicular lesion
Ovaries	Decreased estradiol or progesterone	Organ failure
		Organ dysgenesis
		Antiovarian antibodies
		Malnourishment, very low weight, metabolic disease
Fallopian tubes and uterus	Inadequate endometrium	Low progesterone output
	Tubal scarring and closure	Pelvic inflammatory disease
	Decreased cervical mucus	Cervical infections
Conception	Immobilization and destruction of sperm	Antisperm antibodies
Male		
Hypothalamus and pituitary	Oligospermia to azoospermia (no sperm)	Primary defects in hypothalamic or pituitary glands
		Exogenous androgens
		Testicular dysfunction
Testes	Oligospermia to azoospermia	Orchitis
	Delayed or deficient sexual maturity	Testicular infections (mumps)
	Decreased testosterone	Alcoholism/substance abuse
		Chromosomal defects
Prostate	Decreased seminal fluid	Infections of prostate or seminal vesicles
Urethrogenital tract	Retrograde or absent ejaculation	Physical abnormalities
		Chronic diabetes

GnRH, gonadotropin-releasing hormone; FSH, follicle-stimulating hormone; LH, luteinizing hormone.

multiple causes of male and female infertility are shown in Table 22.4.

The principles underlying the evaluation of disorders of normal menstrual functions, as outlined by the World Health Organization (WHO), are the same for ovarian and pituitary dysfunction (Box 22.2). A diagnostic approach to secondary amenorrhea is outlined in Figure 22.2.

Hypogonadotropic Hypogonadism

Hypogonadotropic hypogonadism, or gonadotropin (FSH and LH) deficiency resulting in decreased sex steroid production, is a common cause of secondary amenorrhea. There are many physiologic and pathologic causes of hypogonadotropic hypogonadism, including weight loss as associated with anorexia nervosa or various disease processes, intense physical exercise (commonly termed *runner's amenorrhea*), and pituitary tumors that disrupt secretion of FSH or LH.[58] Prolactin production by prolactinomas can have similar effects. Any secondary cause of chronic hypogonadism can induce pathologic bone loss, resulting in osteopenia or, if severe, osteoporosis ("*athlete's triad*": constituted by amenorrhea, eating disorder, and osteoporosis).

BOX 22.2 Classification of Amenorrhea by WHO Guidelines

- Type 1. Hypothalamic hypogonadism (low or normal FSH and/or LH)
- Hypothalamic amenorrhea (anorexia nervosa, idiopathic, exercise induced)
- Kallmann's syndrome
- Isolated gonadotropin deficiency
- Type 2. Estrogenic chronic anovulation (normal FSH and LH)
- Polycystic ovarian syndrome (LH > FSH in some patients 2:1 or greater)
- Hyperthecosis
- Type 3. Hyperthalamic hypogonadism (elevated FSH and/or LSH)
- Premature ovarian failure
- Turner's syndrome

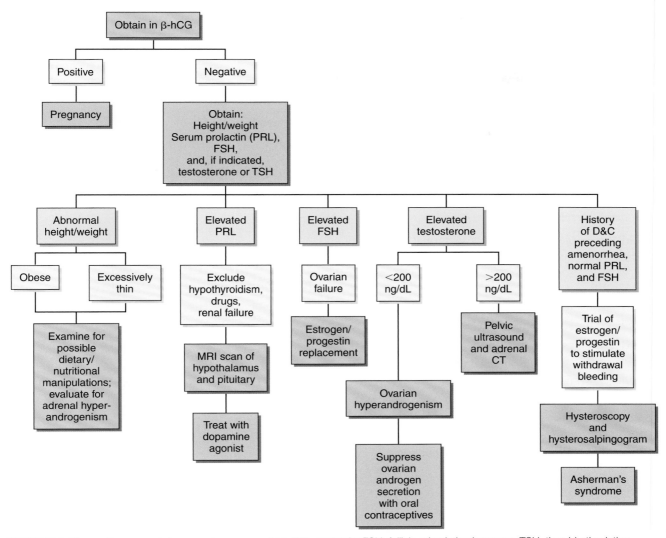

FIGURE 22.2 Diagnostic approach to secondary amenorrhea. PRL, prolactin; FSH, follicle-stimulating hormone; TSH, thyroid-stimulating hormone; hCG, human chorionic gonadotropin.

CASE STUDY 22.2

A 49-year-old woman presented with increased hair growth for the past 6 months that started abruptly; she had male pattern hair loss, as well. On examination, she had temporal loss of hair and clitorimegaly. Laboratory evaluation revealed the following: testosterone, 360 ng/dL; FSH, 12 IU/L; LH, 9 IU/L; and a normal prolactin level.

The next step in the evaluation is one of the following:

1. DHEAS level
2. Repeat FSH and LH levels
3. Fasting blood sugar level
4. Fasting lipid level
5. Computed tomography of adrenal and ovaries

Hypergonadotropic Hypogonadism

Hypergonadotropic hypogonadism is characterized by ovarian failure resulting in elevation of FSH concentrations, with or without LH elevations. Ovarian failure occurs naturally between 45 and 55 years of age in American women. When the depletion of oocytes and follicles occurs at the expected time, it is termed *menopause*. Menopause is a natural, inevitable event that results in elevation of FSH and LH levels, with low levels of estrogen.[57]

Premature ovarian failure is defined as primary hypogonadism in a woman before the age of 40 and can be a result of congenital chromosomal abnormality (e.g., Turner's syndrome[61]) or premature menopause.[62] Patients with Turner's syndrome do not complain of the same hot flashes experienced by patients with secondary hypergonadotropic hypogonadism. Premature menopause can occur in isolation or in association with other endocrine gland failure such as hypoparathyroidism, hypothyroidism, or hypoadrenalism.[62]

CASE STUDY 22.3

A 24-year-old man presented with a history of hay fever, which had been treated with antihistamines. He relates diminished smell. He continues to grow slowly, and pubertal development has been slow. The man denies erections or nocturnal emissions.

Management

Testosterone replacement therapy
Sexual maturity
Later desired fertility

GnRH pulsatile therapy produced a normal sperm count in 4 months and the man's wife became pregnant.

Questions

1. What is the level of the defect?
2. What is the significance of the body measurements?
3. What are the diagnostic considerations?
4. What test(s) might be obtained to make the diagnosis?
5. What constitutes normal fertility?
6. How will you counsel this man when he asks if he can have children?

Physical Exam (PE)	Eunuchoidal Man, Appearing Younger than Age
Height	72 in.
Arm span	75 in.
Weight	180 lb
Blood pressure	130/82 mm Hg
Hair	Spare facial, axillary, and pubic

Genitalia	Penis, 3.1 cm (small)	
Testes	Soft, 1 cm × 1.5 cm × 1.5 cm (normal, 4.5 cm × 3 cm × 3 cm)	
GnRH Stimulation		
Time (min)	LH	Normal
0, GnRH	<2 mU/mL	Pre-, <5
		Adult, 3–18
15	<2	Post-, 2.5 times baseline at some point
30	3	
45	<2	
60	3	
After GnRH Priming		
Time (min)	LH	Normal
0	<2 mU/mL	Pre-, <5
		Adult, 3–18
15	10	LH rise >2.5 times baseline
30	12	
45	16	
60	12	
Laboratory Values		
Testosterone	157 ng/dL (normal, prepubertal <100; adult, 300–1,000)	
LH	<2 mU/mL (normal, prepubertal <5; adult, 3–18)	
Prolactin	6 ng/mL (normal, 5–25)	
TSH	1.2 mU/mL (normal, 0.3–5.0)	

Polycystic Ovary Syndrome

This common disorder can present in many ways: infertility, hirsutism, chronic anovulation, glucose intolerance, hyperlipidemia or dyslipidemia, and hypertension.[50–52] The onset is often perimenarcheal, chronic, and notable for its slow progression. Investigations for this disorder involve estimation of free testosterone, SHBG, FSH, LH, fasting glucose, insulin, lipid levels, DHEAS, prolactin, and ± AMH levels. Ovarian ultrasound reveals multiple cysts in many patients (about 30% of patients do not have ovarian cysts). Most patients with this disorder are overweight; however, some patients with polycystic ovary syndrome (PCOS), especially of eastern Asian or South American descent, are of normal weight. Most symptoms and laboratory abnormalities are reversed with weight loss and increased physical activity. The drug Glucophage (metformin), commonly used for the treatment of diabetes, is useful in this condition, even in the absence of diabetes. Although not U.S. Food and Drug Administration approved for this use, it reportedly can normalize menstrual cycles and improve conception rates.[63]

Hirsutism

Hirsutism is an abnormal, abundant, androgen-sensitive terminal hair growth in areas in which terminal hair follicles are sparsely distributed or not normally found in

BOX 22.3 Classification of Hirsutism[51]

Functional (normal androgen levels with excess hair growth) or true androgen excess (elevated androgens)
Ovarian (LH mediated) or adrenal (adrenocorticotropin hormone mediated)
Peripheral conversion of androgens (obesity)
Tumoral hyperandrogenism (ovarian, adrenal)
Chorionic gonadotropin mediated

TABLE 22.5 Causes of Hirsutism

Common
Idiopathic
Polycystic ovary syndrome

Uncommon
Drugs: danazol, oral contraceptives with androgenic progestins
Congenital adrenal hyperplasia
Hyperprolactinemia
Cushing syndrome
Adrenal tumors
Ovarian tumors

women (Box 22.3). Typical causes of hirsutism are listed in Table 22.5.[51]

Hirsutism should only be considered in the context of a woman's ethnic origin. Women of Italian, eastern European, south Asian, and Irish descent possess more androgen-sensitive terminal hair than do most northern European women, making a careful elicitation of ethnic background important prior to initiation of an extensive laboratory evaluation in a woman born in the United States. It is estimated that about 5% to 10% of American women have hirsutism, which can be quantified using a measurement technique known as the modified Ferriman-Gallwey Scale that identifies nine areas (lip, chin, sideburn region, neck, chest, abdomen, upper and lower back, and thigh) for assessment and allots points on a scale of 1 to 4 based on hair thickness and pigmentation. A score of higher than 8 is consistent with a diagnosis of hirsutism.[64] Hormonal abnormalities associated with hirsutism are summarized in Table 22.6.

Estrogen Replacement Therapy

Estrogen replacement remains a contentious issue. The Women's Health Initiative study enrolled 16,608 postmenopausal women who were placed on conventional hormone replacement combinations. The study showed an overall increased incidence of invasive breast cancer (hazard ratio,

1.26), stroke, venous clot formation, coronary heart disease (CHD) events, and no benefit in cognitive decline, with combined estrogen plus progestin therapy (however, *unopposed estrogen* therapy alone was not associated with increase in either breast cancer or CHD, suggesting that these risks may be conferred by the progestin component). With HRT, reductions in bone loss, colon polyp formation, and menopausal symptoms (hot flashes and vaginal dryness) were noted. The recently published ELITE trial (Early versus Late Intervention Trial with Estradiol) results showed decreased progression of subclinical atherosclerosis (as seen by slower increase in carotid intima–media thickening) in menopausal women who were started on HRT within less than or equal to 6 years of menopause, lending further credence to the "timing hypothesis," that is, younger women may indeed benefit from HRT in terms of decreased CHD risk.[66–69] In large meta-analyses of randomized controlled trials, including the Women's Health Initiative, a significantly lower risk of CHD (hazard ratio, 0.68; 95% CI, 0.48 to 0.96) and of death from any cause (hazard ratio, 0.61; 95% CI, 0.39 to 0.95) was found with hormone therapy than with placebo among women who were younger than 60 years of age, less than 10 years past menopause, or both when they underwent randomization.[70]

TABLE 22.6 Androgen Levels in Hirsutism and Virilization

Analyte Condition	Total Testosterone	Free Testosterone	Dehydroepiandrosterone Sulfate
Idiopathic hirsutism[65]	↑	↑↑↑	↑
Polycystic ovary syndrome	↑	↑↑	↑
Congenital adrenal hyperplasia	↑↑	↑↑	↑↑↑
Virilizing Tumors			
Ovarian	↑↑↑	↑↑↑	↑
Adrenal	↑↑	↑↑	↑↑↑

Modified from Demers LM. *Hirsutism and Virilization, News and Views*. Washington, DC: American Association for Clinical Chemistry; 1989.

CASE STUDY 22.4

A school physical examination of a 17-year-old boy showed less pubic and axillary hair than those of peers, penis and scrotum that were smaller, breast tissue since age 13, no erections or nocturnal emissions, and no adolescent growth spurt. Sleeve and pant lengths increased every 4 to 6 months.

Questions

1. At what level is the defect in this case?

2. What diagnostic possibilities would explain the endocrine data?

3. What treatment(s) would be available to
   a. Treat his androgen deficiency?
   b. Allow him to father children if he wanted fertility?

4. His appearance shows the defect occurred:
   a. Prior to birth (during fetal life)
   b. After birth (postnatal)

PE	
Height	73 in.
Arm span	74 in.
Weight	148 lb
BP	110/70 mm Hg
Pulse	69 bpm
Hair	Scant axillary and pubic
Breasts	Moderate gynecomastia, 3 cm
Genitalia	Penis, 4.5 cm
Testes	1.5 × 1 × 1 cm, bilaterally (normal, >4.5 × 3 × 3 cm)
LABORATORY	
Testosterone, total	115 ng/dL (normal, 300–1,000)
LH	42 mU/mL (normal, adult, 3–18)
Karyotype	47,XXY

For additional student resources, please visit thePoint® at http://thepoint.lww.com

questions

1. If serum levels of estradiol do not increase after injection of hCG, the patient has
   a. Primary ovarian failure
   b. Pituitary failure
   c. Tertiary ovarian failure
   d. Secondary ovarian failure

2. If a patient had a luteal phase defect, which hormone would most likely be deficient?
   a. Progesterone
   b. Estrogen
   c. hCG
   d. FSH
   e. Prolactin

3. Which of the following is the precursor for estradiol formation in the placenta?
   a. Fetal adrenal DHEAS
   b. Maternal testosterone
   c. Maternal progesterone
   d. Placental hCG
   e. Fetal adrenal cholesterol

4. Which of the following target tissues is incapable of producing steroidal hormones?
   a. Adrenal medulla
   b. Placenta
   c. Ovary
   d. Testis
   e. Adrenal cortex

5. The parent substance in the biosynthesis of androgens and estrogens is
   a. Cholesterol
   b. Cortisol
   c. Catecholamines
   d. Progesterone

6. The biologically most active, naturally occurring androgen is
   a. DHEA
   b. Androstenedione
   c. Epiandrosterone
   d. Testosterone

review questions (continued)

7. For the past 3 weeks, serum estriol levels in a pregnant woman have been steadily increasing. This is consistent with
a. A normal pregnancy
b. Hemolytic disease of the newborn
c. Fetal death
d. Congenital cytomegalovirus infection

8. Which of the following is secreted by the placenta and used for the early detection of pregnancy?
a. hCG
b. FSH
c. LH
d. Progesterone

9. Chronic fetal metabolic distress is demonstrated by
a. Decreased urinary estriol excretion and decreased maternal serum estriol
b. Decreased estrogen in maternal plasma and increased estriol in amniotic fluid
c. Increased estradiol in maternal plasma, with a corresponding increase of estriol in amniotic fluid
d. Increased urinary estriol excretion and increased maternal serum estriol

10. Androgen secretion by the testes is stimulated by
a. LH
b. FSH
c. Testosterone
d. Gonadotropins

11. A deficiency in estrogen during the follicular phase will result in
a. A failure of embryo implantation
b. An increased length of the menstrual cycle
c. A lack of graafian follicle release from the ovary
d. An incomplete development of the endometrium

12. Which hormone is responsible for an increase in body temperature at the time of ovulation?
a. Progesterone
b. Estrogen
c. LH
d. FSH
e. Estradiol

13. A midcycle LH surge will stimulate which series of events?
a. An increase in FSH
b. A decrease in FSH
c. Anovulation
d. Amenorrhea
e. A decrease in progesterone production

references

1. Sinisi AA, Pasquali D, Notaro A, et al. Sexual differentiation. *J Endocrinol Invest.* 2003;26(3 suppl):23–28.
2. Dewing P, Bernard P, Vilain E. Disorders of gonadal development. *Semin Reprod Med.* 2002;20:189–198.
3. Gao F, Maiti S, Huff V. The Wilms tumor gene, Wt1, is required for Sox9 expression and maintenance of tubular architecture in the developing testis. *Proc Natl Acad Sci U S A.* 2006;103(32):11987–11992.
4. Nef S, Parada LF. Cryptorchidism in mice mutant for Insl3. *Nat Genet.* 1999;22:295–299.
5. Durlinger AL, Visser JA, Themmen AP. Regulation of ovarian function: the role of anti-Mullerian hormone. *Reproduction.* 2002;124:601–609.
6. Sharpe RM, McKinnell C, Kivlin C, et al. Proliferation and functional maturation of Sertoli cells, and their relevance to disorders of testis function in adulthood. *Reproduction.* 2003;125:769–784.
7. Svechnikov K, Landreh L, Weisser J, et al. Origin, development and regulation of human Leydig cells. *Horm Res Paediatr.* 2010;73:93–101.
8. Rey RA, Grinspon RP. Normal male sexual differentiation and aetiology of disorders of sex development. *Best Pract Res Clin Endocrinol Metab.* 2011;25(2):221–238.
9. Campbell RE, Suter KJ. Redefining the gonadotropin-releasing hormone neurone dendrite. *J Neuroendocrinol.* 2010;22(7):650–658.
10. Grover A, Smith CE, Gregory M, et al. Effects of FSH receptor deletion on epididymal tubules and sperm morphology, numbers, and motility. *Mol Reprod Dev.* 2005;72(2):135–144.
11. Labrie F. Extragonadal synthesis of sex steroids: intracrinology. *Ann Endocrinol (Paris).* 2003;64:95–107.
12. Hiort O, Holterhus PM. Androgen insensitivity and male infertility. *Int J Androl.* 2003;26:16–20.
13. Lee DK, Chang C. Molecular communication between androgen receptor and general transcription machinery. *J Steroid Biochem Mol Biol.* 2003;84:41–49.
14. Sultan C, Gobinet J, Terouanne B, et al. The androgen receptor: molecular pathology. *J Soc Biol.* 2002;196:223–240.
15. Sultan C, Lumbroso S, Paris F, et al. Disorders of androgen action. *Semin Reprod Med.* 2002;20:217–228.
16. Segal TY, Mehta A, Anazodo A, et al. Role of gonadotropin-releasing hormone and human chorionic gonadotropin stimulation tests in differentiating patients with hypogonadotropic hypogonadism from those with constitutional delay of growth and puberty. *J Clin Endocrinol Metab.* 2009;94(3):780–785.

17. Tong S, Wallace EM, Burger HG. Inhibins and activins: clinical advances in reproductive medicine. *Clin Endocrinol (Oxf)*. 2003;58:115–127.

18. Cheng CK, Leung PCK. Molecular biology of gonadotropin-releasing hormone (GnRH)-I, GnRH-II, and their receptors in humans. *Endocr Rev*. 2005;26(2):283–306.

19. Seminara SB, Hayes FJ, Crowley WF Jr. Gonadotropin-releasing hormone deficiency in the human (idiopathic hypogonadotropic hypogonadism and Kallmann's syndrome): pathophysiological and genetic considerations. *Endocr Rev*. 1998;19:521–539.

20. De Rosa M, Zarrilli S, Di Sarno A, et al. Hyperprolactinemia in men: clinical and biochemical features and response to treatment. *Endocrine*. 2003;20:75–82.

21. Heaton JP, Morales A. Endocrine causes of impotence (non-diabetes). *Urol Clin North Am*. 2003;30:73–81.

22. Matsuzaki T, Azuma K, Irahara M, et al. Mechanism of anovulation in hyperprolactinemic amenorrhea determined by pulsatile gonadotropin-releasing hormone injection combined with human chorionic gonadotropin. *Fertil Steril*. 1994;62:1143–1149.

23. Kaiser U. Hyperprolactinemia and infertility: new insights. *J Clin Invest*. 2012;122:3467–3468.

24. Dandona P, Dhindsa S. Update: hypogonadotropic hypogonadism in type 2 diabetes and obesity. *J Clin Endocrinol Metab*. 2011;96(9):2643–2651.

25. Dhindsa S, Prabhakar S, Sethi M, et al. Frequent occurrence of hypogonadotropic hypogonadism in type 2 diabetes. *J Clin Endocrinol Metab*. 2004;89(11):5462–5468.

26. Holt SK, Lopushnyan N, Hotaling J, et al. Prevalence of low testosterone and predisposing risk factors in men with type 1 diabetes mellitus: findings from the DCCT/EDIC. *J Clin Endocrinol Metab*. 2014;99:E1655–E1660.

27. Harman SM, Metter EJ, Tobin JD, et al. Longitudinal effects of aging on serum total and free testosterone levels in healthy men. Baltimore Longitudinal Study of Aging. *J Clin Endocrinol Metab*. 2001;86:724–731.

28. Feldman HA, Longcope C, Derby CA, et al. Age trends in the level of serum testosterone and other hormones in middle-aged men: longitudinal results from the Massachusetts Male Aging Study. *J Clin Endocrinol Metab*. 2002;87(2):589–598.

29. Snyder PJ, Bhasin S, Cunningham GR, et al. Effects of testosterone treatment in older men. *N Engl J Med*. 2016;374(7):611–624. doi: 10.1056/NEJMoa1506119.

30. Agirregoitia E, Valdivia A, Carracedo A, et al. Expression and localization of delta-, kappa-, and mu-opioid receptors in human spermatozoa and implications for sperm motility. *J Clin Endocrinol Metab*. 2006;91:4969–4975.

31. Luboshitzky R, Aviv A, Hefetz A, et al. Decreased pituitary-gonadal secretion in men with obstructive sleep apnea. *J Clin Endocrinol Metab*. 2002;87:3394–3398.

32. Bhasin S, Snyder PJ, Montori VM, et al. Testosterone therapy in adult men with androgen deficiency syndromes: an Endocrine Society clinical practice guideline. *J Clin Endocrinol Metab*. 2006;91(6):1995–2010.

33. Dandona P, Rosenberg MT. A practical guide to male hypogonadism in the primary care setting. *Int J Clin Pract*. 2010;64(6):682–696.

34. Testosterone for 'late-onset hypogonadism' in men? *Drug Ther Bull*. 2010;48:69–72.

35. Srinivas-Shankar U, Wu FC. Drug insight: testosterone preparations. *Nat Rev Urol*. 2006;3:653–665.

36. https://www.aveedrems.com/AveedUI/rems/preHome.action.

37. Friedl KE, Hannan CJ Jr, Jones RE, et al. High-density lipoprotein cholesterol is not decreased if an aromatizable androgen is administered. *Metabolism*. 1990;39:69–74.

38. McGee EA, Hsueh AJW. Initial and cyclic recruitment of ovarian follicles. *Endocr Rev*. 2000;21(2):200–214.

39. Sherman BM, West JH, Korenman SG. The menopausal transition: analysis of LH, FSH, estradiol, and progesterone concentrations during menstrual cycles of older women. *J Clin Endocrinol Metab*. 1976;42:629–636.

40. Jost A, Vigier B, Prepin J, et al. Studies on sex differentiation in mammals. *Recent Prog Horm Res*. 1973;29:1–41.

41. Messinis IE. Ovarian feedback, mechanism of action and possible clinical implications. *Hum Reprod Update*. 2006;12(5):557–571.

42. Filicori M, Santoro N, Merriam GR, et al. Characterization of the physiological pattern of episodic gonadotropin secretion throughout the human menstrual cycle. *J Clin Endocrinol Metab*. 1986;62:1136–1144.

43. Badouraki M, Christoforidis A, Economou I, et al. Sonographic assessment of uterine and ovarian development in normal girls aged 1 to 12 years. *J Clin Ultrasound*. 2008;36(9):539–544.

44. Canipari R, Cellini V, Cecconi S. The ovary feels fine when paracrine and autocrine networks cooperate with gonadotropins in the regulation of folliculogenesis. *Curr Pharm Des*. 2012;18(3):245–255.

45. Peters H, Byskov AG, Grinsted J. Follicular growth in fetal and prepubertal ovaries of humans and other primates. *Clin Endocrinol Metab*. 1978;7:469–485.

46. Gougeon A. Dynamics of follicular growth in the human: a model from preliminary results. *Hum Reprod*. 1986;1:81–87.

47. Fakheri RJ, Javitt NB. Autoregulation of cholesterol synthesis: physiologic and pathophysiologic consequences. *Steroids*. 2011;76(3):211–215.

48. Poutanen M. Understanding the diversity of sex steroid action. *J Endocrinol*. 2012;212:1–2.

49. te Velde ER, Pearson PL. The variability of female reproductive ageing. *Hum Reprod Update*. 2002;8(2):141–154.

50. Carmina E, Campagna AM, Lobo RA. A 20-year follow-up of young women with polycystic ovary syndrome. *Obstet Gynecol*. 2012;119(2):263–269.

51. Escobar-Morreale HF, Carmina E, Dewailly D, et al. Epidemiology, diagnosis and management of hirsutism: a consensus statement by the Androgen Excess and Polycystic Ovary Syndrome Society. *Hum Reprod Update*. 2012;18(2):146–170.

52. Panidis D, Tziomalos K, Misichronis G, et al. Insulin resistance and endocrine characteristics of the different phenotypes of polycystic ovary syndrome: a prospective study. *Hum Reprod*. 2012;27(2):541–549.

53. Sarfati J, Bachelot A, Coussieu C, et al.; Study Group Hyperandrogenism in Postmenopausal Women. Impact of clinical, hormonal, radiological, and immunohistochemical studies on the diagnosis of postmenopausal hyperandrogenism. *Eur J Endocrinol*. 2011;165:779–788.

54. Robertson DM. *Inhibins and activins in blood: predictors of female reproductive health? Mol Cell Endocrinol*. June 2011.

55. Sherwood OD. Relaxin's physiological roles and other diverse actions. *Endocr Rev*. 2004;25(2):205–234.

56. Jabbour HN, Kelly RW, Fraser HM, et al. Endocrine regulation of menstruation. *Endocr Rev*. 2006;27(1):17–46.

57. Broekmans FJ, Soules MR, Fauser BC. Ovarian aging: mechanisms and clinical consequences. *Endocr Rev.* 2009;30(5):465–493.

58. Santoro N. Update in hyper- and hypogonadotropic amenorrhea. *J Clin Endocrinol Metab.* 2011;96(11):3281–3288.

59. Marshall WA, Tanner JM. Variations in pattern of pubertal changes in girls. *Arch Dis Child.* 1969;44:291–303.

60. Lessey BA. Assessment of endometrial receptivity. *Fertil Steril.* 2011;96:522–529.

61. Elsheikh M, Dunger DB, Conway GS, et al. Turner's syndrome in adulthood. *Endocr Rev.* February 2002;23(1):120–140.

62. Hoek A, Schoemaker J, Drexhage HA. Premature ovarian failure and ovarian autoimmunity. *Endocr Rev.* 1997;18(1):107–134.

63. Palomba S, Falbo A, Zullo F, et al. Evidence-based and potential benefits of metformin in the polycystic ovary syndrome: a comprehensive review. *Endocr Rev.* 2009;30(1):1–50.

64. Cook H, Brennan K, Azziz R. Reanalyzing the modified Ferriman-Gallwey score: is there a simpler method for assessing the extent of hirsutism? *Fertil Steril.* 2011;96(5):1266–1270.

65. Azziz R, Carmina E, Sawaya ME. Idiopathic hirsutism. *Endocr Rev.* 2000;21(4):347–362.

66. Chlebowski RT, Wactawski-Wende J, Ritenbaugh C, et al.; Women's Health Initiative Investigators. Estrogen plus progestin and colorectal cancer in postmenopausal women. *N Engl J Med.* 2004;350(10):991–1004.

67. Manson JE, Hsia J, Johnson KC, et al.; Women's Health Initiative Investigators. Estrogen plus progestin and the risk of coronary heart disease. *N Engl J Med.* 2003;349(6):523–534.

68. Hays J, Ockene JK, Brunner RL, et al.; Women's Health Initiative Investigators. Effects of estrogen plus progestin on health-related quality of life. *N Engl J Med.* 2003;348(19):1839–1854.

69. Hodis HN, Mack W, Henderson VW, et al. Vascular effects of early versus late postmenopausal treatment with estradiol. *N Engl J Med.* 2016;374(13):1221–1231. doi: 10.1056/NEJMoa1505241.

70. Boardman HM, Hartley L, Eisinga A, et al. Hormone therapy for preventing cardiovascular disease in post-menopausal women. *Cochrane Database Syst Rev.* 2015;(3):CD002229.

23

The Thyroid Gland

MARISSA GROTZKE

chapter objectives

Upon completion of this chapter, the clinical laboratorian should be able to do the following:

- Discuss the biosynthesis, secretion, transport, and action of the thyroid hormones.
- Know the location of the thyroid gland.
- Describe the hypothalamic–pituitary–thyroid axis and how it regulates thyroid hormone production.
- Explain the principles of each thyroid function test discussed.
- Correlate laboratory information with regard to suspected thyroid disorders, given a patient's clinical data.
- Describe the appropriate laboratory thyroid function testing protocol to use to effectively evaluate or monitor patients with suspected thyroid disease.

For additional student resources, please visit thePoint®
at http://thepoint.lww.com

THE THYROID

The thyroid gland is responsible for the production of two hormones: thyroid hormone and calcitonin. Calcitonin is secreted by parafollicular C cells and is involved in calcium homeostasis. Thyroid hormone is critical in regulating body metabolism, neurologic development, and numerous other body functions. Clinically, conditions affecting thyroid hormone levels are much more common than those affecting calcitonin and are the major focus of this chapter.

Thyroid Anatomy and Development

The thyroid gland is positioned in the lower anterior neck and is shaped like a butterfly. It is made up of two lobes resting on each side of the trachea, bridged by the isthmus, with a band of thyroid tissue running anterior to the trachea. Posterior to the thyroid gland lie the **parathyroid glands**—which regulate serum calcium levels—and the recurrent laryngeal nerves innervating the vocal cords. The locations of these structures become important during thyroid surgery, when injury could lead to hypocalcemia or permanent hoarse voice.

The fetal thyroid develops from an outpouching of the foregut at the base of the tongue that migrates to its final location over the thyroid cartilage in the first 4 to 8 weeks of gestation. By week 11 of gestation, the thyroid gland begins to produce measurable amounts of thyroid hormone.[1] Iodine is an essential component of thyroid hormone. In parts of the world where severe iodine deficiency exists, neither the mother nor the fetus can produce sufficient amounts of thyroid hormone and both develop **hypothyroidism**. As thyroid hormone is critical to fetal neurologic development, hypothyroidism can lead to mental retardation and cretinism. In areas where iodine deficiency is not an issue, other problems with thyroid development may occur, including congenital hypothyroidism, which occurs in 1 of 4,000 live births.[2] If the mother has normal thyroid function, small amounts of maternal thyroid hormone crossing the placenta protect the fetus during development. Immediately postpartum, however, these newborns require initiation of thyroid hormone or their further neurologic development will be significantly impaired. In much of the developed world, screening tests are performed on newborns to detect congenital hypothyroidism.

Thyroid Hormone Synthesis

Thyroid hormone is made primarily of the trace element iodine, making iodine metabolism a key determinant in thyroid function.[1] Iodine is found in seafood, dairy products, iodine-enriched breads, and vitamins. Significantly, iodine is used in high concentrations in the contrast medium used in many radiologic procedures, including computed tomography (CT) scans and heart catheterization. It is also present in amiodarone, a medication used to treat certain heart conditions. The recommended minimum daily intake of iodine is 150 µg, although most individuals in developed countries ingest far more than this

amount. In the United States, the average adult daily intake of iodine has decreased since the 1970s but remains sufficient at an estimated 240 and 740 daily µg, well above the US Institute of Medicine's recommended adult dietary allowance of 150 µg/day.[3,4] If iodine intake drops below 50 µg daily, the thyroid gland is unable to manufacture adequate amounts of thyroid hormone, and thyroid hormone deficiency—hypothyroidism—results.[5]

Thyroid cells are organized into spheres surrounding a central core of fluid called *colloid*. These structures are called follicles. The major component of colloid, **thyroglobulin**, is a glycoprotein manufactured exclusively by thyroid **follicular cells** and rich in the amino acid tyrosine. Some of these tyrosyl residues will be iodinated, producing the building blocks of thyroid hormone. On the outer side of the follicle, iodine is actively transported into the thyroid cell by the Na^+/I^- symporter located on the basement membrane. Inside the thyroid cell, iodide diffuses across the cell to the apical side of the follicle, which abuts the core of colloid. Here, catalyzed by a membrane-bound enzyme called **thyroid peroxidase (TPO)**, concentrated iodide is oxidized and bound with tyrosyl residues on thyroglobulin. This results in production of monoiodothyronine (MIT) and diiodothyronine (DIT). This same enzyme also aids in the coupling of two tyrosyl residues to form **triiodothyronine (T_3)** (one MIT residue + one DIT residue) or **thyroxine (T_4)** (two DIT residues). These are the two active forms of thyroid hormone. This thyroglobulin matrix, with branches now holding T_4 and T_3, is stored in the core of the thyroid follicle. *Thyroid-stimulating hormone (TSH)* signals the follicular cell to ingest a microscopic droplet of colloid by endocytosis. Inside the follicular cell, these droplets are digested by intracellular lysosomes into T_4, T_3, and other products. T_4 and T_3 are then secreted by the thyroid cell into the circulation (Fig. 23.1).

Activity of thyroid hormone depends on the location and number of iodine atoms. Approximately 80% of T_4 is metabolized into either T_3 (35%) or reverse T_3 (rT_3) (45%). Outer-ring deiodination of T_4 (5'-deiodination) leads to production of 3,5,3'-triiodothyronine (T_3). T_3 is three to eight times more metabolically active than is T_4 and often considered to be the active form of thyroid hormone, with T_4 considered the "pre"-hormone (with thyroglobulin being the "prohormone"). In addition to its "pre"-hormone activity, however, inner-ring deiodination of T_4 results in the production of metabolically inactive rT_3 (Fig. 23.2).

There are three forms of iodothyronine 5'-deiodinase. Type 1 iodothyronine 5'-deiodinase, the most abundant form, found mostly in the liver and kidney, is the largest contributor to the circulating T_3 pool. Certain drugs (e.g., propylthiouracil, glucocorticoids, and propranolol) slow the activity of this deiodinase and are used in the treatment of severe thyroid hormone excess, or hyperthyroidism. Type 2 iodothyronine 5'-deiodinase, found in the brain and pituitary gland, functions to maintain constant levels of T_3 in the central nervous system. Its activity is decreased when levels of circulating T_4 are high and increased when

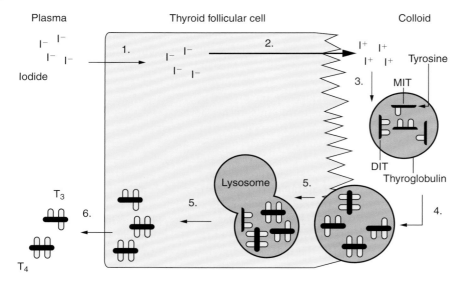

Plasma   Thyroid follicular cell   Colloid

FIGURE 23.1 Biosynthesis of thyroid hormone. Thyroid hormone synthesis includes the following steps: (1) iodide (I^-) trapping by thyroid follicular cells; (2) diffusion of iodide to the apex of the cell and transport into the colloid; (3) oxidation of inorganic iodide to iodine and incorporation of iodine into tyrosine residues within thyroglobulin molecules in the colloid; (4) combination of two diiodotyrosine (DIT) molecules to form tetraiodothyronine (thyroxine, T_4) or of monoiodotyrosine (MIT) with DIT to form triiodothyronine (T_3); (5) uptake of thyroglobulin from the colloid into the follicular cell by endocytosis, fusion of the thyroglobulin with a lysosome, and proteolysis and release of T_4 and T_3; and (6) release of T_4 and T_3 into the circulation.

levels are low. Activity of the deiodination enzymes gives another level of control of thyroid hormone activity beyond the **thyrotropin-releasing hormone (TRH)** and *thyrotropin (TSH)* control of the hypothalamic–pituitary–thyroid axis[1] (Fig. 23.2).

Protein Binding of Thyroid Hormone

When released into the circulation, only 0.04% of T_4 and 0.4% of T_3 are unbound by proteins and available for hormonal activity. The three major binding proteins, in order of significance, are **thyroxine-binding globulin (TBG)**, **thyroxine-binding prealbumin (TBPA)**, and albumin. Alterations to the concentrations of binding proteins significantly affect circulating quantities of T_4 and T_3. For example, high estrogen levels during pregnancy lead to increased TBG production by the liver, which results in higher levels of bound thyroid hormones, leading to high levels of total T_3 and total T_4. Typically, however, levels of the unbound active, or free, thyroid hormones remain in

the normal range and the individual remains euthyroid. In some instances, however, measurement of **free T_4** and **free T_3** may be necessary to eliminate any confusion caused by abnormal binding protein levels.

Control of Thyroid Function

Understanding of the **hypothalamic–pituitary–thyroid axis** is essential for correctly interpreting thyroid function testing. This axis is central to the regulation of thyroid hormone production. TRH is synthesized by neurons in the supraoptic and supraventricular nuclei of the hypothalamus and stored in the median eminence of the hypothalamus. When secreted, this hormone stimulates cells in the anterior pituitary gland to manufacture and release TSH. TSH, in turn, circulates to the thyroid gland and leads to increased production and release of thyroid hormone. When the hypothalamus and pituitary sense that there is an inadequate amount of thyroid hormone in circulation, TRH and TSH secretion increases and

Thyroid hormone
Thyroxine (T_4)

Monodeiodinase

Inactive thyroid hormone
3,3,5′-Triiodothyronine (rT_3)

Active thyroid hormone
3,5,3′-Triiodothyronine (T_3)

FIGURE 23.2 Metabolism of thyroxine.

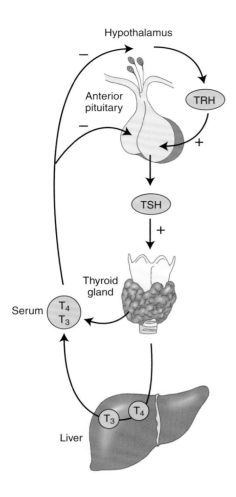

FIGURE 23.3 Hypothalamic–pituitary–thyroid axis. Thyrotropin-releasing hormone (TRH) stimulates the production and release of thyrotropin (TSH). TSH stimulates the thyroid gland to synthesize and secrete thyroid hormone. T_4 that is released by the thyroid gland is mostly converted to T_3 by the liver and kidney. T_3 and T_4 feedback inhibit TSH release directly through action at the pituitary and indirectly by decreasing TRH release from the hypothalamus. (Adapted from Surks MI, Sievert R. Drugs and thyroid function. *N Engl J Med.* 1995;333:1688.)

stimulates increased thyroid hormone production. If thyroid hormone levels are high, TRH and TSH release will be inhibited, leading to lower levels of thyroid hormone production. This feedback loop requires a normally functioning hypothalamus, pituitary, and thyroid gland, as well as an absence of any interfering agents or agents that mimic TSH action (Fig. 23.3).

Actions of Thyroid Hormone

Once released from the thyroid gland, thyroid hormone circulates in the bloodstream where free T_4 and T_3 are available to travel across the cell membrane. In the cytoplasm, T_4 is deiodinated into T_3, the active form of thyroid hormone. T_3 combines with its nuclear receptor on thyroid hormone-responsive genes, leading to production of messenger RNA that, in turn, leads to production of proteins that influence metabolism and development.

Effects of thyroid hormone include tissue growth, brain maturation, increased heat production, increased oxygen consumption, and increased expression of β-adrenergic receptors. Clinically, individuals who have excess thyroid hormone (**thyrotoxicosis**) will have symptoms of increased metabolic activity such as tachycardia and tremor, while individuals with hypothyroidism note symptoms of lowered metabolic activity like edema and constipation.

TESTS FOR THYROID FUNCTION

Blood Tests

Thyroid-Stimulating Hormone

The most useful test for assessing thyroid function is the TSH, currently in its third generation. All the assays are capable of diagnosing primary hypothyroidism (thyroid gland disease leading to low thyroid hormone production) with elevated levels of TSH. Second-generation TSH immunometric assays, with detection limits of 0.1 mU/L, effectively screen for hyperthyroidism, but the third-generation TSH chemiluminometric assays, with increased sensitivity to detection limits of 0.01 mU/L, give fewer false-negative results and more accurately distinguish between euthyroidism and hyperthyroidism. Although a fourth-generation assay exists, it is used for research purposes and the third-generation TSH assays are the preferred method for monitoring and adjusting thyroid hormone replacement therapy and screening for abnormal thyroid hormone production in the clinical setting.[6]

The sensitivity of the third-generation TSH assays led to the ability to detect what is termed subclinical disease—or a mild degree of thyroid dysfunction—due to the large reciprocal change in TSH levels seen for even small changes in free T_4.[7] In **subclinical hypothyroidism**, the TSH is minimally increased while the free T_4 stays within the normal range. Likewise, in **subclinical hyperthyroidism**, the TSH is low while the free T_4 is normal (Table 23.1). The clinical significance of subclinical disease and thresholds for treatment remain somewhat unclear and remain an ongoing topic of investigation.

Serum T_4 and T_3

Serum total T_4 and T_3 levels are usually measured by radioimmunoassay (RIA), chemiluminometric assay, or similar immunometric technique. As previously mentioned, because more than 99.9% of thyroid hormone is protein bound, alteration in thyroid hormone–binding proteins frequently leads to total T_4 and T_3 levels outside of the normal range without representing true clinical thyroid dysfunction. Because of this, assays to measure free T_4 and T_3, the biologically active hormone forms, were developed. At least partially because of lower processing costs and ease of interpretation, free T_4 kits now replace total T_4 assessment at the clinical level.[8] Currently available assay kits for measuring free T_4 levels are not error proof, though, and can still be affected by some binding protein abnormalities.[9] When this is suspected, measurement of

TABLE 23.1	Interpretation of Thyroid Tests		
	Low Free T$_4$	**Normal Free T$_4$**	**High Free T$_4$**
Low TSH	Secondary hypothyroidism Severe nonthyroidal illness	Subclinical hyperthyroidism Nonthyroidal illness	Hyperthyroidism
Normal TSH	Secondary hypothyroidism Severe nonthyroidal illness	Normal	Artifact Pituitary hyperthyroidism Laboratory draw within 6–9 h of thyroxine dose
High TSH	Primary hypothyroidism	Subclinical hypothyroidism	Test artifact Pituitary hyperthyroidism Thyroid hormone resistance

free T$_4$ levels is performed by dialysis. Kits that estimate free T$_3$ levels have theoretical advantages; however, actual clinical utility is yet to be clearly defined.

Thyroglobulin

Thyroglobulin is a protein synthesized and secreted exclusively by thyroid follicular cells. This prohormone in the circulation is proof of the presence of thyroid tissue. This fact makes thyroglobulin an ideal tumor marker thyroid cancer posttreatment surveillance as patients with well-differentiated thyroid cancer successfully treated with surgery and radioactive iodine ablation should have undetectable thyroglobulin levels.

Thyroglobulin is currently measured by double-antibody RIA, enzyme-linked immunoassay (ELISA), immunoradiometric assay (IRMA), and immunochemiluminescent assay (ICMA) methods. The accuracy of the thyroglobulin assay is primarily dependent on the specificity of the antibody used and the absence of antithyroglobulin autoantibodies. Even with modern assays, antithyroglobulin autoantibodies interfere with measurements and lead to unreliable thyroglobulin results. For this reason, it is critically important to screen for autoantibodies whenever thyroglobulin is measured. If antibodies are present, the value of the thyroglobulin assay is marginal. Approximately 25% of patients with well-differentiated thyroid cancer have antithyroglobulin autoantibodies, compared to 10% of the general population. If a patient with well-differentiated thyroid cancer and antithyroglobulin autoantibodies has been successfully treated with surgery and radioactive iodine ablation, autoantibodies should disappear over time.[6]

Thyroid Autoimmunity

Many diseases of the thyroid gland are related to autoimmune processes. In autoimmune thyroid disease, antibodies are directed at thyroid tissue with variable responses. The most common cause of hyperthyroidism is an autoimmune disorder called **Graves' disease**. The antibodies in this condition are directed at the TSH receptor (TSHR), stimulating the receptor and leading to growth of the thyroid gland and production of excessive amounts of thyroid hormone. This condition can be diagnosed with tests that detect TSHR-stimulating antibodies. Two types of assays exist to detect an autoimmune etiology to hyperthyroidism: competition-based assays that detect TSH receptor antibodies (TRAb) based upon their ability to compete for TSHR with a known ligand and thyroid-stimulating immunoglobulin (TSI) assays detecting cAMP production in patients' sera. Tests for **TSH receptor antibodies** (TRAb, TSHRAb) can detect antibodies directed against the TSHR whether they act to stimulate or block the TSHR. Both stimulating and blocking antibody assays will be positive in 70% to 100% of patients with Graves' disease.[10] **Chronic lymphocytic thyroiditis**—commonly known as **Hashimoto's thyroiditis**—is at the other end of the autoimmune continuum. In this condition, antibodies lead to decreased thyroid hormone production by destruction of the thyroid gland, which is the most common cause of hypothyroidism in the developed world. The best test for this condition is the TPO antibody, which is present in 10% to 15% of the general population and 80% to 99% of patients with autoimmune hypothyroidism (Table 23.2).

TABLE 23.2	Prevalence of Thyroid Autoantibodies		
Antibody	**General Population**	**Graves' Disease**	**Autoimmune Hypothyroidism**
Antithyroglobulin	3%	12%–30%	35%–60%
Thyroid peroxidase (previously antimicrosomal)	10%–15%	45%–80%	80%–99%
Anti-TSH receptor	1%–2%	70%–100%	6%–60%

OTHER TOOLS FOR THYROID EVALUATION

Nuclear Medicine Evaluation

Radioactive iodine is useful in assessing the metabolic activity of thyroid tissue and assisting in the evaluation and treatment of thyroid cancer. When radioactive iodine is given orally, a percentage of the dose is taken up by the thyroid gland. This percentage is called the radioactive iodine uptake (RAIU). High uptake suggests that the gland is metabolically active and producing significant amounts of thyroid hormone. Low uptake suggests that the gland is metabolically inactive. Because TSH stimulates iodine uptake by the thyroid gland, it is important to interpret the scan in conjunction with an assessment of TSH levels. An undetectably low TSH should turn off the thyroid gland's uptake of iodine. If the uptake is normal or high despite an undetectably low TSH, the thyroid must be either acting autonomously without regard to the hypothalamus–pituitary–thyroid feedback system or through a TSH surrogate. Such is the case with Graves' disease, where an immunoglobulin activates the TSHR on the thyroid gland, leading to high rates of thyroid hormone production and a high RAIU. The high level of thyroid hormone in the circulation feeds back on the pituitary and hypothalamus, turning off TSH, but this has no effect on the levels of TSI (the TSH surrogate). Conversely, if the RAIU is low in the presences of an undetectably low TSH, the differential diagnosis includes excess exogenous thyroid hormone ingestion, high iodine intake, or a condition in which stored thyroid hormone is leaking from the thyroid gland (typically in a setting known as **subacute thyroiditis**).

Radioactive iodine can also be useful in the evaluation of thyroid nodules in the presence of a low or undetectable TSH. Thyroid nodules that take up significant amounts of radioactive iodine on thyroid scans—termed "hot" nodules—are statistically unlikely to be thyroid cancer. The converse, however, does not hold true as nodules that show little or no radioiodine uptake—indeterminate ("warm") or "cold" nodules, respectively—may be cancerous, but the majority of such nodules are benign.

Thyroid Ultrasound

The significance of thyroid ultrasound in the assessment of thyroid anatomy and characterization of palpable thyroid abnormalities has progressively increased in the last several years. Thyroid ultrasounds are capable of detecting even thyroid nodules of such a small size as to be of unclear or even no clinical significance; depending upon age, in up to 50% of clinically normal thyroid glands, small (<1 cm) thyroid nodules can be seen.[11]

Fine-Needle Aspiration

Thyroid fine-needle aspiration (FNA) biopsy is often the first step and most accurate tool in the evaluation of thyroid nodules in the absence of hyperthyroidism. The routine use of FNA allows prompt identification and treatment of thyroid malignancies and avoids unnecessary surgery in most individuals with benign thyroid lesions. In this procedure, a small-gauge needle is inserted into the nodule and cells are aspirated for cytologic evaluation. The procedure can be performed using palpation if the nodule is palpable, but is becoming more commonly used with the assistance of ultrasound imaging. FNA biopsy results are reported according to the Bethesda System for Reporting Thyroid Cytopathology as falling into one of six categories: nondiagnostic/unsatisfactory, benign, atypia/follicular lesion of undetermined significance, follicular neoplasm/suspicious for follicular neoplasm, suspicious for malignancy, and malignant. These categories dictate subsequent treatment, ranging from routine ultrasound monitoring to surgical excision.[12,13]

CASE STUDY 23.1

A 24-year-old woman presents 2 months postpartum with symptoms of hyperthyroidism. She does not have evidence of Graves' ophthalmopathy. Her TSH level is undetectable, and free T_4 is two times the upper limit of normal.

Questions
1. What are possible causes for her thyrotoxicosis?
2. What tests would be useful to sort out the cause of her thyrotoxicosis?

DISORDERS OF THE THYROID

Hypothyroidism

Hypothyroidism—defined as a low free T_4 level with a normal or high TSH—is one of the most common disorders of the thyroid gland, occurring in 5% to 15% of women over the age of 65. Symptoms of hypothyroidism vary, depending on the degree of hypothyroidism and the rapidity of its onset (Box 23.1). When thyroid hormone is significantly decreased, symptoms of cold intolerance, fatigue, dry skin, constipation, hoarseness, dyspnea on exertion, cognitive dysfunction, hair loss, and weight gain have been reported. On physical examination, those with severe hypothyroidism may have low body temperature, slowed movements, bradycardia, delay in the relaxation phase of deep tendon reflexes, yellow discoloration of the skin (from hypercarotenemia), hair loss, diastolic hypertension, pleural and pericardial effusions, menstrual irregularities, and periorbital edema.

Because of the diffuse distribution of thyroid hormone receptors and the many metabolic effects of thyroid hormone, hypothyroidism can lead to a variety of other abnormalities. Hyponatremia can occur from the combination of increased urinary sodium excretion and an inability to maximally dilute urine due to inappropriate release of

BOX 23.1 Signs and Symptoms of Hypothyroidism

Signs

Delayed relaxation phase of deep tendon reflex testing
Bradycardia
Diastolic hypertension
Coarsened skin, yellowing of skin (carotenemia)
Periorbital edema
Thinning of eyebrows/loss of lateral aspect of brows
Slowed movements/speech
Pleural/pericardial effusion
Ascites

Symptoms

Cold intolerance
Depression
Mental retardation (infants), slowed cognition
Menorrhagia
Growth failure (children)
Pubertal delay
Dry skin
Edema
Constipation
Hoarseness
Dyspnea on exertion

antidiuretic hormone; significant degrees of hypothyroidism can lead to myopathy and elevated levels of creatine kinase (CK); and anemia can also be seen, either as a result of a decreased demand for oxygen carrying capacity or through an associated autoimmune pernicious anemia.[14–16] Fifty percent or more of those with uncorrected hypothyroidism will have hyperlipidemia that improves with thyroid hormone replacement.[17,18] In the presence of these clinical abnormalities (hyponatremia, unexplained elevation of creatine phosphokinase [CPK], anemia, or hyperlipidemia), evaluation for hypothyroidism as a potential secondary cause should be considered.

Hypothyroidism can be divided into primary, secondary, or tertiary disease, dependent on the location of the defect (Box 23.2). The most common cause of hypothyroidism in developed countries is chronic lymphocytic thyroiditis, or Hashimoto's thyroiditis. This disorder is an autoimmune disease targeting the thyroid gland, often associated with an enlarged gland, or goiter. TPO antibody testing is positive in 80% to 99% of patients with chronic lymphocytic thyroiditis. Other common causes of hypothyroidism include iodine deficiency, thyroid surgery, and radioactive iodine treatment (Table 23.3). Occasionally, individuals will experience transient hypothyroidism associated with inflammation of the thyroid gland. Examples of transient hypothyroidism include recovery from nonthyroidal illness

and the hypothyroid phase of any of the forms of subacute thyroiditis (painful thyroiditis, postpartum thyroiditis, and painless thyroiditis).

American Thyroid Association and American Association of Clinical Endocrinologists Guidelines for Hypothyroidism Screening

Measurement of TSH:

- At age 35
- Every 5 years after the age of 35
- Individuals with risk factors or symptoms: goiter, presence of other autoimmune disease, first-degree relative with autoimmune thyroid disease, lithium use, and amiodarone use

Hypothyroidism is treated with thyroid hormone replacement therapy. Levothyroxine (T_4) is the treatment of choice. In primary hypothyroidism, the goal of therapy is to achieve a normal TSH level. If hypothyroidism is of secondary or tertiary origin, TSH levels will not be useful in managing the condition, and a midnormal free T_4 level becomes the treatment target. Levothyroxine has a half-life of approximately 7 days. When doses of thyroid hormone are changed, it is important to wait at least five half-lives before rechecking thyroid function tests in order to achieve a new steady state.[19,20]

Thyrotoxicosis

Thyrotoxicosis is a constellation of findings that result when peripheral tissues are presented with, and respond to, an excess of thyroid hormone. Thyrotoxicosis can be the result of excessive thyroid hormone ingestion, leakage of stored thyroid hormone from storage in the thyroid follicles, or excessive thyroid gland production of thyroid hormone. The manifestations of thyrotoxicosis vary, depending on the degree of thyroid hormone elevation and the status of the affected individual. Symptoms often include anxiety, emotional lability, weakness, tremor, palpitations, heat intolerance, increased perspiration, and weight loss despite a normal or increased appetite (Box 23.3).

BOX 23.2 Types of Hypothyroidism

Primary

Thyroid gland dysfunction

Secondary

Pituitary dysfunction

Tertiary

Hypothalamic dysfunction

TABLE 23.3	**Causes of Hypothyroidism**	
	Condition	**Comments**
Primary	Chronic lymphocytic thyroiditis (Hashimoto's thyroiditis)	TPOAb or TgAb positive in 80%–99% of cases
	Treatment for toxic goiter—subtotal thyroidectomy or radioactive iodine	History and physical exam (neck scar) are key to diagnosis
	Excessive iodine intake	History and urinary iodine measurement useful
	Subacute thyroiditis	Usually transient
Secondary	Hypopituitarism	Caused by adenoma, radiation therapy, or destruction of pituitary
Tertiary	Hypothalamic dysfunction	Rare

TgAb, thyroglobulin antibodies; TPOAb, thyroid peroxidase antibodies.

Graves' Disease

Graves' disease is the most common cause of thyrotoxicosis. It is an autoimmune disease in which antibodies are produced that activate the TSHR. Features of Graves' disease include thyrotoxicosis, goiter, ophthalmopathy (eye changes associated with inflammation and infiltration of periorbital tissue), and dermopathy (skin changes in the lower extremities that have an orange peel texture). There is a strong familial disposition to Graves' disease—15% of patients will have a close relative with this condition—and women are five times more likely to develop it than men. Laboratory testing will usually document a high free T_4 and/or T_3 level with a low or undetectable TSH. TSIs and TSH receptor antibodies are usually positive in this condition. RAIU will be elevated, and the thyroid scan will show diffuse uptake (Table 23.4).

Approximately 20% to 25% of patients with Graves' hyperthyroidism develop clinically obvious Graves' ophthalmopathy, a particularly concerning manifestation.[21] With more sensitive testing, such as orbital CT scanning or magnetic resonance imaging (MRI), most patients with Graves' hyperthyroidism will be shown to have ophthalmopathy.[22] Findings in Graves' ophthalmopathy include orbital soft tissue swelling, injection of the conjunctivae, proptosis (forward protrusion of the eye secondary to infiltration of retro-orbital muscles and fat), double vision (secondary to orbital muscle involvement and fibrosis), and corneal disease (often related to trauma because of difficulty closing the eyelids). Treatment of Graves' ophthalmopathy may include noninvasive modalities such as moisturizing and protecting the cornea with drops and ointment or more invasive therapies such as injection of glucocorticoids retro-orbitally and, less frequently, surgical decompression of the orbits to prevent optic nerve injury and blindness.

Thyroid disease associated with Graves' disease is treated with medication, radioactive iodine, or surgery. Initially, many thyrotoxic patients require β-blockers to control symptoms of adrenergic excess, such as tremor and tachycardia. Propylthiouracil (PTU) or methimazole (MMI) can be added to inhibit thyroid hormone biosynthesis and secretion.[23] The antithyroidal medications, as they are known, carry a risk profile that includes rash and, rarely, hepatotoxicity, agranulocytosis, and aplastic anemia. These medications may have immunomodulatory effects on the underlying autoimmune disease, helping promote remission of the condition after several months of therapy. Long-term remission rates vary but generally run between 20% and 50% in the United States. Women are more likely to achieve remission than are men. Likewise, patients with small goiters and mild hyperthyroidism are more likely to achieve remission. Low dietary iodine increases the chance of staying in long-term remission. Patients experiencing

BOX 23.3 Signs and Symptoms of Thyrotoxicosis

Signs

Tachycardia
Tremor
Warm, moist, flushed, smooth skin
Lid lag, widened palpebral fissures
Ophthalmopathy (Graves' disease)
Goiter
Brisk deep tendon reflexes
Muscle wasting and weakness
Dermopathy/pretibial myxedema (Graves' disease)
Osteopenia, osteoporosis

Symptoms

Nervousness, irritability, anxiety
Tremor
Palpitations
Fatigue, weakness, decreased exercise tolerance
Weight loss
Heat intolerance
Hyperdefecation
Menstrual changes (oligomenorrhea)
Prominence of eyes

	Condition	Pathogenic Mechanism	TSH Level	RAIU	Other Tests
Hyperthyroidism	Graves' disease	TSHRAb	↓	↑	TRAb positive; TSI positive
	Toxic adenoma	Benign nodule	↓	↑	Seen on thyroid scan
	Toxic multinodular goiter	Foci of functional autonomy	↓	↑	Seen on thyroid scan
	TSH-secreting tumor	Benign pituitary tumor	Normal/↑	↑	Pituitary MRI
Nonhyperthyroidism	Painful thyroiditis	Leakage of thyroid hormone	↓	↓	Tg inappropriately high
	Postpartum thyroiditis	Leakage of thyroid hormone	↓	↓	TPOAb often high
	Exogenous hormone	Medication	↓	↓	
	Ectopic thyroid tissue	Metastatic thyroid cancer; struma ovarii	↓	↓	Distant metastasis seen on thyroid scan

TABLE 23.4 Disorders Associated with Thyrotoxicosis

RAIU, radioactive iodine uptake; Tg, thyroglobulin; TSHRAb, TSH receptor antibodies; TSI, thyroid-stimulating immunoglobulin; TPOAb, thyroid peroxidase antibodies.

such a remission do not require therapy with thyroid hormone replacement.

When radioactive iodine or surgery is used, the goal is to destroy or remove enough thyroid tissue so that the patient becomes hypothyroid. Subsequent lifelong treatment with thyroid hormone replacement therapy is usually required. Radioactive iodine therapy has been used for treatment of Graves' disease for more than 50 years and is considered both safe and effective. Surgery is associated with risk of recurrent laryngeal nerve injury, leading to permanent hoarseness, and injury to the parathyroid glands, causing hypoparathyroidism leading to hypocalcemia.

CASE STUDY 23.2

A 67-year-old woman is referred for treatment of hyperlipidemia. Her cholesterol and triglycerides are high, despite treatment with lipid-lowering medication. She is noted to have hair loss (wearing a wig) and hoarseness to her voice. She complains of cold intolerance and fatigue.

Questions

1. What testing would be helpful to screen for thyroid disease?

2. What treatment might she require?

3. What other laboratory abnormalities are commonly seen in hypothyroid patients other than hyperlipidemia and abnormal thyroid function tests?

Because of their comparative risks, radioactive iodine is generally the preferred treatment modality in the United States. Antithyroidal medications are typically used either because of patient preference or during pregnancy and breastfeeding. There are two situations in Graves' disease in which surgery is preferred to other forms of therapy: (1) if there is concern that the patient may have thyroid cancer in addition to Graves' disease, surgery is the best way to ensure removal of the potential cancer, and (2) in patients with severe ophthalmopathy, some experts in Graves' disease management prefer surgery because of concern that radioactive iodine treatment may cause an acute flaring of associated eye problems. Surgery may also be used during the second trimester of pregnancy in women for whom antithyroidal medication is not an option.

Toxic Adenoma and Multinodular Goiter

Toxic adenomas and multinodular goiter are two relatively common causes of hyperthyroidism. These conditions are caused by autonomously functioning thyroid tissue. In these instances, neither TSH nor TSHR-stimulating immunoglobulin is required to stimulate thyroid hormone production. In some toxic nodules, receptor mutations have been identified. These mutations have the same effect as chronic stimulation of the TSHR on thyroid hormone production. Clinically, toxic adenomas present signs and symptoms of hyperthyroidism, possibly with palpable nodule(s). On a thyroid scan, the nodules are "hot"—that is, they avidly take up radioactive iodine. The RAIU within the nodule is also inappropriately high for the suppressed level of TSH. In toxic multinodular goiter, there are multiple areas within the thyroid gland that are autonomously producing thyroid hormone (Table 23.4). Treatment for these two conditions involves surgery, radioactive iodine, or medication (PTU or MMI). Although the medications can block thyroid hormone production, they are not expected to lead to remission in these two conditions. Often, the toxic nodules produce so much thyroid hormone that the rest of the thyroid gland is suppressed and metabolically inactive. When radioactive iodine is given, it tends to destroy only the hyperactive (autonomous) nodules, leaving normal (suppressed) thyroid tissue undamaged. Because the normal thyroid tissue is hypofunctioning and takes up little of the radioactive iodine, when treatment is given, the patient may be left with normal thyroid function without the need for thyroid hormone replacement therapy.

DRUG-INDUCED THYROID DYSFUNCTION

Amiodarone-Induced Thyroid Disease

Several drugs other than PTU and MMI can affect thyroid function. Amiodarone, a drug used to treat cardiac arrhythmias, is a fat-soluble drug with a long half-life (50 days) that interferes with normal thyroid function.[24] The fact that 37% of the molecular weight of amiodarone is iodine accounts for a significant part of the thyroid dysfunction seen. Iodine, when given in large doses, acutely leads to inhibition of thyroid hormone production. This is called the Wolff-Chaikoff effect. Amiodarone also blocks T_4-to-T_3 conversion. The combination of these two actions leads to hypothyroidism in 8% to 20% of patients on chronic amiodarone therapy. Amiodarone can also lead to hyperthyroidism in 3% of patients treated chronically with this medication. Certain patients develop hyperthyroidism as they escape the Wolff-Chaikoff effect and use the excess iodine for thyroid hormone production. In others, the medication may induce inflammation of the gland (subacute thyroiditis) with subsequent leakage of stored thyroid hormone into the circulation.

Subacute Thyroiditis

Several conditions occur that lead to transient changes in thyroid hormone levels.[25] These conditions are associated with inflammation of the thyroid gland, leakage of stored thyroid hormone, followed by repair of the gland. Although nomenclature varies between authors, grouping together postpartum thyroiditis, painless thyroiditis, and painful thyroiditis as forms of subacute thyroiditis is one of the simplest classification schemes. These conditions are often associated with a thyrotoxic phase when thyroid hormone is leaking into the circulation, a hypothyroid phase when the thyroid gland is repairing itself, and a euthyroid phase when the gland is repaired with the duration of these phases lasting from weeks to months.

Postpartum thyroiditis is the most common form of subacute thyroiditis. It occurs in 3% to 16% of women in the postpartum period.[26] It is strongly associated with the presence of TPO antibodies and chronic lymphocytic thyroiditis. Patients may experience a period of thyrotoxicosis followed by hypothyroidism or simply hypothyroidism or hyperthyroidism. Thyroid hormone levels usually return to normal after several months; however, by 4 years postpartum, 25% to 50% of patients have persistent

hypothyroidism, goiter, or both.[27] During the thyrotoxic phase, β-blockers can be used if treatment is necessary. During the hypothyroid phase, thyroid hormone replacement therapy can be given if symptoms require, usually for three to 6 months, with continuation if permanent hypothyroidism develops. The thyrotoxic phase of this condition, as well as other forms of subacute thyroiditis, can be distinguished from Graves' disease by a low RAIU and an absence of TSI or TSH receptor antibodies (Table 23.4). Painless thyroiditis or subacute lymphocytic thyroiditis shares many characteristics of postpartum thyroiditis, except there is no associated pregnancy.

Painful thyroiditis, also called *subacute granulomatous*, *subacute nonsuppurative thyroiditis*, or *de Quervain's thyroiditis*, is characterized by neck pain, low-grade fever, myalgia, a tender diffuse goiter, and swings in thyroid function tests (as discussed earlier). Viral infections are felt to trigger this condition. TPO antibodies are usually absent; erythrocyte sedimentation rate and thyroglobulin levels are often elevated.

NONTHYROIDAL ILLNESS

Hospitalized patients, especially critically ill patients, often have abnormalities in their thyroid function tests without thyroid dysfunction, a condition known as nonthyroidal illness or euthyroid sick syndrome. Typically, the laboratory pattern is one of normal or low TSH, low T_3, and low free T_4.[28] Because illness decreases 5′-monodeiodinase activity, less T_4 is converted to active T_3. This leads to decreased levels of T_3 and higher levels of reverse T_3. There also seems to be an element of central hypothyroidism and thyroid hormone–binding changes associated with severe illness. It is believed that many of these changes are an appropriate adaptation to illness and thyroid hormone replacement therapy is not indicated.

THYROID NODULES

Thyroid nodules are common. Clinically apparent thyroid nodules are present in 6.4% of adult women and 1.5% of adult men, according to Framingham data.[29] Autopsy studies, however, suggest 20% to 76% of women in iodine-replete areas have thyroid nodules, with rates correlating with decade of age and increased use of thyroid ultrasound supports these estimates, with unsuspected nodules, or "incidentalomas" found in 20% to 45% of women and 17% to 25% of men.[30,31] Despite the frequency of thyroid nodules, only 5% to 9% of nonpalpable nodules prove to be thyroid cancer.[32] FNA of these nodules, with cytologic examination of the aspirate, has become a routine practice to help distinguish the nodules that require surgical removal from those that do not.[12]

For additional student resources, please visit **thePoint** at http://thepoint.lww.com

questions

1. All of the following statements about iodine are true EXCEPT
   a. Radioactive iodine treatment of Graves disease is effective in less than 40% of patients treated with this agent.
   b. Iodine deficiency is one of the most common causes of hypothyroidism in the world.
   c. T_4 has four iodine molecules.
   d. RAIU is often useful in determining the cause of thyrotoxicosis.

2. The fetus
   a. Is dependent on thyroid hormone for normal neurologic development
   b. Does not develop a thyroid gland until the third trimester
   c. Is not susceptible to damage from radioactive iodine therapy given to the mother
   d. Will be born with hypothyroidism in approximately 1 of 400 births in developed countries

3. The thyroid gland
   a. Depends on TPO to permit iodination of the tyrosyl residues to make MIT and DIT
   b. Is an ineffective iodine trap
   c. Depends on TPO to permit the joining of two DIT residues to form T_3
   d. Usually functions independent of TSH levels

4. The thyroid gland produces all of the following EXCEPT
   a. TSH
   b. Thyroglobulin
   c. T_3
   d. T_4

5. Hypothyroidism is generally associated with all of the following EXCEPT
   a. TSH receptor antibodies
   b. Depression
   c. An elevation of TSH levels
   d. TPO antibodies

6. A 34-year-old woman presents with goiter, tachycardia, and weight loss of 2 months duration. TSH is undetectable and free T_4 is high. All of the following tests are useful in diagnosing the cause of the hyperthyroidism EXCEPT
   a. FNA biopsy of the thyroid gland
   b. TSH receptor antibodies
   c. RAIU
   d. TSH

7. A 65-year-old woman presents with fatigue, hypothermia, pericardial effusions, and hair loss. Her thyroid function tests show a significantly elevated TSH and a low free T_4. All of the following laboratory test abnormalities may be associated with her underlying condition EXCEPT
   a. Elevated WBC
   b. An elevated cholesterol level
   c. Anemia
   d. Elevated CPK levels

8. A 26-year-old man presents with a 3-cm, right lobe, thyroid nodule and a normal TSH. What is the next test that should be performed?
   a. FNA of the nodule
   b. Free T_4 level
   c. Thyroid ultrasound
   d. Thyroid scan

9. The following are treatment options for hyperthyroidism associated with Graves' disease EXCEPT
   a. Thyroid hormone
   b. PTU
   c. Beta-blockers
   d. Radioactive iodine

10. All of the following abnormalities might be expected in a severely ill patient EXCEPT
    a. Low rT_3
    b. Low T_4
    c. Low T_3
    d. Low TSH

11. Of the following thyroid hormones, which is considered the most biologically active?
    a. T_3 bound to TBG
    b. T_4 bound to TBG
    c. Free T_4
    d. Free T_3
    e. rT_3

12. The primary serum test to screen for thyroid disease is
    a. Free T_4
    b. rT_3
    c. Total T_4
    d. Autoimmune antibodies to thyroid tissue
    e. TSH

13. Of the following, which will MOST likely interfere with quantitation of thyroglobulin?
    a. Antithyroglobulin autoantibodies
    b. Thyroid-stimulating antibodies
    c. TSH receptor antibodies
    d. Thyroid peroxidase antibodies

references

1. Greenspan FS. The thyroid gland. In: Greenspan FS, Strewler GJ, eds. *Basic & Clinical Endocrinology.* 5th ed. New York, NY: Appleton & Lange; 1997.
2. Lavin L. *Manual of Endocrinology.* 2nd ed. Boston, MA: Little, Brown & Co.; 1994:395.
3. Caldwell KL, Makhmudov A, Ely E, et al. Iodine status of the U.S. populations, national health and nutrition examination survey, 2005–2006 and 2007–2008. *Thyroid.* 2001;21:419–427.
4. Institute of Medicine, Food and Nutrition Board. Iodine. In National Academy of Sciences. *Dietary Reference Intakes for Vitamin A, Vitamin K, Arsenic, Boron, Chromium, Copper, Iodine, Iron, Manganese, Molybdenum, Nickel, Silicon, Vanadium, and Zinc.* Washington, DC: National Academies Press; 2001.
5. Kopp P. Thyroid hormone synthesis. In: Braverman LE, Utiger RD, eds. *The Thyroid: Fundamental and Clinical Text.* 9th ed. Philadelphia, PA: Williams and Wilkins; 2005.
6. Ross DS, Ardisson LJ, Meskell MJ. Measurement of thyrotropin in clinical and subclinical hyperthyroidism using a new chemiluminescent assay. *J Clin Endocrinol Metab.* 1989;69(3):684.
7. Spencer CA, LoPresiti JS, Patel A, et al. Applications of a new chemiluminometric thyrotropin assay to subnormal measurement. *J Clin Endocrinol Metab.* 1990;70:453–460.
8. Ekins R. The free hormone hypothesis and measurement of free hormones [editorial]. *Clin Chem.* 1992;38:1289–1293.
9. Wong TK, Pekary AE, Hoo GS, et al. Comparison of methods for measuring free thyroxine in nonthyroidal illness. *Clin Chem.* 1992;38:720–724.
10. Barbesino G, Tomer Y. Clinical utility of TSH receptor antibodies. *J Clin Endocrinol Metab.* 2013;98:2247–2255.
11. Tan GH, Gharib H. Thyroid incidentalomas: management approaches to nonpalpable nodules discovered incidentally on thyroid imaging. *Ann Intern Med.* 1997;126:226.
12. Haugen BR, Alexander EK, Bible KC, et al. 2015 American Thyroid Association management guidelines for adult patients with thyroid nodules and differentiated thyroid cancer: the American Thyroid Association Guidelines Task Force on thyroid nodules and differentiated thyroid cancer. *Thyroid.* 2016;26:1–133.
13. Crippa S, Mazzuchelli L, Cibas ES, et al. The Bethesda System for reporting thyroid fine-needle aspiration specimens. *Am J Clin Pathol.* 2010;134:343–344.
14. Mariani L, Berns J. The renal manifestations of thyroid disease. *J Am Soc Nephrol.* 2012;23:22–26.
15. Khaleeli AA, Gohil K, McPhail G, et al. Muscle morphology and metabolism in hypothyroid myopathy: effects of treatment. *J Clin Pathol.* 1983;36:519–526.
16. Green ST, Ng JP. Hypothyroidism and anaemia. *Biomed Pharmacother.* 1986;40:326–331.
17. Diekman T, Lansberg PJ, Kastelein JJ, et al. Prevalence and correction of hypothyroidism in a large cohort of patients referred for dyslipidemia. *Arch Intern Med.* 1995;155:1490–1495.
18. O'Brien T, Dinneen SF, O'Brien PC, et al. Hyperlipidemia in patients with primary and secondary hypothyroidism. *Mayo Clin Proc.* 1993;68:860–866.
19. Garber J, Cobin R, Gharib H, et al. Clinical practice guidelines for hypothyroidism in adults: cosponsored by the American Association of Clinical Endocrinologists and the American Thyroid Association. *Endocr Pract.* 2012;18:1001.
20. Ladenson PW, Singer PA, Ain KB, et al. American Thyroid Association guidelines for detection of thyroid dysfunction. *Arch Intern Med.* 2000;160:1573–1575.
21. Burch HB, Wartofsky L. Graves' ophthalmopathy: Current concepts regarding pathogenesis and management. *Endocr Rev.* 1993;14:747–793.
22. Villadolid MC, Yokoyama N, Izumi M, et al. Untreated Graves' disease patients without clinical ophthalmopathy demonstrate a high frequency of extraocular muscle (EOM) enlargement by magnetic resonance. *J Clin Endocrinol Metab.* 1995;80:2830–2833.
23. Solomon BL, Evaul JE, Burman KD, et al. Remission rates with antithyroid drug therapy: continuing influence of iodine intake? *Ann Intern Med.* 1987;107:510–512.
24. Nademanee K, Singh BN, Callahan B, et al. Amiodarone, thyroid hormone indexes, and altered thyroid function: long-term serial effects in patients with cardiac arrhythmias. *Am J Cardiol.* 1986;58:981–986.
25. Pearce EN, Farwell AP, Braverman LE. Thyroiditis. *N Engl J Med.* 2003;348(26):2646–2455.
26. Gerstein HC. How common is postpartum thyroiditis? A methodologic overview of the literature. *Arch Intern Med.* 1990;150:1397–1400.
27. Othman S, Phillips DI, Parkes AB, et al. A long-term follow-up of postpartum thyroiditis. *Clin Endocrinol (Oxf).* 1990;32:559–564.
28. DeGroot L. Dangerous dogmas in medicine: the non-thyroidal illness syndrome. *J Clin Endocrinol Metab.* 1999;84:151–164.
29. Vander JB, Gaston EA, Dawber TG. The significance of non-toxic thyroid nodules. *Ann Intern Med.* 1968;69:537.
30. Vanderpump MPJ. The epidemiology of thyroid diseases. In: Braverman LE, Utiger RD, eds. *Werner and Ingbar's the Thyroid: a Fundamental and Clinical Text.* 9th ed. Philadelphia, PA: JB Lippincott-Raven; 2005:398–496.
31. Brander A, Viikinkoski P, Nickels J, et al. Thyroid gland: US screening in a random adult population. *Radiology.* 1991;181:683.
32. Papini E, Guglielmi R, Bianchini A, et al. Risk of malignancy in nonpalpable thyroid nodules: predictive value of ultrasound and color-Doppler features. *J Clin Endocrinol Metab.* 2002;87:1941–1946.

24

Calcium Homeostasis and Hormonal Regulation

JOSEPHINE ABRAHAM and DEV ABRAHAM

chapter outline

key terms

1,25-Dihydroxy vitamin D
25-Hydroxy vitamin D
Bisphosphonates
Bone turnover
Calcium-sensing receptor
Cinacalcet
Cortical bone
Dual-energy x-ray absorptiometry
Fibroblast growth factor 23 (FGF23)
Hypercalcemia
Hypocalcemia
Lithium
Osteoblast
Osteoclast
Osteomalacia
Osteoporosis
Parathyroid hormone
Parathyroid hormone–related protein)
Rickets
Teriparatide
Thiazide diuretics
Trabecular bone
Vitamin D

chapter objectives

Upon completion of this chapter, the clinical laboratorian should be able to do the following:

- Describe the endocrine and organ physiology of calcium metabolism.
- Discuss the laboratory tools used to evaluate calcium metabolism.
- Apply the laboratory tools to clinical disease states of calcium metabolism.

For additional student resources, please visit thePoint® at http://thepoint.lww.com

FIGURE 24.1 Calcium homeostasis. Tissue and organs involved in calcium homeostasis (gut, skeleton, and kidneys) and how they relate to blood calcium. Also shown is the means of getting calcium de novo into the system (GI absorption) and elimination of calcium from the system (renal excretion) under normal physiologic conditions.

CALCIUM HOMEOSTASIS

Serum calcium level is maintained at a constant level for the optimal excitability of neural and muscular tissue and the coordinated functioning of various organ systems in the human body. Calcium levels are maintained with a narrow range for optimal nerve impulse transmission, muscular contraction, blood coagulation, hormone secretion, and intercellular adhesion. Imbalance of calcium can lead to serious clinical consequences.

In this chapter, the regulation of blood calcium and consequences of alterations in calcium balance are discussed. A preview of organs and organ systems involved is as described in Figure 24.1.

An adult human body contains 1,000 g of calcium.[1] About 99% of this is in the form of hydroxyapatite salt (provides structural rigidity along with collagen matrix), and the remainder (1%) is in the extracellular fluids and regulates various biochemical events. In the blood, calcium exists in ionized (50%), protein-bound (40% to plasma proteins), and complexed (10% to citrate and phosphate) forms. The pH of blood influences binding with proteins (binding increases with high pH and decreases with low pH). The ionized calcium is the only relevant fraction from the cellular function standpoint. The principal organs involved in calcium homeostasis are the skin, liver, small intestine, skeleton, parathyroid glands, and kidneys. Diet is the only source of calcium. The skeleton acts as a mineral repository, releasing calcium into blood on demand, especially during times of poor intake. During prolonged low oral intake or malabsorption, the blood levels are maintained at near-normal levels at the expense of the skeletal stores. The only significant loss of calcium from the body is into urine.

HORMONAL REGULATION OF CALCIUM METABOLISM

Vitamin D and **parathyroid hormone (PTH)** are the two most important hormones that regulate calcium and phosphate homeostasis. No clear role for calcitonin has been established in healthy humans.

Vitamin D

Vitamin D is a steroid hormone that is synthesized in the skin following exposure to UVB rays from the sun. Following the photobiosynthesis of vitamin D from cholesterol, it undergoes further hydroxylation in the liver and kidneys (Fig. 24.2).[2]

The hepatic enzyme, 25-hydroxylase, metabolizes vitamin D_3 to 25-hydroxy vitamin D_3. Serum 25-hydroxy vitamin D estimation is the best indicator of body stores; therefore, low 25-hydroxy vitamin D levels in the blood imply deficiency. The renal 1α-hydroxylase, under PTH regulation, completes the formation of the active metabolite, **1,25-dihydroxy vitamin D** (1,25(OH)$_2$D).

Endogenous synthesis of vitamin D is influenced by the amount of sun exposure, available sunlight (less in northern latitudes), skin covering (clothing and sun block), and age of the individual. Older individuals have less effective photobiosynthesis of vitamin D.

Vitamin D_3 (cholecalciferol) is scarcely found in nature. The major dietary sources are internal organs such as liver and sea food. Vitamin D_2 (ergocalciferol) is found in edible mushrooms. Commercially available milk is fortified with vitamin D_3. Breast-fed infants are at risk for vitamin D deficiency, since breast milk is a poor source of vitamin D. Multivitamins contain 400 units of vitamin D_3, about the same amount found in a quart of vitamin D—fortified milk.

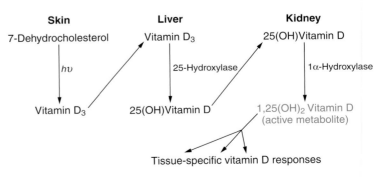

FIGURE 24.2 Vitamin D synthesis. Tissues involved in the synthesis of vitamin D and the steps that each tissue is responsible for. Also shown are enzymes responsible for the two enzymatically mediated steps (hepatic 25-hydroxylation and renal 1α-hydroxylation). The product of this pathway, 1,25(OH)$_2$D, is responsible for the tissue-specific effects of vitamin D.

FIGURE 24.3 Vitamin D mechanism of action. DNA binding and interaction with other components of the transcriptional machinery of the vitamin D–vitamin D receptor complex are shown. Note the striking evolutionary similarity between this mechanism and that of other steroid and thyroid hormones. As prime examples, vitamin D inhibits transcription of the *PTH* gene in parathyroid tissue and stimulates transcription of the calcium transporter in the intestinal brush border epithelium.

Vitamin D is a steroid hormone derived from cholesterol. The same cholesterol biosynthetic pathway that provides the precursors for vitamin D also provides the precursors for other steroid hormones from the adrenal gland and gonads. The steroid receptor supergene family of nuclear receptors carries out its physiologic regulation by directing transcription of specific vitamin D–responsive genes. $1,25(OH)_2D$ is the natural ligand for the vitamin D receptor. Synthetic analogs of vitamin D such as paricalcitol bind to vitamin D receptors with very high affinity and are used to treat secondary hyperparathyroidism due to chronic renal failure.

The $1,25(OH)_2D$–vitamin D receptor complex binds to the vitamin D response element upstream (5′) of the transcription start site of vitamin D genes and induces gene transcription (Fig. 24.3).

Activated vitamin D, $1,25(OH)_2D$, induces active absorption of calcium in the small bowel cells, which is the dominant mechanism of calcium absorption in humans. Only about 5% to 10% of calcium is absorbed passively.[3,4] The lack of active intestinal absorption of calcium induced by activated vitamin D, $1,25(OH)_2D$, results in hypocalcemia. Even though activated $1,25(OH)_2D$ also stimulates absorption of phosphate, a larger fraction of phosphate absorption occurs passively and is much less dependent upon normal $1,25(OH)_2D$ levels. This mechanism is illustrated in chronic renal failure patients.

In the bone, $1,25(OH)_2D$ stimulates differentiation of **osteoclast** precursors to osteoclasts. $1,25(OH)_2D$ also stimulates **osteoblasts** to influence osteoclasts to mobilize bone calcium. $1,25(OH)_2D$ does not directly affect *mature* osteoclast function. $1,25(OH)_2D$ plays an important role in the mineralization of bone, and abnormal bone results when vitamin D is deficient (e.g., celiac sprue) or its metabolism is defective (e.g., renal failure).

As noted earlier, $1,25(OH)_2D$ increases blood calcium by augmenting intestinal absorption of calcium. Blood calcium feeds back to parathyroid glands and regulates the synthesis and secretion of PTH. Also, $1,25(OH)_2D$ has direct control over the *PTH* secretion, and high levels reduce secretion of PTH. Elevated serum phosphate levels reduce $1,25(OH)_2D$ formation (Fig. 24.4).

Parathyroid Hormone

PTH is secreted from four parathyroid glands that are located adjacent to the thyroid gland. The parathyroid glands were first described in 1852 by Sir Richard Owen,[5] when he performed dissection on an Indian Rhinoceros that had died in London Zoo. Normal parathyroid glands are ovoid or bean shaped and measure approximately 3 mm in size. The superior parathyroid glands are smaller than the inferior pair. The parathyroid glands have an anatomically distinct vascular supply from that of the thyroid gland and are enveloped in a pad of anatomically distinct fibrofatty capsule.[6]

One human postmortem examination study revealed that four glands are found in 91% of the subjects, three glands in 5%, and five glands in 4%.[7] The locations of para-

FIGURE 24.4 Calcium, PTH, and vitamin D feedforward and feedback loops. The endocrine response to shifts in blood calcium (rising or falling) is shown. A concerted hormone response, mediated at the organ level by the organs shown in Figure 24.1, helps restore blood calcium toward normal.

thyroid glands vary widely due to the embryonic origination from the third and fourth pharyngeal pouches with eventual migration to the lower neck. The superior parathyroid glands develop in the fourth pharyngeal pouch and migrate caudally along with the ultimobranchial bodies, which give rise to parafollicular (C) cells of the thyroid gland. The superior pair is commonly located along the upper two-thirds of the posterior margin of the thyroid lobe. The superior parathyroid glands are relatively constant in their location along the posterior margin of the thyroid gland. The third bronchial pouches give rise to the inferior pair and the thymus gland, and together, they migrate to the lower neck; in some individuals, the inferior parathyroid glands can migrate into the thorax.

The parathyroid glands have specialized **calcium-sensing receptors** (CSRs) that respond to rising or falling calcium levels by increasing or decreasing PTH secretion, respectively. The primary targets for the PTH are the bone and kidneys. PTH mobilizes calcium from bone by increasing bone resorption. PTH has three effects on the kidneys:

1. Increase the reabsorption of renal tubular calcium
2. Increase phosphate excretion
3. Enhance 1α-hydroxylation of **25-hydroxy vitamin D**

Activated $1,25(OH)_2D$ promotes meal-related intestinal absorption of calcium. In summary, low blood calcium is sensed by the parathyroid CSR, which in turn secretes PTH and sets into motion a cascade of events aimed at restoring normal blood calcium levels.

The multiple actions of PTH described above are mediated via PTH receptor, located on the cell membrane of target tissues. This receptor activates adenylate cyclase and the "second messenger" pathway involving cyclic AMP (cAMP), which modulates protein phosphorylation.

ORGAN SYSTEM REGULATION OF CALCIUM METABOLISM

The three organ systems that regulate calcium metabolism are the gastrointestinal (GI) tract, the kidneys, and the bone.

GI Regulation

Normal intestinal function is required for calcium absorption. Interruptions in intestinal function, as may be seen with short bowel syndromes (following resection), gastric weight loss surgeries, intestinal mucosal disease (celiac disease), genetic defects, and bowel fistula, may affect calcium absorption. Adequate dietary calcium intake, the availability of normal amounts of vitamin D, and metabolism are all necessary for optimal calcium absorption. $1,25(OH)_2D$ controls calcium absorption from the small bowel. Dietary phosphate can bind dietary calcium in the intestinal lumen, forming the insoluble and nonabsorbable precipitate, calcium phosphate. The insolubility of calcium phosphate is the basis for the use of calcium carbonate as a "phosphate binder" in patients with renal failure. Likewise, a diet rich in phosphate will tend to inhibit calcium absorption by the same mechanism.

Role of Kidneys

The kidneys play an essential role in calcium metabolism. This is exemplified in subjects who develop renal failure, leading to markedly disordered calcium and phosphate metabolism.[8] Impaired hydroxylation of 25-hydroxy vitamin D to form the active $1,25(OH)_2D$ results in poor calcium absorption from the gut. Diseased kidneys fail to excrete phosphate, leading to elevated serum phosphate levels. Hyperphosphatemia is a powerful stimulus for PTH and **fibroblast growth factor 23 (FGF23)** secretion. FGF23 is a powerful phosphaturic hormone secreted by the osteocytes that binds to the FGF receptor 1 and coreceptor Klotho in the kidney. FGF23 inhibits 1α-hydroxylation of 25 vitamin D (inactive) to and $1,25(OH)_2D$ (active) but also stimulates 24α-hydroxylation (inactivation) of $1,25(OH)_2D$. The net result is very low $1,25(OH)_2$ D levels, leading to hypocalcemia.

Serum PTH levels can be elevated in chronic renal failure patients. Once a critical calcium/phosphate product is reached, precipitation of these minerals occurs within the tissues, leading to devastating consequences.

In physiological state, PTH increases renal tubular reabsorption of calcium, thereby reducing renal loss. **Hypercalcemia**, whether as a result of autonomous overproduction of PTH, termed *primary hyperparathyroidism (PHPT)*, or from other causes, increases the filtered load of calcium. Even though PTH stimulates tubular reabsorption of calcium, this process is overwhelmed, and the *net* calcium excretion is increased compared with normal state. This is the fundamental mechanism by which PHPT subjects form calcium kidney stones. See Figure 24.5 for organ system integration of calcium homeostasis.

Bone Physiology

Bone contains about 1 kg of calcium and serves as a repository for calcium, phosphate, and magnesium. **Bone turnover** or "remodeling" is a regulated and coupled process of simultaneous bone formation and breakdown that occurs to varying degrees throughout the life and at multiple sites in the skeleton. The process of "coupling" ensures that neither resorption nor formation occurs in excess compared to the other, thereby preventing imbalance between formation and loss of bone. Too much resorption results in weaker bones and too much bone formation can obliterate the marrow space. Bone formation is mediated by osteoblasts, and bone breakdown, or resorption, is mediated by osteoclasts (a cell in the monocyte/macrophage lineage). Interestingly, although osteoclasts are required to mobilize calcium from bone, they do not appear to express receptors for either $1,25(OH)_2D$ or PTH. Rather, these hormones act directly on osteoblasts, which in turn produce a complex array of hormones, which regulate the osteoclast activity, either activating or deactivating them. When the net rates of osteoblast-mediated bone formation and osteoclast-mediated

FIGURE 24.5 Organ system integration of calcium homeostasis.

bone resorption are mismatched, or uncoupled, such that resorption exceeds formation, bone mass will ultimately decrease. Decreased bone mass translates clinically into an increased risk of fracture, as seen in osteoporosis. As bones turn over, several proteins are released into the blood and eventually excreted in the urine, collectively called as bone turnover markers.[9] Bone turnover markers are useful in the monitoring of clinical response to osteoporosis therapies and for predicting fracture risks.

Resorption markers include the following:

- Hydroxyproline
- N-telopeptides
- C telopeptides
- Cross-links
- Tartrate-resistant acid phosphatase (TRAP)

Formation markers include the following:

- Bone-specific alkaline phosphatase (BSAP)
- Osteocalcin
- Procollagen N-terminal extension peptides

There are two main types of bones found in the skeleton: **cortical bone** and **trabecular bone**. Cortical bone is the predominant bone type found in the shaft of long bones, such as the femur. Cortical bone is very strong, yet light in weight and is therefore well suited for the mechanical needs of the extremities. Trabecular bone is the primary bone type found in the axial skeleton, such as the vertebrae. It consists of numerous cross-hair or honeycomb-type connections called *trabeculae*. These interconnected trabeculae

give this type of bone considerable strength for weight bearing. Although the femur is primarily cortical bone and the vertebrae is primarily trabecular bone, sites such as the femoral trochanter and proximal humerus are a mixture of both cortical and trabecular bones. The ends of long bones contain more trabecular bone. The shafts of long bones are predominantly cortical. Certain disease states induce preferential bone loss in specific bone types. Cortical bone is preferentially lost in PHPT, and trabecular bone is mostly lost in postmenopausal osteoporosis. In most conditions, bone loss is diffuse.

In summary, normal calcium homeostasis is achieved by a complex and regulated interplay between vitamin D, PTH, and the target organs. Defects in the function and formation of hormones or organ system disorders can induce disease states, which will be reviewed in the rest of this chapter.

HYPERCALCEMIA

Hypercalcemia results when blood calcium levels in a subject are above the expected normal range of a healthy population. Patients with low serum albumin would be expected to have low total calcium and normal ionized calcium; the opposite is true for patients with high serum albumin. Ionized calcium best correlates with the biological activity of calcium, as well as with symptoms of hypercalcemia or hypocalcemia, and thus, the direct measurement of ionized calcium may often be more valuable clinically. The binding of calcium to proteins should be taken into consideration during assessment of blood calcium levels.

The duration and the level of calcium elevation determine the severity of symptoms and the degree of end-organ damage. Some common symptoms of acute severe hypercalcemia include lethargy, stupor, and coma. Patients with chronic mild hypercalcemia are symptom free. Moderate calcium elevation is associated with intellectual weariness, personality changes, nausea, anorexia, polyuria, kidney stones, hypertension, and electrocardiogram (ECG) changes. In the outpatients setting, PHPT is the most common cause for hypercalcemia.

Cancer-mediated hypercalcemia often presents with profound central nervous system (CNS) symptoms due to rapid and significant calcium elevation at the time of diagnosis.

Causes of Hypercalcemia

1. **Disorders of parathyroid glands and CSRs:**

   - PHPT (autonomous overproduction of PTH): Adenoma (>80%), hyperplasia (5% to 10%), carcinoma (<1%), and familial syndromes (MEN1, MEN2a, and PHPT–jaw tumor syndrome).
   - Secondary and tertiary hyperparathyroidism: In chronic renal failure patients, the sustained hypocalcemic–hyperphosphatemic stimuli result in parathyroid hyperplasia, leading to sustained and autonomous overproduction of PTH with ensuing hypercalcemia.
   - CSR abnormalities (extracellular calcium levels are sensed aberrantly resulting in hypercalcemia): Familial hypocalciuric hypercalcemia (FHH) (inactivating mutation of CSR), calcium receptor antibodies, and lithium carbonate.
   - Other endocrine disorders: adrenal insufficiency, hyperthyroidism, pheochromocytomas, and vipoma.

2. **Cancer-mediated hypercalcemia (paraneoplastic hypercalcemia):**
   - PTHrP production by tumors: Upper GI adenocarcinomas, squamous cell carcinomas of head and neck and lung, renal cell carcinoma, ovarian carcinoma, HTLV-1 lymphoma, adrenal cancer, carcinoid tumor, islet cell cancer, and pheochromocytoma. Prostate and colonic cancers rarely produce PTHrP.
   - 1,25 Hydroxylation of 25-hydroxy vitamin D: Various cell types of lymphomas.
   - Cytokine production by tumor cells leads to activation of bone resorption (myeloma and diffuse bone metastasis): Cytokines such as macrophage inflammatory protein-1 alpha, tumor necrosis factor alpha, prostaglandins, and IL-6, which activate osteoclasts through receptor activator of nuclear factor kappa B (RANK).

3. **Granulomatous diseases:** Sarcoidosis, tuberculosis, leprosy, fungal infections, Crohn disease (granulomas express the hydroxylation enzyme that is required to convert 25-hydroxy vitamin D to active $1,25(OH)_2D$).

4. **Medications:** Hydrochlorothiazide (HCTZ), lithium, vitamin A and/or D toxicity, oral calcium excess (milk alkali syndrome [MAS]), tamoxifen, and aminophylline toxicity.

5. **Miscellaneous:** William's syndrome and chronic immobilization.

The signs and symptoms of hypercalcemia are highly variable and depend upon the rapidity of onset and severity of hypercalcemia. Clinically, the signs and symptoms also vary from patient to patient and comorbid conditions may also influence the development of symptoms. The signs and symptoms are best described by organ systems:

CNS: Impairment of CNS function, including lethargy, decreased alertness, depression, confusion, forgetfulness, obtundation, and coma.

GI: Patients may experience anorexia, constipation, peptic ulcers, and nausea and vomiting.

Renal: Hypercalciuria leading to kidney stone formation and calcification of renal tubules resulting in nephrogenic diabetes insipidus.

Skeletal: Increased bone resorption and demineralization leading to fractures.

Cardiovascular: Hypercalcemia may cause or exacerbate hypertension. The following ECG changes are seen in hypercalcemia: Increased PR interval, wide QRS complex, and short QT syndrome.

Primary Hyperparathyroidism

PHPT is the most common cause of hypercalcemia, with an incidence of 1 in 500 to 1,000 in the general population. Women are affected threefold more commonly than men. The hallmark of this disorder is the autonomous overproduction of PTH, most commonly by a single adenoma in one of the parathyroid glands (>80%), less commonly by multiple gland hyperplasia (~5% to 10%), and very rarely by parathyroid cancer. Parathyroid carcinoma occurs more commonly in a familial syndrome called the hyperparathyroidism–jaw tumor syndrome. PHPT is also encountered in multiple endocrine neoplasia types 1 and 2 (MEN1 and MEN2a). The apparent increase in the incidence of PHPT was traced to the introduction and wide availability of multichannel analyzers in the 1970s. The incidence of PHPT increased from 7.8 cases per 100,000 to 51 cases per 100,000 in Olmsted County, Minnesota, United States, following the introduction of routine calcium testing.[10] Fuller Albright's description of the disease in the 1930s was notable for advanced bone and end-stage kidney disease at the time of diagnosis.[11] This presentation is very uncommon. The fortuitous detection of a large proportion of the prevalent subclinical PHPT subjects, along with early intervention and treatment, has changed the clinical presentation of PHPT. In countries where multichannel analyzers are not available, the disease presentation is severe and with catastrophic renal and skeletal consequences, similar to how it was in the United States in the early 1900s. The dominant clinical phenotype of PHPT in the United States is asymptomatic hypercalcemia, invariably identified fortuitously in patients undergoing yearly physical examination. The apparent increase in the incidence of PHPT was correlated to the wide availability and use of multichannel testing since the 1970s.[12] In the Kaiser Permanente study, involving 3.5 million people, the incidence of PHPT varied from 34 to 124 per 100,000 person years. The incidence increases with advancing age and was highest and Blacks followed by White's with rates for Asians and Hispanics lowest among the ethnicities. Women are affected three-fold more frequently than men.[13] Along with the increase in the diagnosis of patients with PHPT, the surgical case volume increased an astounding 177% in a state-wide health planning study from California between 1999 and 2008.[14]

The diagnosis of PHPT is made by biochemical testing, and elevated serum calcium (or ionized calcium) level with inappropriately normal or elevated PTH level confirms the diagnosis. The biochemical differential diagnosis of hypercalcemia is listed in Table 24.1.

PTH Assays

PTH is a polypeptide hormone with C-terminal and amino (N)-terminal ends composed of 84 amino acid residues. PTH 1 to 84 refer to the entire hormone sequence. n-Truncated PTH (7 to 84 PTH) are deficient in the first few residues of the n-terminal end and hence biologically inactive. The integrity of 1 to 11 amino acid residues in the N-terminal end of PTH is required for the biologic activity of PTH. PTH assays use two antibodies that bind to specific sites (one on each of the C- and N-terminal ends), which enable precise detection of intact PTH. A few commonly available assays include the following:

- Intact PTH: measures 7 to 84 PTH and 1 to 84 PTH.
- Bioactive PTH: measures 1 to 84 PTH.
- CAP assay: cAMP inducible PTH. This assay detects biologically active PTH by its ability to induce formation of cAMP.
- PRHrP assays and PTH assays are exclusive to each other, by design. There is no cross-reactivity. Therefore, PTH levels are low in subjects with cancers producing PTHrP.
- PTH can also be estimated in needle biopsy specimens obtained from parathyroid tumors. Hook effect has not been observed despite massive elevation of PTH levels in these specimens obtained by direct puncture of enlarged parathyroid glands.[15]

CASE STUDY 24.1

A 40-year-old woman presents to her physician complaining of marked left flank pain that began the previous night. She reports that the pain is worse than that of giving birth. She also reports blood in her urine earlier on the day she came to see her doctor. She has felt more fatigued and as if her concentration has not been as good as normal for the last year or so, and she feels more forgetful. She has no significant past medical history. She is taking no medications. Family history contributes no pertinent information. On physical examination, she appears to be in extreme pain. There is marked tenderness on very gentle percussion over the left costovertebral angle. Labs are drawn and are notable for calcium 11.2 mg/dL (normal, 8.5 to 10.2 mg/dL), albumin 3.8 g/dL (normal, 3.5 to 4.8 g/dL), and intact PTH 162 pg/mL (normal, 11 to 54 pg/mL). Renal function is normal (BUN 25 mg/dL and creatinine 0.9 mg/dL). Urine analysis is notable for blood and greater than 50 red blood cells per high-power field. This prompts a 24-hour urine collection, which reveals calcium elevated at 483 mg per 24 hour (normal, 100 to 250 mg per 24 hour).

Questions

1. Which laboratory results are abnormal?
2. What is the presumptive diagnosis for this patient? The differential diagnosis?
3. What treatment is indicated for this disease?

Biochemical Findings in PHPT

1. Hypercalcemia
2. Hypophosphatemia: PTH induces phosphaturia.
3. Elevated PTH relative to serum calcium (inappropriately normal PTH in the face of hypercalcemia).
4. Low-normal 25-OH-D and high normal or elevated (30%) $1,25(OH)_2D$ due to PTH-enhancing renal hydroxylation.
5. Urinary calcium excretion is elevated.
6. Metabolic hyperchloremic acidosis (chloride is exchanged for phosphate).
7. Elevated serum alkaline phosphatase in severe disease.

TABLE 24.1	**Biochemical Differential Diagnosis of Hypercalcemia**					
Causes	**Sr CA**	**Sr PO$_4$**	**PTH**	**PTHrP**	**1,25 Vit D**	**Urine Calcium**
PHPT	↑	↓	↑→	↓	↑	↑↑
Cancer PTHrP	↑↑	↓	↓	↑	↓	↑↑
CRF–3HPT Creatinine ↑	↑↓	↑↑	↑↑	↓	↓	↓
FHH Mg ↑	↑	→	↑→	↓	→	↓↓
Milk alk Vit D	↑	↑↓	↓	↓	↑	↑

PTH, parathyroid hormone; PTHrP, parathyroid hormone–related protein; PHPT, primary hyperparathyroidism; CRF, chronic renal failure; HPT, hyperparathyroidism; FHH, familial hypocalciuric hypercalcemia; milk alk Vit D, milk alkali vitamin D.

Management of PHPT

Surgical resection of the affected gland(s) results in cure. Only about 30% of patients with PHPT need surgery at the time of diagnosis. Therefore, the following consensus criteria were generated by a panel of experts, and some changes to these criteria were adopted later; the goal is for the early identification of subjects that are at risk of developing end-organ damage and to prevent progression. The indications for surgery recommended by the expert panel are as follows:

Parameter	2002	2009	2014
Serum calcium	>1 mg	>1 mg	>1 mg
Urine calcium	>400 mg/d	Not recommended	>400 mg/d and nephrolithiasis or risk
Creatinine clearance	Reduction of 30% or more	<60 mL/min	<60 mL/min
BMD-DXA	T-score <−2.5 at any site	T-score <−2.5 same plus previous fracture	T-score <−2.5 at any site and vertebral fracture by other imaging
Age	<50 y	<50 y	<50 y

Surgical management of PHPT involves neck exploration with removal of the abnormal gland. Minimally invasive surgery (MIS) utilizes presurgical imaging to locate the abnormal gland, thereby guiding the surgeon to the diseased gland. MIS results in smaller incision and shorter recuperation times when compared with traditional exploration. Technetium-99m sestamibi scan (Parathyroid adenomas are rich in mitochondria, which trap this isotope. This scan is also used in cardiac imaging. The heart is another mitochondria-rich organ.) and high-resolution neck ultrasound are the two commonly used imaging tools. Also, with the availability of rapid PTH, once the adenoma is removed, PTH levels plummet (the half-life of PTH is <5 min), which enables biochemical confirmation of adenoma removal.

PHPT: Important Points

Insidious onset and gradual progression
Kidney stones in 20% to 30%
Bone loss—cortical > trabecular bone
Surgery is the only definitive management
Single gland tumor is common (85%)

Medical management of PHPT is practiced in poor surgical candidates and those with mild disease. **Bisphosphonates**, selective estrogen receptor modulators (SERMs), and estrogen are all useful to varying degrees in any given patient. Allosteric calcium receptor modulator such as **cinacalcet** that binds to CaSR is used for controlling calcium levels in select patients with PHPT.

Familial Hypocalciuric Hypercalcemia

FHH is a benign condition that results from germline mutation involving the CSR.[16,17] These inactivating mutations affecting the CSR upset their operating set point ranges (Fig. 24.6). Unlike in PHPT, the PTH production and calcium elevation in this condition are not progressive and result in stable mild hypercalcemia since birth. The hallmarks of this disorder include mild hypercalcemia, hypocalciuria (renal tubular cell calcium sensing is upset resulting in urine 24-hour calcium levels of <100 mg/d), mild PTH elevation (the parathyroid cellular calcium sensing is also abnormal), and mild elevation of magnesium. The hallmark is low urinary calcium excretion. Urinary fractional excretion in this condition is less than 1%, that is, less than 0.01. Magnesium levels are mildly elevated. Inheritance is autosomal dominant with 100% penetrance among carriers, resulting in multiple members in the family being affected.

The following are the salient clinical and diagnostic features:

1. Serum calcium is elevated (mild to moderate elevation).
2. Serum magnesium is mildly elevated.
3. PTH is mildly elevated.
4. Urine calcium levels are typically less than 100 mg in 24 hours, with fractional excretion of urine calcium of less than 1% (i.e., ≤0.01 is highly suggestive of a diagnosis of FHH).
5. Mutant CSR can be demonstrated.
6. End-organ dysfunction (bone and kidney) is uncommon; therefore, surgery should not be performed.

Antibodies to the CSR upset the set point and induce hypercalcemia; these patients have normal calcium receptors. Surgical removal of parathyroid gland(s) should not

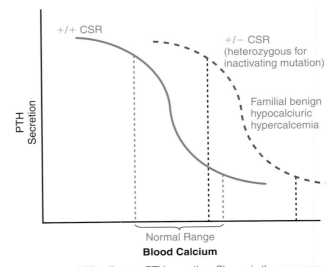

FIGURE 24.6 CSR: effect on PTH secretion. Shown is the response of parathyroid tissue (as demonstrated by PTH secretion) to blood calcium. The *set point* is determined by the parathyroid response mediated by the transmembrane CSR. The *normal curve* is for heterozygosity for the "wild-type" SCR (+/+). The *right-shifted curve* is shown for the case where there is heterozygosity for the receptor (familial benign hypocalciuric hypercalcemia): one wild-type copy of the gene and one inactivating mutation (+/−).

be performed in these patients. Hence, it is very important to differentiate this disorder from PHPT to avoid unnecessary and ineffective surgeries.

Hyperthyroidism

Due to the direct effects of thyroxine on the bones, there is increased resorption and hypercalcemia. PTH levels are low.

FHH: Important Points

Low urine calcium
No end-organ damage
Multiple family members are affected
Mild elevation of magnesium
Surgery is ineffective and should not be performed

Addison's Disease

Hypercalcemia is commonly seen in patients presenting with addisonian crisis. PTH levels are low. It gets corrected promptly with fluid and steroid replacement. It is thought to be a result of hypovolemia and dehydration. The exact mechanism is truly unknown.

Milk Alkali Syndrome

This syndrome in its classic form, described in the 1930s, follows the oral administration of very high (>20 g) amount of calcium and large amounts of milk to control gastric acid levels in patients with peptic ulcer disease. The hallmark of this disorder includes hypercalcemia, alkalosis, and renal impairment. Serum phosphate is often elevated. It is very rare to see the typical form of MAS now because of the use of proton pump inhibitors and H_2 blockers.

The reappearance of MAS in the 1990s follows the supplementation with lower amounts (even 1.5 to 2 g) of calcium carbonate for the treatment of osteoporosis in elderly patients with renal insufficiency. The presenting features are hypercalcemia, alkalosis, dehydration, and renal impairment with mental status changes. Serum phosphate level is low (administered salt is carbonate or citrate). Therapy includes intravenous and oral hydration and cessation of excessive calcium supplementation.

Medications That Cause Hypercalcemia

HCTZ and lithium are the most common of drugs that induce hypercalcemia. HCTZ enhances distal tubular calcium absorption. Lithium affects the formation of intracellular inositol triphosphate, thereby upsetting the CSR function (similar to FHH).

Hypervitaminosis D is a condition that may result from excessive intake of vitamin D. It may also result from aberrant production of $1,25(OH)_2D$ as a result of extrarenal 1α-hydroxylation of 25-hydroxy vitamin D. Granulomatous diseases such as sarcoidosis and tuberculosis and certain lymphomas are capable of this effect. The granulomas or lymphoid tissue that hydroxylates vitamin D is autonomous, and this is not regulated by the normal feedback mechanism; therefore, calcium elevation can be significant. Hypercalcemia

results from increased GI absorption of calcium, without increase in bone resorption; therefore, bisphosphonates are not useful to control blood calcium levels. Also, the normal parathyroid glands respond to the elevation of calcium with reduction of PTH production, resulting in low PTH levels. These subjects also have elevated urine calcium levels.[18]

A variety of cancers may lead to hypercalcemia as a result of production and release of cytokines or PTH-like substances. These tumor-produced humoral substances are not responsive to negative feedback by calcium; therefore, these subjects can have massive elevation of serum calcium levels with low serum PTH levels.[18]

Parathyroid hormone–related protein (PTHrP) is a substance secreted by cancers that shares structural similarities to the N-terminal portion of human PTH molecule. Therefore, it retains functional features of PTH, with some critical differences. Both PTH and PTHrP bind to the same receptor in the kidney and bone as well as a variety of other tissues. In humans, PTHrP functions in the paracrine regulation of cartilage, skin, brain, and lactating breast tissue. In healthy humans, circulating levels of PTHrP are very low or immeasurable. Normal lactating breast tissue is capable of producing PTHrP, which can result in hypercalcemia and resolves following stopping breast-feeding. In most clinical situations of hypercalcemia due to PTHrP secretion, an underlying cancer is the root cause.[19] PTHrP can be secreted by a variety of cancers as described earlier in this chapter. The secretion is not regulated by even very high blood calcium levels, which results in severe hypercalcemia (Fig. 24.7). When humoral hypercalcemia of malignancy is suspected, PTHrP can be measured by specific immunoassay. Also, the intact PTH assay does not cross-react with circulating PTHrP. Normal parathyroid glands sense the elevated calcium levels and markedly reduce the secretion of PTH; therefore, PTH is very low. One salient difference in the biological functions between PTH and PTHrP is the inability of the latter to facilitate renal hydroxylation of 25-hydroxy vitamin D. This dichotomy in function between these otherwise functionally similar protein hormones remains unexplained.

There are a variety of medications that can cause hypercalcemia. **Thiazide diuretics** are used in the treatment of

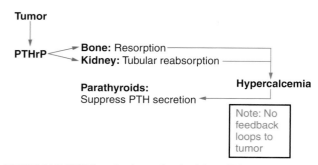

FIGURE 24.7 PTHrP endocrine pathophysiology. This demonstrates the effect of tumors that overproduce PTHrP. The pathophysiologic effect is via the same organ systems used by PTH to increase blood calcium. The difference between PTH and PTHrP is that PTH is subject to feedback regulation, whereas PTHrP is not subject to any feedback regulation by calcium (compare with Fig. 24.4).

hypertension. This agent reduces the renal excretion of calcium, leading to calcium retention and hypercalcemia. At doses routinely used to treat hypertension, hypercalcemia is uncommon in subjects with normal calcium axis. However, when thiazide diuretics are used in subjects with other conditions associated with hypercalcemia such as PHPT, hypercalcemia can be worsened. In patients with subclinical PHPT, hypercalcemia can be precipitated by thiazide diuretics, leading to "unmasking" of PHPT.

Lithium carbonate, when used to treat bipolar disorder, can cause hypercalcemia. Lithium reduces intracellular formation of inositol triphosphate levels altering the "set point" of CSRs, a mechanism similar to FHH mentioned earlier.

High doses of vitamin A, or vitamin A analogs/metabolites in the retinoic acid family, may cause hypercalcemia. Vitamin A is believed to activate osteoclasts and enhance bone resorption, elevating blood calcium. In this condition, both PTH and 1,25(OH)$_2$D are suppressed.

CASE STUDY 24.2

A 58-year-old man has been a smoker since childhood. He has been smoking three packs per day since he can remember but insists his cigarettes "don't hurt me none, doc." He has been feeling ill recently, however, with loss of appetite, malaise, and weight loss. His mental ability has been dulled recently, and he can't remember from "one minute to the next" especially notable during his work as a cowboy. His cigarettes have not been as enjoyable for him as they used to be. His baseline cough has worsened, and he has noticed blood streaking his sputum when he clears sputum from his throat. He has no significant past medical history other than his tobacco abuse. He takes no medications. His family history is only notable for his father dying of lung cancer at age 63 and his mother dying of emphysema at age 68. On physical examination, he is a thin man who looks much older than his chronologic age and appears unwell. When he produces some sputum at the physician's request, it does indeed have a pink tinge and is streaked with blood. Chest examination reveals some scattered wheezing and some rales in the right upper lung region. He is diffusely weak on muscle strength testing. Labs are notable for calcium 16.8 mg/dL (normal, 8.5 to 10.2 mg/dL), albumin 3.4 (normal, 3.5 to 4.8 g/dL), BUN 27 mg/dL, and creatinine 1.3 mg/dL. Chest radiograph reveals a 3-cm proximal right hilar mass with distal streaking. Further testing is prompted and reveals a PTH of less than 1 pg/mL (normal, 11 to 54 pg/mL) and PTHrP elevated at 18.3 pmol/L (normal 0.0 to 1.5 pmol/L).

Questions

1. Do you think this patient's smoking is related to his hypercalcemia?

2. What other laboratory results are abnormal?

3. What is this patient's diagnosis? His prognosis?

HYPOCALCEMIA

Hypocalcemia refers to low blood calcium levels. It can result from a wide variety of conditions, from organ system dysfunction to lack of hormone effect to acid–base disturbances. The signs and symptoms of hypocalcemia are described below:

Neuromuscular: Tetany (involuntary muscle contraction) affecting primarily the muscles in the hands, feet, legs, and back may be seen. Percussion on cranial nerve VII (facial nerve) just anterior to the ear may elicit twitching in the ipsilateral corner of the mouth (Chvostek's sign). Numbness and tingling in the face, hands, and feet may be seen. Inflation of a blood pressure cuff to 20 mm Hg above the patient's systolic blood pressure to induce a state of ischemia in the arm (metabolic acidosis) may cause spasm in the muscles of the wrist and hand (Trousseau's sign).

CNS: Irritability, seizures, personality changes, and impaired intellectual functioning may be seen.

Cardiovascular: Calcium plays a crucial role not only in the slow inward calcium current of the QRS complex of ventricular depolarization but also in electromechanical coupling. In hypocalcemia, QT prolongation may be seen on the ECG. In the extreme, electromechanical dissociation may be seen. Cardiac contractile dysfunction is rare but in the extreme can result in congestive heart failure. Cardiac dysfunction from hypocalcemia should be treated with emergent intravenous calcium.

Causes of Hypocalcemia

1. Endocrine causes: hypoparathyroidism (lack of PTH):
   - Postoperative
   - Autoimmune (isolated or part of polyglandular autoimmune syndrome)
   - Congenital (mutations of CSR, PTH, and parathyroid aplasia)
   - Pseudohypoparathyroidism, types 1a, 1b, and 2
2. Deficiency of vitamin D: malnutrition, malabsorption due to celiac sprue, weight loss, gastric surgeries, short bowel syndrome, abdominal irradiation, pancreatic disease, liver disease, and renal disease.
3. Hypomagnesemia: magnesium depletion leads to lack of PTH synthesis and release.

The causes of hypocalcemia will be discussed in the setting of both endocrine and organ system dysfunction. However, one key concept should be emphasized when considering hypocalcemia: when functioning properly, the parathyroid glands will not only correct falling blood calcium but also *prevent* it, by increasing PTH secretion. The compensatory rise in PTH secretion, in response to factors that would lower blood calcium, is known as *secondary hyperparathyroidism*. Thus, an individual may have an elevated PTH level—for example, in response to low 25-hydroxy vitamin D—and thus maintain normocalcemia.

Secondary hyperparathyroidism is notable for the normal response of parathyroid glands with appropriate and vigorous secretion of PTH. The biochemical constellation includes low blood calcium, elevated PTH, low serum phosphate, elevated alkaline phosphatase, hypocalciuria, phosphaturia, and vitamin D deficiency or lack of vitamin D effect.[20] Treatment of secondary hyperparathyroidism is directed toward correcting the process inducing hypocalcemia and/or vitamin D deficiency.[21]

CASE STUDY 24.3

A 26-year-old man presents to his physician 3 weeks after having his thyroid surgically removed for thyroid cancer. His doctor is certain that she "got it all." However, since the time he went home from the hospital, he has noticed painful, involuntary muscle cramping. He also feels numbness and tingling around his mouth and in his hands and feet. His girlfriend says he has been irritable for the last couple of weeks. His past medical history is notable only for the recent diagnosis of thyroid cancer, and its resection 3 weeks prior to this visit. His only medication is levothyroxine. Family history contributes no relevant information. On physical examination, he has a well-healing thyroidectomy scar. Tapping on the face interior to the ears causes twitching in the ipsilateral corner of the mouth (Chvostek's sign). There are no palpable masses in the thyroid bed. A blood pressure cuff inflated above the systolic pressure induces involuntary muscle contracture in the ipsilateral hand after 60 seconds (Trousseau's sign). Labs are notable for calcium 5.6 mg/dL (normal, 8.5 to 10.2 mg/dL), albumin 4.1 g/dL, BUN 20 mg/dL, and creatinine 1.0 mg/dL. PTH is undetectable at less than 1 pg/mL.

Questions

1. Which laboratory results are abnormal?
2. What condition is he experiencing since his thyroidectomy?
3. What is the cause of this symptomatic condition?
4. What is the treatment for this patient, in addition to thyroxine medication?

Endocrine Causes of Hypocalcemia

Because proper PTH secretion and action are necessary to maintain normocalcemia, any inadequacy of parathyroid gland function will cause hypocalcemia. The most common cause of hypoparathyroidism is neck surgery, especially, after thyroidectomy with lymph node dissection. This results from accidental removal of these glands due to their small size. The most common outcome is temporary hypoparathyroidism following surgery, due to damage of the delicate parathyroid blood supply, which results in full recovery in most subjects. Parathyroid glands can

be reimplanted into pouches created in skeletal muscles (deltoid, sternomastoid, or forearm muscles). Parathyroid glands also survive careful cryopreservation and reimplantation back into its original owner. Additional causes of hypoparathyroidism include autoimmune destruction of parathyroid tissue. This condition is often associated with other autoimmune diseases such as type 1 diabetes, Hashimoto's thyroiditis, and Addison's disease. Magnesium deficiency can inhibit the secretion of PTH and also blunt its actions on target tissues. Following the correction of hypomagnesemia, PTH secretion and function are reestablished. Depending on the cause, hypoparathyroidism can usually be treated with relatively high doses of vitamin D and calcium. In the absence of PTH, even the small fraction of passively absorbed calcium may simply be excreted in the urine. Hypercalciuria increases the risk of development of kidney stones in these subjects. The use of HCTZ reduces urine calcium losses and elevates serum calcium levels in PTH-deficient subjects.

Pseudohypoparathyroidism is a heritable disorder resulting in a lack of responsiveness to PTH in the target tissue. This results from uncoupling of the PTH receptor from adenylate cyclase, due to a mutant stimulatory G protein (G_s). PTH binds its receptor but cannot activate the second messenger, cAMP, and thus, there is no response. Hypocalcemia develops, although unlike other forms of hypoparathyroidism mentioned, those with pseudohypoparathyroidism have markedly elevated levels of PTH. This is an example of a hormone resistance syndrome. Treatment is with calcium and vitamin D supplementation.

Hypovitaminosis D describes a collection of conditions, including low vitamin D availability, defective metabolism of vitamin D, or mutations in the vitamin D receptor, all of which predispose to hypocalcemia.

Organ System Causes of Hypocalcemia

A variety of intestinal disorders can result in malabsorption of calcium or vitamin D resulting in hypocalcemia. Causes include short bowel syndrome, abdominal irradiation, weight loss surgeries, celiac sprue, and bowel fistulation. Treatment end points are normalization of urine calcium excretion and normalization of PTH.

METABOLIC BONE DISEASES

A variety of disease states can affect skeletal architecture, strength, and integrity. Only **rickets**, **osteomalacia**, and osteoporosis are described here.

Rickets and Osteomalacia

Rickets and osteomalacia are diseases caused by abnormal mineralization of bone. They result from vitamin D deficiency. *Rickets* refers to the disease state affecting growing bones (in children); therefore, permanent skeletal deformity can be seen. *Osteomalacia* refers to the abnormal mineralization of bone in adults or after completion of skeletal maturation. Rickets is associated with bony deformities because of bending of long bones under weight loading and effects of gravity. Bone deformity is not seen in adults. Both conditions are associated with similar biochemical findings of secondary hyperparathyroidism. Fractures may result in either case because of poor bone structure. Hypocalcemia may be seen when the response of secondary hyperparathyroidism is inadequate to counteract the threat of hypocalcemia posed by the vitamin D deficiency. Food fortified with Vitamin D is intended to reduce the risk of developing vitamin D deficiency. Despite these attempts, due to poor consumption of dairy and avoidance of sun exposure, deficiency states do occur. However, those of any age who live indoors, with minimal or no sun exposure, or who lack dietary vitamin D, are at risk for developing this condition. As mentioned in the discussion on vitamin D physiology, adequacy of vitamin D in the body can be assessed by measuring the blood level of 25-hydroxy vitamin D. Because secondary hyperparathyroidism is also expected in the setting of rickets or osteomalacia, PTH and calcium should be obtained to further confirm the suspected diagnosis.

CASE STUDY 24.4

An 82-year-old woman living in a nursing home feels unsteady on her feet and does not wander outside anymore. She has lactose intolerance and has never been able to drink milk. She does not take any dietary supplements. She says, "I feel my age, doc," but otherwise has no specific complaints. On her annual laboratory assessment, her calcium level is found to be slightly low at 8.2 mg/dL (normal, 8.5 to 10.2 mg/dL) with albumin 3.5 g/dL (normal, 3.5 to 4.8 g/dL), BUN 28 mg/dL, and creatinine 1.1 mg/dL. This prompts further evaluation, which reveals PTH elevated at 181 pg/mL and 25-hydroxy vitamin D low at 6 ng/mL (normal, 20 to 50 ng/mL).

Questions

1. What diagnostic possibility is suggested from the initial laboratory results of her annual assessment?

2. This patient's differential diagnosis includes two diseases. What are they?

3. Is her renal function related to either of these two diseases?

4. How should this patient be treated?

Rickets can, however, develop under conditions of adequate amounts of vitamin D. This unique situation may develop from genetic defects in vitamin D metabolism or in the vitamin D receptor. Although 25-hydroxy vitamin D level is often normal, $1,25(OH)_2D$ level may be low, normal, or high depending on the genetic defect. Defects in vitamin D metabolism are best treated by supplying the metabolically active compound, $1,25(OH)_2D$ (calcitriol). A wide variety of vitamin D receptor defects have been described, including abnormal ligand binding, abnormal DNA binding, and abnormal transactivation of transcriptional machinery at the regulatory site of vitamin D–responsive genes. The type of defect present determines how well the patient will respond to pharmacologic doses of calcitriol.

Osteoporosis

Osteoporosis is the most prevalent metabolic bone disease in adults. Osteoporosis affects an estimated 20 to 25 million Americans with an estimated 4:1 female-to-male predominance. It is believed to cause approximately 1.5 million fractures annually in the United States. A recent study estimates that 4.5 million women, aged greater than 50 years, have osteoporosis of the hip.[22] The most devastating consequence of osteoporosis is a hip fracture. While as many as half of vertebral compressions may be asymptomatic, a hip fracture carries with it a significant morbidity as well as an increased mortality. Most hip fractures require surgery at the very least. Mortality from hip fracture is increased by about 20% in the first year following the fracture, and it is estimated that the number of deaths related to hip fracture are now on par with those from breast cancer.

Multiple additional conditions have been identified as significant risk factors for reduced bone mass and a consequent increased risk of fracture, although risk factor assessment alone is generally not sufficient to characterize or quantify bone mass and diagnose osteoporosis. The following are validated risk factors for the prediction of fracture, independent of formal bone density evaluation: decreased bone mass due to previous fracture, advanced age, family history of osteoporosis or fracture, body weight less than 127 lb, long-term glucocorticoid therapy, cigarette smoking, or excess alcohol intake. Other conditions known to also alter calcium metabolism and increase fracture risk include Cushing's syndrome, hyperparathyroidism, disorders of vitamin D metabolism, hyperthyroidism, and certain malignancies (mast cell disease). Several medications have negative effects on the skeleton, leading to low bone mass and increase in the risk of fractures. The most notable are the glucocorticoids. They are widely used to treat a variety of inflammatory conditions such as asthma, rheumatoid arthritis, and lupus, as well as to prevent rejection after organ transplantation. First, they limit bone formation by inhibiting the action of osteoblasts while also inducing osteoblast apoptosis. They also increase the bone breakdown by stimulating the formation and action of osteoclasts. Therefore, the net loss of bone mass is compounded. "Glucocorticoid-induced osteoporosis" is a major source of morbidity associated with pharmacologic doses of glucocorticoids. Two bisphosphonates, alendronate and risedronate, are approved by the Food and Drug Administration (FDA) for the treatment of glucocorticoid-induced bone loss. Other medications that induce low bone mass include anticonvulsants (particularly phenytoin) and cyclosporin A.

CASE STUDY 24.5

A 6-year-old girl is brought to a pediatrician by her parents who report that her height is not progressing as they think it should (or like it did for her 8-year-old sister) and her legs look bowed. The patient drinks milk, and other than her shorter stature and bowed legs, she has the normal characteristics of her 6-year-old friends. She takes no medications. Family history is notable for some cousins on the father's side with a similar problem back in the Appalachian Hill country along Virginia/Tennessee border where the family hails from. The pediatrician obtains lab studies that are notable for a calcium level of 7.2 mg/dL (normal, 8.5 to 10.2 mg/dL) with albumin 4.1 g/dL (normal, 3.5 to 4.8 g/dL). Lower extremity radiographs show bowing of the long bones and generalized demineralization. This prompts the measurement of several other laboratory tests, which reveal intact PTH elevated at 866 pg/mL (normal, 11 to 54 pg/mL), 25-hydroxy vitamin D normal at 35 ng/mL (normal, 20 to 57 ng/mL), and 1,25(OH)$_2$D undetectable at less than 1 pg/mL (normal, 20 to 75 pg/mL).

Questions

1. What condition do the preliminary lab tests indicate?
2. What is the significance of 25-hydroxy vitamin D and 1,25(OH)$_2$D levels in the follow-up laboratory tests?
3. Describe the inborn error of metabolism with this patient.
4. What secondary condition will recur if vitamin D treatment is discontinued later in her life?

Diagnosis of Osteoporosis

Several laboratory tests are available and useful for the evaluation of a subject with osteoporosis and other bone disorders. There are no specific laboratory tests that can be used to diagnose osteoporosis. The vast majority of osteoporotic subjects will have normal biochemical tests. The diagnosis rests on clinical risk factors and **dual-energy x-ray absorptiometry (DEXA)** scan. In 2008, the WHO created a well-validated fracture assessment tool, which enables clinicians to identify a given individual's 10-year fracture risk based on simple data, even in the absence of DEXA scan results. The hallmark of osteoporosis is skeletal fragility; therefore, it can be diagnosed without any additional testing when a fracture occurs at an inappropriate degree of trauma or following trivial trauma or no trauma at all. This is termed a *fragility* fracture (Fig. 24.8). The occurrence of one fragility fracture predicts further fragility fractures. Currently, osteoporosis is also diagnosed based upon calculated bone density using DEXA of the lumbar spine and the hip. This imaging technique, commonly referred to as bone mineral densitometry, measures grams of calcium per square centimeter of cross-sectional area of bone (g/cm^2). Density is mass/volume, or g/cm^3, so the term bone *density* is a misnomer. Peak bone mass usually occurs at about the age of 30 years for both men and women and is associated with the lowest risk of fracture. The bone "density," as calculated by DEXA, is then compared with that expected in a healthy 30-year-old individual of the same race and gender. This is reported as SDs above or below the mean peak bone mass using a "T-score." A positive or "+" T-score equates to above the average peak bone mass and negative or "−" is for below the average peak bone mass. Normal bone density is defined as 1 SD from the mean, or a T-score between −1.0 and +1.0. Osteoporosis is defined as a T-score of −2.5 or below. An intermediate between normal and osteoporosis,

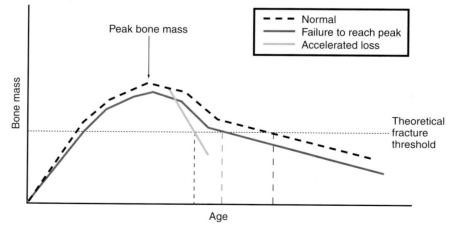

FIGURE 24.8 Bone mass as a function of age; perturbations that can affect bone mass. Shown is the accrual of bone mass with age to a peak that occurs in the mid-twenties to early thirties (for both sexes) and the bone loss that occurs throughout life after the peak. Fracture risk increases as bone mass is lost. The "theoretical fracture threshold" is an artificial notion but may be useful in demonstrating that at a given degree of trauma (varying from the simple act of weight bearing to increasing levels of impact) factors that are associated with low bone mass increase fracture risk and that the age that fracture risk is reached is relatively lower if the lower bone mass is reached earlier.

termed *osteopenia*, is diagnosed as a T-score between −1.0 and −2.5. In summary, osteoporosis is diagnosed by either the occurrence of a fragility fracture or a T-score of −2.5 or below by DEXA imaging.

Treatment of Osteoporosis

Treatment of osteoporosis is directed at prevention of the primary consequence of this disease: fracture. All treatment plans should include modification of preventable risk factors such as smoking and alcohol consumption. They should also include an evaluation of fall risk and consideration of walkers, handrails, night-lights, hip pads, etc. Further, all patients with osteoporosis—or those at high risk for developing osteoporosis—should have adequate dietary calcium (usually 1,200 to 1,500 mg daily) and vitamin D (usually 400 to 800 IU daily). The most commonly used medications for the prevention and treatment of osteoporosis are the antiresorptive agents. Examples of commonly used bisphosphonates include alendronate, risedronate, ibandronate, and zoledronate. The bisphosphonate agents have unusual side effects. They can cause upper GI ulceration if the pill gets retained in the esophagus; therefore, patients are instructed to stay upright after swallowing the pills with water, to prevent retention. Chronic use is associated with osteonecrosis of the jaw and low bone turnover fracture of the thigh bone.[22,23] The most commonly used SERM is raloxifene. Testosterone is commonly used in males with hypogonadism and estrogen ± progestin in women. **Teriparatide** is an anabolic agent, one which forms bone, rather than blocks resorption, unlike bisphosphonates. It is very effective for the treatment of those with osteoporosis. Teriparatide stimulates the formation of both cortical and trabecular bones without increasing the bone resorption. Furthermore, it can be used sequentially with an antiresorptive drug, which can further potentiate the positive effects on the skeleton. Because it is a peptide hormone, it requires subcutaneous injections. Currently, it is only approved for the treatment of severe osteoporosis, and its use for the treatment of hypoparathyroidism is being evaluated. This agent is used for a period of 2 years. A unique side effect in experimental animals is the formation of bone tumor, which has not been observed in human subjects.

CASE STUDY 24.6

A 74-year-old woman slipped while mopping the kitchen floor, fell, and sustained a hip fracture. The hip fracture was treated with open reduction and internal fixation. After discharge from the hospital, she presents to her physician and asks if she has osteoporosis and, if so, what should be done. She only drinks milk on her cereal and takes no dietary supplements of calcium or vitamin D. She has asthma and has been treated with prednisone bursts and tapers about six times in her life (as best she can recall).

She went through menopause at age 49 and never took hormone replacement. Other than her hip, she reports no other fractures in adulthood but does report that she thinks she has lost about 2.5 in. in height. She thinks her mom had osteoporosis, because she had a "dowager's hump." The physician orders bone densitometry, which shows postero-anterior spine T-score −3.8 and hip T-score −3.1 (done on the nonfractured hip!). Labs revealed normal calcium and albumin, renal function, thyroid function, albumin, and CBC. Alkaline phosphatase is slightly elevated, but she has a recent fracture.

Questions

1. What is this patient's diagnosis?
2. Name four or five risk factors for this diagnosis.
3. In addition to adequate calcium and vitamin D supplements, this patient would be a candidate for which new therapeutic drug?

SECONDARY HYPERPARATHYROIDISM IN RENAL FAILURE

The kidney's central role in the regulation of bone and mineral metabolism was discussed earlier. Chronic kidney disease (CKD) results in striking bone mineral and skeletal changes. The diseased kidneys fail to excrete phosphate; this along with the impaired formation of $1,25(OH)_2D$ leads to a vicious cycle of events resulting in parathyroid gland stimulation and hyperplasia. The bone mineral metabolic changes are progressive and proportional to the severity of renal dysfunction and eventually ubiquitous in patients with end-stage renal disease. In severe cases, the ensuing parathyroid hyperplasia results in autonomy of the parathyroid gland leading to hypercalcemia; this is also referred to as tertiary hyperparathyroidism. The difference between secondary and tertiary hyperparathyroidism is the development of sustained hypercalcemia. Patients who develop transient, iatrogenic hypercalcemia encountered in a renal failure patient should not be given the diagnosis of tertiary hyperparathyroidism. The term tertiary is not widely used nowadays. In early stages of CKD, in response to low blood calcium and elevation of phosphate levels, compensatory elevation of PTH and FGF23 maintains near-normal calcium and phosphorus levels.[24] As kidney disease becomes severe, the compensatory mechanisms are overwhelmed, leading to permanent abnormalities of calcium, phosphorus, PTH, vitamin D, bone mineralization, and vascular and soft tissue calcification. These biochemical changes completely resolve following renal transplantation. Renal replacement therapies such as hemodialysis and peritoneal dialysis only induce partial correction of these changes.

One of the earliest changes in CKD is reduction of urinary phosphorus excretion, leading to an increase in serum phosphorus levels. Compensatory increase in the phosphaturic hormones such as FGF23 and PTH helps maintain near-normal serum phosphate levels for a period. When renal function declines to lower than 30 mL/min, hyperphosphatemia is observed. Hyperphosphatemia also stimulates PTH secretion and inhibits 1,25(OH)$_2$D production. Low 1,25(OH)$_2$D leads to poor GI absorption of calcium. Hyperphosphatemia and elevation of FGF23 levels are independent predictors of survival; higher levels are associated with poorer outcomes.[24] Hyperphosphatemia is treated with a combination of dietary restriction of phosphorus and oral phosphate binders. Commonly used phosphate binders include calcium carbonate, calcium acetate, and noncalcium binders including sevelamer and lanthanum. Patients with CKD have low blood calcium levels. The imbalance in calcium and phosphate levels results in extracellular deposition of calcium resulting in vascular and tissue calcification, a condition called calciphylaxis, which results in increased mortality.

Most patients with CKD have low 1,25(OH)$_2$D levels. As phosphorus levels increase, FGF23 levels increase as a compensatory mechanism, which in turn inhibits 1α-hydroxylation of 25-hydroxy vitamin D. The decreased 1,25(OH)$_2$D leads to impaired calcium absorption, and the lower calcium levels stimulate PTH release. This triggers a cascade of bone mineral metabolic events leading to poor bone mineralization.

PTH is secreted in response to hypocalcemia, hyperphosphatemia, and/or low 1,25(OH)$_2$D levels. PTH levels trend up with increasing severity of renal disease. Secondary hyperparathyroidism is treated with vitamin D analogs such as calcitriol, doxercalciferol, and paricalcitol.[25] Calcimimetics are allosteric activators of the extracellular CSR, sensitizing the parathyroid gland to extracellular calcium and decreasing PTH secretion independent of vitamin D. Calcimimetics such as cinacalcet have been shown to decrease PTH, calcium, and phosphorus.[26]

> **For additional student resources, please visit** the Point® **at http://thepoint.lww.com**

questions

1. True or false? PTH and 1,25(OH)$_2$D (vitamin D) are the principal hormones involved in the normal physiologic regulation of calcium homeostasis.

2. The primary organs involved in the maintenance of calcium homeostasis are the intestine, _____, and kidney.

3. Skin, _____, and kidneys are involved in the production of the active metabolite of vitamin D.

4. True or false? Cod liver oil (ugh!) is a source of vitamin D.

5. True or false? 1,25(OH)$_2$D is the best blood test for determining adequacy of vitamin D stores in the body.

6. True or false? PTHrP is produced by some cancers and often leads to cancer-associated hypercalcemia.

7. True or false? 1,25(OH)$_2$D, due to 1-hydroxylase activity in macrophages, may be produced to excess in granulomatous diseases and lymphoid disorders, leading to hypercalcemia.

8. In PHPT, the defect primarily lies in _____. In secondary hyperparathyroidism, the defect primarily lies with the threat of _____ to the body.

9. Development of _____ _____ is the primary complication of hypercalciuria (increased urinary excretion of calcium).

10. _____ _____ is the most common cause of hypoparathyroidism.

11. _____ is a type of bone most rapidly lost in response to hypogonadism and glucocorticoid therapy.

12. _____ cells in bone are responsible for bone resorption, and _____ cells are responsible for bone formation.

13. _____ is the most prevalent metabolic bone disease in the United States.

14. True or false? Hormone replacement does not inhibit bone resorption in osteoporotic patients.

15. True or false? Teriparatide is the only drug currently approved by the FDA for the treatment of osteoporosis that directly stimulates bone formation (i.e., it is not an antiresorptive drug).

references

1. Neer R, Berman M, Fisher L, et al. Multicompartmental analysis of calcium kinetics in normal adult males. *J Clin Invest.* 1967;46:1364–1379.

2. Norman AW, Roth J, Orci L. The vitamin D endocrine system: steroid metabolism, hormone receptors and biological response. *Endocrine Rev.* 1982;3:331–366.

3. Sheikh MD, Ramirez A, Emmett M, et al. Role of vitamin D dependent and vitamin D independent mechanisms in absorption of food calcium. *J Clin Invest.* 1988;81:126–132.

4. Gallagher JC, Riggs BL, Eisman J, et al. Intestinal calcium absorption and serum vitamin D metabolites in normal subjects and osteoporotic patients. *J Clin Invest.* 1979;64:729–736.

5. Owen R. On the anatomy of the Indian Rhinoceros (Rh. Unicornis L.). *Trans Zool Soc Lond.* 1862;4:31–58.

6. Gilmore JR. The gross anatomy of parathyroid glands. *J Pathol.* 1938;46:133.

7. Alveryd A. Parathyroid glands in thyroid surgery. *Acta Chir Scand.* 1968;389:1.

8. Block GA, Klassen PS, Lazarus JM, et al. Mineral metabolism, mortality, and morbidity in maintenance hemodialysis. *J Am Soc Nephrol.* 2004;15(8):2208–2218.

9. Sakou T. Bone morphogenetic proteins: from basic studies to clinical approaches. *Bone.* 1998;22:591–603.

10. Heath H, Hodgson SR, Kennedy MA. Primary hyperparathyroidism: incidence, morbidity and economic impact in a community. *N Eng J Med.* 1980;302:189–193.

11. Albright E, Reifenstein EC. *The Parathyroid Glands and Metabolic Bone Disease.* Baltimore, MD: Williams and Wilkins; 1948.

12. Yeh MW, Ituarte PHG, Zhou HC, et al. Incidence and prevalence of primary hyperparathyroidism in a racially mixed population. *J Clin Endocrinol Metab.* 2013;98(3):1122–1129.

13. Abdulla AG, Ituarte P, Harari A, et al. Trends in the frequency and quality of parathyroid surgery: analysis of 17,082 cases over 10 years. *Ann Surg.* 2015;261(4):746–750.

14. Eastell R, Brandi ML, Costa AG, et al. Diagnosis of asymptomatic primary hyperparathyroidism: Proceedings of the Fourth International Workshop. *J Clin Endocrinol Metab.* 2014;99:3570–3579.

15. Abraham D, Sharma PK, Bentz J, et al. The utility of ultrasound guided FNA of parathyroid adenomas for pre-operative localization prior to minimally invasive parathyroidectomy. *Endocr Pract.* 2007;13(4):333–337.

16. Brown EM, Gamba G, Rccardi D, et al. Cloning and characterization of an extracellular calcium sensing receptor from bovine parathyroid. *Nature.* 1993;366:575.

17. Hendy GN, D'Souza-Li L, Yang B, et al. Mutations of the calcium-sensing receptor (CASR) in familial hypocalciuric hypercalcemia, neonatal severe hyperparathyroidism, and autosomal dominant hypocalcemia. *Hum Mutat.* 2000;16:281.

18. Stewart AF, Horst F, Deftos LJ, et al. Biochemical evaluation of patients with cancer-associated hypercalcemia: evidence for humoral and non-humoral groups. *N Eng J Med.* 1980;303:1377–1383.

19. Lips P, van Schoor NM, Bravenboer N. Vitamin D-related disorders. In: Rosen CJ, ed. *Primer on the Metabolic Bone Diseases and Disorders of Mineral Metabolism.* 7th ed. Washington, DC: American Society of Bone and Mineral Research; 2008:329.

20. Holick MF, Binkley NC, Bischoff-Ferrari HA, et al. Evaluation, treatment, and prevention of vitamin D deficiency: an Endocrine Society clinical practice guideline. *J Clin Endocrinol Metab.* 2011;96:1911.

21. Looker AC, Melton LJ III, Harris TB, et al. Prevalence and trends in low femur bone density among older US adults: NHANES 2005–2006 compared with NHANES III. *J Bone Miner Res.* 2010;25(1):64–71.

22. Watts NB, Diab DL. Long-term use of bisphosphonates in osteoporosis. *J Clin Endocrinol Metab.* 2010;95:1555.

23. Neer RM, Arnaud CD, Zanchetta JR, et al. Effect of parathyroid hormone (1-34) on fractures and bone mineral density in postmenopausal women with osteoporosis. *N Engl J Med.* 2001;344:1434–1441.

24. Gutierrez OM, Mannstadt M, Isakova T, et al. Fibroblast growth factor 23 and mortality among patients undergoing hemodialysis. *N Engl J Med.* 2008;359(6):584–592.

25. Sprague SM, Coyne D. Control of secondary hyperparathyroidism by vitamin D receptor agonists in chronic kidney disease. *Clin J Am Soc Nephrol.* 2010;5(3):512–518.

26. Block GA, Martin KJ, de Francisco AL, et al. Cinacalcet for secondary hyperparathyroidism in patients receiving hemodialysis. *N Engl J Med.* 2004;350(15):1516–1525.

25

Liver Function

JANELLE M. CHIASERA and XIN XU

chapter objectives

Upon completion of this chapter, the clinical laboratorian will be able to do the following:

- Diagram the anatomy of the liver.
- Explain the following functions of the liver: bile secretion, synthetic activity, and detoxification.
- List two important cell types associated with the liver and state the function of each.
- Define jaundice and classify the three different types of jaundice.
- Discuss the basic disorders of the liver and which laboratory tests may be performed to diagnose them.
- Evaluate liver-related data and correlate that data with normal or pathology states.
- Compare and contrast how total and direct bilirubin measurements are performed.
- List the enzymes most commonly used to assess hepatocellular and hepatobiliary disorders.
- Describe the various types of hepatitis to include cause, transmission, occurrence, alternate name, physiology, diagnosis, and treatment.

For additional student resources, please visit thePoint®
at http://thepoint.lww.com

The liver is a very large and complex organ responsible for performing vital tasks that impact all body systems. Its complex functions include metabolism of carbohydrates, lipids, proteins, and bilirubin; detoxification of harmful substances; storage of essential compounds; and excretion of substances to prevent harm. The liver is unique in the sense that it is a relatively resilient organ that can regenerate cells that have been destroyed by some short-term injury or disease or have been removed. However, if the liver is damaged repeatedly over a long period of time, it may undergo irreversible changes that permanently interfere with its essential functions. If the liver becomes completely nonfunctional for any reason, death will occur within approximately 24 hours due to hypoglycemia. This chapter focuses on the normal structure and function of the liver, the pathology associated with it, and the laboratory tests used to aid in the diagnosis of liver disorders.

ANATOMY

Gross Anatomy

Understanding the function and dysfunction of the liver depends on understanding its gross and microscopic structure. The liver is a large and complex organ weighing approximately 1.2 to 1.5 kg in the healthy adult. It is located beneath and attached to the diaphragm, is protected by the lower rib cage, and is held in place by ligamentous attachments. Despite the functional complexity of the liver, it is relatively simple in structure. It is divided unequally into two lobes by the falciform ligament. The right lobe is approximately six times larger than the left lobe. The lobes are functionally insignificant; however, communication flows freely between all areas of the liver (Fig. 25.1).

Unlike most organs, which have a single blood supply, the liver is an extremely vascular organ that receives its blood supply from two major sources: the hepatic artery

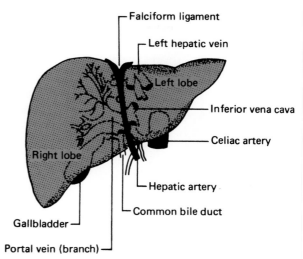

FIGURE 25.2 Blood supply to the liver.

and the portal vein. The hepatic artery, a branch of the aorta, supplies oxygen-rich blood from the heart to the liver and is responsible for providing approximately 25% of the total blood supply to the liver. The portal vein supplies nutrient-rich blood (collected as food is digested) from the digestive tract, and it is responsible for providing approximately 75% of the total blood supply to the liver. The two blood supplies eventually merge into the hepatic sinusoid, which is lined with hepatocytes capable of removing potentially toxic substances from the blood. From the sinusoid, blood flows to the central canal (central vein) of each lobule. It is through the central canal that blood leaves the liver. Approximately 1,500 mL of blood passes through the liver per minute. The liver is drained by a collecting system of veins that empties into the hepatic veins and ultimately into the inferior vena cava (Fig. 25.2).

The excretory system of the liver begins at the bile canaliculi. The bile canaliculi are small spaces between the

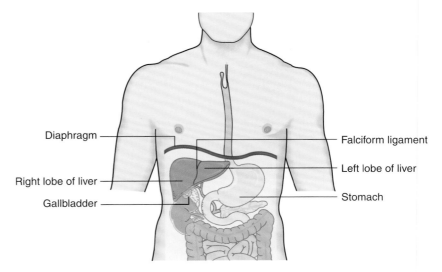

FIGURE 25.1 Gross anatomy of the liver.

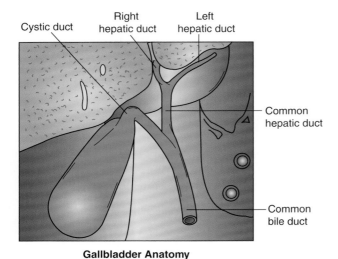

Cystic duct
Right hepatic duct
Left hepatic duct
Common hepatic duct
Common bile duct

Gallbladder Anatomy

FIGURE 25.3 Excretory system of the liver.

hepatocytes that form intrahepatic ducts, where excretory products of the cells can drain. The intrahepatic ducts join to form the right and left hepatic ducts, which drain the secretions from the liver. The right and left hepatic ducts merge to form the common hepatic duct, which is eventually joined with the cystic duct of the gallbladder to form the common bile duct. Combined digestive secretions are then expelled into the duodenum (Fig. 25.3).

Microscopic Anatomy

The liver is divided into microscopic units called **lobules**. The lobules are the functional units of the liver, responsible for all metabolic and excretory functions performed by the liver. Each lobule is roughly a six-sided structure with a centrally located vein (called the *central vein*) with portal

triads at each of the corners. Each portal triad contains a hepatic artery, a portal vein, and a bile duct surrounded by connective tissue. The liver contains two major cell types: hepatocytes and **Kupffer cells**. The hepatocytes, making up approximately 80% of the volume of the organ, are large cells that radiate outward in plates from the central vein to the periphery of the lobule. These cells perform the major functions associated with the liver and are responsible for the regenerative properties of the liver. Kupffer cells are macrophages that line the **sinusoids** of the liver and act as active phagocytes capable of engulfing bacteria, debris, toxins, and other substances flowing through the sinusoids (Fig. 25.4).

BIOCHEMICAL FUNCTIONS

The liver performs four major functions: excretion/secretion, metabolism, detoxification, and storage. The liver is so important that if the liver becomes nonfunctional, death will occur within 24 hours due to hypoglycemia. Although the liver is responsible for a number of functions, this chapter focuses on the four major functions mentioned previously.

Excretory and Secretory

One of the most important functions of the liver is the processing and excretion of endogenous and exogenous substances into the **bile** or urine such as the major heme waste product, **bilirubin**. The liver is the only organ that has the capacity to rid the body of heme waste products. Bile is made up of bile acids or salts, bile pigments, cholesterol, and other substances extracted from the blood. The body produces approximately 3 L of bile per day and excretes 1 L of what is produced. Bilirubin is the principal pigment

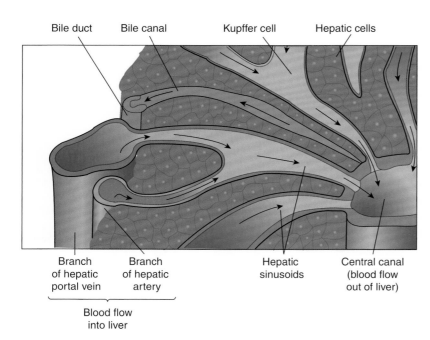

Bile duct
Bile canal
Kupffer cell
Hepatic cells
Branch of hepatic portal vein
Branch of hepatic artery
Hepatic sinusoids
Central canal (blood flow out of liver)
Blood flow into liver

FIGURE 25.4 Microscopic anatomy of the liver.

in bile, and it is derived from the breakdown of red blood cells. Approximately 126 days after the emergence from the reticuloendothelial tissue, red blood cells are phagocytized and hemoglobin is released. Hemoglobin is degraded to heme, globin, and iron. The iron is bound by transferrin and is returned to iron stores in the liver or bone marrow for reuse. The globin is degraded to its constituent amino acids, which are reused by the body. The heme portion of hemoglobin is converted to bilirubin in 2 to 3 hours. Bilirubin is bound by albumin and transported to the liver. This form of bilirubin is referred to as *unconjugated* or *indirect bilirubin.* **Unconjugated** bilirubin is insoluble in water and cannot be removed from the body until it has been conjugated by the liver. Once at the liver cell, unconjugated bilirubin flows into the sinusoidal spaces and is released from albumin so it can be picked up by a carrier protein called *ligandin.* Ligandin, which is located in the hepatocyte, is responsible for transporting unconjugated bilirubin to the endoplasmic reticulum, where it may be rapidly conjugated. The conjugation (esterification) of bilirubin occurs in the presence of the enzyme **uridine diphosphate glucuronosyltransferase** (UDPGT), which transfers a glucuronic acid molecule to each of the two propionic acid side chains of bilirubin to form bilirubin diglucuronide, also known as

conjugated bilirubin. Conjugated bilirubin is water soluble and is able to be secreted from the hepatocyte into the bile canaliculi. Once in the hepatic duct, it combines with secretions from the gallbladder through the cystic duct and is expelled through the common bile duct to the intestines. Intestinal bacteria (especially the bacteria in the lower portion of the intestinal tract) work on conjugated bilirubin to produce mesobilirubin, which is reduced to form mesobilirubinogen and then **urobilinogen** (a colorless product). Most of the urobilinogen formed (roughly 80%) is oxidized to an orange-colored product called *urobilin* (stercobilin) and is excreted in the feces. The urobilin or stercobilin is what gives stool its brown color. There are two things that can happen to the remaining 20% of urobilinogen formed. The majority will be absorbed by extrahepatic circulation to be recycled through the liver and re-excreted. The other very small quantity left will enter systemic circulation and will subsequently be filtered by the kidney and excreted in the urine (Fig. 25.5).[1]

Approximately 200 to 300 mg of bilirubin is produced per day, and it takes a normally functioning liver to process the bilirubin and eliminate it from the body. This, as stated earlier, requires that bilirubin be conjugated. Almost all the bilirubin formed is eliminated in the feces, and a

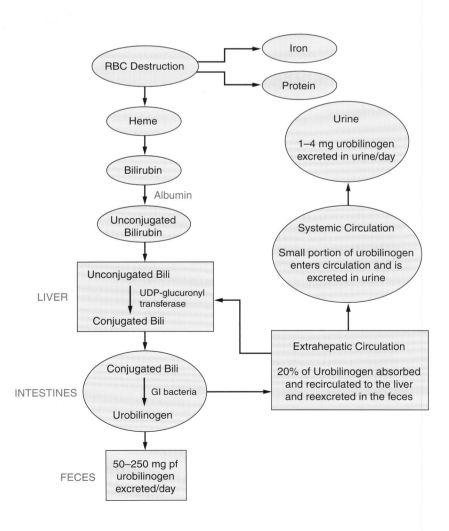

FIGURE 25.5 Metabolism of bilirubin. (Reprinted by permission of Waveland Press, Inc. from Anderson SC, Cockayne S. *Clinical Chemistry/Concepts and Applications/2003.* Long Grove, IL: Waveland Press, Inc.; 2007. All rights reserved.)

small amount of the colorless product, urobilinogen, is excreted in the urine. The healthy adult has very low levels of total bilirubin (0.2 to 1.0 mg/dL) in the serum, and of this amount, the majority is in the unconjugated form.[2]

Metabolism

The liver has extensive metabolic capacity; it is responsible for metabolizing many biological compounds including carbohydrates, lipids, and proteins.

The metabolism of carbohydrates is one of the most important functions of the liver. When carbohydrates are ingested and absorbed, the liver can do three things: (1) use the glucose for its own cellular energy requirements, (2) circulate the glucose for use at the peripheral tissues, or (3) store glucose as glycogen (principal storage form of glucose) within the liver itself or within other tissues. The liver is the major player in maintaining stable glucose concentrations due to its ability to store glucose as glycogen (glycogenesis) and degrade glycogen (glycogenolysis) depending on the body's needs. Under conditions of stress or in a fasting state when there is an increased requirement for glucose, the liver will break down stored glycogen (glycogenolysis), and when the supply of glycogen becomes depleted, the liver will create glucose from nonsugar carbon substrates like pyruvate, lactate, and amino acids (*gluconeogenesis*).

Lipids are metabolized in the liver under normal circumstances when nutrition is adequate and the demand for glucose is being met. The liver is responsible for metabolizing both lipids and the lipoproteins and is responsible for gathering free fatty acids from the diet, and those produced by the liver itself, and breaking them down to produce acetyl-CoA. Acetyl-CoA can then enter several pathways to form triglycerides, phospholipids, or cholesterol. Despite popular belief, the greatest source of cholesterol in the body comes from what is produced by the liver, not from dietary sources. In fact, approximately 70% of the daily production of cholesterol (roughly 1.5 to 2.0 g) is produced by the liver.[3] A more thorough discussion of lipid metabolism may be found in Chapter 15.

Almost all proteins are synthesized by the liver except for the immunoglobulins and adult hemoglobin. The liver plays an essential role in the development of hemoglobin in infants. One of the most important proteins synthesized by the liver is albumin, which carries with it a wide range of important functions. The liver is also responsible for synthesizing the positive and negative acute-phase reactants and coagulation proteins, and it also serves to store a pool of amino acids through protein degradation. The most critical aspect of protein metabolism includes transamination and deamination of amino acids. Transamination (via a transaminase) results in the exchange of an amino group on one acid with a ketone group on another acid. After transamination, deamination degrades them to produce ammonium ions that are consumed in the synthesis of urea and urea is excreted by the kidneys.

Although it would seem logical that any damage to the liver would result in a loss of synthetic and metabolic functions of the liver, that is not the case. The liver must be extensively impaired before it loses its ability to perform these essential functions.

CASE STUDY 25.1

The following laboratory test results were obtained in a patient with severe jaundice, right upper quadrant abdominal pain, fever, and chills (Case Study Table 25.1.1).

CASE STUDY TABLE 25.1.1   Laboratory Results

Serum alkaline	Four times normal phosphatase
Serum cholesterol	Increased
AST (SGOT)	Normal or slightly increased
5′-Nucleotidase	Increased
Total serum bilirubin	25 mg/dL
Conjugated bilirubin	19 mg/dL
Prothrombin time	Prolonged but improves with a vitamin K injection

Questions

1. What is the most likely cause of jaundice in the patient?

Detoxification and Drug Metabolism

The liver serves as a gatekeeper between substances absorbed by the gastrointestinal tract and those released into systemic circulation. Every substance that is absorbed in the gastrointestinal tract must first pass through the liver; this is referred to as *first pass*. This is an important function of the liver because it can allow important substances to reach the systemic circulation and can serve as a barrier to prevent toxic or harmful substances from reaching systemic circulation. The body has two mechanisms for detoxification of foreign materials (drugs and poisons) and metabolic products (bilirubin and ammonia). Either it may bind the material reversibly to inactivate the compound or it may chemically modify the compound so it can be excreted in its chemically modified form. One of the most important functions of the liver is the drug-metabolizing system of the liver. This system is responsible for the detoxification of many drugs through oxidation, reduction, hydrolysis, hydroxylation, carboxylation, and demethylation. Many of these take place in the liver microsomes via the cytochrome P-450 isoenzymes.

LIVER FUNCTION ALTERATIONS DURING DISEASE

Jaundice

The word **jaundice** comes from the French word *jaune*, which means "yellow," and it is one of the oldest known pathologic conditions reported, having been described by Hippocratic physicians.[4] Jaundice, or **icterus**, is used to describe the yellow discoloration of the skin, eyes, and mucous membranes most often resulting from the retention of bilirubin; however, it may also occur due to the retention of other substances. Although the upper limit of normal for total bilirubin is 1.0 to 1.5 mg/dL, jaundice is usually not noticeable to the naked eye (known as *overt jaundice*) until bilirubin levels reach 3.0 to 5.0 mg/dL. Although the terms *jaundice* and *icterus* are used interchangeably, the term *icterus* is most commonly used in the clinical laboratory to refer to a serum or plasma sample with a yellow discoloration due to an elevated bilirubin level. Jaundice is most commonly classified based on the site of the disorder: **prehepatic jaundice, hepatic jaundice,** and **posthepatic jaundice.** This classification is important because knowing the classification of jaundice will aid health care providers in formulating an appropriate treatment or management plan. *Prehepatic* and *posthepatic jaundice*, as the names imply, are caused by abnormalities outside the liver, either before, as in "prehepatic," or after, as in "posthepatic." In these conditions, liver function is normal or it may be functioning at a maximum to compensate for abnormalities occurring elsewhere. This is not the case with hepatic jaundice, where the jaundice is due to a problem with the liver itself—an intrinsic liver defect or disease.

Prehepatic jaundice occurs when the problem causing the jaundice occurs prior to liver metabolism. It is most commonly caused by an increased amount of bilirubin being presented to the liver such as that seen in acute and chronic hemolytic anemias. Hemolytic anemia causes an increased amount of red blood cell destruction and the subsequent release of increased amounts of bilirubin presented to the liver for processing. The liver responds by functioning at maximum capacity; therefore, people with prehepatic jaundice rarely have bilirubin levels that exceed 5.0 mg/dL because the liver is capable of handling the overload. This type of jaundice may also be referred to as *unconjugated hyperbilirubinemia* because the fraction of bilirubin increased in people with prehepatic jaundice is the unconjugated fraction. This fraction of bilirubin (unconjugated bilirubin) is not water soluble, is bound to albumin, is not filtered by the kidneys, and is not seen in the urine.

Hepatic jaundice occurs when the primary problem causing the jaundice resides in the liver (intrinsic liver defect or disease). This intrinsic liver defect or disease can be due to disorders of bilirubin metabolism and transport defects (Crigler-Najjar syndrome, Dubin-Johnson syndrome,

Gilbert's disease, and neonatal physiologic jaundice of the newborn) or due to diseases resulting in hepatocellular injury or destruction. Gilbert's disease, Crigler-Najjar syndrome, and physiologic jaundice of the newborn are hepatic causes of jaundice that result in elevations in unconjugated bilirubin. Conditions such as Dubin-Johnson and Rotor's syndrome are hepatic causes of jaundice that result in elevations in conjugated bilirubin.

Gilbert's syndrome, first described in the early twentieth century, is a benign autosomal recessive hereditary disorder that affects approximately 5% of the US population.[5] Gilbert's syndrome results from a genetic mutation in the UGT1A1 gene that produces the enzyme uridine diphosphate glucuronosyltransferase, one of the enzymes important for bilirubin metabolism. The UGT1A1 gene is located on chromosome 2, and other mutations of this same gene produce Crigler-Najjar syndrome, a more severe and dangerous form of hyperbilirubinemia.[6]

Of the many causes of jaundice, Gilbert's syndrome is the most common cause, and interestingly, it carries no morbidity or mortality in the majority of those affected and carries generally no clinical consequences. It is characterized by intermittent unconjugated hyperbilirubinemia, underlying liver disease due to a defective conjugation system in the absence of hemolysis. The hyperbilirubinemia usually manifests during adolescence or early adulthood. Total serum bilirubin usually fluctuates between 1.5 and 3.0 mg/dL, and it rarely exceeds 4.5 mg/dL. The molecular basis of Gilbert's syndrome (in whites) is related to the UDPGT superfamily, which is responsible for encoding enzymes that catalyze the conjugation of bilirubin. The UGT1A1 (the hepatic 1A1 isoform of UDPGT) contributes substantially to the process of conjugating bilirubin. The UGT1A1 promoter contains the sequence (TA)6TAA. The insertion of an extra TA in the sequence, as seen in Gilbert's syndrome, reduces the expression of the *UGT1A1* gene to 20% to 30% of normal values. That is, the liver's conjugation system in Gilbert's syndrome is working at approximately 30% of normal.[7,8]

Crigler-Najjar syndrome was first described by Crigler and Najjar in 1952 as a syndrome of chronic nonhemolytic unconjugated hyperbilirubinemia.[9] Crigler-Najjar syndrome, like Gilbert's syndrome, is an inherited disorder of bilirubin metabolism resulting from a molecular defect within the gene involved with bilirubin conjugation. Crigler-Najjar syndrome may be divided into two types: type 1, where there is a complete absence of enzymatic bilirubin conjugation, and type II, where there is a mutation causing a severe deficiency of the enzyme responsible for bilirubin conjugation. Unlike Gilbert's syndrome, Crigler-Najjar syndrome is rare and is a more serious disorder that may result in death.[10]

While Gilbert's disease and Crigler-Najjar syndrome are characterized as primarily unconjugated hyperbilirubinemias, Dubin-Johnson syndrome and Rotor's syndrome are characterized as conjugated hyperbilirubinemias. Dubin-Johnson syndrome is a rare autosomal recessive inherited disorder caused by a deficiency of the canalicular multidrug resistance/multispecific organic anionic transporter protein (MDR2/cMOAT). In other words, the liver's ability to uptake and conjugate bilirubin is functional; however, the removal of conjugated bilirubin from the liver cell and the excretion into the bile are defective. This results in accumulation of conjugated and, to some extent, unconjugated bilirubin in the blood, leading to hyperbilirubinemia and bilirubinuria. Dubin-Johnson is a condition that is obstructive in nature, so much of the conjugated bilirubin circulates bound to albumin. This type of bilirubin (conjugated bilirubin bound to albumin) is referred to as *delta bilirubin*. An increase in delta bilirubin poses a problem in laboratory evaluation because the delta bilirubin fraction reacts as conjugated bilirubin in the laboratory method to measure conjugated or direct bilirubin. A distinguishing feature of Dubin-Johnson syndrome is the appearance of dark-stained granules (thought to be pigmented lysosomes) on a liver biopsy sample. Usually, the total bilirubin concentration remains between 2 and 5 mg/dL, with more than 50% due to the conjugated fraction. This syndrome is relatively mild in nature with an excellent prognosis. People with Dubin-Johnson syndrome have a normal life expectancy, so no treatment is necessary.[11,12]

Rotor's syndrome is clinically similar to Dubin-Johnson syndrome, but the defect causing Rotor's syndrome is not known.[13] It is hypothesized to be due to a reduction in the concentration or activity of intracellular binding proteins such as ligandin. Unlike in Dubin-Johnson syndrome, a liver biopsy does not show dark pigmented granules. Rotor's syndrome is seen less commonly than Dubin-Johnson syndrome; it is a relatively benign condition and carries an excellent prognosis, and therefore, treatment is not warranted. However, an accurate diagnosis is required to aid in distinguishing it from more serious liver diseases that require treatment.

Physiologic jaundice of the newborn is a result of a deficiency in the enzyme UDPGT, one of the last liver functions to be activated in prenatal life since bilirubin processing is handled by the mother of the fetus. Premature infants may be born without UDPGT, the enzyme responsible for bilirubin conjugation. This deficiency results in the rapid buildup of unconjugated bilirubin, which can be life threatening. When unconjugated bilirubin builds up in the neonate, it cannot be processed and it is deposited in the nuclei of brain and degenerate nerve cells, causing kernicterus. Kernicterus often results in cell damage and death in the newborn, and this condition will continue until UDPGT is produced. Infants with this type of jaundice are usually treated with phototherapy to destroy the bilirubin as it passes through the capillaries of the skin. Since it was first described in 1958, phototherapy has been effectively used as a relatively inexpensive and noninvasive method of treating neonatal hyperbilirubinemia through photo oxidation. Conventional phototherapy lowers serum bilirubin levels by using halogen or fluorescent lights to transform bilirubin into water-soluble isomers that can be eliminated without conjugation in the liver. During phototherapy, the baby is undressed so that as much of the skin as possible is exposed to the light, his/her eyes are covered to protect the nerve layer at the back of the eye (retina) from the bright light, and the bilirubin levels are measured at least once a day. Alternatively, fiberoptic phototherapy is also available via a blanket, called a bili-blanket, that consists of a pad of woven fibers used to transport light from a light source to the baby's back. The light generated through the bili-blanket breaks down the bilirubin through photo oxidation. The dose of phototherapy is a key factor in how quickly it works and the dose is determined by the wavelength of the light, the intensity of the light (irradiance), the distance between the light and the baby, and the body surface area exposed to the light. Commercially available phototherapy systems include those that deliver light via fluorescent bulbs, halogen quartz lamps, light-emitting diodes, and fiberoptic mattresses. In extreme cases of hyperbilirubinemia, an exchange transfusion may be used as the second-line treatment when phototherapy fails. An exchange transfusion involves removing aliquots of blood and replacing it with donor blood in order to remove abnormal blood components and circulating toxins while maintaining adequate circulating blood volume. Because hyperbilirubinemia is so serious in newborns, bilirubin levels are carefully and frequently monitored so the dangerously high levels of unconjugated bilirubin (approximately 20 mg/dL) can be detected and treated appropriately.[14]

Posthepatic jaundice results from biliary obstructive disease, usually from physical obstructions (gallstones or tumors) that prevent the flow of conjugated bilirubin into the bile canaliculi. Since the liver cell itself is functioning, bilirubin is effectively conjugated; however, it is unable to be properly excreted from the liver. Since bile is not being brought to the intestines, stool loses its source of normal pigmentation and becomes clay-colored. The laboratory findings for bilirubin and its metabolites in the abovementioned types of jaundice are summarized in Table 25.1. Mechanisms of hyperbilirubinemia may be found in Figure 25.6.

Cirrhosis

Cirrhosis is a clinical condition in which scar tissue replaces normal, healthy liver tissue. As the scar tissue replaces the normal liver tissue, it blocks the flow of blood through the organ and prevents the liver from functioning properly. Cirrhosis rarely causes signs and symptoms in its early stages, but as liver function deteriorates, the signs and symptoms appear, including fatigue, nausea, unintended weight loss, jaundice, bleeding from the gastrointestinal tract, intense itching, and swelling in the legs and abdomen. Although some patients with cirrhosis may have prolonged survival, they generally have a poor prognosis. Cirrhosis was the twelfth leading cause of death by disease in 2013, killing just over 36,400 people.[15] In the United States, the most common cause of cirrhosis is chronic alcoholism. Other causes of cirrhosis include chronic hepatitis B (HBV), C (HCV), and D virus (HDV) infection, autoimmune hepatitis, inherited disorders (e.g., α1-antitrypsin deficiency,

TABLE 25.1   Changes in Concentration of Bilirubin in Those with Jaundice

Type of Jaundice	Serum		
	Total Bilirubin	Conjugated Bilirubin	Unconjugated Bilirubin
Prehepatic	↑	↔	↑
Hepatic			
• Gilbert's disease	↑	↔	↑
• Crigler-Najjar syndrome	↑	↓	↑
• Dubin-Johnson	↑	↑	↔
• Rotor's syndrome	↑	↑	↔
• Jaundice of newborn	↑	↔	↑
Posthepatic	↑	↑	↑

Adapted from Table 27.3 of Kaplan LA, Pesce AJ, Kazmierczak S. *Clinical Chemistry: Theory, Analysis, Correlation*. 4th ed. St. Louis, MO: Mosby; 2003.

Wilson's disease, hemochromatosis, and galactosemia), nonalcoholic steatohepatitis, blocked bile ducts, drugs, toxins, and infections.

Liver damage from cirrhosis cannot easily be reversed, but treatment can stop or delay further progression of the disorder. Treatment depends on the cause of cirrhosis and any complications a person is experiencing. For example, cirrhosis caused by alcohol abuse is treated by abstaining from alcohol. Treatment for hepatitis-related cirrhosis involves medications used to treat the different types of hepatitis, such as interferon for viral hepatitis and corticosteroids for autoimmune hepatitis.

Tumors

Cancers of the liver are classified as primary or metastatic. Primary liver cancer is cancer that begins in the liver cells while metastatic cancer occurs when tumors from other parts of the body spread (metastasize) to the liver. Metastatic liver cancer is much more common than primary liver cancer; 90% to 95% of all hepatic malignancies are classified as metastatic. Cancers that commonly spread to the liver include colon, lung, and breast cancer. Tumors of the liver may also be classified as benign or malignant. The common benign tumors of the liver include hepatocellular adenoma (a condition occurring almost exclusively in females of childbearing age) and hemangiomas (masses of blood vessels with no known etiology). Malignant tumors of the liver include **hepatocellular carcinoma** (HCC) (also known as hepatocarcinoma, and **hepatoma**) and bile duct carcinoma. Of those, HCC is the most common malignant tumor of the liver. Hepatoblastoma is an uncommon hepatic malignancy of children.

HCC has become increasingly important in the United States. Approximately 85% of the new cases of this liver cancer occur in developing countries, with the highest incidence of HCC reported in regions where HBV is endemic such as Southeast Asia and sub-Saharan Africa. Approximately 500,000 people are diagnosed annually with HCC worldwide, of which 28,000 new cases and 20,000 deaths were reported in the United States in 2012.[16,17] It is estimated that in the United States, chronic HBV and HCV infections account for approximately 30% and 40% of cases of HCC.[18]

Approximately 80% of cases worldwide are attributable to HBV and HCV; however, the mechanism by which the infection leads to HCC is not well established. While surgical resection of HCC is sometimes possible, currently, orthotopic liver transplantation in people with HCC with underlying cirrhosis who meet the Milan criteria (single tumor ≤5 cm in size or ≤3 tumors each ≤3 cm in size, and no macrovascular invasion) is also available for

FIGURE 25.6 Mechanisms of hyperbilirubinemia. **(A)** Normal bilirubin metabolism, **(B)** hemolytic jaundice, **(C)** Gilbert's disease, **(D)** physiologic jaundice, **(E)** Dubin-Johnson syndrome, and **(F)** intrahepatic or extrahepatic obstruction. (Adapted from Kaplan LA, Pesce AJ, Kazmierczak S. *Clinical Chemistry: Theory, Analysis, Correlation*. 4th ed. St. Louis, MO: Mosby; 2003:449.)

HCC. The estimated 4-year survival rate is 85% and the recurrence-free survival rate is 92%.[19]

Whether primary or metastatic, any malignant tumor in the liver is a serious finding and carries a poor prognosis, with survival times measured in months.

Reye's Syndrome

Reye's syndrome is a term used to describe a group of disorders caused by infectious, metabolic, toxic, or drug-induced disease found almost exclusively in children, although adult cases of Reye's syndrome have been reported.[20] Although the precise cause of Reye's syndrome is unknown, it is often preceded by a viral syndrome such as varicella, gastroenteritis, or an upper respiratory tract infection such as influenza.[21–23] Although not described as the precise cause of Reye's syndrome, studies have demonstrated a strong epidemiologic association between the ingestion of aspirin during a viral syndrome and the subsequent development of Reye's syndrome.[24,25] As a result, the Centers for Disease Control and Prevention (CDC) cautioned physicians and parents to avoid salicylate use in children with a viral syndrome, and the U.S. Surgeon General mandated that a warning label be added to all aspirin-containing medications, beginning in 1986.[26,27] Reye's syndrome is an acute illness characterized by noninflammatory encephalopathy and fatty degeneration of the liver, with a clinical presentation of profuse vomiting accompanied with varying degrees of neurologic impairment such as fluctuating personality changes and deterioration in consciousness. The encephalopathy is characterized by a progression from mild confusion (stage 1) through progressive loss of neurologic function to loss of brain stem reflexes (stage 5). The degeneration of the liver is characterized by a mild hyperbilirubinemia and threefold increases in ammonia and the aminotransferases (aspartate aminotransferase [AST] and alanine aminotransferase [ALT]). Without treatment, rapid clinical deterioration leading to death may occur.[28,29]

Drug- and Alcohol-Related Disorders

Drug-induced liver disease is a major problem in the United States, accounting for one-third to one-half of all reported cases of acute liver failure. The liver is a primary target organ for adverse drug reactions because it plays a central role in drug metabolism. Many drugs are known to cause liver damage, ranging from very mild transient forms to fulminant liver failure. Drugs can cause liver injury by a variety of mechanisms, but the most common mechanism of toxicity is via an immune-mediated injury to the hepatocytes.[30] In this type of mechanism, the drug induces an adverse immune response directed against the liver itself and results in hepatic and/or cholestatic disease.[31]

Of all the drugs associated with hepatic toxicity, the most important is ethanol. In very small amounts, ethanol causes very mild, transient, and unnoticed injury to the liver; however, with heavier and prolonged consumption, it can lead to alcoholic cirrhosis. While the exact amount of alcohol needed to cause cirrhosis is unknown, a small minority of people with alcoholism develop this condition.[32] Approximately 90% of the alcohol absorbed from the stomach and small intestines is transported to the liver for metabolism. Within the liver, the elimination of alcohol requires the enzymes alcohol dehydrogenase and acetaldehyde dehydrogenase to convert alcohol to acetaldehyde and subsequently to acetate. The acetate can then be oxidized to water and carbon dioxide, or it may enter the citric acid cycle.

Long-term excessive consumption of alcohol can result in a spectrum of liver abnormalities that may range from alcoholic fatty liver with inflammation (steatohepatitis) to scar tissue formation, as in hepatic fibrosis, to the destruction of normal liver structure seen in hepatic cirrhosis. Alcohol-induced liver injury may be categorized into three stages: alcoholic fatty liver, alcoholic hepatitis, and alcoholic cirrhosis. The risk for the development of cirrhosis increases proportionally with the consumption of more than 30 g (the equivalent of 3 to 4 drinks) of alcohol per day, with the highest degree of risk seen with the consumption of greater than 120 g (the equivalent of 12 to 16 drinks) per day.[33]

Alcoholic fatty liver represents the mildest category where very few changes in liver function are measurable. This stage is characterized by slight elevations in AST, ALT, and γ-glutamyltransferase (GGT), and on biopsy, fatty infiltrates are noted in the vacuoles of the liver. This stage tends to affect young to middle-aged people with a history of moderate alcohol consumption. A complete recovery within 1 month is seen when the drug is removed. Alcoholic hepatitis presents with common signs and symptoms including fever, ascites, proximal muscle loss, and far more laboratory evidence of liver damage such as moderately elevated AST, ALT, GGT, and alkaline phosphatase (ALP) and elevations in total bilirubin greater than 5 mg/dL. The elevations in AST are more than twice the upper reference of normal but rarely exceed 300 IU/mL. The elevations in ALT are comparatively lower than AST, resulting in an AST/ALT ratio (De Ritis ratio) greater than 2. Serum proteins, especially albumin, are decreased and the international normalized ratio (INR, which is a ratio of coagulation time in the patient compared with a normal coagulation time) is elevated. Prognosis is dependent on the type and severity of damage to the liver, and when serum creatinine levels begin to increase, it is a threatening sign, which may precede the onset of hepatorenal syndrome and death.[34] There are a variety of scoring systems that have been used to assess the severity of alcoholic hepatitis and to guide treatment including the Maddrey's discriminant function,[35] the Glasgow score,[36] and the Model for End-Stage Liver Disease (MELD) score.[37] All three scoring systems use bilirubin, INR, creatinine, age, white cell counts, blood urea nitrogen, and albumin levels to stage and guide treatment. The last and most severe stage is alcoholic cirrhosis. The prognosis associated with alcoholic cirrhosis is dependent on the nature and severity of associated conditions such as a gastrointestinal bleeding or ascites; however, the 5-year survival rate is 60% in those who abstain from alcohol and 30% in those who continue to drink. This condition appears to be more common in males than in females, and the symptoms tend to be nonspecific and include weight loss, weakness, hepatomegaly, splenomegaly, jaundice, ascites, fever, malnutrition, and edema. Laboratory abnormalities include increased liver function tests (AST, ALT, GGT, ALP, and total bilirubin), decreased albumin, and a prolonged prothrombin time. A liver biopsy is the only method by which a definitive diagnosis may be made.[38]

Other drugs, including tranquilizers, some antibiotics, antineoplastic agents, lipid-lowering medication, and anti-inflammatory drugs, may cause liver injury ranging from mild damage to massive hepatic failure and cirrhosis. One of the most common drugs associated with serious hepatic injury is acetaminophen. When acetaminophen is taken in massive doses, it is virtually certain to produce fatal hepatic necrosis unless rapid treatment is initiated.

CASE STUDY 25.2

The following laboratory test results were found in a patient with mild weight loss and nausea and vomiting, who later developed jaundice and an enlarged liver (Case Study Table 25.2.1)

CASE STUDY TABLE 25.2.1   Laboratory Results

Total serum bilirubin	20 mg/dL
Conjugated bilirubin	10 mg/dL
Alkaline phosphatase	Mildly elevated
AST (SGOT)	Significantly elevated
ALT (SGPT)	Moderately elevated
Albumin	Decreased
γ-Globulin	Increased

Questions
1. What disease process is most likely in this patient?

ASSESSMENT OF LIVER FUNCTION/ LIVER FUNCTION TESTS

Bilirubin
Analysis of Bilirubin: A Brief Review

The reaction of bilirubin with a diazotized sulfanilic acid solution to form a colored product was first described by Ehrlich in 1883 using urine samples. Since then, this type of reaction (bilirubin with a diazotized sulfanilic acid solution) has been referred to as the classic *diazo reaction*, a reaction on which all commonly used methods today are based. In 1913, van den Bergh found that the diazo reaction may be applied to serum samples but only in the presence of an accelerator (solubilizer). However, this methodology had errors associated with it. It was not until 1937 that Malloy and Evelyn developed the first clinically useful methodology for the quantitation of bilirubin in serum samples using the classic diazo reaction with a 50% methanol solution as an accelerator. In 1938, Jendrassik and Grof described a method using the diazo reaction with caffeine–benzoate–acetate as an accelerator. Today, all commonly used methods for measuring bilirubin and its fractions are modifications of the technique described by Malloy and Evelyn. Total bilirubin and conjugated bilirubin (direct bilirubin) are measured and unconjugated bilirubin (indirect bilirubin) is determined by subtracting conjugated bilirubin from total bilirubin (see Fig. 25.7).

Bilirubin has also been quantified using bilirubinometry in the neonatal population. This methodology is only useful in the neonatal population because of the presence of carotenoid compounds in adult serum that causes strong positive interference in the adult population. Bilirubinometry involves the measurement of reflected light from the skin using two wavelengths that provide a numerical index based on spectral reflectance. Newer-generation bilirubinometers use microspectrophotometers that determine the optical densities of bilirubin, hemoglobin, and melanin in the subcutaneous layers of the infant's skin. Mathematical isolation of hemoglobin and melanin allows measurement of the optical density created by bilirubin.[39]

When using the several methods described earlier, two of the three fractions of bilirubin were identified: conjugated (direct) and unconjugated (indirect) bilirubin. Unconjugated (indirect) bilirubin is a nonpolar and water-insoluble substance that is found in plasma bound to albumin. Because of these characteristics, unconjugated bilirubin will only react with the diazotized sulfanilic acid solution (diazo reagent) in the presence of an accelerator (solubilizer). Conjugated (direct) bilirubin is a

Bilirubin + diazotized sulfanilic acid + accelerator ⟶ 2 azobilirubin (total bilirubin)

Bilirubin + diazotized sulfanilic acid ⟶ 2 azobilirubin (conjugated bilirubin)

Total bilirubin − conjugated bilirubin = unconjugated bilirubin (indirect bilirubin)

FIGURE 25.7 Methods to measure different fractions of bilirubin.

polar and water-soluble compound that is found in plasma in the free state (not bound to any protein). This type of bilirubin will react with the diazotized sulfanilic acid solution directly (without an accelerator). Thus, conjugated and unconjugated bilirubin fractions have historically been differentiated by solubility of the fractions. Conjugated bilirubin reacts in the absence of an accelerator, whereas unconjugated bilirubin requires an accelerator. While for many years bilirubin results were reported as direct and indirect, this terminology is now outdated. Direct and indirect bilirubin results should be reported as conjugated and unconjugated, respectively.[40]

The third fraction of bilirubin is referred to as **"delta" bilirubin**. Delta bilirubin is conjugated bilirubin that is covalently bound to albumin. This fraction of bilirubin is seen only when there is significant hepatic obstruction. Because the molecule is attached to albumin, it is too large to be filtered by the glomerulus and excreted in the urine. This fraction of bilirubin, when present, will react in most laboratory methods as conjugated bilirubin. Thus, total bilirubin is made up of three fractions: conjugated, unconjugated, and delta bilirubin. The three fractions together are known as *total bilirubin*.

Specimen Collection and Storage

Total bilirubin methods using a diazotized sulfanilic acid solution may be performed on either serum or plasma. Serum, however, is preferred for the Malloy-Evelyn procedure because the addition of the alcohol in the analysis can precipitate proteins and cause interference with the method. A fasting sample is preferred as the presence of lipemia will increase measured bilirubin concentrations. Hemolyzed samples should be avoided as they may decrease the reaction of bilirubin with the diazo reagent. Bilirubin is very sensitive to and is destroyed by light; therefore, specimens should be protected from light. If left unprotected from light, bilirubin values may reduce by 30% to 50% per hour. If serum or plasma is separated from the cells and stored in the dark, it is stable for 2 days at room temperature, 1 week at 4°C, and indefinitely at −20°C.[41]

METHODS

There is no preferred reference method or standardization of bilirubin analysis; however, the American Association for Clinical Chemistry and the National Bureau of Standards have published a candidate reference method for total bilirubin, a modified Jendrassik-Grof procedure using caffeine–benzoate as a solubilizer.[42] Because they both have acceptable precision and are adapted to many automated instruments, the Jendrassik-Grof or Malloy-Evelyn procedure is the most frequently used method to measure bilirubin. The Jendrassik-Grof method is slightly more complex, but it has the following advantages over the Malloy-Evelyn method:

- Not affected by pH changes
- Insensitive to a 50-fold variation in protein concentration of the sample

- Maintains optical sensitivity even at low bilirubin concentrations
- Has minimal turbidity and a relatively constant serum blank
- Is not affected by hemoglobin up to 750 mg/dL

Because this chapter does not allow for a detailed description of all previously mentioned bilirubin test methodologies, only the most widely used principles for measuring bilirubin in the adult and pediatric populations are covered.[43–45]

Malloy-Evelyn Procedure

Bilirubin pigments in serum or plasma are reacted with a diazo reagent. The diazotized sulfanilic acid reacts at the central methylene carbon of bilirubin to split the molecule forming two molecules of azobilirubin. This method is typically performed at pH 1.2 where the azobilirubin produced is red-purple in color with a maximal absorption of 560 nm. The most commonly used accelerator to solubilize unconjugated bilirubin is methanol, although other chemicals have been used.[46]

Jendrassik-Grof Method for Total and Conjugated Bilirubin Determination

Principle

Bilirubin pigments in serum or plasma are reacted with a diazo reagent (sulfanilic acid in hydrochloric acid and sodium nitrite), resulting in the production of the purple product azobilirubin. The product azobilirubin may be measured spectrophotometrically. The individual fractions of bilirubin are determined by taking two aliquots of sample and reacting one aliquot with the diazo reagent only and the other aliquot with the diazo reagent and an accelerator (caffeine–benzoate). The addition of caffeine–benzoate will solubilize the water-insoluble fraction of bilirubin and will yield a total bilirubin value (all fractions). The reaction without the accelerator will yield conjugated bilirubin only. After a short period of time, the reaction of the aliquots with the diazo reagent is terminated by the addition of ascorbic acid. The ascorbic acid destroys the excess diazo reagent. The solution is then alkalinized using an alkaline tartrate solution, which shifts the absorbance spectrum of the azobilirubin to a more intense blue color that is less subject to interfering substances in the sample. The final blue product is measured at 600 nm, with the intensity of color produced directly proportional to bilirubin concentration. Indirect (unconjugated) bilirubin may be calculated by subtracting the conjugated bilirubin concentration from the total bilirubin concentration.

Comments and Sources of Error

Instruments should be frequently standardized to maintain reliable bilirubin results, and careful preparation of bilirubin standards is critical as these are subject to deterioration from exposure to light. Hemolysis and lipemia should be avoided as they will alter bilirubin concentrations. Serious loss of bilirubin occurs after exposure to fluorescent and indirect and direct sunlight; therefore, it is imperative that

Population	Type of Bilirubin	Reference Range
Adults	Conjugated bilirubin	0.0–0.2 mg/dL (0–3 µmol/L)
	Unconjugated bilirubin	0.2–0.8 mg/dL (3–14 µmol/L)
	Total bilirubin	0.2–1.0 mg/dL (3–17 µmol/L)
Premature infants	Total bilirubin at 24 h	1–6 mg/dL (17–103 µmol/L)
	Total bilirubin at 48 h	6–8 mg/dL (103–137 µmol/L)
	Total bilirubin 3–5 d	10–12 mg/dL (171–205 µmol/L)
Full-term infants	Total bilirubin at 24 h	2–6 mg/dL (34–103 µmol/L)
	Total bilirubin at 48 h	6–7 mg/dL (103–120 µmol/L)
	Total bilirubin 3–5 d	4–6 mg/dL (68–103 µmol/L)

TABLE 25.2 Reference Ranges for Bilirubin in Adults and Infants

exposure of samples and standards to light be kept to a minimum. Specimens and standards should be refrigerated in the dark until testing can be performed.

Reference Range
See Table 25.2.

Urobilinogen in Urine and Feces

Urobilinogen is a colorless end product of bilirubin metabolism that is oxidized by intestinal bacteria to the brown pigment urobilin. In the normal individual, part of the urobilinogen is excreted in feces, and the remainder is reabsorbed into the portal blood and returned to the liver. A small portion that is not taken up by the hepatocytes is excreted by the kidney as urobilinogen. Increased levels of urinary urobilinogen are found in hemolytic disease and in defective liver cell function, such as that seen in **hepatitis**. Absence of urobilinogen from the urine and stool is most often seen with complete biliary obstruction. Fecal urobilinogen is also decreased in biliary obstruction, as well as in HCC.[47]

Most quantitative methods for urobilinogen are based on a reaction first described by Ehrlich in 1901: the reaction of urobilinogen with *p*-dimethylaminobenzaldehyde (Ehrlich's reagent) to form a red color. Many modifications of this procedure have been made over the years to improve specificity. However, because the modifications did not completely recover urobilinogen from the urine, most laboratories use the less laborious, more rapid, semiquantitative method described next.

Determination of Urine Urobilinogen (Semiquantitative)

Principle
Urobilinogen reacts with *p*-dimethylaminobenzaldehyde (Ehrlich's reagent) to form a red color, which is then measured spectrophotometrically. Ascorbic acid is added as a reducing agent to maintain urobilinogen in the reduced state. The use of saturated sodium acetate stops the reaction and minimizes the combination of other chromogens with the Ehrlich's reagent.[48]

Specimen
A *fresh* 2-hour urine specimen is collected. This specimen should be kept cool and protected from light.

Comments and Sources of Error
1. The results of this test are reported in Ehrlich units rather than in milligrams of urobilinogen because substances other than urobilinogen account for some of the final color development.
2. Compounds, other than urobilinogen, that may be present in the urine and react with Ehrlich's reagent include porphobilinogen, sulfonamides, procaine, and 5-hydroxyindoleacetic acid. Bilirubin will form a green color and, therefore, must be removed, as previously described.
3. Fresh urine is necessary, and the test must be performed without delay to prevent oxidation of urobilinogen to urobilin. Similarly, the spectrophotometric readings should be made within 5 minutes after color production because the urobilinogen–aldehyde color slowly decreases in intensity.

Reference Range
Urine urobilinogen, 0.1 to 1.0 Ehrlich units every 2 hours or 0.5 to 4.0 Ehrlich units per day (0.86 to 8 mmol/d); 1 Ehrlich unit is equivalent to approximately 1 mg of urobilinogen.

Fecal Urobilinogen

Visual inspection of the feces is usually sufficient to detect decreased urobilinogen. However, the semiquantitative determination of fecal urobilinogen is available and involves the same principle described earlier for the urine. It is carried out in an aqueous extract of fresh feces, and any urobilin present is reduced to urobilinogen by treatment with alkaline ferrous hydroxide before Ehrlich's reagent is added. A range of 75 to 275 Ehrlich units per 100 g of fresh feces or 75 to 400 Ehrlich units per 24-hour specimen is considered a normal reference range.[48]

Serum Bile Acids

Serum bile acid analysis is rarely performed because the methods required are very complex. These involve extraction with organic solvents, partition chromatography, gas chromatography–mass spectrometry, spectrophotometry, ultraviolet light absorption, fluorescence, radioimmunoassay, and enzyme immunoassay (EIA) methods. Although serum bile acid levels are elevated in liver disease, the total concentration is extremely variable and adds no diagnostic value to other tests of liver function. The variability of the type of bile acids present in serum, together with their existence in different conjugated forms, suggests that more relevant information of liver dysfunction may be gained by examining patterns of individual bile acids and their state of conjugation. For example, it has been suggested that the ratio of the trihydroxy to dihydroxy bile acids in serum will differentiate patients with obstructive jaundice from those with hepatocellular injury and that the diagnosis of primary biliary cirrhosis and extrahepatic cholestasis can be made on the basis of the ratio of the cholic to chenodeoxycholic acids. However, the high cost of these tests, the time required to do them, and the current controversy concerning their clinical usefulness render this approach unsatisfactory for routine use.[49,50]

Enzymes

Liver enzymes play an important role in the assessment of liver function because injury to the liver resulting in cytolysis or necrosis will cause the release of enzymes into circulation. Enzymes also play an important role in differentiating hepatocellular (functional) from obstructive (mechanical) liver disease, which is an important clinical distinction because failure to identify an obstruction will result in liver failure if the obstruction is not rapidly treated. Although many enzymes have been identified as useful in the assessment of liver function, the most clinically useful include the aminotransferases (ALT and AST), the phosphatases (ALP and 5′-neucleotidase), GGT, and lactate dehydrogenase (LD).

The methods used to measure these enzymes, the normal reference ranges, and other general aspects of enzymology are discussed in Chapter 13. Discussion in this chapter focuses on the characteristic changes in serum enzyme levels seen in various hepatic disorders. It is important to note that the diagnosis of disease depends on a combination of patient history, physical examination, laboratory testing, and sometimes radiologic studies and biopsy, and therefore, abnormalities in liver enzymes alone are not diagnostic in and of themselves.[51,52]

Aminotransferases

The two most common aminotransferases measured in the clinical laboratory are AST (formerly referred to as serum glutamic oxaloacetic transaminase [SGOT]) and ALT (formerly referred to as serum glutamic pyruvic transaminase [SGPT]). The aminotransferases are responsible for catalyzing the conversion of aspartate and alanine to oxaloacetate and pyruvate, respectively. In the absence of acute necrosis or ischemia of other organs, these enzymes are most useful in the detection of hepatocellular (functional) damage to the liver. ALT is found mainly in the liver (lesser amounts in skeletal muscle and kidney), whereas AST is widely distributed in equal amounts in the heart, skeletal muscle, and liver, making ALT a more "liver-specific" marker than AST. Regardless, the serum activity of both transaminases rises rapidly in almost all diseases of the liver

and may remain elevated for up to 2 to 6 weeks. The highest levels of AST and ALT are found in acute conditions such as viral hepatitis, drug- and toxin-induced liver necrosis, and hepatic ischemia. The increase in ALT activity is usually greater than that for AST. Only moderate increases are found in less severe conditions. AST and ALT are found to be normal or only mildly elevated in cases of obstructive liver damage. Because AST and ALT are present in other tissues besides the liver, elevations in these enzymes may be a result of other organ dysfunction or failure such as acute myocardial infarction, renal infarction, progressive muscular dystrophy, and those conditions that result in secondary liver disease such as infectious mononucleosis, diabetic ketoacidosis, and hyperthyroidism. It is often helpful to conduct serial determinations of aminotransferases when following the course of a patient with acute or chronic hepatitis, and caution should be used in interpreting abnormal levels because serum transaminases may actually decrease in some patients with severe acute hepatitis, owing to the exhaustive release of hepatocellular enzymes.[51,52]

Phosphatases

Alkaline Phosphatase

The ALP family of enzymes are zinc metalloenzymes that are widely distributed in all tissues; however, highest activity is seen in the liver, bone, intestine, kidney, and placenta. The clinical utility of ALP lies in its ability to differentiate hepatobiliary disease from osteogenic bone disease. In the liver, the enzyme is localized to the microvilli of the bile canaliculi, and therefore, it serves as a marker of extrahepatic biliary obstruction, such as a stone in the common bile duct, or in intrahepatic cholestasis, such as drug cholestasis or primary biliary cirrhosis. ALP is found in very high concentrations in cases of extrahepatic obstruction with only slight to moderate increases seen in those with hepatocellular disorders such as hepatitis and cirrhosis. Because bone is also a source of ALP, it may be elevated in bone-related disorders such as Paget's disease, bony metastases, diseases associated with an increase in osteoblastic activity, and rapid bone growth during puberty. ALP is also found elevated in pregnancy due to its release from the placenta, where it may remain elevated up to several weeks postdelivery. As a result, interpretation of ALP concentrations is difficult because enzyme activity of ALP can increase in the absence of liver damage.[51,52]

5′-Nucleotidase

5′-Nucleotidase (5NT) is a phosphatase that is responsible for catalyzing the hydrolysis of nucleoside-5′-phosphate esters. Although 5NT is found in a wide variety of cells, serum levels become significantly elevated in hepatobiliary disease. There is no bone source of 5NT, so it is useful in differentiating ALP elevations due to the liver from other conditions where ALP may be seen in increased concentrations (bone diseases, pregnancy, and childhood growth). Levels of both 5NT and ALP are elevated in liver disease, whereas in primary bone disease, ALP level is elevated, but the 5NT level is usually normal or only slightly elevated. This enzyme is much more sensitive to metastatic liver disease than is ALP because, unlike ALP, its level is not significantly elevated in other conditions, such as in pregnancy or during childhood. In addition, some increase in enzyme activity may be noted after abdominal surgery.[51–54]

γ-Glutamyltransferase
GGT is a membrane-localized enzyme found in high concentrations in the kidney, liver, pancreas, intestine, and prostate but not in bone. Similar to the clinical utility of 5NT (see earlier), GGT plays a role in differentiating the cause of elevated levels of ALP as the highest levels of GGT are seen in biliary obstruction. GGT is a hepatic microsomal enzyme; therefore, ingestion of alcohol or certain drugs (barbiturates, tricyclic antidepressants, and anticonvulsants) elevates GGT. It is a sensitive test for cholestasis caused by chronic alcohol or drug ingestion. Measurement of this enzyme is also useful if jaundice is absent for the confirmation of hepatic neoplasms.[51–55]

Lactate Dehydrogenase
LD is an enzyme with a very wide distribution throughout the body. It is released into circulation when cells of the body are damaged or destroyed, serving as a general, nonspecific marker of cellular injury. Moderate elevations of total serum LD levels are common in acute viral hepatitis and in cirrhosis, whereas biliary tract disease may produce only slight elevations. High serum levels may be found in metastatic carcinoma of the liver. As a result of its wide distribution, LD measurements provide no additional clinical information above that which is provided by the previously mentioned enzymes. However, fractionation of LD into its five tissue-specific isoenzymes may give useful information about the site of origin of the LD elevation.

Tests Measuring Hepatic Synthetic Ability

A healthy functioning liver is required for the synthesis of serum proteins (except the immunoglobulins). The measurement of serum proteins, therefore, can be used to assess the synthetic ability of the liver. Although these tests are not sensitive to minimal liver damage, they may be useful in quantitating the severity of hepatic dysfunction.

A decreased serum albumin may be a result of decreased liver protein synthesis, and the albumin level correlates well with the severity of functional impairment and is found more often in chronic rather than in acute liver disease. The serum α-globulins also tend to decrease with chronic liver disease. However, a low or absent α-globulin suggests α-antitrypsin deficiency as the cause of the chronic liver disease. Serum γ-globulin levels are transiently increased in acute liver disease and remain elevated in chronic liver disease. The highest elevations are found in chronic active hepatitis and postnecrotic cirrhosis. In particular, immunoglobulin G (IgG) and IgM levels are more consistently elevated in chronic active hepatitis; IgM, in primary biliary cirrhosis; and IgA, in alcoholic cirrhosis.

Prothrombin time is commonly increased in liver disease because the liver is unable to manufacture adequate amounts of clotting factor or because the disruption of bile flow results in inadequate absorption of vitamin K from the intestine. However, a prothrombin time is not routinely used to aid in the diagnosis of liver disease. Rather, serial measurements of prothrombin times may be useful in following the progression of disease and the assessment of the risk of bleeding. A marked prolongation of the prothrombin time indicates severe diffuse liver disease and a poor prognosis.

Tests Measuring Nitrogen Metabolism

The liver plays a major role in removing ammonia from the bloodstream and converting it to urea so that it can be removed by the kidneys. A plasma ammonia level, therefore, is a reflection of the liver's ability to perform this conversion. In liver failure, ammonia and other toxins increase in the bloodstream and may ultimately cause hepatic coma. In this condition, the patient becomes increasingly disoriented and gradually lapses into unconsciousness. The cause of hepatic coma is not fully known, although ammonia is presumed to play a major role. However, the correlation between blood ammonia levels and the severity of the hepatic coma is poor. Therefore, ammonia levels are most useful when multiple measurements are made over time.

The most common laboratory determination of ammonia concentrations is based on the following reaction:

$$NH_4 + \alpha\text{-ketoglutarate} + NADH \xrightarrow{\text{Glutamate dehydrogenase (GLDH)}} Glutamate + NAD + H_2O$$

(Eq. 25-1)

The resulting decrease in absorbance at 340 nm is measured and is proportional to ammonia concentration. The sample of choice is plasma collected in ethylenediaminetetraacetic acid (EDTA), lithium heparin, or potassium oxalate, and the samples should be immediately placed on ice to prevent metabolism of other nitrogenous compounds to ammonia in the sample, leading to false elevations in ammonia. If analysis cannot be performed immediately, the plasma should be removed and placed on ice or frozen. Frozen ($-70°C$) samples are stable for several days. Hemolyzed samples should be rejected for analysis as red blood cells have a concentration of ammonia two to three times higher than that of plasma.[56] Lipemic samples and those with high bilirubin concentrations may be unsuitable for analysis in some systems. The glutaminase activity of GGT is a major contributor to the endogenous production of ammonia; therefore, concentrations may be artifactually increased in samples with raised GGT activity.[57]

Hepatitis

Hepatitis implies injury to the liver characterized by the presence of inflammation in the liver tissue. Infectious causes for the inflammation of liver include viral, bacterial, and parasitic infections, as well as noninfectious causes, such as radiation, drugs, chemicals, and autoimmune

TABLE 25.3   The Hepatitis Viruses

	Nucleotide	Incubation Period	Primary Mode of Transmission	Vaccine	Chronic Infection	Serologic Diagnosis Available
Hepatitis A	RNA	2–6 wk	Fecal–oral	Yes	No	Yes
Hepatitis B	DNA	8–26 wk	Parenteral, sexual	Yes	Yes	Yes
Hepatitis C	RNA	2–15 wk	Parenteral, sexual	No	Yes	Yes
Hepatitis D	RNA	—	Parenteral, sexual	Yes	Yes	Yes
Hepatitis E	RNA	3–6 wk	Fecal–oral	No	?	Yes

diseases and toxins. Viral infections account for the majority of hepatitis cases observed in the clinical setting. Major hepatitis subtypes include HAV, HBV, HCV, HDV, and HEV. Infections with these viruses can lead to the onset of acute disease with symptoms, including jaundice, dark urine, fatigue, nausea, vomiting, and abdominal pain. Some subtypes, such as HBV and HCV, can lead to the prolonged elevation of serum transaminase level (longer than 6 months), a condition termed *chronic hepatitis.* Routes of transmission vary from one viral subtype to another. HAV and HEV are typically caused by ingestion of contaminated food or water. HBV, HCV, and HDV usually occur as a result of parenteral contact with infected body fluids (e.g., from blood transfusions or invasive medical procedures using contaminated equipment) and sexual contact. Refer Table 25.3 for a list of hepatitis viruses.

Hepatitis A

HAV, also known as infectious hepatitis or short incubation hepatitis, is the most common form of viral hepatitis worldwide. It is caused by a nonenveloped RNA virus of the picornavirus family. Tens of millions of HAV infections occur annually, with the most common reported source of infection in the household occurring via contaminated or improperly handled food.[58] Because HAV is excreted in bile and shed in the feces, which can contain up to 10^9 infectious virions per gram, the fecal–oral route is the primary means of HAV transmission.[59,60] Patients with HAV infection present with symptoms of fever, malaise, anorexia, nausea, abdominal discomfort, dark urine, and jaundice. Symptoms are generally self-limited and resolve within 3 weeks. However, in rare instances, patients develop fulminant liver failure. Chronic infection with HAV is not found and there is no evidence of a carrier state or long-term sequelae in humans.[58]

Clinical markers for the diagnosis and the progression of HAV infection are measured through the presence of serologic antibodies. IgM antibodies to HAV (IgM anti-HAV) are detectable at or prior to the onset of clinical illness and decline in 3 to 6 months, when it becomes undetectable by commercially available diagnostic tests.[61] IgG antibodies to HAV (IgG anti-HAV) appear soon after IgM, persist for years after infection, and confer lifelong immunity.[62] IgM anti-HAV has been used as the primary marker of acute infection.[63] The presence of elevated titers of IgG anti-HAV

in the absence of IgM indicates a past infection. Another reliable method to detect acute infection in patients is assaying for the presence of viral antigen, which is shed in the feces. However, the antigen is no longer present soon after liver enzymes have reached their peak levels. Another method of detecting HAV infection is amplification of viral RNA by reverse transcription polymerase chain reaction (RT-PCR). Nucleic acid detection techniques are more sensitive than immunoassays for viral antigen to detect HAV in samples of different origins (e.g., clinical specimens, environmental samples, or food). Because of the high proportion of asymptomatic HAV infections, nucleic acid amplification techniques are useful to determine the extent to which unidentified infection occurs.[64]

The availability of vaccines to provide long-term immunity against HAV infection has the potential to significantly reduce the incidence of disease and possibly eliminate the transmission of this virus worldwide.[65–68] In 2006, following the approval of the HAV vaccine for children in the United States, the U.S. Food and Drug Administration (FDA)/CDC recommended that all children receive the HAV vaccine as early as age 12 to 23 months. The use of this vaccine has significantly reduced the incidence of HAV in the United States and has therefore changed the epidemiology of this infection. In addition to children, the HAV vaccine is recommended for the following people: those traveling to countries where hepatitis A is common, those who are family and caregivers of adoptees from countries where hepatitis A is common, those who have sexual encounters with other men, those who are users of recreational drugs (injected or not), those with chronic or long-term liver disease (including hepatitis B or hepatitis C), and those with clotting factor disorders.[69]

Hepatitis B

Known as *serum hepatitis* or *long-incubation hepatitis*, HBV can cause both acute and chronic hepatitis and is the most ubiquitous of the hepatitis viruses. Two billion individuals are infected globally and between 350 and 400 million persons are carriers of the virus. In the United States, 12 million people have been infected with 2 million of those individuals estimated to be chronic carriers of the virus.[58] The highest incidence of acute HBV was among adults aged 25 to 45 years.[70] HBV is comparatively stable in the environment and remains viable for longer than 7 days on environmental surfaces at room temperature.[71] It is detected in virtually all body fluids, including blood, feces, urine, saliva, semen, tears, and breast milk; the three major routes of transmission are parenteral, perinatal, and sexual. Persons at high risk for infection in the United States include persons who engage in the sharing of body fluids, such as high-risk sexual behaviors (e.g., prostitution and male homosexuality), and the sharing of drug injection needles. Children born to mothers who are hepatitis B surface antigen (HBsAg) positive at the time of delivery, immigrants from endemic areas, and sexual partners and household contacts of patients who have HBV are high-risk groups for HBV infection. Although transmission of HBV by blood transfusion occurs, effective screening tests now make this transmission route rare. Health care workers, including laboratory personnel, may be at increased risk for developing HBV, depending on their degree of exposure to blood and body fluids.[72]

Serologic Markers of HBV Infection

HBV is a 42-nm DNA virus classified in the Hepadnaviridae family. The liver is the primary site of HBV replication. Following an HBV infection, the core of the antigen is synthesized in the nuclei of hepatocytes and then passed into the cytoplasm of the liver cell, where it is surrounded by the protein coat. An antigen present in the core of the virus (HBcAg) and a surface antigen present on the surface protein (HBsAg) have been identified by serologic studies. Another antigen, called the e antigen (HBeAg), has also been identified.[73]

Hepatitis B Surface Antigen

Previously known as the Australia antigen and hepatitis-associated antigen, HBsAg is the antigen for which routine testing is performed on all donated units of blood. HBsAg is a useful serologic marker in patients before the onset of clinical symptoms because it is present during the prodrome of acute HBV. HBsAg is not infectious; however, its presence in the serum may indicate the presence of the hepatitis virus.

Therefore, persons who chronically carry HBsAg in their serum must be considered potentially infectious because the presence of the intact virus cannot be excluded. HBsAg is the only serologic marker detected during the first 3 to 5 weeks after infection in newly infected patients. The average time from exposure to detection of HBsAg is 30 days (range 6 to 60 days).[74–76] Highly sensitive single-sample nucleic acid tests can detect HBV DNA in the serum of an infected person 10 to 20 days before detection of HBsAg.[76] HBsAg positivity has been reported for up to 18 days after HBV vaccination and is clinically insignificant.[77,78] Patients who achieve complete viral clearance develop the antibody to the HBsAg, following the disappearance of the HBsAg (Fig. 25.8). The presence of anti-HBs antibody in patients is frequently observed in the general population, suggestive of past infection. Patients who have developed the antibody to the HBsAg are not susceptible to future reinfection with HBV.[72]

Hepatitis B Core Antigen

HBcAg has not been demonstrated to be present in the plasma of hepatitis victims or blood donors. This antigen is present only in the nuclei of hepatocytes during an acute infection with HBV. The antibody to the core antigen, anti-HBc, usually develops earlier in the course of infection than the antibody to the surface antigen (Fig. 25.8). A test for the IgM antibody to HBcAg was developed as a serologic marker for clinical use. The presence of this IgM antibody is specific for acute HBV infection. In patients who have chronic HBV infection, the IgM anti-HBc antibody titer can persist during chronic viral replication at low levels that typically are not detectable by assays used in the United States. However, persons with exacerbation of chronic infection can test positive for IgM anti-HBc.[78] Another marker for acute infection is a viral DNA-dependent DNA polymerase that is closely associated with the presence of the core antigen. This viral enzyme is required for viral replication and is detectable in serum early in the course of viral hepatitis, during the phase of active viral replication.[79]

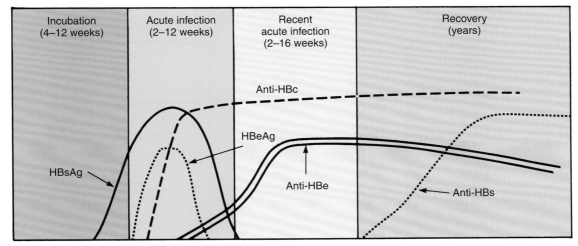

Sequence of HBV Markers

FIGURE 25.8 Serology of hepatitis B infection with recovery.

CASE STUDY 25.3

The following laboratory results were obtained from a 19-year-old college student who consulted the Student Health Service because of fatigue and lack of appetite. She adds that she recently noted that her sclera appears somewhat yellowish and that her urine has become dark (Case Study Table 25.3.1).

CASE STUDY TABLE 25.3.1 Laboratory Results

ALT (SGPT)	Elevated
AST (SGOT)	Elevated
Alkaline phosphatase	Minimally elevated
Lactate dehydrogenase	Elevated
Serum bilirubin	5 mg/dL
Urine bilirubin	Increased
Hepatitis A antibody (IgG)	Negative
Hepatitis A antibody (IgM)	Positive
Hepatitis B surface antigen	Negative
Hepatitis B surface antibody	Negative
Hepatitis C antibody	Negative

Questions

1. What is the most likely diagnosis?
2. What additional factors in the patient's history should be sought?
3. What is the prognosis?

Hepatitis B e Antigen

The e antigen, an antigen closely associated with the core of the viral particle, is detected in the serum of persons with acute or chronic HBV infection. The presence of the e antigen appears to correlate well with both the number of infectious virus particles and the degree of infectivity of HBsAg-positive sera. The presence of HBeAg in HBsAg carriers is an unfavorable prognostic sign and predicts a severe course and chronic liver disease. Conversely, the presence of anti-HBe antibody in carriers indicates a low infectivity of the serum (Fig. 25.9). The e antigen is detected in serum only when surface antigen is present (Fig. 25.10).

The serologic markers of HBV infection typically used to differentiate among acute, resolving, and chronic infections are HBsAg, anti-HBc, and anti-HBs (Table 25.4). Persons who recover from natural infection typically will be positive for both anti-HBs and anti-HBc, whereas persons who respond to HBV vaccine have only anti-HBs. Persons who become chronically infected fail to develop antibody to the HBsAg, resulting in the persistent presence of HBsAg as well as the presence of anti-HBc in patient serum, typically for life.[80–83] HBeAg and anti-HBe screenings typically are used for the management of patients with chronic infection. Serologic assays are available commercially for all markers except HBcAg because no free HBcAg circulates in blood.[70]

Nucleic acid hybridization or PCR technique is used to detect HBV DNA in the blood and is another method used to measure disease progression. This technique provides a more sensitive measurement of infectivity and disease progression than serology. It may be used to monitor the effectiveness of antiviral therapy in patients with chronic HBV infection, but it supplements rather than replaces current HBV serologic assays.[84–86]

Chronic Infection with HBV

Approximately 90% of patients infected with HBV recover within 6 months. Recovery is accompanied by the development of the antibody to the HBsAg. However, about 10% of patients progress to a chronic hepatitis infection.

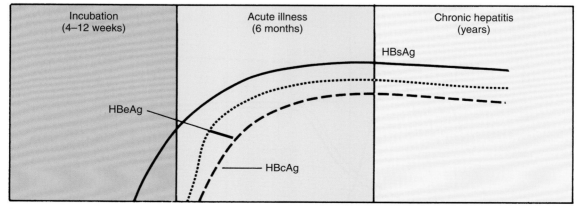

FIGURE 25.9 No antibody is formed against HBsAg. The persistence of HBeAg implies high infectivity and a generally poor prognosis. This patient would likely develop cirrhosis unless seroconversion occurs or treatment is given.

Sequence of HBV Surface Markers
Chronic Hepatitis

FIGURE 25.10 Serology of chronic hepatitis with formation of antibody to HBeAg. This is a favorable sign and suggests that the chronic hepatitis may resolve. Complete recovery would be heralded by the disappearance of HBsAg and formation of its corresponding antibody.

The likelihood of developing chronic HBV infection is higher in individuals infected perinatally (90%) and during childhood (20% to 30%), when the immune system is thought to be less developed and unable to achieve efficient viral clearance, than in adult immunocompetent subjects (<1%).[87] Approximately 25% of persons who were chronically infected since childhood and 15% of those who were chronically infected since adulthood die prematurely from cirrhosis or liver cancer. In the majority of cases, patients remain asymptomatic until the onset of cirrhosis.[88]

Patients with chronic HBV display the characteristic serologic profile as shown in Figure 25.10. The presence of HBsAg in chronically infected patients is an indication that they are infectious and at risk for developing complications, including cirrhosis and HCC. The natural course of chronic HBV infection is divided into four phases based on the virus–host interaction: immune tolerance, immune clearance (HBeAg-positive chronic hepatitis), low or non-replication (inactive HBsAg carrier), and reactivation (HBeAg-negative chronic hepatitis).[89–91] Patients can be

HBSAG[a]	Total Anti-HBC[b]	IGM[c] Anti-HBC	Anti-HBS[d]	Interpretation
–[e]	–	–	–	Never infected
+[f,g]	–	–	–	Early acute infection; transient (up to 18 d) after vaccination
+	+	+	–	Acute infection
–	+	+	+ or –	Acute resolving infection
–	+	–	+	Recovered from past infection and immune
+	+	–	–	Chronic infection
–	+	–	–	False positive (i.e., susceptible); past infection, "low-level" chronic infection[h]; or passive transfer of anti-HBc to infant born to HBsAg-positive mother
–	–	–	+	Immune if concentration is ≥10 mIU/mL after vaccine series completion; passive transfer after hepatitis B immune globulin administration

TABLE 25.4 **Typical Interpretation of Serologic Test Results for Hepatitis B Virus Infection**
Serologic Marker

[a]Hepatitis B surface antigen.
[b]Antibody to hepatitis B core antigen.
[c]Immunoglobulin M.
[d]Antibody to HBsAg.
[e]Negative test result.
[f]Positive test result.
[g]To ensure that an HBsAg-positive test result is not a false positive, samples with reactive HBsAg results should be tested with a licensed neutralizing confirmatory test if recommended in the manufacturer's package insert.
[h]Persons positive only for anti-HBc are unlikely to be infectious except under unusual circumstances in which they are the source for direct percutaneous exposure of susceptible recipients to large quantities of virus (e.g., blood transfusion or organ transplant).

						HBV DNA	
Phase	**Serum ALT**	**HBeAg**	**Anti-HBe**			**Copies/mL**	**IU/mL**
Immune tolerance	Normal or minimally	Positive	Negative	Very high levels		10^8–10^{11} elevated	20 million– 20 billion
HBeAg-positive chronic	Persistently elevated hepatitis	Positive	Negative	High levels		10^6–10^{10}	200,000– 2 billion
HBeAg-negative chronic hepatitis	Elevated and often fluctuating	Negative	Positive	Moderate levels, often fluctuating		10^4–10^8	2,000– 20 million
Inactive carrier	Normal	Negative	Positive	Low or no detectable levels		$<10^4$	$<2,000$

TABLE 25.5 **Serological Profiles of Chronic Hepatitis B Virus Infection**

ALT, alanine aminotransferase; HBV, hepatitis B virus.
Adapted from Fattovich G, Bortolotti F, Donato F. Natural history of chronic hepatitis B: special emphasis on disease progression and prognostic factors. *J Hepatol.* 2008;48:335–352.

classified according to their serologic status as shown in Table 25.5.[87]

HBV Treatment and Prevention

Persons who have chronic HBV infection require medical evaluation and regular monitoring.[92–94] The FDA has approved several drugs for the treatment of chronic HBV that can achieve sustained suppression of HBV replication and remission of liver disease in certain persons.[93]

HBV vaccination is the most effective measure to prevent HBV infection and its consequences, including cirrhosis of the liver, liver cancer, liver failure, and death. HBsAg is the antigen used for HBV vaccination.[95,96] The vaccine is highly effective in stimulating the production of hepatitis B surface antibody and thereby rendering the recipient immune. As a result of the national program of childhood immunization, by 2005, a 98% decline in HBV infection was reported among children aged 13 years or younger, as well as a 97% decline among adolescents aged 12 to 19 years.[58] In 2006, the Advisory Committee on Immunization Practices (ACIP) recommended universal HBV vaccination for all unvaccinated adults at risk for HBV infection and for all adults requesting protection from HBV infection. All health care workers who handle blood products and are in close proximity to body fluids should have the hepatitis vaccine. The hepatitis B immune globulin (HBIG) provides passively acquired anti-HBs and temporary protection (i.e., 3 to 6 months) when administered in standard doses. HBIG typically is used as an adjunct to HBV vaccine for postexposure immunoprophylaxis to prevent HBV infection. For nonresponders to HBV vaccination, HBIG administered alone is the primary means of protection after an HBV exposure.[70]

Hepatitis C

HCV (originally "non-A non-B hepatitis") is caused by a virus with an RNA genome that is a member of the Flaviviridae family. HCV is transmitted parenterally. Although the sexual and fecal–oral routes as modes of transmission have been documented, the virus is transmitted primarily by blood transfusion of inappropriately screened blood products.[97–99] Approximately 3% of the world population is infected by the virus and most infections become chronic and may lead to cirrhosis, end-stage liver disease, HCC, and death. In the United States, HCV infection is present in about 1.6% of the noninstitutionalized population.[100] As many as 4 million Americans are chronically infected.[58] Clinically, acute HCV infection presents only mild infection and patients may remain completely asymptomatic. However, HCV infection has a high rate of progression to chronic hepatitis, cirrhosis, and liver carcinoma, making HCV a major cause of chronic hepatitis in the United States.[99,101] In addition, HCV infection is a leading cause of liver transplantation in this country.[102]

Laboratory Tests for Hepatitis C

The hepatitis C antibody is usually not detected in the first few months of infection but will almost always be present in the later stages. The antibody is not protective against reinfection and sometimes disappears several years following resolution of the infection. Laboratory testing for the diagnosis of HCV infection in the clinical setting is relatively straightforward. Currently, two laboratory tests are commonly used to diagnose HCV infection in clinical practice: anti-HCV detection by EIA and quantitative nucleic acid PCR assays for serum HCV RNA.[103–108] In clinical practice, the most common approach is initially to test a patient's serum for the presence of anti-HCV by EIA. If this test gives a positive result, the next step is to test for serum HCV RNA by PCR.[105] The HCV antibody test is designed to detect antibodies generated in response to HCV infection.[105,107] Although a positive HCV antibody test result generally indicates that the patient has been exposed to the HCV virus, this test cannot determine whether the patient is currently infected with HCV or has recovered from HCV infection.[103,107] Some patients with a positive HCV antibody test result have spontaneously cleared HCV. These patients (anti-HCV positive but HCV RNA negative) are recommended to retake the test for HCV RNA on a second occasion, 3 to 6 months after the first HCV RNA test.[107]

Chronic HCV Infection

Most patients with HCV infection progress to chronic infection. Although patients with chronic HCV infection appear to be at high risk for liver cirrhosis, the role of HCV in the development of HCC is not clear. Most chronically infected patients are asymptomatic and manifest only mild elevations of liver function tests, especially transaminases. The degree of elevation in liver enzymes has little predictive value toward disease progression. About 80% of infected patients develop chronic hepatitis, although, in most cases, the disease does not progress. The percentage of patients progressing to liver cirrhosis varies widely in different studies but has been estimated to be as high as 40% after 40 years. Alcohol consumption concomitant with chronic HCV infection significantly increases the risk of cirrhosis. Liver biopsies are performed periodically in these patients, with the degree of inflammation and fibrosis correlating with the risk of cirrhosis.[109–112]

Patients with chronic HCV infection are usually treated with pegylated interferon and ribavirin. Therapeutic efficacy is monitored by using PCR to determine the number of viral copies in serum.[113] A prototypic envelope peptide-based vaccine has been reported to induce antibodies in human subjects, but there is no evidence for the presence of a neutralizing antibody against HCV.[114] Likely, an effective and safe vaccine against HCV will not be available soon.

Hepatitis D

HDV is a unique subviral satellite virus infection. It is a small, defective RNA-containing virus that cannot replicate independently but rather requires the HBsAg of HBV for replication. Therefore, it is incapable of causing any illness in patients who do not have HBV infection. Modes of transmission are generally similar to those of HBV.

Approximately 5% of the global HBV carriers are coinfected with HDV, leading to a total of 10 to 15 million HDV carriers worldwide.[115,116] Each year, 7,500 new cases of HDV infections are estimated to occur in the United States.[117] Chronic HDV infection is estimated to be responsible for more than 1,000 deaths each year in the United States.[118]

HDV virions possess an outer envelope composed of HBsAg proteins and host membrane lipids and an inner nucleocapsid consisting of viral RNA and hepatitis delta antigen (HDAg). It is believed that HBsAg-mediated binding to a cellular receptor helps HDV penetrate the hepatocyte.[119] Nuclear localization signal domain on the HDAg facilitates transit of its genome into the nucleus, where viral replication takes place.[120] HDV infection can occur concurrently with HBV infection (coinfection) or in a patient with established HBV infection (superinfection) (Table 25.6). The rate of chronicity following coinfection with HBV and HDV is equal to that of HBV infection alone.[121] HDV superinfection is likely to become chronic simply because HBV infection is already chronic. In general, in the acute phase, HDV superinfected carriers may develop severe hepatitis, and around 70% to 90% will progress to chronicity.[122]

The diagnosis of HDV relies on detection of antibodies against HDAg and serum HDV RNA, as well as HBV markers.[123] Clinical symptoms of HDV cannot be distinguished from those of other hepatic viruses. Accurate diagnosis is made by a negative test for IgM anti-HBc and confirmed by the detection of HDV markers.[124] Widespread use of the HBV vaccine has resulted in a decline in the incidence of HDV.[125] Interferon-α is currently the therapy used for treating chronic HDV infection. Compared with chronic HBV or HCV, chronic HDV treatment requires a higher dosage and a longer duration of treatment, and posttreatment relapses are common.[124]

TABLE 25.6	Clinical Features of Hepatitis D Virus (HDV) Coinfection and Superinfection in Hepatitis B Virus (HBV)	
	Coinfection	**Superinfection**
HBV infection	Acute	Chronic
Outcomes	Recovery with seroclearance	Usually persistent infection
Markers		
HBsAg	Positive, early and transient	Positive and persistent
IgM anti-HBc	Positive	Negative
Anti-HBs	Positive in recovery phase	Negative
HDV infection	Acute	Acute or chronic
Outcomes	Recovery with seroclearance	Usually persistent infection
Markers		
Serum HDAg[a]	Early and short-lived	Early and transient, undetectable later
Liver HDAg	Positive and transient	Positive, maybe negative in late stage
Serum HDV RNA	Positive, early and transient	Positive, early and persistent
Anti-HDV	Late acute phase, low titer	Rapidly increasing, high titers
IgM anti-HDV	Positive, transient, pentameric	Rapidly increasing, high titers, monomeric

[a]Using immunoblot assay, detection rate of serum HDAg may be comparable to Northern blot detection of HDV RNA using cDNA probe.
IgM, immunoglobulin M; HDAg, hepatitis delta antigen.
Adapted from Hsieh TH, Liu CJ, Chen DS, et al. Natural course and treatment of hepatitis D virus infection. *J Formos Med Assoc.* 2006;105:869–881.

CASE STUDY 25.4

The following results were obtained in the patient from Case Study 25.2 (Case Study Table 25.4.1).

CASE STUDY TABLE 25.4.1 Laboratory Results

Hepatitis A antibody (IgG)	Positive
Hepatitis A antibody (IgM)	Negative
Hepatitis B surface antigen	Positive
Hepatitis B surface antibody	Negative
Hepatitis core antibody (IgM)	Positive
Hepatitis C antibody	Negative

Questions

1. What is the most likely diagnosis?
2. What is the prognosis?
3. What complications may develop?

Hepatitis E

The RNA-containing HEV, a nonenveloped RNA virus that is only 27 to 34 nm in diameter, is the sole member of the genus *Hepevirus* in the family Hepeviridae. After infection, the incubation period is short, generally between 21 and 42 days prior to the onset of symptoms. The virus may be detected in feces and bile by about 7 days after infection. HEV is transmitted primarily by the fecal–oral route, and waterborne epidemics are characteristic of HEV in many developing countries. However, in industrialized countries, several nonhuman mammals such as pigs, cows, and sheep are susceptible to infection with HEV, leading to the potential spread of the virus through zoonosis.[126] The clinical presentation of HEV is comparable to that of HAV. The severity of an HEV infection is generally greater than the severity of an HAV infection.[127] In general, HEV infection is mild, except in pregnant women, in whom it may be a devastating illness.[128]

Because cases of HEV are not clinically distinguishable from cases of other types of acute viral hepatitis, diagnosis is made by biochemical assessment of liver function. Acute HEV is diagnosed when the presence of IgM anti-HEV is detected.[127,129] The presence of a high or increasing anti-HEV IgG titer may support the diagnosis of acute HEV infection, and in such cases, acute HEV can be presumed even in the absence of IgM anti-HEV.[130] EIA and immuno-chromatography are most convenient for the detection of IgM and/or IgG anti-HEV. Additional testing by RT-PCR has a limited confirmatory role. Acute-phase HEV RNA can be detected in feces by PCR in approximately 50% of cases.

In most instances, there is a very good positive correlation between the results assayed by RT-PCR and EIA.[127] HEV should be suspected in outbreaks of waterborne hepatitis occurring in developing countries, especially if the disease is more severe in pregnant women or if HAV has been excluded. If laboratory tests are not available, epidemiologic evidence can help in establishing a diagnosis.[131]

At present, no commercially available vaccines exist for the prevention of HEV. Experimental immune prophylaxis against HEV based on recombinant antigens appears to confer short-term protection and may be useful for pregnant women in endemic areas and travelers coming into these regions.

Other Forms of Hepatitis

Five forms of viral hepatitis (A, B, C, D, and E) are well recognized. The role of G viruses is currently unclear. Hepatitis F is an enteric agent that may be transmitted to primates. Again, more needs to be learned about this agent and its role, if any, in human disease. Other forms of viral hepatitis, such as TT virus and SEN virus, may exist. The GB group of flavo-like viruses, GBV-A, GBV-B, and GBV-C, are also associated with acute and chronic hepatitis. Little is known about these diseases, and no diagnostic tests for them are commercially available at this time.[132–135] Cytomegalovirus, Epstein-Barr virus, and probably several other agents can also cause hepatitis.

CASE STUDY 25.5

A 36-year-old man consulted his family physician because of liver function abnormalities, which had been noted initially during a preinsurance physical examination 6 months earlier. The following laboratory results were obtained, which were identical to those obtained 6 months ago (Case Study Table 25.5.1).

CASE STUDY TABLE 25.5.1 Laboratory Results

Hepatitis A antibody (IgG)	Positive
Hepatitis A antibody (IgM)	Negative
Hepatitis B surface antigen	Positive
Hepatitis B surface antibody	Negative
Hepatitis B core antibody (IgM)	Positive
Hepatitis C antibody	Negative

Questions

1. What is the most likely diagnosis?
2. What is the prognosis?
3. What complications may develop?
4. What additional tests should be done?

For additional student resources, please visit the **Point**® at http://thepoint.lww.com

questions

1. Which of the following enzymes would best aid in identifying hepatobiliary disease?
   a. Alkaline phosphatase (ALP)
   b. Aspartate aminotransferase (AST)
   c. Alanine aminotransferase (ALT)
   d. Ammonia

2. In which of the following types of cells does the conjugation of bilirubin take place?
   a. Hepatocytes
   b. Kupffer cells
   c. Macrophages
   d. Phagocytic cells

3. Which of the following enzymes is responsible for the conjugation of bilirubin?
   e. UDP-glucuronosyltransferase
   a. Alkaline phosphatase
   b. Glutamate dehydrogenase
   c. Leucine aminopeptidase

4. Which of the following fractions of bilirubin is water soluble and reacts with a diazo reagent without the addition of an accelerator?
   a. Conjugated bilirubin
   b. Unconjugated bilirubin
   c. Total bilirubin
   d. Indirect bilirubin

5. Which form of hepatitis is caused by a DNA virus?
   a. Hepatitis B
   b. Hepatitis A
   c. Hepatitis C
   d. Hepatitis D

6. Which of the following enzymes is most useful in establishing the hepatic origin of an elevated serum alkaline phosphatase?
   a. 5′-Nucleotidase
   b. Alanine aminotransferase (ALT)
   c. Aspartate aminotransferase (AST)
   d. Lactate dehydrogenase

7. Hepatitis E is likely to cause serious consequences in
   a. Pregnant women
   b. Children
   c. Travelers in Third World countries
   d. Older people

8. Worldwide, most primary malignant tumors of the liver are related to
   a. Alcoholism
   b. Gallstones
   c. Reye's syndrome
   d. Malaria

9. The reagent *p*-dimethylaminobenzaldehyde is used to measure which of the following?
   a. Urobilinogen
   b. Total bilirubin
   c. Ammonia
   d. Alkaline phosphatase

10. Which of the following conditions would result in elevations in primarily conjugated bilirubin?
    a. Dubin-Johnson syndrome
    b. Physiologic jaundice of the newborn
    c. Crigler-Najjar syndrome
    d. Gilbert's syndrome

11. A urinalysis dipstick test indicated that urobilinogen was absent. Which condition does this support?
    a. Biliary obstruction.
    b. Hepatitis A acute infection.
    c. Defective liver cell function.
    d. Hepatocellular disease.
    e. This would support all of the above conditions.

12. Measuring serum ammonia levels has the potential to be fraught with preanalytical errors that may interfere with achieving an accurate result. Of the following preanalytical steps, which is incorrect?
    a. After phlebotomy, the patient's blood should be immediately placed on ice.
    b. The blood should be collected in a red clot tube without anticoagulant.
    c. Hemolyzed samples should be rejected as this interferes by falsely increasing ammonia levels.
    d. Lipemia may also interfere with plasma ammonia measurements.
    e. All of the above are correct.

13. A patient presents with elevated levels of IgG anti-HAV, while levels of IgM anti-HAV are nondetectable. This patient is likely to
    a. Have an acute infection of HAV
    b. Have a chronic infection of HAV

(continues on page 526)

review questions (continued)

c. Have an immunity to HAV

d. Be a carrier of HAV

14. The product produced and *measured* when reacting bilirubin with a diazo reagent is

a. NADPH

b. NAD

c. Azobilirubin

d. Bilirubin diglucuronide

15. A healthy 28-year-old female sees her physician for a routine examination and has received a "relatively" clean bill of health except for the results below.

Total bilirubin	2.8 mg/dL
Direct bilirubin	0.1 mg/dL
Indirect bilirubin	2.7 mg/dL

These results most likely indicate?

a. Normal bilirubin metabolism

b. Extrahepatic obstruction

c. Dubin-Johnson syndrome

d. Gilbert's disease

16. Which of the following is measured using glutamate dehydrogenase and is a measure of advanced stages, poor prognosis, and coma in liver disease?

a. Total bilirubin

b. Ammonia

c. Unconjugated bilirubin

d. Urea

17. In which of the following disease states would you see an elevation in total bilirubin and conjugated bilirubin only?

a. Biliary obstruction

b. Hemolysis

c. Neonatal jaundice

d. Gilbert's disease

18. As a reduction product of bilirubin catabolism, this compound is partially reabsorbed from the intestines through the portal circulation for reexcretion by the liver. What is this compound?

a. Urobilinogen

b. Azobilirubin

c. Biliverdin

d. Urobilin

e. Bilirubin

19. You are the technologist on duty and you are performing the following assay:

Patient sample + Diazo reagent + Accelerator → Product

Which fraction(s) of bilirubin will react in the above reaction?

a. Conjugated

b. Delta

c. Unconjugated

d. All of the above

20. Choose the diagnosis most consistent with the following laboratory findings:

Serum: total bilirubin 5.8 mg/dL
Direct bilirubin 0.1 mg/dL
Indirect bilirubin 5.7 mg/dL

a. Physiologic jaundice of the newborn

b. Posthepatic bile obstruction

c. Dubin-Johnson syndrome

d. Rotor's syndrome

e. None of the above

references

1. Wang X, Chowdhury JR, Chowdhury NR. Bilirubin metabolism: applied physiology. *Curr Paediatr.* 2006;16:70–74.
2. Ahlfors CE. Measurement of plasma unbound unconjugated bilirubin. *Anal Biochem.* 2000;279:130–135.
3. McNamara JR, Warnick GR, Wu LL. Lipids and lipoproteins. In: Bishop ML, Duben-Engellkirk JL, Fody EP, eds. *Clinical Chemistry: Principles, Procedures, Correlations*. Philadelphia, PA: Lippincott Williams & Wilkins; 2000:323.
4. Papavramidou N, Fee E, Christopoulou-Aletra H. Jaundice in the hippocratic corpus. *J Gastrointest Surg.* 2007;11:1728–1731.
5. Pashankar D, Schreiber RA. Jaundice in older children and adolescents. *Pediatr Rev.* 2001;22:219–226.
6. Monaghan G, Ryan M, Seddon R, et al. Genetic variation in bilirubin UDP-glucuronosyltransferase gene promoter and Gilbert's syndrome. *Lancet.* 1996;347:578–581.
7. Black M, Billing BH. Hepatic bilirubin UDP-glucuronyl transferase activity in liver disease and Gilbert's syndrome. *N Engl J Med.* 1969;280:1266–1271.
8. Kaplan M, Hammerman C. Bilirubin and the genome: the hereditary basis of unconjugated neonatal hyperbilirubinemia. *Curr Pharmacogenomics.* 2005;3:21–42.
9. Crigler JF Jr, Najjar VA. Congenital familial nonhemolytic jaundice with kernicterus. *Pediatrics.* 1952;10:169–180.
10. Berk PD, Noyer C. The familial unconjugated hyperbilirubinemia. *Semin Liver Dis.* 1994;14:346–351.
11. Berk PD. Bilirubin metabolism and the hereditary hyperbilirubinemias. *Semin Liver Dis.* 1994;14:321–322.
12. Berk PD, Noyer C. The familial conjugated hyperbilirubinemia. *Semin Liver Dis.* 1994;14:386–394.
13. Zimniak P. Dubin-Johnson and Rotor syndromes: molecular basis and pathogenesis. *Semin Liver Dis.* 1993;13:248–260.

14. Dennery PA, Seidman DS, Stevenson DK. Neonatal hyperbilirubinemia. *N Engl J Med.* 2001;344:581–590.

15. Xu J, Murphy SL, Kochanek KD, et al. Deaths: final data for 2013. *Natl Vital Stat Rep.* 2016;64(2):1–119.

16. Ferlay J, Soerjomataram I, Ervik M, et al. *GLOBOCAN 2012 v1.0, Cancer Incidence and Mortality Worldwide: IARC Cancer Base No. 11 [Internet].* Lyon, France: International Agency for Research on Cancer; 2013. Available from: http://globocan.iarc.fr. Accessed May 1, 2016.

17. El-Serag HB. Hepatocellular carcinoma. *N Engl J Med.* 2011;365:1118–1127.

18. American Cancer Society. *Cancer Facts & Figures 2012.* Atlanta, GA: American Cancer Society; 2012. Available from: http://www.cancer.org/acs/groups/content/@epidemiologysurveilance/documents/document/acspc-031941.pdf. Accessed February 22, 2012.

19. Mazzaferro V, Regalia E, Doci R, et al. Liver transplantation for the treatment of small hepatocellular carcinomas in patients with cirrhosis. *N Engl J Med.* 1996;334:693–699.

20. Peters LJ, Wiener GJ, Gilliam J, et al. Reye's syndrome in adults. A case report and review of the literature. *Arch Intern Med.* 1986;146:2401–2403.

21. Preblud SR, Orenstein WA, Bart KJ. Varicella: clinical manifestations, epidemiology and health impact in children. *Pediatr Infect Dis.* 1984;3:505–509.

22. Edwards KM, Bennett SR, Garner WL, et al. Reye's syndrome associated with adenovirus infections in infants. *Am J Dis Child.* 1985;139:343–346.

23. Johnson GM, Scurletis TD, Carroll NB. A study of sixteen fatal cases of encephalitis. *N C Med J.* 1963;24:464–473.

24. Starko KM, Ray CG, Dominguez LB, et al. Reye's syndrome and salicylate use. *Pediatrics.* 1980;66:859–864.

25. Waldman RJ, Hall WN, McGee H, et al. Aspirin as a risk factor in Reye's syndrome. *JAMA.* 1982;247:3089–3094.

26. Surgeon General's advisory on the use of salicylates and Reye syndrome. *MMWR Morb Mortal Wkly Rep.* 1982;31:289–290.

27. Davis DL, Buffler P. Reduction of deaths after drug labelling for risk of Reye's syndrome. *Lancet.* 1992;340:1042.

28. Daugherty CC, Gartside PS, Heubi JE, et al. A morphometric study of Reye's syndrome. Correlation of reduced mitochondrial numbers and increased mitochondrial size with clinical manifestations. *Am J Pathol.* 1987;129:313–326.

29. Belay ED, Bresee JS, Holman RC, et al. Reye's syndrome in the United States from 1981 through 1997. *N Engl J Med.* 1999;340:1377–1382.

30. Liu ZX, Kaplowitz N. Immune-mediated drug-induced liver disease. *Clin Liver Dis.* 2002;6:755–774.

31. Lieber CS. Alcohol and the liver: metabolism of alcohol and its role in hepatic and extrahepatic diseases. *Mt Sinai J Med.* 2000;67:84–94.

32. Bissell DM, Gores GJ, Laskin DL, et al. Drug-induced liver injury: mechanisms and test systems. *Hepatology.* 2001;33:1009–1013.

33. Bellentani S, Saccoccio G, Costa G, et al. Drinking habits as cofactors of risk for alcohol induced liver damage. *Gut.* 1997;41:845–850.

34. Mutimer DJ, Burra P, Neuberger JM, et al. Managing severe alcoholic hepatitis complicated by renal failure. *Q J Med.* 1993;86:649–656.

35. Maddrey WC, Boitnott JK, Bedine MS, et al. Corticosteroid therapy of alcoholic hepatitis. *Gastroenterology.* 1978;75:193–199.

36. Forrest EH, Evans CD, Stewart S, et al. Analysis of factors predictive of mortality in alcoholic hepatitis and derivation and validation of the Glasgow alcoholic hepatitis score. *Gut.* 2005;54:1174–1179.

37. Dunn W, Jamil LH, Brown LS, et al. MELD accurately predicts mortality in patients with alcoholic hepatitis. *Hepatology.* 2005;41:353–358.

38. Nagata K, Suzuki H, Sakaguchi S. Common pathogenic mechanism in development progression of liver injury caused by non-alcoholic or alcoholic steatohepatitis. *J Toxicol Sci.* 2007;32:453–468.

39. Bertini G, Rubaltelli FF. Non-invasive bilirubinometry in neonatal jaundice. *Semin Neonatol.* 2002;7:129–133.

40. Lott JA, Doumas BT. "Direct" and total bilirubin tests: contemporary problems. *Clin Chem.* 1993;39:641–647.

41. Wilding P, Zilva JF, Wilde CE. Transport of specimens for clinical chemistry analysis. *Ann Clin Biochem.* 1977;14:301–306.

42. Doumas BT, Kwok-Cheung PP, Perry BW, et al. Candidate reference method for determination of total bilirubin in serum: development and validation. *Clin Chem.* 1985;31:1779–1789.

43. Doumas BT, Wu TW. The measurement of bilirubin fractions in serum. *Crit Rev Clin Lab Sci.* 1991;28:415–445.

44. Ross JW, Miller WG, Myers GL, et al. The accuracy of laboratory measurements in clinical chemistry: a study of 11 routine chemistry analytes in the College of American Pathologists Chemistry Survey with fresh frozen serum, definitive methods, and reference methods. *Arch Pathol Lab Med.* 1998;122:587–608.

45. Slaughter MR. Sensitivity of conventional methods for bilirubin measurements. *J Lab Clin Med.* 1996;127:233.

46. Malloy HT, Evelyn KA. The determination of bilirubin with the photoelectric colorimeter. *J Biol Chem.* 1937;119:481–490.

47. Hofmann AF. Bile acid secretion, bile flow and biliary lipid secretion in humans. *Hepatology.* 1990;12(3 pt 2):17S–22S.

48. Kotal P, Fevery J. Quantitation of urobilinogen in feces, urine, bile and serum by direct spectrophotometry of zinc complex. *Clin Chim Acta.* 1991;202:1–9.

49. Azer SA, Klaassen CD, Stacey NH. Biochemical assay of serum bile acids: methods and applications. *Br J Biomed Sci.* 1997;54:118–132.

50. Polkowska G, Polkowski W, Kudlicka A, et al. Range of serum bile acid concentrations in neonates, infants, older children, and in adults. *Med Sci Monit.* 2001;7(suppl 1):268–270.

51. Green RM, Flamm S. AGA technical review on the evaluation of liver chemistry tests. *Gastroenterology.* 2002;123:1367–1384.

52. American Gastroenterological Association medical position statement: evaluation of liver chemistry tests. *Gastroenterology.* 2002;123:1364–1366.

53. Pagani F, Panteghini M. 5′-Neucleotidase in the detection of increased activity of the liver form of alkaline phosphatase in serum. *Clin Chem.* 2001;47:2046–2048.

54. Sunderman FW. The clinical biochemistry of 5′-nucleotidase. *Ann Clin Lab Sci.* 1990;20:123–139.

55. Conigrave KM, Dengenhardt LJ, Whitfield JB. CDT, GGT and AST as markers of alcohol use: the WHO/ISBRA collaborative project. *Alcohol Clin Exp Res.* 2002;25:332–339.

56. Jay DW. Nonprotein nitrogen. In: Bishop ML, Duben-Englekirk JL, Fody EP, eds. *Clinical Chemistry: Principles, Procedures, Correlations.* Philadelphia, PA: Lippincott Williams & Wilkins; 2000:260–274.

57. da Fonseca-Wollheim F. Deamidation of glutamine by increased plasma gamma-glutamyltransferase is a source of rapid ammonia formation in blood and plasma specimens. *Clin Chem.* 1990;36:1479–1482.

58. Koff RS. Review article: vaccination and viral hepatitis—current status and future prospects. *Aliment Pharmacol Ther.* 2007;26:1285–1292.

59. Skinhoj P, Mathiesen LR, Kiryger P, et al. Faecal excretion of hepatitis A virus in patients with symptomatic hepatitis A infection. *Scand J Gastroenterol.* 1981;16:1057–1059.

60. Tassopoulos NC, Papaevangelou GJ, Ticehurst JR, et al. Fecal excretion of Greek strains of hepatitis A virus in patients with hepatitis A and in experimentally infected chimpanzees. *J Infect Dis.* 1986;154:231–237.

61. Kao HW, Ashcavai M, Redeker AG. The persistence of hepatitis A IgM antibody after acute clinical hepatitis A. *Hepatology.* 1984;4:933–936.

62. Skinhoj P, Mikkelsen F, Hollinger FB. Hepatitis A in Greenland: importance of specific antibody testing in epidemiologic surveillance. *Am J Epidemiol.* 1977;105:140–147.

63. Cuthbert JA. Hepatitis A: old and new. *Clin Microbiol Rev.* 2001;14:38–58.

64. Nainan OV, Xia G, Vaughan G, et al. Diagnosis of hepatitis A virus infection: a molecular approach. *Clin Microbiol Rev.* 2006;19:63–79.

65. Bell BP, Feinstone SM. Hepatitis A vaccine. In: Plotkin SA, Orenstein WA, Offit PA, eds. *Vaccine.* 4th ed. Philadelphia, PA: WB Saunders; 2004:269–297.

66. Centers for Disease Control and Prevention (CDC). Prevention of hepatitis A through active or passive immunization: recommendations of the Advisory Committee on Immunization Practices (ACIP). *MMWR Morb Mortal Wkly Rep.* 1999;48(RR-12):1–37.

67. Hollinger FB, Emerson SU. Hepatitis A virus. In: Knipe SM, Howley PM, eds. *Fields Virology.* 4th ed. New York, NY: Lippincott Williams & Wilkins; 2001:799–840.

68. Margolis HS. Viral hepatitis. In: Wallace RB, Doebbeling BN, eds. *Maxcy-Rosenau-Last Public Health and Preventive Medicine.* 14th ed. Stamford, CT: Appleton & Lange; 2000:174–188.

69. Centers for Disease Control and Prevention. General Recommendations on Immunization: Recommendations of the ACIP. *MMWR Morb Mortal Wkly Rep.* 2011;60(RR-02):1–64.

70. Centers for Disease Control and Prevention. A comprehensive immunization strategy to eliminate transmission of hepatitis B virus infection in the United States. Recommendations of the Advisory Committee on Immunization Practices (ACIP) Part II: immunization of adults. *MMWR Morb Mortal Wkly Rep.* 2006;55(RR-16):1–25.

71. Bond WW, Favero MS, Petersen NJ, et al. Survival of hepatitis B virus after drying and storage for one week. *Lancet.* 1981;1:550–551.

72. Davis GL. Hepatitis B: diagnosis and treatment. *South Med J.* 1997;90:866–870.

73. Neuschwander-Tetri BA. Common blood tests for liver disease. Which ones are most useful? *Postgrad Med.* 1995;98:49–56, 59, 63.

74. Krugman S, Overby LR, Mushahwar IK, et al. Viral hepatitis, type B. Studies on natural history and prevention re-examined. *N Engl J Med.* 1979;300:101–106.

75. Hoofnagle JH, DiBisceglie AM. Serologic diagnosis of acute and chronic viral hepatitis. *Semin Liver Dis.* 1991;11:73–83.

76. Biswas R, Tabor E, Hsia CC, et al. Comparative sensitivity of HBV NATs and HBsAg assays for detection of acute HBV infection. *Transfusion* 2003;43:788–798.

77. Lunn ER, Hoggarth BJ, Cook WJ. Prolonged hepatitis B surface antigenemia after vaccination. *Pediatrics.* 2000;105:E81.

78. Kao JH, Chen PJ, Lai MY, et al. Acute exacerbations of chronic hepatitis B are rarely associated with superinfection of hepatitis B virus. *Hepatology.* 2001;34(4 pt 1):817–823.

79. Kurstak C, Kurstak E, Hossain A. Progress in diagnosis of viral hepatitis A, B, C, D and E. *Acta Virol.* 1996;40:107–115.

80. Alward WL, McMahon BJ, Hall DB, et al. The long-term serological course of asymptomatic hepatitis B virus carriers and the development of primary hepatocellular carcinoma. *J Infect Dis.* 1985;151:604–609.

81. Liaw YF, Sheen IS, Chen TJ, et al. Incidence, determinants and significance of delayed clearance of serum HBsAg in chronic hepatitis B virus infection: a prospective study. *Hepatology.* 1991;13:627–631.

82. Adachi H, Kaneko S, Matsushita E, et al. Clearance of HBsAg in seven patients with chronic hepatitis B. *Hepatology.* 1992;16:1334–1337.

83. McMahon BJ, Holck P, Bulkow L, et al. Serologic and clinical outcomes of 1536 Alaska Natives chronically infected with hepatitis B virus. *Ann Intern Med.* 2001;135:759–768.

84. Jalava T, Ranki M, Bengtström M, et al. A rapid and quantitative solution hybridization method for detection of HBV DNA in serum. *J Virol Methods.* 1992;36:171–180.

85. Malavé Lara C, Gorriño MT, Campelo C, et al. Detection of hepatitis B virus DNA in chronic carriers by the polymerase chain reaction. *Eur J Clin Microbiol Infect Dis.* 1992;11:740–744.

86. Aspinall S, Steele AD, Peenze I, et al. Detection and quantitation of hepatitis B virus DNA: comparison of two commercial hybridization assays with polymerase chain reaction. *J Viral Hepat.* 1995;2:107–111.

87. Fattovich G, Bortolotti F, Donato F. Natural history of chronic hepatitis B: special emphasis on disease progression and prognostic factors. *J Hepatol.* 2008;48:335–352.

88. Hadziyannis S, Papatheodoridis GV. Hepatitis B e antigen-negative chronic hepatitis: natural history and treatment. *Semin Liver Dis.* 2006;26:130–141.

89. EASL International Consensus Conference on Hepatitis B. Consensus statement. *J Hepatol.* 2003;38:533–540.

90. Perz JF, Armstrong GL, Farrington LA, et al. The contribution of hepatitis B virus and hepatitis C virus infections to cirrhosis and primary liver cancer worldwide. *J Hepatol.* 2006;45:529–538.

91. Lok ASF, McMahon BJ. Chronic hepatitis B. *Hepatology.* 2007;45:507–539.

92. Lok AS, McMahon BJ; Practice Guidelines Committee, American Association for the Study of Liver Disease (AASLD). Chronic hepatitis B. *Hepatology.* 2001;34:1225–1241.

93. Lok AS, McMahon BJ; Practice Guidelines Committee, American Association for the Study of Liver Disease (AASLD). Chronic hepatitis B: update of recommendations. *Hepatology.* 2004;39:857–861.

94. Bruix J, Sherman M; Practice Guidelines Committee, American Association for the Study of Liver Disease (AASLD). Management of hepatocellular carcinoma. *Hepatology.* 2005;42:1208–1236.

95. Purcell RH, Gerin JL. Hepatitis B subunit vaccine: a preliminary report of safety and efficacy tests in chimpanzees. *Am J Med Sci.* 1975;270:395–399.

96. Hilleman MR, McAleer WJ, Buynak EB, et al. Quality and safety of human hepatitis B vaccine. *Dev Biol Stand.* 1983;54:3–12.

97. Alter MJ, Margolis HS, Krawczynski K, et al. The natural history of community-acquired hepatitis C in the United States. *N Engl J Med.* 1992;327:1899–1905.

98. Yen T, Keeffe EB, Ahmed A. The epidemiology of hepatitis C virus infections. *J Clin Gastroenterol.* 2003;36:47–53.

99. Koerner K, Cardoso M, Dengler T, et al. Estimated risk of transmission of hepatitis C virus by blood transfusion. *Vox Sang.* 1998;74:213–216.

100. Armstrong GL, Wasley A, Simard EP, et al. The prevalence of hepatitis C virus infection in the United States, 1999 through 2002. *Ann Intern Med.* 2006;144:705–714.

101. Holland PV. Post-transfusion hepatitis: current risks and causes. *Vox Sang.* 1998;74(suppl 2):135–141.

102. Rustgi VK. The epidemiology of hepatitis C infection in the United States. *J Gastroenterol.* 2007;42:513–521.

103. Strader DB, Wright T, Thomas DL, et al. American Association for the Study of Liver Diseases practice guideline: diagnosis, management, and treatment of hepatitis C. *Hepatology.* 2004;39:1147–1171.

104. Dal Molin G, Tiribelli C, Campello C. A rational use of laboratory tests in the diagnosis and management of hepatitis C virus infection. *Ann Hepatol.* 2003;2:76–83.

105. Pawlotsky J-M. Diagnostic testing in hepatitis C virus infection: viral kinetics and genomics. *Semin Liver Dis.* 2003;23(suppl 1):3–11.

106. Pawlotsky JM, Lonjon I, Hezode C, et al. What strategy should be used for diagnosis of hepatitis C virus infection in clinical laboratories? *Hepatology.* 1998;27:1700–1702.

107. Alter MJ, Kuhnert WL, Finelli L. Guidelines for laboratory testing and result reporting of antibody to hepatitis C virus. *MMWR Recomm Rep.* 2003;52(RR-03):1–16.

108. CDC. Recommendations for prevention and control of hepatitis C virus (HCV) infection and HCV-related chronic disease. *MMWR Recomm Rep.* 1998;47(RR-19):1–39.

109. Corrao G, Arico S. Independent and combined action of hepatitis C virus infection and alcohol consumption on the risk of symptomatic liver cirrhosis. *Hepatology.* 1994;20:1115–1120.

110. Seeff LB. The natural history of chronic hepatitis C virus infection. *Clin Liver Dis.* 1997;1:587–602.

111. Poynard T, Ratziu V, Charlotte F, et al. Rates and risk factors of liver fibrosis progression in patients with chronic hepatitis C. *J Hepatol.* 2001;34:730–739.

112. Forns X, Ampurdanès S, Sanchez-Tapias JM, et al. Long-term follow-up of chronic hepatitis C in patients diagnosed at a tertiary-care center. *J Hepatol.* 2001;35:265–271.

113. Mast EE, Kuramoto IK, Favorov MO, et al. Prevalence of and risk factors for antibody to hepatitis E virus seroreactivity among blood donors in Northern California. *J Infect Dis.* 1997;176:34–40.

114. Di Bisceglie AM, Frey S, Gorse GJ. A phase I safety and immunogenicity trial of a novel E1E2/MF59C.1 hepatitis C vaccine candidate in healthy HCV-negative adults [abstract]. *Hepatology.* 2005;42(suppl 1):750A.

115. Hadziyannis SJ. Decreasing prevalence of hepatitis D virus infection. *J Gastroenterol Hepatol* 1997;12:745–746.

116. Farci P. Delta hepatitis: an update. *J Hepatol.* 2003;39(suppl 1):S212–S219.

117. Centers for Disease Control and Prevention. Hepatitis surveillance report. *MMWR Morb Mortal Wkly Rep.* 1990;53:23.

118. di Bisceglie AM. Interferon therapy for chronic viral hepatitis. *N Engl J Med* 1994;330:137–138.

119. Sureau C, Moriarty AM, Thornton GB, et al. Production of infectious hepatitis delta virus in vitro and neutralization with antibodies directed against hepatitis B virus pre-S antigens. *J Virol.* 1992;66:1241–1245.

120. Taylor JM. The structure and replication of hepatitis delta virus. *Annu Rev Microbiol.* 1992;46:253–276.

121. Caredda F, d'Arminio Monforte A, Rossi E, et al. Prospective study of epidemic delta infection in drug addicts. *Prog Clin Biol Res.* 1983;143:245–250.

122. Wu JC, Chen TZ, Huang YS, et al. Natural history of hepatitis D viral superinfection: significance of viremia detected by polymerase chain reaction. *Gastroenterology.* 1995;108:796–802.

123. Macagno S, Smedile A, Caredda F, et al. Monomeric (7S) immunoglobulin M antibodies to hepatitis delta virus in hepatitis type D. *Gastroenterology.* 1990;98:1582–1586.

124. Hsieh TH, Liu CJ, Chen DS, et al. Natural course and treatment of hepatitis D virus infection. *J Formos Med Assoc.* 2006;105:869–881.

125. Mele A, Mariano A, Tosti ME, et al. Acute hepatitis delta virus infection in Italy: incidence and risk factors after the introduction of the universal anti-hepatitis B vaccination campaign. *Clin Infect Dis.* 2007;44:e17–e24.

126. Okamoto H. Genetic variability and evolution of hepatitis E virus. *Virus Res.* 2007;127:216–228.

127. Purcell RH. Hepatitis E virus. In: Fields BN, Knipe DM, et al., eds. *Fields Virology.* 3rd ed. Philadelphia, PA: Lippincott-Raven; 1996:2831–2843.

128. Khuroo MS, Teli MR, Skidmore S, et al. Incidence and severity of viral hepatitis in pregnancy. *Am J Med.* 1981;70:252–255.

129. Ticehurst JR. Hepatitis E virus. In: Murray PR, Baron EJ, Pfaller MA, et al., eds. *Manual of Clinical Microbiology.* 7th ed. Washington, DC: American Society for Microbiology Press; 1999:1053–1069.

130. Panda SK, Thakral D, Rehman S. Hepatitis E virus. *Rev Med Virol.* 2007;17:151–180.

131. Harrison TJ. Hepatitis E virus: an update. *Liver.* 1999;19:171–176.

132. Frider B, Sookoian S, Castaño G, et al. Detection of hepatitis G virus RNA in patients with acute non-A-E hepatitis. *J Viral Hepat.* 1998;5:161–164.

133. Loya F. Does the hepatitis G virus cause hepatitis? *Tex Med.* 1996;92:68–73.

134. Doo EC, Lian TJ, Shiffs ER, et al. The hepatitis viruses. In: Schiff ER, Sorrell MF, Maddrey WC, eds. *Schiff's Diseases of the Liver.* Philadelphia, PA: Lippincott Williams & Wilkins; 2003:917–940.

135. Alter HJ, Umemura T, Tanaka Y. Putative new hepatitis virus. In: Schiff ER, Sorrell MF, Maddrey WC, eds. *Schiff's Diseases of the Liver.* Philadelphia, PA: Lippincott Williams & Wilkins; 2003:891–905.

26

Laboratory Markers of Cardiac Damage and Function

RONALD R. HENRIQUEZ, MICHAEL DURANDO, BRIAN C. JENSEN,
CHRISTOPER R. McCUDDEN, and MONTE S. WILLIS

chapter outline

key terms

Acute coronary syndromes
Angina pectoris
Arrhythmias
Atherosclerosis
Cardiac markers
CK-MB
Congestive heart failure
Creatine kinase (CK)
D-Dimer
Heart-type fatty acid–binding
  protein
Homocysteine
Ischemia-modified albumin
Myocardial infarction
Myocarditis
Myoglobin
Troponin I (TnI)
Troponin T (TnT)

chapter objectives

Upon completion of this chapter, the clinical laboratorian should be able to do the following:

- Diagram the anatomy of the heart.
- Explain the origin of general symptoms of cardiac disease.
- Discuss the etiology and physiologic effects of the following cardiac conditions:
  - Congenital heart disease
  - Hypertensive heart disease
  - Infectious heart diseases
  - Coronary heart disease
  - Congestive heart failure
- Identify risk factors for coronary heart disease.

For additional student resources, please visit thePoint®
at http://thepoint.lww.com

chapter objectives (continued)

- List features of an ideal cardiac marker.
- List and briefly describe three novel markers of inflammation currently under investigation.
- Compare and contrast the specificity and sensitivity of the most commonly used serum cardiac markers.
- Assess the clinical utility of the various cardiac markers to assess myocardial infarction.
- Analyze the role of the clinical laboratory in the assessment of a patient with cardiac disease.

Cardiovascular disease (CVD) commonly occurs in the general population and affects the majority of people older than 60 years. This includes four major types of CVD based on the location in which it occurs: (1) coronary heart disease (CHD), (2) cerebrovascular disease, (3) peripheral arterial disease, and (4) aortic atherosclerotic disease. CHD manifests as **myocardial infarction (MI)** (heart attack), **angina pectoris** (chest pain), heart failure, and sudden cardiac death. Cerebrovascular disease manifests as a stroke or transient ischemic attack (short, "reversible strokes"), while peripheral arterial disease manifests by intermittent claudication (acute localized pain to the arms and legs). Aortic atherosclerosis manifests as aneurysms (abnormal widening of an artery) or dissection (tears in thoracic or abdominal aorta), which are acute life-threatening events. There are common themes in the pathogenesis of these CVDs, including the presence of **atherosclerosis**, which increases the likelihood of ischemia (lack of blood supply) localized to different parts of the body. CHD, in which atherosclerosis and ischemia are localized to the vasculature of the heart, accounts for one-third of the total cases of CVD. The critical role of laboratory testing in diagnosing CHD will be the focus of this chapter.

One of the most common reasons people go to the emergency department is for the acute onset of chest pain. While nearly seven million people end up in emergency departments for this reason, only 15% to 25% of them actually have **acute coronary syndrome (ACS)** resulting from CHD.[1,2] There are a number of noncardiac reasons for having chest pain, including common maladies such as esophageal reflux ("heartburn") due to stomach acid moving retrograde into the esophagus. It is critical to differentiate cardiac from noncardiac causes, but differentiating patients with ACS or other life-threatening conditions from patients with non–life-threatening diseases from noncardiac causes is challenging. This is evidenced by the fact that the diagnosis of ACS is missed in approximately 2% of patients, which results in substantial morbidity and mortality.[2] Several advances in risk-stratifying patients with chest pain have been made, including better laboratory markers of cardiac injury,[3] which allows for rapid identification of those patients whose chest pain is due to CHD. Such patients

benefit from rapid initiation of therapy directed at ACS. Patients without elevated **cardiac markers** are typically at lower risk and may undergo further evaluation of the cause of their symptoms, including through radionuclide imaging and computed tomography (CT).

The lack of an adequate blood supply to the heart leads to ischemia. Since the heart depends upon a constant supply of oxygen and nutrients supplied by the coronary arteries, any disruption in the balance of oxygen supply and cardiac demand puts the heart at serious risk. Adequate supply of blood to the heart is compromised by a number of factors, most commonly the formation of a thrombus in the context of underlying atherosclerosis, which is the underlying cause for MI (narrowing of the coronary arteries). Atherosclerosis is a chronic process involving damage to the endothelium and the buildup of cholesterol-rich lesions that threaten to occlude the vasculature.

CARDIAC ISCHEMIA, ANGINA, AND HEART ATTACKS

Cardiac ischemia can lead to activity-related chest pain (stable angina) or an ACS. Stable angina predictably occurs with a given amount of activity and resolves with rest, whereas ACS frequently occurs unpredictably and does not respond to cessation of activity. ACS is further classified as unstable angina or the more severe acute MI, also known as a heart attack. Cardiac biomarkers are normal in the setting of unstable angina, but elevated in MI. The "classic" manifestation of cardiac ischemia is angina, described as a squeezing of the chest, heavy chest pressure, a burning feeling, or difficulty breathing.[4] This "classic" manifestation often radiates to the left shoulder, neck, or arm and typically increases in intensity over a period of minutes and gets worse with either physical or psychological stress. However, the symptoms often arise in the absence of situations that precipitate it. Nonclassic symptoms, more commonly experienced by women, include a more stabbing, pulsating, or sharp chest pain rather than the typical viselike pressure, nausea, shortness of breath, or abdominal pain.[5–7] In addition to these heart-related symptoms, the American Heart Association (AHA) and the American College of Cardiology (ACC) have also defined

TABLE 26.1	**Symptoms not Related to Cardiac Ischemia-Induced Angina (Chest Pain)[8]**

Pleuritic pain (sharp/knifelike pain brought on by respiratory movements/cough)
Epigastric pain (primary/sole location in the abdomen)
Indigestion
Increasing dyspnea in the absence of chest pain
Psychiatric disorders (e.g., somatoform disorders, panic attack, anxiety disorders)
Severe noncardiac conditions such as sepsis, burns, respiratory failure, acute neurological diseases, and drug toxicity (including cancer chemotherapy). Pain that can mimic ACS

chest-related symptoms that are not indicative of cardiac involvement (see Table 26.1).

Guidelines from the ACC and the AHA categorize patients into two classes: class I, patients with suspected ACS and high-risk features (chest pain, syncope/presyncope, or palpitations), and class IIb, patients with less severe symptoms.[8] Class I patients should be immediately transported to ED by emergency medical services.[8] Class IIb patients may be considered for referral to the ED, a chest pain unit, or a facility capable of performing evaluation.[8] If a patient does not need immediate intervention because of circulatory collapse (i.e., the patient is conscious), a history is taken to evaluate the chest pain for its likelihood of being an MI. Risk factors for atherosclerosis should also be solicited, including advanced age, male gender, diabetes, and any previous history of MI. Younger patients with a low risk of

ACS should be carefully screened for cocaine use, as it can cause vascular spasm of the coronary arteries, resulting in ischemia and chest pain.[8] Patients with chest pain are initially evaluated by a physical examination, an electrocardiogram (ECG), a chest x-ray, and the detection of biomarkers by laboratory tests. The physical examination identifies possible causes of precipitating myocardial ischemia (high blood pressure, pulmonary disease, and heart failure or cardiac valve disease)[8] and may identify a noncardiac cause for the symptom. An ECG should be obtained within the first 10 minutes after presentation for further risk stratification. The presence of new or transient changes (>1 mm) in the ST segment of the ECG is strongly suggestive of acute ischemia.[8] Less specific ST-segment changes or T-wave abnormalities can also be helpful in risk-stratifying patients.[8] A normal ECG, however, does not rule out the presence of ACS. Chest radiography can also assist in the evaluation of a patient with chest pain by identifying a noncardiac source of the pain (e.g., pneumonia, pneumothorax, and aortic dissection) or sequelae of underlying cardiac causes (e.g., pulmonary edema caused by cardiac dysfunction).[8]

The use of biomarkers is critical in the evaluation of acute chest pain to identify angina (chest pain) as an MI (heart attack). Universal definitions of MI were recently published in 2008 outlining the consensus reached by the joint European Society of Cardiology/ACC/AHA/World Health Federation Task Force (see Table 26.2). These guidelines emphasized the use of the term MI only in the setting of myocardial ischemia and not as a result of any other cause[9] and designated several types of MI (Table 26.3). The 2014 ACC/AHA guidelines emphasize cardiac troponins as the most sensitive and specific biomarkers for non–ST-segment elevation ACS.[8]

TABLE 26.2	**Universal Definition of MI Released by the Joint European Society of Cardiology/American College of Cardiology/American Heart Association/World Health Federation Task Force (2007)[9]**

Any One of the Following:

1. Typical rise and fall of troponin with at least one value above the 99th percentile of the URL, plus one of the following:
   a. Ischemic symptoms
   b. Development of pathologic Q waves on ECG
   c. ECG changes indicative of ischemia (ST-segment changes)
   d. Coronary artery intervention
2. Sudden, unexplained cardiac death before blood samples can be obtained or before biomarkers can appear in the blood, and accompanied by evidence of symptoms, ECG, coronary angiogram, or autopsy
3. For PCI patients with normal baseline troponin levels, troponin >99th percentile of URL is indicative of periprocedural myocardial necrosis
4. For CABG patients with normal baseline, troponin >99th percentile of URL is indicative of periprocedural myocardial necrosis
5. Pathologic findings of an acute MI

ECG, electrocardiogram; PCI, percutaneous coronary intervention (also known as "coronary angioplasty" or "angioplasty"); CABG, coronary artery bypass graft (also known as "bypass surgery"); URL, upper reference limit.

TABLE 26.3	Classification of MI According to the Universal Definition of Myocardial Infarction Released by the Joint European Society of Cardiology/American College of Cardiology/ American Heart Association/World Health Federation Task Force (2007)[9]
Type 1:	Spontaneous MI related to ischemia due to a primary coronary event such as plaque erosion and/or rupture, fissuring, or dissection
Type 2:	MI secondary to ischemia due to either increased oxygen demand or decreased supply, e.g., coronary artery spasm, coronary embolism, anemia, **arrhythmias**, hypertension, and hypotension
Type 3:	Sudden unexpected cardiac death, including cardiac arrest, often with symptoms suggestive of MI, accompanied by presumably new ST elevation or new LBBB or evidence of fresh thrombus in a coronary artery by angiography and/or at autopsy, but death occurring before blood samples could be obtained or at a time before the appearance of cardiac biomarkers in the blood
Type 4a:	MI associated with PCI
Type 4b:	MI associated with stent thrombosis as documented by angiography or at autopsy
Type 5:	MI associated with CABG

MI, myocardial infarction; LBBB, left bundle branch block; PCI, percutaneous coronary intervention (also known as "coronary angioplasty" or "angioplasty"); CABG, coronary artery bypass graft (also known as "bypass surgery").

CASE STUDY 26.1

A 15-month-old girl with a heart murmur since birth was evaluated for repeated pulmonary infections, failure to grow, cyanosis, and mild clubbing of fingers and toes. She had been on digitalis therapy by the referring physician. The radiograph showed a moderately enlarged heart and an enlarged pulmonary artery. Pertinent laboratory data were obtained.

Total protein (6.0–8.3 g/dL)	5.4
Albumin (3.5–5.2 g/dL)	3.0
Hemoglobin (14–18 g/dL)	19.2
Hematocrit (40%–54%)	59
Erythrocyte count (4.3–5.7 × 10^6/mm^3)	6.4

A cardiac catheterization was performed, and a large ventricular septal defect was found.

Questions

1. How does this congenital defect affect the body's circulation?

2. Why are the red cell measurements increased in this patient?

3. What treatment will be suggested for this patient?

4. What is this patient's prognosis?

THE PATHOPHYSIOLOGY OF ATHEROSCLEROSIS, THE DISEASE PROCESS UNDERLYING MI

Atherosclerosis is a chronic disease process that occurs over a number of years and contributes to approximately 50% of all deaths in modern Western societies.[10] Evidence of atherosclerosis can often be found in the human aorta before the age of 10,[11] but atherosclerosis becomes pathologic with the development of atherosclerotic plaques (atheromas), which predispose the vasculature to thrombosis, leading to organ ischemia and infarction (Fig. 26.1). The pathophysiology of atherosclerosis is gradual and complicated, involving a progressive accumulation of lipids, smooth muscle cells, macrophages, and connective tissue within the intima of large- and medium-sized arteries, ultimately causing luminal narrowing and decreased perfusion (Fig. 26.1). Although the exact etiology of atherosclerosis remains unclear, the *reaction to injury* hypothesis is strongly favored by current evidence, proposing that atherosclerosis is due to a chronic inflammatory response to an accumulation of subtle vascular wall injuries.[12]

Pathohistological evidence from human and experimental studies demonstrates that endothelial and inflammatory cells interact with chemical and inflammatory mediators to promote the development of atherosclerotic plaques. This process begins with vascular injury, which is initiated when endothelial cells are damaged or rendered dysfunctional by vascular abnormalities, such as turbulent blood flow, hyperlipidemia, and hyperhomocysteinemia. A damaged vascular endothelium has an increased permeability to circulating lipids, so having high cholesterol (hyperlipidemia) in the wake of a damaged endothelium favors the accumulation of lipoproteins, predominantly low-density lipoprotein (LDL),

Normal artery

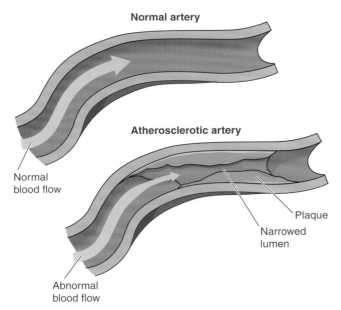

Atherosclerotic artery

Normal
blood flow

Plaque

Narrowed
lumen

Abnormal
blood flow

FIGURE 26.1 Comparison of normal and atherosclerotic arteries. Narrowing the arterial lumen due to atherosclerotic plaque leads to abnormal blood flow, contributing to progression of atherosclerosis. (Adapted from NHLBI Atherosclerosis homepage, http://www.nhlbi.nih.gov/health/health-topics/topics/atherosclerosis/)

FIGURE 26.2 LDL deposition and oxidation within the vessel wall leads to monocyte recruitment and differentiation into activated macrophages that phagocytose oxidized LDL (oxLDL) to become foam cells. Foam cells release HDL and proinflammatory mediators, and their rupture contributes to lesion progression. (Adapted from Glass CK, Witztum JL. Atherosclerosis: the road ahead. *Cell.* 2001;104(4):503–516, Ref.[10].)

and very–low density lipoprotein (VLDL), within the arterial intima (Fig. 26.1).[13] In addition, apoB-containing LDL has high affinity for arterial wall proteoglycans.[14] Retention of lipids in arterial walls due to hypercholesterolemia and/or elevated levels of apoB-containing lipoproteins is thus a crucial step in the pathogenesis of atherosclerotic lesions. The central role of cholesterol accumulation (i.e., LDL and VLDL) in the progression of atherosclerosis is the reason treating high cholesterol is such a priority in preventing and attenuating heart disease.

Once lesion initiation has begun, LDL deposited within the intima is oxidized by endothelial cells, lipoxygenase, and free radicals generated by the auto-oxidation of **homocysteine.**[11] The formation of oxidized LDL is central to lesion progression. Oxidized LDL is toxic to endothelial cells, causing additional intimal damage and subsequent retention of cholesterol-rich lipoproteins, and it elicits an inflammatory response that releases proinflammatory cytokines and recruits inflammatory cells to the early lesion. Among the earliest recruited leukocytes are neutrophils and monocytes, which play critical roles in early atherogenesis by maintaining a proinflammatory state around the initial lesion (Fig. 26.2).[10]

Maturation of monocytes into activated macrophages is a key step in lesion progression. Macrophage scavenger receptors recognize oxidized LDL, but not native LDL, and activated macrophages rapidly phagocytose cholesterol-rich lipoproteins that have been oxidized within the vessel wall (Fig. 26.2).[11] Excessive uptake of oxidized LDL transforms macrophages into bloated, cholesterol-filled cells called *foam cells.*[15] Filled with cytoplasmic lipid droplets, foam cells exhibit a variety of functions that both promote

lesion progression, including the production of proinflammatory signals, and counter lesion progression, such as the secretion of HDL (Fig. 26.2). Foam cells also display numerous metabolic abnormalities, including activation of inflammasomes and the NF-kB pathway, and it is generally agreed that foam cells play a harmful role in lesion progression.[15] In addition, rupture of foam cells and release of their contents cause further damage to the vascular endothelium, stimulating more inflammation. Intimal deposition and subsequent oxidation of LDL and its effects on monocyte differentiation are thus of key importance in the early development of an atherosclerotic lesion.

As the cycle of endothelial cell damage progresses, additional cell types are recruited to the plaque, in particular T and B lymphocytes and macrophages (Fig. 26.3). These cells are activated by a stream of cytokines, such as interleukin (IL)-1 and tumor necrosis factor-α, that are released by endothelial cells within the plaque.[16] Interactions between T cells and foam cells promote a chronic inflammatory state and help recruit smooth muscle cells into the intima (Fig. 26.3).[10] Additionally, growth factors, such as platelet-derived growth factor, fibroblast growth factor, and tissue growth factor-α, are released by lymphocytes and endothelial cells, further stimulating smooth muscle cell migration and activation.[16]

Once smooth muscle cells migrate into the core of the atheroma, they proliferate and deposit extracellular matrix

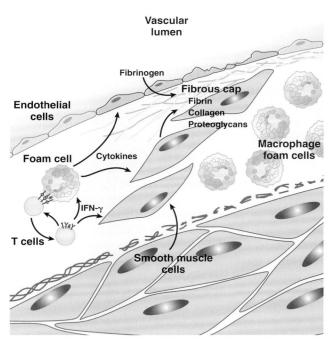

Vascular lumen

Fibrinogen

Fibrous cap
Fibrin
Collagen
Proteoglycans

Endothelial cells

Macrophage foam cells

Foam cell
Cytokines

IFN-γ

T cells

Smooth muscle cells

FIGURE 26.3 T cells and foam cells maintain a proinflammatory state that induces the migration of smooth muscle cells into the intima, where they secrete collagen, proteoglycans, and fibrin that form a fibrous cap around the atheroma. (Adapted from Glass CK, Witztum JL. Atherosclerosis: the road ahead. *Cell.* 2001;104(4):503–516, Ref.[10].)

components that give stability and strength to the plaque.[10] Cytokines released from T cells, such as interferon-γ, exert a number of both pro- and antiatherogenic effects on macrophages and smooth muscle cells, but the net effect of this cytokine release is proinflammatory and proatherogenic. Smooth muscle cells are induced to secrete collagen, elastin, and proteoglycans that form a fibrous backbone and outer shell that fix the plaque firmly in the vessel wall (Fig. 26.3). As the atheroma grows, its core becomes increasingly isolated from surrounding blood supply, leading to hypoxia that stimulates release of proangiogenic cytokines. This causes aberrant neovascularization around the periphery of the plaque, which predisposes to hemorrhage and deposition of erythrocyte components, such as hemosiderin and lipids, within the plaque core.[17] Microvasculature hemorrhage and subsequent deposition of additional debris provokes further inflammation, leukocyte recruitment, and remodeling of the plaque.

The steps described above—beginning with lipid and cellular infiltration following vascular injury and progressing to chronic inflammation and fibrosis—continue in a feed-forward cycle that ultimately culminates in complete vessel occlusion, thrombosis, plaque rupture, or some combination of the three. Each of these possible outcomes predisposes to organ ischemia. In the context of the heart, coronary artery ischemia and resultant hypoxia pose an immediate risk of cellular injury due to the high metabolic activity and oxygen demand of the myocardium. The ultimate outcome of such injury is ischemic heart disease,

varying in severity from angina to MI, the symptoms of which are dependent on the extent of coronary artery atherosclerosis. The most common locations for symptomatic cardiac atheroma formation are the proximal left anterior descending, the proximal left main coronary, and the entire right coronary arteries. Coronary atherosclerosis typically becomes symptomatic only after atherosclerotic plaques obstruct approximately 75% (or >50% in the left main) of the cross-sectional area of the vessel.[10]

MARKERS OF CARDIAC DAMAGE

Initial Markers of Cardiac Damage

The first biochemical markers of cardiac damage were discovered in 1954 when Karmen et al.[18] hypothesized that "destruction of cardiac muscle, reported rich in transaminase activity, might result in a release of this enzyme into the blood stream and might thus increase the serum transaminase activity." Today, serum biomarkers have become the centerpiece of evaluation and management of patients presenting with chest pain. The underlying principle behind serum biomarkers of cardiac damage relies on the fact that cell death releases intracellular proteins from the myocardium into the circulation. Detection of cardiac proteins in plasma provides insight into the occurrence, extent, and timing of MI, all of which are critical for proper medical management.

The first cardiac markers to be used extensively in clinical practice were glutamic oxaloacetic transaminase, lactic dehydrogenase, and malic dehydrogenase. The first, glutamic oxaloacetic transaminase, now known as aspartate transaminase (AST), became widely used in the diagnosis of MI shortly after its discovery as a serum marker by Ladue et al. in 1954.[19] But because of the high false-negative rate of AST, the labor-intensive nature of the AST assay, and the short window of AST elevation, AST was soon replaced by lactate dehydrogenase (LD) as the marker of choice.[20]

Compared with AST, LD was found to be a more sensitive marker of MI that remains elevated for significantly longer post-MI, up to 2 weeks. But LD is involved in NADH-dependent reactions in the glycolytic pathway, which takes place in nearly all cells in the body, and its specificity to cardiac muscle is thus quite low. Early researchers observed that serum LD levels were elevated in other conditions such as cancer and anemia.[20] These pitfalls were overcome to some extent through assays that differentiate between LD of cardiac and noncardiac origin.[21] Specifically, five different isoforms of LD (LD1 to LD5) are found in human plasma,[22] which correspond to the organ from where the enzyme originates. LD1 is most abundant in the myocardium, and LD5 is expressed mainly in the skeletal muscle and liver. Therefore, the diagnosis of MI was made by comparing plasma LD1 and LD2 levels. Because LD1 is specific to the myocardium, plasma normally contains greater levels of LD2 than LD1; however, damage to the myocardium and subsequent release of LD1 can cause plasma LD1 levels to surpass LD2.[23] Early studies demonstrated that the plasma LD1:LD2 ratio exceeds approximately 0.75 24 to 48 hours past the onset of symptoms of MI and remains elevated for up to 2 weeks.[23] The LD1:LD2 ratio was thus of great utility as an early biomarker in the management of patients presenting several days after possible MI.

Creatine kinase (CK) was the next marker to gain favor. Like LD, CK is found in nearly all cells in the body, but unlike LD, CK catalyzes a reaction important for high-energy phosphate production (the conversion of creatine to creatine phosphate), which is greatly upregulated in the muscle cells and brain. High levels of CK are thus found in all muscle cells, in particular striated muscle. Damage to the muscle or brain results in rapidly detectable increases in plasma CK, which can be readily detected in plasma with a high sensitivity at short times after muscle injury. After the discovery in 1960 of elevated levels of plasma CK post-MI,[24] CK became an important marker of cardiac damage. In a typical patient with acute MI, serum CK levels were found to exceed the normal range within 6 to 8 hours, to reach a peak of two- to tenfold normal by 24 hours, and then decline to the normal range after 3 to 4 days (Fig. 26.4).[26] A CK plasma concentration greater than two times normal was shown to correlate with MI,[25,27] and an elevation in serum CK, together with elevated AST and LD, was used as the primary means of enzymatic detection of MI for many years.

Unfortunately, the ubiquitous expression of CK in all striated muscle was a problem for specificity of CK as a marker for MI, in spite of its high sensitivity. CK elevations were readily detected in conditions such as stroke, pulmonary disease, and chronic alcoholism and after strenuous exercise.[28] This obstacle was initially overcome through the discovery that CK exists in three cytoplasmic isoenzymes. The cytoplasmic isoenzymes are dimers composed of combinations of M and B subunits (where M is for muscle and B is for brain). Dimers of 2 M subunits are called CK-MM, 2 B subunits as CK-BB, and 1 M and 1 B subunit as **creatine kinase MB (CK-MB)**. Elevated plasma levels of CK-MM or CK-BB can be found after injury to the muscle or brain, respectively. After it was found that 15% to 30% of CK in the myocardium is MB, compared with 1% to 3% in normal striated muscle,

detection of elevated CK-MB was shown to be highly specific to myocardial damage.[29] Additionally, elevations in serum CK-MB could be detected at 4 to 6 hours after the onset of MI symptoms, significantly less than the 24 to 48 hours necessary to detect peak LD plasma levels (Fig. 26.4). Like its rapid rise post-MI, CK-MB levels quickly drop to baseline levels by 2 to 4 days post-MI, compared with 10 to 14 days for LD.[30] Because of its higher specificity and its rapid elevation post-MI, CK-MB was long considered the most reliable serum marker of MI and is still widely used today.[31,32]

Use of these three markers—AST, LD, and CK—was the cornerstone of post-MI management for several decades. Each had its individual applications: CK for the early presentation, LD for the late presentation, and AST for the intermediate.[33] But their lack of specificity to the myocardium and to myocardial injury fueled the search for better markers. Extensive research in the 1970s led to the discovery that muscle cells express structural and regulatory proteins, such as troponin and tropomyosin, in a pattern that is tissue specific.[32] The subsequent development of rapid and sensitive techniques for detection of the tissue-specific forms of troponin quickly made troponin a promising marker of cardiac injury.[34]

Cardiac Troponins

Troponin is a complex of three proteins that regulate the calcium-dependent interactions of myosin heads with actin filaments during striated muscle contraction. **Troponin T (TnT)** binds the troponin complex to tropomyosin, **troponin I (TnI)** inhibits the binding of actin and myosin, and troponin C (TnC) binds to calcium to reverse the inhibitory activity of TnI.[35] The troponin complex is responsible for transmitting the calcium signal that triggers muscle contraction (Fig. 26.5). Several properties of troponin made it attractive as a marker of myocardial damage.

In contrast to other cardiac markers, troponins were found to have tissue-specific isoforms that could be used to detect damage to the heart. Although the same isoform of TnC is expressed in slow-twitch (type 2) and cardiac muscle, unique isoforms of TnI and TnT are expressed in fast-twitch

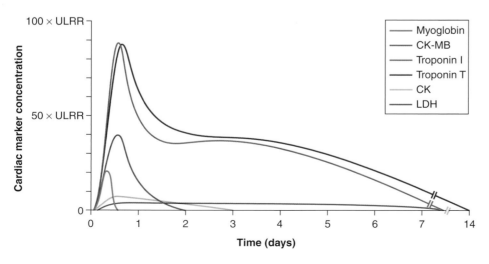

FIGURE 26.4 Temporal elevations of important markers of myocardial damage post-MI. ULRR, upper limit of reference range. (Adapted from French JK, White HD. Clinical implications of the new definition of myocardial infarction. *Heart.* 2004;90(1):99–106, Ref.[25].)

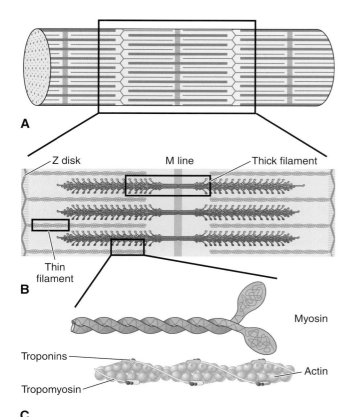

A

Z disk   M line   Thick filament

B

Thin filament

Myosin

Troponins

Actin

Tropomyosin

C

FIGURE 26.5 Regulatory proteins in the contractile apparatus of striated muscle. Striated muscle is composed of bundles of myofibril-containing fibers, made up of repeating units of cross-striations called sarcomeres (**A**). The sarcomere is composed of thick and thin myofilaments, which tether the Z disk to the M line (**B**). Thick filaments are composed primarily of large molecules of myosin, which have a rodlike tail region and a protruding head region (**C**). Thin filaments are composed of actin, which plays a structural role, and troponin and tropomyosin, which line actin filaments and regulate calcium-dependent interactions with myosin on thick filaments to stimulate contraction.

(type 1), slow-twitch, and cardiac muscle.[35] Each TnI, TnT, and TnC isoform is encoded by a separate gene and expressed in a muscle-type–specific manner.[36] This allows for highly specific detection of troponin of cardiac origin (e.g., cardiac TnI [cTnI]). Further increasing the sensitivity of troponin detection was the demonstration that cardiac troponins are very tightly complexed to the contractile apparatus, such that circulating levels of cardiac troponins are normally extremely low.[35] Early studies demonstrated that normal levels of circulating cTnI are below 10 ng/mL, but patients with acute MI can have serum cTnI levels well over 100 ng/mL,[37] demonstrating the specificity of cardiac troponins as indicators of myocardial cell damage.

The development of sensitive detection methods was the next step toward integrating cardiac troponins into the diagnostic workup of MI. Because the skeletal and cardiac isoforms of TnT and TnI contain differing amino acid sequences, monoclonal antibodies can be raised against cardiac-specific epitopes. This allowed for the development of sensitive immunoassays for cardiac troponins that have

a far greater specificity than other markers. For example, detection of cTnI was specific for cardiac injury even in acute muscle disease, chronic muscle disease, chronic renal failure, and following intense exercise, such as running a marathon.[38] Additionally, measurement of plasma troponin levels allows for the detection of myocardial cell injury in syndromes, such as acute ischemic syndrome or **myocarditis**, that is undetectable using other markers.[39]

Finally, troponins offer additional advantages due to the timing of their release. CK-MB levels elevate rapidly post-MI (4 to 6 hours) but return to baseline after 2 to 4 days; CK-MB can thus only be used within a short window of time after a suspected MI. Conversely, LD levels remain elevated for up to 1 week but are not detectable until 24 to 48 hours post-MI (Fig. 26.4). Cardiac troponins, on the other hand, are detectable in the plasma at 3 to 12 hours after myocardial injury, peaking at 12 to 24 hours and remaining elevated for more than 1 week: 8 to 21 days for TnT and 7 to 14 days for TnI (Fig. 26.4).[39] Cardiac troponins thus offer the widest window for detection post-MI and with the highest sensitivity and specificity.

Taken together, the characteristics of specific, sensitive, and rapid detection propelled cardiac troponins to the center of MI diagnosis, where they still remain. Cardiac troponin (I or T) is currently the preferred biomarker for myocardial necrosis, recognized to have nearly absolute myocardial tissue specificity as well as high clinical sensitivity, detecting even minor cardiac damage (as utilized in the universal definition of MI).[9] An elevated plasma cardiac troponin level is defined as a measurement greater than the 99th percentile of a normal reference value range, specified as the upper limit of the reference range (Fig. 26.4). Current guidelines recommend drawing blood for the measurement of troponin as soon as possible after onset of symptoms of a possible MI (universal definition of MI).[9] If troponin assays are not available, the next best alternative is CK-MB, and measurement of total CK is no longer recommended for the diagnosis of MI for the reasons outlined above (universal definition of MI).[9]

CK-MB and Troponin I/Troponin T Considerations in Kidney Disease Patients

Prognosis in chronic kidney disease. Increases in cTnI/cTnT are associated with increases in short-term cardiac outcomes in patients with chronic kidney disease diagnosed with acute MI.[40–42] Stably increased serum troponin levels predict worse long-term cardiovascular outcomes and worse survival in asymptomatic CKD patients in the absence of acute MI.[43–54]

Dialysis patients. In a recent meta-analysis of 11 studies, elevated cTnT was associated with an increase in all-cause mortality (95% confidence interval [CI] 2.4 to 43).[42] Few studies here used the high-sensitivity assay; cTnT measured with high-sensitive assay has also been reported as an independent predictor of all-cause mortality in dialysis patients.[55,56]

Effect of hemodialysis. In kidney failure, the need to dialyze patients is common when failure is severe. Hemodialysis involves filtering the blood to remove the built-up toxins and results in altering the concentration of cardiac enzymes. Studies have yielded conflicting results. Dialysis minimally changes CK-MB and did not change cTnI concentrations.[57] Decreased cTnI and cTnT levels decreased 27% to 37% following dialysis with a high-flux membrane (but not low-flux membrane).[58] cTnT rose after dialysis in patients with CVD, suggesting the rise in cTnT resulting from cardiac injury.[59] While the cut-offs for the diagnosis for AMI should be the same for dialysis patients and nondialysis chronic kidney disease patients, considerations above are important with the growing number of patients surviving with chronic kidney disease.

Other Markers of Cardiac Damage

In spite of the nearly universal use of troponin and CK-MB in diagnosing cardiac damage, it is worthwhile mentioning additional markers of cardiac damage that have been used in the past and/or proposed experimentally. These include **myoglobin**, **heart-type fatty acid–binding protein (H-FABP)**, **ischemia-modified albumin (IMA)**, myeloperoxidase (MPO), C-reactive protein (CRP), myeloid-related protein (MRP)-8/14, and pregnancy-associated plasma protein A (PAPP-A). While their clinical utility has not been universally established, they are discussed frequently as potential alternatives, so they have been discussed here briefly.

CASE STUDY 26.2

A 59-year-old woman came to the emergency department of a local hospital complaining of pain and a feeling of heaviness in her abdomen for several days. She reported no weakness, chest pain, or left arm pain. She has no chronic health problems except for seasonal allergies and slightly elevated total cholesterol.

Cardiac Enzymes	8:30 PM, April 11	6:30 AM, April 12
Total CK (54–186 U/L)	170	106
CK-MB (0–5 ng/mL)	6.3	3.8
% CK-MB (<6%)	3.7	3.6
Myoglobin (<70 µg/L)	52	41
Troponin T (0–0.1 µg/L)	0.8	2.3

Questions

1. Do the symptoms and personal history of this patient suggest acute MI?
2. Based on the preceding laboratory data, would this diagnosis be acute MI?
3. Why or why not?

Myoglobin

Myoglobin is an iron- and oxygen-binding protein found exclusively in the muscle and is normally absent from the circulation. The myoglobin found in the muscle forms pigments, giving the muscle its characteristic red color. The exact color of the muscle depends on the oxidation state of the iron atom in myoglobin and the amount of oxygen attached to it. Myoglobin is a small protein, which is released quickly when the muscle is damaged (see Fig. 26.4 for serum release pattern).[60] It has a very short half-life of 9 minutes.[61] Because myoglobin is released so quickly, it has been proposed as an adjunct marker for troponin or CK-MB in the early diagnosis of MI.[62] There are limitations to using myoglobin as a marker of cardiac damage. It is not specific for the heart, being elevated with any cause of skeletal muscle damage, and is cleared in an irregular pattern.[63] Recent studies have also shown that high-sensitivity troponin assays can detect elevated troponin levels prior to elevations in myoglobin,[64–66] making myoglobin's use less attractive.

Heart-Type Fatty Acid–Binding Protein

H-FABP is a small protein, which behaves much like myoglobin in its kinetics and release. It is found in all muscles, but in contrast to myoglobin, H-FABP is found relatively more abundantly in the heart.[67] The utility of H-FABP has been described for the diagnosis of early acute MI. The sensitivity for the diagnosis of an acute MI has been reported to be higher than cardiac TnT (cTnT) or myoglobin.[68] However, cTnT has a higher specificity than H-FABP (94% vs. 52%) indicating that elevated H-FABP was found in patients without disease.[68] Recent studies have confirmed the utility of using both H-FABP and cTnI for the early diagnosis of MI/ACS.[69] Using both markers may also be a valuable rule-out test for patients presenting between 3 and 6 hours after chest pain,[69] though H-FABP is not used in the routine evaluation of chest pain.

Ischemia-Modified Albumin

In contrast to the markers described above that detect myocardial tissue damage, the IMA test does not. Instead, it measures changes that occur in albumin in the presence of ischemia, giving it the advantage that it might detect ischemia before damage has occurred to the heart. The free radical formation that occurs during tissue ischemia is believed to modify albumin within minutes of ischemia and lasts for about 6 hours.[70–73] These modifications in albumin alter its ability to bind transition metals, such as cobalt, by its N-terminal domain.[72] The amount of IMA is measured by the spectrophotometric determination of albumin's binding to cobalt.[70] While IMA is not specific for cardiac damage, it does have a clinical sensitivity for ACS of 50% to 90%.[74,75] Additional studies will be necessary to determine the utility of IMA in the early diagnosis of ACS; its use will complement, not replace, troponin and CK-MB detection.

Novel Markers of Plaque Instability: MPO, CRP, MRP-8/14, and PAPP-A

MPO, CRP, MRP-8/14, and PAPP-A have been studied in international multicenter studies for their utility in the early diagnosis and risk stratification of acute MI in emergency departments in patients with acute chest pain.[76] The concentration of all four markers was significantly higher in patients with acute MI compared with patients with other diagnoses.[76] But these markers were all inferior to troponins in detecting acute MI.[76] MPO, MRP-8/14, and CRP were able to predict all-cause mortality and these provided independent prognostic information apart from clinical risk factors and high-sensitive cTnT; PAPP-A did not.[76] Interestingly, these plaque instability markers did not correlate with each other or myocardial cell death determined by troponin.[76] The exact mechanisms leading to plaque instability, plaque fissure, and subsequent rupture are not fully understood, but all are expressed in atherosclerotic plaques and contribute to vessel inflammation.[77–80]

CASE STUDY 26.3

An 83-year-old man with known severe coronary artery disease, diffuse small vessel disease, and significant stenosis distal to a vein graft from previous CABG surgery was admitted when his physician referred him to the hospital after a routine office visit. His symptoms included 3+ pedal edema, jugular vein distention, and heart sound abnormalities. Significant laboratory data obtained on admission were as follows:

Urea nitrogen (6–24 mg/dL)	53
Creatinine (0.5–1.4 mg/dL)	2.2
Total protein (6.0–8.3 g/dL)	5.8
Albumin (3.5–5.3 g/dL)	3.2
Glucose (60–110 mg/dL)	312
Calcium (4.3–5.3 mmol/L)	4.1
Phosphorus (2.5–4.5 mg/dL)	2.4
Total CK (54–186 U/L)	134
CK-MB (0–5 ng/L)	4
% CK-MB (<6%)	3
Myoglobin (<70 µg/L)	62
Troponin T (0–0.1 µg/L)	0.2

Questions

1. Do the symptoms of this patient suggest acute MI?
2. Based on the preceding laboratory data, would this diagnosis be acute MI? Why or why not?
3. Based on the preceding laboratory data, are there other organ system abnormalities present?
4. What are the indicators of these organ system abnormalities?
5. Is there a specific laboratory test that might indicate congestive heart failure in this patient?

CARDIAC INJURY OCCURS IN MANY DISEASE PROCESSES, BEYOND MI

The damage that occurs in the context of MI is due to cardiac muscle cell (myocyte) death. A spectrum of cell death occurs in myocytes, ranging from apoptosis to necrosis to a mixture between the two. Apoptotic cell death is characterized by decreasing cell size, membrane blebbing, nuclear aggregation of chromosomal DNA, and purposeful degradation of DNA. The resulting apoptotic bodies formed from the process of apoptosis are recognized by macrophage, which then remove the debris in an effort to minimize the immune response.[81] Apoptosis requires energy, so as ischemia progresses, the apoptotic process stalls and necrosis occurs if energy supply fails to meet the energy demand, which occurs rapidly in the heart. Thus, a rapid clinical response to myocardial ischemia is essential to limiting the extent of necrosis that occurs and is a central tenet of treating MI. The faster cardiac interventions are performed to restore perfusion (along with oxygen) to the heart, the greater the reduction in infarct size. The strategies for reperfusion include percutaneous interventions using intravascular balloons and stents to clear coronary artery blockages and prevent their recurrence, coronary artery bypass grafting (CABG or "bypass surgery"), and the use of chemical thrombolytics, such as tissue plasminogen activator (aka tPA or tenecteplase).

Despite our focus here on the use of cardiac biomarkers in MI, a number of other causes of myocardial injury result in increased biomarker release. Like MI, these disease processes also have myocyte apoptosis and necrosis as part of their pathophysiology, which explains why these biomarkers may be elevated in these patients. Cell death, in the form of apoptosis and/or necrosis, is a key feature of cardiomyopathies due to genetic causes and/or stress-related causes and contributes to the worsening function that occurs with the disease[82–85] (Fig. 26.6). Cell death also occurs in decompensated heart failure and volume overload.[86] In the cardiac hypertrophy "pre–heart failure state," angiotensin II, catecholamine production, and cytokines release play a role in inducing cardiomyocyte apoptosis[87–89] (Fig. 26.6),

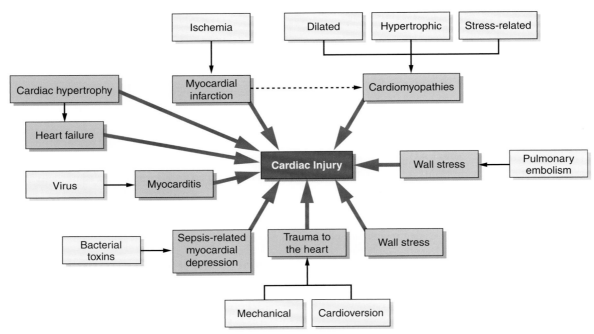

FIGURE 26.6 Common cardiac insults that result in cardiac injury and elevated cardiac biomarkers. (Adapted from McLean A, Huang S. Biomarkers of cardiac injury. In: Vaidya V, Bonventre J, eds. *Biomarkers: In Medicine, Drug Discovery, and Environmental Health*. New York, NY: John Wiley & Sons, Inc.; 2010:119–155, Ref.[85].)

which can lead to low-level release of cardiac biomarkers. Cardiomyocyte cell death is also induced in myocarditis, whereby viruses and bacteria induce an autoimmune response, which recognizes cardiac-specific proteins as foreign and induces cardiac cells to die.[90] Similarly, bacterial toxins in sepsis can cause apoptosis and myocardial depression. Certain drugs are also capable of causing apoptosis and myocardial dysfunction, including doxorubicin and cyclophosphamide[91–93] (Fig. 26.6), as well as alcohol, cocaine, and methamphetamines.

THE LABORATORY WORKUP OF PATIENTS SUSPECTED OF HEART FAILURE AND THE USE OF CARDIAC BIOMARKERS IN HEART FAILURE

Heart failure is a pathological state in which the heart fails to adequately supply the metabolic needs of the body, typically due to a decrease in pumping function. The clinical manifestations of heart failure result largely from the retention of fluid, which is one of the body's maladaptive responses to decreased cardiac output. The most common symptoms of heart failure are shortness of breath, fatigue, and lower extremity edema.

The ACC/AHA/Heart Failure Society of America and the European Society of Cardiology have recommended specific laboratory and clinical tests for patients with suspected heart failure (see Table 26.4).[97–99] Many of these tests may be familiar as routine laboratory tests; others are more specific to the atherosclerotic process and compensatory cardiac function mechanisms.

The ACC/AHA recommendations also suggest determining a cTnI or cTnT if the clinical presentation is suggestive of an ACS; elevated troponin levels may also indicate the severity of the heart failure (discussed in the next section).[97–99] A chest x-ray, 2D echocardiographic analysis, and Doppler flow studies to identify ventricular and/or valvular abnormalities are also recommended in evaluating patients with suspected heart failure.[100,101] As CHD is the most common cause of heart failure, some evaluation for ischemic burden is indicated. To this end, coronary angiography or exercise stress testing may be used depending on the clinical scenario. Pulmonary function testing is generally not helpful in the diagnosis of heart failure as cardiogenic pulmonary edema and intrinsic lung disease can result in similar patterns of abnormalities.[99]

THE USE OF NATRIURETIC PEPTIDES AND TROPONINS IN THE DIAGNOSIS AND RISK STRATIFICATION OF HEART FAILURE

Though shortness of breath is the most common presentation of heart failure, it is a relatively nonspecific symptom. Measurement of circulating B-type natriuretic peptide (BNP), or its precursor N-terminal pro-B–type natriuretic peptide (NT-proBNP), can be particularly helpful in distinguishing cardiac from noncardiac causes of dyspnea and is widely used in emergency departments and other clinical settings.[97–99,102–105]

Natriuretic peptides are secreted from the heart in response to increased pressure and volume load. They play an important

TABLE 26.4	American College of Cardiology/American Heart Association/European Society of Cardiology Recommended Laboratory and Clinical Tests for Patients with Suspected Heart Failure

Complete blood count. A complete blood count can help determine if anemia or infection may be the cause of heart failure.

Serum electrolyte levels. An imbalance of electrolytes can cause fluid retention, and it may play a role in the severity of heart failure.

BUN/creatinine. Determination of BUN/creatinine can determine if damage to the kidneys, due to hypoperfusion, may be occurring secondary to heart failure.

Fasting glucose. Increased glucose levels in both diabetic patients and nondiabetic patients put them at an increased risk for heart failure.[94]

Liver function tests. Elevated liver enzymes (AST, ALT, and LD) may indicate if liver function is affected due to heart failure; congestion of the liver can occur secondary to the inefficiency with which the heart is able to move the venous circulation.

BNP/NT-proBNP levels. Both BNP and its precursor NT-proBNP are elevated after being released in the heart secondary to the stretch induced by heart failure. Their levels correlate closely with the severity of heart failure and can be used to differentiate cardiac causes of shortness of breath from primary lung disease.

ECG. A 12-lead ECG can detect ischemia, infarction, and arrhythmias as a cause for heart failure.

Urinalysis. Recent studies have described a relationship between the amount of protein excreted in urine and cardiovascular risk.[95] The specific relationship between urine protein and CV risk may be due to the common manifestation of vascular endothelial cell dysfunction.[96]

Lipid profile. The lipid profile, including total cholesterol, LDL, HDL, and triglyceride determination, should be performed to determine the risk of CHD.

TSH. Thyroid hormone function tests, in particular TSH levels, should be measured as both hyperthyroidism and hypothyroidism can be a primary cause of heart failure or can contribute to its severity.[97]

BUN, blood urea nitrogen; AST, aspartate aminotransferase; ALT, alanine aminotransferase; LD, lactate dehydrogenase; BNP, B-type natriuretic peptide; NT-proBNP, N-terminal pro-B–type natriuretic peptide; ECG, electrocardiogram; CV, cardiovascular; LDL, low-density lipoprotein; HDL, high-density lipoprotein; TSH, thyroid-stimulating hormone.

role in reducing intravascular volume by promoting natriuresis, diuresis, and vasodilation and inhibiting sympathetic nervous system signaling.[106,107] The proBNP is released by myocardial cells in response to increased volume, increased pressure, and cardiac hypertrophy; this precursor is cleaved by the protease enzyme furin into the active BNP and the inactive NT-proBNP. Both NT-proBNP and BNP are elevated in patients with ventricular dysfunction and strongly predict morbidity and mortality in patients with heart failure.[108–111] Multiple clinical studies have assessed the utility of both NT-proBNP and BNP for ruling out heart failure as a cause of dyspnea (shortness of breath) in the acute clinical setting.[111] Meta-analysis of these studies have found that the pooled estimates of sensitivity and specificity are equivalent for NT-proBNP and BNP. However, the optimum cutoff value for each peptide remains difficult to determine across all populations.[111]

Vasodilation and natriuresis are beneficial in the setting of heart failure, and thus, BNP was pursued as a target for drug development. Scios (later Johnson & Johnson) developed recombinant BNP as nesiritide. It is the first in a new class of therapies designed to treat heart failure, acting as a neurohormonal suppressor just as endogenous BNP.[112] The importance of mentioning that recombinant BNP is used therapeutically is that it can be picked up by laboratory tests for BNP, but not NT-proBNP. Therefore, there are clinical situations wherein NT-proBNP may be the more appropriate test to use to follow heart failure patients.

Cardiac Troponins

While used primarily for the diagnosis of myocardial injury caused by ischemia, elevations of cTnT and cTnI levels were recognized in heart failure patients more than a decade ago.[113–115] The precise reason for elevated troponins in the non-ACS setting of heart failure is not clear. Ongoing cell death including apoptosis and necrosis may be one of the reasons, occurring as a result of increased myocardial wall stress[116] resulting in subendocardial ischemia due to increased myocardial oxygen demand. Diminished cardiac perfusion and oxygen delivery to the heart itself and impaired renal clearance of troponins may also contribute.[116]

While the detection of troponins in heart failure is not diagnostic, it has been reported to add prognostic value. In acute heart failure patients without ACS, elevations in cTnI occur more often than cTnT elevations, although increases in either were related to increased mortality.[116] Other studies have described a 2.6-fold increased risk of in-hospital mortality for heart failure patients with elevated troponin levels at the time of admission.[117] Elevated cardiac troponin has also been associated with lower systolic blood pressure and lower left ventricular ejection fraction at the time of admission,[117] both of which are markers for worse outcome. In outpatients with more severe chronic heart failure (New York Heart Failure Class III or IV), the presence of elevated cardiac troponin was also associated with lower ejection fraction and deteriorating clinical course.[115] Troponin levels were one of the strongest predictors of mortality, particularly if used in conjunction with BNP levels.[118] In general, concomitant elevations in multiple markers (cardiac troponin, high-sensitivity CRP [hsCRP], along with NT-proBNP) are associated with escalating risks of adverse events.[119] Few studies, however, have investigated how troponin levels may be helpful in the initial diagnosis of heart failure, so their current role in heart failure patients is limited to risk stratification.

MARKERS OF CHD RISK

C-Reactive Protein

Inflammation plays an important role in the development and progression of atherosclerosis and CHD. CRP is an acute marker of inflammation that is currently used clinically in the evaluation of CVD risk. CRP is a pentameric protein consisting of five identical subunits that bind to specific ligands, such as LDL cholesterol, in a calcium-dependent manner. CRP is normally present in human plasma at levels less than 10 mg/L, but its rapid synthesis in the liver after stimulus from a variety of inflammatory cytokines may increase plasma levels by 1,000-fold, thus serving as a sensitive biomarker of systemic inflammation.[120] Because atherosclerosis and CHD derive largely from an inflammatory etiology, CRP has long been targeted as a biomarker for CHD, but it has recently gained widest acceptance as a marker of CHD risk.

CASE STUDY 26.4

A 68-year-old man presented to the emergency department with sudden onset of chest pain, left arm pain, dyspnea, and weakness while away from home on a business trip. His prior medical history is not available, but he admits to being a 2-pack per day smoker for longer than 20 years.

Cardiac markers were performed at admission and 8 hours postadmission with the following results:

Cardiac Markers	7:30 AM; September 26	4:00 PM; September 26
CK-MB (0–5 ng/L)	5.3	9.2
Myoglobin	76	124 (<70 µg/L)
Troponin T	<0.1	1.3 (0–0.1 µg/L)

Questions

1. Do these results indicate a specific diagnosis?
2. If so, what is the diagnosis?
3. What myoglobin, CK-MB, and TnT results would be expected if assayed at 4 PM on September 27?
4. Can any assumptions be made about the patient's lifestyle/habits/health that would increase his risk for this condition?
5. Are there any assays that might indicate his risk for further events of this type?

CRP was first described in 1930 when physicians studying the serum from patients with pneumonia observed high seroreactivity with pneumococcal bacterial extracts.[121] After separating the extracts into discrete fractions, only one fraction—arbitrarily designated fraction C—was found to react heavily with serum from acutely ill patients. This fraction contained "nonprotein material" that appeared "to be a carbohydrate common to the *Pneumococcus* species," which was later called C polysaccharide.[121] Only serum from acutely ill patients reacted with the pneumococcal C polysaccharide, and this reactivity disappeared after resolution of their illness. In the early 1940s, a protein requiring calcium ions was identified to be present exclusively in the serum of acutely ill patients. This protein, called "reactive protein," was responsible for reactivity with C polysaccharide.[122,123]

Although first observed in patients afflicted with pneumococcal pneumonia, it became clear that serum CRP was present in many more pathological conditions, and elevated CRP became associated with systemic inflammation.[122] As a biomarker, CRP originally gained the widespread use as an index of acute rheumatic fever.[124] Its association with heart disease was first demonstrated in 1947 when the serum of patients with **congestive heart failure** was found to contain detectable CRP.[125] In the 1950s, the discovery of elevated CRP after MI supported the hypothesis that MI is associated with systemic inflammation,[126] as did the subsequent finding of elevated CRP in patients with CHD.[127] Despite these findings, interest in CRP as a marker of CVD did not develop until the 1980s, when it was shown that CRP levels correlated remarkably well not only with serum CK-MB post-MI but also with the symptoms of cardiac disease, such as chest pain,[128] unstable angina, and chronic atherothrombotic disease.[129] All of these findings helped support the long-held hypothesis that vascular injury and inflammation play important roles in CVD, but CRP failed to provide significant benefit over the other clinically used markers of CVD or MI.

In the 1990s, extensive analysis of epidemiological data revealed that CRP could be applied clinically in a prognostic manner, rather than as a serum biomarker post-MI. This prognostic value was evaluated through several prospective cohort studies that compared baseline CRP levels in healthy individuals with CRP levels after cardiac events.[130] The most influential data were extracted from the Physicians Health Study (PHS), which found that baseline CRP levels were significantly higher in individuals that eventually experienced MI than those who did not.[131] These results showed that baseline plasma levels of CRP in apparently healthy individuals could help predict the risk of first MI, thus demonstrating a novel and substantial application of CRP as a prognostic marker. CRP data from the PHS also demonstrated that the use of anti-inflammatory medication (aspirin) reduced the risk of vascular events, which supported the hypothesis that chronic inflammation contributes to atherosclerosis and CHD.[130] In the late 1990s, the Cholesterol and Recurrent Events (CARE) trial showed that lipid-lowering drugs, such as statins, reduce CRP levels in a largely LDL-dependent manner, suggesting that CRP evaluation may help determine the efficacy of pharmacologic interventions used to treat CVD.[132]

These studies demonstrated that CRP had immense clinical value as a potential novel biomarker for both cardiovascular risk and cardiovascular therapy management. Importantly, the CRP levels in these and later studies were baseline values that were orders of magnitude less than the CRP levels typically present during acute inflammation. Whereas CRP levels present during acute inflammation are readily detectible using common clinical laboratory methods, the levels of CRP reported in these studies were far below the threshold of detection in most standard clinical assays. Because these studies demonstrated substantial prognostic value of monitoring CRP values at baseline levels, it was thus necessary to develop more sensitive methods of CRP measurement. Specifically, it was necessary to measure CRP levels with extremely high sensitivity (hs), in the range of 0.15 and 10 mg/L.[120] In the early 2000s, such methods for hsCRP measurement were developed and validated,[120] and the first set of clinical guidelines for the use of hsCRP as a marker of cardiovascular risk prediction was published by the AHA and the Centers for Disease Control and Prevention in early 2003.[133] These guidelines recommended that hsCRP be the inflammatory marker of choice in the evaluation of cardiac heart disease risk, and they stated that hsCRP concentrations of less than 1, 1 to 3, and greater than 3 correspond clinically to low, moderate, and high relative risk of CVD, respectively.[133]

Homocysteine

Homocysteine is a sulfur-containing amino acid formed in plasma from the metabolic demethylation of methionine, which is derived from dietary protein.[134] Plasma homocysteine circulates in four forms: (1) free thiol (homocysteine, Hcys; ~1%), (2) disulfide (homocystine; 5% to 10%), (3) mixed disulfide (Hcys-Cys; 5% to 10%), and (4) protein-bound thiol groups (80% to 90%).[135] Total plasma homocysteine refers to the combined pool of all forms of homocysteine. Normal total plasma homocysteine ranges from 5 to 15 µmol/L, moderate is 16 to 30 µmol/L, intermediate is 31 to 100 µmol/L, and severe hyperhomocystinemia is greater than 100 µmol/L.

Homocysteine was first isolated in 1932 but connections between homocysteine and vascular disease were not made until 1964, when a high incidence of vascular anomalies and arterial thromboses was observed in patients with homocystinuria.[136] Five years later, a physician studying vascular abnormalities in homocystinuria found an association between homocysteine and atherosclerosis, concluding that "elevated concentration of homocysteine, homocystine, or a derivative of homocysteine is the common factor leading to arterial damage."[137] Later studies demonstrated that premature vascular disease is extremely common in patients with homocystinuria, such that advanced atherosclerosis is frequently found in children with homocystinuria and approximately 50% of patients experience thromboembolic events in their lifetime.[138]

These early studies demonstrated a clear link between extremely high levels of plasma homocysteine (>100 µmol/L [>13.5 mg/L]) and CVD, but mildly elevated homocysteine was later shown to pose a risk of CVD as well. A 1976 study found that "a reduced ability to metabolize homocysteine" may contribute to premature coronary artery disease,[139] and numerous cross-sectional, case–control, and prospective cohort studies further evaluated this relationship. Most, but not all, of these epidemiologic studies indicated that hyperhomocystinemia increases the risk of CVD, but the results varied significantly between studies and study type. Whereas cross-sectional and case–control studies consistently found that hyperhomocystinemia increases the risk of CVD, most prospective studies demonstrated little or no increased risk.[140] One meta-analysis, for example, found that case–control studies estimate approximately an 80% risk of developing CVD due to hyperhomocystinemia, whereas prospective cohort studies estimate only 20% risk.[141] Such variation in clinical and epidemiological data raised questions about what role, if any, homocysteine actually plays in the development of CVD.

Many of these questions have been addressed through a wide body of basic research investigating the mechanisms through which homocysteine may contribute to CVD. Potential mechanisms that have been proposed include homocysteine-induced damage to vascular endothelium,[142] accelerated thrombin formation,[143] promotion of lipid peroxidation,[144] vascular smooth muscle proliferation,[145] and attraction of monocytes to the vascular endothelium.[146] Animal models have shown that mild hyperhomocystinemia contributes to atherosclerotic lesion development and to early lipid accumulation in vascular endothelium.[147] And studies in rats have shown that hyperhomocystinemia stimulates the expression of vascular adhesion molecules, such as monocyte chemoattractant protein (MCP-1), vascular cell adhesion molecule 1, and E-selectin, which increases the binding of monocytes to the endothelium.[148] Treatment of cultured human endothelial and smooth muscle cells with homocysteine also induces the expression of MCP-1, as well as expression of IL-8, a T lymphocyte and neutrophil chemoattractant.[149] Homocysteine-induced expression of these chemokines promotes a proinflammatory state that may contribute to general vascular inflammation that drives atherosclerosis.[150] Together, evidence from in vitro and animal models supports the hypothesis that hyperhomocystinemia promotes atherosclerotic lesion development, thereby increasing the risk of CVD.

Collectively, there is a growing body of evidence implicating hyperhomocysteinemia as an independent risk factor of CVD. Clinically, it has been estimated that up to 40% of patients diagnosed with premature coronary artery disease, peripheral vascular disease, or recurrent venous thrombosis exhibit some extent of hyperhomocystinemia.[150] Several recent meta-analyses found that for every 5 μmol/L (0.7 mg/L) increase in serum homocysteine concentration, the risk of ischemic heart disease increased 20% to 30%[151,152] and that decreasing plasma homocysteine by 3 μmol/L (0.4 mg/L) (through folate supplementation) can reduce the risk of ischemic heart disease by 16%, deep vein thrombosis (DVT) by 25%, and stroke by 24%.[152] The clinical, epidemiological, and biochemical data support a role for homocysteine in the development of atherosclerosis and CVD, but further research will be necessary to delineate the exact mechanisms through which it exerts this effect.

MARKERS OF PULMONARY EMBOLISM

An embolus is a circulating mass of solid, liquid, or gas, and pulmonary embolism (PE) is an acute and serious condition in which an embolus becomes lodged within the pulmonary arteries, impairing blood flow through the pulmonary vasculature and increasing right ventricular pressure. The extent of pulmonary vascular occlusion and subsequent symptoms is a function of the size and location of the embolus. Although most pulmonary emboli involve a pulmonary vessel of second, third, or fourth order yielding mild or no clinical symptoms, extremely large emboli can lodge at the bifurcation of the main pulmonary artery to form *saddle emboli* that can rapidly block pulmonary circulation.[153] Saddle emboli and other emboli that occlude over 60% of the pulmonary circulation greatly increase the risk of right heart failure, cardiovascular collapse, and sudden death. The coincidence of DVT and PE is quite high; approximately half of venous thromboemboli will develop into pulmonary emboli,[154] and approximately 95% of pulmonary emboli originate from deep veins of the legs[155] (Fig. 26.7).

The incidence of PE increases almost exponentially with age, ranging from approximately 5 per 100,000 in childhood to nearly 600 per 100,000 in persons over 75 years old[156] (Fig. 26.8). Women of reproductive age are at a greater risk for PE because of the associations between venous thromboembolism and pregnancy and the use of oral contraceptives. If left untreated, PE-related mortality can exceed 25%, but adequate treatment in the form of anticoagulation decreases this risk to approximately 5%.[158] Initial therapy after diagnoses of PE involves low molecular weight heparin, unfractionated heparin, or fondaparinux (trade name Arixtra), and long-term treatment includes oral vitamin K antagonists.[159]

Diagnosis of PE is inherently challenging because of the similarity of its symptoms to other more common conditions, such as ACS, and because signs and symptoms are frequently not present.[153] The classical presentation of a patient with PE includes chest pain, dyspnea, tachycardia, tachypnea, and coughing.[156] Unilateral leg swelling and redness may indicate DVT and increases the likelihood of PE. Syncope due to circulatory collapse is present in approximately 15% of patients with a large PE, and crackles or decreased breath sounds are common.[156] Vital signs may reveal tachycardia or mild hypoxia. Evidence of increased venous pressure, such as neck vein distension, or increased right ventricular pressure, such as a loud P2 (pulmonic valve closure sound), increases the diagnostic suspicion for PE.[156] Distinction between PE and ACS is particularly difficult because of their similar presentation, in particular chest pain, dyspnea, and ECG abnormalities.

Use of D-Dimer Detection in PE

The first step in the diagnostic workup of patients with suspected PE is determining the pretest clinical probability of PE using one of several decision rules.[156] The most widely used set of decision rules is the Wells score, which considers seven clinical variables obtained solely from medical history and physical examination, as well as the physician's judgment on the likelihood of PE versus other diagnoses.[160]

When the pretest probability of PE is low or intermediate, it is reasonable to order a D-dimer blood test.[156] D-Dimer is a product of plasmin-mediated fibrin degradation that consists of two D-domains from adjacent fibrin monomers that are cross-linked by activated factor XIII. Because D-dimer is derived from cross-linked fibrin, not fibrinogen, the presence of D-dimer in the bloodstream is indicative of current or recent coagulation and subsequent fibrinolysis. D-Dimer thus serves as an indirect marker of coagulation and fibrinolysis.[156] The choice of D-dimer assay is important as the sensitivity of various tests varies greatly. Enzyme-linked fluorescent assay, enzyme-linked immunosorbent assay (ELISA), and latex quantitative assay are highly sensitive quantitative assays for circulating D-dimer levels and are the tests of choice in the workup patients with suspected PE.[161]

D-Dimer levels are abnormal in approximately 90% of patients with PE,[162] and numerous studies have shown that a normal D-dimer results can rule out PE safely in patients with low or intermediate clinical probabilities.[156] However, D-dimer levels are normal in only 40% to 68% of patients without PE. Abnormal levels are often seen in patients with malignancy, recent surgery, renal dysfunction, or increased age.[162] The low specificity of D-dimer testing results in a poor positive predictive value and limited utility in patients with a high clinical probability of PE,[161] for whom CT and ventilation–perfusion scanning are reasonable initial diagnostic tests. However, the high sensitivity of the test translates to a valuable negative predictive value, meaning that D-dimer testing is most useful for excluding PE rather than diagnosing it. One study found that the sensitivity of the D-dimer (by high-sensitivity ELISA) for acute PE was 96.4% and the negative predictive value was 99.6%,[153] thus further evaluation of PE is not indicated for most patients with normal D-dimer levels.[153]

FIGURE 26.7 Thromboemboli originating from the deep veins of the legs travel through venous circulation through the heart and into the pulmonary vasculature, where they lodge in vessels of decreasing diameter and occlude blood flow. (Adapted from Douma RA, Kamphuisen PW, Büller HR. Acute pulmonary embolism. Part 1: epidemiology and diagnosis. *Nat Rev Cardiol.* 2010;7(10):585–596, Ref.[156].)

Value of Assaying Troponin and BNP in Acute PE

A recent meta-analysis was performed to determine the prognostic value of elevated troponin levels in patients with acute PE.[163] Based on publications from January 1998 to November 2006, 122 of 618 patients were found to have elevated troponin levels (19.7%) compared with 51 of 1,367 patients with normal troponin levels.[161] An elevated troponin level was associated significantly with a short-term mortality (odds ratio 5.24), resulting from PE (odds ratio 9.44) and with adverse outcome events (odds ratio 7.03).[161] These results were consistent between TnI and TnT and in both prospective and retrospective studies. Therefore,

an elevated troponin measurement in patients presenting with PE does appear to have utility in determining their short-term mortality outcome. This information can drive the clinician's clinical management as to whether a more aggressive management approach is necessary, such as the use of thrombolysis.

Similarly, BNP has been used as a predictor of adverse outcome in patients with PE. In a study of 110 consecutive patients with PE, the positive and negative predictive values of BNP levels were determined.[164] The risk of death related to PE if BNP > 21.7 pmol/L was 17%; the negative predictive value for uneventful outcome of a BNP < 21.7 pmol/L was 99%.[164] A larger meta-analysis of 12 studies, including 868

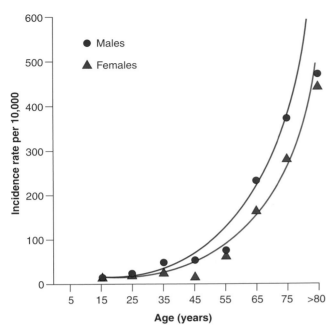

FIGURE 26.8 The incidence of pulmonary embolism (PE) as a function of age in the US population. (Adapted from Anderson FA, Wheeler HB, Goldberg RJ, et al. A population-based perspective of the hospital incidence and case-fatality rates of deep vein thrombosis and pulmonary embolism. The Worcester DVT Study. *Arch Intern Med.* 1991;151(5):933–938, Ref.[157].)

patients with acute PE, determined that elevated BNP levels were significantly associated with an increase in short-term mortality from all causes (odds ratio 6.57) and with death resulting from PE (odds ratio 6.10) or serious adverse events (odds ratio 7.47) with positive predictive values of 14% and negative predictive values of 95%.[165] Together these studies suggest a role for elevated BNP in helping to identify patients with acute PE at high risk for an adverse outcome, in order to drive a more aggressive management approach such as thrombolysis. The high negative predictive value of a normal BNP is also a particularly useful piece of data used to select patients with an uneventful clinical course.

SUMMARY

CHD is an extremely common condition that causes substantial morbidity and death worldwide. CHD is due in large part to atherosclerosis, which is best defined as a proinflammatory process in which cells, lipids, and connective tissue cause intimal thickening within large- and medium-sized arteries. This process impairs normal blood flow and may progress to occlude the entire vessel diameter. This narrowing of the coronary arteries leads to cardiac ischemia, which may manifest as activity-induced chest pain (stable angina), or ACS. Severe occlusion of coronary vessels causes complete ischemia and subsequent necrosis of surrounding tissue, which is known as MI. The extent of MI and subsequent morbidity can vary tremendously, ranging from undetected infarction with little consequence to sudden death. Because of the physiological and pathological responses that take

place within the myocardium immediately after infarction, rapid diagnosis is extremely important. Methods of rapidly diagnosing MI with a high sensitivity and specificity are thus extremely important for the management and potentially the survival of a patient that presents with symptoms of MI.

CASE STUDY 26.5

A 48-year-old woman was seen by her primary physician for a routine physical examination. Her father and his brother died before the age of 55 with acute MI and another uncle had CABG surgery at age 52. Because of this family history, she requested for any testing that might indicate a predisposition or increased risk factors for early cardiac disease. She does not smoke, does not have hypertension, is approximately 20 lb overweight, and exercises moderately. The following test results were obtained.

Total cholesterol (<200 mg/dL)	187 mg/dL
HDL cholesterol (30–75 mg/dL)	52 mg/dL
LDL cholesterol (60–130 mg/dL)	95 mg/dL
Lipoprotein(a) (<30 mg/dL)	34 mg/dL
Triglycerides (60–160 mg/dL)	203 mg/dL
Glucose (60–110 mg/dL)	83 mg/dL
Total CK (15–130 IU/L)	65 IU/L
CK-MB (<8 IU/L)	1.9 IU/L
% CK-MB (0%–6%)	3
Homocysteine (<15 μmol/L)	18 μmol/L
Fibrinogen (2–4.5 mg/dL)	4.3 mg/dL
D-Dimer (0–250 μg/mL)	160 μg/mL
hsCRP (0.016–0.76 mg/dL)	0.91 mg/dL

Questions

1. Do any of the results obtained indicate a high risk for development of cardiac disease? If so, which results?

2. Does this patient have risk factors for early cardiac disease that can be modified by diet or lifestyle modifications? If so, what changes can be made?

3. Is there any specific treatment that can be instituted to reduce this patient's risk?

4. How should this patient be monitored?

| TABLE 26.5 | Comparison of Past and Present Biomarkers for Cardiac Damage and Function with a Summary of Their Current Clinical Utility |

Marker	Currently Used to Diagnose ACS/Acute MI	Currently Used to Differentiate Heart failure From Lung Disease	Currently Used to Diagnose Pulmonary Embolism/Risk Stratification	Used for Cardiovascular Risk Stratification	No Longer Used/ Used Less Commonly/ Experimental
LD					X
CK-MB	X				
Myoglobin					X
IMA					X
H-FABP					X
TnI, TnT	X		X	X	
hsTn	X				X
hsCRP				X	
Homocysteine				X	
BNP		X	X		
NT-proBNP		X	X		
D-Dimer			X		

LD, lactate dehydrogenase; CK-MB, creatine kinase MB; IMA, ischemia-modified albumin; H-FABP, heart-type fatty acid–binding protein; TnI, troponin I; TnT, troponin T; hsTn, high-sensitive troponin; BNP, B-type natriuretic peptide; NT-proBNP, N-terminal pro-B–type natriuretic peptide.

Plasma biomarkers have become the centerpiece of evaluation and diagnosis of such patients (Table 26.5). AST, LD, and CK-MB were widely used biomarkers in the diagnosis of MI but have largely been replaced by high-sensitivity troponin assays. cTnI and cTnT assays have extremely high specificity to cardiac tissue, and detection methods are sensitive enough to pick up even very minor cardiac tissue damage. Current guidelines therefore recommend measurement of cardiac troponins in the circulation as soon as possible after symptoms of MI. Other experimental markers, such as myoglobin, H-FABP, and IMA, lack the specificity of troponin testing but may be useful when assayed together with troponins.

Plasma biomarkers of cardiac disease risk are also an important factor in the management of patients at risk for CHD, in particular CRP and homocysteine, both of which indicate systemic inflammation and correlate with the elevated risk of CHD and MI. Similarly, the management and diagnosis of heart failure is facilitated by the analysis of circulating biomarkers, most importantly cardiac troponins and BNP.

For additional student resources, please visit thePoint® at http://thepoint.lww.com

questions

1. A serum TnT concentration is of most value to the patient with an MI when
   a. The CK-MB has already peaked and returned to normal concentrations
   b. The onset of symptoms is within 3 to 6 hours of the sample being drawn
   c. The myoglobin concentration is extremely elevated
   d. The TnI concentration has returned to normal concentrations

2. A normal myoglobin concentration 8 hours after the onset of symptoms of a suspected MI will
   a. Essentially rule out an acute MI
   b. Provide a definitive diagnosis of acute MI
   c. Be interpreted with careful consideration of the TnT concentration
   d. Give the same information as a total CK-MB

(continues on page 548)

review questions (continued)

3. Which of the following analytes has the highest specificity for cardiac injury?
a. TnI
b. CK-MB mass assays
c. Total CK-MB
d. AST

4. Which of the following newer markers of inflammation circulates in serum bound to LD and HDL?
a. Lipoprotein-associated phospholipase A2
b. CK-MB
c. cTnI
d. hsCRP

5. A person with a confirmed blood pressure of 125/87 would be classified as
a. Prehypertension
b. Normal
c. Stage 1 hypertension
d. Stage 2 hypertension

6. Rheumatic heart disease is a result of infection with which of the following organisms?
a. Group A streptococci
b. *Staphylococcus aureus*
c. *Pseudomonas aeruginosa*
d. *Chlamydia pneumoniae*

7. Which of the following defects is the most common type of congenital CVD encountered?
a. Ventricular septal defects (VSD)
b. Tetralogy of Fallot
c. Coarctation of the aorta
d. Transposition of the great arteries

8. Which of the following cardiac markers is the most useful indicator of congestive heart failure?
a. BNP
b. TnI
c. CK-MB
d. Glycogen phosphorylase isoenzyme BB

9. Which of the following is the preferred biomarker for the assessment of myocardial necrosis?
a. CK
b. AST
c. CK-MB
d. TnI

10. Which of the following is NOT a feature of an ideal cardiac marker?
a. Ability to predict future occurrence of cardiac disease
b. Absolute specificity
c. High sensitivity
d. Close estimation of the magnitude of cardiac damage

references

1. Lindsell C, Anantharaman V, Diercks D, et al. The Internet Tracking Registry of Acute Coronary Syndromes (i*trACS): a multicenter registry of patients with suspicion of acute coronary syndromes reported using the standardized reporting guidelines for emergency department chest pain studies. *Ann Emerg Med.* 2006;48(6):666–677.
2. Pope JH, Aufderheide TP, Ruthazer R, et al. Missed diagnoses of acute cardiac ischemia in the emergency department. *N Engl J Med.* 2000;342(16):1163–1170.
3. Morrow DA. Clinical application of sensitive troponin assays. *N Engl J Med.* 2009;361(9):913–915.
4. Runge M, Ohman M, Stouffer G. The history and physical exam. In: Runge M, Stouffer G, Patterson C, eds. *Netter's Cardiology.* 2nd ed. Philadelphia, PA: Saunders Elsevier; 2010.
5. Mosca L, Manson JE, Sutherland SE, et al. Cardiovascular disease in women: a statement for healthcare professionals from the American Heart Association. Writing Group. *Circulation.* 1997;96(7):2468–2482.
6. Douglas PS, Ginsburg GS. The evaluation of chest pain in women. *N Engl J Med.* 1996;334(20):1311–1315.
7. Kudenchuk PJ, Maynard C, Martin JS, et al. Comparison of presentation, treatment, and outcome of acute myocardial infarction in men versus women (the Myocardial Infarction Triage and Intervention Registry). *Am J Cardiol.* 1996;78(1):9–14.
8. Amsterdam EA, Wenger NK, Brindis RG, et al. 2014 AHA/ACC guideline for the management of patients with non-ST-elevation acute coronary syndromes: a report of the American College of Cardiology/American Heart Association Task Force on Practice Guidelines. *Circulation.* 2014;130(25):e344–e426.
9. Thygesen K, Alpert J, White H, et al. Universal definition of myocardial infarction. *Circulation.* 2007;116(22):2634–2653.
10. Glass CK, Witztum JL. Atherosclerosis. the road ahead. *Cell.* 2001;104(4):503–516.
11. Lusis AJ. Atherosclerosis. *Nature.* 2000;407(6801):233–241.
12. Ross R. The pathogenesis of atherosclerosis—an update. *N Engl J Med.* 1986;314(8):488–500.
13. Nakashima Y, Wight TN, Sueishi K. Early atherosclerosis in humans: role of diffuse intimal thickening and extracellular matrix proteoglycans. *Cardiovasc Res.* 2008;79(1):14–23.
14. Skålén K, Gustafsson M, Rydberg EK, et al. Subendothelial retention of atherogenic lipoproteins in early atherosclerosis. *Nature.* 2002;417(6890):750–754.

15. Moore KJ, Tabas I. Macrophages in the pathogenesis of atherosclerosis. *Cell.* 2011;145(3):341–355.

16. Libby P. Changing concepts of atherogenesis. *J Intern Med.* 2000;247(3):349–358.

17. Virmani R, Kolodgie FD, Burke AP, et al. Atherosclerotic plaque progression and vulnerability to rupture: angiogenesis as a source of intraplaque hemorrhage. *Arterioscler Thromb Vasc Biol.* 2005;25(10):2054–2061.

18. Karmen A, Wroblewski F, Ladue JS. Transaminase activity in human blood. *J Clin Invest.* 1955;34(1):126–131.

19. Ladue JS, Wroblewski F, Karmen A. Serum glutamic oxaloacetic transaminase activity in human acute transmural myocardial infarction. *Science.* 1954;120(3117):497–499.

20. King J, Waind AP. Lactic dehydrogenase activity in acute myocardial infarction. *Br Med J.* 1960;2(5209):1361–1363.

21. Warburton FG, Bernstein A, Wright AC. Serum creatine phosphokinase estimations in myocardial infarction. *Br Heart J.* 1965;27(5):740–747.

22. Wroblewski F, Gregory KF. Lactic dehydrogenase isozymes and their distribution in normal tissues and plasma and in disease states. *Ann N Y Acad Sci.* 1961;94:912–932.

23. Vasudevan G, Mercer DW, Varat MA. Lactic dehydrogenase isoenzyme determination in the diagnosis of acute myocardial infarction. *Circulation.* 1978;57(6):1055–1057.

24. Dreyfus JC, Schapira G, Resnais J, et al. [Serum creatine kinase in the diagnosis of myocardial infarct]. *Rev Fr Etud Clin Biol.* 1960;5:386–387.

25. French JK, White HD. Clinical implications of the new definition of myocardial infarction. *Heart.* 2004;90(1):99–106.

26. Sobel BE, Shell WE. Serum enzyme determinations in the diagnosis and assessment of myocardial infarction. *Circulation.* 1972;45(2):471–482.

27. Dillon MC, Calbreath DF, Dixon AM, et al. Diagnostic problem in acute myocardial infarction: CK-MB in the absence of abnormally elevated total creatine kinase levels. *Arch Intern Med.* 1982;142(1):33–38.

28. Wagner GS, Roe CR, Limbird LE, et al. The importance of identification of the myocardial-specific isoenzyme of creatine phosphokinase (MB form) in the diagnosis of acute myocardial infarction. *Circulation.* 1973;47(2):263–269.

29. Malasky BR, Alpert JS. Diagnosis of myocardial injury by biochemical markers: problems and promises. *Cardiol Rev.* 2002;10(5):306–317.

30. Robinson DJ, Christenson RH. Creatine kinase and its CK-MB isoenzyme: the conventional marker for the diagnosis of acute myocardial infarction. *J Emerg Med.* 1999;17(1):95–104.

31. Scott BB, Simmons AV, Newton KE, et al. Interpretation of serum creatine kinase in suspected myocardial infarction. *Br Med J.* 1974;4(5946):691–693.

32. Goldberg DM, Winfield DA. Diagnostic accuracy of serum enzyme assays for myocardial infarction in a general hospital population. *Br Heart J.* 1972;34(6):597–604.

33. Goldberg DM. Clinical enzymology: an autobiographical history. *Clin Chim Acta.* 2005;357(2):93–112.

34. Cummins P, Perry SV. Troponin I from human skeletal and cardiac muscles. *Biochem J.* 1978;171(1):251–259.

35. Adams JE, Abendschein DR, Jaffe AS. Biochemical markers of myocardial injury. Is MB creatine kinase the choice for the 1990s? *Circulation.* 1993;88(2):750–763.

36. MacGeoch C, Barton PJ, Vallins WJ, et al. The human cardiac troponin I locus: assignment to chromosome 19p13.2-19q13.2. *Hum Genet.* 1991;88(1):101–104.

37. Cummins B, Auckland ML, Cummins P. Cardiac-specific troponin-I radioimmunoassay in the diagnosis of acute myocardial infarction. *Am Heart J.* 1987;113(6):1333–1344.

38. Adams JE, Bodor GS, Dávila-Román VG, et al. Cardiac troponin I. A marker with high specificity for cardiac injury. *Circulation.* 1993;88(1):101–106.

39. Coudrey L. The troponins. *Arch Intern Med.* 1998;158(11):1173–1180.

40. Stacy SR, Suarez-Cuervo C, Berger Z, et al. Role of troponin in patients with chronic kidney disease and suspected acute coronary syndrome: a systematic review. *Ann Intern Med.* 2014;161(7):502–512.

41. Aviles RJ, Askari AT, Lindahl B, et al. Troponin T levels in patients with acute coronary syndromes, with or without renal dysfunction. *N Engl J Med.* 2002;346(26):2047–2052.

42. Michos ED, Wilson LM, Yeh HC, et al. Prognostic value of cardiac troponin in patients with chronic kidney disease without suspected acute coronary syndrome: a systematic review and meta-analysis. *Ann Intern Med.* 2014;161(7):491–501.

43. Dierkes J, Domröse U, Westphal S, et al. Cardiac troponin T predicts mortality in patients with end-stage renal disease. *Circulation.* 2000;102(16):1964–1969.

44. Deegan PB, Lafferty ME, Blumsohn A, et al. Prognostic value of troponin T in hemodialysis patients is independent of comorbidity. *Kidney Int.* 2001;60(6):2399–2405.

45. deFilippi C, Wasserman S, Rosanio S, et al. Cardiac troponin T and C-reactive protein for predicting prognosis, coronary atherosclerosis, and cardiomyopathy in patients undergoing long-term hemodialysis. *JAMA.* 2003;290(3):353–359.

46. Wood GN, Keevil B, Gupta J, et al. Serum troponin T measurement in patients with chronic renal impairment predicts survival and vascular disease: a 2 year prospective study. *Nephrol Dial Transplant.* 2003;18(8):1610–1615.

47. Boulier A, Jaussent I, Terrier N, et al. Measurement of circulating troponin Ic enhances the prognostic value of C-reactive protein in haemodialysis patients. *Nephrol Dial Transplant.* 2004;19(9):2313–2318.

48. Iliou MC, Fumeron C, Benoit MO, et al. Prognostic value of cardiac markers in ESRD: Chronic Hemodialysis and New Cardiac Markers Evaluation (CHANCE) study. *Am J Kidney Dis.* 2003;42(3):513–523.

49. Conway B, McLaughlin M, Sharpe P, et al. Use of cardiac troponin T in diagnosis and prognosis of cardiac events in patients on chronic haemodialysis. *Nephrol Dial Transplant.* 2005;20(12):2759–2764.

50. Khan NA, Hemmelgarn BR, Tonelli M, et al. Prognostic value of troponin T and I among asymptomatic patients with end-stage renal disease: a meta-analysis. *Circulation.* 2005;112(20):3088–3096.

51. Havekes B, van Manen JG, Krediet RT, et al. Serum troponin T concentration as a predictor of mortality in hemodialysis and peritoneal dialysis patients. *Am J Kidney Dis.* 2006;47(5):823–829.

52. Wang AY, Lam CW, Yu CM, et al. Troponin T, left ventricular mass, and function are excellent predictors of cardiovascular congestion in peritoneal dialysis. *Kidney Int.* 2006;70(3):444–452.

53. Hickson LJ, Cosio FG, El-Zoghby ZM, et al. Survival of patients on the kidney transplant wait list: relationship to cardiac troponin T. *Am J Transplant.* 2008;8(11):2352–2359.

54. Hayashi T, Obi Y, Kimura T, et al. Cardiac troponin T predicts occult coronary artery stenosis in patients with chronic kidney disease at the start of renal replacement therapy. *Nephrol Dial Transplant.* 2008;23(9):2936–2942.

55. Hassan HC, Howlin K, Jefferys A, et al. High-sensitivity troponin as a predictor of cardiac events and mortality in the stable dialysis population. *Clin Chem.* 2014;60(2):389–398.

56. McGill D, Talaulikar G, Potter JM, et al. Over time, high-sensitivity TnT replaces NT-proBNP as the most powerful predictor of death in patients with dialysis-dependent chronic renal failure. *Clin Chim Acta.* 2010;411(13–14):936–939.

57. Tun A, Khan IA, Win MT, et al. Specificity of cardiac troponin I and creatine kinase-MB isoenzyme in asymptomatic long-term hemodialysis patients and effect of hemodialysis on these cardiac markers. *Cardiology.* 1998;90(4):280–285.

58. Lippi G, Tessitore N, Montagnana M, et al. Influence of sampling time and ultrafiltration coefficient of the dialysis membrane on cardiac troponin I and T. *Arch Pathol Lab Med.* 2008;132(1):72–76.

59. Wayand D, Baum H, Schätzle G, et al. Cardiac troponin T and I in end-stage renal failure. *Clin Chem.* 2000;46(9):1345–1350.

60. Kagen L. *Myoglobin: Biochemical, Physiological, and Clinical Aspects.* New York, NY: Columbia University Press; 1973.

61. Klocke FJ, Copley DP, Krawczyk JA, et al. Rapid renal clearance of immunoreactive canine plasma myoglobin. *Circulation.* 1982;65(7):1522–1528.

62. McCord J, Nowak RM, McCullough PA, et al. Ninety-minute exclusion of acute myocardial infarction by use of quantitative point-of-care testing of myoglobin and troponin I. *Circulation.* 2001;104(13):1483–1488.

63. Kagen L, Scheidt S, Butt A. Serum myoglobin in myocardial infarction: the "staccato phenomenon." Is acute myocardial infarction in man an intermittent event? *Am J Med.* 1977;62(1):86–92.

64. Kavsak PA, MacRae AR, Newman AM, et al. Effects of contemporary troponin assay sensitivity on the utility of the early markers myoglobin and CKMB isoforms in evaluating patients with possible acute myocardial infarction. *Clin Chim Acta.* 2007;380(1–2):213–216.

65. Eggers KM, Oldgren J, Nordenskjöld A, et al. Diagnostic value of serial measurement of cardiac markers in patients with chest pain: limited value of adding myoglobin to troponin I for exclusion of myocardial infarction. *Am Heart J.* 2004;148(4):574–581.

66. Ilva T, Eriksson S, Lund J, et al. Improved early risk stratification and diagnosis of myocardial infarction, using a novel troponin I assay concept. *Eur J Clin Invest.* 2005;35(2):112–116.

67. Van Nieuwenhoven FA, Kleine AH, Wodzig WH, et al. Discrimination between myocardial and skeletal muscle injury by assessment of the plasma ratio of myoglobin over fatty acid-binding protein. *Circulation.* 1995;92(10):2848–2854.

68. Seino Y, Ogata K, Takano T, et al. Use of a whole blood rapid panel test for heart-type fatty acid-binding protein in patients with acute chest pain: comparison with rapid troponin T and myoglobin tests. *Am J Med.* 2003;115(3):185–190.

69. McMahon CG, Lamont JV, Curtin E, et al. Diagnostic accuracy of heart-type fatty acid-binding protein for the early diagnosis of acute myocardial infarction. *Am J Emerg Med.* 2012;30(2):267–274.

70. Bhagavan NV, Lai EM, Rios PA, et al. Evaluation of human serum albumin cobalt binding assay for the assessment of myocardial ischemia and myocardial infarction. *Clin Chem.* 2003;49(4):581–585.

71. Christenson RH, Duh SH, Sanhai WR, et al. Characteristics of an Albumin Cobalt Binding Test for assessment of acute coronary syndrome patients: a multicenter study. *Clin Chem.* 2001;47(3):464–470.

72. Bar-Or D, Curtis G, Rao N, et al. Characterization of the Co(2+) and Ni(2+) binding amino-acid residues of the N-terminus of human albumin. An insight into the mechanism of a new assay for myocardial ischemia. *Eur J Biochem.* 2001;268(1):42–47.

73. Bar-Or D, Lau E, Winkler JV. A novel assay for cobalt-albumin binding and its potential as a marker for myocardial ischemia-a preliminary report. *J Emerg Med.* 2000;19(4):311–315.

74. Roy D, Quiles J, Aldama G, et al. Ischemia Modified Albumin for the assessment of patients presenting to the emergency department with acute chest pain but normal or non-diagnostic 12-lead electrocardiograms and negative cardiac troponin T. *Int J Cardiol.* 2004;97(2):297–301.

75. Sinha MK, Roy D, Gaze DC, et al. Role of "Ischemia modified albumin", a new biochemical marker of myocardial ischaemia, in the early diagnosis of acute coronary syndromes. *Emerg Med J.* 2004;21(1):29–34.

76. Schaub N, Reichlin T, Meune C, et al. Markers of plaque instability in the early diagnosis and risk stratification of acute myocardial infarction. *Clin Chem.* 2012;58(1):246–256.

77. Nicholls SJ, Hazen SL. Myeloperoxidase and cardiovascular disease. *Arterioscler Thromb Vasc Biol.* 2005;25(6):1102–1111.

78. Ionita MG, Vink A, Dijke IE, et al. High levels of myeloid-related protein 14 in human atherosclerotic plaques correlate with the characteristics of rupture-prone lesions. *Arterioscler Thromb Vasc Biol.* 2009;29(8):1220–1227.

79. Bayes-Genis A, Conover CA, Overgaard MT, et al. Pregnancy-associated plasma protein A as a marker of acute coronary syndromes. *N Engl J Med.* 2001;345(14):1022–1029.

80. Mueller C, Buettner HJ, Hodgson JM, et al. Inflammation and long-term mortality after non-ST elevation acute coronary syndrome treated with a very early invasive strategy in 1042 consecutive patients. *Circulation.* 2002;105(12):1412–1415.

81. Krysko DV, Denecker G, Festjens N, et al. Macrophages use different internalization mechanisms to clear apoptotic and necrotic cells. *Cell Death Differ.* 2006;13(12):2011–2022.

82. Yaoita H, Maruyama Y. Intervention for apoptosis in cardiomyopathy. *Heart Fail Rev.* 2008;13(2):181–191.

83. Olivetti G, Abbi R, Quaini F, et al. Apoptosis in the failing human heart. *N Engl J Med.* 1997;336(16):1131–1141.

84. Ibe W, Saraste A, Lindemann S, et al. Cardiomyocyte apoptosis is related to left ventricular dysfunction and remodelling in dilated cardiomyopathy, but is not affected by growth hormone treatment. *Eur J Heart Fail.* 2007;9(2):160–167.

85. McLean A, Huang S. Biomarkers of cardiac injury. In: Vaidya V, Bonventre J, eds. *Biomarkers: In Medicine, Drug Discovery, and Environmental Health.* New York, NY: John Wiley & Sons, Inc.; 2010:119–155.

86. Dent MR, Das S, Dhalla NS. Alterations in both death and survival signals for apoptosis in heart failure due to volume overload. *J Mol Cell Cardiol.* 2007;43(6):726–732.

87. Anselmi A, Gaudino M, Baldi A, et al. Role of apoptosis in pressure-overload cardiomyopathy. *J Cardiovasc Med (Hagerstown).* 2008;9(3):227–232.

88. Leri A, Claudio PP, Li Q, et al. Stretch-mediated release of angiotensin II induces myocyte apoptosis by activating p53 that enhances the local renin-angiotensin system and decreases the Bcl-2-to-Bax protein ratio in the cell. *J Clin Invest.* 1998;101(7):1326–1342.

89. Colucci WS, Sawyer DB, Singh K, et al. Adrenergic overload and apoptosis in heart failure: implications for therapy. *J Card Fail.* 2000;6(2 suppl 1):1–7.

90. Cooper LT. Myocarditis. *N Engl J Med.* 2009;360(15):1526–1538.

91. Lai HC, Yeh YC, Ting CT, et al. Doxycycline suppresses doxorubicin-induced oxidative stress and cellular apoptosis in mouse hearts. *Eur J Pharmacol.* 2010;644(1–3):176–187.

92. Shi J, Abdelwahid E, Wei L. Apoptosis in Anthracycline Cardiomyopathy. *Curr Pediatr Rev.* 2011;7(4):329–336.

93. Asiri YA. Probucol attenuates cyclophosphamide-induced oxidative apoptosis, p53 and Bax signal expression in rat cardiac tissues. *Oxid Med Cell Longev.* 2010;3(5):308–316.

94. Haffner SJ, Cassells H. Hyperglycemia as a cardiovascular risk factor. *Am J Med.* 2003;115(Suppl 8A):6S–11S.

95. Buckalew VM, Freedman BI. Effects of race on albuminuria and risk of cardiovascular and kidney disease. *Expert Rev Cardiovasc Ther.* 2011;9(2):245–249.

96. Ochodnicky P, Henning RH, van Dokkum RP, et al. Microalbuminuria and endothelial dysfunction: emerging targets for primary prevention of end-organ damage. *J Cardiovasc Pharmacol.* 2006;47(suppl 2):S151–S162; discussion S172–S156.

97. Hunt SA, Abraham WT, Chin MH, et al. 2009 Focused update incorporated into the ACC/AHA 2005 Guidelines for the Diagnosis and Management of Heart Failure in Adults A Report of the American College of Cardiology Foundation/American Heart Association Task Force on Practice Guidelines Developed in Collaboration With the International Society for Heart and Lung Transplantation. *J Am Coll Cardiol.* 2009;53(15):e1–e90.

98. Lindenfeld J, Albert NM, Boehmer JP, et al. HFSA 2010 Comprehensive Heart Failure Practice Guideline. *J Card Fail.* 2010;16(6):e1–e194.

99. Dickstein K, Cohen-Solal A, Filippatos G, et al. ESC Guidelines for the diagnosis and treatment of acute and chronic heart failure 2008: the Task Force for the Diagnosis and Treatment of Acute and Chronic Heart Failure 2008 of the European Society of Cardiology. Developed in collaboration with the Heart Failure Association of the ESC (HFA) and endorsed by the European Society of Intensive Care Medicine (ESICM). *Eur Heart J.* 2008;29(19):2388–2442.

100. Pinamonti B, Di Lenarda A, Sinagra G, et al. Restrictive left ventricular filling pattern in dilated cardiomyopathy assessed by Doppler echocardiography: clinical, echocardiographic and hemodynamic correlations and prognostic implications. Heart Muscle Disease Study Group. *J Am Coll Cardiol.* 1993;22(3):808–815.

101. Temporelli PL, Scapellato F, Eleuteri E, et al. Doppler echocardiography in advanced systolic heart failure: a noninvasive alternative to Swan-Ganz catheter. *Circ Heart Fail.* 2010;3(3):387–394.

102. Maisel AS, Krishnaswamy P, Nowak RM, et al. Rapid measurement of B-type natriuretic peptide in the emergency diagnosis of heart failure. *N Engl J Med.* 2002;347(3):161–167.

103. Januzzi JL, Camargo CA, Anwaruddin S, et al. The N-terminal Pro-BNP investigation of dyspnea in the emergency department (PRIDE) study. *Am J Cardiol.* 2005;95(8):948–954.

104. Maisel AS, McCord J, Nowak RM, et al. Bedside B-Type natriuretic peptide in the emergency diagnosis of heart failure with reduced or preserved ejection fraction. Results from the Breathing Not Properly Multinational Study. *J Am Coll Cardiol.* 2003;41(11):2010–2017.

105. Januzzi JL, van Kimmenade R, Lainchbury J, et al. NT-proBNP testing for diagnosis and short-term prognosis in acute destabilized heart failure: an international pooled analysis of 1256 patients: the International Collaborative of NT-proBNP Study. *Eur Heart J.* 2006;27(3):330–337.

106. de Lemos JA, Morrow DA, Bentley JH, et al. The prognostic value of B-type natriuretic peptide in patients with acute coronary syndromes. *N Engl J Med.* 2001;345(14):1014–1021.

107. McFarlane SI, Winer N, Sowers JR. Role of the natriuretic peptide system in cardiorenal protection. *Arch Intern Med.* 2003;163(22):2696–2704.

108. Wang TJ, Larson MG, Levy D, et al. Plasma natriuretic peptide levels and the risk of cardiovascular events and death. *N Engl J Med.* 2004;350(7):655–663.

109. Bibbins-Domingo K, Gupta R, Na B, et al. N-terminal fragment of the prohormone brain-type natriuretic peptide (NT-proBNP), cardiovascular events, and mortality in patients with stable coronary heart disease. *JAMA.* 2007;297(2):169–176.

110. Cowie MR, Jourdain P, Maisel A, et al. Clinical applications of B-type natriuretic peptide (BNP) testing. *Eur Heart J.* 2003;24(19):1710–1718.

111. Worster A, Balion CM, Hill SA, et al. Diagnostic accuracy of BNP and NT-proBNP in patients presenting to acute care settings with dyspnea: a systematic review. *Clin Biochem.* 2008;41(4–5):250–259.

112. Fonarow GC. B-type natriuretic peptide: spectrum of application. Nesiritide (recombinant BNP) for heart failure. *Heart Fail Rev.* 2003;8(4):321–325.

113. Güler N, Bilge M, Eryonucu B, et al. Cardiac troponin I levels in patients with left heart failure and cor pulmonale. *Angiology.* 2001;52(5):317–322.

114. Logeart D, Beyne P, Cusson C, et al. Evidence of cardiac myolysis in severe nonischemic heart failure and the potential role of increased wall strain. *Am Heart J.* 2001;141(2):247–253.

115. La Vecchia L, Mezzena G, Zanolla L, et al. Cardiac troponin I as diagnostic and prognostic marker in severe heart failure. *J Heart Lung Transplant.* 2000;19(7):644–652.

116. Nagarajan V, Tang WH. Biomarkers in advanced heart failure: diagnostic and therapeutic insights. *Congest Heart Fail.* 2011;17(4):169–174.

117. Peacock WF, De Marco T, Fonarow GC, et al. Cardiac troponin and outcome in acute heart failure. *N Engl J Med.* 2008;358(20):2117–2126.

118. Horwich TB, Patel J, MacLellan WR, et al. Cardiac troponin I is associated with impaired hemodynamics, progressive left ventricular dysfunction, and increased mortality rates in advanced heart failure. *Circulation.* 2003;108(7):833–838.

119. Yin WH, Chen JW, Feng AN, et al. Multimarker approach to risk stratification among patients with advanced chronic heart failure. *Clin Cardiol.* 2007;30(8):397–402.

120. Ledue TB, Rifai N. High sensitivity immunoassays for C-reactive protein: promises and pitfalls. *Clin Chem Lab Med.* 2001;39(11):1171–1176.

121. Tillett WS, Francis T. Serological reactions in pneumonia with a non-protein somatic fraction of pneumococcus. *J Exp Med.* 1930;52(4):561–571.

122. Abernethy TJ, Avery OT. The occurrence during acute infections of a protein not normally present in the blood: I. Distribution of the reactive protein in patients' sera and the effect of calcium on the flocculation reaction with C polysaccharide of pneumococcus. *J Exp Med.* 1941;73(2):173–182.

123. Macleod CM, Avery OT. The Occurrence during acute infections of a protein not normally present in the blood: II. isolation and properties of the reactive protein. *J Exp Med.* 1941;73(2):183–190.

124. Elster SK, Braunwald E, Wood HF. A study of C-reactive protein in the serum of patients with congestive heart failure. *Am Heart J.* 1956;51(4):533–541.

125. Hedlund P. The appearance of acute phase protein in various diseases. *Acta Med Scand.* 1947;128(suppl 196):579–601.

126. Kroop IG, Shackman NH. Level of C-reactive protein as a measure of acute myocardial infarction. *Proc Soc Exp Biol Med.* 1954;86(1):95–97.

127. Kroop IG, Shackman NH. The C-reactive protein determination as an index of myocardial necrosis in coronary artery disease. *Am J Med.* 1957;22(1):90–98.

128. de Beer FC, Hind CR, Fox KM, et al. Measurement of serum C-reactive protein concentration in myocardial ischaemia and infarction. *Br Heart J.* 1982;47(3):239–243.

129. Liuzzo G, Biasucci LM, Gallimore JR, et al. The prognostic value of C-reactive protein and serum amyloid a protein in severe unstable angina. *N Engl J Med.* 1994;331(7):417–424.

130. Ridker PM. C-reactive protein: eighty years from discovery to emergence as a major risk marker for cardiovascular disease. *Clin Chem.* 2009;55(2):209–215.

131. Ridker PM, Cushman M, Stampfer MJ, et al. Inflammation, aspirin, and the risk of cardiovascular disease in apparently healthy men. *N Engl J Med.* 1997;336(14):973–979.

132. Ridker PM, Rifai N, Pfeffer MA, et al. Inflammation, pravastatin, and the risk of coronary events after myocardial infarction in patients with average cholesterol levels. Cholesterol and Recurrent Events (CARE) Investigators. *Circulation.* 1998;98(9):839–844.

133. Pearson TA, Mensah GA, Alexander RW, et al. Markers of inflammation and cardiovascular disease: application to clinical and public health practice: A statement for healthcare professionals from the Centers for Disease Control and Prevention and the American Heart Association. *Circulation.* 2003;107(3):499–511.

134. Abraham JM, Cho L. The homocysteine hypothesis: still relevant to the prevention and treatment of cardiovascular disease? *Cleve Clin J Med.* 2010;77(12):911–918.

135. Hankey GJ, Eikelboom JW. Homocysteine and vascular disease. *Lancet.* 1999;354(9176):407–413.

136. Gibson JB, Carson NA, Neill DW. Pathological findings in homocystinuria. *J Clin Pathol* 1964;17:427–437.

137. McCully KS. Vascular pathology of homocysteinemia: implications for the pathogenesis of arteriosclerosis. *Am J Pathol.* 1969;56(1):111–128.

138. Nygård O, Nordrehaug JE, Refsum H, et al. Plasma homocysteine levels and mortality in patients with coronary artery disease. *N Engl J Med.* 1997;337(4):230–236.

139. Wilcken DE, Wilcken B. The pathogenesis of coronary artery disease. A possible role for methionine metabolism. *J Clin Invest.* 1976;57(4):1079–1082.

140. Christen WG, Ajani UA, Glynn RJ, et al. Blood levels of homocysteine and increased risks of cardiovascular disease: causal or casual? *Arch Intern Med.* 2000;160(4):422–434.

141. Splaver A, Lamas GA, Hennekens CH. Homocysteine and cardiovascular disease: biological mechanisms, observational epidemiology, and the need for randomized trials. *Am Heart J.* 2004;148(1):34–40.

142. Blundell G, Jones BG, Rose FA, et al. Homocysteine mediated endothelial cell toxicity and its amelioration. *Atherosclerosis.* 1996;122(2):163–172.

143. Loscalzo J. Homocysteine-mediated thrombosis and angiostasis in vascular pathobiology. *J Clin Invest.* 2009;119(11):3203–3205.

144. Heinecke JW. Biochemical evidence for a link between elevated levels of homocysteine and lipid peroxidation in vivo. *Curr Atheroscler Rep.* 1999;1(2):87–89.

145. Tsai JC, Perrella MA, Yoshizumi M, et al. Promotion of vascular smooth muscle cell growth by homocysteine: a link to atherosclerosis. *Proc Natl Acad Sci U S A.* 1994;91(14):6369–6373.

146. Sung FL, Slow YL, Wang G, et al, Homocysteine stimulates the expression of monocyte chemoattractant protein-1 in endothelial cells leading to enhanced monocyte chemotaxis. *Mol Cell Biochem.* 2001;216(1–2):121–128.

147. Chen Z, Karaplis AC, Ackerman SL, et al. Mice deficient in methylenetetrahydrofolate reductase exhibit hyperhomocysteinemia and decreased methylation capacity, with neuropathology and aortic lipid deposition. *Hum Mol Genet.* 2001;10(5):433–443.

148. Wang G, Woo CW, Sung FL, et al. Increased monocyte adhesion to aortic endothelium in rats with hyperhomocysteinemia: role of chemokine and adhesion molecules. *Arterioscler Thromb Vasc Biol.* 2002;22(11):1777–1783.

149. Poddar R, Sivasubramanian N, DiBello PM, et al. Homocysteine induces expression and secretion of monocyte chemoattractant protein-1 and interleukin-8 in human aortic endothelial cells: implications for vascular disease. *Circulation.* 2001;103(22):2717–2723.

150. Austin RC, Lentz SR, Werstuck GH. Role of hyperhomocysteinemia in endothelial dysfunction and atherothrombotic disease. *Cell Death Differ.* 2004;11(suppl 1):S56–S64.

151. Humphrey LL, Fu R, Rogers K, et al. Homocysteine level and coronary heart disease incidence: a systematic review and meta-analysis. *Mayo Clin Proc.* 2008;83(11):1203–1212.

152. Wald DS, Law M, Morris JK. Homocysteine and cardiovascular disease: evidence on causality from a meta-analysis. *BMJ.* 2002;325(7374):1202.

153. Goldhaber SZ. Pulmonary embolism. *Lancet.* 2004;363(9417):1295–1305.

154. Silverstein MD, Heit JA, Mohr DN, et al. Trends in the incidence of deep vein thrombosis and pulmonary embolism: a 25-year population-based study. *Arch Intern Med.* 1998;158(6):585–593.

155. Kumar V, Fausto N, Abbas A. *Robbins and Cotran Pathologic Basis of Disease.* 7th ed. Philadelphia, PA: W.B. Saunders Company; 2004.

156. Douma RA, Kamphuisen PW, Büller HR. Acute pulmonary embolism. Part 1: epidemiology and diagnosis. *Nat Rev Cardiol.* 2010;7(10):585–596.

157. Anderson FA, Wheeler HB, Goldberg RJ, et al. A population-based perspective of the hospital incidence and case-fatality rates of deep vein thrombosis and pulmonary embolism. The Worcester DVT Study. *Arch Intern Med.* 1991;151(5):933–938.

158. Douketis JD, Kearon C, Bates S, et al. Risk of fatal pulmonary embolism in patients with treated venous thromboembolism. *JAMA.* 1998;279(6):458–462.

159. van Es J, Douma RA, Gerdes VE, et al. Acute pulmonary embolism. Part 2: treatment. *Nat Rev Cardiol.* 2010;7(11):613–622.

160. Wells PS, Anderson DR, Rodger M, et al. Excluding pulmonary embolism at the bedside without diagnostic imaging: management of patients with suspected pulmonary embolism presenting to the emergency department by using a simple clinical model and D-dimer. *Ann Intern Med.* 2001;135(2):98–107.

161. Agnelli G, Becattini C. Acute pulmonary embolism. *N Engl J Med.* 2010;363(3):266–274.

162. Stein PD, Hull RD, Patel KC, et al. D-Dimer for the exclusion of acute venous thrombosis and pulmonary embolism: a systematic review. *Ann Intern Med.* 2004;140(8):589–602.

163. Becattini C, Vedovati MC, Agnelli G. Prognostic value of troponins in acute pulmonary embolism: a meta-analysis. *Circulation.* 2007;116(4):427–433.

164. ten Wolde M, Tulevski II, Mulder JW, et al. Brain natriuretic peptide as a predictor of adverse outcome in patients with pulmonary embolism. *Circulation.* 2003;107(16):2082–2084.

165. Coutance G, Le Page O, Lo T, et al. Prognostic value of brain natriuretic peptide in acute pulmonary embolism. *Crit Care.* 2008;12(4):R109.

27

Renal Function

KARA L. LYNCH and ALAN H. B. WU

key terms

Acute kidney injury
Albuminuria
Aldosterone
Antidiuretic hormone (ADH)
Chronic kidney disease
Countercurrent multiplier system
Creatinine clearance
Cystatin C
Diabetes mellitus
Erythropoietin
Estimated glomerular filtration
rate (eGFR)
Glomerular filtration rate (GFR)
Glomerulonephritis
Glomerulus
Hemodialysis
Hemofiltration
Loop of Henle
β_2-Microglobulin (β2-M)
Myoglobin
Nephrotic syndrome
Prostaglandin
Renin
Rhabdomyolysis
Tubular reabsorption
Tubular secretion
Tubule
Vitamin D

chapter objectives

Upon completion of this chapter, the clinical laboratorian should be able to do the following:

- Diagram the anatomy of the nephron.
- Describe the physiologic role of each part of the nephron: glomerulus, proximal tubule, loop of Henle, distal tubule, and collecting duct.
- Describe the mechanisms by which the kidney maintains fluid and electrolyte balance in conjunction with hormones.
- Discuss the significance and calculation of glomerular filtration rate and estimated glomerular filtration rate.
- Relate the clinical significance of total urine proteins, albuminuria, myoglobin clearance, serum β2-microglobulin, and cystatin C.
- List the tests in a urinalysis and microscopy profile and understand the clinical significance of each.
- Describe diseases of the glomerulus and tubules and how laboratory tests are used in these disorders.
- Distinguish between acute kidney injury and chronic kidney disease.
- Discuss the therapy of chronic renal failure with regard to renal dialysis and transplantation.

For additional student resources, please visit thePoint
at http://thepoint.lww.com

The kidneys are vital organs that perform a variety of important functions (Table 27.1). The most prominent functions are removal of unwanted substances from plasma (both waste and surplus); homeostasis (maintenance of equilibrium) of the body's water, electrolyte, and acid–base status; and participation in hormonal regulation. In the clinical laboratory, kidney function tests are used in the assessment of renal disease, water balance, and acid–base disorders and in situations of trauma, head injury, surgery, and infectious disease. This chapter focuses on renal anatomy and physiology and the analytic procedures available to diagnose, monitor, and treat kidney dysfunction.

RENAL ANATOMY

The kidneys are paired, bean-shaped organs located retroperitoneally on either side of the spinal column. Macroscopically, a fibrous capsule of connective tissue encloses each kidney. When dissected longitudinally, two regions can be clearly discerned—an outer region called the cortex and an inner region called the medulla (Fig. 27.1). The pelvis can also be seen. It is a basin-like cavity at the upper end of the ureter into which newly formed urine passes. The bilateral ureters are thick-walled canals, connecting the kidneys to the urinary bladder.

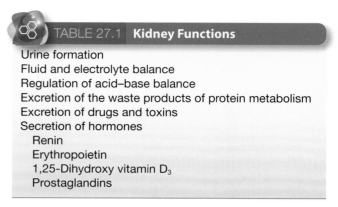

TABLE 27.1	Kidney Functions

Urine formation
Fluid and electrolyte balance
Regulation of acid–base balance
Excretion of the waste products of protein metabolism
Excretion of drugs and toxins
Secretion of hormones
  Renin
  Erythropoietin
  1,25-Dihydroxy vitamin D_3
  Prostaglandins

Urine is temporarily stored in the bladder until voided from the body by way of the urethra. The highlighted section in Figure 27.1 shows the arrangement of nephrons in the kidney, functional units of the kidney that can only be seen microscopically. Each kidney contains approximately 1 million nephrons. Each nephron is a complex apparatus composed of five basic parts, expressed diagrammatically in Figure 27.2.

- The **glomerulus**—a capillary tuft surrounded by the expanded end of a renal **tubule** known as Bowman's capsule. Each glomerulus is supplied by an afferent arteriole carrying the blood in and an efferent arteriole carrying the

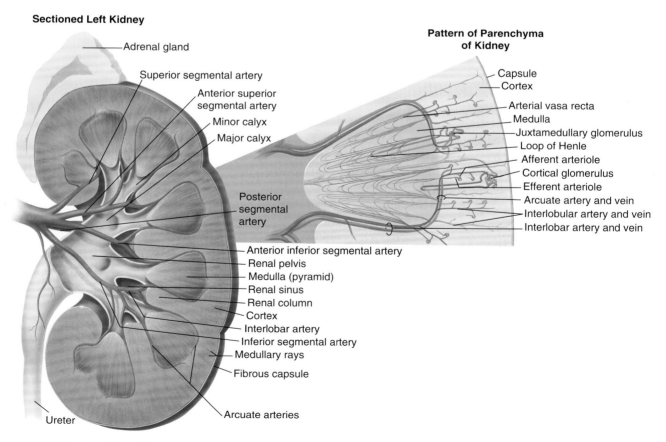

FIGURE 27.1 Anatomy of the kidney.

Distal convoluted tubule
Proximal convoluted tubule
Bowman's capsule
Glomerulus
Afferent arteriole
Efferent arteriole
Collecting tubule
Artery
Vein
Peritubular capillaries
Loop of Henle

FIGURE 27.2 Representation of a nephron and its blood supply.

blood out. The efferent arteriole branches into peritubular capillaries that supply the tubule.
- The proximal convoluted tubule—located in the cortex.
- The long loop of Henle—composed of the thin descending limb, which spans the medulla, and the ascending limb, which is located in both the medulla and the cortex, composed of a region that is thin and then thick.
- The distal convoluted tubule—located in the cortex.
- The collecting duct—formed by two or more distal convoluted tubules as they pass back down through the cortex and the medulla to collect the urine that drains from each nephron. Collecting ducts eventually merge and empty their contents into the renal pelvis.

The following section describes how each part of the nephron normally functions.

RENAL PHYSIOLOGY

There are three basic renal processes:

1. Glomerular filtration
2. Tubular reabsorption
3. Tubular secretion

Figure 27.3 illustrates how three different substances are variably processed by the nephron. Substance A is filtered and secreted, but not reabsorbed; substance B is filtered and a portion reabsorbed; and substance C is filtered and completely reabsorbed.[1] The following is a description of how specific substances are regulated in this manner to maintain homeostasis.

Glomerular Filtration

The glomerulus is the first part of the nephron and functions to filter incoming blood. Several factors facilitate filtration. One factor is the unusually high pressure in the glomerular capillaries, which is a result of their position between two arterioles. This sets up a steep pressure difference across the walls. Another factor is the semipermeable glomerular basement membrane, which has a molecular size cutoff value of approximately 66,000 Da, about the molecular size of albumin. This means that water, electrolytes, and small dissolved solutes, such as glucose, amino acids, low-molecular-weight proteins, urea, and creatinine, pass freely through the basement membrane and enter the proximal convoluted tubule. Other blood constituents, such as albumin; many plasma proteins; cellular elements; and protein-bound substances, such as lipids and bilirubin, are too large to be filtered. In addition, because the basement membrane is negatively charged, negatively charged molecules, such as proteins, are repelled. Of the 1,200 to 1,500 mL of blood that the kidneys receive each minute (approximately one-quarter of the total cardiac output), the glomerulus filters out 125 to 130 mL of an essentially protein-free, cell-free fluid, called *glomerular filtrate*. The volume of blood filtered per minute is the **glomerular filtration rate (GFR)**, and its determination is

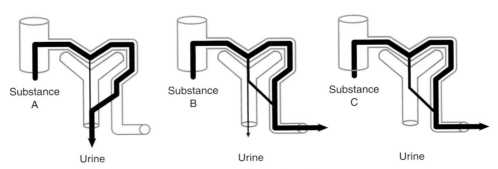

Substance A   Substance B   Substance C

Urine   Urine   Urine

FIGURE 27.3 Renal processes of filtration, reabsorption, and secretion.

essential in evaluating renal function, as discussed in the section on Analytic Procedures.

Tubular Function

Proximal Convoluted Tubule

The proximal tubule is the next part of the nephron to receive the now cell-free and essentially protein-free blood. This filtrate contains waste products, which are toxic to the body above a certain concentration, and substances that are valuable to the body. One function of the proximal tubule is to return the bulk of each valuable substance back to the blood circulation. Thus, 75% of the water, sodium, and chloride; 100% of the glucose (up to the renal threshold); almost all of the amino acids, vitamins, and proteins; and varying amounts of urea, uric acid, and ions, such as magnesium, calcium, potassium, and bicarbonate, are reabsorbed. Almost all (98% to 100%) of uric acid, a waste product, is actively reabsorbed, only to be secreted at the distal end of the proximal tubule.

When the substances move from the tubular lumen to the peritubular capillary plasma, the process is called **tubular reabsorption**. With the exception of water and chloride ions, the process is active; that is, the tubular epithelial cells use energy to bind and transport the substances across the plasma membrane to the blood. The transport processes that are involved normally have sufficient reserve for efficient reabsorption, but they are saturable. When the concentration of the filtered substance exceeds the capacity of the transport system, the substance is then excreted in the urine. The plasma concentration above which the substance appears in urine is known as the renal threshold, and its determination is useful in assessing both tubular function and nonrenal disease states. A renal threshold does not exist for water because it is always transported passively through diffusion down a concentration gradient. Chloride ions in this instance diffuse in the wake of sodium.

A second function of the proximal tubule is to secrete products of kidney tubular cell metabolism, such as hydrogen ions, and drugs, such as penicillin. The term **tubular secretion** is used in two ways: (1) tubular secretion describes the movement of substances from peritubular capillary plasma to the tubular lumen, and (2) tubular secretion also describes when tubule cells secrete products of their own cellular metabolism into the filtrate in the tubular lumen. Transport across the membrane of the cell is again either active or passive.

Loop of Henle

The osmolality in the medulla in this portion of the nephron increases steadily from the corticomedullary junction inward and facilitates the reabsorption of water, sodium, and chloride. The hyperosmolality that develops in the medulla is continuously maintained by the **loop of Henle**, a hairpin-like loop between the proximal tubule and the distal convoluted tubule. The opposing flows in the loop, the downward flow in the descending limb, and the upward flow in the ascending limb are termed a countercurrent

flow. To understand how the hyperosmolality is maintained in the medulla, it is best to look first at what happens in the ascending limb. Sodium and chloride are actively and passively reabsorbed into the medullary interstitial fluid along the entire length of the ascending limb. Because the ascending limb is relatively impermeable to water, little water follows, and the medullary interstitial fluid becomes hyperosmotic compared with the fluid in the ascending limb. The fluid in the ascending limb becomes hypotonic or dilute as sodium and chloride ions are reabsorbed without the loss of water, so the ascending limb is often called the diluting segment. The descending limb, in contrast to the ascending limb, is highly permeable to water and does not reabsorb sodium and chloride. The high osmolality of the surrounding interstitial medulla fluid is the physical force that accelerates the reabsorption of water from the filtrate in the descending limb. Interstitial hyperosmolality is maintained because the ascending limb continues to pump sodium and chloride ions into it. This interaction of water leaving the descending loop and sodium and chloride leaving the ascending loop to maintain a high osmolality within the kidney medulla produces hypo-osmolal urine as it leaves the loop. This process is called the **countercurrent multiplier system**.[2]

Distal Convoluted Tubule

The distal convoluted tubule is much shorter than the proximal tubule, with two or three coils that connect to a collecting duct. The filtrate entering this section of the nephron is close to its final composition. About 95% of the sodium and chloride ions and 90% of water have already been reabsorbed from the original glomerular filtrate. The function of the distal tubule is to effect small adjustments to achieve electrolyte and acid–base homeostasis. These adjustments occur under the hormonal control of both **antidiuretic hormone (ADH)** and **aldosterone**. Figure 27.4 describes the action of these hormones.

Antidiuretic Hormone

ADH is a peptide hormone secreted by the posterior pituitary, mainly in response to increased blood osmolality; ADH is also released when blood volume decreases by more than 5% to 10%. Large decreases of blood volume will stimulate ADH secretion even when plasma osmolality is decreased. ADH stimulates water reabsorption. The walls of the distal collecting tubules are normally impermeable to water (like the ascending loop of Henle), but they become permeable to water in ADH. Water diffuses passively from the lumen of the tubules, resulting in more concentrated urine and decreased plasma osmolality.

Aldosterone

This hormone is produced by the adrenal cortex under the influence of the **renin**–angiotensin mechanism. Its secretion is triggered by decreased blood flow or blood pressure in the afferent renal arteriole and by decreased plasma sodium. Aldosterone stimulates sodium reabsorption in the distal tubules and potassium and hydrogen ion

FIGURE 27.4 Antidiuretic hormone (ADH) and aldosterone control of the renal reabsorption of water and Na⁺. (Reprinted with permission from Kaplan A, et al. The kidney and tests of renal function. In: Kaplan A, Jack R, Orpheum KE, et al., eds. *Clinical Chemistry: Interpretation and Techniques.* 4th ed. Baltimore, MD: Williams & Wilkins; 1995:158, Figure 6.2.).

secretion. Hydrogen ion secretion is linked to bicarbonate regeneration and ammonia secretion, which also occur here. In addition to these ions, small amounts of chloride ions are reabsorbed.

Collecting Duct

The collecting ducts are the final site for either concentrating or diluting urine. The hormones ADH and aldosterone act on this segment of the nephron to control reabsorption of water and sodium. Chloride and urea are also reabsorbed here. Urea plays an important role in maintaining the hyperosmolality of the renal medulla. Because the collecting ducts in the medulla are highly permeable to urea, urea diffuses down its concentration gradient out of the tubule and into the medulla interstitium, increasing its osmolality.[3]

Elimination of Nonprotein Nitrogen Compounds

Nonprotein nitrogen compounds (NPNs) are waste products formed in the body as a result of the degradative metabolism of nucleic acids, amino acids, and proteins. Excretion of these compounds is an important function of the kidneys. The three principal compounds are urea, creatinine, and uric acid.[4,5] For a more detailed treatment of their biochemistry and disease correlations, see Chapter 12.

Urea

Urea makes up the majority (more than 75%) of the NPN waste excreted daily as a result of the oxidative catabolism of protein. Urea synthesis occurs in the liver. Proteins are broken down into amino acids, which are then deaminated

to form ammonia. Ammonia is readily converted to urea, avoiding toxicity. The kidney is the only significant route of excretion for urea. It has a molecular weight of 60 Da and, therefore, is readily filtered by the glomerulus. In the collecting ducts, 40% to 60% of urea is reabsorbed. The reabsorbed urea contributes to the high osmolality in the medulla, which is one of the processes of urinary concentration mentioned earlier (see loop of Henle).

Creatinine

Muscle contains creatine phosphate, a high-energy compound for the rapid formation of adenosine triphosphate (ATP). This reaction is catalyzed by creatine kinase (CK) and is the first source of metabolic fuel used in muscle contraction. Every day, up to 20% of total muscle creatine (and its phosphate) spontaneously dehydrates and cycles to form the waste product creatinine. Therefore, creatinine levels are a function of muscle mass and remain approximately the same in an individual from day to day unless muscle mass or renal function changes. Creatinine has a molecular weight of 113 Da and is, therefore, readily filtered by the glomerulus. Unlike urea, creatinine is not reabsorbed by the tubules. However, a small amount of creatinine is secreted by the kidney tubules at high serum concentrations.

Uric Acid

Uric acid is the primary waste product of purine metabolism. The purines, adenine and guanine, are precursors of nucleic acids ATP and guanosine triphosphate, respectively. Uric acid has a molecular weight of 168 Da. Like creatinine, it is readily filtered by the glomerulus, but it then undergoes a complex cycle of reabsorption and secretion as it courses through the nephron. Only 6% to 12% of the original filtered uric acid is finally excreted. Uric acid exists in its ionized and more soluble form, usually sodium urate, at urinary pH > 5.75 (the first pK_a of uric acid). At pH < 5.75, it is undissociated. This fact has clinical significance in the development of urolithiasis (formation of calculi) and gout.

Water, Electrolyte, and Acid–Base Homeostasis

Water Balance

The kidney's contribution to water balance in the body is through water loss or water conservation, which is regulated by the hormone ADH. ADH responds primarily to changes in osmolality and intravascular volume. Increased plasma osmolality or decreased intravascular volume stimulates secretion of ADH from the posterior pituitary. ADH then increases the permeability of the distal convoluted tubules and collecting ducts to water, resulting in increased water reabsorption and excretion of more concentrated urine. In contrast, the major system regulating water intake is thirst, which appears to be triggered by the same stimuli that trigger ADH secretion.

In states of dehydration, the renal tubules reabsorb water at their maximal rate, resulting in production of a small amount of maximally concentrated urine (high urine osmolality, 1,200 mOsm/L).[6] In states of water excess, the tubules reabsorb water at only a minimal rate, resulting in excretion of a large volume of extremely dilute urine (low urine osmolality, down to 50 mOsm/L).[7,8] The continuous fine-tuning possible between these two extreme states results in the precise control of fluid balance in the body (Fig. 27.5).

Electrolyte Balance

The following is a brief overview of the notable ions involved in maintenance of electrolyte balance within the body. For a more comprehensive treatment of this subject, refer Chapter 16.

Sodium

Sodium is the primary extracellular cation in the human body and is excreted principally through the kidneys. Sodium balance in the body is controlled only through excretion. The renin–angiotensin–aldosterone hormonal system is the major mechanism for the control of sodium balance.

Potassium

Potassium is the main intracellular cation in the body. The precise regulation of its concentration is of extreme importance to cellular metabolism and is controlled chiefly by renal means. Like sodium, it is freely filtered by the glomerulus and then actively reabsorbed throughout the entire nephron (except for the descending limb of the loop of Henle). Both the distal convoluted tubule and the collecting ducts can reabsorb and excrete potassium, and this excretion is controlled by aldosterone. Potassium ions can compete with hydrogen ions in their exchange with sodium (in the proximal convoluted tubule); this process

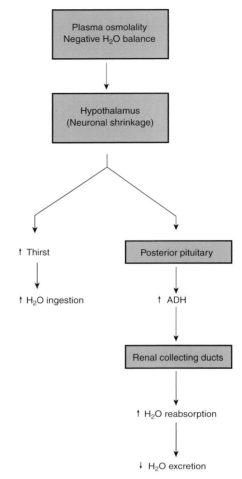

FIGURE 27.5 Antidiuretic hormone (ADH) control of thirst mechanism.

is used by the body to conserve hydrogen ions and, thereby, compensate in states of metabolic alkalosis.

Chloride

Chloride is the principal extracellular anion and is involved in the maintenance of extracellular fluid balance. It is readily filtered by the glomerulus and is passively reabsorbed as a counterion when sodium is reabsorbed in the proximal convoluted tubule. In the ascending limb of the loop of Henle, potassium is actively reabsorbed by a distinct chloride "pump," which also reabsorbs sodium. This pump can be inhibited by loop diuretics, such as furosemide. As expected, the regulation of chloride is controlled by the same forces that regulate sodium.[6,8]

Phosphate, Calcium, and Magnesium

The phosphate ion occurs in higher concentrations in the intracellular than in the extracellular fluid environments. It exists as either a protein-bound or a non–protein-bound form; homeostatic balance is chiefly determined by proximal tubular reabsorption under the control of parathyroid hormone (PTH). Calcium, the second most predominant intracellular cation, is the most important inorganic messenger in the cell. It also exists in protein-bound and non–protein-bound states. Calcium in the non–protein-bound form is either ionized and physiologically active or nonionized and complexed to small, diffusible ions, such as phosphate and bicarbonate. The ionized form is freely filtered by the glomerulus and reabsorbed in the tubules under the control of PTH. However, renal control of calcium concentration is not the major means of regulation. PTH- and calcitonin-controlled regulation of calcium absorption from the gut and bone stores is more important than renal secretion or reabsorption. Magnesium, a major intracellular cation, is important as an enzymatic cofactor. Like phosphate and calcium, it exists in both protein-bound and ionized states. The ionized fraction is easily filtered by the glomerulus and reabsorbed in the tubules under the influence of PTH. See Chapter 24 for more detailed information.

Acid–Base Balance

Many nonvolatile acidic waste products are formed by normal body metabolism each day. Carbonic acid, lactic acid, ketoacids, and others must be continually transported in the plasma and excreted from the body, causing only minor alterations in physiologic pH. The renal system constitutes one of three means by which constant control of overall body pH is accomplished. The other two strategies involved in this regulation are the respiratory system and the acid–base buffering system.[9]

The kidneys manage their share of the responsibility for controlling body pH by dual means: conserving bicarbonate ions and removing metabolic acids. For a more in-depth examination of these processes, refer Chapter 17.

Regeneration of Bicarbonate Ions

In a complicated process, bicarbonate ions are first filtered out of the plasma by the glomerulus. In the lumen of the renal tubules, this bicarbonate combines with hydrogen ions to form carbonic acid, which subsequently degrades to carbon dioxide (CO_2) and water. This CO_2 then diffuses into the brush border of the proximal tubular cells, where it is reconverted by carbonic anhydrase to carbonic acid and then degrades back to hydrogen ions and regenerated bicarbonate ions. This regenerated bicarbonate is transported into the blood to replace what was depleted by metabolism; the accompanying hydrogen ions are secreted back into the tubular lumen, and from there, they enter the urine. Filtered bicarbonate is "reabsorbed" into the circulation, helping to return blood pH to its optimal level and effectively functioning as another buffering system.

Excretion of Metabolic Acids

Hydrogen ions are manufactured in the renal tubules as part of the regeneration mechanism for bicarbonate. These hydrogen ions, as well as others that are dissociated from nonvolatile organic acids, are disposed of by several different reactions with buffer bases.

Reaction with Ammonia (NH$_3$)

The glomerulus does not filter NH_3. However, this substance is formed in the renal tubules when the amino acid glutamine is deaminated by glutaminase. This NH_3 then reacts with secreted hydrogen ions to form ammonium ions (NH_4^+), which are unable to readily diffuse out of the tubular lumen and, therefore, are excreted into the urine. This mode of acid excretion is the primary means by which the kidneys compensate for states of metabolic acidosis.

Reaction with Monohydrogen Phosphate (HPO$_4^{2-}$)

Phosphate ions filtered by the glomerulus can exist in the tubular fluid as disodium hydrogen phosphate (Na_2HPO_4) (dibasic). This compound can react with hydrogen ions to yield dihydrogen phosphate (monobasic), which is then excreted. The released sodium then combines with bicarbonate to yield sodium bicarbonate and is reabsorbed. These mechanisms can excrete increasing amounts of metabolic acid until a maximum urine pH of approximately 4.4 is reached. After this, renal compensation is unable to adjust to any further decreases in blood pH, and metabolic acidosis ensues. Few free hydrogen ions are excreted directly in the urine.

Endocrine Function

In addition to numerous excretory and regulatory functions, the kidney has endocrine functions as well. It is both a primary endocrine site, as the producer of its own hormones, and a secondary site, as the target locus for hormones manufactured by other endocrine organs. The kidneys synthesize renin, **erythropoietin**, 1,25-dihydroxy vitamin D$_3$, and the **prostaglandins**.

Renin

Renin is the initial component of the renin–angiotensin–aldosterone system. Renin is produced by the juxtaglomerular cells of the renal medulla when extracellular fluid volume or blood pressure decreases. It catalyzes the synthesis of angiotensin by cleavage of the circulating plasma precursor angiotensinogen. Angiotensin is converted to angiotensin II by angiotensin-converting enzyme. Angiotensin II is a powerful vasoconstrictor that increases blood pressure and stimulates release of aldosterone from the adrenal cortex. Aldosterone, in turn, promotes sodium reabsorption and water conservation.[7,8] For a more detailed look at the complexities of this feedback loop, see Chapter 21.

Erythropoietin

Erythropoietin is a single-chain polypeptide produced by cells close to the proximal tubules, and its production is regulated by blood oxygen levels. Hypoxia produces increased serum concentrations within 2 hours. Erythropoietin acts on the erythroid progenitor cells in the bone marrow, increasing the number of red blood cells (RBCs). In chronic renal insufficiency, erythropoietin production is significantly reduced. The routine administration of recombinant human erythropoietin is common in chronic renal failure patients. Before this therapy was available, anemia was a clinical reality in these patients.[4,7] Erythropoietin concentrations in blood can be measured by immunoassays. Recombinant human erythropoietin has also been used in sports doping to stimulate erythrocyte production and increase the oxygen-carrying capacity in the blood of endurance athletes. Assays capable of detecting posttranslational modifications on erythropoietin have been produced and are capable of distinguishing exogenous from endogenous erythropoietin.

1,25-Dihydroxy Vitamin D₃

The kidneys are the sites of formation of the active form of **vitamin D**, $1,25\text{-}(OH)_2$ vitamin D_3. This form of vitamin D is one of three major hormones that determine phosphate and calcium balance and bone calcification in the human body. Chronic renal insufficiency is, therefore, often associated with osteomalacia (inadequate bone calcification, the adult form of rickets), owing to the continual distortion of normal vitamin D metabolism.

Prostaglandins

The prostaglandins are a group of potent cyclic fatty acids formed from essential (dietary) fatty acids, primarily arachidonic acid. They are formed in almost all tissue and their actions are diverse. The prostaglandins produced by the kidneys increase renal blood flow, sodium and water excretion, and renin release. They act to oppose renal vasoconstriction due to angiotensin and norepinephrine.

ANALYTIC PROCEDURES

All laboratory methods used for the evaluation of renal function rely on the measurement of waste products in blood, usually urea and creatinine, which accumulate when the kidneys begin to fail. Renal failure must be advanced, with only about 20% to 30% of the nephrons still functioning, before the concentration of either substance begins to increase in the blood. The rate at which creatinine and urea are removed or cleared from the blood into the urine is termed clearance. Clearance is defined as that volume of plasma from which a measured amount of substance can be completely eliminated into the urine per unit of time expressed in milliliters per minute.[5] Calculation of creatinine clearance has become the standard laboratory method for determining the GFR. Urea clearance was one of the first clearance tests performed; however, it is no longer widely used since it does not accurately provide a full clearance assessment. Older tests used administration of insulin, sodium [^{125}I] iothalamate, or p-aminohippurate to assess glomerular filtration or tubular secretion. These tests are difficult to administer and are no longer common.

Creatinine Clearance

Creatinine is a nearly ideal substance for the measurement of clearance. It is an endogenous metabolic product synthesized at a constant rate for a given individual and cleared essentially only by glomerular filtration. It is not reabsorbed and is only slightly secreted by the proximal tubule. Serum creatinine levels are higher in males than in females due to the direct correlation with muscle mass. Analysis of creatinine is simple and inexpensive using colorimetric assays; however, different methods for assaying plasma creatinine, such as kinetic or enzymatic assays, have varying degrees of accuracy and imprecision (see Chapter 12).

Creatinine clearance is derived by mathematically relating the serum creatinine concentration to the urine creatinine concentration excreted during a period of time, usually 24 hours. Specimen collection, therefore, must include both a 24-hour urine specimen and a serum creatinine value, ideally collected at the midpoint of the 24-hour urine collection. The urine container must be kept refrigerated throughout the duration of both the collection procedure and the subsequent storage period until laboratory analysis can be performed. The concentration of creatinine in both serum and urine is measured by the applicable methods discussed in Chapter 12. The total volume of urine is carefully measured, and the creatinine clearance is calculated using the following formula:

$$\frac{U_{Cr}\,(mg/dL) \times V_{Ur}\,(mL/24\ hours)}{P_{Cr}\,(mg/dL) \times 1,440\ minutes/24\ hours} \times \frac{1.73}{A}$$

(Eq. 27-1)

where Cr is creatinine clearance, U_{Cr} is urine creatinine clearance, V_{Ur} is urine volume excreted in 24 hours, P_{Cr} is serum creatinine concentration, and $1.73/A$ is normalization factor for body surface area (1.73 is the generally accepted average body surface in square meters, and A is the actual body surface area of the individual determined from height and weight). If the patient's body surface area varies greatly from the average (e.g., obese or pediatric patients), this correction for body mass must be included in the formula. The reference range for creatinine clearance is lower in females compared with males and normally decreases with age.

Estimated GFR

The National Kidney Foundation recommends that estimated GFR (eGFR) be calculated each time a serum creatinine level is reported. (Additional information is available at the National Kidney Foundation Web site at http://www.kidney.org/.) The equation is used to predict GFR and is based on serum creatinine, age, body size, gender, and race, without the need of a urine creatinine. Because the calculation does not require a timed urine collection, it should be used more often than the traditional creatinine clearance and result in earlier detection of **chronic kidney disease** (CKD). There are a number of formulas that can be used to estimate GFR on the basis of serum creatinine levels.

Cockcroft-Gault Formula

The Cockcroft-Gault formula is one of the first formulas used to estimate GFR. This formula predicts creatinine clearance, and the results are not corrected for body surface area. This equation assumes that women will have a 15% lower **creatinine** clearance than men at the same level of serum creatinine.

$$GFR\,(mL/min) = \frac{(140 - Age) \times Weight\,(kg)}{72 \times S_{Cr}\,(mg/dL)}$$
$$\times (0.85\ if\ female)$$

(Eq. 27-2)

Modification of Diet in Renal Disease Formula

The modification of diet in renal disease (MDRD) formula was developed in the Modification of Diet in Renal Disease Study of chronic renal insufficiency. The study showed that the MDRD formula provided a more accurate assessment of GFR than the Cockcroft-Gault formula. The MDRD formula was validated in a large population that included European Americans and African Americans. It does not require patient weight and is corrected for body surface area. The MDRD formula is known to underestimate the GFR in healthy patients with GFRs over 60 mL/min and to overestimate GFR in underweight patients. The four-variable MDRD equation includes age, race, gender, and serum creatinine as variables.

$$GFR\left(mL/min/1.73m^2\right) = 186 \times S_{Cr}\left(mg/dL\right)^{-1.154}$$
$$\times Age^{-0.203} \times \left(1.212 \text{ if Black}\right)$$
$$\times \left(0.742 \text{ if female}\right) \quad \text{(Eq. 27-3)}$$

CKD-EPI Formula

The CKD-EPI (Chronic Kidney Disease Epidemiology Collaboration) formula was published in 2009.[10] It was developed in an effort to create a formula more accurate than the MDRD formula. Multiple studies have shown the CKD-EPI formula to perform better and with less bias than the MDRD formula, especially in patients with higher GFR. Many laboratories still use the MDRD formula; however, some have converted to the CKD-EPI formula.

$$eGFR\left(mL/min/1.73\,m^2\right) = 141 \times \min\left(S_{Cr}/k,l\right)^a$$
$$\times \max\left(S_{Cr}/k,l\right)^{-1.209} \times 0.993^{Age}$$
$$\times \left(1.018 \text{ if female}\right)$$
$$\times \left(1.159 \text{ if Black}\right) \quad \text{(Eq. 27-4)}$$

k is 0.7 for females and 0.9 for males, a is −0.329 for females and −0.411 for males, min indicates the minimum of S_{Cr}/k or 1, and max indicates the maximum of S_{Cr}/k or 1.

Cystatin C

Cystatin C is a low-molecular-weight protein produced at a steady rate by most body tissues. It is freely filtered by the glomerulus, reabsorbed, and catabolized by the proximal tubule. Levels of cystatin C rise more quickly than creatinine levels in acute kidney injury (AKI). Plasma concentrations appear to be unaffected by diet, gender, race, age, and muscle mass. Studies have shown measurement of cystatin C to be at least as useful as serum creatinine and creatinine clearance in detecting early changes in kidney function. A rise in cystatin C is often detectable before there is a measureable decrease in the GFR or increase in creatinine. Cystatin C can be measured by immunoassay methods.[11] Some findings suggest that an equation that uses both serum creatinine and cystatin C with age, sex, and race would be better than equations that use only one of these serum markers.[12,13]

Biologic Variation

When the same test is performed on various individuals, we find that the mean of each person's results is not the same, showing that individual homeostatic setting points often vary. Biologic variation is defined as the random fluctuation around a homeostatic setting point.[14] This includes the fluctuation around the homeostatic setting point for a single individual, termed within-subject biologic variation, and differences between the homeostatic setting points of multiple individuals, termed between-subject biologic variation. In the case of creatinine, levels for an individual differ slightly over time, and the mean values of all individuals vary significantly from each other. Therefore, each individual's results span only a small portion of the population-based reference interval. This means that for creatinine, within-subject biologic variation is less than between-subject biologic variation. When this is true of a given analyte, the analyte is said to have marked individuality. Interestingly, the between-subject biologic variation is much smaller for cystatin C compared with creatinine, showing that population-based reference values are more useful for cystatin C compared with creatinine. However, the within-subject variation is greater for cystatin C compared with creatinine. As a result, creatinine is more helpful in monitoring renal function over time for a given individual, whereas cystatin C is potentially more useful for detecting minor renal impairment.

β₂-Microglobulin

β₂-Microglobulin (β2-M) is a small, nonglycosylated peptide (molecular weight, 11,800 Da) found on the surface of most nucleated cells. The plasma membrane sheds β2-M at a constant rate, as a relatively intact molecule. β2-M is easily filtered by the glomerulus, and 99.9% is reabsorbed by the proximal tubules and catabolized. Elevated levels in serum indicate increased cellular turnover as seen in myeloproliferative and lymphoproliferative disorders, inflammation, and renal failure. Both blood and urine β2-M tests may be ordered to evaluate kidney damage and to distinguish between disorders that affect the glomeruli and the renal tubules. Measurement of serum β2-M is used clinically to assess renal tubular function in renal transplant patients, with elevated levels indicating organ rejection.

Myoglobin

Myoglobin is a low-molecular-weight protein (16,900 Da) associated with acute skeletal and cardiac muscle injury. Myoglobin functions to bind and transport oxygen from the plasma membrane to the mitochondria in muscle cells. Blood levels of myoglobin can rise very quickly with severe muscle injury. In **rhabdomyolysis**, myoglobin release from skeletal muscle is sufficient to overload the proximal tubules and cause acute renal failure. Early diagnosis and aggressive treatment of elevated myoglobin may prevent or lessen the severity of renal failure. Serum and urine myoglobin can be measured easily and rapidly by immunoassays.

Albuminuria

The term **albuminuria**, previously referred to as microalbuminuria, describes the presence of albumin in the urine. Urine albumin measurement is important in the management of patients with **diabetes mellitus**, who are at serious risk for developing nephropathy over their lifetime. In the early stages of nephropathy, there is renal hypertrophy, hyperfunction, and increased thickness of the glomerular and tubular basement membranes. In this early stage, there are no overt signs of renal dysfunction. In the next 7 to 10 years, there is progression to glomerulosclerosis, with increased glomerular capillary permeability. This permeability allows small (micro) amounts of albumin to pass into the urine. If detected in this early phase, rigid glucose control, along with treatment to prevent hypertension, can be instituted and progression to kidney failure prevented. Quantitative albumin-specific immunoassays, usually using nephelometry or immunoturbidimetry, are widely used. For a 24-hour urine collection, 30 to 300 mg of albumin is diagnostic of albuminuria. A 24-hour urine collection is preferred, but a random urine sample in which the ratio of albumin to creatinine is measured, is common. An albumin to creatinine ratio (ACR) of greater than 30 mg/g is diagnostic of albuminuria.

Neutrophil Gelatinase–Associated Lipocalin

Neutrophil gelatinase–associated lipocalin (NGAL) is a 25-kDa protein expressed by neutrophils and epithelial cells including those of the proximal tubule. The gene encoding NGAL is upregulated in the presence of renal ischemia, tubule injury, and nephrotoxicity.[15] It can be measured in plasma and urine and is elevated within 2 to 6 hours of AKI. NGAL has been shown to be a useful early predictor of AKI and has prognostic value for clinical endpoints, such as initiation of dialysis and mortality. However, urinary NGAL excretion may also arise from systemic stress in the absence of AKI, limiting its specificity.

NephroCheck

NephroCheck is the first FDA-cleared test used to determine if critically ill patients are at risk for developing moderate to severe AKI in the 12 hours following administration of the test. NephroCheck quantifies concentrations of tissue inhibitor of metalloproteinase 2 (TIMP-2) and insulin-like growth factor binding protein 7 (IGFBP-7) in urine specimens and multiplies the results to generate a quantitative AKI risk index (AKIRisk Score). The two biomarkers invoke cell cycle arrest in response to tissue insults that cause AKI.[16] Elevation of these two biomarkers is thought to signal the kidney's attempt to protect itself from harmful insults and signal the increased risk for imminent AKI. The biomarker concentrations have been shown to correspond to severity across all stages of AKI.

Urinalysis

Urinalysis (UA) permits a detailed, in-depth assessment of renal status with an easily obtained specimen. UA also serves as a quick indicator of an individual's glucose status and hepatic–biliary function. Routine UA includes assessment of physical characteristics, chemical analyses, and a microscopic examination of the sediment from a (random) urine specimen.

Specimen Collection

The importance of a properly collected and stored specimen for UA cannot be overemphasized. Initial morning specimens are preferred, particularly for protein analyses, because they are more concentrated from overnight retention in the bladder. The specimen should be obtained by a clean midstream catch or catheterization. The urine should be freshly collected into a clean, dry container with a tight-fitting cover. It must be analyzed within 1 hour of collection if held at room temperature or else refrigerated at 2°C to 8°C for not more than 8 hours before analysis. If not assayed within these time limits, several changes will occur. Bacterial multiplication will cause false-positive nitrite tests, and urease-producing organisms will degrade urea to ammonia and alkalinize the pH. Loss of CO_2 by diffusion into the air adds to this pH elevation, which, in turn, causes cast degeneration and red cell lysis.

Physical Characteristics

Visual Appearance

Color intensity of urine correlates with concentration: the darker the color, the more concentrated is the specimen. The various colors observed in urine are a result of different excreted pigments. Yellow and amber are generally due to urochromes (derivatives of urobilin, the end product of bilirubin degradation), whereas a yellowish-brown to green color is a result of bile pigment oxidation. Red and brown after standing are due to porphyrins, whereas reddish-brown in fresh specimens comes from hemoglobin or red cells. Brownish-black after standing is seen in alkaptonuria (a result of excreted homogentisic acid) and in malignant melanoma (in which the precursor melanogen oxidizes in the air to melanin). Drugs and some foods, such as beets, may also alter urine color.

Odor

Odor ordinarily has little diagnostic significance. The characteristic pungent odor of fresh urine is due to volatile aromatic acids, in contrast to the typical ammonia odor of urine that has been allowed to stand. Urinary tract infections impart a noxious, fecal smell to urine, whereas the urine of diabetics often smells fruity as a result of ketones. Certain inborn errors of metabolism, such as maple sugar urine disease, are associated with characteristic urine odors.

Turbidity

The cloudiness of a urine specimen depends on pH and dissolved solids composition. Turbidity generally may be due to gross bacteriuria, whereas a smoky appearance is seen in hematuria. Threadlike cloudiness is observed when the specimen is full of mucus. In alkaline urine, suspended precipitates of amorphous phosphates and carbonates may be responsible for turbidity, whereas in acidic urine, amorphous urates may be the cause.[17]

Volume

The volume of urine excreted indicates the balance between fluid ingestion and water lost from the lungs, sweat, and intestine. Most adults produce from 750 to 2,000 mL every 24 hours, averaging about 1.5 L per person. Polyuria is observed in diabetes mellitus and insipidus (in insipidus, as a result of lack of ADH), as well as in chronic renal disease, acromegaly (overproduction of the growth hormone somatostatin), and myxedema (hypothyroid edema). Anuria or oliguria (<200 mL/d) is found in nephritis, urinary tract obstruction, AKI, and kidney failure.

Specific Gravity

The specific gravity (SG) of urine is the weight of 1 mL of urine in grams divided by the weight of 1 mL of water. SG gives an indication of the density of a fluid that depends on the concentration of dissolved total solids. SG varies with the solute load to be excreted (consisting primarily of NaCl and urea), as well as with the urine volume. It is used to assess the state of hydration/dehydration of an individual or as an indicator of the concentrating ability of the kidneys.

The most commonly encountered analytic method consists of a refractometer, or total solids meter. This operates on the principle that the refractive index of a urine specimen will vary directly with the total amount of dissolved solids in the sample. This instrument measures the refractive index of the urine as compared with water on a scale that is calibrated directly into the ocular and viewed while held up to a light source. Correct calibration is vital for accuracy. Most recently, an indirect colorimetric reagent strip method for assaying SG has been added to most dipstick screens. Unlike the refractometer, dipsticks measure only ionic solutes and do not take into account glucose or protein.

The normal range for urinary SG is 1.003 to 1.035 g/mL. SG can vary in pathologic states. Low SG can occur in diabetes insipidus, pyelonephritis, and **glomerulonephritis**, in which the renal concentrating ability has become dysfunctional. High SG can be seen in diabetes mellitus, congestive heart failure, dehydration, adrenal insufficiency, liver disease, and nephrosis. SG will increase about 0.004 units for every 1% change in glucose concentration and about 0.003 units for every 1% change in protein. Fixed SG (isosthenuria) around 1.010 is observed in severe renal damage, in which the kidney excretes urine that is iso-osmotic with the plasma. This generally occurs after an initial period of anuria because the damaged tubules are unable to concentrate or dilute the glomerular filtrate.[16]

pH

Determinations of urinary pH must be performed on fresh specimens because of the significant tendency of urine to alkalinize on standing. Normal urine pH falls within the range of 4.7 to 7.8. Acidity in urine (pH < 7.0) is primarily caused by phosphates, which are excreted as salts conjugated to Na^+, K^+, Ca^{2+}, and NH_4^+. Acidity also reflects the excretion of the nonvolatile metabolic acids pyruvate, lactate, and citrate. Owing to the Na^+/H^+ exchange pump mechanism of the renal tubules, pH (H^+ concentration) increases as sodium is retained. Pathologic states, in which increased acidity is observed, include systemic acidosis, as seen in diabetes mellitus, and renal tubular acidosis (RTA). In RTA, the tubules are unable to excrete excess H^+ even though the body is in metabolic acidosis, and urinary pH remains around 6.

Alkaline urine (pH > 7.0) is observed postprandially as a normal reaction to the acidity of gastric HCl dumped into the duodenum and then into the circulation or following ingestion of alkaline food or medications. Urinary tract infections and bacterial contamination also will alkalinize pH. Medications such as potassium citrate and sodium bicarbonate will reduce urine pH. Alkaline urine is also found in Fanconi syndrome, a congenital generalized aminoaciduria resulting from defective proximal tubular function.

Chemical Analyses

Routine urine chemical analysis is rapid and easily performed with commercially available reagent strips or dipsticks. These strips are plastic coated with different reagent bands directed toward different analytes. When dipped into urine, a color change signals a deviation from normality. Colors on the dipstick bands are matched against a color chart provided with the reagents. Automated and semiautomated instruments that detect by reflectance photometry provide an alternative to the color chart and offer better precision and standardization. Abnormal results are followed up by specific quantitative or confirmatory urine assays. The analytes routinely tested are glucose, protein, ketones, nitrite, leukocyte esterase, bilirubin/urobilinogen, and hemoglobin/blood.

Glucose and Ketones

These constituents are normally absent in urine. The clinical significance of these analytes and their testing methods are discussed in Chapter 14.

Protein

Reagent strips for UA are used as a general qualitative screen for proteinuria. They are primarily specific for albumin, but they may give false-positive results in specimens that are alkaline and highly buffered. Positive dipstick results should be confirmed by more specific chemical assays, as described in Chapter 11, or more commonly by microscopic evaluation to detect casts.

Nitrite

This assay semiquantitates the amount of urinary reduction of nitrate (on the reagent strip pad) to nitrite by the enzymes of gram-negative bacteria. A negative result does not mean that no bacteriuria is present. A gram-positive pathogen, such as *Staphylococcus*, *Enterococcus*, or *Streptococcus*, may not produce nitrate-reducing enzymes; alternatively, a spot urine sample may not have been retained in the bladder long enough to pick up a sufficient number of organisms to register on the reagent strip.[16]

Leukocyte Esterase

White blood cells (WBCs), especially phagocytes, contain esterases. A positive dipstick for esterases indicates possible WBCs in urine.

Bilirubin/Urobilinogen

Hemoglobin degradation ultimately results in the formation of the waste product bilirubin, which is then converted to urobilinogen in the gut through bacterial action. Although most of this urobilinogen is excreted as urobilin in the feces, some is excreted in urine as a colorless waste product. This amount is normally too small to be detected as a positive dipstick reaction. In conditions of prehepatic, hepatic, and posthepatic jaundice, however, urine dipstick tests for urobilinogen and bilirubin may be positive or negative, depending on the nature of the patient's jaundice. A more in-depth view of bilirubin metabolism and assay methods is given in Chapter 25. Reagent strip tests for bilirubin involve diazotization and formation of a color change. Dipstick methods for urobilinogen differ, but most rely on a modification of the Ehrlich reaction with *p*-dimethylaminobenzaldehyde.[16]

Hemoglobin/Blood

Intact or lysed RBCs produce a positive dipstick result. The dipstick will be positive in cases of renal trauma/injury, infection, and obstruction that result from calculi or neoplasms.

Sediment Examination

Centrifuged, decanted urine aliquot leaves behind a sediment of formed elements that is used for microscopic examination.

Cells

For cellular elements, evaluation is best accomplished by counting and then taking the average of at least 10 microscopic fields.

Red Blood Cells

Erythrocytes greater in number than 0 to 2/high-power field (HPF) are considered abnormal. Such hematuria may result simply from severe exercise or menstrual blood contamination. However, it may also be indicative of trauma, particularly vascular injury, renal/urinary calculi obstruction, pyelonephritis, or cystitis. Hematuria in conjunction with leukocytes is diagnostic of infection.

White Blood Cells

Leukocytes greater in number than 0 to 1/HPF are considered abnormal. These cells are usually polymorphonuclear phagocytes, commonly known as segmented neutrophils. They are observed when there is acute glomerulonephritis, urinary tract infection, or inflammation of any type. In hypotonic urine (low osmotic concentration), WBCs can become enlarged, exhibiting a sparkling effect in their cytoplasmic granules. These cells possess a noticeable Brownian motion and are called glitter cells, but they have no pathologic significance.

Epithelial Cells

Several types of epithelial cells are frequently encountered in normal urine because they are continuously sloughed off the lining of the nephrons and urinary tract. Large, flat, squamous vaginal epithelia are often seen in urine specimens from female patients, and samples heavily contaminated with vaginal discharge may show clumps or sheets of these cells. Renal epithelial cells are round, uninucleated cells and, if present in numbers greater than 2/HPF, indicate clinically significant active tubular injury or degeneration. Transitional bladder epithelial cells (urothelial cells) may be flat, cuboidal, or columnar and also can be observed in urine on occasion. Large numbers will be seen only in cases of urinary catheterization, bladder inflammation, or neoplasm.

Miscellaneous Elements

Spermatozoa are often seen in the urine of both males and females. They are usually not reported because they are of no pathologic significance. In males, however, their presence may indicate prostate abnormalities. Yeast cells are also frequently found in urine specimens. Because they are extremely refractile and of a similar size to RBCs, they can easily be mistaken under low magnification. Higher power examination for budding or mycelial forms differentiates these fungal elements from erythrocytes. Parasites found in urine are generally contaminants from fecal or vaginal material. In fecal contaminant category, the most commonly encountered organism is *Enterobius vermicularis* (pinworm) infestation in children. In the vaginal contaminant category, the most common is the intensely motile flagellate, *Trichomonas vaginalis*. A true urinary parasite, sometimes seen in patients from endemic areas of the world, is the ova of the trematode *Schistosoma haematobium*. This condition will usually occur in conjunction with a significant hematuria.[16]

Bacteria

Normal urine is sterile and contains no bacteria. Small numbers of organisms seen in a fresh urine specimen usually represent skin or air contamination. In fresh specimens, however, large numbers of organisms, or small numbers accompanied by WBCs and the symptoms of urinary tract infection, are highly diagnostic for true infection. Clinically significant bacteriuria is considered to be more than 20 organisms/HPF or, alternatively, 10^5 or greater registered on a microbiologic colony count. Most pathogens seen in urine are gram-negative coliforms (microscopic "rods") such as *Escherichia coli* and *Proteus* spp. Asymptomatic bacteriuria, in which there are significant numbers of bacteria without appreciable clinical symptoms, occurs somewhat commonly in young girls, pregnant women, and patients with diabetes. This condition must be taken seriously because, if left untreated, it may result in pyelonephritis and, subsequently, permanent renal damage.

Casts

Casts are precipitated, cylindrical impressions of the nephrons. They comprise Tamm-Horsfall mucoprotein (uromucoid) from the tubular epithelia in the ascending limb of the loop of Henle. Casts form whenever there is sufficient renal stasis, increased urine salt or protein concentration, and decreased urine pH. In patients with severe renal disease, truly accurate classification of casts may require use of "cytospin" centrifugation and Papanicolaou staining for adequate differentiation. Unlike cells, casts should be examined under low power and are most often located around the edges of the coverslip.

Hyaline

The matrix of these casts is clear and gelatinous, without embedded cellular or particulate matter. They may be difficult to visualize unless a high-intensity lamp is used. Their presence indicates glomerular leakage of protein. This leakage may be temporary (as a result of fever, upright posture, dehydration, or emotional stress) or may be permanent. Their occasional presence is not considered pathologic.

Granular

These casts are descriptively classified as either coarse or finely granular. The type of embedded particulate matter is simply a matter of the amount of degeneration that the epithelial cell inclusions have undergone. Their occasional presence is not pathologic; however, large numbers may be found in chronic lead toxicity and pyelonephritis.

Cellular

Several different types of casts are included in this category. RBC or erythrocytic casts are always considered pathologic because they are diagnostic for glomerular inflammation that results in renal hematuria. They are seen in subacute bacterial endocarditis, kidney infarcts, collagen diseases, and acute glomerulonephritis. WBC or leukocytic casts are also always considered pathologic because they are diagnostic for inflammation of the nephrons. They are observed in pyelonephritis, **nephrotic syndrome**, and acute glomerulonephritis. In asymptomatic pyelonephritis, these casts may be the only clue to detection. Epithelial cell casts are sometimes formed by fusion of renal tubular epithelia after desquamation; occasional presence is normal. Many, however, are observed in severe desquamative processes and renal stases that occur in heavy metal poisoning, renal toxicity, eclampsia, nephrotic syndrome, and amyloidosis. Waxy casts are uniformly yellowish, refractile, and brittle appearing, with sharply defined, often broken edges. They are almost always pathologic because they indicate tubular inflammation or deterioration. They are formed by renal stasis in the collecting ducts and are, therefore, found in chronic renal diseases. Fatty casts are abnormal, coarse, granular casts with lipid inclusions that appear as refractile globules of different sizes. Broad (renal failure) casts may be up to two to six times wider than "regular" casts and may be cellular, waxy, or granular in composition. Like waxy casts, they are derived from the collecting ducts in severe renal stasis.

Crystals

Acid Environment

Crystals seen in urine with pH values of less than 7 include calcium oxalate, which are normal colorless octahedrons or "envelopes"; they may have an almost starlike appearance. Also seen are amorphous urates, normal yellow-red masses with a grain of sand appearance. Uric acid crystals

found in this environment are normal yellow to red-brown crystals that appear in extremely irregular shapes, such as rosettes, prisms, or rhomboids. Cholesterol crystals in acid urine are clear, flat, rectangular plates with notched corners. They may be seen in nephrotic syndrome and in conditions producing chyluria and are always considered abnormal. Cystine crystals are also sometimes observed in acid urine; they are highly pathologic and appear as colorless, refractile, nearly flat hexagons, somewhat similar to uric acid. These are observed in homocystinuria (an aminoaciduria resulting in mental retardation) and cystinuria (an inherited defect of cystine reabsorption resulting in renal calculi).

Alkaline Environment

Crystals seen in urine with pH values greater than 7 include amorphous phosphates, which are normal crystals that appear as fine, colorless masses, resembling sand. Also seen are calcium carbonate crystals, which are normal forms that appear as small, colorless dumbbells or spheres. Triple phosphate crystals are also observed in alkaline urines; they are colorless prisms of three to six sides, resembling "coffin lids." Ammonium biurate crystals are normal forms occasionally found in this environment, appearing as spiny, yellow-brown spheres, or "thorn apples."

Other

Sulfonamide crystals are abnormal precipitates shaped like yellow-brown sheaves, clusters, or needles, formed in patients undergoing antimicrobial therapy with sulfa drugs. These drugs are seldom used today. Tyrosine/leucine crystals are abnormal types shaped like clusters of smooth, yellow needles or spheres. These are sometimes seen in patients with severe liver disease.[16]

PATHOPHYSIOLOGY

Glomerular Diseases

Disorders or diseases that directly damage the renal glomeruli may, at least initially, exhibit normal tubular function. With time, however, disease progression involves the renal tubules as well. The following syndromes have discrete symptoms that are recognizable by their patterns of clinical laboratory findings.

Acute Glomerulonephritis

Pathologic lesions in acute glomerulonephritis primarily involve the glomerulus. Histologic examination shows large, inflamed glomeruli with a decreased capillary lumen. Abnormal laboratory findings usually include rapid onset of hematuria and proteinuria (usually albumin and generally <3 g/d). The rapid development of a decreased GFR, anemia, elevated blood urea nitrogen (BUN) and serum creatinine, oliguria, sodium and water retention (with consequent hypertension and some localized edema), and, sometimes, congestive heart failure is typical. Numerous hyaline and granular casts are generally seen on UA. The actual RBC casts are regarded as highly suggestive of this syndrome. Acute glomerulonephritis is often related to recent infection by group A β-hemolytic streptococci. It is theorized that circulating immune complexes trigger a strong inflammatory response in the glomerular basement membrane, resulting in a direct injury to the glomerulus itself. Other possible causes include drug-related exposures, acute kidney infections due to other bacterial (and, possibly, viral) agents, and other systemic immune complex diseases, such as systemic lupus erythematosus and bacterial endocarditis.

Chronic Glomerulonephritis

Lengthy glomerular inflammation may lead to glomerular scarring and the eventual loss of functioning nephrons. This process often goes undetected for lengthy periods because only minor decreases in renal function occur at first and only slight proteinuria and hematuria are observed. Gradual development of uremia (or azotemia, excess nitrogen compounds in the blood) may be the first sign of this process.

Nephrotic Syndrome

Nephrotic syndrome (Fig. 27.6) can be caused by several different diseases that result in injury and increased permeability of the glomerular basement membrane. This defect almost always yields several abnormal findings, such as massive proteinuria (>3.5 g/d) and resultant hypoalbuminemia. The subsequent decreased plasma oncotic pressure causes a generalized edema as a result of the movement of body fluids out of vascular and into interstitial spaces. Other hallmarks of this syndrome are hyperlipidemia and lipiduria. Lipiduria takes the form of oval fat bodies in the urine. These bodies are degenerated renal tubular cells containing reabsorbed lipoproteins. Primary causes are associated directly with glomerular disease states.

Tubular Diseases

Tubular defects occur to a certain extent in the progression of all renal diseases as the GFR falls. In some instances, however, this aspect of the overall dysfunction becomes predominant. The result is decreased excretion/reabsorption of certain substances or reduced urinary concentrating capability. Clinically, the most important defect is RTA, the primary tubular disorder affecting acid–base balance. This disease can

be classified into two types, depending on the nature of the tubular defect. In distal RTA, the renal tubules are unable to keep up the vital pH gradient between the blood and tubular fluid. In proximal RTA, there is decreased bicarbonate reabsorption, resulting in hyperchloremic acidosis. In general, reduced reabsorption in the proximal tubule is manifested by findings of abnormally low serum values for phosphorus and uric acid and by glucose and amino acids in the urine. In addition, there may be some proteinuria (usually <2 g/d).

Acute or chronic inflammation of the tubules and surrounding interstitium also may occur as a result of radiation toxicity, renal transplant rejection, viral–fungal–bacterial infections, and a reaction to medications. This is known as interstitial nephritis. Characteristic clinical findings in these cases are decreases in GFR, urinary concentrating ability, and metabolic acid excretion; leukocyte casts in the urine; and inappropriate control of sodium balance.[4,7]

Urinary Tract Infection/Obstruction

Infection

The site of infection may be either in the kidneys (pyelonephritis) or in the urinary bladder (cystitis). In general, a microbiologic colony count of more than 10^5 colonies/mL is considered diagnostic for infection in either locale. Bacteriuria (as evidenced by positive nitrite dipstick findings for some organisms), hematuria, and pyuria (leukocytes in the urine, as shown by positive leukocyte esterase dipstick) are all frequently encountered abnormal laboratory results in these cases. In particular, WBC (leukocyte) casts in the urine is considered diagnostic for pyelonephritis.[4,7,16]

Obstruction

Renal obstructions can cause disease in one of two ways. Either they may gradually raise the intratubular pressure until nephrons necrose and chronic renal failure ensues or they may predispose the urinary tract to repeated infections.

Obstructions may be located in the upper or lower urinary tract. Blockages in the upper tract are characterized by a constricting lesion below a dilated collecting duct. Obstructions of the lower tract are evidenced by the

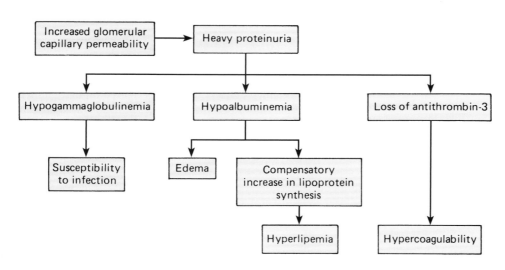

FIGURE 27.6 Pathophysiology of nephrotic syndrome.

TABLE 27.2 Types of Kidney Stones

Stone Composition	Cause of Stone Formation
Calcium oxalate	Hyperparathyroidism High urine calcium Vitamin D toxicity Sarcoidosis Osteoporosis
Magnesium ammonium phosphate	Infectious processes
Calcium phosphate	Excess alkali consumption Infection with urease-producing organisms
Uric acid	Gout High levels of uric acid in blood and urine
Cystine	Inherited cystinuria

residual urine in the bladder after cessation of micturition (urination); symptoms include slowness of voiding, both initially and throughout urination. Causes of obstructions can include neoplasms (e.g., prostate/bladder carcinoma or lymph node tumors constricting ureters), acquired diseases (e.g., urethral strictures or renal calculi), and congenital deformities of the lower urinary tract. The clinical symptoms of advancing obstructive disease include decreased urinary concentrating capability, diminished metabolic acid excretion, decreased GFR, and reduced renal blood flow. Laboratory tests useful in determining the nature of the blockage are UA, urine culture, BUN, serum creatinine, and CBC. Final diagnosis is usually made by radiologic imaging techniques.[5,8]

Renal Calculi

Renal calculi, or kidney stones, are formed by the combination of various crystallized substances, which are listed in Table 27.2. Of these, calcium oxalate stones are by far the most commonly encountered, particularly in the tropics and subtropics.

It is currently believed that recurrence of calculi in susceptible individuals is a result of several causes but mainly a reduced urine flow rate (related to a decreased fluid intake) and saturation of the urine with large amounts of essentially insoluble substances. Chemical analysis of stones is important in determining the cause of the condition. Specialized x-ray diffraction and infrared spectroscopy techniques are widely used for this purpose. Clinical symptoms are, of course, similar to those encountered in other obstructive processes: hematuria, urinary tract infections, and characteristic abdominal pain.[4,7,16]

Renal Failure
Acute Kidney Injury

Acute kidney injury (AKI) is a sudden, sharp decline in renal function as a result of an acute toxic or hypoxic insult to the kidneys. AKI is a common and serious condition that occurs in approximately 50% of patients admitted to the intensive care unit.[18] The risk, injury, failure, loss of function, end-stage renal disease (RIFLE), and the Acute Kidney Injury Network definitions of AKI are based on changes in both serum creatinine and urinary output; however, both display poor specificity and sensitivity for the early detection of AKI.[19] Novel urine and plasma biomarkers, such as NGAL and NephroCheck (TIMP-2 and IGFBP-7), have emerged as excellent biomarkers for the early prediction and prognosis of AKI. AKI is subdivided into three types, depending on the location of the precipitating defect.

Prerenal AKI: The defect lies in the blood supply before it reaches the kidney. Causes can include cardiovascular system failure and consequent hypovolemia.

Intrinsic AKI: The defect involves the kidney. The most common cause is acute tubular necrosis; other causes include vascular obstructions/inflammations and glomerulonephritis.

Postrenal AKI: The defect lies in the urinary tract after it exits the kidney. Generally, acute renal failure occurs as a consequence of lower urinary tract obstruction or rupture of the urinary bladder.

CASE STUDY 27.1

A 52-year-old man with a history of AIDS, hypertension, diabetes mellitus, and alcohol abuse was found unconscious in his home by his roommate. In the emergency department, he was hypotensive (103/60 mm Hg), febrile (temperature 101°F), and unresponsive. Computed tomography scan of the abdomen showed cholecystitis and gallstones. Laboratory data are listed.

The patient was diagnosed with acute renal failure. He was administered intravenous fluids; BUN fell to 68 mg/dL and creatinine fell to 2.2 mg/dL. The patient's blood culture report was positive for *E. coli*. He was treated with tobramycin and cefepime. The patient continued to deteriorate

and died 5 days after admission. Cause of death was multiorgan failure secondary to AIDS, sepsis, and alcoholic cirrhosis.

Questions

1. What is the significance of the patient's elevated CK? Explain why the physician ordered a CK-MB and troponin level. What can you conclude about the patient's cardiac status?

2. What is the cause of his acute renal failure?

3. What is the significance of the patient's large urine hemoglobin?

4. How would you interpret this patient's liver function tests considering his clinical history?

(*continues on page 568*)

CASE STUDY 27.1 (continued)

Drugs of Abuse	Negative	Urinalysis	
Serum ethanol	84 mg/dL	Hemoglobin	Positive
		WBC	4 HPF (0–4)
		RBC	2 HPF (0–4)
CK	3,308 U/L (24–204)	BUN	71 mg/dL (8–21)
CK-MB	15 ng/mL (0–7.5)	Creatinine	4.1 mg/dL (0.9–1.5)
Troponin T	<0.01 ng/mL (0–0.4)	Alkaline phosphatase	443 U/L (45–122)
pH	7.50	Aspartate aminotransferase	305 U/L (9–45)
pCO_2	27 mm Hg	Alanine aminotransferase	78 U/L (8–63)
Total CO_2	15 mmol/L	Gamma glutamyl transpeptidase	724 U/L (11–50)
		Total bilirubin	2.7 mg/dL (0.2–1.0)
		Direct bilirubin	2.4 mg/dL (0–0.2)

Toxic insults to the kidney that are severe enough to initiate AKI include hemolytic transfusion reactions, myoglobinuria due to rhabdomyolysis, heavy metal/solvent poisonings, antifreeze ingestion, and analgesic and aminoglycoside toxicities. These conditions directly damage the renal tubules. Hypoxic insults include conditions that severely compromise renal blood flow, such as septic/hemorrhagic shock, burns, and cardiac failure. The most commonly observed symptoms of acute renal failure are oliguria and anuria (<400 mL/d). The diminished ability to excrete electrolytes and water results in a significant increase in extracellular fluid volume, leading to peripheral edema, hypertension, and congestive heart failure. Most prominent, however, is the onset of the uremic syndrome or kidney failure, in which increased BUN and serum creatinine values are observed along with the preceding symptoms. The outcome of this disease is either recovery or, in the case of irreversible renal damage, progression to chronic renal failure.[4,7]

Chronic Kidney Disease

CKD is a clinical syndrome that occurs when there is a gradual decline in renal function over time (Fig. 27.7). It is defined by the presence of kidney damage or decreased kidney function for three or more months, irrespective of the cause. According to the Center for Disease Control, 1 in 10 US adults has some level of CKD. Early detection and treatment are needed to prevent progression to kidney failure and complications such as coronary vascular disease.

The National Kidney Foundation formulated guidelines for earlier diagnosis, treatment, and prevention of further disease progression in 2002. See Table 27.3 for the five stages of CKD. Since the original classification was published, stage 3 CKD has been subdivided into GFR stages 3a and 3b to more accurately reflect the continuous association between lower GFR and risk for mortality and adverse kidney outcomes. Patients receiving treatment with dialysis are subclassified as GFR stage 5D to highlight the level of care required. GFR and evidence of kidney damage based on measurement of proteinuria or other markers form the basis of the classifications.[20]

In recent years, albuminuria staging has been added to eGFR staging due to the graded increase in risk for mortality, progression of CKD, and end-stage renal disease at higher levels of albuminuria, independent of eGFR. The three stages include A1 (ACR < 30 mg/g) optimal to mild increase with increased risk between being associated with levels between 10 and 29 mg/g, A2 (ACR 30 to 299 mg/g) moderate increase, and A3 (ACR ≥ 300 mg/g) severe increase.

The conditions that can precipitate AKI also may lead to chronic renal failure. Several other causes for this syndrome are listed in Table 27.4.

Increasing Incidence of CKD

There is an increasing incidence of CKD in the United States due to the increase in diabetes, the aging population, obesity, and metabolic syndrome. Diabetes mellitus

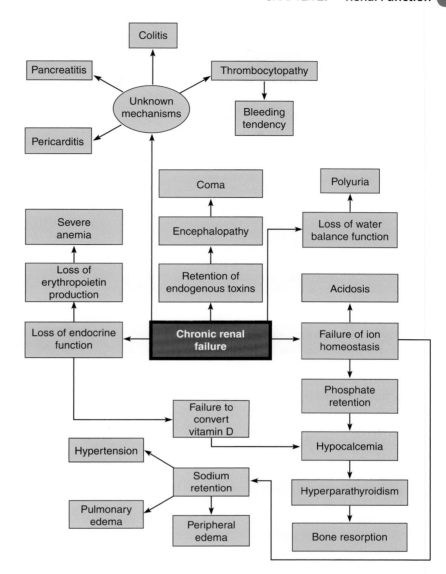

FIGURE 27.7 Pathophysiology of chronic kidney disease.

can have profound effects on the renal system. According to the National Kidney Foundation, diabetes is the leading cause of CKD and accounts for 45% of people diagnosed with kidney failure each year (www.kidney.org). The effects are primarily glomerular, but they may affect all kidney structures as well and are theorized to be caused by the abnormally hyperglycemic environment that constantly bathes the vascular system.[4,7]

Typically, diabetes affects the kidneys by causing them to become glucosuric, polyuric, and nocturic. These states are caused by the heavy demands made on the kidneys to diurese hyperosmotic urine. In addition, a mild

TABLE 27.3	Systematic Classification of CKD Stages	
Stage	**Description**	**GFR (mL/min per 1.73 m²)**
1	Kidney damage with normal or ↑GFR	>90
2	Kidney damage with normal or ↓GFR	60–89
3A	Moderate ↓ GFR	45–59
3B	Moderate to severe ↓ GFR	30–44
4	Severe ↓ GFR	15–29
5	Kidney failure	<15

GFR, glomerular filtration rate; CKD, chronic kidney disease.
Stages 1 to 5 illustrate the progression of CKD.
Source: National Kidney Foundation. *K/DOQI Clinical Practice Guidelines for Chronic Kidney Disease: Executive Summary*. New York, NY: National Kidney Foundation; 2002:16.

TABLE 27.4 Etiology of Chronic Renal Failure

Etiology	Examples
Renal circulatory diseases	Renal vein thrombosis, malignant hypertension
Primary glomerular diseases	Systemic lupus erythematosus, chronic glomerulonephritis
Renal sequelae to metabolic disease	Gout, diabetes mellitus, amyloidosis
Inflammatory diseases	Tuberculosis, chronic pyelonephritis
Renal obstructions	Prostatic enlargement, calculi
Congenital renal deformity	Polycystic kidneys, renal hypoplasia
Miscellaneous conditions	Radiation nephritis

proteinuria (microalbuminuria) often develops between 10 and 15 years after the original diagnosis (see the section "Microalbumin"). Hypertension often manifests next, further exacerbating the renal damage. Eventually, chronic renal insufficiency or nephrotic syndrome may evolve, and each may be identified by their characteristic symptoms and laboratory findings. Early treatment of diabetes that focuses on tight control of blood glucose and prevention of high blood pressure may prolong the onset of chronic renal failure.

Aside from hypertension and diabetes, age is the key predictor of CDK. Due to the decline in fertility and increase in the average life span, the percentage of the population aged 65 years or older is projected to increase from 12.4% in 2000 to 19.6% in 2030, according to the U.S. Census Bureau. This continual rise, over the previous decade and those to come, contributes significantly to the increasing incidence of CKD.

Epidemiologic evidence links obesity to CKD and kidney failure. However, diabetes mellitus and hypertension have potential confounding roles because obesity is a risk factor for diabetes and hypertension, the two most common causes of CKD and kidney failure. Recent studies show that obesity itself increases the risk of kidney injury.[21] As an individual gains weight, the nephron number remains the same; however, the GFR increases to meet the higher metabolic demands, which results in damage to the kidney.

The metabolic syndrome, characterized by the presence of at least three of the following risk factors—abdominal obesity, hypertension, low high-density lipoprotein cholesterol level, hypertriglyceridemia, or hyperglycemia—is a prevalent disorder in the United States. In a population study of a representative sample of the US general population, the risk of CKD and microalbuminuria increased progressively with a greater number of components of metabolic syndrome.[22] Individuals with metabolic syndrome had a 2.6-fold increased risk of developing CKD

compared with individuals without metabolic syndrome.[22] Interventions that target biochemical components of metabolic syndrome may reduce the risk of CDK.

Renal Hypertension

Renal disease–induced hypertension can be caused by decreased perfusion to all or part of the kidney (ischemia). Lack of perfusion may be caused by traumatic injury or narrowing of an artery or intrarenal arterioles. Chronic ischemia of any kind results in nephron dysfunction and eventual necrosis. The resulting changes in blood and body fluid volumes within the kidney trigger the activation of the renin–angiotensin–aldosterone system, setting off vasoconstriction that is manifested as persistent hypertension.

Renal hypertension can be evaluated by monitoring serum aldosterone, Na^+, and renin levels. As a result of the effect of aldosterone, there will be increased serum Na^+, decreased serum K^+, and increased urine K^+.

CASE STUDY 27.2

A 42-year-old man presented to the hospital admitting to have ingested three cups of antifreeze and a rodenticide product 10 hours prior. Upon arrival to the hospital, the patient was somnolent and afebrile and vitals were within normal limits. His chemistry results are shown below. Calcium oxalate crystals were found in his urine (pH 5). His urine toxicology screen was negative.

Na^+	139 mmol/L	Osmolality (serum)	416 mOsm/kg
K^+	4.3 mmol/L	Blood gases (arterial)	
Cl^-	94 mmol/L	pH	7.26
CO_2	10 mmol/L	pCO_2	13 mm Hg
BUN	9 mg/dL	pO_2	129 mm Hg
Creatinine	2.2 mg/dL	HCO_3^-	18 mmol/L
Glucose	167 mg/dL	Prothrombin time	12.8 s
Ca^{2+}	9.9 mg/dL	International normalized ratio	1.1
Albumin	4.5 g/dL		

Treatment with fomepizole (4-MP) was initiated to prevent further metabolism of ethylene glycol. The patient became agitated and was intubated for airway protection and placed on a propofol (sedative–hypnotic) drip. Nephrology was called and hemodialysis was started. Laboratory test results the morning after the first hemodialysis are listed below. The initial ethylene glycol level from time of presentation to the emergency room was received at this time and is included.

Na⁺	143 mmol/L	Albumin	3.1 g/dL
K⁺	4.1 mmol/L	Mg²⁺	1.6 mg/dL
Cl⁻	108 mmol/L	CK	405 U/L
CO₂	18 mmol/L	Osmolality	364 mOsm/kg
BUN	8 mg/dL	Blood gases (arterial)	
Creatinine	3.1 mg/dL	pH	7.4
Glucose	194 mg/dL	pCO_2	26 mm Hg
Ca²⁺	7.7 mg/dL	pO_2	192 mm Hg
Ethylene glycol	499.4 mg/dL	HCO₃⁻	15 mmol/L

The patient remained intubated and sedated. He continued to receive hemodialysis two times a day for 4 hours at a time. The patient also continued to receive fomepizole every 12 hours and following each round of hemodialysis. This treatment continued until the osmolar and anion gaps were normalized.

Questions

1. What caused the formation of the calcium oxalate crystals? What is the clinical significance of calcium oxalate crystal formation?

2. Calculate the anion and osmolar gaps for both sets of laboratory results. In this case, what is the cause of the anion and osmolar gaps? How are these values clinically significant?

3. What are other common drugs and toxins that can cause acute renal failure?

Therapy for AKI
Dialysis
In patients with AKI, uremic symptoms, uncontrolled hyperkalemia, and acidosis have traditionally been indications that the kidneys are unable to excrete the body's waste products and a substitute method in the form of dialysis was necessary. Dialysis is often instituted before this stage, however. Several forms of dialysis are available; however,

they all use a semipermeable membrane surrounded by a dialysate bath.

In traditional **hemodialysis** (removal of waste from blood), the membrane is synthetic and outside the body. Arterial blood and dialysate are pumped at high rates (150 to 250 and 500 mL/min, respectively) in opposite directions. The blood is returned to the venous circulation and the dialysate discarded. The diffusion of low-molecular-weight solutes (<500 Da) into the dialysate is favored by this process, but mid-molecular-weight solutes (500 to 2,000 Da) are inadequately cleared. Creatinine clearance is about 150 to 160 mL/min.

In peritoneal dialysis, the peritoneal wall acts as the dialysate membrane, and gravity is used to introduce and remove the dialysate. Two variations of this form are available, continuous ambulatory peritoneal dialysis (CAPD) and continuous cycling peritoneal dialysis; however, the process is continuous in both, being performed 24 hours a day, 7 days a week. This method is not as rigorous as the traditional method. Small solutes (e.g., potassium) have significantly lower clearance rates compared with the traditional method, but more large solutes are cleared and steady-state levels of blood analytes are maintained.

Continuous arteriovenous **hemofiltration** (ultrafiltration of blood), continuous venovenous hemofiltration, continuous arteriovenous hemodialysis, and continuous venovenous hemodialysis together make up the slow continuous renal replacement therapies developed to treat AKI in critically ill patients in intensive care settings. In these methods, the semipermeable membrane is again outside the body. Solutes up to 5,000 Da (the pore size of the membranes) and water are slowly (10 mL/min) and continuously filtered from the blood in the first two methods, causing minimal changes in plasma osmolality. Volume loss can be replaced in the form of parenteral nutrition and intravenous medications. The final two methods are similar to the filtration methods, but a continuous trickle of dialysis fluid is pumped past the dialysis membrane, resulting in continuous diffusion and a doubling of the urea clearance.

Therapy for Kidney Failure
For patients with irreversible renal failure, dialysis and transplantation are the only two therapeutic options. Initiation of either treatment occurs when the GFR falls to 5 mL/min (10 to 15 mL/min in patients with diabetic nephropathy).

Dialysis
Traditional hemodialysis or its more recent, high-efficiency form and peritoneal dialysis are the available methods. The clinical laboratory used in conjunction with a hemodialysis facility must be able to adequately monitor procedural efficiency in a wide variety of areas. Renal dialysis has basic goals, and specific laboratory tests should be performed to evaluate the achievement of each goal.

Transplantation
The most efficient hemodialysis techniques provide only 10% to 12% of the small solute removal of two normal kidneys and considerably less removal of larger solutes. Even patients who

are well dialyzed have physical disabilities and decreased quality of life. Kidney transplantation offers the greatest chance for full return to a healthy, productive life. However, this option is limited by the significant shortage of donor organs. For kidney failure patients, waiting for an organ donation can vary from several months to several years.

Renal transplantation is from a compatible donor to a recipient suffering from irreversible renal failure. The organ can be from a cadaver or a live individual (80% and 20%, respectively, of all kidney transplants in the United States). For this procedure to be successful, the body's immune response to the transplanted organ must be suppressed. Therefore, the donor and recipient are carefully screened for ABO blood group, human leukocyte antigen (HLA) compatibility, and preformed HLA antibodies. The HLA system is the major inhibitor to transplantation.

Although kidney transplants have the capacity to function for decades, the mean half-life of a cadaveric transplant is approximately 7 years. The mortality rate is not significantly different from hemodialysis. Three-year graft survival figures vary from 65% to 85%, with live grafts doing better. It has been reported that there is no difference in

CASE STUDY 27.3

A 78-year-old woman with a history of hypertension, aortic thoracic graft, and esophageal reflux disease complained of fever (100°F) and weakness. She had been treated 3 weeks before at the hospital for a urinary tract infection. She was admitted to the hospital for a diagnostic workup and transfusion. Her laboratory results are as follows:

Na+	129 mmol/L	Hct	25.6%
K+	3.7 mmol/L	Hgb	8.5 g/dL
Cl-	97 mmol/L	WBC	9,700
CO2	19 mmol/L		
BUN	52 mg/dL		
Creatinine	3.2 mg/dL		

Urine culture was positive for *Citrobacter*. UA results are listed:

Color	Hazy/yellow
Specific gravity	1.015
pH	5
Blood	Large
Protein	2
Glucose	Negative
Ketones	Negative
Nitrates	Negative
RBC	>25
WBC	1–4
Casts	Granular, 1–4

The patient's renal function continued to decline, and she was put on hemodialysis. A renal biopsy was performed that showed end-stage crescentic glomerulonephritis. Two days later, the patient sustained a perforated duodenal ulcer, which required surgery and blood transfusion. Subsequently, she developed coagulopathy and liver failure. Her condition continued to deteriorate in the next few days, and she died following removal of life support.

Questions

1. Looking at the UA, what is the significance of the results of 2+ protein and greater than 25 RBCs?
2. What is the most likely cause of glomerulonephritis?
3. Why was the patient put on hemodialysis?

patient survival among hemodialysis, CAPD, and cadaveric kidney transplantation. Live related donor transplantation is associated with a better patient survival than other therapeutic options for kidney failure.

questions

1. Calculate creatinine clearance, given the following information: serum creatinine, 1.2 mg/dL; urine creatinine, 120 mg/dL; urine volume, 1,750 mL/24 h; body surface area, 1.80 m².

2. Predict GFR in a 50-year-old woman who weighs 60 kg using the Cockcroft-Gault equation. Her serum creatinine level is 2.5 mg/dL.

3. The measurement of serum cystatin C, a small protein produced by nucleated cells, is useful for
  a. Detecting an early decrease in kidney function
  b. Calculating creatinine clearance
  c. Diagnosing end-stage renal disease
  d. Monitoring dialysis patients

4. Acute renal failure can be classified into three types. List each type and give an example of each.
  a. _____
  b. _____
  c. _____

5. The proximal tubule functions to
  a. Reabsorb 75% of salt and water
  b. Concentrate salts
  c. Form the renal threshold
  d. Reabsorb urea

6. Renal clearance is the
  a. Volume of plasma from which a substance is removed per unit of time
  b. Volume of urine produced per day
  c. Amount of creatinine in urine
  d. Urine concentration of a substance divided by the urine volume per unit of time

7. Renin release by the kidney is stimulated by
  a. A decrease in extracellular fluid volume or pressure
  b. Increased plasma sodium concentration
  c. Increased dietary sodium
  d. Renal tubular reabsorption

8. The set of results that most accurately reflects severe renal disease is
  a. *Serum creatinine*, 3.7 mg/dL; *creatinine clearance*, 44 mL/min; *BUN*, 88 mg/dL
  b. *Serum creatinine*, 1.0 mg/dL; *creatinine clearance*, 110 mL/min; *BUN*, 17 mg/dL
  c. *Serum creatinine*, 2.0 mg/dL; *creatinine clearance*, 120 mL/min; *BUN*, 14 mg/dL
  d. *Serum creatinine*, 1.0 mg/dL; *creatinine clearance*, 95 mL/min; *BUN*, 43 mg/dL

9. Creatinine clearance results are corrected using a patient's body surface area to account for differences in
  a. Muscle mass
  b. Age
  c. Dietary intake
  d. Sex

10. A patient is suffering from an acute bleed. What is the most accurate way to describe the subsequent acute kidney injury?
  a. Prerenal acute kidney injury.
  b. Renal acute kidney injury.
  c. Postrenal acute kidney injury.
  d. None of the above apply.

references

1. Vander A, Sherman JH, Luciano DS. *Human Physiology: The Mechanisms of Body Function.* 7th ed. New York, NY: McGraw-Hill; 1998:503, 508, 519.
2. Kaplan A, Szabo LL, Jack R, et al. *Clinical Chemistry: Interpretation and Techniques.* 4th ed. Baltimore, MD: Williams & Wilkins; 1995:156–157.
3. Davies A, Blakely A, Kidd C. *Human Physiology.* London: Harcourt Publishers; 2001:747.
4. Rock RC, Walker WG, Jennings CD. Nitrogen metabolites and renal function. In: Tietz NW, ed. *Fundamentals of Clinical Chemistry.* 3rd ed. Philadelphia, PA: WB Saunders; 1987:669.
5. Russell PT, Sherwin JE, Obernolte R, et al. Nonprotein nitrogenous compounds. In: Kaplan LA, Pesce AJ, eds. *Clinical Chemistry: Theory, Analysis, and Correlation.* 2nd ed. St. Louis, MO: CV Mosby; 1989:1005.
6. Fraser D, Jones G, Kooh SW, et al. Calcium and phosphate metabolism. In: Tietz NW, ed. *Fundamentals of Clinical Chemistry.* 3rd ed. Philadelphia, PA: WB Saunders; 1987:705.
7. First MR. Renal function. In: Kaplan LA, Pesce AJ, eds. *Clinical Chemistry: Theory, Analysis, and Correlation.* 4th ed. St. Louis, MO: CV Mosby; 2003:477–491.
8. Kleinman LI, Lorenz JM. Physiology and pathophysiology of body water and electrolytes. In: Kaplan LA, Pesce AJ, eds. *Clinical Chemistry: Theory, Analysis, and Correlation.* 4th ed. St. Louis, MO: CV Mosby; 2003:441–461.
9. Sherwin JE, Bruegger BB. Acid–base control and acid–base disorders. In: Kaplan LA, Pesce AJ, eds. *Clinical Chemistry: Theory, Analysis, and Correlation.* 4th ed. St. Louis, MO: CV Mosby; 2003:462–476.

10. Levey AS, Stevens LA, Schmid CH, et al. A new equation to estimate glomerular filtration rate. *Ann Intern Med.* 2009;150:604–612.

11. Lab Tests Online. Cystatin C at a glance. http://www.labtestsonline.org/understanding/analytes/cystatin_c/glance.html

12. Stevens LA, Coresh J, Schmid CH, et al. Estimated GFR using serum cystatin C alone and in combination with serum creatinine: a pooled analysis of 3418 individuals with CKD. *Am J Kidney Dis.* 2008;51:395–406.

13. Schwartz GJ, Munoz A, Schneide MF, et al. New equations to estimate GFR in children with CKD. *J Am Soc Nephrol.* 2009;20:629–637.

14. Fraser CG. *Biological Variation: From Principles to Practice.* Washington, DC: AACC Press; 2001.

15. Haase M, Bellomo R, Haase-Fielitz A. Neutrophil gelatinase-associated lipocalin. *Curr Opin Crit Care.* 2010;16:526–532.

16. Kashani K, Al-Khafaji A, Ardiles T, et al. Discovery and validation of cell cycle arrest biomarkers in human acute kidney injury. *Crit Care.* 2013;17:R25.

17. Kaplan LA, Pesce AJ. Examination of urine. In: Kaplan LA, Pesce AJ, eds. *Clinical Chemistry: Theory, Analysis, and Correlation.* 4th ed. St. Louis, MO: CV Mosby; 2003:1092–1109.

18. Mandelbaum T, Scott DJ, Lee J, et al. Outcome of critically ill patients with acute kidney injury using the Acute Kidney Injury Network criteria. *Crit Care Med.* 2011;39(12):2659–2664.

19. Mehta RL, Kellum JA, Shah SV, et al. Acute Kidney Injury Network: report of an initiative to improve outcomes in acute kidney injury. *Crit Care.* 2007;11:R31.

20. Mitchum C. Implementing the new kidney disease testing guidelines. *Clin Lab News.* 2002;September:14.

21. Kramer H, Luke A. Obesity and kidney disease: a big dilemma. *Curr Opin Nephrol Hypertens.* 2007;16:237–241.

22. Chen J, Muntner P, Hamm LL, et al. The metabolic syndrome and chronic kidney disease in U.S. adults. *Ann Intern Med.* 2004;140:167–174.

28

Pancreatic Function and Gastrointestinal Function

EDWARD P. FODY

chapter outline

key terms

Cholecystokinin (CCK)
D-Xylose absorption test
Fecal elastase
Gastrin
Intrinsic factor
Islets of Langerhans
Lactose tolerance test
Pancreatitis
Pepsin
Secretagogues
Secretin
Steatorrhea
Zollinger-Ellison syndrome

chapter objectives

Upon completion of this chapter, the clinical laboratorian should be able to do the following:

• Discuss the physiologic role of the pancreas in the digestive process.
• List the hormones excreted by the pancreas, together with their physiologic roles.
• Describe the following pancreatic disorders and list the associated laboratory tests that would aid in diagnosis: acute pancreatitis, chronic pancreatitis, pancreatic carcinoma, cystic fibrosis, and pancreatic malabsorption.
• Describe the physiology and biochemistry of gastric secretion.
• List the tests used to assess gastric and intestinal function.
• Explain the clinical aspects of gastric analysis.
• Evaluate a patient's condition, given clinical data.

For additional student resources, please visit thePoint® at http://thepoint.lww.com

The gastrointestinal (GI) system is composed of the mouth, esophagus, stomach, small intestine, and large intestine. Digestion, which is primarily a function of the small intestine, is the process by which starches, proteins, lipids, nucleic acids, and other complex molecules are degraded to simple constituents (molecules) for absorption and use in the body. This chapter discusses the physiology and biochemistry of gastric secretion, intestinal physiology, pathologic aspects of intestinal function, and tests of gastric and intestinal function.

The pancreas is a large gland that is involved in the digestive process but located outside of the GI system. It is composed of both endocrine and exocrine tissues. The liver is the other major external gland that is involved in the digestive process, and it is covered in Chapter 25. The endocrine functions of the pancreas include production of insulin and glucagon; both hormones are involved in carbohydrate metabolism. Exocrine function involves the production of many enzymes used in the digestive process. This chapter discusses the physiology of pancreatic function, diseases of the pancreas, and tests of pancreatic function.

PHYSIOLOGY OF PANCREATIC FUNCTION

As a digestive gland, the pancreas is only second in size to the liver, weighing about 70 to 105 g. It is located behind the peritoneal cavity across the upper abdomen at about the level of the first and second lumbar vertebrae, about 1 to 2 in. above the umbilicus. It is located in the curve made by the duodenum (Fig. 28.1). The pancreas is composed of two morphologically and functionally different tissues: endocrine tissue and exocrine tissue. The *endocrine* (hormone-releasing) component is by far the smaller of the two and consists of the **islets of Langerhans**, which are well-delineated, spherical or ovoid clusters composed of at least four different cell types. The islet cells secrete at least four hormones into the blood: insulin, glucagon, gastrin, and somatostatin. The larger, *exocrine* pancreatic (enzyme-secreting) component secretes about 1.5 to 2 L/d of fluid, which is rich in digestive enzymes, into ducts that ultimately empty into the duodenum.

This digestive fluid is produced by pancreatic acinar cells (grape-like clusters), which line the pancreas and are connected by small ducts. These small ducts empty into progressively larger ducts, eventually forming one major pancreatic duct and a smaller accessory duct. The major pancreatic duct and the common bile duct open into the duodenum at the major duodenal papilla (Fig. 28.2). Normal, protein-rich, pancreatic fluid is clear, colorless, and watery, with an alkaline pH that can reach up to 8.3. This alkalinity is caused by the high concentration of sodium bicarbonate present in pancreatic fluid, which is used eventually to neutralize the hydrochloric acid in gastric fluid from the stomach as it enters the duodenum. The bicarbonate and chloride concentrations vary reciprocally so that they total about 150 mmol/L.

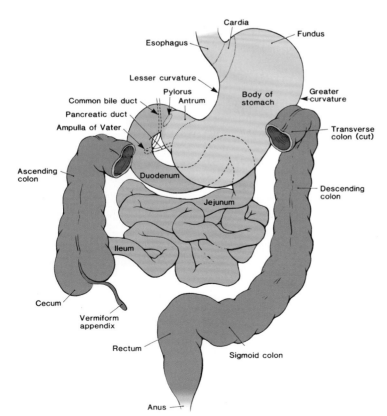

FIGURE 28.1 Peritoneum and mesenteries. The parietal peritoneum lines the abdominal cavity, and the visceral peritoneum covers abdominal organs. Retroperitoneal organs are covered by the parietal peritoneum. The mesenteries are membranes that connect abdominal organs to each other and to the body wall. (Reprinted from Thompson JS, Akesson EJ, eds. *Thompson's Core Textbook of Anatomy*. 2nd ed. Philadelphia, PA: JB Lippincott; 1990:115, with permission.)

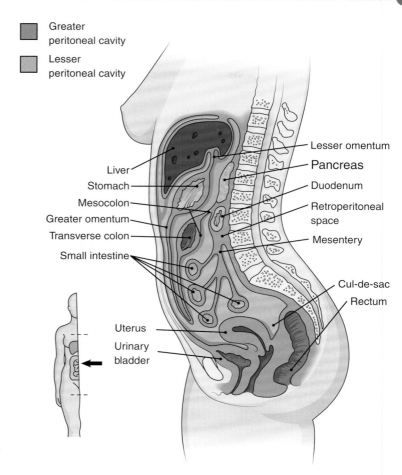

Greater
peritoneal cavity

Lesser
peritoneal cavity

Liver
Stomach
Mesocolon
Greater omentum
Transverse colon
Small intestine

Lesser omentum
Pancreas
Duodenum
Retroperitoneal
space
Mesentery

Cul-de-sac
Rectum

Uterus
Urinary
bladder

FIGURE 28.2 Diagram of the pancreas and its relationship
to the duodenum.

Pancreatic fluid has about the same concentrations of potassium and sodium as serum. The digestive enzymes, or their proenzymes secreted by the pancreas, are capable of digesting the three major classes of food substances (proteins, carbohydrates, and fats) and include (1) the proteolytic enzymes trypsin, chymotrypsin, elastase, collagenase, leucine aminopeptidase, and some carboxypeptidases; (2) lipid-digesting enzymes, primarily lipase and lecithinase; (3) carbohydrate-splitting pancreatic amylase; and (4) several nucleases (ribonuclease), which separate the nitrogen-containing bases from their sugar-phosphate strands.

Pancreatic activity is under both nervous and endocrine control. Branches of the vagus nerve can cause a small amount of pancreatic fluid secretion when food is smelled or seen, and these secretions may increase as the bolus of food reaches the stomach. Most of the pancreatic action, however, is under the hormonal control of **secretin** and **cholecystokinin** (**CCK**; formerly called *pancreozymin*). Secretin is responsible for the production of bicarbonate-rich and, therefore, alkaline pancreatic fluid, which protects the lining of the intestine from damage. Secretin is synthesized in response to the acidic contents of the stomach reaching the duodenum. It can also affect gastrin activity in the stomach. This pancreatic fluid contains few digestive enzymes. CCK, in the presence of fats or amino acids in the

duodenum, is produced by the cells of the intestinal mucosa and is responsible for release of enzymes from the acinar cells by the pancreas into the pancreatic fluid.

DISEASES OF THE PANCREAS

Other than trauma, only three diseases cause more than 95% of the medical attention devoted to the pancreas. If they affect the endocrine function of the pancreas, these diseases can result in altered digestion and nutrient metabolism. The role of the pancreas in diabetes mellitus is discussed in Chapter 14.

Cystic fibrosis (known by various other terms, such as *fibrocystic disease of the pancreas* and *mucoviscidosis*) is an inherited autosomal recessive disorder characterized by dysfunction of mucous and exocrine glands throughout the body. The disease is relatively common and occurs in about 1 of 1,600 live births. It has various manifestations and can initially present in such widely varying ways as intestinal obstruction of the newborn, excessive pulmonary infections in childhood, or, uncommonly, as pancreatogenous malabsorption in adults. The disease causes the small and large ducts and the acini to dilate and convert into small cysts filled with mucus, eventually resulting in the prevention of pancreatic secretions reaching the duodenum or, depending on the age of the patient, a plug that blocks the lumen of the bowel, leading to obstruction. As the disease progresses, there is increased destruction and fibrous scarring of the pancreas and a corresponding decrease in function. Cystic fibrosis is transmitted as an autosomal recessive disorder with a high degree of penetrance. It occurs primarily in persons of Northern European descent. The cystic fibrosis gene known as *CFTR* occurs on chromosome 7, and more than 900 mutations causing this disorder have been identified; however, some occur more commonly than others. In areas of high frequency, such as Brittany in Western France, more than 10% of the population may carry a cystic fibrosis mutation, and 1 in 3,000 infants may be affected, making it the most common genetic disorder in these populations. Genetic screening is now widely carried out.[1-3]

Pancreatic carcinoma is the fourth most frequent form of fatal cancer and causes about 38,000 deaths each year in the United States, which represents about 7% of all deaths from malignant neoplasms. The disease is slightly more common in males than in females and in African Americans than in Whites. The 5-year survival rate is about 6%, and most patients die within 1 year of diagnosis. Most pancreatic tumors arise as adenocarcinomas of the ductal epithelium. Because the pancreas has a rich supply of nerves, pain is a prominent feature of the disease. If the tumor arises in the body or tail of the pancreas, detection does not often occur until an advanced stage of the disease because of its central location and the associated vague symptoms. Cancer of the head of the pancreas is usually detected earlier because of its proximity to the common bile duct. Signs of these tumors are jaundice, weight loss, anorexia, and nausea. Jaundice is associated with signs of posthepatic hyperbilirubinemia (intrahepatic cholestasis) and low levels of fecal bilirubin, resulting in clay-colored stools. However, findings are not specific for pancreatic tumors, and other causes of obstruction must be ruled out.

Islet cell tumors of the pancreas affect the endocrine capability of the pancreas. If the tumor occurs in beta cells, hyperinsulinism is often seen, resulting in low blood glucose levels, sometimes followed by hypoglycemic shock. Pancreatic cell tumors, which overproduce gastrin, are called *gastrinomas*; they cause **Zollinger-Ellison syndrome** and can be duodenal in origin. These tumors are associated with watery diarrhea, recurring peptic ulcer, and significant gastric hypersecretion and hyperacidity. Pancreatic cell glucagon-secreting tumors are rare; the hypersecretion of glucagon is associated with diabetes mellitus.

Pancreatitis, or inflammation of the pancreas, is ultimately caused by autodigestion of the pancreas as a result of reflux of bile or duodenal contents into the pancreatic duct. Pathologic changes can include acute edema, with large amounts of fluid accumulating in the retroperitoneal space and an associated decrease in effective circulating blood volume; cellular infiltration, leading to necrosis of the acinar cells, with hemorrhage as a possible result of necrotic blood vessels; and intrahepatic and extrahepatic pancreatic fat necrosis. Pancreatitis is generally classified as acute (no permanent damage to the pancreas), chronic

(irreversible injury), or relapsing/recurrent, which can also be acute or chronic. It commonly occurs in midlife. Painful episodes can occur intermittently, usually reaching a maximum within minutes or hours, lasting for several days or weeks, and frequently accompanied by nausea and vomiting. Pancreatitis is often associated with alcohol abuse or biliary tract diseases such as gallstones, but patients with hyperlipoproteinemia and those with hyperparathyroidism are also at a significantly increased risk for this disease.

Other etiologic factors associated with acute pancreatitis include mumps, obstruction caused by biliary tract disease, gallstones, pancreatic tumors, tissue injury, atherosclerotic disease, shock, pregnancy, hypercalcemia, hereditary pancreatitis, immunologic factors associated with postrenal transplantation, and hypersensitivity. Symptoms of acute pancreatitis include severe abdominal pain that is generalized or in the upper quadrants and often radiates toward the back or down the right or left flank. The etiology of chronic pancreatitis is similar to that of acute pancreatitis, but chronic excessive alcohol consumption appears to be the most common predisposing factor.

Laboratory findings include increased amylase, lipase, triglycerides, and hypercalcemia, which is often associated with underlying hyperparathyroidism. Hypocalcemia may be found and has been attributed to the sudden removal of large amounts of calcium from the extracellular fluid because of impaired mobilization or as a result of calcium fixation by fatty acids liberated by increased lipase action on triglycerides. Hypoproteinemia is attributable mainly to the notable loss of plasma into the retroperitoneal space. A shift of arterial blood flow from the inflamed pancreatic cells to less affected or normal cells causes oxygen deprivation and tissue hypoxia in the area of damage, including the surrounding organs and tissue.

All three conditions can result in severely diminished pancreatic exocrine function, which can significantly compromise digestion and absorption of ingested nutrients. This is the essence of the general malabsorption syndrome, which embodies abdominal bloating and discomfort; the frequent passage of bulky, malodorous feces; and weight loss. Failure to digest or absorb fats, known as **steatorrhea**, renders a greasy appearance to feces (more than 5 g of fecal fat per 24 hours). The malabsorption syndrome typically involves abnormal digestion or absorption of proteins, polysaccharides, carbohydrates, and other complex molecules, as well as lipids. Severely deranged absorption and metabolism of electrolytes, water, vitamins (particularly fat-soluble vitamins A, D, E, and K), and minerals can also occur. Malabsorption can involve a single substance, such as vitamin B_{12}, which results in a megaloblastic anemia (pernicious anemia), or lactose caused by a lactase deficiency. In addition to pancreatic exocrine deficiency, the malabsorption syndrome can be caused by biliary obstruction, which deprives the small intestine of the emulsifying effect of bile, and various diseases of the small intestine, which inhibit absorption of digested products.

TESTS OF PANCREATIC FUNCTION

Depending on etiology and clinical picture, pancreatic function may be suspect when there is evidence of increased amylase and lipase.[4–7] The reader is referred to Chapter 13 for an in-depth discussion of these enzymes. Other laboratory tests of pancreatic function include those used for detection of malabsorption (e.g., examination of stool for excess fat, D-xylose test, and fecal fat analysis), tests measuring other exocrine function (e.g., secretin, CCK, fecal fat, trypsin, and chymotrypsin), tests assessing changes associated with extrahepatic obstruction (e.g., bilirubin), and endocrine-related tests (e.g., gastrin, insulin, and glucose) that reflect changes in the endocrine cells of the pancreas.

Direct evaluation of pancreatic fluid may include measurement of the total volume of pancreatic fluid and the amount or concentration of bicarbonate and enzymes, which requires pancreatic stimulation. Stimulation may be accomplished using a predescribed meal or administration of secretin, which allows for volume and bicarbonate evaluation, or secretin stimulation followed by CCK stimulation, which adds enzymes to the pancreatic fluid evaluation. The advantage of these tests, both of which require intubation of the patient, is that the chemical and cytologic examinations are performed on actual pancreatic secretions. Cytologic examination of the fluid can often establish the presence, or at least the suspicion, of malignant neoplasms, although the precise localization of the primary organ of involvement (i.e., pancreas, biliary system, ampulla of Vater, or duodenum) is not possible by duodenal aspiration.

Because of advances in imaging techniques, these stimulation tests are used less often; none have proved especially useful in diagnosis of mild or acute pancreatic disease in which the acute phase has subsided. Most of the tests have found clinical utility in excluding the pancreas from diagnosis. The sweat test, used for screening cystic fibrosis, is not specific for assessing pancreatic involvement but, when used along with the clinical picture at the time of testing, can provide important diagnostic information. The following pancreatic function tests are reviewed briefly: secretin/CCK test, fecal fat analysis, sweat chloride determinations, and amylase and lipase interpretation.

CASE STUDY 28.1

A 38-year-old man entered the emergency department with the complaint of severe, midabdominal pain of 6 hours' duration. A friend, who had driven him to the hospital, stated that the patient fainted three times as he was being helped into the automobile. The patient had a 15-year history of alcoholism and drank 1 to 2 pints of whiskey everyday. He had last been hospitalized for acute alcoholism 3 months ago, at which time he had relatively minor abnormalities of liver function. On this admission, his blood pressure was 80/40 mm Hg; pulse, 110 beats/min and thready; and respirations, 24 breaths per minute and shallow. Clinical laboratory test results are shown in Case Study Table 28.1.1.

CASE STUDY TABLE 28.1.1	Laboratory Results
Serum amylase	640 units (3.5–260 units)
Serum sodium	133 mmol/L (135–145 mmol/L)
Potassium	3.4 mmol/L (3.8–5.5 mmol/L)
Calcium	4.0 mmol/L (4.5–5.5 mmol/L)
Blood urea nitrogen	32 mg/dL (8–25 mg/dL)
White blood cell count	16,500/μL
Hemoglobin	12 g/dL

Questions

1. What is the probable disease?
2. What is the cause for the low serum calcium?
3. What is the cause for the increased blood urea nitrogen?

Secretin/CCK Test

The secretin/CCK test is a direct determination of the exocrine secretory capacity of the pancreas. The test involves intubation of the duodenum without contamination by gastric fluid, which would neutralize any bicarbonate. The test is performed after a 6-hour or overnight fast. Pancreatic secretion is stimulated by intravenously administered secretin in a dose varying from 2 to 3 U/kg of body weight, followed by CCK administration. If a simple secretin test is desired, the higher dose of secretin is given alone.

No single protocol has been uniformly established for the test. Pancreatic secretions are collected variously for 30, 60, or 80 minutes after administration of the stimulants, either as 10-minute specimens or as a single, pooled collection. The pH, secretory rate, enzyme activities (e.g., trypsin, amylase, or lipase), and amount of bicarbonate are determined. The average amount of bicarbonate excreted per hour is about 15 mmol/L for men and 12 mmol/L for women, with an average flow of 2 mL/kg. Assessment of enzymes must be taken in view of total volume output. Decreased pancreatic flow is associated with pancreatic obstruction and increase in enzyme concentrations. Low concentrations of bicarbonate and enzymes are associated with cystic fibrosis, chronic pancreatitis, pancreatic cysts, calcification, and edema of the pancreas.

CASE STUDY 28.2

A 56-year-old man who is an alcoholic presents with a 2-week history of midabdominal pain. He also describes clay-colored stools, mild icterus, nausea, vomiting, and a 10-lb weight loss. Laboratory findings are shown in Case Study Table 28.2.1.

CASE STUDY TABLE 28.2.1   Laboratory Results

Test	Result	Reference Range
Serum bilirubin	4.2 mg/dL	0.3–1.0 mg/dL
Serum lactate dehydrogenase	625 IU/L	0–200 IU/L
Serum alanine aminotransferase	76 IU/L	0–46 IU/L
Serum alkaline phosphatase	462 IU/L	0–80 IU/L
Serum amylase	80 IU/L	0–85 IU/L
Urine bilirubin	3+	Negative

Questions

1. What organ system is primarily involved?

2. What are the major diagnostic considerations?

3. What do the laboratory results mean? What additional laboratory tests would be useful in establishing a diagnosis?

4. What other studies or procedures might be required?

Fecal Fat Analysis

Fecal lipids are derived from four sources: unabsorbed ingested lipids, lipids excreted into the intestine (predominantly in the bile), cells shed into the intestine, and metabolism of intestinal bacteria. Patients on a lipid-free diet still excrete 1 to 4 g of lipid in the feces in a 24-hour period. Even with a lipid-rich diet, the fecal fat does not normally exceed about 7 g in a 24-hour period. Normal fecal lipid is composed of about 60% fatty acids; 30% sterols, higher alcohols, and carotenoids; 10% triglycerides; and small amounts of cholesterol and phospholipids. Although significantly increased fecal fat can be caused by biliary obstruction, severe steatorrhea is usually associated with exocrine pancreatic insufficiency or disease of the small intestine.

Qualitative Screening Test for Fecal Fat

Various screening tests have been devised for detecting steatorrhea. These tests commonly use fat-soluble stains (e.g., Sudan III, Sudan IV, Oil Red O, or Nile blue sulfate), which dissolve in and color lipid droplets. Of greater importance than the particular technical procedure is the level of experience and dependability of the clinical laboratorian performing the test.

Sudan Staining for Fecal Fat

Neutral fats (triglycerides) and many other lipids stain yellow-orange to red with Sudan III because the dye is much more soluble in lipid than in water or ethanol.[8,9] Free fatty acids do not stain appreciably unless the specimen is heated in the presence of the stain with 36% acetic acid. The slide may be examined warm or cool and the number of fat droplets assessed. As the slide cools, the fatty acids crystallize out in long, colorless, needle-like sheaves. Detection of meat fiber is accomplished by a third aliquot of fecal sample mixed on the slide with 10% alcohol and a solution of eosin stained for 3 minutes. The meat fiber should stain as rectangular cross-striated fibers. Splitting the sample and detecting neutral fats, fatty acids, and undigested meat fibers can provide diagnostic information. Increases in fats and undigested meat fibers are indicative of patients with steatorrhea of pancreatic origin. A representative fecal specimen is used for analysis.

Normal feces can have up to 40 or 50 small (1 to 5 mm), neutral lipid droplets per high-power microscope field. Steatorrhea is characterized by an increase in the number and size of stainable droplets, often with some fat globules in the 50- to 100-mm range. Fatty acid assessment greater than 100 stained small droplets, along with the presence of meat fiber, is expected in patients with steatorrhea.

Quantitative Fecal Fat Analysis

The definitive test for steatorrhea is the quantitative fecal fat determination, usually on a 72-hour stool collection, although the collection period may be increased to up to 5 days. Traditional methods for fecal fat determination are the gravimetric and titrimetric methods. Newer methods involve the use of infrared and nuclear magnetic resonance spectroscopy.[10,11] In the gravimetric method, fatty acid soaps (predominantly calcium and magnesium salts of fatty acids) are converted to free fatty acids, followed by extraction of most of the lipids into an organic solvent, which is then evaporated so that the lipid residue can be weighed. In titrimetric methods, lipids are saponified with hydroxide, and the fatty acid salts are converted to free fatty acids using acid. The free fatty acids, along with various unsaponified lipids, are then extracted with an organic solvent, and the fatty acids are titrated with hydroxide after evaporation of the solvent and redissolving of the residue in ethanol. The titration methods obviously measure only saponifiable fatty acids and, consequently, render results about 20% lower than those from gravimetric methods. A further objection is that titrimetric methods use an assumed average molecular weight for fatty acids to convert moles of fatty acids to grams of lipid.

At one time, it was common to measure the amount of free fatty acids as a percentage of total lipids on the presumption that a high percentage of free fatty acids indicates adequate pancreatic lipase activity. This method is no longer considered reliable because of spurious results, particularly caused by lipase produced by intestinal bacteria.

It is essential that patients be placed on a lipid-rich diet for at least 2 days before instituting the fecal collection. The diet must contain at least 50 g, and preferably 100 g, of lipids each day. Fecal collections should extend for 3 or more successive days.

There are various ways to express fecal lipid excretion. Expressing lipid excretion as a percentage of wet or dry fecal weight is open to serious challenge because of wide variations in both fecal water content and dry residue as a result of dietary intake. The most widely accepted approach is to report the grams of fecal fat excreted in a 24-hour period.

Gravimetric Method for Fecal Fat Determination

The entire fecal specimen is emulsified with water. An aliquot is acidified to convert all fatty acid soaps to free fatty acids, which are then extracted with other soluble lipids into petroleum ether and ethanol. After evaporation of the organic solvents, the lipid residue is weighed. All feces for a 3-day period are collected in tared containers. The containers *must not* have a wax coating. The specimen must be kept refrigerated.

Total lipid does not change significantly during 5 days' storage of the specimen at refrigerator temperatures. Patients must not ingest castor oil, mineral oil, or other oily laxatives and must not use rectal suppositories containing oil or lipid for 2 days before the test and during the test.

The reference range for fecal lipids in adults is 1 to 7 g per 24 hours.

Sweat Electrolyte Determinations

Measurement of the sodium and chloride concentration in sweat is the most useful test for the diagnosis of cystic fibrosis.[12–14] Significantly elevated concentrations of both ions occur in more than 99% of affected patients. The twofold to fivefold increases in sweat sodium and chloride are diagnostic of cystic fibrosis in children. Even in adults, no other condition causes increases in sweat chloride and sodium above 80 mmol/L. Sweat potassium is also increased, but less significantly so, and is not generally relied on for diagnosis. Contrary to some assertions, sweat electrolyte determinations do not distinguish heterozygote carriers of cystic fibrosis from normal homozygotes.

Older methods for acquiring sweat specimens required skilled technologists who frequently performed the test. Induction of sweat included applying plastic bags or wrapping the patient in blankets, which was fraught with serious risks of dehydration, electrolyte disturbances, and hyperpyrexia. In 1959, pilocarpine administration by iontophoresis was reported as an efficient method for sweat collection and stimulation. Iontophoresis uses an electric current that causes pilocarpine to migrate into a limited skin area, usually the inside of the forearm, toward the negative electrode from a moistened pad on the positive electrode. A collection vessel is then applied to the skin. The sweat is then analyzed for chloride. For confirmation, the test should be repeated. Commercially available surface electrodes that analyze the sweat chloride are readily available. For details, the reader is referred to Chapter 29.

It is widely accepted that sweat chloride concentrations greater than 60 mmol/L are diagnostic of cystic fibrosis in children. Sweat sodium and chloride concentrations in female patients undergo fluctuation with the menstrual cycle and reach a peak 5 to 10 days before the onset of menstruation but do not overlap with the ranges associated with cystic fibrosis.

Serum Enzymes

Amylase is the serum enzyme most commonly relied on for detecting pancreatic disease.[15,16] It is not, however, a function test. Amylase is particularly useful in the diagnosis of acute pancreatitis, in which significant increases in serum concentrations occur in about 75% of patients. Typically, amylase in serum increases within a few hours of the onset of the disease, reaches a peak in about 24 hours, and because of its clearance by the kidneys returns to normal within 3 to 5 days, often making urine amylase a more sensitive indicator of acute pancreatitis. The magnitude of the enzyme elevation cannot be correlated with the severity of the disease.

CASE STUDY 28.3

Parents brought their 7-year-old son to the pediatrician with the complaint of frequent fevers and failure to grow. The child had three bouts of pneumonia during the past 2 years and was bothered by chronic bronchitis, which caused him to cough up copious amounts of thick, yellow, mucoid sputum. Despite a big appetite, he had gained only 1 to 2 lb in the past 2 years and was of short, frail stature. He especially liked salty foods. He usually had three or four bulky, foul-smelling bowel movements daily. A 9-year-old sister was in excellent health.

Questions

1. What is the most likely disease?
2. What clinical laboratory test would be most informative, and what results would be expected?
3. What other clinical laboratory tests would likely be abnormal?

Determination of the renal clearance of amylase is useful in detecting minor or intermittent increases in the serum concentration of this enzyme. To correct for diminished glomerular function, the most useful expression is the ratio of amylase clearance to creatinine clearance, as follows:

$$\frac{\% \text{ Amylase clearance}}{\text{Creatinine}} = 100 \times \frac{\text{UA}}{\text{SA}} \times \frac{\text{SC}}{\text{UC}} \quad \text{(Eq. 28-1)}$$

where UA is urine amylase, SA is serum amylase, SC is serum creatinine, and UC is urine creatinine.

Normal values are less than 3.1%. Significantly increased values, averaging about 8% or 9%, occur in acute pancreatitis but may also occur in other conditions, such as burns, sepsis, and diabetic ketoacidosis.

The use of serum lipase in the clinical detection of pancreatic disease has been compromised in the past by technical problems inherent in the various analytic methods. Improved analytic methods appear to indicate that lipase increases in serum about as soon as amylase in acute pancreatitis and that increased levels persist somewhat longer than those of amylase. Consequently, some physicians consider lipase more sensitive than amylase as an indicator of acute pancreatitis or other causes of pancreatic necrosis.

Both amylase and lipase may be significantly increased in serum in many other conditions (e.g., opiate administration, pancreatic carcinoma, intestinal infarction, obstruction or perforation, and pancreatic trauma). Amylase levels are also frequently increased in mumps, cholecystitis, hepatitis, cirrhosis, ruptured ectopic pregnancy, and macroamylasemia, which is a benign condition in which amylase binds to an immunoglobulin molecule, causing chronic elevation of serum amylase values but normal urine amylase levels. Lipase levels are often significantly increased in bone fractures and in association with fat embolism.

FECAL ELASTASE

Elastase-1 is a chymotrypsin-like enzyme secreted by the pancreas. The measurement of this enzyme in stool has been proposed as a sensitive test of pancreatic function.[17–19] **Fecal elastase** is performed on random stool samples and has the advantage of being noninvasive. It has been shown to be useful in the diagnosis of cystic fibrosis in children.[20,21]

The reference range for fecal elastase for normal greater than 200 μg/g, moderate pancreatic insufficiency is between 100 and 200 μg/g and severe pancreatic insufficiency is less than 100 μg/g.

PHYSIOLOGY AND BIOCHEMISTRY OF GASTRIC SECRETION

Gastric secretion occurs in response to various stimuli[22]:

- Neurogenic impulses from the brain transmitted by means of the vagal nerves (e.g., responses to the sight, smell, or anticipation of food)
- Distention of the stomach with food or fluid
- Contact of protein breakdown products, termed **secretagogues**, with the gastric mucosa
- The hormone **gastrin** is the most potent stimulus to gastric secretion; it is secreted by specialized G cells in the gastric mucosa and the duodenum in response to vagal stimulation and contact with secretagogues.

Inhibitory influences include high gastric acidity, which decreases the release of gastrin by the gastric G cells. Gastric inhibitory polypeptide is secreted by K cells in the middle and distal duodenum and proximal jejunum in response to food products such as fats, glucose, and amino acids. Vasoactive intestinal polypeptide, produced by H cells in the intestinal mucosa, directly inhibits gastric secretion, gastrin release, and gastric motility.

Gastric fluid has a high content of hydrochloric acid, pepsin, and mucus. Hydrochloric acid is secreted against a hydrogen ion gradient as great as 1 million times the concentration in plasma (i.e., gastric fluid can reach a pH of 1.2 to 1.3 under conditions of augmented or maximal stimulation). **Pepsin** refers to a group of relatively weak proteolytic enzymes, with pH optima from about 1.6 to 3.6, that catalyze all native proteins except mucus. The most important component of gastric secretion in terms of body physiology is **intrinsic factor**, which greatly facilitates the absorption of vitamin B_{12} in the ileum.

CLINICAL ASPECTS OF GASTRIC ANALYSIS

Gastric analysis is used in clinical medicine mainly for the following purposes[23,24]:

- Gastric analysis was once widely used in clinical medicine but has now been largely replaced by fiberoptic endoscopy and improved radiologic procedures.
- Gastric analysis is used clinically mainly to detect hypersecretion characteristics of the *Zollinger-Ellison syndrome*. This syndrome involves a gastrin-secreting neoplasm, usually located in the pancreatic islets, and exceptionally high plasma gastrin concentrations. Basal 1-hour secretion usually exceeds 10 mmol, and the ratio of basal 1-hour to maximal secretion usually exceeds 60% (i.e., the stomach is not really in the basal state but rather is pathologically stimulated by the high plasma gastrin level).

Gastric analysis is also used occasionally to evaluate pernicious anemia in adults. Gastric atrophy is present in this condition, and the stomach fails to secrete intrinsic factor, which binds to vitamin B_{12} to prevent its degradation by gastric acid. The pH of gastric fluid in this condition typically does not fall below 6, even with maximum stimulation. Rarely, gastric analysis may aid in determining the type of surgical procedure required for ulcer treatment.

Previously, various substances were used to stimulate gastric secretion (e.g., caffeine, alcohol, and test meals), but these are submaximal stimuli and obsolete. From 1953 until the late 1970s, histamine acid phosphate was used as a maximal stimulus to gastric secretion. Because of adverse effects, some of them severe, histamine has now been replaced by pentagastrin, which is a synthetic pentapeptide composed of the four C-terminal amino acids of gastrin linked to a substituted alanine derivative.

Normal gastric fluid is translucent, pale gray, and slightly viscous and often has a faintly acrid odor. Residual volume should not exceed 75 mL. Residual specimens occasionally contain flecks of blood or are green, brown, or yellow from reflux of bile during the intubation procedure. The presence of food particles is abnormal and indicates obstruction.

TESTS OF GASTRIC FUNCTION

Measuring Gastric Acid in Basal and Maximal Secretory Tests

After an overnight fast, gastric analysis is usually performed as a 1-hour basal test, followed by a 1-hour stimulated test subsequent to pentagastrin administration (6 μg/kg subcutaneously).[25,26] Test results reveal wide overlap among healthy subjects and diseased patients, except for anacidity (e.g., in pernicious anemia) and the extreme hypersecretion found in Zollinger-Ellison syndrome. Gastric peptic ulcer is usually associated with normal secretory volume and acid output. Duodenal peptic ulcer is usually associated with increased secretory volume in both the basal and maximal secretory tests; considerable overlap occurs, nevertheless, with the normal range.

Measuring Gastric Acid

In stimulated secretion specimens, the ability of the stomach to secrete against a hydrogen ion gradient is determined by measuring the pH. The total acid output in a timed interval is determined from the titratable acidities and volumes of the component specimens. After intubation, the residual secretion is aspirated and retained. Secretion for the subsequent 10 to 30 minutes is discarded to allow for adjustment of the patient to the intubation procedure. Specimens are ordinarily obtained as 15-minute collections for a period of 1 hour.

The gastrin response to intravenous secretin stimulation may be used to investigate patients with mildly elevated serum gastrin levels. In this test, pure porcine secretin is injected intravenously, and gastrin levels are collected at 5-minute intervals for the next 30 minutes. In patients with Zollinger-Ellison syndrome, the gastrin level increases at least 100 pg/mL over the basal level. Patients with ordinary peptic ulceration, achlorhydria, or other conditions show a slight decrease in gastrin concentration.

The volume, pH, and titratable acidity and the calculated acid output of each specimen are reported, as are the total volume and acid output for each test period (sum of the component specimens). There is considerable variation in gastric acid output among healthy subjects in both the basal and maximal secretory tests. Nevertheless, in the basal test, most healthy subjects secrete 0 to 6 mmol of acid in a total volume of 10 to 100 mL. In the maximal 1-hour test, using histamine or pentagastrin as the stimulus, most men secrete 1 to 40 mmol of acid in a total volume of 40 to 350 mL. Women and older persons usually secrete somewhat less acid than do young men.

Plasma Gastrin

Measurement of plasma gastrin levels is invaluable in diagnosing Zollinger-Ellison syndrome, in which fasting levels typically exceed 1,000 pg/mL and can reach 400,000 pg/mL, compared with the normal range of 50 to 150 pg/mL.[23,27] Gastrin is usually not increased in simple peptic ulcer disease. Increased plasma gastrin levels do occur in most pernicious anemia patients but decrease toward normal when hydrochloric acid is artificially instilled into the stomach.

INTESTINAL PHYSIOLOGY

Digestion, predominantly a function of the small intestine, is the process in which starches, proteins, lipids, nucleic acids, and other complex molecules are degraded to monosaccharides, amino acids and oligopeptides, fatty acids, purines, pyrimidines, and other simple constituents. For most large molecules, digestion is necessary for absorption to occur. Each day, the duodenum receives about 7 to 10 L of ingested water and food and secretion from the salivary glands, stomach, pancreas, and biliary tract. The materials then enter the jejunum and ileum, where another 1 to 1.5 L of secretion is added. Ultimately, however, only about 1.5 L of fluid material reaches the *cecum*, which is the first portion of the colon or large intestines. This considerable absorptive capability is possible because the small intestine (about 20 ft long) has numerous mucosal folds, minute projections from the luminal surface called *villi*, and microscopic projections on the mucosal cells called *microvilli*, all of which greatly increase the secretory and absorptive surface to an estimated 200 m². Absorption takes place by passive diffusion for some substances and by active transport for others. In addition, the small intestine actively secretes electrolytes and other metabolic products. The large intestine (about 5 ft long) has two major functions: water resorption, in which the 1.5 L of fluid received by the cecum is reduced to about 100 to 300 mL of feces, and storage of feces before defecation. The abdominal structures that constitute the alimentary tract are shown diagrammatically in Figure 28.3.

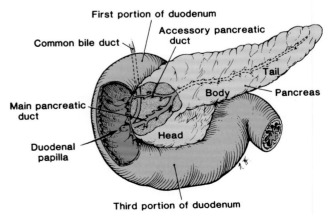

FIGURE 28.3 The abdominal structures of the alimentary tract.

CLINICOPATHOLOGIC ASPECTS OF INTESTINAL FUNCTION

Clinical chemistry testing of intestinal function focuses almost entirely on the evaluation of absorption and its derangements in various disease states. As discussed in the Pancreatic Function section of this chapter, diseases of the exocrine pancreas and biliary tract may also cause malabsorption. Intestinal diseases that may cause the malabsorption syndrome are highly varied in their etiology, pathogenesis, and severity. These intestinal diseases and disorders include tropical and nontropical or celiac sprue, Whipple's disease, Crohn's disease, primary intestinal lymphoma, small intestinal resection, intestinal lymphangiectasia, ischemia, amyloidosis, and giardiasis. In addition to the malabsorption syndrome, which ordinarily causes impaired absorption of fats, proteins, carbohydrates, and other substances, specific malabsorption states also occur (e.g., acquired deficiency of lactase, which prevents normal absorption of lactose, and Hartnup syndrome, a genetic disorder that involves deficient intestinal transport of phenylalanine and leucine).

CASE STUDY 28.4

A 34-year-old man was admitted for diagnostic evaluation with the complaint of epigastric pain of 2 years' duration, which was variously described as gnawing or burning. He had been diagnosed with a duodenal peptic ulcer 18 months ago; at that time, therapy of antacids and dietary revision provided considerable alleviation of symptoms. More recently, the pain had become more persistent and awakened the patient 4 to 6 times each night. Radiologic studies revealed a 2.5-cm ulcer crater in the first portion of the duodenum and a 0.5-cm ulcer in the antrum of the stomach. Serum electrolytes were normal. Hemoglobin was 8.3 g/dL with normal red blood cell indices. White blood count was 13,100. Gastric analysis revealed 640 mL of secretion in the basal hour, with an acid output of 38 mmol, and 780 mL of secretion in the 1-hour pentagastrin stimulation test, with an acid output of 48 mmol.

Questions

1. What is the probable disease?
2. In view of existing data, what other test would be virtually diagnostic for this disease?
3. What is the explanation for decreased hemoglobin and increased white blood cell count?

TESTS OF INTESTINAL FUNCTION

Lactose Tolerance Test

The disaccharidases, lactase (which cleaves lactose into glucose and galactose) and sucrase (which cleaves sucrose into glucose and fructose), are produced by the mucosal cells of the small intestine.[28,29] Congenital deficiencies of these enzymes are rare, but acquired deficiencies of lactase are commonly found in adults. Affected patients experience abdominal discomfort, cramps, and diarrhea after ingesting milk or milk products. About 10% to 20% of white Americans and 75% of African Americans are affected.

Lactose tolerance testing was used to establish this diagnosis, but the test is subject to many false-positive and false-negative results. This test has largely been replaced by hydrogen breath testing.

D-Xylose Absorption Test

D-Xylose is a pentose sugar that is ordinarily not present in the blood in any significant amount.[30,31] As with other monosaccharides, pentose sugars are absorbed unaltered in the proximal small intestine and do not require the intervention of pancreatic lytic enzymes. Therefore, the ability to absorb D-xylose is of value in differentiating malabsorption of intestinal etiology from that of exocrine pancreatic insufficiency. Because only about one-half of orally administered D-xylose is metabolized or lost by action of intestinal bacteria, significant amounts are excreted unchanged in the urine. Some protocols have used the measurement of only the D-xylose excreted in the urine during the 5 hours following ingestion of a 25-g dose by a fasting adult (0.5 g/kg in a child). Even with normal renal function, false-positive and false-negative results frequently occur. Blood levels measured one or more times after ingestion of D-xylose (e.g., at 30 minutes, 1 hour, or 2 hours) significantly improve the diagnostic reliability of the test. Some protocols use smaller doses of D-xylose to avoid abdominal cramps, intestinal hypermotility, and osmotic diarrhea that frequently accompany the 25-g dose.

D-Xylose Test

After ingestion of a specified solution of D-xylose, blood specimens are obtained and urine is collected for a 5-hour period to determine the extent of D-xylose absorption. The concentration of D-xylose is determined by heating protein-free supernates of urine and plasma to convert xylose to furfural, which is then reacted with *p*-bromoaniline to form a pink product, the absorbance of which is measured at 520 nm. Thiourea is added as an antioxidant to prevent the formation of interfering chromogens. After an overnight fast, the patient voids and drinks a D-xylose solution: 25 g of D-xylose in 250 mL of water for adults and 0.5 g/kg for children, or other dose as established. The patient drinks an equivalent amount of water during the next hour. No additional food or fluids are to be taken until the test is completed. Urine is collected for 5 hours after the D-xylose ingestion. A blood specimen is collected in potassium oxalate at 2 hours (commonly, 1 hour is chosen for children).

Normal blood concentrations of D-xylose in association with decreased urine excretion suggest impairment of renal function or incomplete urine collection. Aspirin therapy diminishes renal excretion of D-xylose, whereas indomethacin decreases intestinal absorption. After ingestion of a 25-g dose of D-xylose, healthy adults should excrete at least 4 g in the 5-hour period. For infants and children, the excretion following a dose of 0.5 g/kg for various ages expressed as

TABLE 28.1 D-Xylose Results for Pediatric Patients[2,4]

Age	Reference Range
Younger than 6 mo	11%–33%
6–12 mo	20%–32%
1–3 y	20%–42%
3–10 y	25%–45%
Older than 10 y	25%–50%

percentages of ingested dose are shown in Table 28.1. Blood levels for healthy adults vary widely, but a blood concentration of less than 25 mg/dL at 2 hours should be considered abnormal after the 25-g dose. With the 0.5 g/kg dose, infants younger than 6 months should have a blood concentration of at least 15 mg/dL at 1 hour, infants older than 6 months and children should achieve levels of at least 30 mg/dL.

Serum Carotenoids

Carotenoids are various yellow to orange or purple pigments that are widely distributed in animal tissue; they are synthesized by many plants and impart a yellow color to some vegetables and fruits. The major carotenoids in human serum are lycopene, xanthophyll, and beta carotene, the chief precursor of vitamin A in humans. Being fat soluble, carotenoids are absorbed in the small intestine in association with lipids. Malabsorption of lipids typically results in a serum concentration of carotenoids lower than the reference range of 50 to 250 mg/dL. Starvation, dietary idiosyncrasies, and fever also cause diminished serum concentrations. The test does not distinguish among the various etiologies of malabsorption.

Other Tests of Intestinal Malabsorption

Deficiencies of numerous analytes can occur in association with intestinal malabsorption. Measurement of these analytes is usually of value, not so much in confirming the diagnosis of malabsorption as in determining the extent of nutritional deficiency and, thus, the need for replacement therapy. Diminished appetite and dietary intake are usually more severe in patients who have malabsorption with an intestinal etiology. Body wasting or cachexia may be severe. Frequently, because loss of albumin into the intestinal lumen and diminished dietary intake of protein accompany the diminished absorption of oligopeptides and amino acids, a negative nitrogen balance occurs together with decreased serum total proteins and albumin. A serum albumin of less than 2.5 g/dL is much more characteristic of intestinal disease than of pancreatic disease. In association with severe disease of the small intestine, deficiencies of fat-soluble vitamins A, D, E, and K occur. Vitamin K deficiency, in turn, causes deficiencies of vitamin K–dependent coagulation factors II (prothrombin), VII (proconvertin), IX (plasma thromboplastin component), and X (Stuart-Prower factor), which are reflected in abnormal prothrombin time and partial thromboplastin time tests.

In severe small intestinal disease, such as tropical or celiac sprue, malabsorption of folate and vitamin B_{12} can occur, and megaloblastic anemia is rather common and is of some

benefit in distinguishing intestinal from pancreatic disease. Absorption of iron is usually diminished, and the tendency toward low serum iron levels may be aggravated by intestinal blood loss. Intestinal absorption of calcium is often diminished as a result of calcium binding by unabsorbed fatty acids and accompanying vitamin D deficiency and decreased serum magnesium. Because sodium, potassium, water absorption, and metabolism may also be seriously deranged, serum sodium and potassium levels are decreased and dehydration occurs. Impaired absorption of carbohydrates in intestinal diseases, such as sprue, results in decreased to flat blood concentration curves in glucose, lactose, and sucrose tolerance tests.

CASE STUDY 28.5

A 26-year-old woman appeared in the outpatient clinic with the complaint of abdominal discomfort, diarrhea, and an 18-lb, unintentional weight loss during the past 2 to 3 years. She related a similar period of 5 or 6 years of abdominal distress and diarrhea in childhood, but this essentially disappeared when she was about 12 to 13 years old. She was now having three to five bowel movements daily, which were described as bulky, malodorous, and floating. She weighed 106 lb and was 67 in. tall. She never had surgical procedures. Physical examination revealed poor skin turgor, general pallor, and a protuberant abdomen. Abnormal clinical laboratory values included those in Case Study Table 28.5.1.

Fecal examination revealed no ova or parasites, and bacteriologic culture revealed no pathogens.

CASE STUDY TABLE 28.5.1   Laboratory Results

Analyte	Result
Hemoglobin	8.1 g/dL
Hematocrit	30%
RBC count	$4.1 \times 10^6/\mu L$
Serum sodium	134 mmol/L
Potassium	3.4 mmol/L
Serum carotenoids	14 µg/dL
Fecal fat	22 g/24 h
D-Xylose absorption test (25-g dose)	5-h excretion of 1.3 g and blood level at 2 h of 8 mg/dL
Prothrombin time	15.8 s (12–14 s)
Activated partial thromboplastin time	56 s (30–45 s)

Questions

1. What is the disease process?
2. What is the probable etiology in this case?
3. What is the cause of the abnormal coagulation tests?
4. What is the probable major cause for the anemia, and what are other possible contributing causes?

For additional student resources, please visit thePoint® at http://thepoint.lww.com

questions

1. Laboratory findings in pancreatitis include all of the following EXCEPT
   a. Increased cortisol
   b. Increased amylase
   c. Increased lipase
   d. Increased triglycerides

2. Which of the following tests is a direct determination of the exocrine secretory capacity of the pancreas?
   a. Secretin/CCK test
   b. Amylase
   c. Quantitative fecal fat analysis
   d. D-Xylose test
   e. Lactose tolerance test

3. Which of the following statements concerning cystic fibrosis is NOT correct?
   a. Affects males and females about equally
   b. Occurs predominantly in populations of Northern European extraction
   c. Frequently diagnosed by measurement of sweat chloride
   d. Caused by a variety of mutations on chromosome 7
   e. Genetic screening is usually unsuccessful

4. The proper time period for the collection of a fecal fat specimen is
   a. 72 hours
   b. 24 hours
   c. 36 hours
   d. 48 hours
   e. 96 hours

5. Which of the following tests is only of the absorptive ability of the intestine?
   a. D-Xylose test
   b. Lactose tolerance test

   c. Fecal fat (72-hour collection)
   d. Serum carotenoids
   e. Serum albumin

6. A serum albumin of less than 2.5 g/dL would be most indicative of
   a. Intestinal disease
   b. Pancreatitis
   c. Peptic ulcer
   d. Pancreatic carcinoma

7. Which of the following is accurate when describing or diagnosing Zollinger-Ellison syndrome?
   a. Extreme hyposecretion of gastrin in the stomach
   b. Extreme hypersecretion of gastrin in the duodenum
   c. An increase in serum gastrin levels of 100 pg/mL following intravenous exposure to secretin
   d. A decrease in serum gastrin levels of 100 pg/mL following intravenous exposure to secretin
   e. Is confirmed when the hydrogen breath test is positive

8. The D-xylose absorption test is particularly helpful in differentiating malabsorption of intestinal etiology from exocrine pancreatic insufficiency because:
   a. D-Xylose is mostly absorbed in the stomach and then secreted via the kidney in its unaltered monosaccharide form.
   b. D-Xylose is mostly altered in the small intestine to facilitate its absorption across this membrane and metabolized by the liver so its metabolites may be excreted via the kidney.
   c. D-Xylose is mostly absorbed, not typically found in the blood, unaltered in the small intestine, and excreted unaltered via the kidney.
   d. None of the above describe why the D-xylose test is useful in identifying malabsorption diseases.

suggested reading

Berger HG, Buchler M, Kozarek R, et al. *An Integrated Textbook of Basic Science, Medicine and Surgery*. Indianapolis, IN: Wiley-Blackwell; 2008.

Feldman M, Friedman LS, Brandt LJ. *Sleisenger and Fordtran's Gastrointestinal and Liver Disease: Pathophysiology, Diagnosis, Management*. St. Louis, MO: WB Saunders; 2006.

references

1. Scotet V, Gillet D, Dugueperoux I, et al. Spatial and temporal distribution of cystic fibrosis and of its mutations in Brittany, France: a retrospective study from 1960. *Hum Genet.* 2002;111:247–254.

2. Corbetta C, Seia M, Bassotti A, et al. Screening for cystic fibrosis in newborn infants: results of a pilot programme based on a two tier protocol (IRT/DNA/IRT) in the Italian population. *J Med Screen.* 2002;9:60–63.

3. Gregg AR, Simpson JL. Genetic screening for cystic fibrosis. *Obstet Gynecol Clin North Am.* 2002;29:329–340.
4. Walsh MK. Diagnosis, prognosis, and treatment of acute pancreatitis. *Am Fam Physician.* 2008;77:594.
5. Lankish PG. Chronic pancreatitis. *Curr Opin Gastroenterol.* 2007;23:502–507.
6. Schibli S, Corey M, Gaskin KJ, et al. Towards the ideal quantitative pancreatic function test: analysis of test variables that influence validity. *Clin Gastroenterol Hepatol.* 2006;4:90–97.
7. Leus J, Van Biervliet S, Robberecht E. Detection and follow up of exocrine pancreatic insufficiency in cystic fibrosis: a review. *Eur J Pediatr.* 2000;159:563–568.
8. Simko V. Sudan stain and quantitative fecal fat. *Gastroenterology.* 1990;98:1722–1723.
9. Huang G, Khouri MR, Shiau YF. Sudan stain of fecal fat: new insight into an old test. *Gastroenterology.* 1989;96 (2 pt 1):421–427.
10. Kunz P, Künnecke B, Kunz I, et al. Natural abundance 13C-NMR spectroscopy for the quantitative determination of fecal fat. *Clin Biochem.* 2003;36:505–510.
11. Voortman G, Gerrits J, Altavilla M, et al. Quantitative determination of fecal fatty acids and triglycerides by Fourier transform infrared analysis with a sodium chloride transmission flow cell. *Clin Chem Lab Med.* 2002;40:795–798.
12. Baumer JH. Evidence based guidelines for the performance of the sweat test for the investigation of cystic fibrosis in the UK. *Arch Dis Child.* 2003;88:1126–1127.
13. Wang L, Freedman SD. Laboratory tests for the diagnosis of cystic fibrosis. *Am J Clin Pathol.* 2002;117(suppl):S109–S115.
14. De Boeck K, Wilschanski M, Castellani C, et al. Diagnostic Working Group. Cystic fibrosis: terminology and diagnostic algorithms. *Thorax.* 2006;61:627–635.
15. Matull WR, Pereira SP, O'Donohue JW. Biochemical markers of acute pancreatitis. *J Clin Pathol.* 2006;59:340–344.
16. Kylänpää-Bäck ML, Repo H, Kemppainen E. New laboratory tests in acute pancreatitis. *Addict Biol.* 2002;7:181–190.
17. Lüth S, Teyssen S, Forssmann K, et al. Fecal elastase-1 determination—"Gold Standard" of indirect pancreatic function tests? *Scand J Gastroenterol.* 2001;36(10):1092–1099.
18. Erickson JA, Aldeen WE, Grenache DG, et al. Evaluation of a fecal pancreatic elastase-1 enzyme-linked immunosorbent assay: assessment versus an established assay and

implication in classifying pancreatic function. *Clin Chim Acta.* 2008;397(1–2):87–91.
19. Qualia CM, Villalona JF, Ren C, et al. Specificity of the polyclonal antibody test system for human elastase in stool. *J Pediatr Gastroenterol Nutr.* 2007;45:E26–E66.
20. Daftary A, Acton J, Heubi J, et al. Fecal elastase-1: utility in pancreatic function in cystic fibrosis. *J Cystic Fibrosis.* 2006;2(5):71–76.
21. Keim V, Teich N, Moessner J. Value of polyclonal elastase ELISA for diagnosis of chronic pancreatitis. *Pancreas.* 2000;21(4):484.
22. Schubert ML. Gastric secretion. *Curr Opin Gastroenterol.* 2007;23:595–601.
23. Hung PD, Schubert ML, Mihas AA. Zollinger-Ellison syndrome. *Curr Treat Options Gastroenterol.* 2003;6:163–170.
24. Metz DC, Starr JA. A retrospective study of the usefulness of acid secretory testing. *Aliment Pharmacol Ther.* 2000;14:103–111.
25. Hirschowitz BI, Simmons J, Mohnen J. Long-term lansoprazole control of gastric acid and pepsin secretion in ZE and non-ZE hypersecretors: a prospective 10-year study. *Aliment Pharmacol Ther.* 2001;15:1795–1806.
26. Berger AC, Gibril F, Venzon DJ, et al. Prognostic value of initial fasting serum gastrin levels in patients with Zollinger-Ellison syndrome. *J Clin Oncol.* 2001;19:3051–3057.
27. Metz DC, Buchanan M, Purich E, et al. A randomized controlled crossover study comparing synthetic porcine and human secretions with biologically derived porcine secretin to diagnose Zollinger-Ellison syndrome. *Aliment Pharmacol Ther.* 2001;15:669–676.
28. Korpela R, Peuhkuri K, Poussa T. Comparison of a portable breath hydrogen analyser (Micro H2) with a Quintron MicroLyzer in measuring lactose maldigestion, and the evaluation of a Micro H2 for diagnosing hypolactasia. *Scand J Clin Lab Invest.* 1998;58:217–224.
29. Matthews SB, Waud JP, Roberts AG, et al. Systemic lactose intolerance: a new perspective on an old problem. *Postgrad Med J.* 2005;81:167–173.
30. Farrell RJ, Kelly CP. Diagnosis of celiac sprue. *Am J Gastroenterol.* 2001;96:3237–3246.
31. Uil JJ, van Elburg RM, van Overbeek FM, et al. Clinical implications of the sugar absorption test: intestinal permeability test to assess mucosal barrier function. *Scand J Gastroenterol Suppl.* 1997;223:70–78.

29

Body Fluid Analysis

KYLE B. RIDING

chapter outline

Cerebrospinal Fluid
Serous Fluids
  Pleural Fluid
  Pericardial Fluid
  Peritoneal Fluid
Amniotic Fluid
  Hemolytic Disease of the Newborn
  Neural Tube Defects

Fetal Lung Maturity
Phosphatidylglycerol
Lamellar Body Counts
Sweat
Synovial Fluid
Questions
References

chapter objectives

Upon completion of this chapter, the clinical laboratorian should be able to do the following:

- Identify the source of amniotic fluid, cerebrospinal fluid, sweat, synovial fluid, pleural fluid, pericardial fluid, and peritoneal fluid.
- Describe the physiologic purpose of amniotic fluid, cerebrospinal fluid, sweat, synovial fluid, pleural fluid, pericardial fluid, and peritoneal fluid.
- Discuss the clinical utility and methods used to test amniotic fluid, cerebrospinal fluid, sweat, synovial fluid, pleural fluid, pericardial fluid, and peritoneal fluid.
- Correlate patient status when given appropriate laboratory results obtained from amniotic fluid, cerebrospinal fluid, sweat, synovial fluid, pleural fluid, pericardial fluid, and peritoneal fluid.
- Differentiate between a transudate and an exudate both in terms of their respective causes and laboratory results associated with each.

For additional student resources, please visit thePoint® at http://thepoint.lww.com

588

This chapter is designed to acquaint the reader with bodily fluids that are frequently analyzed in the clinical chemistry laboratory. The source, method of collection, physiologic purpose, and clinical utility of laboratory measurements for each of these body fluids are emphasized.

CEREBROSPINAL FLUID

Cerebrospinal fluid (CSF) is the liquid that surrounds the brain and spinal cord. The brain and spinal cord are covered by the meninges that consist of three layers: the dura mater, arachnoid, and pia mater (Fig. 29.1). The CSF flows between the arachnoid mater and the pia mater in an area referred to as the subarachnoid space. The three functions of the CSF are (1) physical support and protection, (2) provision of a controlled chemical environment to supply nutrients to the tissues and removal of wastes, and (3) intracerebral and extracerebral transport (Fig. 29.2).

The major and most obvious function of CSF is as a buoyant cushion for the brain. The denser brain floats in the less dense fluid, allowing movement within the skull. The significance of the cushion function is demonstrated by the result of a blow to the head. The initial shock is transferred to the entire brain, instead of inflicting damage to one area. The brain may be bruised at the side opposite the blow, depending on the force imparted.

The second major function of CSF is the maintenance of a constant chemical matrix for the CNS. Serum components may vary greatly, but constituent levels of CSF are maintained within narrow limits.

The transport function is described as a neuroendocrine role. The CSF is involved in the distribution of hypophyseal hormones within the brain and the clearance of hormones from the brain to the blood.

The total CSF volume is about 150 mL or about 8% of the total CNS cavity volume. The fluid is formed predominantly

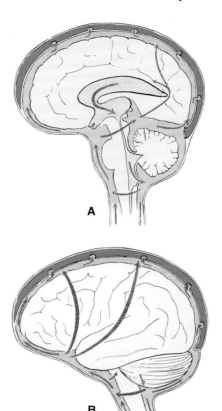

FIGURE 29.2 Major pathways of CSF. **(A)** Sagittal view. **(B)** Lateral view. (Reprinted from Milhorat TH. *Hydrocephalus and the Cerebrospinal Fluid*. Baltimore, MD: Lippincott Williams & Wilkins; 1972:25, with permission.)

at the choroid plexus deep within the brain and by the ependymal cells lining the ventricles. The endothelial cells of the choroid plexuses have very tight-fitting junctures to control the passage of substances across their membranes. This is termed the **blood–brain barrier**. Damage to the

Skin
Galea aponeurotica
Bone
Epidural space
Superior sagittal sinus
Dura mater
Subdural space
Arachnoid
Subarachnoid space
Pia mater

Falx cerebri
Cerebral hemisphere

FIGURE 29.1 Meninges of the brain.

blood–brain barrier is frequently the reason for abnormal chemistry results in CSF analysis.

CSF is formed at an average rate of about 0.4 mL/min or 500 mL/d. Formation is a result of selective ultrafiltration of plasma and active secretion by the epithelial membranes. Absorption of CSF occurs at outpouchings in the dura called **arachnoid villi**, also known as **granulations**, that protrude through the dura to the venous sinuses of the brain and into the bloodstream. The granulations act as one-way valves to maintain an excretion volume equal to the production volume.

Specimens of CSF are obtained by lumbar puncture, usually at the interspace of vertebrae L3 to L4 or lower, using aseptic technique (Fig. 29.3). The fluid obtained is usually separated into three numbered aliquots: (1) for chemistry and serology, (2) for microbiology, and (3) for hematology. In some instances, a fourth tube may be collected for cytology analysis. The order of the tubes reflects the presumed order for minimization of interference from less than optimal collection technique, with tube 3 presumably least contaminated by cells of intervening tissue. It is paramount to remember that this specimen is of limited volume and should be analyzed immediately. Any remaining sample should be preserved because of its limited availability.

Laboratory investigation of CSF is indicated for cases of suspected CNS infection, demyelinating disease, malignancy, and hemorrhage in the CNS. As with all patient samples entering the laboratory, physical examination of the specimen is the first and often the most important observation made. Normal CSF is clear, colorless, free of clots, and free of blood. Differences from these standards indicate a probable pathology and merit further examination. Cloudy fluids usually require microscopic examination, with a yellow to brown or red color indicating the presence of blood.

The two most common reasons for blood and hemoglobin pigments to be found in CSF are **traumatic tap** and **subarachnoid hemorrhage**. Traumatic tap is the artifactual presence of blood or derivatives due to interdiction of blood vessels during the lumbar puncture. Hemorrhage results from a breakdown of the barrier of the CNS and circulatory system from trauma, for example. Because of the life-threatening complications associated with hemorrhage, it must be differentiated from traumatic tap.

There are several ways to differentiate a traumatic tap from a subarachnoid hemorrhage. The first method involves comparing the amount of blood present between the collected tubes. If there is a significant difference in the amount of blood present between the first and last

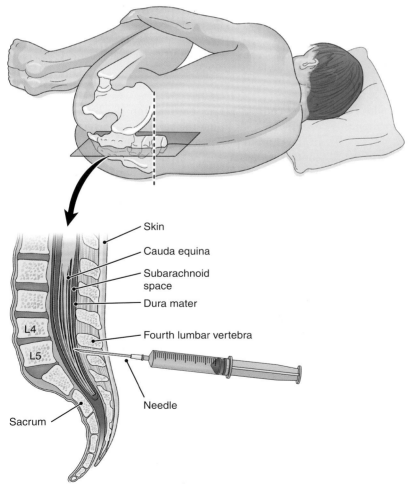

Skin
Cauda equina
Subarachnoid space
Dura mater
Fourth lumbar vertebra
L4
L5
Needle
Sacrum

FIGURE 29.3 Placement of the needle for CSF collection.

tubes collected (i.e., later tubes gradually clearing and less bloody), then the puncture was traumatic. If all tubes collected show the same degree of blood, then a subarachnoid hemorrhage is most likely. Figure 29.4 demonstrates the difference in appearance of normal clear CSF, red CSF in hemorrhage, xanthochromic CSF from an old hemorrhage, and CSF from a traumatic tap.[1]

A second method of discriminating between a traumatic tap and subarachnoid hemorrhage involves comparison of the appearance of the CSF precentrifugation and postcentrifugation. If the supernatant of the postcentrifugation sample appears colorless, the presence of blood is likely due to a traumatic tap. If the supernatant appears pink, red, or xanthochromic, hemorrhage should be suspected. This is due to red blood cells lysing easily in CSF due to the low level of proteins and lipids compared to that of plasma. The resultant in vivo hemolysis causes the release of free oxyhemoglobin that eventually changes to methemoglobin, and then after about 12 hours, bilirubin is formed (accounting for the xanthochromia). Gradual decrease in CSF color after a hemorrhage occurs over the first 2 days, clearing in about 2 to 4 weeks.[2]

FIGURE 29.4 Comparison of CSF appearance between **(A)** normal CSF (all three tubes with the same clarity), **(B)** red CSF from fresh hemorrhage (all three tubes with the same *red* color and opaqueness), **(C)** xanthochromic CSF from old hemorrhage (all three tubes with the same *yellow* color and clear), and **(D)** CSF from a traumatic tap (decreasing amounts of redness in each successive tube). Note: Full color image on thePoint at http://thepoint.lww.com/.

Differentiation of a traumatic tap from a hemorrhage may also involve checking for the presence of a clot and/or hemosiderin-containing macrophages. Samples exhibiting signs of a traumatic tap may have clots present within the CSF and will exhibit no hemosiderin. Conversely, samples from a patient experiencing a subarachnoid hemorrhage will show no signs of fibrin clots but may contain hemosiderin-laden macrophages.

A wide variety of biochemical markers with CSF samples may be measured. However, in routine practice, the number of useful indicators involves only four analytes. The tests of interest are glucose, protein (total and specific), lactate, and glutamine. Before any chemical analysis, the sample should be centrifuged to avoid contamination by cellular elements.

Glucose enters the spinal fluid predominantly via a facilitative transport compared with a passive (diffusional) or an active (energy-dependent) transport. It is carried across the epithelial membrane by a stereospecific carrier species. The carrier mechanism is responsible for transport of lipid-insoluble materials across the membrane into the CSF. Generally, this is a "downhill" process consistent with a concentration gradient. This mechanism causes the CSF glucose concentration to be about two-thirds that of plasma.

Due to its dependence on plasma glucose concentrations, an isolated CSF glucose concentration may be misleading, and it is recommended that a plasma sample be obtained 2 to 4 hours prior to the tap so that plasma and CSF glucose levels can equilibrate. Normal CSF glucose is considered to be 60% to 70% that of the blood glucose. Increased glucose levels are not clinically significant, usually providing only confirmation of hyperglycemia. It is important to note that as hyperglycemia progresses and exceeds 600 mg/dL, the CSF glucose level does not remain at 60% to 70% of plasma values most likely due to cellular carriers being saturated and incapable of further transport. This saturation will cause the plasma/CSF glucose to decrease. For this reason, caution should be taken when comparing the plasma and CSF glucose values in a patient with severe hyperglycemia.

Decreased CSF glucose levels (**hypoglycorrhachia**) can be the result of (1) disorder in carrier-mediated transport of glucose into CSF, (2) active metabolism of glucose by cells or organisms, or (3) increased metabolism by the CNS. The pathophysiological mechanism of altered transport remains unclear, but it is speculated to be the cause of hypoglycorrhachia in tubercular meningitis and sarcoidosis. Acute bacterial, amebic, fungal, and trichinosis meningitis are examples of glucose consumption by organisms, whereas diffuse meningeal neoplasia and brain tumor are examples of glucose consumption by CNS tissue. Consumption of glucose is usually accompanied by an increased lactate level due to anaerobic glycolysis by organisms or cerebral tissue.

Protein levels in CSF reflect the selective ultrafiltration of the CSF blood–brain barrier. All protein usually found in plasma is found in CSF but at much lower levels. Total protein is about 0.5%, or 1%, that of plasma but the specific protein concentrations in CSF are not proportional to the plasma levels because of the specificity of the ultrafiltration process.

Because of this relationship of CSF and serum proteins, serum analysis should accompany CSF protein analysis.

A decreased level of CSF total protein can arise from (1) decreased dialysis from plasma, (2) increased protein loss (e.g., removal of excessive volumes of CSF), or (3) leakage from a tear in the dura, CSF otorrhea, or CSF rhinorrhea. The last reason is most common. A dural tear can occur as a result of a previous lumbar puncture or from severe trauma. **Otorrhea** and **rhinorrhea** refer to the leakage of CSF from the ear or into the nose, respectively. Identification of CSF leakage is best done by an analysis for β-transferrin, a protein unique to the CSF.

An increased level of CSF total protein is a useful nonspecific indicator of pathologic states. Increases may be caused by (1) lysis of contaminant blood from traumatic tap, (2) increased permeability of the epithelial membrane, (3) increased production by CNS tissue, or (4) obstruction. The presence of any amount of blood can elevate CSF protein levels because of the 200:1 concentration ratio. The blood–brain barrier becomes more permeable from bacterial or fungal infections. An increase in CNS production occurs in subacute sclerosing panencephalitis (SSPE) or multiple sclerosis (MS). There may also be combinations of permeability and production, with the collagen vascular diseases. An obstructive process, such as tumor or abscess, would also cause increased protein.

Diagnostically more sensitive information can be obtained by analysis of the protein fractions present. A comparison to the serum pattern is necessary for accurate conclusions. Under normal conditions, prealbumin is present in CSF in higher concentration than in serum. Although the respective proteins can be determined in both serum and CSF, the proteins of greatest interest are albumin and immunoglobulin G (IgG). Because albumin is produced solely in the liver, its presence in CSF must occur by means of blood–brain barrier passage. IgG, however, can arise by local synthesis from plasma cells within the CSF. The measurement of albumin in both serum and CSF is then used to normalize the IgG values from each matrix to determine the source of the IgG.

To determine the integrity of the blood–brain barrier, a CSF/serum albumin index is calculated as follows:

$$\frac{\text{CSF albumin (mg/dL)}}{\text{Serum albumin (g/dL)}} = \frac{\text{CSF serum}}{\text{albumin index}} \quad \text{(Eq. 29-1)}$$

An index value less than 9 indicates an intact blood–brain barrier.

This index can then be used to calculate the IgG index to determine CNS synthesis of IgG to aid the diagnosis of demyelinating diseases, such as MS and SSPE. MS is the most common inflammatory demyelinating disease of the CNS:

$$\frac{\text{CSF IgG/serum IgG}}{\text{CSF albumin serum albumin}} = \frac{\text{CSF IgG}}{\text{index}} \quad \text{(Eq. 29-2)}$$

The normal value is less than 0.73.

Increases in serum albumin cause increases in the CSF levels because of membrane permeability. However, increased CSF IgG, without concomitant CSF albumin increase, suggests local production (MS or SSPE). Increases in permeability and production are found with bacterial meningitis. Methods to analyze IgG and albumin CSF levels are the same as for serum but are optimized for the lower levels found.

Increased CSF protein levels or clinical suspicion usually indicates the need for electrophoretic separation of the respective proteins. At times, this separation demonstrates multiple banding of the IgG band. This observation is referred to as **oligoclonal bands** (a small number of clones of IgG from the same cell type with nearly identical electrophoretic properties). This occurrence is usually associated with inflammatory diseases and MS or SSPE. These types of disorders would stimulate the immunocompetent cells. The recognition of an oligoclonal pattern supersedes the report of normal protein levels and is a cause for concern if the corresponding serum separation does not demonstrate identical banding.

Another protein thought to be specific for MS is myelin basic protein (MBP). Initial reports suggested high specificity, but MBP has also been found in nondemyelinating disorders and does not always occur in demyelinating disorders. MBP levels are used to monitor therapy of MS. Current international guidelines for the diagnosis of MS recognize both an elevated IgG index and the presence of CSF oligoclonal bands that are not found in the serum as supporting evidence. Immunoassay procedures are available for analyzing MBP.[3]

Lactate is a useful indicator of anaerobic metabolism within the CSF. While the level of lactate in the CSF can potentially parallel that of the plasma, CSF elevations can occur independent of plasma concentrations under situations where anaerobic metabolism is occurring at an increased rate solely within the CNS. An increased lactate level with a normal to decreased glucose level has been suggested as a readily accessible indicator for bacterial meningitis. This finding is helpful in differentiating bacterial meningitis and other forms of infectious meningitis.[4] Analysis of glucose and lactate in CSF is easily accomplished by techniques used for plasma and serum. It is important that provision for the analysis of glucose or lactate in CSF be immediate or that the specimen be preserved with an antiglycolytic, such as sodium fluoride.

Glutamine is formed by the combination of ammonia and glutamate. It is hypothesized that the synthesis of glutamine is a means to reduce ammonia levels within the central nervous system. While the level of ammonia within CSF is difficult to accurately determine due to its relative instability, the level of glutamine within a CSF samples is reflective of the amount of ammonia present within the central nervous system. Glutamate elevations are frequently seen in patients with hepatic encephalopathy along with various other pathologies.

CASE STUDY 29.1

A 31-year-old man was in good health until about 1 year ago, after he began working as an accountant. Within the last year, he began to notice episodic blurring of vision, diplopia, mild vertigo, and headache. He complained of sensory loss in his hands and a feeling of weakness after physical exertion but thought that was just "out of shape." He went to his physician after suffering leg and shoulder weakness accompanied by a feeling of paralysis, which was followed by a sensation of "pins and needles" in his left leg. Neurologic examination led to a spinal tap being performed for laboratory findings and a brain and spinal cord magnetic resonance imaging (MRI). His MRI showed demyelinating lesions, and other ancillary tests showed demyelinating damage to the auditory and visual pathway. The laboratory results were as follows:

CSF	Clear, colorless fluid, apparently free of debris; culture yields no growth
WBC	Normal
Glucose	60 mg/dL (plasma = 80 mg/dL)
Total protein	59 mg/dL
Albumin index	1.7
IgG index	0.97
Electrophoresis	Oligoclonal bands present

Questions

1. What is the significance of the albumin index? The IgG index?
2. What pathology is consistent with these results?

SEROUS FLUIDS

The lungs, heart, and abdominal cavities are surrounded by two serous membranes: the parietal membrane lining the cavity wall and the visceral membrane lining the organs. Serous fluids, an ultrafiltrate of plasma, are located between the membranes. When *serum* dialyzes across these membranes, the fluid formed is called **serous fluid**—specifically, pleural (lung), pericardial (heart), and peritoneal (abdominal) fluid.

The formation of serous fluid is a continuous process driven by the hydrostatic pressure of the systemic circulation and maintenance of oncotic pressure due to protein. The potential space is usually fluid filled with no gases present. The fluid reduces or eliminates friction caused by expansion and contraction of the encased organs.

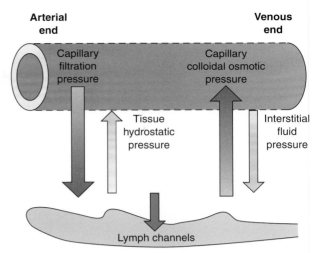

FIGURE 29.5 Forces governing the exchange of fluid at the capillary level.

Serous fluids, along with other extracellular fluids, account for 45% of the body's water volume and share common characteristics in regard to their chemical composition.[5] Various forces control the movement of fluids within the different extracellular compartments of the body. The tissue's colloidal osmotic pressure (interstitial fluid pressure), along with the capillary's hydrostatic pressure (filtration pressure), regulates the outward flow of fluid from the capillary. The colloidal osmotic pressure of the capillary and the tissue's hydrostatic pressure regulate the inward flow of fluid into the capillary from the tissue.[6] Figure 29.5 illustrates the direction of these forces. Furthermore, the lymphatic system removes the fluids entering into the interstitial space. Figure 29.6 shows the normal flow of fluids among the bloodstream, tissues, and lymphatic vessels.

Examining these biochemical and cellular alterations that occur to serous fluids can assist in diagnosing and monitoring the patient's condition.[7] Such alterations occur due to an imbalance in pressures that lead to excessive egress of fluid into tissue spaces that cause an accumulation of fluid that when noted is the typical indication for analysis of the serous fluid. This accumulation is called an **effusion**. Effusions are further classified as **transudate** or **exudate**. Proper classification of effusions is critical to patient care.

A transudate may occur during various systemic disorders that disrupt fluid filtration, fluid reabsorption, or both. Conditions such as congestive heart failure, hepatic cirrhosis, and nephrotic syndrome are examples of systemic disorders that may result in the formation of transudates. Exudate effusions occur during inflammatory processes that result in damage to blood vessel walls, body cavity membrane damage, or decreased reabsorption by the lymphatic system. Infections, inflammations, hemorrhages, and malignancies are examples of pathologic processes that can cause the formation of exudates. The formation of transudates and exudates can damage tissues and body cavity membranes and alter lymphatic function.

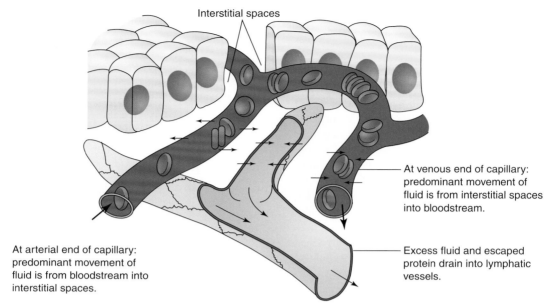

Interstitial spaces

At venous end of capillary: predominant movement of fluid is from interstitial spaces into bloodstream.

At arterial end of capillary: predominant movement of fluid is from bloodstream into interstitial spaces.

Excess fluid and escaped protein drain into lymphatic vessels.

FIGURE 29.6 Exchanges through capillary membranes in the formation and removal of interstitial fluid.

Various laboratory tests are used to differentiate between transudates and exudates, including fluid appearance, specific gravity, amylase, glucose, lactate dehydrogenase (LD), and proteins. Additional tests such as ammonia, lipids, and pH may be useful in confirming the cause of an effusion for specific body sites.

Pleural Fluid

The outer layer of the pleural space, the parietal layer, is served by the systemic circulation and the inner layer, the visceral layer, by the bronchial circulation. As with all serous fluids, pleural fluid is formed by the ultrafiltration of plasma through the parietal layer and is essentially interstitial fluid of the systemic circulation. With normal conditions, there is 3 to 20 mL of pleural fluid in the pleural space. The fluid exits by drainage into the lymphatics of the visceral pleura and the visceral circulation. Any alteration in the rate of formation or removal of the pleural fluid affects the volume, causing an effusion.

Once an effusion is identified, it is then necessary to classify the nature of the effusion by analysis of the pleural fluid. The fluid is removed from the pleural space by needle and syringe after visualization by radiology. This procedure is called **thoracentesis**; the fluid is called *thoracentesis fluid* or **pleural fluid** (Fig. 29.7). Samples are collected as follows: a heparinized tube for culture, an ethylenediaminetetraacetic acid (EDTA) tube for microscopy, a sodium fluorescein (NaF) tube for glucose and lactate, and a nonanticoagulated tube for further biochemical testing.

Transudates are secondary to remote (nonpleural) systemic pathologies and exhibit biochemical and cellular abnormalities consistent with noninflammatory changes in fluid dynamics within the pleural space. An example would be hypoproteinemia due to malnutrition leading to

decreased oncotic pressure and subsequent decrease in fluid reabsorption into the capillaries. An exudate indicates primary involvement of the pleura and lung, such as infection, and demands immediate attention. An example of an exudative process would be infection-mediated damage to the membranes, allowing increased fluid entry into the pleural space (Table 29.1).

The assignment of fluid to either the transudate or exudate category had previously been based on the protein concentration of the fluid. This criterion has been replaced

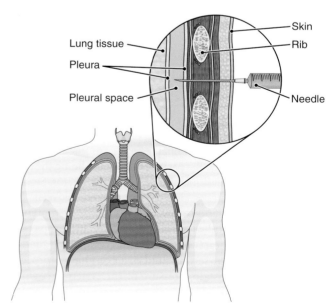

Lung tissue

Pleura

Pleural space

Skin

Rib

Needle

FIGURE 29.7 Thoracentesis. A needle is inserted into the pleural space to withdraw fluid. (From Cohen BJ. *Medical Terminology*. 4th ed. Philadelphia, PA: Lippincott Williams & Wilkins; 2004.)

TABLE 29.1	Causes of Pleural Effusions
Transudative	**Exudative**
Congestive heart failure[a]	Bacterial pneumonia[a]
Nephrotic syndrome	Tuberculosis
Hypoproteinemia	Pulmonary abscess
Hepatic cirrhosis	Malignancy (lymphatic obstruction)
Chronic renal failure	Viral/fungal infection
	Pulmonary infarction
	Pleurisy
	Pulmonary malignancy
	Lymphoma
	Pleural mesothelioma

[a]Most common cause.

by the use of a series of fluid/plasma (F/P) ratios known as Light's criteria. This criteria specifically state that if the F/P ratio for total protein is greater than 0.5 or the ratio for LD is greater than 0.6 (or the pleural fluid LD/upper limit serum LD ratio reference interval is >0.67), the fluid is an exudate. For pleural fluid, an additional characterization can be made by determining the pleural fluid cholesterol, the fluid-to-serum cholesterol ratio, and the fluid-to-serum bilirubin ratio. Exudates are indicated by fluid cholesterol greater than 60 mg/dL, fluid-to-serum cholesterol ratio greater than 0.3, and fluid-to-bilirubin ratio of 0.6 or higher.

Further characterization of the exudate by the chemistry laboratory may involve analysis for glucose, lactate, amylase, triglyceride, or pH. A decrease in glucose or increase in lactate would suggest infection or inflammation. An increase in amylase compared with that of serum suggests pancreatitis. Grossly elevated triglyceride levels (2 to 10× serum) could indicate thoracic duct leakage. The use of pH measurements, performed as one would perform a blood–gas level determination, has gained favor. Succinctly, pH less than 7.2 suggests infection, and pH close to 6.0 indicates esophageal rupture. The methodologies for these analyses are the same as those employed for the serum and blood constituents and, therefore, are feasible in the clinical laboratory.

Pericardial Fluid

The relationship of the pericardium, **pericardial fluid**, and the heart is similar to that with the lungs and pleural fluid. Mechanisms of formation and drainage are the same. Pericardial effusions are an accumulation of fluid around the heart caused by damage to the mesothelium and are usually always exudates. Figure 29.8 illustrates the pericardium surrounding the heart. Normally, the pericardium contains less than 50 mL of fluid. The procedure for removing excess pericardial fluid, pericardiocentesis, is dangerous and therefore rarely performed (Fig. 29.8). However, this procedure is necessary to obtain a sample if cultures are needed to investigate an infection or if cytology is needed for suspected malignancy.[8] Adenosine deaminase testing may also be requested in suspected cases of tubercular effusions.

FIGURE 29.8 Aspirating pericardial fluid. In pericardiocentesis, a needle and a syringe are inserted through the chest wall into the pericardial sac (as shown below). Electrocardiographic monitoring, with a lead wire attached to the needle and electrodes placed on the limbs (right arm, left arm, and left leg), helps ensure proper needle placement and avoids damage to the heart. (From *Nursing Procedures*. 4th ed. Ambler, PA: Lippincott Williams & Wilkins; 2004.)

CASE STUDY 29.2

A 65-year-old female patient was admitted with a progressive increase in breathlessness, orthopnea, jugular venous distention, chest pain, ankle edema, sacral edema, and swollen legs, arms, and hands over the previous 4 weeks. She suffered from dyspepsia, increasing over recent weeks, and the general practitioner had noted new heart murmurs. A pansystolic murmur was audible, and inspiratory crackles were heard throughout both lung fields. Muffled heart sounds were heard, possibly due to the muffling effect of fluid surrounding the heart. She could not walk a block to the grocery store without being totally exhausted and short of breath. She was afebrile with rapid breathing, with a low-volume pulse. Her sitting blood pressure was 100/60 mm Hg.

The ECG indicated sinus tachycardia with anterolateral Q waves indicating a previous infarction. Chest x-ray indicated cardiomegaly, interstitial edema, and fluid in the lower lungs. Routine chemistry showed serum Na^+ 129 mmol/L, K^+ 5.9 mmol/L, creatinine 157 mmol/L, and urea 9.1 mmol/L. Brain natriuretic peptide was elevated and troponin level was unremarkable.

The physician suspected progressive systolic dysfunction after myocardial infarction. An abnormality of the ECG in a breathless patient is a supportive evidence for a cardiac cause of dyspnea, while a normal ECG usually suggests another diagnosis.[9] Also, radiological cardiomegaly most often represents significant ventricular dilation or hypertrophy. A complication is the presence of increased

CASE STUDY 29.2 (continued)

pericardial fluid. Echocardiography provides definitive diagnosis. Echocardiography showed a dilated heart (left ventricular end-diastolic distention [LVEDD]) with apical dilation, compatible with previous anterior infarction, and with increased pericardial fluid.

Questions

1. Is this pericardial fluid most likely an exudate or a transudate? Under what conditions will the physician want to perform a pericardiocentesis to collect the fluid?
2. What condition does the patient most likely have?

Peritoneal Fluid

Excess fluid (>50 mL) in the peritoneal cavity indicates disease. The presence of excess **peritoneal fluid** is called **ascites**, and the fluid is called *ascitic fluid*. The process of obtaining samples of this fluid by needle aspiration is paracentesis (Fig. 29.9). Usually, the fluid is visualized by ultrasound to confirm its presence and volume before paracentesis is attempted.

The same mechanisms that cause serous effusions in other body cavities are operative for the peritoneal cavity. Specifically, a disturbance in the rate of dialysis secondary to a remote pathology is a transudate, compared with a primary pathology of the peritoneal membrane causing an exudate. The multiple factors that apply to this large space, such as renal and hepatic function, tend to cloud the distinction. The most common cause of transudative ascites is portal hypertension. Obstructions to hepatic flow, such as cirrhosis, congestive heart failure, and hypoalbuminemia for any reason also, demonstrate high incidence.

The exudative causes of ascites are predominantly metastatic ovarian, prostate, and colon cancer and infective peritonitis. The recommended method for differentiating transudates and exudates is the serum–ascites albumin gradient (SAAG). The SAAG is calculated by subtracting the fluid albumin level from the serum albumin level. A difference of 1.1 g/dL or more is used to indicate a transudative process while a difference of less than 1.1 g/dL indicates an exudative process. A neutrophil count greater than 250 cells/µm indicates peritonitis. Measurement of the tumor markers CEA and CA125 is indicated in suspected cases of malignancy.

CASE STUDY 29.3

A 47-year-old man was brought to the hospital by the police after falling to the pavement and being unable to rise. His admission laboratory values revealed the following:

Laboratory Values

Sodium 133 mmol/L (135–146 mmol/L)	A nonreactive acute hepatitis panel
Potassium 3.1 mmol/L (3.6–5.2 mmol/L)	Ammonia level 71 µmol/L (9–35 µmol/L)
Chloride 93 mmol/L (96–110 mmol/L)	White blood cell count was 6.9×10^3/µL (4.5–11×10^3/µL)
Creatinine 0.7 mg/dL (0.8–1.5 mg/dL)	Platelet count 101×10^3/µL (130–400×10^3/µL)
Blood urea nitrogen < 5 mg/dL (7–25 mg/dL)	Hemoglobin and hematocrit 13.4 g/dL (13.5–17.5 g/dL) and 38.7% (40%–51%)
Glucose 128 mg/dL (65–99 mg/dL)	Prothrombin time of 14.3 s (9.5–12.5 s), with an INR of 1.3 (0.9–1.1)
Total protein 6.9 g/dL (6–8 g/dL)	Normal partial thromboplastin time of 31.6 s
Albumin 2.4 g/dL (3.4–5.4 g/dL)	Alkaline phosphatase 241 U/L (20–120 U/L)
Total bilirubin of 8.0 mg/dL (<1.3 mg/dL)	AST 103 U/L (<45 U/L)
Acetaminophen level <10 µg/mL (10–20 µg/mL)	ALT 40 U/L (<46 U/L)

CASE STUDY 29.3 (continued)

An abdominal ultrasound was significant for the presence of ascites and a cirrhotic-appearing liver. The patient was admitted to the hospital for further evaluation and subsequent treatment of alcohol withdrawal and decompensated cirrhosis. He was put on a salt and protein-restricted diet and diuretics to manage ascites (accumulated fluid in the peritoneal cavity). He was treated with benzodiazepines and lactulose and placed on a diuretic regimen of furosemide 40 mg orally daily along with spironolactone 100 mg orally daily.

Ascitic fluid should be sampled in all inpatients and outpatients with new-onset ascites. If uncomplicated cirrhotic ascites is suspected, the initial specimen of ascitic fluid should be sent for cell count and differential, albumin, and total protein concentration. With the results of the above tests, the SAAG can be calculated.

Peritoneal Fluid	
White blood cell count of 8/µL with 26% segmented neutrophils	Total protein <3.0 g/dL
Albumin of <1.0 g/dL	Fluid culture = no growth

Alcoholic hepatitis is a syndrome of progressive inflammatory liver injury associated with long-term heavy intake of ethanol. Patients who are severely affected present with subacute onset of fever, hepatomegaly, leukocytosis, marked impairment of liver function (e.g., jaundice and coagulopathy), and manifestations of portal hypertension (e.g., ascites, hepatic encephalopathy, and variceal hemorrhage). However, milder forms of alcoholic hepatitis often may not cause any symptoms.

Questions

1. What lab tests are abnormal?
2. What will the SAAG value be, and how is it calculated?
3. How will diuretics reduce this excess fluid?
4. Why is his diet salt restricted?

AMNIOTIC FLUID

The amniotic sac provides an enclosed environment for fetal development. This sac is bilayered as the result of a fusion of the amniotic (inner) and chorionic (outer) membranes at an early stage of fetal development. The fetus is suspended in **amniotic fluid** (AF) within the sac. The AF provides a cushioning medium for the fetus, regulates the temperature of the fetal environment, allows fetal movement, and serves as a matrix for influx and efflux of constituents such as glucose, sodium, and potassium.

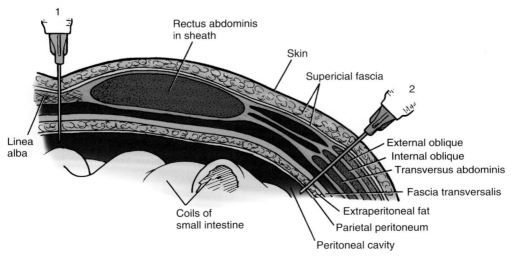

FIGURE 29.9 Paracentesis of the abdominal cavity in midline. (From Snell RS. *Clinical Anatomy*. 7th ed. Philadelphia, PA: Lippincott Williams & Wilkins; 2003.)

Depending on the interval of the gestational period, the fluid may be derived from different sources, but ultimately, the mother is the source of the AF. At the initiation of pregnancy, some maternal secretions cross the amnion and contribute to the volume. Shortly after formation of the placenta and embryo and fusion of membranes, AF is largely derived by transudation across the fetal skin. In the last half of pregnancy, the skin becomes substantially less permeable, and fetal micturition, or urination, becomes the major volume source.

The fate of the fluid also varies with the period of gestation. A bidirectional exchange is presumed to occur across the membranes and at the placenta. Similarly, during early pregnancy, the fetal skin is involved in exchange of AF. In the last half of pregnancy, the mechanism of fetal swallowing is the major fate of AF.

There is a dynamic balance established between production and clearance; fetal urination and swallowing maintain this balance. The continual swallowing maintains intimate contact of the AF with the fetal gastrointestinal tract, buccal cavity, and bronchotracheal tree. This contact is evidenced by the sloughed cellular material from the fetus that provides us with an indication of various fetal developmental milestones and functional stages.

A sample of fluid is obtained to analyze the cellular material and the biochemical constituents of the AF. This fluid is collected via transabdominal **amniocentesis** (amniotic sac puncture), which is performed under aseptic conditions. Before an attempt is made to obtain fluid, the positions of the placenta, fetus, and fluid pockets are visualized using ultrasonography. Aspiration of anything except fluid could lead to erroneous conclusions, as well as possible harm to the fetus (Fig. 29.10).

Amniocentesis and subsequent AF analysis are performed to test for congenital diseases, neural tube defects (NTDs), hemolytic disease, and fetal pulmonary development. Emphasis is placed on those conditions diagnosed or monitored using the clinical biochemistry laboratory.

Hemolytic Disease of the Newborn

The analysis of AF to screen for hemolytic disease of the newborn (erythroblastosis fetalis) was the first recognized laboratory procedure performed on AF. Hemolytic disease of the newborn is a syndrome of the fetus resulting from incompatibility between maternal and fetal blood, because of differences in either the ABO or Rh blood group systems. Maternal antibodies to fetal erythrocytes cause a hemolytic reaction that can vary in severity. The resultant hemoglobin breakdown products, predominantly bilirubin, appear in the AF and provide a measure of the severity of the incompatibility reaction.

The most commonly used method is a direct spectrophotometric scan of undiluted AF and subsequent calculation of the relative bilirubin amount. Classically, absorbance due to bilirubin is reported instead of a concentration of bilirubin. The method consisted of scanning AF from 550 to 350 nm against a water blank. The common method, the method of Liley,[10] requires the plotting of the absorbances at 5 nm intervals against wavelength, using semilogarithmic paper. A baseline is constructed by creating a line between the absorbance readings at 550 and 350 nm. An absorbance peak seen at 450 nm is a result of bilirubin within the AF. The larger the difference between baseline absorbance and peak absorbance at 450 nm is an indication of the level of bilirubin present within the AF. This direct observation is referred to as the ΔA_{450} (Fig. 29.11).

To avoid interference in the spectrophotometric scan, specimens should be immediately centrifuged and the fluid separated from the sediment. This will prevent not only particulate interference but also the possibility of increased lysis of red blood cells in the specimen producing hemoglobin in the AF. As with all specimens for bilirubin analysis,

FIGURE 29.10 Amniocentesis. A sample is removed from the amniotic sac for fetal abnormality testing.

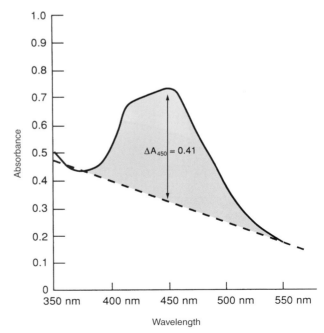

FIGURE 29.11 Change in A_{450} nm from AF bilirubin scan.

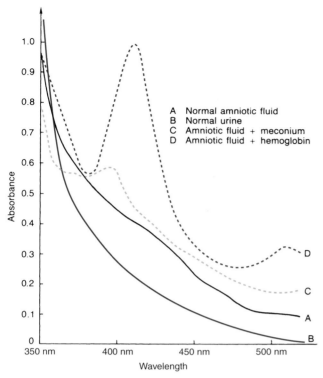

FIGURE 29.12 Amniotic fluid absorbance scans.

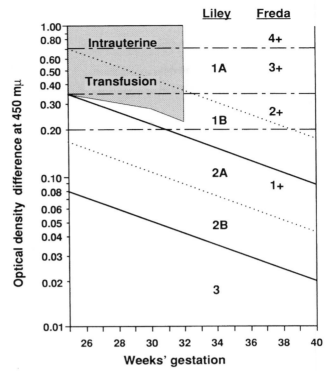

FIGURE 29.13 Assessment of fetal prognosis. Liley method: *1A*, *above broken line*, condition desperate, immediate delivery or transfusion; *1B*, between *broken* and *continuous lines*, hemoglobin greater than 8 g/100 mL, delivery or transfusion (*stippled area*) urgent; *2A*, between *continuous* and *broken lines*, hemoglobin 8 to 10 g/100 mL, delivery 36 to 37 weeks; *2B*, between *broken* and *continuous lines*, hemoglobin 11 to 13.9 g/100 mL, delivery 37 to 39 weeks; *3*, below *continuous line*, not anemic, delivery at term. Freda method: *4+*, above *upper horizontal line*, fetal death imminent, immediate delivery or transfusion; *3+*, between *upper* and *middle horizontal lines*, fetus in jeopardy, death within 3 weeks, delivery or transfusion as soon as possible; *2+*, between *middle* and *lower horizontal lines*, fetal survival for at least 7 to 10 days, repeat test, possible indication for transfusion; *1+*, below *lower horizontal line*, fetus in no immediate danger of death. (Adapted from Robertson JG. Evaluation of the reported methods of interpreting spectrophotometric tracings of amniotic fluid in rhesus isoimmunization. *Am J Obstet Gynecol.* 1966;95:120.)

AF specimens for bilirubin scans must be protected from light. Specimens are routinely collected in amber-colored tubes. Exposure to light results in the photo-oxidation of bilirubin to biliverdin that will not be detected at 450 nm, resulting in underestimation of the hemolytic disease severity.

Examples of interferences, compared with a normal specimen, are given in Figure 29.12. Each laboratory should compile its own catalog of real examples for spectrophotometric analysis. The presence of hemoglobin is identified by its peak absorbance at 410 to 415 nm; the presence of urine is identified by the broad curve and confirmed by creatinine and urea analyses; and the presence of meconium is identified by the distinctly greenish color of the AF and flat absorbance curve.

Care must be used in the interpretation of the spectra. A decision for treatment can be made based on the degree of hemolysis and gestational age. The rather limited treatment options are immediate delivery, intrauterine transfusion, and observation. The transfusion can be accomplished by means of the umbilical artery and titrated to the desired hematocrit. Several algorithms have been proposed to aid in decision making and are outlined in Figure 29.13.

Neural Tube Defects

Screening for NTDs is initially performed using maternal serum. The presence of elevated levels of α-fetoprotein (AFP) is primarily associated with NTDs such as spina bifida and anencephaly. Elevated maternal serum AFP is also found with abdominal hernias into the umbilical cord, cystic hygroma, and poor pregnancy outcome. Low maternal serum AFP is associated with an increased incidence of Down's syndrome and other aneuploidy states.

AFP is a product of, first, the fetal yolk sac and, then, the fetal liver. It is released into the fetal circulation and presumably enters the AF by transudation. Entry into the maternal circulation could be by placenta crossover or from the AF. An open NTD (e.g., spina bifida) that causes an increase in amniotic fluid α-fetoprotein (AFAFP) is accompanied by an increase in maternal serum AFP. Under normal conditions, AFAFP would be cleared by fetal swallowing and metabolism. An increased presence overloads this mechanism, causing AFAFP elevation. Both serum and AF are routinely analyzed using immunologic methods. Results are reported as multiples of the median. Because of the variety of demographics involved in determining normal values, each laboratory should establish its own median values for gestational weeks (usually weeks 15 to 21). Results can then be calculated using the formula:

$$MoM = \frac{\text{Specimen AFP concentration}}{\text{Medium AFP concentration for gestational week}} \quad \text{(Eq. 29-3)}$$

The protocol for AFP testing to determine the presence of an NTD is generally the following:

1. Maternal serum AFP, usually in conjunction with hCG, unconjugated estriol, and inhibin A assays
2. Repeat the AFP, if elevated
3. Diagnostic ultrasound
4. Amniocentesis for confirmation

Interpretation of maternal serum AFP testing is complex, being a function of age, race, weight, gestational age, and level of nutrition. Therefore, the material serum AFP can only be used as a screening tool and should not be considered diagnostics for any of the conditions it is associated with and are listed above. Testing of AFAFP is the confirmatory procedure to detect NTDs.

Concern over the difficulty in interpreting AFP tests generated the need for a second test to confirm NTDs and abdominal wall defects. The secondary method used is the assay for a central nervous system (CNS)-specific acetylcholinesterase (AChE). The NTD allows direct or, at least less difficult, passage of AChE into the AF. Analysis for CNS-specific AChE in the AF then offers a degree of confirmation for AFAFP. The methods used for CNS AChE include enzymatic, immunologic, and electrophoretic with inhibition. The latter includes the use of acetylthiocholine as substrate and BW284C51, a specific CNS inhibitor, to differentiate the serum pseudocholinesterase from the CNS-specific AChE.

Fetal Lung Maturity

The primary reason for AF testing is the need to assess fetal pulmonary maturity. All the organ systems are at jeopardy from prematurity, but the state of the fetal lungs is a priority from the clinical perspective. Consequently, the laboratory is asked whether sufficient specific phospholipids are reflected in the AF to prevent atelectasis (alveolar collapse) if the fetus were to be delivered. This question is important when preterm delivery is contemplated because of other risk factors in pregnancy, such as preeclampsia and premature rupture of membranes. Risk factors to fetus or mother can be weighed against interventions, such as delay of delivery with steroid administration to the mother to enhance fetal **surfactant** production, or against at-risk postdelivery therapies, such as exogenous surfactant therapy, high-frequency ventilation, and extracorporeal membrane oxygenation.

Alveolar collapse in the neonatal lung may occur during the changeover from placental oxygen to air as an oxygen source at birth if the proper quantity and type of phospholipid (surfactant) is not present. The ensuing condition,

which may vary in the degree of severity, is called **respiratory distress syndrome (RDS)**. It has also been referred to as *hyaline membrane disease* because of the hyaline membrane found in affected lungs. Lung maturation is a function of differentiation of alveolar epithelial cells (pneumocytes) into type I and type II cells beginning near the 24th week of pregnancy. The type I cells form the alveolar–capillary membrane for exchange of gases. The type II cells produce and store the surfactants needed for alveolar stability in the form of lamellar bodies.

As the lungs mature, increases occur in phospholipid concentration—particularly the compounds phosphatidylglycerol (PG) and lecithin[11] (Fig. 29.14). These two compounds, comprising 10% and 70%, of total phospholipid concentration, respectively, are most important as surfactants. Their presence in high enough levels acts in concert to allow contraction and re-expansion of the neonatal alveoli. Insufficient surfactant allows alveoli to collapse, requiring a great deal of energy to re-expand the alveoli upon inspiration. This not only creates an extreme energy demand on a newborn but probably also causes physical damage to the alveoli with each collapse. The damage may lead to "hyaline" deposition, or the newborn may not have the strength to continue inspiration at the energy cost. The result of either can be fatal.

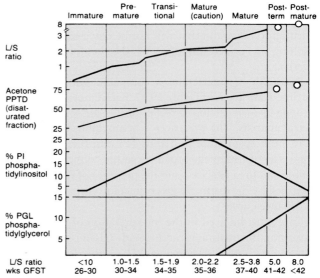

FIGURE 29.14 The form used to report the lung profile. The four determinations are plotted on the *ordinate*, and the weeks of gestation are plotted on the *abscissa* (as well as the *L/S ratio* as an "internal standard"). When plotted, these fall with a high frequency into a given grid that then identifies the stage of development of the lung as shown in the upper part of the form. The designation "mature (caution)" refers to patients other than those with diabetes who can be delivered *if necessary* at this time; if the patient has diabetes, she can be delivered with safety when the values fall in the "mature" grid. (Reprinted from Kulovich MV, Hallman MB, Gluck L. The lung profile. I. Normal pregnancy. *Am J Obstet Gynecol.* 1979;135:57, with permission. Copyright 1977 by the Regents of the University of California.)

Tests for assessing fetal lung maturity (FLM) include functional assays and quantitative assays. Functional assays provide a direct physical measure of AF in an attempt to assess surfactant ability to decrease surface tension. These include the "bubble or shake" test and the foam stability index (FSI). Quantitative tests include the lecithin–sphingomyelin ratio (**L/S ratio**), PG, and lamellar body counts.

The FSI,[12] a variant of Clements' original "bubble test"[13] that was performed at the bedside, appears acceptable as a rapid, inexpensive, and informative assay. This qualitative, technique-dependent test requires only common equipment. The assay is based on the ability of surfactant to generate a surface tension lower than that of a 0.47 mol fraction ethanol–water solution. If sufficient surfactant is present, a stable ring of foam bubbles remains at the air–liquid interface. As surfactant increases (FLM probability increases), a larger mole fraction of ethanol is required to overcome the surfactant-controlled surface tension. The highest mole fraction used while still maintaining a stable ring of bubbles at the air–liquid interface is reported as the FSI (Table 29.2). The test is dependent on technique and can also be skewed by contamination of any kind in the AF (e.g., blood or meconium contamination). Interpretation of the FSI bubble patterns is difficult and technique dependent. Results can vary among clinical laboratorians. Most laboratories have found that an FSI of 0.47 correlates well with an L/S ratio of 2.0.

The quantitative tests were given emphasis primarily by the work of Gluck et al.[14] The phospholipids of importance in these tests are PG, lecithin, and sphingomyelin (SP). Relative amounts of PG and lecithin increase dramatically with pulmonary maturity, whereas SP concentration is relatively constant and provides a baseline for the L/S ratio. Increases in PG and lecithin correspond to the larger amounts of surfactant being produced by the type II pneumocytes as fetal lungs mature.

The classic technique for separation and evaluation of the lipids involves thin-layer chromatography (TLC) of an extract of the AF. The extraction procedure removes most interfering substances and results in a concentrated lipid solution. Current practices use either one- or two-dimensional TLC for identification. Laboratory needs determine if a one-dimensional or a two-dimensional method is performed. An example of the phospholipids separation by one-dimensional TLC is shown in Figure 29.15.[15]

The classic breakpoint for judgment of maturity has been an L/S ratio of 2.0. As a result of the time-consuming requirements of performing the L/S ratio, several additional

FIGURE 29.15 Thin-layer chromatogram of AF phospholipids. Standard phospholipids (*ST*), total extract (*T*), and acetone-precipitable compounds (*A*) in AF are shown. The phospholipid standards contained, per liter, 2 g each of lecithin and P1, 1 g each of PG and SP, and 0.3 g each of PS and PE; 10 mL of the standard was spotted. (Reprinted from Tsai MY, Marshall JG. Phosphatidylglycerol in 261 samples of amniotic fluid. *Clin Chem.* 1979;25(5):683, with permission. Copyright 1979 American Association for Clinical Chemistry.)

tests have been developed to allow faster determination of FLM. The L/S ratio, however, remains the "gold standard" by which all methods are compared.

Phosphatidylglycerol

As mentioned previously, an additional phospholipid essential for FLM is PG that increases in proportion to lecithin. In the case of diabetic mothers, however, development of PG is delayed. Therefore, using an L/S ratio of 2.0 as an indicator of FLM cannot be relied upon to ensure that RDS will not occur unless PG is also included in interpretation of the L/S ratio. With the current trend toward less labor-intensive techniques, an immunologic assay using antibody specific for PG can be used to determine FLM.

The AmnioStat-FLM (Irvine Scientific, Santa Ana, CA) immunologic test is designed to measure the adequate presence of PG in AF. Because lecithin production is not affected in diabetic mothers and the levels of PG and lecithin rise at the same rate in unaffected pregnancies, the AmnioStat-FLM can be used to determine whether adequate FLM is present. Good correlation has been shown compared with the L/S ratio. The antibody-specific immunologic assay offers the additional advantage, not present in other assays, of being unaffected by specimen debris such as meconium and blood.

Lamellar Body Counts

The phospholipids produced and secreted by the type II alveolar cells are released in the form of lamellar bodies. As FLM increases, these lamellated packets of surfactant also exhibit an increased presence in the AF. The fact that lamellar bodies are approximately the same size as platelets provides a convenient method to determine their concentration

TABLE 29.2	**FSI Determination**		
	Tube 1	Tube 2	Tube 3
Vol AF	0.50	0.50	0.50
Vol 95% EtOH	0.51	0.53	0.55
FSI	0.47	0.48	0.49

using the platelet channel on automated hematology analyzers.[16] Based on the model of analyzer used, the number of lamellar bodies needed to ensure FLM can vary. This variation occurs as a result of different instrumental methods used to detect the bodies. Acceptable counts must be correlated with the specific instrumentation.[17] A standardized protocol has been developed in an effort to make the assay transferable between laboratories and has allowed a greater incorporation of this assay into practice.[18]

CASE STUDY 29.4

A 28-year-old woman is pregnant for the second time, having miscarried a year ago. At the time she miscarried, she was working as a volunteer in Haiti and did not seek medical care. Her doctor is concerned that the baby that she is carrying now may have hemolytic disease due to Rh incompatibility. She also has diabetes. She has an increase in optical density at 450 nm on her amniotic fluid screen with a Liley graph reading of 0.6 and is at approximately 34 weeks of gestation. Her L/S ratio was 2.1. The physician is considering inducing labor. Further testing of the amniotic fluid shows an FLM II reading of 55 mg surfactant/g of albumin.

Questions

1. What do the tests reveal? Why was the FLM II reading ordered in this case when the patient already had the L/S ratio performed?

2. Why is the physician considering inducing labor?

SWEAT

The common eccrine sweat glands function in the regulation of body temperature. They are innervated by cholinergic nerve fibers and are a type of exocrine gland. Sweat has been analyzed for its multiple inorganic and organic contents but, with one notable exception, has not been proved as a clinically useful model. That exception is the analysis of sweat for chloride levels in the diagnosis of cystic fibrosis (CF). The sweat test is the single most accepted common diagnostic tool for the clinical identification of this disease. Normally, the coiled lower part of the sweat gland secretes a "presweat" upon cholinergic stimulation. As the presweat traverses the ductal part of the gland going through the dermis, various constituents are resorbed. In CF, the electrolytes, most notably chloride and sodium ions, are improperly resorbed owing to a mutation in the cystic fibrosis transmembrane conductance regulator (*CFTR*) gene, which controls a cyclic AMP–regulated chloride channel.

CF (mucoviscidosis) is an autosomal recessive inherited disease that affects the exocrine glands and causes electrolyte and mucous secretion abnormalities. This exocrinopathy is present only in the homozygous state. The frequency of the carrier (heterozygous) state is estimated at 1 of 20 in the United States. The disease predominantly affects those of non-Hispanic Caucasian decent. The observed rate of expression ranks CF as the most common lethal hereditary disease in the United States, with death usually occurring by the third decade. The primary cause of death is pneumonia, secondary to the heavy, abnormally viscous secretion in the lungs. These heavy secretions cause obstruction of the microairways, predisposing the CF patient to repeated episodes of pneumonia. Patients also experience pancreatic insufficiency due to abnormally viscous secretions obstructing pancreatic ducts. This obstruction ostensibly causes pooling and autoactivation of the pancreatic enzymes. The enzymes then cause destruction of the exocrine pancreatic tissue.

Diagnostic algorithms for CF continue to rely on abnormal sweat electrolytes, pancreatic or bronchial abnormalities, and family history. The use of blood immunoreactive trypsin, a pancreatic product, is now prevalent in newborn screening programs. The rapidly developing area of molecular genetics provides the definitive methodology. The gene defect causing CF has been localized on chromosome 7, and the most frequent mutations have been characterized. However, approximately 1,550 mutations of the *CFTR* gene have been cataloged with the majority of patients found to be homozygous or heterozygous for the most common mutation.

The sweat glands remain structurally unaffected by CF. Analysis of sweat for both sodium and chloride is valid but, historically, chloride was and is the major element, leading to use of the sweat chloride test. Because of its importance, a standard method has been suggested by the Cystic Fibrosis Foundation. This method is based on the pilocarpine nitrate iontophoresis method of Gibson and Cooke.[19] Pilocarpine is a cholinergic-like drug used to stimulate the sweat glands. The sweat is absorbed on a gauze pad during the procedure. After collecting sweat by iontophoresis, chloride analysis is performed. Many methods have been suggested, and all are dependent on laboratory requirements. Generally, the sweat is leached into a known volume of distilled water and analyzed for chloride (chloridometer). In general, values greater than 60 mmol/L are considered positive.

Other tests including osmolarity, conductivity, and chloride electrodes or patches placed on the skin are available but are considered screening tests with abnormal results followed by the Gibson-Cooke reference method. A variety of instrumentation is available for these screening tests.

Although a value of 60 mmol/L is generally recognized for the quantitative pilocarpine iontophoretic test, it is important to consider several factors in interpretation. Not only will there be analytic variation around the cutoff, an epidemiologic borderline area will also occur. Considering this, the range of 45 to 65 mmol/L for chloride would be more appropriate in determining the need for repetition. Some patients with *CFTR* mutations have been found to have values below 60 mmol/L. Other variables must be considered. Age generally increases the limit—so much so that it is increasingly difficult to classify adults. Obviously, the patient's state of hydration also affects sweat levels. Because the complete procedure is technically demanding, expertise should be developed before the test is clinically available. A complete description of sweat collection and analysis, including procedural justifications, is available for review.[20]

SYNOVIAL FLUID

Joints are classified as movable or immovable. The movable joint contains a cavity that is enclosed by a capsule; the inner lining of the capsule is the synovial membrane (Fig. 29.16). This cavity contains **synovial fluid**, which is formed by ultrafiltration of plasma across the synovial membrane. Along with ultrafiltration of the plasma, the membrane also secretes a mucoprotein rich in hyaluronic acid. This mucoprotein is what causes the synovial fluid to be viscous. Synovial fluid functions as a lubricant for the joints and as a transport medium for delivery of nutrients and removal of cell wastes. The volume of fluid found in a large joint, such as the knee, rarely exceeds 3 mL. Normal fluid is clear, colorless to pale yellow, viscous, and non-clotting. Variations are indicative of pathologic conditions and are summarized in Table 29.3. Collection of a synovial fluid sample is accomplished by arthrocentesis of the joint under aseptic conditions (Fig. 29.17). The sample should be collected in a heparin tube for culture, a heparin or liquid EDTA for microscopic analysis, and a fluoride tube for glucose analysis. The viscosity of the fluid often requires the use of hyaluronidase to break down the mucoprotein matrix and allow for appropriate manual or automated aspiration and delivery into reaction vessels.

Chemical analysis of synovial fluid includes the testing of several different analytes. These analytes include total protein, glucose, uric acid, and LD. Total protein within the synovial fluid can be measured using the most common methods performed on serum samples. The normal range for synovial fluid protein is 1 to 3 g/dL. Increased synovial fluid protein levels are seen in ankylosing spondylitis, arthritis, arthropathies that accompany Crohn's disease, gout, psoriasis, Reiter's syndrome, and ulcerative colitis.

Synovial fluid glucose levels are interpreted using serum glucose levels after a 6- to 8-hour fast. Normally, synovial fluid glucose levels are less than 10 mg/dL lower than serum levels. Infectious disorders of the joint demonstrate large decreases in synovial fluid glucose and can be as much as 20 to 100 mg/dL less than serum levels. Other groups of joint disorders typically demonstrate a less degree of decrease in synovial fluid glucose.[19] The ratio of synovial fluid to plasma glucose (normally 0.9:1) remains the most useful mechanism to evaluate glucose levels within the synovial fluid. Decreased ratios are found in inflammatory (e.g., gout, rheumatoid arthritis [RA], and systemic lupus erythematosus) and septic (e.g., bacterial and viral arthritis) conditions. Standard methods for glucose analysis can be used for synovial fluid analysis.

Synovial fluid uric acid levels should be determined in patients with a monoarthritic episode to confirm or rule out the presence of gouty arthritis since plasma uric acid levels do not correlate with synovial fluid levels. While identifying the presence of uric acid crystals via microscopic methods is diagnostic of gouty arthritis, the determination of synovial fluid uric acid levels can be used in laboratories where crystal identification is not a routine procedure. Synovial fluid uric acid levels normally ranges from 6 to 8 mg/dL.

Although rarely performed, lactic acid measurements can be helpful in diagnosing septic arthritis. Normally, synovial fluid lactate is less than 25 mg/dL but can be as high as 1,000 mg/dL in septic arthritis. LD can be elevated in synovial fluid,

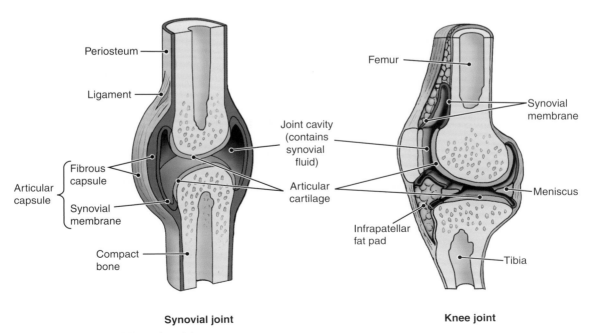

FIGURE 29.16 Synovial joint and model.

TABLE 29.3   **Classification of Synovial Fluids**

Group	Category	Visual	Viscosity	Mucin Clot	Cell Count	Glucose Blood: SF	Other
Clear	Normal High	Colorless—straw Good	<150 WBCs <25% neutrophils	0–10			
I	Noninflammatory	Yellow Slightly cloudy	Decreased	Fair	< –1,000 WBCs <30% neutrophils	0–10	
II	Inflammatory	White, gray, yellow Cloudy, turbid	Absent	Poor	<100,000 WBCs >50% neutrophils	0–4	
III	Septic	White, gray, yellow, or green Cloudy, purulent	Absent	Poor	50,000–200,000 WBCs >90% neutrophils	20–100	Positive cultures
IV	Crystal induced	White Cloudy, turbid, opaque, milky	Absent	Poor	500–200,000 WBCs <90% neutrophils	0–80	Crystals present
V	Hemorrhagic	Sanguinous, xanthochromic, red, or brown Cloudy	Absent	Poor	50–10,000 WBCs <50% neutrophils	0–20	RBCs present

Source: Mundt L, Shanahan K. *Graff's Textbook of Routine Urinalysis and Body Fluids*. 2nd ed. Philadelphia, PA: Lippincott Williams & Wilkins; 2011:268.

while serum levels remain normal. Synovial fluid LD levels are usually increased in RA, infectious arthritis, and gout.

Rheumatoid factor (RF) is an antibody to immunoglobulins. Most patients with RA have RF in their serum, whereas more than half of these patients will demonstrate RF in synovial fluid. Determining synovial fluid RF is important to diagnose cases where RF is only being produced by joint tissue. In these cases, synovial fluid RF may be positive while the serum RF is negative.[20]

FIGURE 29.17 Placement of needle in arthrocentesis of knee joint.

CASE STUDY 29.5

A 57-year-old female has had joint pain for 4 years. Her joints are becoming progressively deformed with swelling. Her doctor orders a synovial fluid analysis cell count, differential, synovial fluid RF serology, protein, glucose, LD, serum glucose level, serum RF, and fluid crystal analysis. Her results are as follows:

Fluid appearance: yellow/cloudy

WBC count, differential: greater than 25,000 WBCs/µL and greater than 50% polymorphonuclear neutrophils (PMNs) with ragocytes seen

Synovial Fluid	Serum Chemistries
Protein: 3.7 g/dL	
Glucose: 81 mg/dL	Glucose: 100 mg/dL (ratio 0.81 fluid:1.0 serum)
LD: 100 mg/dL	
RF: positive	RF: positive
Crystals: none seen	

Questions

1. What is the most probable diagnosis for this patient? What laboratory findings support your conclusion?

2. Name another condition that could have similar symptoms but was ruled out based upon the presented laboratory findings? What results would have been different in the condition you listed?

For additional student resources, please visit the Point® at http://thepoint.lww.com

questions

1. Clinical chemistry laboratory testing for the assessment of infectious meningitis may include all of the following tests on a CSF sample EXCEPT
   a. Glucose.
   b. Total protein.
   c. Lactate.
   d. Glutamine.
   e. All of the above would be used to confirm a suspected case of infectious meningitis.

2. Cerebrospinal fluid performs which of the following functions?
   a. Buoyant cushion for the brain
   b. Supplies nutrients to the central nervous system
   c. Removes wastes
   d. Intracerebral and extracerebral transport
   e. All of the above

3. Assessing the integrity of the blood–brain barrier can be accomplished using which of the following ratios?
   a. CSF IgG/CSF albumin
   b. CSF albumin/CSF IgG
   c. CSF albumin/serum albumin
   d. Serum albumin/CSF albumin
   e. CSF total protein/serum total protein

4. A red CSF indicates
   a. Cerebral hemorrhage
   b. Traumatic tap
   c. Bacterial meningitis
   d. Viral meningitis
   e. Cerebral hemorrhage or traumatic tap

5. Lamellar body counts indicate
   a. Surfactant phospholipid packets
   b. A ratio of lecithin to sphingomyelin
   c. Direct measure of phosphatidylglycerol levels
   d. Amniotic fluid bilirubin levels
   e. Meconium count of the fetus

6. A transudate could be caused by all of the following EXCEPT
   a. Congestive heart failure
   b. Lymphoma
   c. Renal failure
   d. Hepatic cirrhosis
   e. Nephrotic syndrome

7. CF is characterized by
   a. Elevated sweat chloride levels
   b. Homozygous expression of an autosomal recessive trait
   c. Pancreatic insufficiency
   d. All of these
   e. None of these

8. The high viscosity characteristic of normal synovial fluid samples is caused by
   a. Hyaluronic acid
   b. Hyaluronidase
   c. Elevated white blood cell counts
   d. The presence of crystals
   e. All of the above

9. An exudative pleural effusion would exhibit which of the following laboratory results?
   a. F/P total protein ratio of 0.4
   b. F/P LD ratio of 0.7
   c. Fluid cholesterol of 35 mg/dL
   d. F/P cholesterol ratio of 0.1
   e. F/P bilirubin ratio of 0.3

10. Pleural fluid is collected via
    a. Thoracentesis
    b. Paracentesis
    c. Pericardiocentesis
    d. Spinal tap
    e. None of the above

references

1. Brunzel NA. *Fundamentals of Urine and Body Fluid Analysis.* 2nd ed. Philadelphia, PA: Saunders; 2004:327–328.
2. McBride LJ. *Textbook of Urinalysis and Body Fluids: a Clinical Approach.* New York, NY: Lippincott; 1998:200–201.
3. Okta M, Okta K, et al. Clinical and analytical evaluation of an enzyme immunoassay for myelin basic protein in cerebrospinal fluid. *Clin Chem.* 2000;46:1336–1330.
4. Bailey EM, Domenico P, Cunha BA. Bacterial or viral meningitis. *Postgrad Med.* 1990;88:217.

5. Calbreath DF. *Clinical Chemistry: a Fundamental Textbook.* Philadelphia, PA: Saunders; 1992:370.

6. Ross DL, Neeley AE. *Textbook of Urinalysis and Body Fluids.* New York, NY: Appleton-Century-Crofts; 1983:275.

7. Calbreath DF. *Clinical Chemistry: A Fundamental Textbook.* Philadelphia, PA: Saunders; 1992:371.

8. Ross DL, Neeley AE. *Textbook of Urinalysis and Body Fluids.* New York, NY: Appleton-Century-Crofts; 1983:280.

9. Davie AP, Francis CM, Love MP, et al. Value of the electrocardiogram in identifying heart failure due to left ventricular systolic dysfunction. *Br Med J.* 1996;312:222–224.

10. Liley AW. Liquor amnil analysis in the management of the pregnancy complicated by rhesus sensitization. *Am J Obstet Gynecol.* 1961;82:1359.

11. Kulovich MV, Hallman MB, Gluck L. The lung profile. I. Normal pregnancy. *Am J Obstet Gynecol.* 1979;135:157.

12. Statland BE, Freer DE. Evaluation of two assays of functional surfactant in amniotic fluid: surface-tension lowering ability and the foam stability index test. *Clin Chem.* 1979;25:1770.

13. Clements JA, Plataker ACG, Tierney DF, et al. Assessment of the risk of the respiratory distress syndrome by a rapid test for surfactant in amniotic fluid. *N Engl J Med.* 1972;286:1077.

14. Gluck L, Kulovich MV, Borer RC Jr, et al. Diagnosis of the respiratory distress syndrome by amniocentesis. *Am J Obstet Gynecol.* 1971;109:440.

15. Tsai MY, Marshall JG. Phosphatidylglycerol in 261 samples of amniotic fluid from normal and diabetic pregnancies, as measured by one-dimensional thin layer chromatography. *Clin Chem.* 1979;25:682.

16. Khazardoost H, Yakazadeh S, Borna F, et al. Amniotic fluid lamellar body count and its sensitivity and specificity evaluating fetal lung maturity. *J Obstet Gynecol.* 2005;25:257–259.

17. Szallasi A, Gronowski AM, Eby CS. Lamellar body count in amniotic fluid: a comparison of four different hematology analyzers. *Clin Chem.* 2003;49:994–997.

18. Neerhof ME, Dohnal JC, Ashwood ER, et al. Lamellar body counts: a consensus on protocol. *Obstet Gynecol.* 2001;97:318–320.

19. Gibson LE, Cooke RE. A test for concentration of electrolytes in cystic fibrosis of the pancreas utilizing pilocarpine by iontophoresis. *Pediatrics.* 1959;23:545.

20. Clinical Laboratory Standards Institute. *Sweat Testing: Sample Collection and Quantitative Analysis Approved Guidelines.* Villanova, PA: Clinical Laboratory Standards Institute, reaffirmed 2005. (CLSI document C34-A2.)

PART four

Specialty Areas of Clinical Chemistry

30

Therapeutic Drug Monitoring

TAKARA L. BLAMIRES

key terms

Bioavailability
Distribution
Peak drug concentration
Pharmacogenomics
Pharmacokinetics
Standard dosage
Therapeutic drug monitoring
Therapeutic range
Trough drug concentration

chapter objectives

Upon completion of this chapter, the clinical laboratorian should be able to the following:

- Discuss drug characteristics that make therapeutic drug monitoring essential.
- Identify factors that influence the absorption of an orally administered drug.
- List factors that influence the rate of drug elimination.
- Define drug distribution and discuss factors that influence it.

(continues on page 610)

For additional student resources, please visit thePoint® at http://thepoint.lww.com

chapter objectives (continued)

- Calculate volume of distribution, elimination constant, and drug half-life.
- Relate the concentration of a circulating drug to pharmacokinetic parameters.
- Discuss collection of appropriate specimens for therapeutic drug monitoring.
- Identify the therapeutic category or use of each drug presented in this chapter.
- Describe complications that result from major toxicity of drugs presented in this chapter.
- Identify key features of each drug presented in this chapter that may influence its blood concentration.

OVERVIEW

Therapeutic drug monitoring (TDM) involves the coordinated effort of several health care professionals to accurately monitor circulating drug concentrations in serum, plasma, and whole blood specimens. Laboratory personnel play an essential role in TDM. Appropriate timing of specimen collection, accurate measurement of drug concentrations, and timely reporting of results are necessary to achieve safe and effective patient drug therapy. The main purposes for TDM are to (1) ensure drug dosage is within a range that produces maximal therapeutic benefit known as the **therapeutic range** and (2) identify when the drug is outside the therapeutic range, which may lead to drug inefficacy or toxicity. For most drug therapies, safe and effective dosage regimens for the majority of the population have been established, and TDM is unnecessary. However, for some therapeutic drugs, there is a narrow window between therapeutic efficacy and toxicity. Therefore, careful monitoring and appropriate dosage adjustments are necessary to maintain therapeutic concentrations.

The **standard dosage** for a drug is the dose providing therapeutic benefits as statistically derived from observations in a healthy population. Disease states may produce altered physiologic conditions in which the standard dose does not produce the predicted concentration and must be adjusted accordingly. Patient age, gender, genetics, diet, prescription drugs, self-administered over-the-counter drugs, and even naturopathic agents can influence drug concentrations and efficacy. For these reasons, it is important to establish a dosage regimen to fit individual situations and needs. This is achieved with TDM.

TDM may also be used to identify patients who are noncompliant or to reoptimize a dosing regimen based on drug–drug interactions or a change in the patient's physiologic state that has unpredictably affected circulating drug concentrations.

The basis of TDM includes consideration of the route of administration, rate of absorption, distribution of drug within the body, and rate of elimination (Fig. 30.1). There are many factors that influence drug absorption, distribution, and elimination; therefore, the process of achieving therapeutic drug concentrations is by no means straightforward. This chapter introduces these concepts and their influence on circulating drug concentrations as well as briefly discussing some drugs commonly monitored by TDM testing in the clinical laboratory.

ROUTES OF ADMINISTRATION

To achieve maximum therapeutic benefit, a drug must be at an appropriate concentration at its site of action. For instance, a cardioactive drug might need to reach myocytes at a dosage concentration that is effectively maintained in the therapeutic range for days to weeks. Intravenous (IV) administration into the circulatory system offers the most direct and effective delivery to their sites of action. The fraction of the administered dose that eventually reaches its site of action is defined as its **bioavailability**. In addition to IV, drugs can be administered by several other routes. Drugs can be injected directly into muscle tissue through intramuscular (IM) injections or just under the skin with a subcutaneous (SC) injection. They can also be inhaled or absorbed through the skin (transcutaneous) through use of a transdermal patch. Rectal delivery through a suppository is commonly used in infants and in situations in which oral delivery is not possible. Oral administration is the most common route of delivery as it is the least invasive for patients. Each method of administration presents with different characteristics that can affect circulating drug concentrations. As oral administration is the most common, the following discussions of drug absorption, distribution, metabolism, and elimination will focus on this method of administration.

FIGURE 30.1 Overview of factors that influence the circulating concentration of an orally administered drug. GI, gastrointestinal.

DRUG ABSORPTION

For orally administered drugs, the efficiency of absorption from the gastrointestinal tract is dependent on several factors including (1) dissociation from its administered form, (2) solubility in gastrointestinal fluids, and (3) diffusion across gastrointestinal membranes. Tablets and capsules require dissolution before being absorbed, whereas liquid solutions tend to be more rapidly absorbed. Some drugs are subject to uptake by active transport mechanisms intended for dietary constituents; however, most are absorbed by passive diffusion from the gastrointestinal tract into the bloodstream. This process requires that the drug be in a hydrophobic, or nonionized, state. Because of gastric acidity, weak acids are efficiently absorbed in the stomach, but weak bases are preferentially absorbed in the intestine where the pH is more alkaline. For most drugs, absorption from the gastrointestinal tract occurs in a predictable manner in healthy people; however, changes in intestinal motility, pH, inflammation, as well as the presence of food or other drugs may dramatically alter absorption rates. For instance, a patient with inflammatory bowel syndrome may have a compromised gastrointestinal tract, which may affect normal absorption of some drugs. Absorption can also be affected by coadministration of drugs that affect gastrointestinal function such as antacids, kaolin, sucralfate, cholestyramine, and antiulcer medications. Morphine may also slow gastrointestinal motility, thereby influencing the rate of drug absorption.

Additionally, drug absorption rates may change with age, pregnancy, or pathologic conditions. In these instances, predicting the final circulating concentration in blood from a standard oral dose can be difficult. However, with the use of TDM, effective oral dosage regimens can be determined.

DRUG DISTRIBUTION

The free fraction of circulating drug is subject to diffusion out of the vasculature and into interstitial and intracellular spaces. The relative proportion between circulation and the tissues defines the drug's **distribution**. The ability to leave circulation is largely dependent on the lipid solubility of the drug. Drugs that are highly hydrophobic can easily cross cellular membranes and partition into lipid compartments, such as adipose tissue and nerve cells. Drugs that are polar and not ionized can also cross cell membranes, but do not sequester into lipid compartments. Ionized species diffuse out of the vasculature, but at a slow rate. The volume of distribution index is used to describe the distribution characteristics of a drug and is expressed mathematically as follows:

$$V_d = D/C \qquad \text{(Eq. 30-1)}$$

where V_d is the volume of distribution in liters, D is an IV injected dose of the drug in milligrams (mg) or grams (g), and C is the drug concentration in plasma (mg/L or g/L). Drugs that are hydrophobic can have large V_d values due to partitioning into hydrophilic compartments. Substances that are ionized or are primarily bound in plasma have small V_d values due to sequestration in the vasculature.

FREE VERSUS BOUND DRUGS

Most drugs in circulation are subject to binding with serum constituents. Although many potential bonds may be formed, most are drug–protein complexes. An important aspect regarding drug dynamics is that typically only the free or unbound fraction can interact with its site of action and result in a biologic response. For this reason, the free drug fraction is also termed *active*. At a standard dose, the total plasma drug concentration may be within the therapeutic range, but the patient experiences toxic adverse effects due to a high free fraction or does not realize a therapeutic benefit due to a low free fraction. This may occur secondary to changes in blood protein content as might occur during inflammation, malignancies, pregnancy, hepatic disease, nephrotic syndrome, malnutrition, and acid–base disturbances. Albumin represents the majority of protein constituents in plasma, and changes in its concentration can affect the free versus bound status of many drugs. Additionally, increases in plasma alpha-1-acid glycoprotein during acute phase reactions will lead to increased binding of drugs such as propranolol, quinidine, chlorpromazine, cocaine, and benzodiazepines. The fraction of free drug may also be influenced by the concentration of substances that compete for binding sites, which may be other drugs or endogenous substances, such as urea, bilirubin, or hormones. Measurement of the free drug fraction should be considered for drugs that are highly protein bound or when clinical signs are inconsistent with the total drug measurement.

DRUG METABOLISM

All substances absorbed from the intestine (except the rectum) enter the hepatic portal system. In this system, circulating blood from the gastrointestinal tract is routed through the liver before it enters into general circulation. Certain drugs are subject to significant hepatic uptake and metabolism during passage through the liver. This process is known as *first-pass metabolism*. Liver metabolism may not be the same in every patient as it can be influenced by an individual's genetics. These variations in drug metabolism related to genetics are examined in the discipline of **pharmacogenomics**. In addition to genetic variation, a patient with impaired liver function may have reduced capacity to metabolize drugs. This is a particularly important consideration if the efficacy of a drug depends on metabolic generation of a therapeutically active metabolite. This enzymatic process is referred to as *biotransformation*. Patients with liver disorders may require reduced dosages of the drug as the rate of metabolism and the subsequent elimination process may be slowed.

Most drugs are *xenobiotics*, which are exogenous substances that are capable of entering biochemical pathways intended for endogenous substances. There are many potential biochemical pathways in which drugs can be acted on or biotransformed. The biochemical pathway responsible for a large portion of drug metabolism is the hepatic mixed-function oxidase (MFO) system. The basic function of this system involves taking hydrophobic substances and, through a series of enzymatic reactions, converting them into water-soluble products. These products can then either be transported into the bile or released into general circulation for elimination by renal filtration.

There are many enzymes involved in the MFO system and are commonly divided into two functional groups or phases. Phase I reactions produce reactive intermediates. Phase II reactions conjugate functional groups, such as glutathione, glycine, phosphate, and sulfate, to reactive sites on the intermediates resulting in water-soluble products. The MFO system is nonspecific and allows many different endogenous and exogenous substances to go through this series of reactions. Although there are many potential substrates for this pathway, the products formed from an individual substance are specific. For example, acetaminophen is metabolized in the MFO pathway ultimately leading to the formation of a glutathione conjugate following phase II reactions. In the presence of too much acetaminophen, as in the case of an overdose, the MFO system may be overwhelmed and cannot effectively metabolize it to a safe, water-soluble end product for elimination by the kidneys. In this case, the conjugating group for a given drug can become depleted in phase II reactions and an accumulation of phase I products occurs. Excessive phase I products may result in toxic effects, and in the case of acetaminophen, irreversible damage to hepatocytes may occur.

It is also noteworthy that the MFO system can be induced. This is seen as an increase in the synthesis and activity of the rate-limiting enzymes within this pathway. The most common inducers are xenobiotics that are MFO substrates. Thus, certain drugs may affect their own rate of elimination. Due to biologic variability in the degree of induction, TDM is commonly used to establish an appropriate dosage regimen for these drugs.

Because many potential substrates enter the MFO system, competitive and noncompetitive drug–drug interactions can result in altered rates of elimination of the involved drugs. Interactions are not limited to drug–drug, but may also include drug–food (i.e., grapefruit) or drug–beverage (i.e., alcohol and caffeine). For example, metabolism of acetaminophen by the MFO system is altered in the presence of alcohol rendering it more toxic. In most instances, the degree of alteration is unpredictable.

Changes in hepatic status can also affect the concentration of circulating drugs eliminated by this pathway. Induction of the MFO system typically results in accelerated clearance and a corresponding shorter drug half-life. Hepatic disease states characterized by a loss of functional tissue may result in slower rates of clearance and a corresponding longer drug half-life. For example, cirrhosis results in irreversible damage and fibrosis of the liver, rendering hepatocytes nonfunctional. Consequently, xenobiotics may not be effectively metabolized by the MFO system, thereby reducing the rate of metabolism and elimination while increasing the opportunity for toxicity. In these situations, TDM aids in appropriate dosage adjustment.

For some drugs, there is considerable variance in the rate of hepatic and nonhepatic drug metabolism within a normal population. This results in a highly variable rate of clearance, even in the absence of disease. Establishing dosage regimens for these drugs is, in many instances, aided by the use of TDM. With the use of molecular genetics, it is now also possible to identify common genetic variants of some drug-metabolizing pathways, and identification of these individuals may assist in establishing an individualized dosage regimen.

DRUG ELIMINATION

Drugs can be cleared from the body by various mechanisms. The plasma free fraction of a parent drug or its metabolites is subject to glomerular filtration, renal secretion, or both. For those drugs not secreted or subject to reabsorption, the elimination rate of free drug directly relates to the glomerular filtration rate. Decreases in glomerular filtration rate directly result in an increased drug half-life and elevated plasma concentration. Aminoglycoside antibiotics and cyclosporine, an immunosuppressant drug, are examples of drugs that are not secreted or reabsorbed by the renal tubules.

Independent of the clearance mechanism, decreases in the plasma drug concentration most often occur as a first-order process indicating an exponential rate of loss. This implies that the rate of change of drug concentration over time varies continuously in relation to the concentration of the drug. First-order elimination follows the following general equation:

$$\Delta C / \Delta T = -kC \qquad \text{(Eq. 30-2)}$$

This equation defines how the change in concentration per unit time ($\Delta C / \Delta T$) is directly related to the concentration of drug (C) and the constant (k). The k value is a proportionality factor that describes the percent change per unit time. It is commonly referred to as the *elimination constant* or the *rate of elimination* and is negative because it is a decreasing value. The graphic solution to this equation is an exponential function that declines in the predicted curvilinear manner, asymptotically approaching zero (Fig. 30.2). The graph shown in Figure 30.2 illustrates a large change at high drug concentrations and a smaller change at low drug concentrations; however, the rate, or percent lost, remains the same. Plotting it in semilogarithmic dimensions (Fig. 30.3) can linearize this function.

Drugs are eliminated through hepatic metabolism, renal filtration, or a combination of the two. For some drugs, elimination by these routes is highly variable and functional changes in either organ system may result in changes in the rate of elimination. In these situations, information regarding elimination rate and estimating the circulating concentration of a drug after a given time period are important factors in establishing an effective and safe

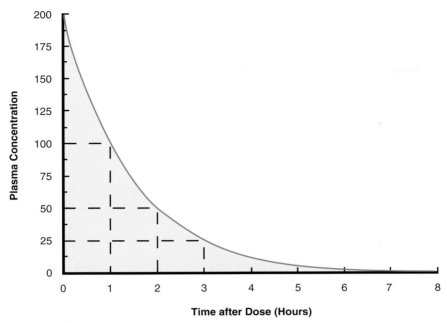

FIGURE 30.2 First-order drug elimination. This graph demonstrates exponential rate of loss on a linear scale. *Hash-marked lines* are representative of half-life.

dosage regimen. Equation 30-2 and Figures 30.2 and 30.3 are useful in determining the rate of elimination and concentration of a drug after a given time period. The following equation illustrates how the concentration of drug can be estimated based on initial concentration, the elimination constant, and time since the initial dose was administered:

$$C_T = C_0 e^{-kt} \qquad \text{(Eq. 30-3)}$$

where C_0 is the initial concentration of drug, C_T is the concentration of drug after the time period (T), k is the elimination constant, and T is the time period evaluated. This is the most useful form of the elimination equation. By measuring the initial drug concentration and the concentration after time (T), the elimination constant can be determined. Once k is known, the amount of drug that will be present after a certain time period can be determined.

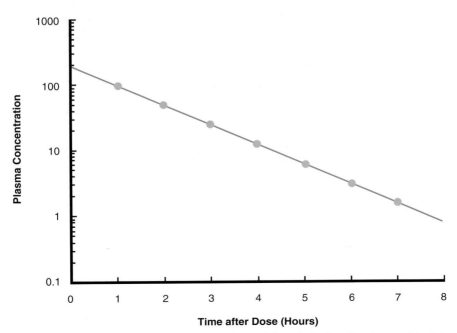

FIGURE 30.3 Semilogarithmic plot of exponential rate of drug elimination. The slope of this plot is equal to the rate of elimination (k).

Example

The concentration of gentamicin is 10 µg/mL at 12:00. At 16:00, the gentamicin concentration is 6 µg/mL. What is the elimination constant (k) for gentamicin in this patient? Using Eq. 30-3:

$$C_T = C_0 e^{-kt}$$

$$C_0 = 10\,\mu g/mL, C_T = 6\,\mu g/mL, T = 4\ hours, k = ?$$

Substituting these values into the elimination equation (Eq. 30-3) yields:

$$6\mu g/mL = \left(10\,\mu g/mL\right) e^{-k(4\,hours)}$$

Divide both sides by 10 µg/mL and note that the concentration units can be cancelled:

$$0.6 = e^{-k(4\,hours)}$$

To eliminate the exponent, take the natural logarithm of both sides:

$$\ln 0.6 = \ln\left(e^{-k(4\ hours)}\right)$$

Solve the natural log:

$$-0.51 = -k\left(4\ hours\right)$$

Multiply both sides by −1:

$$0.51 = k\left(4\ hours\right)$$

Divide both sides by 4 hours:

$$0.13/hours = k$$

The calculated value for k indicates the patient is eliminating gentamicin at a rate of 13% per hour.

In this same patient on the same day, what would the predicted blood concentration of gentamicin be at midnight (24:00)?

For C_0, either the 12:00 or 16:00 value can be used as long as the correct corresponding time duration is used. In this example, the 16:00 value of 6 µg/mL will be used.

$$C_0 = 6\mu g/mL, T = 8\ hours, k = 0.13/hours, C_T = ?$$

Substituting these values into the elimination equation (Eq. 30-3) yields:

$$C_T = \left(6\,\mu g/mL\right) e^{-0.13/hours(8\,hours)}$$

Solve for the exponent and note that the time unit can be cancelled:

$$C_T = \left(6\,\mu g/mL\right) e^{-1.04}$$

$$C_T = \left(6\,\mu g/mL\right)(0.35)$$

$$C_T = 2.1\mu g/mL$$

The calculated C_T value indicates the patient would have a serum gentamicin concentration of 2.1 µg/mL at midnight (24:00).

Although the elimination constant (k) is a useful value, it is not common nomenclature in the clinical setting. Instead, the term *half-life (T½)* is used. One half-life is the time needed for the serum concentration to decrease by one-half. It can be determined graphically (Fig. 30.2) or by conversion of the elimination constant (k) to half-life ($T½$) using the formula given in Eq. 30-4. Of these two methods, the calculation provides the easiest and most accurate way to determine the drug half-life. Referring to the example above, the half-life of gentamicin in this patient would be calculated as follows:

$$T\,\tfrac{1}{2} = 0.693/k \qquad \text{(Eq. 30-4)}$$

$$T\,\tfrac{1}{2} = 0.693/\left(0.13/hours\right)$$

$$T\,\tfrac{1}{2} = 5.33\ hours$$

The gentamicin half-life value for this patient indicates that after 5.33 hours, the concentration of drug in their blood would be one-half the initial concentration.

PHARMACOKINETICS

Pharmacokinetics is the activity of a drug in the body as influenced by absorption, distribution, metabolism, and excretion. Evaluation of pharmacokinetics assists in establishing or modifying a dosage regimen as it takes into consideration in vivo factors that affect the concentration of the drug and its rate of change. Figure 30.3 is an idealized plot of elimination after an IV bolus assuming there is no previous distribution of the drug. A drug that distributes outside of the vascular space would produce an elimination graph such as in Figure 30.4. The rapid rate of change seen immediately after the initial IV bolus is a result of distribution and elimination. The rate of elimination (k) can be determined only after distribution is complete. Figure 30.5 is a plot of serum drug concentration as it would appear after oral administration of a drug. As absorbed drug enters the circulation, it is subject to simultaneous distribution and elimination. Serum concentrations rise when the rate of absorption exceeds the rate of distribution and elimination and declines as elimination and distribution exceed the rate of absorption. The rate of elimination can only be determined after absorption and distribution are complete.

Most drugs are not administered as a single bolus, but are delivered on a scheduled basis (e.g., once every 8 hours). With this type of administration, the blood drug concentration oscillates between a maximum and a minimum referred to as the **peak drug concentration** and the **trough drug concentration**, respectively. The goal of a multiple-dosage regimen is to achieve trough and peak concentrations in the therapeutic range and to ensure that the peak is not in the toxic range. Evaluation of this oscillating function cannot be done immediately after initiation of a scheduled dosage

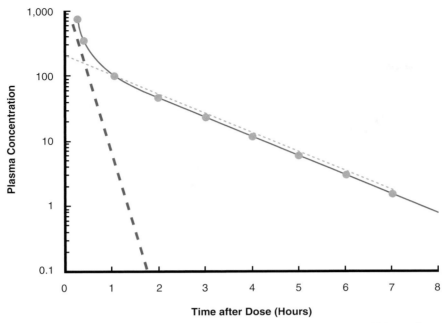

FIGURE 30.4 Semilogarithmic elimination plot of a drug subject to distribution. Initial rate of elimination is influenced by distribution (*dashed line*) and terminal elimination rate (*dotted line*). After distribution is complete (1.5 hours), elimination is first order.

regimen. Approximately five to seven doses are required before a *steady-state* oscillation is achieved as demonstrated in Figure 30.6.

After the first oral dose, absorption and distribution occur, followed only by elimination. Before the concentration of drug drops significantly, the second dose is given. The peak of the second dose is additive to what remained from the first dose. Because elimination is first order, the higher concentration results in a larger amount eliminated. The third through seventh scheduled doses all have the same effect, increasing serum concentration and the amount eliminated. By the end of the seventh dose, the amount of drug administered in a

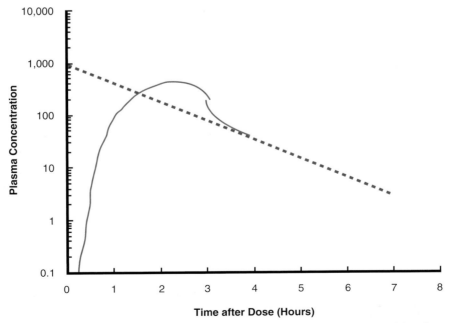

FIGURE 30.5 Plasma concentration of a drug after oral administration. After oral administration at time 0, serum concentration increases (*solid line*) after a brief lag period. Plasma concentrations peak when rate of elimination and distribution exceed rate of absorption. First-order elimination (*dotted line*) occurs when absorption and distribution are complete.

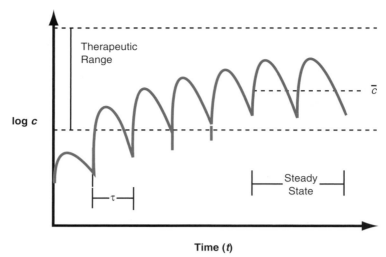

FIGURE 30.6 Steady-state kinetics in a multiple-dosage regimen. The character τ indicates the dosage interval. Equal doses at this interval reach steady state after six or seven dosage intervals. $\bar{c}$ mean drug concentration.

single dose is equal to the amount eliminated during the dosage period. At this point, steady state is established and peak and trough concentrations can be evaluated.

SPECIMEN COLLECTION

Accurate timing of specimen collection is the single most important factor in TDM. In general, trough concentrations are drawn right before the next dose, and peak concentrations are drawn 1 hour after an orally administered dose. This rule of thumb must always be used within the clinical context of the situation. Drugs that are absorbed at a slower rate may require several hours before peak drug concentrations can be evaluated. In all situations, determination of serum drug concentrations should be performed only after steady state has been achieved.

Serum or plasma is the specimen of choice for the determination of circulating concentrations of most drugs. Care must be taken that the appropriate container is used when collecting these specimens as some drugs have a tendency to be absorbed into the gel of certain separator collection tubes. It is necessary to follow manufacturer recommendations when this preanalytical effect is possible as failure to do so may result in falsely low values. Heparinized plasma is generally suitable for most drug analyses. Calcium-binding anticoagulants add a variety of anions and cations that may interfere with analysis or cause a drug to distribute differently between cells and plasma. As a result, specimen tubes that contain ethylenediaminetetraacetic acid (EDTA), citrate, or oxalate are generally considered unacceptable specimen types for TDM.

PHARMACOGENOMICS

The effectiveness of a drug within a population can be divided into two categories: patients who are *responders* and patients who are *nonresponders*. Responders are patients benefiting from the therapeutic and desired effects of the drug, while nonresponders do not demonstrate a beneficial effect from the initiation of a given drug regimen. The therapeutic effectiveness of drugs in responders and nonresponders has recently been attributed to the interindividual variation in genetic polymorphisms of the patients' drug metabolism pathways. As previously mentioned, pharmacogenomics is the science of studying these variations and developing drug therapies to compensate for the genetic differences impacting therapy regimens.

One of the most prominent gene families that affect drug metabolism is the cytochrome P-450 (CYP450) family, which is a family of enzymes within the MFO system previously described. The differences in rates of drug metabolism in a population are attributed to the variations in the enzymes as a result of genetic polymorphism. The three variations most often linked to differences in drug metabolism are CYP2D6, CYP2C9, and CYP3A4. This information can be used to personalize drug doses to the degree that is appropriate for the CYP450 profile of the patient. For example, if the patient's CYP450 profile indicates he or she has genes known to metabolize more slowly, they would be given lower doses of the drug to avoid toxic concentrations. Alternatively, if a patient's CYP450 profile indicates he or she has genes predisposing the patient to an increased rate of metabolism, he or she would need an increased dose to maintain therapeutic drug concentrations. Pharmacogenetic profiling can also be used to predict drug–drug interactions or as an indicator if the drug will provide any therapeutic benefit at all.[1]

CARDIOACTIVE DRUGS

Many cardiac conditions are treated with drugs, of which, only a few require TDM. The cardiac glycosides and antiarrhythmics are two classes of cardioactive drugs for which TDM aids in achieving an appropriate dosage regimen.

Digoxin

Digoxin (Lanoxin) is a cardiac glycoside used in the treatment of congestive heart failure. It functions by inhibiting membrane Na^+, K^+-ATPase. This causes a decrease in intracellular potassium, which results in increased intracellular calcium in cardiac myocytes. The increased intracellular calcium improves cardiac contractility. This effect is seen in the serum concentration range of 0.8 to 2 ng/mL (1 to 2.6 nmol/L).[2] Higher serum concentrations (>3 ng/mL [3.8 nmol/L]) decrease the rate of ventricular depolarization. Although this level can be used to control ventricular tachycardia, it is not frequently used because of toxic adverse effects, including nausea, vomiting, and visual disturbances, that occur at plasma concentrations greater than 2 ng/mL. Adverse cardiac effects, such as premature ventricular contractions (PVCs) and atrioventricular node blockage, are also common.

Absorption of orally administered digoxin is variable and influenced by dietary factors, gastrointestinal motility, and formulation of the drug. In circulation, about 25% is protein bound. The unbound or free form of digoxin is sequestered into muscle cells, and at equilibrium, the tissue concentration is 15 to 30 times greater than that of plasma. Elimination of digoxin occurs primarily by renal filtration of unbound digoxin. The remainder is metabolized into several products by the liver. The half-life of plasma digoxin is 38 hours in an average adult. The major contributing factor to the extended half-life is the slow release of tissue digoxin back into circulation.

Because of variable gastrointestinal absorption, establishing a dosage regimen usually requires assessment of plasma concentrations after initial dosing to ensure that effective and nontoxic plasma concentrations are achieved. In addition, changes in glomerular filtration rate can have a dramatic effect on plasma concentrations. Frequent dosage adjustments, in conjunction with measurement of plasma digoxin concentrations, should be performed in patients with renal disease. The therapeutic benefits and toxicities of digoxin can also be influenced by the concentration of electrolytes in the plasma. Low potassium and magnesium potentiate digoxin actions.[2] In these conditions, adjustment of plasma concentrations below the therapeutic range may be necessary to avoid toxicity. Thyroid status may also influence the actions of digoxin. Hyperthyroid patients display a resistance to digoxin actions, and hypothyroid patients are more sensitive.[3]

The timing for evaluation of peak digoxin concentrations is crucial. In an average adult, plasma concentrations peak between 2 and 3 hours after an oral dose; however, uptake into the tissues is a relatively slow process. As a result, peak plasma concentrations do not correlate well with tissue concentrations. It has been established that the plasma concentration 8 to 10 hours after an orally administered dose correlates well with the tissue concentration, and specimens should be drawn within this window. Specimens collected before this time are misleading and are not considered a valid representation of the patient's drug status.

Immunoassays are used to measure total digoxin concentration in serum.[2] With most commercial assays, cross-reactivity with hepatic metabolites is minimal; however, newborns, pregnant women, and patients with uremia or late-stage liver disease produce an endogenous substance that cross-reacts with the antibodies used to measure serum digoxin. In patients with these digoxin-like immunoreactive substances, falsely elevated concentrations are common and should be considered along with the clinical context.

Quinidine

Quinidine (Quinidex Extentabs, Cardioquin, Quinora) is a naturally occurring drug used to treat various cardiac arrhythmias. The two most common formulations are quinidine sulfate and quinidine gluconate. Quinidine is generally administered orally as gastrointestinal absorption is complete and rapid for quinidine sulfate with peak serum concentrations achieved 2 hours post dose. Quinidine gluconate is a slow-release formulation with peak serum concentrations 4 to 5 hours after an oral dose.[2] Because of its slow rate of absorption, trough levels of quinidine gluconate are usually drawn 1 hour post dose. The most common adverse effects of quinidine toxicity are nausea, vomiting, and abdominal discomfort though more serious complications such as thrombocytopenia and tinnitus can occur. Signs of cardiovascular toxicity, such as PVCs, may be seen when blood concentrations are twice the upper limit of the therapeutic range. In most instances, monitoring of quinidine therapy only involves measurement of trough specimens to ensure serum concentrations are within the therapeutic range. Assessment of peak specimens is performed only when symptoms of toxicity are present.

Approximately 70% to 80% of absorbed quinidine is bound to plasma proteins.[2] Quinidine has a half-life of 6 to 8 hours and is primarily eliminated by hepatic metabolism. Induction of hepatic metabolism, such as by barbiturates, increases the clearance rate of quinidine, whereas impairment of this system, as seen in late-stage liver disease, may extend the half-life of quinidine in circulation. Plasma quinidine concentrations can be determined by chromatographic methods or immunoassays and the therapeutic range for quinidine is 2 to 5 μg/mL. Manufactured quinidine may contain bioactive contaminants such as dihydroquinidine. Early immunoassays detected quinidine only, but most current immunoassays cross-react with these bioactive contaminants and serum measurements represent the total quinidine potential.

Procainamide

Like quinidine, procainamide (Procanbid, Procan SR, Pronestyl) is used to treat cardiac arrhythmias. Oral administration is common as gastrointestinal absorption is rapid and complete with peak plasma concentrations at about 1 hour post dose.[2] Approximately 20% of absorbed procainamide is bound to plasma proteins. Procainamide has a half-life of approximately 4 hours and is eliminated by a combination of both renal filtration and hepatic metabolism. *N*-acetylprocainamide, a hepatic metabolite of the parent drug, demonstrates antiarrhythmic activity similar to procainamide, and measurements of the total antiarrhythmic drug potential must take into consideration the parent drug and its metabolite. The therapeutic range for procainamide is 4 to 8 μg/mL. Alteration in either renal or hepatic function can lead to increased plasma concentrations of the parent drug and metabolites. An increased concentration can result in myocardial depression and arrhythmia. Both procainamide and its active metabolite can be measured by immunoassay to determine the total drug potential.

CASE STUDY 30.1

A patient with congestive heart failure has been successfully treated with digoxin for several years, but recently developed renal failure. Laboratory records indicate semiannual peak digoxin concentrations that have all been within the therapeutic range. A serum specimen was collected upon admission and results are shown in the ase Study Table 30.1.1. Although the digoxin concentration is elevated, the physician indicates the patient is not exhibiting signs or symptoms of toxicity.

CASE STUDY TABLE 30.1.1

Laboratory Results

Test	Result	Reference Interval
Sodium	129	135–145 mmol/L
Potassium	5.5	3.5–5 mmol/L
Chloride	113	97–107 mmol/L
Blood pH	7.25	7.35–7.45
tCO_2	16	21–31 mmol/L
Urea nitrogen	180	5–20 mg/dL
Creatinine	4.5	0.6–1 mg/dL
Osmolality	275	282–300 mOsm/kg
Digoxin	2.5	0.9–2 ng/mL

Questions

1. If the specimen was collected without consideration of the time of the patient's last digoxin dose, how might this affect the interpretation of the result?

2. Other than the time relative to dose administration, what additional factors should be taken into consideration when interpreting the digoxin result?

3. What additional laboratory test would aid in the interpretation of this case?

Disopyramide

Disopyramide (Norpace) is another antiarrhythmic agent used in the treatment of cardiac abnormalities. Disopyramide may be administered as a quinidine substitute when the adverse effects of quinidine are unacceptable. It is most commonly administered as an oral preparation as gastrointestinal absorption is complete and rapid with plasma concentrations peaking at about 1 to 2 hours post dose.[2] Disopyramide binds to several plasma proteins, but binding is highly variable between individuals and is concentration dependent. As a result, it is difficult to correlate total plasma drug concentration with therapeutic benefit and toxicity. In most patients, total blood concentrations in the range of 3 to 7.5 μg/mL (8.8 to 22.1 μmol/L) have been determined to be effective and nontoxic; however, interpretation of disopyramide results should take the clinical perspective into consideration. The adverse effects of disopyramide therapy are dose dependent.[2] Anticholinergic effects, such as dry mouth and constipation, may be seen at concentrations greater than 4.5 μg/mL (13.3 μmol/L). Cardiac effects of drug toxicity, such as bradycardia and atrioventricular node blockage, are usually seen at concentrations greater than 10 μg/mL (29.5 μmol/L). Disopyramide has a half-life of approximately 7 hours and is primarily eliminated by renal filtration and, to a lesser extent, by hepatic metabolism. In conditions with a decreased glomerular filtration rate, the drug half-life is prolonged and expected concentrations are elevated. Plasma disopyramide concentrations are commonly determined by chromatographic methods or immunoassay.

CASE STUDY 30.2

A patient receiving procainamide therapy for cardiac arrhythmia is given an IV loading dose resulting in a serum concentration of 6 μg/mL. The therapeutic range for procainamide is 4 to 8 μg/mL, and its half-life is 4 hours. Four hours after the initial loading dose, another equivalent dose is given as an IV bolus resulting in a serum concentration of 7.5 μg/mL.

Questions

1. Does the serum concentration after the second dose seem appropriate? If not, what would be the predicted serum concentration at this time?

2. What factors would influence the rate of elimination of this drug?

ANTIBIOTICS

Aminoglycosides

Aminoglycosides are a group of chemically related antibiotics used to treat gram-negative bacterial infections that are resistant to other less-toxic antibiotics. There are many individual antibiotics within this classification, but the most frequently encountered ones in a clinical setting are gentamicin, tobramycin, amikacin, and kanamycin. These antibiotics share a common mechanism of action, but vary in effectiveness against different strains of bacteria. The most serious effects of aminoglycoside toxicity are nephrotoxicity and ototoxicity. The ototoxic effects are irreversible and involve disruption of inner ear cochlear and vestibular membranes, which results in hearing and balance impairment. Cumulative effects may be seen with repeated high-level exposure. Nephrotoxicity is also a major concern for patients on this type of antibiotic therapy as aminoglycosides impair the function of the proximal renal tubules, which can result in electrolyte imbalance and proteinuria. These effects are usually reversible; however, extended high-level exposure may result in necrosis of renal tubular cells and subsequent renal failure.[4] Toxic concentrations for this type of drug are usually considered as any concentration above the therapeutic range.

Because aminoglycosides are poorly absorbed in the gastrointestinal tract, administration is generally limited to IV or IM injection; therefore, these drugs are not used in an outpatient setting. Peak concentrations are achieved 1 to 2 hours post dose, and approximately 10% of the drug is bound to plasma proteins in circulation. Aminoglycosides have a half-life of approximately 2 to 3 hours, depending on the specific antibiotic, and are eliminated by renal filtration. In patients with compromised renal function, appropriate dosage adjustments must be made based on plasma concentrations. Chromatography and immunoassay are the primary methods used for aminoglycoside determinations.

Teicoplanin

Teicoplanin is a bactericidal antibiotic effective against both aerobic and anaerobic gram-positive bacilli as well as gram-positive cocci that cannot be treated with less-toxic antibiotics. Of note, teicoplanin has proven effective in the treatment of methicillin-resistant *Staphylococcus aureus* (MRSA) infections. This antibiotic has very poor absorption when administered orally and should be given through IV or IM injection. Teicoplanin has a long half-life of 70 to 100 hours, and 90% to 95% is bound to plasma proteins in circulation. It is not metabolized in the liver, but is eliminated by renal filtration and secretion. TDM is not routinely performed for teicoplanin as a relationship between plasma concentrations and toxicity has not been established; however, monitoring may assist in dosage optimization. When trough specimens are measured, the therapeutic range for teicoplanin is 10 to 60 mg/L for the treatment of endocarditis and 20 to 60 mg/L for staphylococci infections. Adverse effects associated with teicoplanin toxicity include nausea, vomiting, fever, diarrhea, and mild hearing loss.

Vancomycin

Vancomycin (Vancocin HCl) is a glycopeptide antibiotic effective against gram-positive cocci and bacilli infections. Because of poor gastrointestinal absorption, vancomycin should be administered by IV infusion allowing peak concentrations to be achieved 1 hour post dose. In circulation, approximately 55% is bound to plasma proteins. Unlike other drugs, a clear relationship between blood concentration and toxic adverse effects has not been firmly established. Indeed, many of the toxic effects occur in the therapeutic range (5 to 10 μg/mL [3.45 to 6.9 μmol/L]).[4] Major toxicities of vancomycin include red man syndrome, nephrotoxicity, and ototoxicity. Red man syndrome is characterized by an erythemic flushing of the extremities. The nephrotoxic and ototoxic effects are similar to those of the aminoglycosides. It appears that nephrotoxic effects occur more frequently at trough concentrations greater than 10 μg/mL (6.9 μmol/L) and ototoxic effects occur more frequently when peak concentrations exceed 40 μg/mL (27.6 μmol/L). Because vancomycin has a long distribution phase, generally only trough concentrations are monitored to ensure the drug concentration is within the therapeutic range. Vancomycin has a half-life of 4 to 6 hours and is primarily eliminated by renal filtration and secretion. Vancomycin concentrations are routinely determined by immunoassay and chromatographic methods.

ANTIEPILEPTIC DRUGS

Epilepsy, convulsions, and seizures are prevalent neurologic disorders. Because antiepileptic drugs (AEDs) are used as prophylactics, therapeutic ranges are considered guidelines and should be interpreted in accordance with the presenting clinical context.[5] Effective concentrations are determined as the concentration that provides therapeutic benefit with no or acceptable adverse effects. In recent years, a second generation of anti-AEDs have been introduced in clinical practice as supplemental therapy to more traditional drugs' first-generation AEDs such as phenobarbital and phenytoin. Unlike first-generation AEDs, optimal concentration ranges have not been firmly established. For these drugs, TDM may be used to establish individual baseline concentrations at which the patient is responding well.[5] It is important to take these individual therapeutic ranges into account as physiologic conditions change (age related, pregnancy, kidney or liver disease, etc.) and in reassessing concentrations when other AEDs are added to an established regimen.[5] Most AEDs are analyzed by immunoassay or chromatography and measure the free or bound drug in a serum or plasma sample. In a normal physiologic state, the total drug concentration may be sufficient for therapeutic monitoring purposes; however, a free drug measurement may be necessary when there is cause for alteration in patient plasma protein, such as in the later stages of pregnancy, in late-stage renal or hepatic disease, malnutrition, or when a known drug–drug interaction may occur.[6] As with all TDM, specimen collection timing must be consistent, and the preferred specimen is generally a trough specimen collected at the end of the dosing interval.[6]

Phenobarbital and Primidone

Phenobarbital (Luminal or Solfoton) is a slow-acting barbiturate that effectively controls several types of seizures. Absorption of oral phenobarbital is slow, but complete.

For most patients, peak plasma concentrations are reached about 10 hours after an oral dose, and approximately 50% of circulating phenobarbital is bound to plasma proteins. The half-life of phenobarbital is 70 to 100 hours. It is eliminated primarily by hepatic metabolism; however, renal filtration is also significant. With compromised renal or hepatic function, the rate of elimination is decreased. Because of the slow rate of absorption and long half-life, blood concentrations of phenobarbital do not change dramatically within a dosing interval; therefore, only trough concentrations are typically evaluated unless toxicity is suspected. Toxic adverse effects of phenobarbital include drowsiness, fatigue, depression, and reduced mental capacity.

Phenobarbital clearance occurs by the hepatic MFO system. It is also important to note that phenobarbital is a potent inducer of the MFO system. After initiation of therapy, dose adjustment is usually required after the induction period is complete. For most individuals, this occurs within 10 to 15 days after the initial dose.

Primidone is an inactive proform of phenobarbital. Primidone is rapidly absorbed in the gastrointestinal tract and converted to its active form, phenobarbital. Primidone is preferred over phenobarbital when steady-state kinetics need to be established quickly. Both primidone and phenobarbital are measured to assess the total AED potential in circulation with a therapeutic range of 10 to 40 mg/L.

CASE STUDY 30.3

A patient on successful oral phenytoin therapy for seizure disorders presents with severe diarrhea for the past 2 weeks. Subsequent to the prolonged diarrhea, the patient had a seizure. Evaluation of the serum phenytoin concentration at the time of the seizure revealed a low value. The dose was increased until the serum concentration was within the therapeutic range. The diarrhea resolved; however, several days after the dose adjustment, the patient had another seizure.

Questions

1. What is the most probable cause of the initial low serum phenytoin concentration?

2. Would determination of free serum phenytoin aid in resolving the cause of the initial seizure?

3. What assays other than the determination of serum phenytoin would aid in this situation?

4. What is the most probable cause of the seizure after the diarrhea had been resolved?

Phenytoin and Fosphenytoin

Phenytoin (Dilantin) is a common therapeutic agent used in the treatment of seizure disorders. It is also used as a short-term prophylactic agent in brain injury to prevent loss of functional tissue. Phenytoin is primarily administered as an oral preparation though gastrointestinal absorption is variable and sometimes incomplete. Peak concentrations are achieved 3 to 12 hours post dose. Circulating phenytoin has a high but variable degree of protein binding (87% to 97%) and can be easily displaced by other highly protein-bound drugs.[7] Like most drugs, the unbound, or free, fraction is the biologically active form of the drug. Reduced protein binding may occur with anemia, hypoalbuminemia, and as a result of coadministration of other drugs with similar binding properties. In these situations, symptoms of toxicity may be observed even though the total drug concentration is within the therapeutic range. The most significant adverse effect of phenytoin toxicity is initiation of seizures. Thus, seizures in a patient receiving phenytoin therapy may be a result of subtherapeutic or toxic concentrations. Additional adverse effects of phenytoin include hirsutism, gingival hyperplasia, vitamin D deficiency, and folate deficiency. Phenytoin has a half-life of 6 to 24 hours and is eliminated by hepatic metabolism. At therapeutic concentrations, the elimination pathway may become saturated (zero-order kinetics); therefore, relatively small changes in dosage or elimination can have dramatic effects on plasma drug concentrations. Phenytoin is also an inducer of the hepatic MFO pathway, which reduces the half-life of concurrently administered drugs that are eliminated by this pathway.[5]

For most patients, total blood concentrations of 10 to 20 μg/mL (20 to 80 μmol/L) are considered effective. In many situations, however, the therapeutic range must be individualized to suit the clinical situation. The therapeutic range for free serum phenytoin is 1 to 2 μg/mL (4 to 8 μmol/L). This has been well correlated with the pharmacologic actions of this drug. In patients with altered plasma protein binding, determination of the free fraction aids in dosage adjustment.

Fosphenytoin is an injectable proform of phenytoin that is rapidly metabolized (~75 minutes) to form the parent drug. Most immunoassays for phenytoin do not detect fosphenytoin so peak concentrations should only be measured after conversion to the active form is complete.

Valproic Acid

Valproic acid, or valproate (Depakote), is used in the treatment of petit mal and absence seizures.[7] It is administered as an oral preparation as gastrointestinal absorption is rapid and complete. Circulating valproic acid is highly protein bound (93%), and peak concentrations are reached 1 to 4 hours post dose. The percent of valproic acid bound to plasma proteins decreases in renal failure, in late liver disease, and with coadministration of drugs that compete for its binding sites. Valproic acid is eliminated by hepatic metabolism, which may be induced by coadministration of other AEDs, but is inhibited by administration of felbamate, which is another AED.[7] Without coadministration of these drugs, valproic acid has a half-life of 11 to 17 hours. The therapeutic range for valproic acid is relatively wide (50 to 120 μg/mL [347 to 832 μmol/L]), and determination of blood concentrations is primarily performed to ensure that toxic levels (>120 µg/mL) are not present. Nausea, lethargy, and weight gain are the most common adverse effects of valproic acid toxicity; however, pancreatitis, hyperammonemia, and hallucinations have been associated with significantly elevated concentrations (>200 µg/mL [>1387 µmol/L]). Hepatic dysfunction occasionally occurs in some patients even at therapeutic concentrations; therefore, hepatic markers should be checked frequently during the first 6 months of therapy. Many factors influence the portion of valproic acid bound to plasma proteins so measurement of the free fraction provides a more reliable index of therapeutic and toxic concentrations.

Carbamazepine

Carbamazepine (Tegretol) is an effective treatment for various seizure disorders; however, because of its serious adverse effects, it is only used when patients do not respond well to other AEDs. Orally administered carbamazepine is absorbed with a high degree of variability, and approximately 70% to 80% of circulating carbamazepine is bound to plasma proteins. Peak concentrations are achieved 4 to 8 hours post dose, and the half-life for carbamazepine is 10 to 20 hours. It is eliminated primarily by hepatic metabolism so liver dysfunction can result in accumulation of carbamazepine. Carbamazepine is an inducer of hepatic metabolism so frequent monitoring of plasma concentrations must be performed after initiation of therapy until the induction period has come to completion.

Carbamazepine toxicity is diverse and variable. Certain effects occur in a dose-dependent manner, while others do not. There are several idiosyncratic effects of carbamazepine, which affect a portion of the population at therapeutic concentrations including rashes, leukopenia, nausea, vertigo, and febrile reactions. Of these, leukopenia is the most serious. Leukocyte counts are commonly assessed during the first 2 weeks of therapy to detect this possible toxic effect. Liver function tests should also be evaluated during this time period as mild, transient liver dysfunction is commonly seen during initiation of therapy. Persistent increases in liver markers or significant leukopenia commonly result in discontinuation of carbamazepine therapy. The therapeutic range for carbamazepine is 4 to 12 µg/mL (16.9 to 50.8 µmol/L), and plasma concentrations greater than 15 µg/mL (63.5 µmol/L) are associated with hematologic disorders and possible aplastic anemia.

Ethosuximide

Ethosuximide (Zarontin) is used for controlling petit mal seizures. It is administered as an oral preparation with peak concentrations achieved within 2 to 4 hours. The therapeutic range for ethosuximide is 40 to 100 µg/mL (283 to 708 µmol/L). Toxicities associated with high plasma concentrations are rare, tolerable, and generally self-limiting. Common adverse effects of toxicity include nausea, vomiting, anorexia, dizziness, and lethargy. Less than 5% of circulating drug is bound to proteins in the plasma. Ethosuximide is metabolized in the liver; however, approximately 20% is excreted through renal filtration. The half-life for ethosuximide is 40 to 60 hours. TDM for ethosuximide is performed to ensure that blood concentrations are in the therapeutic range.

Felbamate

Felbamate (Felbatol) is primarily indicated for use in severe epilepsies such as in children with the mixed seizure disorder, Lennox-Gastaut syndrome, and in adults with refractory epilepsy.[5–7] Felbamate is most commonly administered orally as it is nearly completely absorbed by the gastrointestinal tract, and peak serum concentrations can be achieved within 1 to 4 hours.[8] In circulation, approximately 30% of felbamate is bound to plasma proteins and has a half-life of 14 to 22 hours in adults. Felbamate is eliminated by renal and hepatic metabolism so impairment of hepatic or renal function can significantly increase the half-life of the drug in circulation. Hepatic metabolism is enhanced by enzyme inducers such as phenobarbital, primidone, phenytoin, and carbamazepine and results in a decreased half-life.

TDM may be indicated due to a narrow therapeutic range, but should only be considered after steady state has been reached. In patients receiving therapeutic doses, felbamate concentrations are typically in the range of 30 to 60 µg/mL (126 to 252 µmol/L).[8] Documented adverse side effects of felbamate toxicity include fatal aplastic anemia and hepatic failure.[5,7]

Gabapentin

Gabapentin (Neurontin) is administered orally with a maximum bioavailability of 60%, which is reduced when antacids are administered concurrently. This drug may be administered as a monotherapy or in conjunction with other AEDs for patients suffering from complex partial seizures with or without generalized seizures.[5,7] Peak concentrations for gabapentin are achieved 2 to 3 hours following dosage. Gabapentin does not bind to plasma proteins and is not metabolized in the liver. It is eliminated unchanged by the kidneys and has a half-life of approximately 5 to 9 hours in patients with normal renal function.[8] Children require a higher dose than adults to maintain a comparable half-life as they eliminate the drug faster than adults. Due to exclusive renal clearance of this drug, impaired kidney function increases the half-life of the circulating drug in a linear manner.[8] Therapeutic concentrations are reported to be between 12 and 20 µg/mL (70.1 and 116.8 µmol/L) although a wide range of serum concentrations have been reported in association with seizure control. Multiple daily doses may be the preferred dosage regimen as excessively high blood concentrations may lead to adverse drug effects, while low-level trough concentrations may lead to breakthrough seizures.[5] Adverse effects associated with gabapentin toxicity are generally mild and may include fatigue, ataxia, dizziness, and weight gain. Gabapentin is the most frequently used AED in patients with liver disease and in treating partial-onset seizures in patients with acute intermittent porphyria.[5]

Lamotrigine

Lamotrigine (Lamictal) is orally administered and is rapidly and completely absorbed from the gastrointestinal tract reaching peak concentrations 3 hours after administration. It is used to treat patients with partial and generalized seizures.[5] Once in circulation, approximately 55% of lamotrigine is protein bound and biologically inactive.[8] Hepatic metabolism accounts for the majority of elimination and in patients undergoing monotherapy, its half-life is 15 to 30 hours.[7,8] The rate of elimination for lamotrigine is highly dependent on patient age and physiologic condition. Younger infants tend to metabolize this drug slower than older infants, and children metabolize lamotrigine twice as quickly as adults. Marked increases in clearance occur during pregnancy, peaking at 32 weeks of gestation.[5]

Lamotrigine clearance is increased by enzyme-inducing AEDs such as phenobarbital, primidone, phenytoin, and carbamazepine; however, valproic acid is an inhibitor of lamotrigine metabolism and may increase its half-life to 60 hours. Because of these drug–drug interactions, TDM is essential to maintain therapeutic drug concentrations. Individual therapeutic ranges may vary, but a concentration range of 2.5 to 15 µg/mL has been noted as efficacious and an increasing concentration seems to correlate well with increased risk of toxicity.[8] A small percentage of patients taking lamotrigine develop a rash. Other adverse effects associated with toxicity include neurological effects, such as dizziness, and gastrointestinal disturbances.

Levetiracetam

Levetiracetam (Keppra) is an orally administered AED that does not bind to plasma proteins so it is almost completely bioavailable and reaches peak concentration by 1 hour post dose.[5,7,8] Use of levetiracetam is indicated in partial and generalized seizures. Sixty-five percent of levetiracetam is excreted unchanged by the kidneys, and it has a half-life of 6 to 8 hours, although the rate of elimination is increased in children and pregnant females and decreased in the elderly. The rate of clearance for this drug correlates well with glomerular filtration rate, which may be of use in monitoring patients with renal impairment. The need for TDM of levetiracetam is not as pronounced as in other AEDs due to its lack of pharmacokinetic variability, but may be useful in monitoring compliance and fluctuating concentrations during pregnancy.[5] Therapeutic concentrations have been reported at 8 to 26 µg/mL. Adverse effects are minimal but include dizziness and weakness.

Oxcarbazepine

Oxcarbazepine (Trileptal) is an orally administered prodrug that is almost immediately metabolized to licarbazepine.[7,8] It is indicated for treatment of partial seizures and secondarily in generalized tonic–clonic seizures. In circulation, almost 40% is bound to plasma proteins, and peak concentrations are achieved at about 8 hours post dose. It is metabolized by the liver into two pharmacologically active, equipotent enantiomers via keto reduction followed

by glucuronide conjugation of the active licarbazepine derivative.[7,8] In adults, the half-life of this drug is 8 to 10 hours. In children, there is a higher clearance rate; therefore, a need exists for a higher dosing regimen to obtain the optimal serum concentration per kilogram of body weight compared with adults. In the elderly population, the drug clearance is reduced by 30% so a lower dosing regimen is needed to maintain therapeutic concentrations.[8] Clearance of the drug and its metabolite is reduced in patients with marked renal dysfunction, and appropriate dosage adjustments must be made to avoid toxicity. The metabolism of licarbazepine is sensitive to enzyme inducers such as phenytoin and phenobarbital, which may decrease the blood concentration by 20% to 40%.[8] TDM may be indicated when therapeutic benefits are not being met, when drug–drug interactions are possible, and during pregnancy. Although not well defined, therapeutic effects of licarbazepine have been reported at serum concentrations of 12 to 35 µg/mL. Adverse effects of toxicity are similar to those of carbamazepine.

Tiagabine

Tiagabine (Gabitril) is used in the treatment of partial seizures.[7] Gastrointestinal absorption of tiagabine is rapid and nearly complete resulting in peak concentrations at 1 to 2 hours post dose. Approximately 96% of circulating tiagabine is protein bound and its half-life is variable, but in the range of 4 to 13 hours. Due to its significant protein binding, the ratio of free to bound drug is affected by other protein-binding drugs such as valproic acid, naproxen, and salicylates and by pregnancy.[8] It is highly metabolized by the hepatic MFO pathway[5,8] so hepatic dysfunction can prolong the half-life of the drug. TDM may be indicated due to intraindividual and interindividual variations. Therapeutic benefits of the drug have been observed at concentrations of 20 to 100 ng/mL.[8] Adverse central nervous system (CNS) side effects have been noted including confusion, difficulty in speaking clearly (stuttering), mild sedation, and a tingling sensation in the body's extremities, or paresthesia, especially in the hands and fingers.[5,9]

Topiramate

Only 15% of topiramate (Topamax) is bound to plasma proteins and is almost completely bioavailable after oral administration. Peak concentrations are achieved within 1 to 4 hours.[7,8] The half-life of topiramate is 20 to 30 hours, and the majority of this drug is eliminated by renal filtration though some is eliminated by hepatic metabolism. Topiramate is used in the treatment of partial and generalized seizures.[5] The dose-to-serum concentration ratio in children is less than that of adults per kilogram of body mass such that they require a higher dose to maintain plasma topiramate concentrations comparable to adults.[8] Plasma concentrations are increased secondary to renal insufficiency, but may be decreased when used with other enzyme-inducing AEDs. The therapeutic range for topiramate is based on collection of trough specimens and is reported to be less than 25 mg/L (75 µmol/L). Adverse CNS side effects of topiramate include change of taste with particular foods (e.g., diet soda and beer) and a sensation of "pins and needles" in the extremities.[5,9] TDM may be indicated when steady state is achieved to provide the clinician with an effective individual baseline concentration and may also be employed when therapeutic benefits are not realized or to monitor drug–drug interactions.[8]

Zonisamide

Zonisamide (Zonegran) is an anticonvulsant used in adjunctive therapy for partial and generalized seizures. This drug is administered orally and absorbed from the gastrointestinal tract on the order of 65% or higher. Peak serum concentrations are reached 4 to 7 hours post dose, and approximately 60% of the drug is bound to plasma proteins and accumulates extensively in erthyrocytes.[8] The majority of zonisamide is metabolized by the liver via glucuronide conjugation, acetylation, and oxidation and then renal excretion. The half-life of zonisamide is 50 to 70 hours in patients receiving monotherapy and may be reduced to 25 to 35 hours when other enzyme-inducing AEDs are being administered concomitantly.[8] Children require higher doses to achieve therapeutic plasma concentrations comparable to that of an adult.[8] Clinicians treating patients with liver or kidney disease should exercise caution as plasma zonisamide concentrations may increase proportionally with the level and type of organ impairment. There is documented overlap in zonisamide blood concentrations between those experiencing therapeutic effectiveness and those experiencing toxic side effects.[8] Symptoms of zonisamide toxicity include difficulty breathing, low blood pressure, slow heart rate, and possible loss of consciousness. TDM may be indicated to establish a baseline level after steady state has been achieved, to detect drug–drug interactions, and at therapeutic failure. Therapeutic doses have been reported in patients with blood concentrations of 10 to 38 µg/mL.

PSYCHOACTIVE DRUGS

Lithium

Lithium (Eskalith, Lithobid) is a mood-altering drug primarily used in the treatment of bipolar disorder, recurrent depression, and aggressive or self-mutilating behavior though it may also be used as a preventative treatment for migraines and cluster headaches. Gastrointestinal absorption is complete and rapid so this drug is administered orally and peak plasma concentrations are reached 2 to 4 hours after the dose was administered. Lithium is a cationic metal that does not bind to proteins. Lithium has a half-life of 10 to 35 hours and is eliminated predominately by renal filtration, but is subject to reabsorption in the renal tubules and compromises in renal function usually result in lithium accumulation. Correlations between plasma lithium concentration and therapeutic response have not been well established; however, plasma concentrations

in the range of 0.5 to 1.2 mmol/L are effective in a large portion of the patient population.[10] The purpose of TDM for lithium is to avoid plasma concentrations associated with toxic effects. Concentrations in the range of 1.5 to 2 mmol/L may cause apathy, lethargy, speech difficulties, and muscle weakness.[10] Concentrations greater than 2 mmol/L are associated with renal impairment, hypothyroidism, and CNS disturbances such as muscle rigidity, seizures, and possible coma. Determination of serum lithium concentrations is commonly done by ion-selective electrode though flame emission photometry and atomic absorption are also viable methods.

Tricyclic Antidepressants

Tricyclic antidepressants (TCAs) are a class of drug used to treat depression, insomnia, extreme apathy, and loss of libido. From a clinical laboratory perspective, imipramine, amitriptyline, and doxepin are the most relevant.[10] Desipramine and nortriptyline are active metabolites of imipramine and amitriptyline, respectively. The TCAs are orally administered and demonstrate a varying degree of absorption. In many patients, they slow gastric emptying and intestinal motility, which significantly slows the rate of absorption. As a result, peak concentrations are reached in the range of 2 to 12 hours. Approximately 85% to 95% of TCAs are protein bound. For most TCAs, therapeutic effects are not seen for the first 2 to 4 weeks after initiation of therapy and the correlation between serum concentration and therapeutic effects of most TCAs is moderate to weak. TCAs are eliminated by hepatic metabolism, and many of their metabolic products have therapeutic actions. The rate of metabolism of these agents is variable and influenced by a wide variety of factors. As a result, the half-life of TCAs varies considerably among patients (17 to 40 hours). The rate of elimination can also be influenced by coadministration of other drugs that are eliminated by hepatic metabolism. The toxicity of TCAs is dose dependent; serum concentrations twice the upper limit of the therapeutic range can lead to drowsiness, constipation, blurred vision, and memory loss. Higher levels may cause seizure, cardiac arrhythmia, and unconsciousness.

Because of the high variability in half-life and absorption, plasma concentrations of the TCAs should not be evaluated until a steady state has been achieved. At this point, therapeutic efficacy is determined from clinical evaluation of the patient, and potential toxicity is determined by TDM. Many of the immunoassays for TCAs use polyclonal antibodies, which cross-react among the different TCAs and their metabolites. These immunoassays are used for TCA screening rather than TDM, and the results are reported out as "total tricyclics."[10] Some immunoassays employ an extraction step to separate the parent drugs from their metabolites prior to analysis, and interpretation of these results requires an in-depth understanding of the assay. Chromatographic methods provide simultaneous evaluation of both the parent drugs and their metabolites, which provides a basis for unambiguous interpretation of results.[10]

Clozapine

Clozapine (Clozaril, FazaClo) is an antipsychotic used in the treatment of otherwise treatment-refractory schizophrenia. Absorption is rapid and almost complete, and approximately 97% of circulating drug is bound to plasma proteins. Peak concentrations are achieved within 2 hours of administration. Clozapine is metabolized in the liver and has a half-life of 8 to 16 hours. Research has shown that although there is not a well-established clinical serum concentration, beneficial effects of the drug have been demonstrated at 350 to 420 ng/mL. TDM may be indicated to check for compliance and in patients with altered pharmacokinetics. TDM may also be used to avoid toxicity, which can result in seizures.[11]

Olanzapine

Olanzapine (Zyprexa) is a thienobenzodiazepine derivative that effectively treats schizophrenia, acute manic episodes, and the recurrence of bipolar disorders.[11] It can be administered as a fast-acting IM injection, but is more commonly administered orally. The drug is absorbed well in the gastrointestinal tract; however, an estimated 40% is inactivated by first-pass metabolism. Peak concentrations are reached 5 to 8 hours post dose, and approximately 93% is bound to plasma proteins in circulation. Olanzapine is metabolized in the liver and has a variable half-life of 21 to 54 hours. Women and nonsmokers tend to have lower clearance and thus higher blood concentrations of olanzapine compared with men and smokers.[11] There is indication that plasma concentration correlates well with clinical outcomes and that TDM may help to optimize clinical response while balancing the occurrence of adverse effects in a therapeutic range of 20 to 50 ng/mL.[11] Adverse effects of olanzapine toxicity include tachycardia, decreased consciousness, and possible coma.

IMMUNOSUPPRESSIVE DRUGS

Transplantation medicine is a rapidly emerging discipline within clinical medicine. The clinical laboratory plays many important roles that determine the success of any transplantation program. Among these responsibilities, monitoring of immunosuppressive drugs used to prevent rejection is of key concern. Most immunosuppressive drugs require establishment of individual dosage regimens to optimize therapeutic outcomes and minimize toxicity.

Cyclosporine

Cyclosporine (Gengraf, Neoral, Sandimmune) is a cyclic polypeptide that has potent immunosuppressive activity. Its primary clinical use is suppression of host-versus-graft rejection of heterotopic transplanted organs. It is administered as an oral preparation with absorption in the range of 5% to 50% and peak concentrations within 1 to 6 hours. Because of this high variability, the relationship between oral dosage and blood concentration is poor; therefore, TDM is an important part of establishing a

dosage regimen. More than 98% of circulating cyclosporine is protein bound, and cyclosporine appears to sequester in cells, including erythrocytes.[12] Erythrocyte content is highly temperature dependent; therefore, evaluation of plasma cyclosporine concentrations requires rigorous control of specimen temperature. To avoid this preanalytic variable, whole blood specimens are used. Correlations have been established between cyclosporine whole blood concentration and therapeutic and toxic effects. Cyclosporine is eliminated by hepatic metabolism to inactive products and has a half-life of approximately 12 hours.

The therapeutic range for cyclosporine is dependent on the organ transplanted and the time after transplantation. Whole blood concentrations in the range of 350 to 400 ng/mL (291 to 333 nmol/L) have been associated with cyclosporine toxicity. The adverse effects of cyclosporine are primarily renal tubular and glomerular dysfunction, which may result in hypertension.[13] Several immunoassays are available for the determination of whole blood cyclosporine concentration though many show cross-reactivity with inactive metabolites. Chromatographic methods are available and provide separation and quantitation of the parent drug from its metabolites.[14]

Tacrolimus

Tacrolimus FK-506 (Astagraf, Envarsus, Hecoria, Prograf) is an orally administered immunosuppressive drug that is 100 times more potent than cyclosporine.[15] Early use of tacrolimus suggested a low degree of toxicity compared with cyclosporine at therapeutic concentrations; however, after extensive use in clinical practice, both drugs appear to have comparable degrees of nephrotoxicity. Tacrolimus has been associated with thrombus formation at concentrations above the therapeutic range.

Many aspects of tacrolimus pharmacokinetics are similar to those of cyclosporine. Gastrointestinal uptake is highly variable with peak plasma concentrations achieved in 1 to 3 hours. More than 98% of circulating tacrolimus is bound to proteins in the plasma. Tacrolimus has a half-life of 10 to 12 hours; it is eliminated almost exclusively by hepatic metabolism, and its metabolic products are primarily secreted into bile for excretion. Increases in immunoreactive tacrolimus may be seen in cholestasis as a result of cross-reactivity with several of these products. Because of the high potency of tacrolimus, circulating therapeutic concentrations are low. This limits the methodologies capable of measuring whole blood concentrations. Currently, the most common method is high-performance liquid chromatography–tandem mass spectrometry; however, several immunoassays are also available. Similar to cyclosporine, therapeutic ranges for tacrolimus are dependent on the transplant type and time from transplantation. Whole blood concentrations correlate well with therapeutic and toxic effects and are the preferred specimen for tacrolimus TDM. Some of the adverse effects associated with tacrolimus toxicity include anemia, leukopenia, thrombocytopenia, and hyperlipidemia.

Sirolimus

Sirolimus (Rapamune) is an antifungal agent with immunosuppressive activity that is used to prevent graft rejection in patients receiving a kidney transplant. Sirolimus is rapidly absorbed after once-daily oral administration, and peak blood concentrations are achieved 1 to 2 hours post dose. Plasma concentrations are affected extensively by intestinal and hepatic first-pass metabolism. To increase the therapeutic efficacy, sirolimus is commonly coadministered with cyclosporine or tacrolimus as the bioavailability for sirolimus is 15% when taken in conjunction with cyclosporine.[14,16,17] Sirolimus has a long half-life of 62 hours and is predominantly metabolized in the liver. Plasma concentrations are affected by individual differences in absorption, distribution, metabolism, and excretion demonstrating the need for TDM. This drug is also extremely potent and requires TDM due to its inherent toxicity. Adverse effects associated with toxicity include thrombocytopenia, anemia, leukopenia, infections, and hyperlipidemia.[16,17] Sirolimus binds more readily to lipoproteins than plasma proteins making whole blood the ideal specimen for analysis.[17] Approximately 92% of circulating sirolimus is bound. Initial TDM is performed using a trough specimen drawn during steady state. Subsequent monitoring is performed by collecting trough specimens on a weekly basis for the first month followed by a biweekly sampling pattern in the second month. These specimens are analyzed and used to establish a safe and effective therapeutic range. A therapeutic range of 4 to 12 µg/L is used when sirolimus is administered in conjunction with cyclosporine, and a range of 12 to 20 µg/L is used if cyclosporine therapy is not used or discontinued.[17] Sirolimus concentrations can be measured using chromatographic methods or by high-performance liquid chromatography–tandem mass spectrometry.[14,16]

Mycophenolic Acid

Mycophenolate mofetil (Myfortic) is a prodrug that is rapidly converted in the liver to its active form, mycophenolic acid (MPA).[13] MPA is a lymphocyte proliferation inhibitor that is used most commonly as supplemental therapy with cyclosporine and tacrolimus in renal transplant patients.[8] As with the other antirejection drugs, low trough concentrations of MPA increase the risk of acute rejection, while high concentrations imply toxicity. MPA is administered orally and absorbed under neutral pH conditions in the intestine.[18] Interindividual variation of gastrointestinal tract physiology influences the degree of absorption of MPA; however, peak concentrations are generally achieved 1 to 2 hours post dose. Once in circulation, MPA is 95% protein bound. The degree to which MPA is protein bound varies both intraindividually and interindividually and is dependent on circulating albumin concentrations, renal function, and the concentration of other drugs that may competitively bind to plasma albumin.[18] MPA is primarily eliminated by renal excretion (>90%) and has a half-life of approximately 17 hours. The therapeutic range for MPA is reported to be 1 to 3.5 µg/mL; toxicity may cause nausea, vomiting, diarrhea, and abdominal pain. Plasma MPA and its metabolites' concentrations can be assayed using chromatography or, more commonly, immunoassay, though immunoassays are generally considered less specific.[18] As with most immunoassay methods, cross-reactivity between MPA and its active metabolite (AcMPAG) should be taken into account along with the clinical picture when evaluating a dosage regimen.

ANTINEOPLASTICS

Assessment of the therapeutic benefit and toxicity of most antineoplastic drugs is not aided by TDM because correlations between plasma concentration and therapeutic benefit are hard to establish. Many of these agents are rapidly metabolized or incorporated into cellular macromolecular structures within seconds to minutes of their administration. In addition, the therapeutic range for many of these drugs includes concentrations associated with toxic effects. Considering that most antineoplastic agents are administered intravenously as a single bolus, the actual delivered dose is more relevant than circulating concentrations.

Methotrexate

Methotrexate (Otrexup, Rasuvo) is one of the few antineoplastic drugs in which TDM may offer some benefit to determining a therapeutic regimen. High-dose methotrexate followed by leucovorin rescue has been shown to be an effective therapy for various neoplastic conditions.[19] The basis for this therapy involves the relative rate of mitosis of normal versus neoplastic cells. In general, neoplastic cells divide more rapidly than normal cells. Methotrexate inhibits DNA synthesis in all cells. Neoplastic cells, as a result of their rapid rate of division, have a higher requirement for DNA and are susceptible to depravation of this essential constituent before normal cells. The efficacy of methotrexate therapy is dependent on a controlled period of inhibition, one that is selectively detrimental to neoplastic cells. This is accomplished by administration of leucovorin, which reverses the action of methotrexate at a specific time after methotrexate infusion. This is referred to as *leucovorin rescue*. Failure to stop the action of methotrexate results in cytotoxic effects to most cells. Evaluation of serum methotrexate concentration, after the inhibitory time period has passed, is used to determine how much leucovorin is needed to counteract many of the toxic effects of methotrexate.[19]

Methotrexate is administered orally with peak plasma concentrations 1 hour post dose. Approximately 50% of methotrexate is bound to plasma proteins in circulation. Methotrexate has a half-life of 5 to 9 hours and is predominantly excreted through the renal system. Trough specimens are preferred for determination of plasma methotrexate concentrations. The therapeutic range for trough specimens is less than 1 µmol/L.

BRONCHODILATORS

Theophylline

Theophylline (Theo-Dur, Theo-24, Uniphyl) is used in the treatment of respiratory disorders, such as asthma and stable chronic obstructive pulmonary disease, for patients that have difficulty using an inhaler or those with nocturnal symptoms. Absorption can be variable with peak blood concentrations achieved after 1 to 2 hours post dose when a rapid-release formation is administered or within 4 to 8 hours for a modified-release preparation. Approximately 50% to 65% of circulating drug is bound to plasma proteins, primarily albumin. Theophylline has a half-life of 3 to 8 hours. It is predominantly metabolized in the liver; however, about 20% is eliminated through the renal system. Beneficial effects have been demonstrated at 10 to 20 mg/L (55 to 110 µmol/L). Though infrequent, concentrations above 20 mg/L may lead to serious adverse effects including insomnia, tachycardia, seizures, arrhythmias, and possible cardiorespiratory arrest. There is poor correlation between dosage and plasma concentrations; however, TDM may initially be useful in optimizing the dosage and used to confirm toxicity when suspected.

For additional student resources, please visit thePoint® at http://thepoint.lww.com

questions

1. If drug X has a half-life ($T_{1/2}$) of 2 days (48 hours) and the concentration at 12:00 today was 10 µg/mL, what would the expected concentration of drug X be at 12:00 tomorrow?
   a. 7 µg/mL
   b. 7.5 µg/mL
   c. 5 µg/mL
   d. 3.5 µg/mL

2. If a drug is administered orally, which of the following would affect the efficiency of its absorption in the gastrointestinal tract?
   a. Dissociation of the drug from its administered form
   b. The drug's solubility in gastrointestinal fluid
   c. Diffusion of the drug across gastrointestinal membranes
   d. All of the above

3. If a trough specimen is required for therapeutic drug monitoring, the most appropriate time to collect the specimen would be:
   a. Eight hours after the last dose was given
   b. Three days after the dose was administered
   c. Immediately after the dose is administered
   d. Immediately before the next dose is given

4. Which of the following statements concerning procainamide is TRUE?
   a. Procainamide should be administered intravenously due to poor absorption.
   b. Procainamide is an antibiotic used to treat gram-positive bacterial infections.
   c. Procainamide is metabolized into an active metabolite with similar antiarrhythmic activity.
   d. Procainamide is eliminated entirely through renal filtration.

5. Which of the following statements concerning lithium is TRUE?
   a. Lithium is used to treat depression, self-mutilating behavior, and bipolar disorder.
   b. Lithium toxicity has been associated with ototoxicity and nephrotoxicity.
   c. Lithium is completely metabolized in the liver with no renal elimination.
   d. Lithium is used in conjunction with cyclosporine to prevent transplant rejection.

6. Which of the following is the primary purpose for measuring serum concentrations of methotrexate?
   a. To determine the optimum dosage for oral administration of methotrexate
   b. To ensure that serum concentrations are within the therapeutic range
   c. To confirm serum concentrations when toxicity is suspected
   d. To determine the amount of leucovorin needed to halt methotrexate action

7. Primidone is an inactive preform of which of the following antiepileptic drugs?
   a. Gabapentin
   b. Clozapine
   c. Phenobarbital
   d. Ethosuximide

8. Bilirubin competes with some drugs for the same binding site on plasma proteins. What effect would an increased concentration of bilirubin in the blood (bilirubinemia) have on the potential activity of this drug?
   a. The fraction of bound drug would increase thereby increasing potential activity.
   b. The fraction of bound drug would decrease thereby decreasing potential activity.
   c. The fraction of bound drug would decrease thereby increasing potential activity.
   d. The fraction of bound drug would increase thereby decreasing potential activity.

review questions (continued)

9. Twenty milligrams (mg) of drug Y is injected intravenously. One hour after the injection, blood is collected and assayed for the concentration of drug Y. If the concentration of drug Y in this specimen was 0.4 mg/L, what is the volume of distribution for this drug?
a. 0.8 L
b. 8 L
c. 20 L
d. 50 L

10. A new orally administered drug has been introduced in your institution. It is unclear whether TDM is needed for this drug. What factors should be taken into consideration when addressing this question?
a. Proximity of the toxic range to the therapeutic range.
b. Consequences of a subtherapeutic concentration.
c. Predictability of serum concentrations after a standard oral dose.
d. All of the above should be taken into consideration.

suggested readings

Birkett DJ. *Pharmacokinetics Made Easy*. New York: McGraw-Hill; 2003.

Broussard L, Tuckler V. The value of TDM, toxicology. *Adv Admin Clin Lab*. 2004;13:32.

Graham K. Lab limelight: TDM: applications for pharmacogenetics. *Adv Admin Clin Lab*. 2007;16:81.

Hardman JG, Limbird LE, Gillman AG, eds. *Goodman & Gilman's The Pharmacological Basis of Therapeutics*. 10th ed. New York: Pergamon Press; 2002.

references

1. Abbot A. With your genes? Take one of these, three times a day. *Nature*. 2003;425:760–762.
2. Campbell TJ, Williams MK. Therapeutic drug monitoring: antiarrhythmic drugs. *Br J Clin Pharmacol*. 2001;52: 21S–34S.
3. Jurgens G, Graudal NA, Kampmann JP. Therapeutic drug monitoring of antiarrhythmic drugs. *Clin Pharmacokinet*. 2003;42:647–663.
4. Winston L, Benowitz N. Once-daily dosing of aminoglycosides: how much monitoring is truly required? *Am J Med*. 2003;114:239–240.
5. Perucca E. An introduction to antiepileptic drugs. *Epilepsia*. 2005;46:31–37.
6. Eadie MJ. Therapeutic drug monitoring—antiepileptic drugs. *Br J Clin Pharmacol*. 2001;52:11S–19S.
7. Israni RK, Kasbekar N, Haynes K, et al. Use of antiepileptic drugs in patients with kidney disease. *Semin Dial*. 2006;19:408–416.
8. Johannessen SI, Tomson T. Pharmacokinetic variability of newer antiepileptic drugs. *Clin Pharmacokinet*. 2006;45:1061–1075.
9. Wikipedia Online. Searched Tiagabine. http://en.wikipedia.org/wiki/Tiagabine. Accessed February 17, 2008.
10. Mitchell PB. Therapeutic drug monitoring of psychotropic medications. *Br J Clin Pharmacol*. 2001;52:45S–54S.
11. Mauri MC, Volonteri LS, Colasanti A, et al. Clinical pharmacokinetics of atypical antipsychotics. *Clin Pharmacokinet*. 2007;46:359–388.
12. Masuda S, Inui K. An update review on individualized dosage of calcineurin inhibitors in organ transplant recipients. *Pharmacol Ther*. 2006;112:184–198.
13. Taylor AL, Watson CJE, Bradley JA. Immunosuppressive agents in solid organ transplantation: mechanisms of action and therapeutic efficacy. *Crit Rev Oncol Hematol*. 2005;56:23–46.
14. Johnston A, Holt DW. Immunosuppressant drugs—the role of therapeutic drug monitoring. *Br J Clin Pharmacol*. 2001;52:61S–73S.
15. Baraldo M, Furlanut M. Chronopharmacokinetics of cyclosporine and tacrolimus. *Clin Pharmacokinet*. 2006;45:775–788.
16. Wong SHY. Therapeutic drug monitoring for immunosuppressants. *Clin Chim Acta*. 2001;313:241–253.
17. Stenton SB, Partovi N, Ensom MHH. Sirolimus: the evidence for clinical pharmacokinetic monitoring. *Clin Pharmacokinet*. 2005;44:769–786.
18. Elbarbry FA, Shoker AS. Therapeutic drug measurement of mycophenolic acid derivatives in transplant patients. *Clin Biochem*. 2007;40:752–764.
19. Lennard L. Therapeutic drug monitoring of cytotoxic drugs. *Br J Pharmacol*. 2001;52:75S–87S.

31

Toxicology

TAKARA L. BLAMIRES

chapter outline

key terms

Bioaccumulation
Body burden
Dose–response relationship
Drugs of abuse
ED_{50}
Individual dose–response relationship
LD_{50}
Poisons
Quantal dose–response relationship
TD_{50}
Therapeutic index
Toxicokinetics
Toxicology
Toxins
Xenobiotics

chapter objectives

Upon completion of this chapter, the clinical laboratorian should be able to do the following:

- Define the following terms: poison, toxicant, toxicology, toxin, xenobiotic, ED_{50}, LD_{50}, TD_{50}.
- Identify the primary routes for exposure and discuss factors that influence the absorption of an ingested toxin.
- Compare and contrast acute and chronic toxicity.
- List major toxicants.
- Define the pathologic mechanisms of the major toxicants.
- Identify common specimen types used in toxicology and discuss the benefits and drawbacks of each.
- Discuss the challenges of properly collecting and handling specimens for toxicology testing.
- Explain the differences between quantitative and qualitative tests in toxicology.
- Identify common qualitative and quantitative test methods used to evaluate toxicity in the clinical laboratory.

For additional student resources, please visit thePoint®
at http://thepoint.lww.com

chapter objectives (continued)

- Explain how the osmolal gap is calculated and used to evaluate the presence of osmotically active substances in blood and urine.
- Discuss the role of the clinical laboratory in the evaluation of exposure to toxins and poisons.
- Evaluate clinical laboratory data in suspected poisoning cases and provide recommendations for further testing.

Toxicology is the study of the adverse effects of xenobiotics in humans. **Xenobiotics** are chemicals and drugs that are not normally found in or produced by the body. The scope of toxicology is very broad and includes three major disciplines: mechanistic, descriptive, and regulatory toxicology. *Mechanistic toxicology* elucidates the cellular, molecular, and biochemical effects of xenobiotics within the context of a dose–response relationship between the xenobiotic and its adverse effect(s). Mechanistic studies provide a basis for rational therapy design and the development of laboratory tests to assess the degree of exposure in individuals. *Descriptive toxicology* uses the results from animal experiments to predict what level of exposure will cause harm in humans. This process is known as *risk assessment*. In *regulatory toxicology*, combined data from mechanistic and descriptive studies are used to establish standards that define the level of exposure that will not pose a risk to public health or safety. Typically, regulatory toxicologists work for, or in conjunction with, government agencies. The Food and Drug Administration (FDA) oversees human safety issues associated with therapeutic drugs, cosmetics, and food additives. The U.S. Environmental Protection Agency (EPA) has regulatory oversight with regard to pesticides, fungicides, rodenticides, and industry-related chemicals that may threaten safe drinking water and clean air. The Occupational Safety and Health Administration (OSHA) is responsible for ensuring safe and healthy work environments. The Consumer Product Safety Commission (CPSC) regulates household chemicals, while the Department of Transportation (DOT) oversees transportation of hazardous chemicals.

There are also a number of specialties within toxicology, including forensic, clinical, and environmental toxicology. *Forensic toxicology* is primarily concerned with the medical and legal consequences of exposure to chemicals or drugs. A major focus of forensic toxicology is establishing and validating the analytic performance of test methods used to generate evidence in legal situations, including cause of death. *Clinical toxicology* focuses on the relationships between xenobiotics and disease states. This area emphasizes not only diagnostic testing but also therapeutic intervention. *Environmental toxicology* includes the evaluation of environmental chemical pollutants and their impact on human health. This is a growing area of concern as we learn more about the mechanisms of action of these chemicals and their adverse effects on

human health. Another goal of environmental toxicology is to monitor occupational health issues and to increase public health biomonitoring efforts nationwide.

Within the organizational structure of a typical clinical laboratory, toxicology is usually considered a specialty of clinical chemistry because the qualitative and quantitative methodologies used to measure xenobiotics overlap with this discipline. However, appropriate diagnosis and management of patients with acute poisoning or chronic exposure to xenobiotics requires an integrated approach from all sections of the clinical laboratory.

XENOBIOTICS, POISONS, AND TOXINS

The terms, xenobiotic, poison, and toxin are often used interchangeably; however, there are some important distinctions that should be made between them. Xenobiotics, as previously mentioned, are defined as exogenous agents that can have an adverse effect on a living organism. This term is more often used to describe environmental exposure to chemicals or drugs. Examples of environmental drug exposures include antibiotics and antidepressants; chemical exposures might include perfluorinated and brominated compounds. Similarly, **poisons** are also exogenous agents that have an adverse effect on a biological system; however, this term is more often used when describing substances from an animal, plant, mineral, or gas. Examples include venoms from poisonous snakes or spiders, poison hemlock, arsenic, lead, and carbon monoxide. **Toxins**, however, are endogenous substances biologically synthesized either in living cells or in microorganisms. Examples include botulinum toxin produced from the microorganism, *Clostridium botulinum*, hemotoxins produced from venomous snakes, and mycotoxins produced from fungus. The terms *toxicant* and *toxic* refer to substances that are not produced within a living cell or microorganism and are more commonly used to describe environmental chemicals.

From a clinical standpoint, almost 50% of poisoning cases are intentional suicide attempts, accidental exposure accounts for about 30%, and the remaining cases are a result of homicide or occupational exposure. Of these, suicide has the highest mortality rate. Accidental exposure occurs most frequently in children; however, accidental drug overdose of either therapeutic or illicit drugs is relatively common in adolescents and adults. Occupational exposure primarily occurs in industrial and agricultural settings, but is an expanding area of concern as we learn more about the role of various chemical agents and their contribution to disease.

ROUTES OF EXPOSURE

Toxins can enter the body via several routes, with ingestion, inhalation, and transdermal absorption being the most common. Of these, ingestion is most often observed in the clinical setting. For most toxins to exert a systemic effect, they must be absorbed into circulation. Absorption of toxins from the gastrointestinal tract occurs via several mechanisms. Some toxins are taken up by processes intended for dietary nutrients; however, most are passively absorbed through diffusion. Diffusion requires that the substance be able to cross the cellular barriers of the gastrointestinal tract. Hydrophobic substances do have the ability to diffuse across cell membranes and, therefore, can be absorbed anywhere along the gastrointestinal tract. Ionized substances, however, cannot passively diffuse across the membranes. Weak acids can become protonated in gastric acid resulting in a nonionized species, which can be absorbed in the stomach. In a similar manner, weak bases can be absorbed in the intestine where the pH is largely neutral or slightly alkaline. Other factors that influence the absorbance of toxins from the gastrointestinal tract include the rate of dissolution, gastrointestinal motility, resistance to degradation in the gastrointestinal tract, and interaction with other substances. Toxins that are not absorbed from the gastrointestinal tract do not produce systemic effects, but may produce local effects, such as diarrhea, bleeding, and malabsorption, which may cause systemic effects secondary to toxin exposure.

DOSE–RESPONSE RELATIONSHIP

The concept that all substances have the potential to cause harm, even water, is a central theme in toxicology. Paracelsus (1493 to 1591) pioneered the use of chemicals in medicine and coined the term "the dose makes the poison." Understanding this, **dose–response relationship** is fundamental and essential to modern toxicology. To enable assessment of substances' potential to cause pathologic effects, it is necessary to establish an index of the relative toxicities of the substances. Several systems are available, but most correlate the dose of a xenobiotic that will result in harmful effects. One such system correlates a single acute oral dose range with the probability of a lethal outcome in an average 70-kg man (Table 31.1). This is a useful system to compare the relative toxicities of substances as the predicted response is death, which is valid. However, most xenobiotics can express pathologic effects other than death at lower degrees of exposure; therefore, other indices have been developed.

A more in-depth characterization can be acquired by evaluating data from a cumulative frequency histogram of toxic responses over a range of doses. This experimental approach is typically used to evaluate responses over a

TABLE 31.1	Toxicity Rating System
Toxicity Rating	**Lethal Oral Dose in Average Adult**
Super toxic	<5 mg/kg
Extremely toxic	5–50 mg/kg
Very toxic	50–500 mg/kg
Moderately toxic	0.5–5 g/kg
Slightly toxic	5–15 g/kg
Practically nontoxic	>15 g/kg

Adapted from Klaassen CD. Principles of toxicology. In: Klaassen CD, Amdur MO, Doull J, eds. *Toxicology: the Basic Science of Poisons*. 3rd ed. New York, NY: Macmillan; 1986:13.

wide range of concentrations. One response monitored is the toxic response or the response associated with an early pathologic effect at lower than lethal doses. This response has been determined to be an indicator of the toxic effects specific for that toxin. For a substance that exerts early toxic effects by damaging liver cells, the response monitored may be increases in serum alanine aminotransferase (ALT) or γ-glutamyltransferase (GGT) activity. The dose–response relationship implies that there will be an increase in the toxic response as the dose is increased. It should be noted that not all individuals display a toxic response at the same dose. The population variance can be seen in a cumulative frequency histogram of the percentage of people producing a toxic response over a range of concentrations (Fig. 31.1). The **TD_{50}** is the predicted dose that would produce a toxic response in 50% of the population. If the monitored response is death, the **LD_{50}** is the predicted dose that would result in death in 50% of the population. Similar experiments can be used to evaluate the doses of therapeutic drugs. The **ED_{50}** is the dose that would be predicted to be effective or have a therapeutic benefit in 50% of the population. The **therapeutic index** is the ratio of the TD_{50} (or LD_{50}) to the ED_{50}. Drugs with a large therapeutic index demonstrate fewer toxic adverse effects when the dose of the drug is in the therapeutic range.

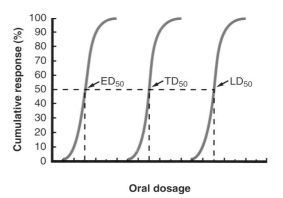

FIGURE 31.1 Dose–response relationship. Comparison of responses of a therapeutic drug over a range of doses. The ED_{50} is the dose of drug in which 50% of treated individuals will experience benefit. The TD_{50} is the dose of drug in which 50% of individuals will experience toxic adverse effects. The LD_{50} is the dose of drug in which 50% of individuals will result in mortality.

Dose–response relationships may apply to an individual or a population. The **individual dose–response relationship** relates to the individual's health status as well as changes in xenobiotic exposure levels. A **quantal dose–response relationship** describes the change in health effects of a defined population based on changes in the exposure to the xenobiotic.

Acute and Chronic Toxicity

Acute toxicity and *chronic toxicity* are terms used to relate the duration and frequency of exposure to observed toxic effects. Acute toxicity is usually associated with a single, short-term exposure to a substance in which the dose is sufficient to cause immediate toxic effects. Chronic toxicity is generally associated with repeated and frequent exposure for extended periods of time (months to years) at doses that are insufficient to cause an immediate acute response. In many instances, chronic exposure is related to an accumulation of the toxicant or the toxic effects within the individual. Chronic toxicity may affect different systems than those associated with acute toxicity; therefore, dose–response relationships may differ for acute and chronic exposures for the same xenobiotic.

ANALYSIS OF TOXIC AGENTS

Toxicology testing may be performed to screen for the presence of a number of agents that might be present (e.g., drug screens, heavy metal panels) or as targeted testing. Targeted testing might be performed when an environmental risk of exposure is known (e.g., industrial workers, chemical plants), to support the investigation of an exposure (e.g., chemical spill, suicide attempt), to comply with occupational regulations or guidelines (e.g., OSHA), or to confirm clinical suspicions of poisoning (e.g., arsenic, cyanide). Due to nonspecific signs and symptoms of toxicity and that frequently the duration and extent of exposure are unknown, diagnosis of most toxic element exposures depends heavily on laboratory testing.

In general, toxicology testing is performed on urine or blood specimens. In selecting the best specimen for a specific test, it is important to recognize that toxic agents exhibit unique absorption, distribution, metabolism, and elimination kinetics or **toxicokinetics**. As such, the predicted toxicokinetics of the individual element(s) being tested must be coordinated with the selection of specimen type and timing of collection relative to the time of exposure. An exposure could be missed entirely if testing is performed on an inappropriate specimen. For example, exposure to methylmercury could be missed if testing is performed on urine as methylmercury is primarily excreted in fecal material. An exposure to arsenic could be missed if testing is performed with blood collected a few days after the exposure due to the short half of arsenic in blood.

Preanalytical variables such as elimination patterns, analyte stability, and specimen collection procedures must be considered. For urine testing, 24-hour collections are preferred in order to compensate for variable elimination patterns throughout the day. Reporting results per gram of creatinine is also common to account for variable excretion and renal function. Random urine collections may not provide the most accurate profile of exposure when compared to a 24-hour collection, but they are useful for screening and qualitative detection of exposure to several potentially toxic agents. Any elevated result that is inconsistent with clinical expectations should be confirmed by testing a second specimen collection or a second specimen type.

One challenge of specimen collection for toxicological studies is that several aspects of the collection, handling, and storage can introduce external contamination into the sample. Common sources of external contamination include patient clothing, skin, hair, collection environment (e.g., dust, aerosols, antiseptic wipes), and specimen handling variables (e.g., container, lid, preservatives). Concentrated acids are commonly used as urine preservatives; however, contaminants may also be introduced in either the acid itself or in the process used to add the acid to the urine (e.g., pipette tips). Specimen containers and lids should also be devoid of contaminating organic and inorganic agents that may interfere with analytical testing. For example, certified "trace element-free" blood collection tubes are available; these tubes commonly have a royal blue top and can be used for most trace elements testing though a tan-top tube is manufactured specifically for lead determinations. Another consideration when handling biological specimens for metals testing is the use of acid-washed pipette tips, containers, and other supplies to prevent contamination. Laboratories may also need to exercise precautions to prevent loss of toxic agents due to in vitro volatilization and metabolism. For instance, mercury and arsenic are particularly vulnerable to loss and metabolism, respectively, during sample processing and storage. These scenarios represent only a fraction of the many specimen handling considerations necessary to reduce preanalytical error in toxicology testing.

Analysis of toxic agents in a clinical setting is typically a two-step process. The first step is a screening test, which is a rapid, simple, qualitative procedure intended to detect the presence of specific substances or classes of toxicants. In general, these procedures have good analytic sensitivity but lack specificity. A negative result can rule out a drug or toxicant; however, a positive result should be considered a presumptive positive until confirmed by a second, more specific method, which is the second step of the test process, or a confirmatory test. Confirmatory tests are generally quantitative and report the concentration of the substance in the specimen in contrast to qualitative screening tests that provide a result of positive (drug is present) or negative (drug is absent). A variety of analytical methods can be used for screening and confirmatory testing though immunoassays are the commonly used for drug screens. In some instances, these assays are specific for a single drug (e.g., tetrahydrocannabinol [THC]), but in most cases, the assay is to detect drugs within a general class (e.g., barbiturates and opiates). Thin-layer chromatography (TLC) is a relatively simple, inexpensive method for detecting various drugs and other organic compounds; gas chromatography (GC) is widely used and a well-established technique for qualitative and quantitative determination of many volatile substances. The reference method for quantitative identification of most organic compounds is gas chromatography coupled with a mass spectrometer (GC–MS) as the detector. Inorganic compounds, including speciation, may be quantitated using inductively coupled plasma-mass spectrometry (ICP-MS) or atomic absorption (AA) methods.

TOXICOLOGY OF SPECIFIC AGENTS

Many chemical agents encountered on a regular basis have potential for toxicity. The focus of this section is to discuss some of the most commonly encountered nondrug toxins seen in a clinical setting, as well as those that present as medical emergencies with acute exposure.[1]

Alcohols

The toxic effects of alcohol are both general and specific. Exposure to alcohol, like exposure to most volatile organic solvents, initially causes disorientation, confusion, and euphoria, but can progress to unconsciousness, paralysis, and, with high-level exposure, even death. Most alcohols display these effects at about equivalent molar concentrations. This similarity suggests a common depressant effect on the central nervous system (CNS) that appears to be mediated by changes in membrane properties. In most cases, recovery from CNS effects is rapid and complete after cessation of exposure.

Distinct from the general CNS effects are the specific toxicities of each type of alcohol, which are usually mediated by biotransformation of alcohols to toxic products. There are several pathways by which short-chain aliphatic alcohols can be metabolized. Of these, hepatic conversion to an aldehyde, by alcohol dehydrogenase (ADH), and further conversion to an acid, by hepatic aldehyde dehydrogenase (ALDH), is the most significant.

$$\text{Alcohol} \xrightarrow{\text{ADH}} \text{Aldehyde} \xrightarrow{\text{ALDH}} \text{Acid} \qquad \text{(Eq. 31-1)}$$

Ethanol

Ethanol exposure is common, and excessive consumption, with its associated consequences, is a leading cause of economic, social, and medical problems throughout the world.[2] The economic impact is estimated to exceed $100 billion per year in terms of lost wages and productivity. Many social and family problems are associated with excessive ethanol consumption, and the burden to the health care system is significant. Ethanol-related disorders are consistently one of the top ten causes of hospital admissions, and approximately 20% of all hospital admissions have some degree of alcohol-related problems. It is estimated that 80,000 Americans die each year, either directly or indirectly, as a result of abusive alcohol consumption. This correlates to about a fivefold increase in premature mortality. In addition, consumption of ethanol during pregnancy may lead to fetal alcohol syndrome or fetal alcohol effects, both of which are associated with delayed motor and mental development in children.

Correlations have been established between blood alcohol concentration and the clinical signs and symptoms of acute intoxication. A blood alcohol concentration of 80 mg/dL has been established as the statutory limit for operation of a motor vehicle in the United States as this concentration is associated with a diminution of judgment and motor function. Determinations of blood ethanol concentration by the laboratory may be used in litigation of drunken driving cases and requires appropriate chain-of-custody procedures for specimen collection and documentation of acceptable quality control performance, instrument maintenance procedures, and proficiency testing records. Approximately 50% of the 40,000 to 50,000 annual automobile-related fatalities in the United States involve alcohol as a factor.

Besides the short-term effects of ethanol, most pathophysiologic consequences of ethanol abuse are associated with chronic consumption. In an average adult, this correlates to the consumption of about 50 g of ethanol per day for about 10 years. This pattern of consumption has been associated with compromised function of various organs, tissues, and cell types; however, the liver appears to be affected the most. The pathologic sequence starts with the accumulation of lipids in hepatocytes. With continued consumption, this may progress to alcoholic hepatitis. In about 20% of individuals with long-term, high-level alcohol intake, this develops into a toxic form of hepatitis. Of those who do not progress to toxic hepatitis, progression to liver cirrhosis is common. Cirrhosis of the liver can be characterized as fibrosis leading to functional loss of the hepatocytes. Progress through this sequence is associated with changes in many laboratory tests related to hepatic function including liver enzymes. Several laboratory indicators have the required diagnostic sensitivity and specificity to identify excessive ethanol consumption and most correlate well to the progression of ethanol-induced liver disease. Table 31.2 lists common laboratory indicators of prolonged ethanol consumption.

Several mechanisms have been proposed to mediate the pathologic effects of long-term ethanol consumption. Of these, adduct formation with acetaldehyde appears to play a key role. Hepatic metabolism of ethanol is a two-step enzymatic reaction with acetaldehyde as a reactive intermediate. Most ethanol is converted to acetate, or acetic acid, in this pathway; however, a significant portion of the acetaldehyde intermediate is released in the free state.

$$\text{Ethanol} \rightarrow \text{Acetaldehyde} \rightarrow \text{Acetate} \atop \rightarrow \text{Acetaldehyde adducts} \qquad \text{(Eq. 31-2)}$$

Extracellular acetaldehyde is a transient species as a result of rapid adduct formation with amine groups of proteins. Many of the pathologic effects of ethanol have been correlated with the formation of these adducts, and formation of acetaldehyde adducts has also been shown to change the structure and function of various proteins.

TABLE 31.2	Common Indicators of Ethanol Abuse
Test	**Comments**
GGT	Increases can be seen before the onset of pathologic consequences
	Increases in serum activity can occur in many non–ethanol-related conditions
AST	Increases in serum activity can occur in many non–ethanol-related conditions
AST/ALT ratio	A ratio of >2.0 is highly specific for ethanol-related liver disease
HDL	High serum HDL is specific for ethanol consumption
MCV	Increased erythrocyte MCV is commonly seen with excessive ethanol consumption
	Increases are not related to folate or vitamin B_{12} deficiency

GGT, γ-glutamyltransferase; AST, aspartate aminotransferase; ALT, alanine aminotransferase; HDL, high-density lipoprotein; MCV, mean cell volume.

Methanol

Methanol is a common laboratory solvent that is also found in many household cleaners. It may be ingested accidentally as a component of many commercial products or as a contaminant of homemade liquors. Methanol is initially metabolized by hepatic ADH to the intermediate formaldehyde. Formaldehyde is then rapidly converted to formic acid by hepatic ALDH. The formation of formic acid causes severe metabolic acidosis, which can lead to tissue injury and possible death. Formic acid is also responsible for optic neuropathy that can lead to blindness.

Isopropanol

Isopropanol, also known as rubbing alcohol, is also commercially available. It is metabolized by hepatic ADH to acetone, which is its primary metabolic end product. Both isopropanol and acetone have CNS depressant effects similar to ethanol; however, acetone has a long half-life, and intoxication with isopropanol can therefore result in severe acute-phase ethanol-like symptoms that persist for an extended period.

Ethylene Glycol

Ethylene glycol (1,2-ethanediol) is a common component of hydraulic fluid and antifreeze. Ingestion by children is relatively common because of its sweet taste. The immediate effects of ethylene glycol ingestion are similar to those of ethanol; however, metabolism by hepatic ADH and ALDH results in the formation of several toxic species including oxalic acid and glycolic acid, which result in severe metabolic acidosis. This is complicated by the rapid formation and deposition of calcium oxalate crystals in the renal tubules. With high levels of consumption, calcium oxalate crystal formation in the kidneys may result in renal tubular damage.

Determination of Alcohols

From a medicolegal perspective, determinations of blood ethanol concentrations must be accurate and precise. Serum, plasma, and whole blood are acceptable specimens, and correlations have been established between ethanol concentration in these specimens and impairment of psychomotor function. Because ethanol uniformly distributes in total body water, serum, which has greater water content than whole blood, has a higher concentration per unit volume. Because of this difference in distribution, most states have standardized the acceptable specimen types admissible

as evidence, and some jurisdictions even mandate a specific method (often GC) be used for legal ethanol determination.

When acquiring a specimen for ethanol determination, several preanalytical issues must be considered to ensure the integrity of the sample. One of these requirements is that the venipuncture site should only be cleaned with an alcohol-free disinfectant. Also, because of the volatile nature of short-chain aliphatic alcohols, specimens must be capped at all times to avoid evaporation. Sealed specimens can be refrigerated or stored at room temperature for up to 14 days without loss of ethanol. Nonsterile specimens or those intended to be stored for longer periods of time should be preserved with sodium fluoride to avoid increases in ethanol content resulting from contamination due to bacterial fermentation.

CASE STUDY 31.1

A patient with a provisional diagnosis of depression was sent to the laboratory for a routine workup. The complete blood cell count was unremarkable except for an elevated erythrocyte mean cell volume. Results of the urinalysis were unremarkable. The serum chemistry testing revealed slightly increased aspartate aminotransferase (AST), total bilirubin, and high-density lipoproteins (HDL). All other chemistry results, including glucose, urea, creatinine, cholesterol, pH, bicarbonate/carbon dioxide (pCO_2), alanine aminotransferase (ALT), sodium, and potassium, were within the reference intervals. The physician suspects ethanol abuse; however, the patient denies an alcohol use. Subsequent testing revealed a serum γ-glutamyltransferase (GGT) three times the upper limit of the reference interval. No ethanol was detected in serum, and screening tests for infectious forms of hepatitis were negative.

Questions

1. Are these results consistent with a patient who is consuming hazardous quantities of ethanol?

2. What additional testing would you recommend to rule ethanol abuse in or out?

Several analytic methods can be used to determine the concentration of ethanol in serum. Among these, osmometric, chromatographic, and enzymatic methods are the most commonly used. When osmolality is measured by freezing point depression, increases in serum osmolality correlate well with increases in serum ethanol concentration. The degree of increase in osmolality due to the presence of ethanol is expressed as the difference between the measured and the calculated osmolality otherwise referred to as the *osmolal gap*. It has been established that serum osmolality increases by approximately 10 mOsm/kg for each 60 mg/dL increase in serum ethanol; therefore, the osmolal gap is useful for estimating the amount of ethanol present in the serum. The osmolal gap can be calculated as follows:

$$\text{Osmolal gap} = \text{measured osmolality} - \text{calculated osmolality} \quad \text{(Eq. 31-3)}$$

This relationship, however, is not specific to ethanol, and increases in the osmolal gap also occur with certain metabolic imbalances. Therefore, use of the osmolal gap for determination of serum or blood ethanol concentration lacks analytic specificity; however, it is a useful screening test.

GC is the established reference method for ethanol determinations and is quite useful as it can simultaneously quantitate other alcohols as well, such as methanol and isopropanol. Analysis begins with dilution of the serum or blood sample with a saturated solution of sodium chloride in a closed container. Volatiles within the liquid specimen partition into the airspace (head space) of the closed container. Sampling of the head space provides a clean specimen with little or no matrix effect. Quantitation can be performed by constructing a standard curve or calculating the concentration based on relative changes to an internal standard (*n*-propanol) as shown in Figure 31.2.

Enzymatic methods for ethanol determination use a nonhuman form of ADH to oxidize ethanol in the specimen to acetaldehyde with simultaneous reduction of NAD$^+$ to NADH.

$$\text{Ethanol} + \text{NAD}^+ \xrightarrow{\text{ADH}} \text{Acetaldehyde} + \text{NADH} \quad \text{(Eq. 31-4)}$$

The NADH produced can be monitored directly by absorbance at 340 nm or can be coupled to an indicator reaction. This form of ADH is relatively specific for ethanol (Table 31.1), and intoxication with methanol or isopropanol produces a negative or low result; therefore, a negative result by this method does not rule out ingestion of other alcohols. There is good agreement between the enzymatic reactions of ethanol and GC. The enzymatic reactions can be fully automated and do not require specialized instrumentation.

Carbon Monoxide

Carbon monoxide is produced by incomplete combustion of carbon-containing substances. The primary environmental sources of carbon monoxide include gasoline engines, improperly ventilated furnaces, and wood or plastic fires. Carbon monoxide is a colorless, odorless, and tasteless gas that is rapidly absorbed into circulation from inspired air.

When carbon monoxide binds to hemoglobin, it is called *carboxyhemoglobin (COHb)*. The affinity of carbon monoxide for hemoglobin is 200 to 225 times greater than for oxygen.[3,4] Air is approximately 20% oxygen by volume. If inspired air contained 0.1% carbon monoxide by volume, this would result in 50% carboxyhemoglobinemia at equilibrium. Because both carbon monoxide and oxygen compete for the same binding site, exposure to carbon monoxide results in a decrease in the concentration of oxyhemoglobin, and, for this reason, carbon monoxide is considered a very toxic substance.

Carbon monoxide expresses its toxic effects by causing a leftward shift in the oxygen–hemoglobin dissociation curve resulting in a decrease in the amount of oxygen delivered to the tissue.[3] The net decrease in the amount of oxygen delivered to the tissue results in hypoxia. The major toxic effects of carbon monoxide exposure are seen in organs with high oxygen demand, such as the brain and heart. The concentration of COHb, expressed as the percentage of COHb, presents relative to the capacity of the specimen to form COHb, and the corresponding symptoms are detailed in Table 31.3. The only treatment for carbon monoxide poisoning is 100% oxygen therapy. In severe cases, hyperbaric oxygen may be used to promote distribution of oxygen to the tissues. The half-life of COHb is roughly 60 to 90 minutes in a patient with normal respiratory function breathing 100% oxygen.

Several methods are available for the evaluation of carbon monoxide poisoning. One screening test for COHb relies on the fact that it has a cherry-red appearance. In this qualitative test, excessive carbon monoxide exposure is evaluated by adding 5 mL of 40% NaOH to 5 mL of an aqueous dilution of the whole blood specimen. Persistence of a pink color of the solution is consistent with a COHb level of 20% or greater.

Retention Time (Minutes)	Analyte
0.675	Methanol
0.911	Acetone
1.098	Ethanol
1.611	Isopropanol
2.430	*n*-Propanol

FIGURE 31.2 Headspace gas chromatography of alcohol. The concentration of each alcohol can be determined by comparison to the response from the internal standard *n*-propanol.

TABLE 31.3	Symptoms of Carboxy-hemoglobinemia
COHb (%)	**Symptoms and Comments**
0.5	Typical in nonsmokers
5–15	Range of values seen in smokers
10	Shortness of breath with vigorous exercise
20	Shortness of breath with moderate exercise
30	Severe headaches, fatigue, impairment of judgment
40–50	Confusion, fainting on exertion
60–70	Unconsciousness, respiratory failure, death with continuous exposure
80	Immediately fatal

COHb, carboxyhemoglobin.

There are two primary quantitative assays for COHb: differential spectrophotometry and GC. Spectrophotometric methods work on the principle that different forms of hemoglobin present with different spectral absorbance curves. By measuring the absorbance at four to six different wavelengths, the concentration of the different species of hemoglobin, including COHb, can be determined by calculation. This is the most common method used for COHb and is the basis for several automated systems. GC methods, however, are considered the reference method for determination of COHb due to their high accuracy and precision. Carbon monoxide is released from hemoglobin after treatment with potassium ferricyanide. After analytic separation, carbon monoxide is detected by changes in thermal conductivity, and the COHb concentration can be determined.

Caustic Agents

Caustic agents are found in many household products and occupational settings. Even though any exposure to a strong acid or alkaline substance is associated with injury, aspiration and ingestion present the greatest hazards. Aspiration is usually associated with pulmonary edema and shock, which can rapidly progress to death. Ingestion produces lesions in the esophagus and gastrointestinal tract, which may produce perforations. This results in hematemesis, abdominal pain, and possibly shock. The onset of metabolic acidosis or alkalosis occurs rapidly after ingestion of caustic agents and corrective therapy for ingestion is usually by dilution.

Cyanide

Cyanide is classified as a supertoxic substance that can exist as a gas, solid, or in solution. Because of the various forms, cyanide exposure can occur by inhalation, ingestion, or transdermal absorption. Cyanide is used in many industrial processes and is a component of some insecticides and rodenticides. It is also produced as a pyrolysis product from the burning of some plastics, including urea foams that are used as insulation in homes. Thus, carbon monoxide and cyanide exposure may account for a significant portion of the toxicities associated with fires and smoke inhalation. Ingestion of cyanide is also a common suicide agent.

Cyanide expresses toxicity by binding to heme iron. Binding to mitochondrial cytochrome oxidase causes an uncoupling of oxidative phosphorylation. This leads to rapid depletion of cellular adenosine triphosphate as a result of the inability of oxygen to accept electrons. Increases in cellular oxygen tension and venous pO_2 occur as a result of lack of oxygen utilization. At low levels of exposure, patients experience headaches, dizziness, and respiratory depression, which can rapidly progress to seizure, coma, and death at greater doses. Cyanide clearance is primarily mediated by rapid enzymatic conversion to thiocyanate, a nontoxic product rapidly cleared by renal filtration. Cyanide toxicity is associated with acute exposure at concentrations sufficient to exceed the rate of clearance by this enzymatic process.

Evaluation of cyanide exposure requires a rapid turnaround time, and several test methods are available. Ion-specific electrode (ISE) methods and photometric analysis following two-well microdiffusion separation are the most common methods. Chronic low-level exposure to cyanide is generally evaluated by determining a urinary thiocyanate concentration.

Metals and Metalloids
Arsenic

Arsenic is a metalloid that may exist bound to or as a primary constituent of many different organic and inorganic compounds. It exists in both naturally occurring and manmade substances; therefore, exposure to arsenic occurs in various settings. Environmental exposure through air and water is prevalent in many industrialized areas, and occupational exposure occurs in agriculture and smelting industries. Arsenic is also a common homicide and suicide agent. Ingestion of less harmful organic forms of arsenic, such as arsenobetaine and arsenocholine, can occur with foods such as clams, oysters, scallops, mussels, crustaceans (crabs and lobsters), and some bottom-feeding finfish.

Arsenic toxicity is largely dependent on the valence state, solubility, and rate of absorption and elimination. The three major groups for arsenic include arsine gas (arsine trioxide), inorganic forms (trivalent and pentavalent), and organic forms (arsenobetaine and arsenocholine). The rate of absorption largely depends on the form of arsenic. Inhalation of arsine gas demonstrates the most acute toxicity. Organic arsenic-containing compounds, such as those found in seafood, are rapidly absorbed by passive diffusion in the gastrointestinal tract. Other forms are absorbed at a slower rate. Clearance of arsenic is primarily by renal filtration of the free, ionized state. Arsenic is rapidly cleared from the blood, such that blood levels may be normal even when urine levels remain markedly elevated. The "fish arsenic" such as arsenobetaine and arsenocholine is cleared in urine within 48 hours; however, the initial half-life of inorganic arsenic is close to 10 hours. Approximately 70% of inorganic arsenic is secreted in urine, of which, 50% of excreted inorganic arsenic has been transformed to the organic form. However, these patterns may vary with the dose and clinical status of the patient. Chronic toxicity of arsenic can be due to low level, persistent exposure that may lead to **bioaccumulation** or increased body burden of this metal. Arsenic expresses toxic effects by high-affinity binding to the thiol groups in proteins; therefore, this can reduce the portion available for renal filtration and elimination. Because many proteins are capable of binding arsenic, the toxic symptoms of arsenic poisoning are nonspecific, and arsenic binding to proteins often results in a change in protein structure and function.[5] Many cellular and organ systems are affected with arsenic toxicity; fever, anorexia, and gastrointestinal distress are often seen with chronic or acute arsenic ingestion at low levels. Peripheral and central damage to the nervous system, renal effects, hemopoietic effects, and vascular disease leading to death are associated with high levels of exposure.

Analysis of arsenic is most commonly performed by atomic absorption spectrophotometry (AAS). Most forms of arsenic are only detectable in the blood for a few hours. More than 90% of an arsenic exposure is recovered in the urine within 6 days making urine the specimen of choice for an exposure occurring in the previous week.

Some toxins can bind to sulfhydryl groups in keratin found in hair and fingernails. For this reason, long-term exposure to some toxins may also be assessed in these tissues. Typically, toxic element deposition in hair and fingernails is demonstrated 2 weeks after an exposure, and in arsenic poisoning cases, distinct white lines can be observed in the fingernails, which are referred to as Mees' lines.

Cadmium

Cadmium is a metal found in many industrial processes, with its main use being in electroplating and galvanizing though it is also commonly encountered during the mining and processing of many other metals. Cadmium is a pigment found in paints and plastics and is the cathodal material of nickel–cadmium batteries. Due to its widespread industrial applications, this element has become a significant environmental pollutant. In the environment, cadmium binds strongly to organic matter where it is immobilized in soil and can be taken up by agricultural crops. Since tobacco leaves accumulate cadmium from the soil, regular use of tobacco-containing products is a common route of human exposure. Smoking is estimated to at least double the lifetime **body burden** of cadmium. For nonsmokers, human exposure to cadmium is largely through the consumption of shellfish, organ meats, lettuce, spinach, potatoes, grains, peanuts, soybeans, and sunflower seeds.

Cadmium expresses its toxicity primarily by binding to proteins; however, it can also bind to other cellular constituents. Cadmium distributes throughout the body, but has a tendency to accumulate in the kidney, where most of its toxic effects are expressed. An early finding of cadmium toxicity is manifested by renal tubular dysfunction in which

tubular proteinuria, glucosuria, and aminoaciduria are typically seen. In addition to renal dysfunction, concomitant parathyroid dysfunction and vitamin D deficiency may also occur. *Itai-itai* disease is characterized by severe osteomalacia and osteoporosis from the long-term consumption of cadmium-contaminated rice. Elimination of cadmium is very slow, as the biological half-life of cadmium is 10 to 30 years. Evaluation of excessive cadmium is most commonly accomplished by the determination of whole blood or urinary content using AAS.

Lead

Lead is a by-product or component of many industrial processes, which has contributed to its widespread presence in the environment. It was a common constituent of household paints before 1972 and is still found in commercial paints and art supplies. Plumbing constructed of lead pipes or joined with leaded connectors has contributed to the lead concentration of water. Gasoline contained tetraethyl lead until 1978. The long-term utilization of leaded gasoline, lead-based paint, and lead-based construction materials has resulted in airborne lead, contaminated soil, and leaded dust.

The lead content of foods is highly variable. In the United States, the average daily intake for an adult is between 75 and 120 µg. This level of intake is not associated with overt toxicity. Because lead is present in all biological systems and because no physiologic or biochemical function has been found, the key issue is identifying the threshold dose that causes toxic effects. Exposure to lead can occur by any route; however, ingestion of contaminated dietary constituents accounts for most exposures.[5] Gastrointestinal absorption is influenced by various factors though the exact factors controlling the rate of absorption are unclear. However, susceptibility to lead toxicity appears to be primarily dependent on age. Adults absorb 5% to 15% of ingested lead, whereas children have a greater degree of absorption, and infants absorb nearly 30% to 40%. Absorbed lead binds with high affinity to many macromolecular structures and is widely distributed throughout the body. Lead distributes into two theoretical compartments: bone and soft tissue, with bone being the largest pool. Lead combines with the matrix of bone and can persist in this compartment for a long period due to its long half-life of almost 20 years. The half-life of lead in soft tissue is somewhat variable though the reported average half-life is 120 days.

Elimination of lead occurs primarily by renal filtration, but because only a small fraction of total body lead is present in circulation, the elimination rate is slow. Considering the relatively constant rate of exposure and the slow elimination rate, total body lead accumulates over a lifetime. As mentioned, the largest accumulation occurs in bone, but there is also significant accumulation in the kidneys, bone marrow, circulating erythrocytes, and peripheral and central nerves.

Lead toxicity is multifaceted and occurs in a dose-dependent manner (Fig. 31.3). Abdominal or neurological

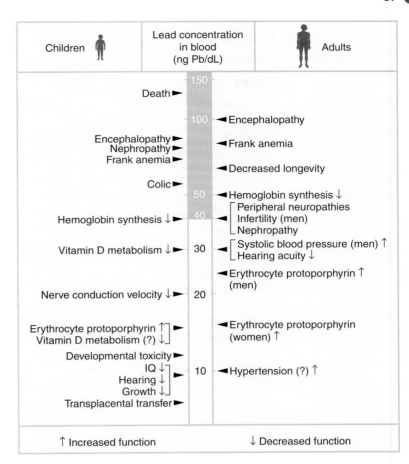

Children 🚶	Lead concentration in blood (ng Pb/dL)	Adults 🧍
Death ►	150	
	100	◄ Encephalopathy
Encephalopathy ► Nephropathy ► Frank anemia ►		◄ Frank anemia
		◄ Decreased longevity
Colic ►	50	◄ Hemoglobin synthesis ↓
Hemoglobin synthesis ↓ ►	40	◄ ⌈ Peripheral neuropathies Infertility (men) Nephropathy
Vitamin D metabolism ↓ ►	30	◄ ⌈ Systolic blood pressure (men) ↑ Hearing acuity ↓
		◄ Erythrocyte protoporphyrin ↑ (men)
Nerve conduction velocity ↓ ►	20	
Erythrocyte protoporphyrin ↑ ⌉ ► Vitamin D metabolism (?) ↓ ⌋		◄ Erythrocyte protoporphyrin (women) ↑
Developmental toxicity ► IQ ↓ ⌉ Hearing ↓ Growth ↓ ⌋ Transplacental transfer ►	10	◄ Hypertension (?) ↑
↑ Increased function		↓ Decreased function

FIGURE 31.3 Comparison of effects of lead on children and adults. (Reprinted from Royce SE, Needleman HL, eds. *Case Studies in Environmental Medicine: Lead Toxicity*. Washington, DC: U.S. Public Health Service, ATSDR; 1990.)

symptoms manifest after acute exposure only. The neurologic effects of lead are of particular importance. Lead exposure causes encephalopathy characterized by cerebral edema and ischemia. Severe lead poisoning can result in stupor, convulsions, and coma. Lower levels of exposure may not present with these symptoms; however, low-level exposure may result in subclinical effects characterized by behavioral changes, hyperactivity, attention deficit disorder and a decrease in intelligence quotient (IQ) scores. Higher levels of exposure have also been associated with demyelinization of peripheral nerves resulting in a decrease in nerve conduction velocity.

Children appear particularly sensitive to these effects and are now evaluated for lead poisoning before entry into school. The normal threshold for blood lead levels (BLL) set by the Centers for Disease Control and Prevention is 10 μg/dL. Growth deficits are seen in children with BLL greater than 10 μg/dL, and anemia may occur at a BLL of 20 μg/dL. Children with a BLL less than 10 μg/dL have been reported to suffer from permanent IQ and hearing deficits. As a result, many states have lowered the upper limit to 5 μg/dL. A threshold to identify permanent effects of lead poisoning is not currently known.

Lead is also a potent inhibitor of many enzymes, which leads to many of the toxic effects of lead exposure. The most noteworthy effects are on vitamin D metabolism and the heme synthetic pathway. Decreased serum concentrations of both 25-hydroxy and 1,25-dihydroxy vitamin D are seen in excessive lead exposure resulting in changes in bone and calcium metabolism. Anemia is the result of the inhibition of the heme synthetic pathway, which results in increases in the concentration of several intermediates in this pathway, including aminolevulinic acid and protoporphyrin. Increases in protoporphyrin result in high concentrations of zinc protoporphyrin in circulating erythrocytes. Zinc protoporphyrin is a highly fluorescent compound, and measurement of this fluorescence has been used to screen for lead toxicity in the clinical laboratory. Increased urinary aminolevulinic acid is a highly sensitive and specific indicator of lead toxicity that correlates well with blood levels. Another hematologic finding of lead poisoning is the presence of basophilic stippling in erythrocytes as a result of inhibition of erythrocytic pyrimidine nucleotidase. This enzyme is responsible for the removal of residual DNA after extrusion of the nucleus. When identified, basophilic stippling is a key indicator of lead toxicity.

Excessive lead exposure has also been associated with hypertension, carcinogenesis, birth defects, compromised immunity, and several renal effects. Early stages of toxicity are associated with renal tubular dysfunction, resulting in glycosuria, aminoaciduria, and hyperphosphaturia. Late stages are associated with tubular atrophy and glomerular fibrosis, which may result in a decreased glomerular filtration rate.

Treatment of lead poisoning involves cessation of exposure and treatment with therapeutic chelators, such as ethylenediaminetetraacetic acid and dimercaptosuccinic acid. These substances are capable of removing lead from soft tissue and bone by forming low molecular weight, high-affinity complexes that can be cleared by renal filtration. The efficacy of this therapy is monitored by determining the urinary concentration of lead.

The assessment of total body burden of lead poisoning is best evaluated by the quantitative determination of lead concentration in whole blood. The use of urine is also valid but correlates closer to the level of recent exposure. Care must be taken during specimen collection to ensure that the specimen does not become contaminated from exogenous sources, and lead-free containers (tan-top K_2EDTA tube) are recommended for this purpose.

Several methods can be used to measure lead concentration. Chromogenic reactions and anodic stripping voltammetry methods have been used, but lack sufficient analytical sensitivity. Point-of-care units have employed these methodologies to screen for lead exposure in children or adults in the workplace. X-ray fluorescence is used to measure environmental levels of lead in nonbiological samples such as soil and foods. For biological specimens, graphite furnace AAS has been used to confirm whole BLLs, but a new standard of measurement has been set with quantitative ICP-MS.

Mercury

Mercury is a metal that exists in three forms: elemental, which is a liquid at room temperature; as inorganic salts; and as a component of organic compounds. Inhalation and accidental ingestion of inorganic and organic forms in industrial settings is the most common reason for toxic levels. Consumption of contaminated foods is the major source of exposure in the general population. Each form of mercury has different toxic characteristics. Elemental mercury (Hg^0) can be ingested without significant effects, and inhalation of elemental mercury is insignificant due to its low vapor pressure. Cationic mercury (Hg^{2+}) is moderately toxic; whereas, organic mercury, such as methylmercury (CH_3Hg^+), is extremely toxic.

Considering that the most common route of exposure to mercury is via ingestion, the primary factor determining toxicity is gastrointestinal absorbance. Elemental mercury is not absorbed well because of its viscous nature. Inorganic mercury is only partially absorbed, but has significant local toxicity in the gastrointestinal tract. The portion that is absorbed distributes uniformly throughout the body. The organic forms of mercury are rapidly and efficiently absorbed by passive diffusion and partitions into hydrophobic compartments. This results in high concentrations in the brain and peripheral nerves.[5] In these lipophilic compartments, organic mercury is biotransformed to its divalent state, allowing it to bind to neuronal proteins. Elimination of systemic mercury occurs primarily via renal filtration of bound low molecular weight species or the free, ionized state. Considering that most mercury is bound to protein, the elimination rate is slow, and chronic exposure, therefore, exerts a cumulative effect.

Mercury toxicity is a result of protein binding, which leads to a change of protein structure and function. The most significant result of this interaction is the inhibition of many enzymes. After ingestion of inorganic mercury, binding to intestinal proteins results in acute gastrointestinal disturbances. Ingestion of moderate amounts may result in severe bloody diarrhea because of ulceration and necrosis of the gastrointestinal tract. In severe cases, this may lead to shock and death. The absorbed portion of ingested inorganic mercury affects many organs. Clinical findings include tachycardia, tremors, thyroiditis, and, most significantly, a disruption of renal function. The renal effect is associated with glomerular proteinuria and loss of tubular function. Organic mercury may also have a renal effect at high levels of exposure; however, neurological symptoms are the primary toxic effects of this hydrophobic form. Low levels of exposure cause tremors, behavioral changes, mumbling speech, and loss of balance. Higher levels of exposure may result in hyporeflexia, hypotension, bradycardia, and renal dysfunction and can lead to death. Analysis of mercury is by AAS using whole blood or an aliquot of a 24-hour urine specimen or anodal stripping voltammetry. Analysis of mercury by AAS requires special techniques as a result of the volatility of elemental mercury.

Pesticides

Pesticides are substances that have been intentionally added to the environment to kill or harm an undesirable life form. Pesticides can be classified into several categories including insecticides, herbicides, fungicides, rodenticides, etc. These agents are generally applied to control vector-borne disease and urban pests and to improve agricultural productivity. Pesticides can be found in occupational settings and in the home; therefore, there are frequent opportunities for exposure. Contamination of food is the major route of exposure for the general population. Inhalation, transdermal absorption, and ingestion as a result of hand-to-mouth contact are common occupational and accidental routes of exposure.

Ideally, the actions of pesticides would be target specific. Unfortunately, most are nonselective and result in toxic effects to many nontarget species, including humans. Pesticides come in many different forms with a wide range of potential toxic effects. The health effects of short-term, low-level exposure to most of these agents have yet to be well elucidated. Extended low-level exposure may result in chronic disease states. Of primary concern, though, is high-level exposure, which may result in acute disease states or death. The most common victims of acute poisoning are people who are applying pesticides without taking appropriate safety precautions to avoid exposure. Ingestion by children at home is also common, and ingestion of pesticides is also a common in suicide attempts.

There is a wide variation in the chemical configuration of pesticides, ranging from simple salts of heavy metals to complex high molecular weight organic compounds. Insecticides are the most prevalent of pesticides. Based on chemical configuration, the organophosphates, carbamates, and halogenated hydrocarbons are the most common insecticides. Organophosphates are the most abundant and are responsible for about one-third of all pesticide poisonings.

Organophosphates and carbamates function by inhibiting acetylcholinesterase, an enzyme present in both insects and mammals. In mammals, acetylcholine is a neurotransmitter found in both central and peripheral nerves. It is also responsible for the stimulation of muscle cells and several endocrine/exocrine glands. The actions of acetylcholine are terminated by the actions of membrane-bound, postsynaptic acetylcholinesterase. Inhibition of this enzyme results in the prolonged presence of acetylcholine on its receptor, which produces a wide range of systemic effects. Low levels of exposure are associated with salivation, lacrimation, and involuntary urination and defecation. Higher levels of exposure result in bradycardia, muscular twitching, cramps, apathy, slurred speech, and behavioral changes. Death due to respiratory failure may also occur.

Absorbed organophosphates bind with high affinity to several proteins, including acetylcholinesterase. Protein binding prevents the direct analysis of organophosphates; thus, exposure is evaluated indirectly by the measurement of acetylcholinesterase inhibition. Inhibition of this enzyme has been found to be a sensitive and specific indicator of organophosphate exposure, but because acetylcholinesterase is a membrane-bound enzyme, serum activity is low. To increase the analytic sensitivity of this assay, erythrocytes that have high surface activity are commonly used. Evaluation of erythrocytic acetylcholinesterase activity for detection of organophosphate exposure, however, is not commonly performed in most laboratories because of low demand and the lack of an automated method.

An alternative test that has become more widely available is the measurement of serum pseudocholinesterase (SChE) activity. SChE is inhibited by organophosphates in a similar manner to the erythrocytic enzyme. Unlike the erythrocytic enzyme, however, changes in the serum activity of SChE lack sensitivity and specificity for organophosphate exposure. SChE is found in the liver, pancreas, brain, and serum though its biological function is not well defined. Decreased levels of SChE can occur in acute infection, pulmonary embolism, hepatitis, and cirrhosis. There are also several variants of this enzyme that demonstrate diminished activity; therefore, decreases in SChE are not specific to organophosphate poisoning. The reference interval for SChE is between 4,000 and 12,000 U/L with intraindividual variation, the degree of variance within an average individual, of about 700 U/L. Symptoms associated with organophosphate toxicity occur at about a 40% reduction in activity. An individual whose normal SChE is on the high side of the reference interval and who has been exposed to toxic levels of organophosphates may still have SChE activity within the reference interval. Because of these factors, determination of SChE activity lacks sensitivity in the diagnosis of organophosphate poisoning and should only be used as a screening test. Immediate antidotal therapy can be initiated in cases of suspected organophosphate poisoning

with a decreased activity of SChE; however, continuation of therapy and documentation of such poisoning should be confirmed by testing of the erythrocytic enzyme.

TOXICOLOGY OF THERAPEUTIC DRUGS

In some cases, toxicity is the result of accidental or intentional overdosage of pharmaceutical drugs. All drugs are capable of toxic effects when improperly administered. This discussion focuses on the therapeutic drugs most commonly tested for in the clinical laboratory.

Salicylates

Acetylsalicylic acid, or aspirin, is a commonly used analgesic, antipyretic, and anti-inflammatory drug. It functions by decreasing thromboxane and prostaglandin formation through the inhibition of cyclooxygenase. At recommended doses, there are several noteworthy adverse effects, including interference with platelet aggregation and gastrointestinal function. There is also an epidemiologic relationship between aspirin, childhood viral infections (e.g., varicella, influenza), and the onset of Reye's syndrome.

Acute ingestion of high doses of aspirin is associated with various toxic effects through several different mechanisms.[1] Because it is an acid, excessive salicylate ingestion is associated with nonrespiratory (metabolic) acidosis. Salicylate is also a direct stimulator of the respiratory center, and hyperventilation can result in respiratory alkalosis. In many instances, the net result of the combined effects is an immediate mixed acid–base disturbance. Salicylates also inhibit the Kreb's cycle resulting in excess conversion of pyruvate to lactic acid. In addition, at high levels of exposure, salicylates stimulate mobilization and use of free fatty acid, resulting in excess ketone body formation. These factors all contribute to nonrespiratory (metabolic) acidosis that may lead to death. Treatment for aspirin overdose involves neutralizing and eliminating the excess acid and maintaining the electrolyte balance.

Correlations have been established between serum concentrations of salicylates and toxic outcomes. Several methods are available for the quantitative determination of salicylate in serum. GC and liquid chromatography (LC) methods provide the highest analytical sensitivity and specificity, but are not widely used due to high equipment expense and required technical skill. Several immunoassay methods are available; however, the most commonly used method is a chromogenic assay known as the Trinder reaction. In this reaction, salicylate reacts with ferric nitrate to form a colored complex that is then measured spectrophotometrically.

Acetaminophen

Acetaminophen (Tylenol), either solely or in combination with other compounds, is a commonly used analgesic drug. In healthy subjects, therapeutic dosages have few adverse effects. Overdose of acetaminophen, however, is associated with severe hepatotoxicity (Fig. 31.4).

Absorbed acetaminophen is bound with high affinity to various proteins, resulting in a low free fraction. Thus, renal

FIGURE 31.4 Rumack-Matthew nomogram.Prediction of acetaminophen-induced hepatic damage based on serum concentration. (Reprinted from Rumack BH, Matthew H. Acetaminophen poisoning and toxicity. *Pediatrics.* 1975;55:871, with permission)

filtration of the parent drug is minimal, and most is eliminated by hepatic uptake, biotransformation, conjugation, and excretion. Acetaminophen can follow several different pathways through this process, each forming a different product. The pathway of major concern is the hepatic mixed-function oxidase (MFO) system. In this system, acetaminophen is first transformed to reactive intermediates, which are then conjugated with reduced glutathione. In overdose situations, glutathione can become depleted, yet reactive intermediates continue to be produced. This results in an accumulation of reactive intermediates inside the cell. Because some intermediates are free radicals, this results in a toxic effect to the cell leading to necrosis of the liver, the organ in which these reactions are occurring.

The time frame for the onset of hepatocyte damage is relatively long. In an average adult, serum indicators of hepatic damage do not become abnormal until 3 to 5 days after ingestion of a toxic dose. The initial symptoms of acetaminophen toxicity are vague and not predictive of hepatic necrosis.[6] The serum concentration of acetaminophen that results in depletion of glutathione has been determined for an average adult. Unfortunately, acetaminophen is rapidly cleared from serum, and determinations are often made many hours after ingestion, making this information of little utility. To aid in this situation, nomograms (Fig. 31.4) are available that predict hepatotoxicity based on serum concentrations of acetaminophen at a known time after ingestion. It is also worth noting that chronic, heavy consumers of ethanol metabolize acetaminophen at a faster rate than average, resulting in a more rapid formation of reactive intermediates and increased possibility of depleting glutathione. Therefore, alcoholic patients are more susceptible to acetaminophen toxicity, and using the nomogram for interpretation in these patients is inappropriate.

The reference method for the quantitation of acetaminophen in serum is high-performance liquid chromatography (HPLC). This method, however, is not widely used in clinical laboratories because of equipment expense and the level of experience required to operate the instruments. Immunoassays are currently the most common analytical methods used for serum acetaminophen determinations with competitive enzyme or fluorescence polarization systems being most frequently used.

TOXICOLOGY OF DRUGS OF ABUSE

Assessment of drug abuse is of medical interest for many reasons. In drug overdose, it is essential to identify the responsible agent to ensure appropriate and timely treatment. In a similar manner, identification of drug abuse in nonoverdose situations provides a rationale for the treatment of addiction. For these reasons, testing for **drugs of abuse** is commonly performed. This typically involves screening a single urine specimen for many substances by qualitative test procedures. In most instances, this procedure only detects recent drug use; therefore, with abstinence of relatively short duration, many abusing patients can avoid detection. In addition, a positive drug screen cannot discriminate between single casual use and chronic abuse. Identification of chronic abuse usually involves several positive test results in conjunction with clinical evaluation. In a similar manner, a positive drug screen does not determine the time frame or dose of the drug taken. Drug abuse or overdose can occur with prescription, over-the-counter, or illicit drugs. The focus of this discussion is on substances with addictive potential.

The use of drugs for recreational or performance enhancement purposes is relatively common. The National Institute on Drug Abuse (NIDA) reports that approximately 30% of the adult population (older than high-school age) have used an illicit drug. Drug abuse testing has become commonplace in professional, industrial, and athletic settings. The potential punitive measures associated with this testing may involve or result in civil or criminal litigation. Therefore, the laboratory must ensure that all results are accurate and all procedures have been properly documented as these results may be used in court as evidence. This requires the use of analytical methods that have been validated as accurate and precise. It also requires scrupulous documentation of specimen security. Protocols and procedures must be established to prevent and detect specimen adulteration. Measurement of urinary temperature, pH, specific gravity, and creatinine is commonly performed to ensure that specimens have not been diluted or treated with substances that may interfere with testing. Specimen collection should be monitored and a chain of custody established to guard against specimen exchange.

Testing for drugs of abuse can be done by several methods. A two-tiered approach of screening and confirmation is usually used. Screening procedures should be simple, rapid, inexpensive, and capable of being automated. They are often referred to as *spot tests*. In general, screening procedures have good analytic sensitivity with marginal specificity meaning that a negative result can rule out an analyte with a reasonable degree of certainty. These methods usually detect classes of drugs based on similarities in chemical configuration, which allows the detection of parent compounds and congeners that have similar effects. Considering that many designer drugs are modified forms of established drugs of abuse, these methods increase the scope of the screening process. A drawback to this type of analysis is that it may also detect chemically related substances that have no or low abuse potential; therefore, interpretation of positive test results requires integration of clinical context and further testing. Confirmation testing must use methods with high sensitivity and specificity; many of these tests provide quantitative as well as qualitative information. Confirmatory testing requires the use of a method different from that used in the screening procedure. GC–MS is the reference method for confirmation of most analytes.

There are several general analytic procedures commonly used for the analysis of drugs of abuse. Chromogenic reactions are occasionally used for screening procedures, but immunoassays are more widely used for screening and confirmatory testing. In general, immunoassays offer a high degree of sensitivity and are easily automated. A wide variety of chromatographic techniques are used for qualitative identification and quantitation of drugs of abuse. TLC is an inexpensive method for screening many drugs simultaneously and has the advantage that no instrumentation is required. GC and LC allow complex mixtures of drugs to be separated and quantitated, but these methods are generally labor intensive and not well suited to screening.

Trends in drug abuse vary geographically and between different socioeconomic groups. For a clinical laboratory to provide effective service requires knowledge of the drug or drug groups likely to be found within the patient population it serves. Fortunately, the process of selecting which drugs to test for has been aided by national studies that have identified the drugs of abuse most commonly seen in various populations (Table 31.4). This provides the basis for test selection in most situations. The following discussion focuses on select drugs with a high potential for abuse.

Amphetamines

Amphetamine and methamphetamine are therapeutic drugs used for narcolepsy and attention deficit disorder. These drugs are stimulants with a high abuse potential as they produce an initial sense of increased mental and physical capacity along with a perception of well-being. These initial effects are followed by restlessness, irritability, and possibly psychosis. Abatement of these late effects is often countered with repeated use; drug tolerance and psychological dependence develop with chronic use. Overdose, although rare in experienced users, results in hypertension, cardiac arrhythmias, convulsions, and possibly death. Various compounds chemically related to amphetamines are components of over-the-counter medications, including ephedrine, pseudoephedrine, and phenylpropanolamine. These amphetamine-like compounds are common in allergy and cold medications.

TABLE 31.4	Prevalence of Common Drugs of Abuse
Substance	**Prevalence (%)**
Alcohol	58
Marijuana	16
Cocaine	2–3
Benzodiazepines	?
Barbiturates	?
Opiates (heroin only)	0.2
Phencyclidine	0
MDMA	1
Amphetamines	0.1–1
Other stimulants	1.3
Other sedatives–hypnotics	0.2

MDMA, methylenedioxymethamphetamine.
This table provides approximate frequencies of relevant drugs of abuse as surveyed from national data. The percentage values estimate the prevalence of use in individuals aged 18–25, the most common users, who by survey claim to have used drugs within the past 30 days. Adapted from Department of Health and Human Services, Substance Abuse and Mental Health Administration, and Office of Applied Studies. *Results from the 2006 National Survey on Drug Use and Health: National Findings.* Retrieved February 8, 2008, from http://www.drugabusestatistics.samhsa.gov/nsduh/2k6nsduh/2k6Results.pdf.

Identification of amphetamine abuse involves analysis of urine for the parent drugs. Immunoassay systems are commonly used as the screening procedure. Because of variable cross-reactivity with over-the-counter medications that contain amphetamine-like compounds, a positive result by immunoassay is considered presumptive positive only. Confirmation of immunoassay-positive tests is most commonly made with LC or GC methods.

Methylenedioxymethamphetamine

Methylenedioxymethamphetamine (MDMA) is an illicit amphetamine derivative commonly referred to as "ecstasy."[7,8] Although it was strongly associated with club culture in the 1990s, its use has continued to grow. There are as many as 200 "designer" analogues that have been developed to produce effects comparable to those of MDMA. MDMA and its analogues are primarily administered orally in tablets of 50 to 150 mg. Other, less-frequent routes of administration are inhalation, injection, or smoking. MDMA has a circulating half-life of approximately 8 to 9 hours. The majority of the drug is eliminated by hepatic metabolism, although 20% is eliminated unchanged in the urine.

CASE STUDY 31.2

An emergency department patient with a provisional diagnosis of overdose with an over-the-counter cold medicine undergoes a drug screen. Test results from immunoassay screening were negative for opiates, barbiturates, benzodiazepines, THC, and cocaine, but positive for

CASE STUDY 31.2 (continued)

amphetamines. The salicylate level was 15 times the upper limit of the therapeutic range. Results for acetaminophen and ethanol were negative.

Questions

1. What would be the expected results of arterial blood gas analysis?
2. What would be the expected results of a routine urinalysis?
3. What are some of the possible reasons the amphetamine screen is positive?

The onset of effect is 30 to 60 minutes, and duration is about 3.5 hours. The desired effects include hallucination, euphoria, empathic and emotional responses, and increased visual and tactile sensitivity. Adverse effects include headaches, nausea, vomiting, anxiety, agitation, impaired memory, violent behavior, tachycardia, hypertension, respiratory depression, seizures, hyperthermia, cardiac toxicity, liver toxicity, and renal failure. The presenting symptoms along with patient behavior and history must be taken into account as routine drug screening by immunoassay of a urine specimen will usually not test positive. Further analysis and confirmation of MDMA are generally performed using GC–MS.

Anabolic Steroids

Anabolic steroids are a group of compounds that are chemically related to the male sex hormone testosterone. These artificial substances were developed in the 1930s as a therapy for male hypogonadism though it was soon discovered that the use of these compounds in healthy subjects increases muscle mass. In many instances, this results in an improvement in athletic performance. Recent studies have reported that 6.5% of adolescent boys and 1.9% of adolescent girls reported the use of steroids without a prescription.

Most illicit steroids are obtained through the black market from underground laboratories and foreign sources. The quality and purity of these drugs are highly variable. In most instances, the acute toxic effects of these drugs are related to inconsistent formulation, which may result in high dosages and impurities. A variety of both physical and psychological effects have been associated with steroid abuse. Chronic use has been associated with toxic hepatitis as well as accelerated atherosclerosis and abnormal aggregation of platelets, both of which predispose individuals to stroke and myocardial infarction. In addition, steroid abuse causes an enlargement of the heart. In this condition, heart muscle cells develop faster than the associated vasculature, which may lead to ischemia of heart muscle cells. This predisposes the individual to cardiac arrhythmias and possible death. In males, chronic

steroid use is associated with testicular atrophy, sterility, and impotence. In females, steroid abuse causes the development of masculine traits, breast reduction, and sterility.

Evaluation of anabolic steroid use can be challenging. Until recently, the primary forms abused were animal derived or synthetic forms. There are several, well-established methods for the detection of the parent drug and its metabolite for the majority of these; however, the newer forms may be difficult to detect. To address this and related issues, the ratio of testosterone to epitestosterone is commonly used as a screening test; high ratios are associated with exogenous testosterone administration.[9]

Cannabinoids

Cannabinoids are a group of psychoactive compounds found in marijuana. Of these, THC is the most potent and abundant. Marijuana, or its processed product, hashish, can be smoked or ingested. A sense of well-being and euphoria are the subjective effect of exposure. It is also associated with an impairment of short-term memory and intellectual function. Effects of chronic use have not been well established though tolerance, and a mild dependence may develop over time. THC overdose has not been associated with any specific adverse effects. THC is a lipophilic substance, which is rapidly removed from circulation by passive distribution into hydrophobic compartments, such as the brain and fat. This results in slow elimination as a result of redistribution back into circulation and subsequent hepatic metabolism.

The half-life of THC in circulation is 1 day after a single use and 3 to 5 days for chronic, heavy consumers. Hepatic metabolism of THC produces several products that are primarily eliminated in urine. The major urinary metabolite is 11-nor-tetrahydrocannabinol-9-carboxylic acid (THC-COOH). This metabolite can be detected in urine for up to 5 days after a single use or up to 4 weeks following chronic, heavy use. Immunoassay tests for THC-COOH are used to screen for marijuana consumption, and GC–MS is used for confirmation. Both methods are sensitive and specific and because of the low limit of detection of both methods, it is possible to find THC-COOH in urine as a result of passive inhalation. Urinary concentration standards have been established to discriminate between passive and direct inhalation.

Cocaine

Cocaine is an effective local anesthetic with few adverse effects at therapeutic concentrations. At higher circulating concentrations, it is a potent CNS stimulator that elicits a sense of excitement and euphoria. Cocaine is an alkaloid salt that can be administered directly (e.g., by insufflation or intravenous injection) or inhaled as a vapor when smoked in the free base form known as crack. The half-life of circulating cocaine is brief; approximately 30 minutes to 1 hour. Acute cocaine toxicity is associated with hypertension, arrhythmia, seizure, and myocardial infarction. Because of its short half-life, maintaining the subjective effects over a single extended period requires repeated dosages of increasing quantity; therefore, correlations between serum concentration and the subjective or toxic effects cannot be established. Because the rate of change is more important than the serum concentration, a primary factor that determines the toxicity of cocaine is the dose and route of administration. Intravenous administration presents with the greatest hazard, closely followed by smoking.

Cocaine's short half-life is a result of rapid hepatic hydrolysis to inactive metabolites, which is the major route of elimination for cocaine. Only a small portion of the parent drug can be found in urine after an administered dose and the primary product of hepatic metabolism is benzoylecgonine, which is largely eliminated in urine. The half-life of benzoylecgonine is 4 to 7 hours; however, it can be detected in urine for up to 3 days after a single use. The presence of this metabolite in urine is a sensitive and specific indicator of cocaine use. In chronic heavy abusers, it can be detected in urine for up to 20 days after the last dose. The primary screening test for detection of cocaine use is measurement of benzoylecgonine in urine by immunoassay. Confirmation testing is most commonly performed using GC–MS.

Opiates

Opiates are a class of substances capable of analgesia, sedation, and anesthesia. All are derived from or chemically related to substances derived from the opium poppy. The naturally occurring substances include opium, morphine, and codeine. Heroin, hydromorphone (Dilaudid), and oxycodone (Percodan) are chemically modified forms of the naturally occurring opiates. Meperidine (Demerol), methadone (Dolophine), propoxyphene (Darvon), pentazocine (Talwin), and fentanyl (Sublimaze) are the common synthetic opiates. Opiates have a high abuse potential, and chronic use leads to tolerance with physical and psychological dependence. Acute overdose presents with respiratory acidosis due to depression of respiratory centers, myoglobinuria, and possibly an increase in serum indicators of cardiac damage (e.g., CKMB, troponin). High-level opiate overdose may lead to death caused by cardiopulmonary failure. Treatment of overdose includes the use of the antagonist naloxone.

Laboratory testing for opiates usually involves initial screening by immunoassay. Most immunoassays are designed to detect the presence of morphine and codeine; however, cross-reactivity allows for detection of many of the opiates including naturally occurring, chemically modified,

and synthetic forms. GC–MS is the method of choice for confirmation testing.

Phencyclidine

Phencyclidine (PCP) is an illicit drug with stimulant, depressant, anesthetic, and hallucinogenic properties. Adverse effects are commonly noted at doses that produce the desired subjective effects, such as agitation, hostility, and paranoia. Overdose is generally associated with stupor and coma. PCP can be ingested or inhaled by smoking PCP-laced tobacco or marijuana. It is a lipophilic drug that rapidly distributes into fat and brain tissue. Elimination is slow as a result of redistribution into circulation and hepatic metabolism. Approximately 10% to 15% of an administered dose is eliminated and unchanged in urine, which allows for identification of the parent drug in urine. In chronic, heavy users, PCP can be detected up to 30 days after abstinence. Immunoassay is used as the screening procedure with GC–MS as the confirmatory method.

Sedatives–Hypnotics

Many therapeutic drugs can be classified as sedatives–hypnotics or tranquilizers, and all members of this class are CNS depressants. They have a wide range of approved therapeutic roles, but they also have high abuse potential, ranging from high to low. These drugs often become available for illegal use through diversion from approved sources. Barbiturates and benzodiazepines are the most common types of sedative–hypnotics abused. Although barbiturates have a higher abuse potential, benzodiazepines are more commonly found in abuse and overdose situations. This appears to be a result of availability. There are many individual drugs within the barbiturate and benzodiazepine classification. Secobarbital, pentobarbital, and phenobarbital are the more commonly abused barbiturates. Diazepam (Valium), chlordiazepoxide (Librium), and lorazepam (Ativan) are the most commonly abused benzodiazepines. Overdose with sedatives–hypnotics initially presents with lethargy and slurred speech, which can rapidly progress to coma. Respiratory depression is the most serious toxic effect of most of these agents though hypotension can occur with barbiturates as well. The toxicity of many of these agents is potentiated by ethanol use.

Immunoassay is the most common screening procedure for both barbiturates and benzodiazepines. Broad cross-reactivity within members of each group allows for the detection of many individual drugs. GC or LC methods can be used for confirmatory testing.

questions

1. Compound A is reported to have an oral LD_{50} of 5 mg/kg body weight. Compound B is reported to have an LD_{50} of 50 mg/kg body weight. Of the following statements regarding the relative toxicity of these two compounds, which is TRUE?
   a. Ingestion of low amounts of compound A would be predicted to cause more deaths than an equal dose of compound B.
   b. Ingestion of compound B would be expected to produce nontoxic effects at a dose greater than 100 mg/kg body weight.
   c. Neither compound A nor compound B is toxic at any level of oral exposure.
   d. Compound A is more rapidly adsorbed from the gastrointestinal tract than compound B.
   e. Compound B would be predicted to be more toxic than compound A if the exposure route were transdermal.

2. Which of the following statements best describes the TD_{50} of a compound?
   a. The dosage of a substance that would be predicted to cause a toxic effect in 50% of the population
   b. The dosage of a substance that is lethal to 50% of the population
   c. The dosage of a substance that would produce therapeutic benefit in 50% of the population
   d. The percentage of individuals who would experience a toxic response at 50% of the lethal dose
   e. The percentage of the population who would experience a toxic response after an oral dosage of 50 mg

3. Of the following analytic methods, which is most commonly used as the confirmatory method for identification of drugs of abuse?
   a. GC with mass spectrometry
   b. Scanning differential calorimetry
   c. Ion-specific electrode
   d. Immunoassay
   e. Nephelometry

4. A weakly acidic toxin ($pK_a = 4.0$) that is ingested will
   a. Be passively absorbed in the stomach (pH = 3.0)
   b. Not be absorbed because it is ionized
   c. Not be absorbed unless a specific transporter is present
   d. Be passively absorbed in the colon (pH = 7.5)
   e. Be absorbed only if a weak base is ingested at the same time

5. What is the primary product of methanol metabolism by the ADH and ALDH system?
   a. Formic acid
   b. Acetone
   c. Acetaldehyde

d. Oxalic acid
e. Formaldehyde

6. Which of the following statements concerning cyanide toxicity is TRUE?
   a. Inhalation of smoke from burning plastic is a common cause of cyanide exposure, and cyanide expresses its toxicity by inhibition of oxidative phosphorylation.
   b. Inhalation of smoke from burning plastic is a common cause of cyanide exposure.
   c. Cyanide is a relatively nontoxic compound that requires chronic exposure to produce a toxic effect.
   d. Cyanide expresses its toxicity by inhibition of oxidative phosphorylation.
   e. All of these are true.

7. Which of the following laboratory results would be consistent with acute high-level oral exposure to an inorganic form of mercury (Hg^{2+})?
   a. All of these
   b. High concentrations of mercury in whole blood and urine
   c. Proteinuria
   d. Positive occult blood in stool
   e. None of these

8. A child presents with microcytic, hypochromic anemia. The physician suspects iron deficiency anemia. Further laboratory testing reveals a normal total serum iron and iron-binding capacity; however, the zinc protoporphyrin level was very high. A urinary screen for porphyrins was positive. Erythrocytic basophilic stippling was noted on the peripheral smear. Which of the following laboratory tests would be best applied to this case?
   a. Whole blood lead
   b. Urinary thiocyanate
   c. COHb
   d. Urinary anabolic steroids
   e. Urinary benzoylecgonine

9. A patient with suspected organophosphate poisoning presents with a low SChE level. However, the confirmatory test, erythrocyte acetylcholinesterase, presents with a normal result. Excluding analytic error, which of the following may explain these conflicting results?
   a. The patient has late-stage hepatic cirrhosis or the patient has a variant of SChE that displays low activity.
   b. The patient has late-stage hepatic cirrhosis.
   c. The patient was exposed to low levels of organophosphates.
   d. The patient has a variant of SChE that displays low activity.
   e. All of these are correct.

review questions (continued)

10. A patient enters the emergency department in a coma. The physician suspects a drug overdose. Immunoassay screening tests for opiates, barbiturates, benzodiazepines, THC, amphetamines, and PCP were all negative. No ethanol was detected in serum. Can the physician rule out drug overdose as the cause of this coma with these results?
   a. No
   b. Yes
   c. Maybe

references

1. Eldridge DL, Holstege CP. Utilizing the laboratory in the poisoned patient. *Clin Lab Med.* 2006;26:13–30.
2. Thorne D, Kaplan KJ. Laboratory indicators of ethanol consumption. *Clin Lab Sci.* 1999;120:343.
3. Kao LW, Nanagas KA. Toxicity associated with carbon monoxide. *Clin Lab Med.* 2006;26:99–125.
4. Widdop B. Analysis of carbon monoxide. *Ann Clin Biochem.* 2002;39:378–391.
5. Ibrahim D, Froberg B, Wolf A, et al. Heavy metal poisoning: clinical presentations and pathophysiology. *Clin Lab Med.* 2006;26:67–97.
6. Rowden AK, Norvell J, Eldridge DL, et al. Acetaminophen poisoning. *Clin Lab Med.* 2006;26:49–65.
7. Haroz R, Greenberg MI. New drugs of abuse in North America. *Clin Lab Med.* 2006;26:147–164.
8. Nyberg Karlsen S, Spigset O, Slordal L. The dark side of ecstasy: neuropsychiatric symptoms after exposure to 3,4-methylenedioxymethamphetamine. *Basic Clin Pharmacol Toxicol.* 2007;102:15–24.
9. Green G. Doping control for the team physician: a review of drug testing procedures in sport. *Am J Sports Med.* 2006;34:1690–1698.

32

Circulating Tumor Markers: Basic Concepts and Clinical Applications

CHRISTOPER R. McCUDDEN and MONTE S. WILLIS

chapter outline

key terms

Cancer
Neoplasm
Oncofetal antigens
Oncogene
Staging
Tumor marker

chapter objectives

Upon completion of this chapter, the clinical laboratorian should be able to do the following:

- Discuss the incidence of cancer.
- Explain the role of tumor markers in cancer management.
- Identify the characteristics or properties of an ideal tumor marker.
- State the major clinical value of tumor markers.
- Name the major tumor types and their associated markers.
- Describe the major properties, methods of analysis, and clinical use of α-fetoprotein, cancer antigen 125, carcinoembryonic antigen, β-human chorionic gonadotropin, and prostate-specific antigen.
- Explain the use of enzymes and hormones as tumor markers.

For additional student resources, please visit thePoint®
at http://thepoint.lww.com

Cancer remains the second leading cause of mortality in developed countries, accounting for 23% of deaths in the United States and approximately 3 million deaths/year globally. Approximately 42% of males and 38% of females will develop invasive cancer in their lifetime; males have a lifetime risk of dying from cancer of 23%, whereas females have a 19% risk.[1] Cancer is a broad term used to describe more than 200 different malignancies that affect more than 50 tissue types. Despite considerable efforts to reduce the incidence of malignancies, it is estimated that there were 1.6 million new cases of cancer in the United States in 2015 (Table 32.1; see additional current global cancer statistics at http://globocan.iarc.fr/factsheet.asp).

Biologically, *cancer* refers to the uncontrolled growth of cells that often forms a solid mass or tumor (**neoplasm**) and spreads to other areas of the body. A complex combination of inherited and acquired genetic mutations lead to tumor formation (*tumorigenesis*) and spreading (*metastasis*) (for comprehensive reviews, see refs [2,3]). During tumorigenesis, mutations activate growth factors (e.g., epidermal growth factor) and **oncogenes** (e.g., K-ras), in combination with inhibition of apoptosis, tumor suppressor, and cell cycle regulation genes (e.g., *BRCA1*, *p53*, and cyclins). As cancer progresses toward metastasis, additional genetic changes are required, such as loss of cell adhesion proteins (e.g., β-catenin and E-cadherin) and activation of angiogenesis genes (e.g., vascular endothelial growth factor) (Fig. 32.1). An understanding of these genetic mechanisms is the basis for many current and future cancer treatments.

A combination of factors determines cancer severity and are used to classify its stage. Depending on the type of cancer, these factors include tumor size, histology, regional lymph node involvement, and presence of metastasis. For most solid tumors (e.g., breast, lung, and kidney), cancer is broadly classified (using roman numerals I to IV) into four stages (Fig. 32.2). Stages correlate with disease severity, where higher stages are indicative of larger tumors and/or significant spreading and severe systemic disease. With disease progression, both proliferation and metastasis occur at the expense of normal organ processes, which is usually the ultimate cause of cancer-associated morbidity and mortality.

TYPES OF TUMOR MARKERS

Cancer can be detected and monitored using biologically relevant **tumor markers**. Tumor markers are produced either directly by the tumor or as an effect of the tumor on healthy tissue (*host*). Tumor markers encompass an array of diverse molecules such as serum proteins, **oncofetal antigens**, hormones, metabolites, receptors, and enzymes.

A variety of enzymes are elevated nonspecifically in tumors (Table 32.2). These elevated enzymes are largely a result of the high metabolic demand of these proliferative cells. Accordingly, enzyme levels tend to correlate with tumor burden, making them clinically useful for monitoring the success of therapy. Serum proteins, such as β_2-microglobulin and immunoglobulins, are also used to monitor cancer therapy (Table 32.3). β_2-Microglobulin is found on the surface of all nucleated cells and can, therefore, be used as a nonspecific marker of the high cell turnover common in tumors. In hematologic malignancies such as multiple myeloma, immunoglobulins provide a relatively specific measure of plasma cell production of monoclonal proteins. In endocrine malignancies, hormones and hormone metabolites are widely used as specific markers of secreting tumors (Table 32.4). Hormones

TABLE 32.1 **Estimated New Cases of Cancer and Deaths From Cancer in the United States**

Primary Site	Estimated New Cases			Estimated Deaths		
	Total	Males	Females	Total	Males	Females
All sites	1,658,370	848,200	810,170	589,430	312,150	277,280
Genital organs	329,330	231,050	98,280	58,670	28,230	30,440
Digestive system	291,150	163,050	128,100	149,300	86,540	62,760
Respiratory system	240,390	130,260	110,130	162,460	89,750	72,710
Breast	234,190	2,350	231,840	40,730	440	40,290
Urinary system	138,710	96,580	42,130	30,970	21,110	9,860
Lymphoma	80,900	44,950	35,950	20,940	12,140	8,800
Skin	80,100	42,670	46,610	13,340	9,120	4,220
Endocrine system	64,860	16,520	48,340	2,890	1,350	1,540
Leukemia	54,270	30,900	23,370	24,450	14,210	10,240
Oral cavity and pharynx	45,780	32,670	13,110	8,650	6,010	2,640
Myeloma	26,850	14,090	12,760	11,240	6,240	5,000
Brain and nervous system	22,850	12,900	9,950	15,320	8,940	6,380
Soft tissue	11,930	6,610	5,320	4,870	2,600	2,270
Bones and joints	2,970	1,640	1,330	1,490	850	640
Eye and orbit	2,580	1,360	1,220	270	140	130

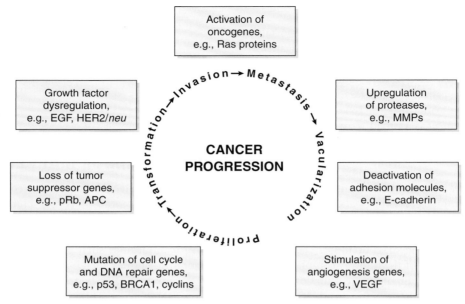

FIGURE 32.1 Genetic changes associated with cancer. A combination of acquired and/or hereditary defects causes tumor formation and metastasis. These processes begin with unregulated proliferation and transformation, followed by invasion and loss of cellular adhesion. A rich vascular supply of oxygen and nutrients is necessary to facilitate growth of a tumor larger than 100 to 200 µm. APC, familial adenomatous polyposis coli, mutated in colorectal cancers; BRCA1, breast cancer susceptibility gene; E-cadherin, adhesion molecule; EGF, epithelial growth factor; MMP, matrix metalloproteinase; p53, cell cycle regulator, mutated in 50% of cancers; pRB, retinoblastoma protein, mutated in many cancers; Ras, small G protein, mutated in many cancers; TIMP, tissue inhibitor of metalloproteinase; VEGF, vascular endothelial growth factor, drug target for inhibin of angiogenesis.

Cancer Staging and Progression

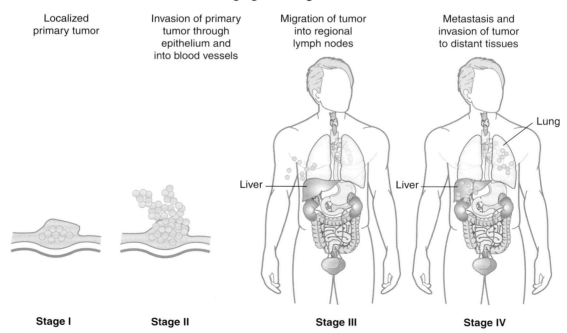

FIGURE 32.2 Generalized cancer staging and progression. Numerous factors are used in combination to define cancer stage; these include tumor size, extent of invasion, lymph node involvement, metastasis, and histologic assessments (basis for the TNM staging system). In this simplified diagram, stage is presented as a function of invasion and spreading regionally and to other tissues; the primary tumor is not shown.

TABLE 32.2 — Enzyme Tumor Markers

Tumor Marker	Tumor Type	Method	Specimen	Clinical Utility
Prostate-specific antigen	Prostate cancer	IA	Serum	Prostate cancer screening, therapy monitoring, and recurrence
Lactate dehydrogenase	Hematologic malignancies	EA	Serum	Prognostic indicator; elevated nonspecifically in numerous cancers
Alkaline phosphatase	Metastatic carcinoma of bone, hepatocellular carcinoma, osteosarcoma, lymphoma, leukemia	EA	Serum	Determination of liver and bone involvement; nonspecific elevation in many bone-related and liver cancers
Neuron-specific enolase	Neuroendocrine tumors	RIA, IHC	Serum	Prognostic indicator and monitoring disease progression for neuroendocrine tumors

EA, enzyme assay; IA, immunoassay; IHC, immunohistochemistry; RIA, radioimmunoassay.

TABLE 32.3 — Serum Protein Tumor Markers

Tumor Marker	Tumor Type	Method	Specimen	Clinical Utility
Serum M-protein	Plasma cell dyscrasias	SPE/IFE	Serum	Diagnosis, therapeutic monitoring of plasma cell malignancies
Serum-free light chains	Plasma cell dyscrasias	IA	Serum	Diagnosis, therapeutic monitoring of plasma cell malignancies
β_2-Microglobulin	Hematologic malignancies	IA	Serum	Prognostic marker for lymphoproliferative disorders

IA, immunoassay; IFE, immunofixation electrophoresis; SPE, serum protein electrophoresis.

TABLE 32.4 — Endocrine Tumor Markers

Tumor Marker	Tumor Type	Method	Specimen	Clinical Utility
ACTH	Pituitary adenoma, ectopic ACTH-producing tumor	IA	Serum	Diagnosis of ectopic ACTH-producing tumor
ADH	Posterior pituitary tumors	IA	Serum	Diagnosis of SIADH
C-peptide	Insulin-secreting tumors	ELISA, IA	Serum	Diagnosis of insulinoma
Calcitonin	MTC and neuroendocrine tumors	IA	Serum	Screening,[a] response to therapy, and monitoring recurrence of MTC
Chromogranin A	Pheochromocytoma, neuroblastoma, carcinoid tumors, small cell lung cancers	ELISA, RIA	Serum	Aid in diagnosis of carcinoid tumors, pheochromocytomas, and neuroblastomas
Cortisol	Adrenal tumors	IA	Serum or urine	Diagnosis of Cushing's syndrome, adrenal adenoma
Gastrin	Neuroendocrine tumor	IA	Serum	Zollinger-Ellison syndrome; gastrinoma
GH	Pituitary adenoma, ectopic GH-secreting tumors	IA	Serum	Diagnosis and post monitoring of acromegaly
HVA	Neuroblastoma, pheochromocytoma, paraganglioma	HPLC	24-h urine	Diagnosis of neuroblastoma[b]
5-HIAA	Carcinoid tumors	HPLC	24-h urine	Diagnosis of carcinoid tumors
Metanephrines (fractionated)[c]	Pheochromocytoma, paraganglioma, neuroblastoma	HPLC	24-h urine or plasma	Screening and diagnosis of pheochromocytoma
PTH	Parathyroid adenoma	IA	Serum	Diagnosis and postsurgical monitoring of parathyroid adenoma
PRL	Pituitary adenoma	IA	Serum	Diagnosis and postsurgical monitoring of prolactinoma
VMA	Pheochromocytoma, paraganglioma, neuroblastoma	HPLC	24-h urine	Diagnosis of neuroblastoma[b]

ACTH, adrenocorticotropic hormone; ADH, antidiuretic hormone; GH, growth hormone; HVA, homovanillic acid; 5-HIAA, hydroxyindoleacetic acid; PTH, parathyroid hormone; PRL, prolactin; VMA, vanillylmandelic acid; ELISA, enzyme-linked immunosorbent assay; HPLC, high-performance liquid chromatography; IA, immunoassay; LC-MS/MS, liquid chromatography–TANDEM mass spectrometry; MTC, medullary thyroid carcinoma; RIA, radioimmunoassay; SIADH, syndrome of inappropriate antidiuretic hormone secretion.
[a]Screening family members for MTC.
[b]HVA and VMA are used in combination for diagnosis of neuroblastomas.
[c]Metanephrine, normetanephrine.

TABLE 32.5   **Use of Serum α-Fetoprotein and Human Chorionic Gonadotropin for Testicular Cancer Classification**

	Germ Cell Tumor	AFP	hCG
Nonseminomatous tumors	Yolk sac tumor (endodermal sinus tumor)	Increased	No
	Choriocarcinoma	No	Increased
	Embryonal carcinoma	Increased	±
	Teratoma	No	No
Seminoma		Not elevated in pure tumors	±

AFP, α-fetoprotein; hCG, human chorionic gonadotropin.

can be valuable in diagnosing neuroblastomas, as well as pituitary and adrenal adenomas. One of the first classes of tumor markers discovered was the oncofetal antigens. Oncofetal antigens such as carcinoembryonic antigen (CEA) and α-fetoprotein (AFP) are expressed transiently during normal development and are then turned on again in the formation of tumors (see Table 32.5 for use of oncofetal antigens). Other tumor markers include monoclonal defined antigens identified from human tumor extracts and cell lines. While these antibodies are directed toward specific carbohydrate or cancer antigens and are best used for monitoring treatment of tumors that secrete these epitopes (Table 32.6). Finally, receptors are used to classify tumors for therapy (Table 32.7). These "nonserologic" markers are outside the scope of the chapter, but they are an important example of the diversity of tumor markers. Prototypic examples of such a marker are estrogen and progesterone receptors and growth factors (HER-2), which are used to choose between endocrine and cytotoxic therapy; endocrine therapy, such as tamoxifen, typically is more effective in patient with ER- and PR-positive patients.

Tumor markers are an invaluable set of tools that health care providers can use for a variety of clinical modalities. Depending on the marker and the type of malignancy, tumor markers for screening, diagnosis, prognosis, therapy monitoring, and detecting recurrence applications are in routine clinical use (Fig. 32.3).

APPLICATIONS OF TUMOR MARKER DETECTION

The ideal tumor marker would be tumor specific, absent in healthy individuals, and readily detectable in body fluids. Unfortunately, all of the presently available tumor markers do not fit this ideal model. However, numerous tumor markers have been identified that have a high enough specificity and sensitivity to be used on a targeted basis for aiding diagnosis, prognosis, detection of recurrence, and monitoring the response to treatment (Fig. 32.3). Clinically, tumor markers are used in combination with clinical signs, symptoms, and histology to facilitate clinical decision making.

Screening and Susceptibility Testing

With the possible exception of prostate-specific antigen (PSA),* no tumor marker identified to date can be used to effectively screen asymptomatic populations. This is because most of the clinically used tumor markers are found in normal cells and benign conditions in addition to cancer. Screening asymptomatic populations would therefore result in detection of false positives (patients without disease with

---

*Screening for prostate cancer remains controversial. Currently strategies focus on informed decision-making support to enable patients to weight the benefits of detecting disease early against the harms of overtreatment.

TABLE 32.6   **Carbohydrate and Cancer Antigen Tumor Markers**

Tumor Marker	Tumor Type	Method	Specimen	Clinical Utility
CA 19-9	Gastrointestinal cancer and adenocarcinoma	Immunoassay	Serum	Monitoring pancreatic cancer
CA 15-3	Metastatic breast cancer	Immunoassay	Serum	Response to therapy and detecting recurrence
CA 27-29	Metastatic breast carcinoma	Immunoassay	Serum	Response to therapy and detecting recurrence
CA-125	Ovarian cancer	Immunoassay	Serum	Monitoring therapy

CA, cancer antigen.

TABLE 32.7   Receptor Tumor Markers

Tumor Marker	Tumor Type	Method	Specimen	Clinical Utility
Estrogen receptor	Breast cancer	IHC	Biopsy	Hormonal therapy indicator
Progesterone receptor	Breast cancer	IHC	Biopsy	Hormonal therapy indicator
Her-2/*neu*	Breast, ovarian, gastrointestinal tumors	IHC, FISH, ELISA	Biopsy	Prognostic and hormonal therapy indicator
Epidermal growth factor receptor	Head, neck, ovarian, cervical cancers	IHC	Biopsy	Prognostic indicator

ELISA, enzyme-linked immunosorbent assay; FISH, fluorescence in situ hybridization; IHC, immunohistochemistry.

detectable tumor marker), leading to undue alarm and risk to patients (e.g., unnecessary imaging, biopsy, and surgery). Presently, only a few tumor markers are used to screen populations with high incidence (targeted screening).

Susceptibility to cancer can be determined using molecular diagnostics in patients with breast, ovarian, or colon cancer by identifying germ-line mutations in patients with a family history of these diseases. Screening for susceptibility to breast and ovarian cancers is done by identifying germ-line *BRCA1* and *BRCA2* mutations. Similarly, familial colon cancers can be identified by the presence of the adenomatous polyposis coli (*APC*) gene. Since greater than 99% of people with familial APC develop colon cancer by the age of 40 years, prophylactic colectomy is routinely performed on APC+ patients. While gene testing can be done from blood

samples, these are not really considered circulating tumor markers and therefore not discussed further.

Prognosis

Tumor marker concentration generally increases with tumor progression, reaching their highest levels when tumors metastasize. Therefore, serum tumor marker levels at diagnosis can reflect the aggressiveness of a tumor and help predict the outcome for patients. High concentrations of a serum tumor marker at diagnosis might indicate the presence of malignancy and possible metastasis, which is associated with a poorer prognosis. In other instances, the mere presence or absence of a particular marker may be valuable. Such is the case with some of the receptors used to base chemotherapeutic treatment in breast cancer as

FIGURE 32.3 Tumor markers are used for screening, prognosis, treatment monitoring, and detecting recurrence of several types of cancer. Whereas few markers are used for screening, many are used to monitor therapy. Endocrine and hormone metabolite markers are often used to aid in diagnosis of secreting tumors. List is not comprehensive but provides examples of the most commonly used markers. Note: PSA screening remains controversial, see text.

described above, where endocrine therapy is indicated only in the presence of given markers.

Monitoring Effectiveness of Therapy and Disease Recurrence

One of the most useful and common applications of tumor markers is monitoring therapy efficacy and detecting disease recurrence. After surgical resection, radiation, or drug therapy of cancer (chemotherapy), tumor markers are routinely followed serially. In patients with elevated tumor markers at diagnosis, effective therapy results in a dramatic decrease or disappearance of the tumor marker. If the initial treatment is effective, the appearance of circulating tumor markers can then be used as a highly sensitive marker of recurrence. Many tumor markers have a lead time of several months before disease would be detected by other modalities (e.g., imaging), allowing for earlier identification and treatment in cases of relapse.

LABORATORY CONSIDERATIONS FOR TUMOR MARKER MEASUREMENT

The unique characteristics and concentrations of tumor makers require special laboratory considerations. Two major considerations are the size and variability of the tumor marker concentration between different manufacturers due to the lack of harmonization and standardization. Lack of standardization makes comparison of serial patient results using different assays treacherous. There are multiple reasons why these assays are not comparable, including differences in antibody specificity, analyte heterogeneity, assay design, lack of standard reference material, calibration, kinetics, and variation in reference ranges. To most accurately monitor tumor marker concentrations in a patient, it is important to use the same methodology (or kit). It is also important to perform diligent quality control during lot changes. This includes a careful comparison of QC material and patient samples because detection of tumor markers can vary widely between reagent lots; this is particularly a concern where polyclonal antibodies are used as reagents (e.g., serum free light chains).

The other main consideration for tumor marker measurement is the wide range of concentrations encountered clinically. Tumor markers often vary in concentration by orders of magnitude, making accurate measurement challenging compared with routine chemistry analytes (e.g., concentration extremes for sodium are between 120 and 160 mmol/L, whereas human chorionic gonadotropin [hCG] may vary between 10 and 10,000,000 mIU/mL!). Handling these ranges requires careful attention to dilution protocols and the risk of antigen excess. These considerations are discussed in the context of specific methodology in the following sections.

Immunoassays

Immunoassays are the most commonly used method to measure tumor markers. There are many advantages to this method, such as the ability to automate testing and relative ease of use. Many tumor markers are amenable to automation and relatively rapid analysis using large immunoassay or integrated chemistry test platforms. However, there are some unique factors to be considered when using immunoassays to measure tumor markers including assay linearity, antigen excess (hook effect), and the potential for heterophile antibodies.

COMMON CANCER TERMS

Angiogenesis: Development of new blood vessels to supply oxygen and nutrients to cells

Apoptosis: Programmed cell death

Cell cycle: Phases of cell activity divided into G, S, and M (growth, DNA synthesis, and mitosis, respectively)

Neoplasm: Synonymous with "tumor," it refers to uncontrolled tissue growth; it may be cancerous (malignant) or noncancerous (benign). Derived from Greek meaning "new formation."

Oncogene: Encodes a protein that, when mutated, promotes uncontrolled cell growth

Tumor suppressor gene: Encodes a protein involved in protecting cells from unregulated growth

---

Linearity

The *linear range* is the span of analyte concentrations over which a linear relationship exists between the analyte and signal. Linearity is determined by analyzing (in replicates) specimens spanning the reportable range. Guidelines for this determination are outlined in the Clinical Laboratory Improvement Amendments (CLIA) guidelines for linearity.[4] Samples exceeding the linear range, which is much more likely to occur in the detection of tumor markers, need to be systemically diluted to determine values within the reportable linear range. Dilutions must be done with careful consideration of the diluent and awareness of the risk of error if using manual calculations (it is common practice to have manual calculations reviewed by another individual). Excessively high tumor marker concentrations can result in falsely low measurements, a phenomenon known as *antigen excess* or *hook effect*.

Hook Effect

When analyte concentrations exceed the analytical range excessively, there is potential for *antigen excess* or *hook effect*. When very high antigen concentrations are present, capture and/or label antibodies can be saturated, resulting in a lack of "sandwich" formation and thus in a significant decrease in signal. The name hook effect refers to the shape of the concentration–signal curve when the reagents are saturated with excess antigen (Fig. 32.4). But the practical understanding of the hook effect is that it causes the actual tumor marker concentration to be grossly underestimated. If clinical suspicion is high for an elevated tumor marker, it

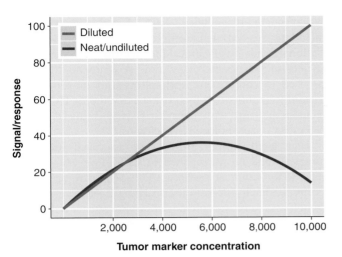

FIGURE 32.4 Hook effect (antigen excess) can occur with tumor markers because they may be found at very high concentrations. When reagents are depleted by excess antigen (the tumor marker), falsely low results may occur (represented by the "neat" curve). Dilution of samples can be used to detect and account for hook effect (represented by the "diluted" line).

can be identified by the laboratory with dilution and repeat testing. Samples displaying hook effect will yield higher (accurate) values on dilution (Fig. 32.4). This phenomenon typically only affects sandwich-type immunoassays.

Heterophile Antibodies

Significant interference can be seen in immunoassays if an individual has circulating antibodies against human or animal immunoglobulin reagents. A subset of heterophilic antibodies are human antianimal antibodies or human antimouse antibodies (HAMAs). HAMAs are most commonly encountered in patients who have been given mouse monoclonal antibodies for therapeutic reasons or who have been exposed to mice,[5] but they may be idiopathic. In patients, these antibodies can cause false-positive or, less commonly, false-negative results by cross-linking the capture/label antibody (see Chapter 8). To confirm that heterophilic antibodies are present, samples may be diluted and the linearity of the dilutions is analyzed (similar to eliminating hook effect). Samples with heterophilic antibodies do not give linear results upon dilution. The presence of antianimal immunoglobulins can also be detected directly with commercial reagents. Nonimmune animal serum is often added to immunoassays to minimize the effects of heterophilic antibodies, and there are commercial blocking reagents that can be used to remove HAMAs. Many monoclonal therapeutic agents are now derived to include only fragments of an antibody so that patients do not develop heterophilic antibodies to the full antibody. In the laboratory, heterophile antibodies can be detected by investigating results that are inconsistent with history and clinical scenario.

Common Analytical Concerns Applied to Tumor Marker Immunoassays

Immunoassays for tumor markers can be affected by interference from icterus, lipemia, hemolysis, and antibody cross-reactivity in the same manner as other immunoassays.

As with all automated tests, the potential for carryover with high levels of tumor marker analytes can also be a concern, leading to falsely elevated levels in patients if adequate washing steps are not included between patient samples.

High-Performance Liquid Chromatography

High-performance liquid chromatography (HPLC) is commonly used to detect small molecules, such as endocrine metabolites. With respect to tumor markers, HPLC is used to detect catecholamine metabolites in plasma and urine. Generally, there is an extraction process, by which the analytes of interest are separated from either plasma or urine. Extractions are applied to a column where they are separated by their physical characteristics (charge, size, and polarity). Catecholamines and catecholamine metabolites are used to help diagnose carcinoid tumors, pheochromocytoma, and neuroblastoma. Neuroblastoma is a common malignant tumor occurring in approximately 7.5% of children under 15 years of age. Neuroblastoma is diagnosed by the detection of high levels of plasma epinephrine, norepinephrine, and dopamine (catecholamines). Pheochromocytoma, a rare tumor associated with hypertension, is diagnosed by detecting elevated plasma metanephrines (along with urine vanillylmandelic acid and free catecholamines). Carcinoid tumors are serotonin-secreting tumors that arise from the small intestine, appendix, or rectum leading to a host of symptoms (carcinoid syndrome), including pronounced flushing, bronchial constriction, cardiac valve lesions, and diarrhea. The diagnosis of carcinoid tumors involves the detection of 5-hydroxyindoleacetic acid, which is a serotonin metabolite. In all of these cases, HPLC is used to detect the hormones and metabolites secreted by these tumors for diagnosis, therapeutic monitoring, and recurrence. HPLC is not subject to hook effect, lot-to-lot antibody variation, and heterophile antibodies but is more labor intensive and requires more experience and skill than automated immunoassays.

Immunohistochemistry and Immunofluorescence

While not found in circulation, it is important for laboratorians to be familiar with solid tissue tumor markers. These are identified in tissue sections typically from a fine-needle aspirate or biopsy samples. Specific antibodies (and the proper control antibodies) are incubated with tissue sections to detect the presence (or absence) of antigens using colorimetric or fluorescent secondary antibodies. In many ways, this is similar to detection by immunoassay, but the added value is the ability to determine whether the antigen in question is in a particular cell type (such as a tumor), in the specific subcellular location. A good example of the use of a tumor marker that is detected by immunohistochemistry is the identification of estrogen and progesterone receptors in breast cancer. When breast tumors are positive for estrogen and progesterone receptors at the cell surface, they tend to respond to hormonal therapy, while tumors lacking these receptors are treated with other chemotherapeutic modalities.[6]

Enzyme Assays

The detection of elevated circulating enzymes generally cannot be used to identify a specific tumor or site of tumor. One key exception to this is the PSA, which is in fact an enzyme; PSA is a serine protease of the kallikrein family, found in both diseased and benign prostate glands (it is also found in low concentrations in amniotic fluid, breast milk, and some other cancers). Before the widespread use of immunoassays and the discovery of oncofetal antigens, enzyme detection use was widespread. When cells die (autolysis/necrosis) or undergo changes in membrane permeability, enzymes are released from intracellular pools into circulation where they are readily detected. Examples of enzymes that have been used as tumor markers include alkaline phosphatase (bone, liver, leukemia, and sarcoma), lactate dehydrogenase (liver, lymphomas, leukemia, and others), and of course PSA (prostate). Enzyme activity assays (see also Chapter 13) are used to quantify all of these enzymes, with the exception of PSA, which is measured by immunoassay.

FREQUENTLY ORDERED TUMOR MARKERS

α-Fetoprotein

AFP is an abundant serum protein normally synthesized by the fetal liver that is reexpressed in certain types of tumors. This reexpression during malignancy classifies AFP as a carcinoembryonic protein. AFP is often elevated in patients with hepatocellular carcinoma (HCC) and germ cell tumors.

Regulation and Physiology

AFP is a 70-kD glycoprotein related to albumin that normally functions as a transport protein. Like albumin, it is involved in regulating fetal oncotic pressure. During development, AFP peaks at approximately one-tenth the concentration of albumin at 30 weeks of gestation. The upper normal limit for serum AFP is approximately 15 ng/mL (reference intervals are method dependent) in healthy adults. Infants initially have high serum AFP values that decline to adult levels at an age of 7 to 10 months.[7]

Clinical Application and Interpretation

AFP is used for the diagnosis, **staging**, prognosis, and treatment monitoring of HCC. Also known as hepatoma, HCC is a tumor that originates in the liver, often due to chronic diseases, such as hepatitis and cirrhosis. Patients with HCC frequently have elevated serum AFP. However, as with most tumor markers, AFP is not completely specific. For example, AFP can also be increased in benign conditions such as pregnancy and other nonmalignant liver disease, as well as other types of malignancies (e.g., testicular cancer—see below).

Although it is not widely used for screening in Europe and North America, AFP has been used to detect HCC in populations with high disease prevalence such as in China. When used for screening high-risk populations, AFP has a sensitivity ranging from 40% to 65% and specificity of 80% to 95% (at cutoffs ranging from 20 to 30 ng/mL).[8] Very high levels of AFP (>500 ng/mL) in high-risk individuals are considered diagnostic of HCC.[9] Several expert groups, including the National Comprehensive Cancer Network, National Academy of Clinical Biochemistry, and the British Society of Gastroenterology, now recommend that AFP be used in conjunction with ultrasound imaging every 6 months in patients at high risk for developing HCC. This includes patients with hepatitis B virus–induced and/or hepatitis C virus–induced liver cirrhosis.[10]

High levels of AFP in HCC are associated with poor prognosis and are exemplified in individuals who do not respond to therapy or have residual disease following surgery. Correspondingly, a decrease in circulating AFP levels after treatment is associated with prolonged survival rates. It is therefore recommended that serial measurements of AFP be used to monitor treatment and postsurgery in patients with HCC.

The other major use for AFP as a tumor marker is for classification and monitoring therapy for testicular cancer. Testicular cancer includes several subtypes broadly classified into seminomatous and nonseminomatous tumors. Seminomatous tumors form directly from malignant germ cells, whereas nonseminomatous tumors differentiate into embryonal carcinoma, teratoma, choriocarcinoma, and yolk sac tumors (endodermal sinus tumor).[11] AFP is used in combination with β-human chorionic gonadotropin (β-hCG) to classify nonseminomatous tumors (Table 32.5). Serum AFP is also useful for tumor staging; AFP is increased in 10% to 20% of stage I tumors, 50% to 80% of stage II tumors, and 90% to 100% of stage III nonseminomatous testicular cancer. As with HCC, AFP can be used serially to monitor therapy efficacy and disease progression, where increases are indicative of relapse or resistance.

METHODOLOGY

AFP is measured using any of a variety of commercially available automated immunoassays. These are typically sandwich immunoassays relying on monoclonal or polyclonal antibodies directed toward different regions of AFP. Serial monitoring of AFP should be done using the same laboratory and assay method to ensure changes (or lack of change) are due to the tumor and not assay variation. As with other glycoproteins, AFP displays some heterogeneity where certain isoforms are preferentially produced by malignant cells; AFP isoforms differ in their glycosylation and sialyation. Antibodies against these isoforms produced by malignant cells may in the future be used to improve the specificity of AFP immunoassays.

Application and Pathophysiology

The primary applications of AFP as a tumor marker are for HCC and nonseminomatous testicular cancer. AFP is typically used as a marker to monitor therapy, detect residual tumor, or detect relapse; AFP is also used as part of maternal serum screening for neural tube defects and chromosomal abnormalities.

Cancer Antigen 125

Cancer antigen 125 (CA-125) was first defined by a murine monoclonal antibody raised against a serous ovarian carcinoma cell line.[10] CA-125 may be useful for detecting ovarian tumors at an early stage and for monitoring treatments without surgical restaging.

Regulation and Physiology

CA-125 is expressed in the ovary, in other tissues of müllerian duct origin, and in human ovarian carcinoma cells. The CA-125 gene encodes a high molecular weight (200,000 to 1,000,000 kDa) mucin protein containing a putative transmembrane region and a tyrosine phosphorylation site.[12] Although it is not usually found in serum, CA-125 may be elevated in patients with endometriosis, during the first trimester of pregnancy, or during menstruation.

Clinical Application and Interpretation

CA-125 is a serologic marker of ovarian cancer. Ovarian cancer accounts for approximately 3% of the newly diagnosed malignancies in women and is among the top five causes of cancer-related death (Table 32.1). Ovarian cancer includes a broad range of categories, including sex cord tumors, stromal tumors, germ cell tumors, and, most commonly, epithelial cell tumors. As with most other tumor markers, CA-125 should not be used to screen for ovarian cancer in asymptomatic individuals. However, CA-125 *is* elevated in a high percentage of ovarian tumors and is recommended as an annual test for women with a family or prior history of ovarian cancer. CA-125 levels also correlate with ovarian cancer stage. CA-125 is elevated in 50% of patients with stage I disease, 90% of patients with stage II, and more than 90% of patients with stage III or IV.

Other tumor markers for ovarian cancer are under development. Human epididymis protein 4 (HE4) is another Food and Drug Administration (FDA)–cleared test for ovarian cancer. HE4 offers improved specificity over CA-125, due to the presence of elevated CA-125 found in nonmalignant conditions, such as endometriosis. Tumor marker identification is still commonly published, with new markers on their way.

CASE STUDY 32.1

A 33-year-old man with a history of chronic liver disease presents with edema, abdominal pain, and recent weight loss. Laboratory examination reveals a low platelet count, hypoalbuminemia, and prolonged prothrombin time and partial thromboplastin time.

Questions

1. Which tumor marker may aid in diagnosing this patient?

2. What additional laboratory tests would be useful in diagnosing this patient?

3. The patient is treated with surgery; how should tumor markers be used to determine the success of surgery?

Methodology

CA-125 can be detected by immunoassays that use OC125 and M11 antibodies. These monoclonal antibodies recognize distinct nonoverlapping regions of the CA-125 epitope. CA-125 is available on many automated platforms. However, results from different platforms are not interchangeable due to differences between reagent detection methods.

Application and Pathophysiology

CA-125 is predominantly used to monitor therapy and to distinguish benign masses from ovarian cancer.[13] For example, in postmenopausal women with a palpable abdominal mass, a high level (>95 U/mL) of CA-125 has a 90% positive predictive value for ovarian cancer. For therapy monitoring, CA-125 is useful both for predicting the success of surgery (debulking procedures) and for determining the efficacy of chemotherapy. Therefore, patients with elevated CA-125 following either treatment modality have a poor prognosis. Prognosis and CA-125 half-life are related; a CA-125 half-life of less than 20 days is associated with longer survival; the average half-life of CA-125 is 4.5 days.[14,15] The upper normal range for serum CA-125 is typically 35 U/mL.

Carcinoembryonic Antigen

CEA was discovered in the 1960s and is a prototypical example of an oncofetal antigen; it is expressed during development and then reexpressed in tumors. CEA is the most widely used tumor marker for colorectal cancer and is also frequently elevated in lung, breast, and gastrointestinal tumors. CEA can be used to aid in the diagnosis, prognosis, and therapy monitoring of colorectal cancer. Although high levels of CEA (>10 ng/mL) are frequently associated with malignancy, high levels of CEA are not specific for colorectal cancer, and therefore, CEA is not used for screening.

Regulation and Physiology

CEA is a large heterogeneous glycoprotein with a molecular weight of approximately 200 kDa. It is part of the immunoglobulin superfamily and is involved in apoptosis, immunity, and cell adhesion. Because of its role in cell adhesion, CEA has been postulated to be involved in metastasis. Akin to other serologic tumor markers, CEA may be elevated nonspecifically because of impaired clearance or through increased production. Increased CEA concentrations have been observed in heavy smokers and in some patients following radiation treatment and chemotherapy. CEA may also be elevated in patients with liver damage due to prolonged clearance. The upper normal range for serum CEA is 3 to 5 ng/mL depending on the assay.

Clinical Application and Interpretation

The main clinical use of CEA is as a marker for colorectal cancer. In colon cancer, CEA is used for prognosis, in postsurgery surveillance, and to monitor response to chemotherapy. For prognosis, CEA can be used in combination with histology and the TNM (see definition box) staging system to establish the need for adjuvant therapy (addition of chemotherapy or treatment after surgery). Adjuvant therapy is indicated in patients with stage II disease (i.e., tumor has spread beyond immediate colon but not to lymph nodes) who have high levels of CEA.[16]

Methodology

Although CEA assays historically used polyclonal antibodies, these have largely been replaced by the use of monoclonal anti-CEA antibodies. CEA is available on numerous commercial automated platforms. Due to the high heterogeneity of CEA, it is essential that the same assay method is applied to serial monitoring.

Application and Pathophysiology

Before surgical resection, baseline CEA values are typically obtained to confirm successful removal of the tumor burden. After surgery and during chemotherapy, it is recommended that CEA levels be serially monitored every 2 to 3 months to detect recurrence and determine therapy efficacy; the half-life of CEA is approximately 2 to 8 days depending on the assay and the individual. If treatment is successful, CEA levels should drop into the reference interval in 1 to 4 months. CEA is not recommended for screening asymptomatic individuals for colorectal cancer. While there are no specific guidelines recommending the use of CEA in other types of cancer, it may be of value for detecting recurrence of antigen-positive breast and gastrointestinal cancers and medullary thyroid carcinoma and to aid in the diagnosis of non–small cell lung cancer.

TNM STAGING SYSTEM

T—tumor size and involvement/invasion of nearby tissue; scale 0–4

N—regional lymph nodes involvement; scale 0–3

M—metastasis; extent of tumor spreading from one tissue to another; scale 0–1

Example grading of a tumor:

T1 N0 M0 = small tumor, no nodal involvement, and no metastasis

---

Human Chorionic Gonadotropin

hCG is a dimeric hormone normally secreted by trophoblasts to promote implantation of the blastocyst and the placenta to maintain the corpus luteum through the first trimester of pregnancy. Some types of tumor invasion are actually similar to uterine implantation, except that implantation in pregnancy is regulated and limited. hCG is elevated in trophoblastic tumors, mainly choriocarcinoma, and germ cell tumors of the ovary and testis.

Regulation and Physiology

hCG is a 45-kD glycoprotein consisting of α- and β-subunits. A unique aspect of hCG is that it is degraded into multiple

fragments. In serum, this results in the presence of the intact molecule, nicked hCG, the free β-subunit (β-hCG), and a hyperglycosylated intact form. Either intact hCG or the free β-subunit may be elevated in malignancies, and most assays detect multiple fragments of hCG.

CASE STUDY 32.2

A 65-year-old man presents to the emergency department after he had abnormally tarry-colored stool on multiple occasions. He has had gastrointestinal discomfort and has felt increasingly tired during the past 2 months. Physical examination reveals a guaiac-positive stool. A subsequently colonoscopy identified a circumferential mass in the sigmoid colon. A biopsy was performed, which identified the mass as an adenocarcinoma. CEA level was obtained as part of the presurgery workup.

Questions

1. Is the CEA test useful as a screening test for colon carcinoma?
2. What other conditions can result in elevated CEA levels?
3. How is CEA used to monitor patients after surgery for colon cancer?

Clinical Application and Interpretation

hCG has several clinical applications as a tumor marker. It is a prognostic indicator for ovarian cancer, a diagnostic marker for classification of testicular cancer, and the most useful marker for detection of gestational trophoblastic diseases (GTDs).[2] GTDs include four distinct types of tumors (hydatidiform mole, persistent/invasive gestational trophoblastic neoplasia, choriocarcinoma, and placental site trophoblastic tumors) that are classified by clinical history, ultrasound, histology, and hCG levels. hCG is invariably elevated in women with GTDs[17] and is often found at higher levels than are observed in normal pregnancy (i.e., >100,000 mIU/mL). It is particularly a helpful marker for monitoring GTD therapy, as levels of hCG correlate with tumor mass and prognosis; hCG is not actually cleared by the FDA for use as a tumor marker despite its widespread utility.

Methodology

hCG can be measured by using any of a variety of widely available automated immunoassays. Typical assays use monoclonal capture and tracer antibodies targeted toward epitopes in the β-subunit and intact hCG. Total β-hCG assays are the most useful assays because they detect both intact hormone and free β-hCG. Due to the variability in hCG assays,[18] it is imperative that patients be monitored with the same technique. It is also important for laboratories to be aware of the relative cross-reactivity of their assay with different hCG isoforms; because hCG assays are designed to detect pregnancy, they are not all equivalent for application as tumor markers.

Application and Pathophysiology

In testicular cancer, the free β-hCG subunit is elevated in 60% to 70% of patients with nonseminomas. hCG can be used in combination with AFP and biopsies to diagnose subtypes of testicular cancer (Table 32.5). Ectopic β-hCG is also occasionally elevated in ovarian cancer and some lung cancers. In practice, free β-hCG is sensitive and specific for aggressive neoplasms; the free β-hCG is not detectable in the serum of healthy subjects.

Prostate-Specific Antigen

PSA is a 28-kD glycoprotein produced in the epithelial cells of the acini and ducts of the prostatic ducts in the prostate. It is a serine protease of the kallikrein gene family. It functionally regulates seminal fluid viscosity and is instrumental in dissolving the cervical mucus cap, allowing sperm to enter.

Regulation and Physiology

In healthy men, low circulating levels of PSA can be detected in the serum. There are two major forms of PSA that are found circulating in the blood: (1) free and (2) complexed. Most of the circulating PSA is complexed to α_1-antichymotrypsin or α_2-macroglobulin. Assays to detect total and free PSA have been developed. While the detection of total PSA has been used in screening for and in monitoring of prostate cancer, evidence for the usefulness in detecting free PSA as a fraction of total has been identified. Patients with malignancy have a lower percentage of free PSA. As with other tumor markers, PSA is not entirely specific. Men with benign prostatic hyperplasia (BPH) and prostatitis can also have high PSA levels. Additional markers, such as prostate cancer gene-3 (PCA-3), are starting to be used to address this lack of specificity, though at this time prostate cancer tumor markers remain controversial and actively researched to improve the sensitivity and specificity.

CASE STUDY 32.3

A 25-year-old man with a history of testicular cancer is followed post surgery over the course of 10 months, with β-hCG and AFP monitored. The patient is treated with radiation at 2 months, followed by chemotherapy (taxol, ifosfamide, and cisplatin) from months 6 through 9 (see Case Study Fig. 32.3.1).

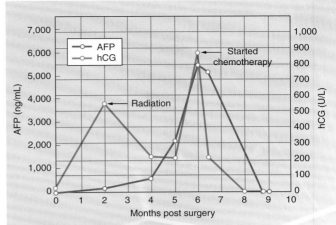

CASE STUDY FIGURE 32.3.1 Time course of hCG and AFP in patient with testicular cancer. The patient was treated with radiation at 2 months and then again with chemotherapy (taxol, ifosfamide, and cisplatin) from months 6 through 9. Reference range for AFP is less than 10 μg/L and that for hCG is less than 5 U/L.

Questions

1. What type of germ cell tumor might this patient have based on the serum AFP and β-hCG levels?

2. Explain the pattern of AFP and hCG observed in the graph.

3. Can a final diagnosis be made based only on the tumor marker findings? If not, why not?

Clinical Application and Interpretation

Several large clinical trials have shown that although PSA can reduce mortality from prostate cancer, it is only a small reduction in overall risk.[19–21] Moreover, harm from screening in the form of biopsies and treatment may outweigh the benefits. Thus, current recommendations focus on informed decision making, where the risks and benefits are outlined and individual patients decide whether or not to be screened.[22–24] Conversations about screening should begin at age 50 (American Cancer Society and American Urological Association).[25] Men at higher risk (first-degree relative with prostate cancer or African American) may consider screening at between 40 to 45 years of age. Serial monitoring is appropriate with a 2-year screening interval may be for men with PSA levels less than 2.0 ng/mL. Screening should always include a digital rectal examination (DRE). Screening utility decreases with age and is not appropriate for men with less than a 10-year life expectancy. In addition to the use of standard cutoff values of total PSA (<4 ng/mL is generally considered normal), other measurements of PSA have been used to test for prostate malignancy; age-adjusted cutoff values of PSA, PSA velocity (rate of rise over time), and free PSA/total PSA ratios have been used to increase the accuracy of PSA testing.[26] Patients with a total PSA greater than 4 ng/mL and/or a clinical suspicion of cancer by DRE undergo biopsy to confirm the presence of prostate cancer, and they are followed closely over time.

TABLE 32.8	Prevalence of Prostate Cancer at Different Prostate-Specific Antigen Concentrations
PSA Concentration (ng/mL)	**Prevalence of Prostate Cancer (%)**
<1	6–10
1–4	17–25
4–10	20–30
>20	>80

Prostate infection, irritation, and BPH (enlargement) can result in increased PSA. Moreover, recent ejaculation or DRE can also lead to increases in circulating PSA.[27–31] It has also been recognized that cancer can be present at all concentrations of PSA (Table 32.8).[32,33] Taken together, these studies urge the interpretation of PSA in the context of the clinical picture (including DRE, imaging, and family history).

Methodology

PSA is measured by immunoassay, which detects both free PSA and PSA complexed with α_1-antichymotrypsin but not α_2-macroglobulin. Most immunoassays commercially available use enzyme, fluorescence, or chemiluminescence on an automated immunoassay platform. Because antibodies recognizing different epitopes may recognize the multiple forms of PSA variably, there can be some discrepant PSA results between manufacturers. Known interferences that have been reported for PSA include both the Hook effect[34] and HAMAs (see above).[35,36]

Application and Pathophysiology

The best clinical use and first clinical application of PSA testing were to monitor for the progression of prostate cancer after therapy. After radical prostatectomy, serum PSA should become undetectable if the cancer is localized. In a series of men treated by radical prostatectomy from 1982 through 1997, biochemical recurrence was found to proceed any evidence of metastatic disease by nearly 8 years.[37] This use of PSA to monitor cancer progression has also been found useful after radiation or endocrine therapy.[38]

CASE STUDY 32.4

A 52-year-old man presented for an annual physical, where a screening PSA and DRE were performed. A serum PSA of 7.0 was detected, and on DRE, asymmetric nodules were detected (see Case Study Fig. 32.4.1). A transrectal biopsy, the gold standard for prostate cancer diagnosis, revealed the presence of carcinoma. A radical prostatectomy was performed a month later, where the preoperative PSA level was 7.1.

CASE STUDY FIGURE 32.4.1 Time course of serum PSA after radical prostatectomy. Because PSA is produced exclusively in the prostate gland, radical prostatectomy in this patient resulted in PSA levels below the level of detection of the assay. The half-life of PSA is 2 to 3 days, which generally requires approximately 1 month for this drop to occur. At 3 months after prostatectomy, this patient's PSA levels were undetectable (generally <0.1 to 0.3 ng/mL), indicating that residual disease was not present. After the first year of surgery, PSA levels should be taken every 3 months (as shown). During the 2nd year, it will be taken every 4 months and after that, every 6 months. Any increase in PSA strongly indicates the recurrence of disease, with a delay in clinical symptoms 1 to 5 years.

Questions

1. Was a prostatectomy performed on this patient because of an elevated PSA?

2. Is there any evidence for residual disease or recurrence in this patient?

3. Why was PSA testing delayed for 1 month after the prostatectomy?

FUTURE DIRECTIONS

Serological tumor markers provide an adjunct to clinical findings and imaging studies for diagnosis, monitoring, and treatment of cancer. Individual markers are not sufficiently sensitive or specific enough to be used in isolation. Tumor markers are an area of active research, such that laboratorians should remain aware of new guidelines and the development of new tests.

questions

1. What is the lifetime risk for women dying of cancer?
   a. 19%
   b. 23%
   c. 43%
   d. 59%

2. Select the appropriate letter regarding tumor marker tests:
   i. Screen for cancer
   ii. Aid in staging of cancer
   iii. Monitor response to therapy
   iv. Detect recurrent disease
   a. All of the above
   b. i, ii, and iii
   c. ii, iii, and iv
   d. i, ii, and iv
   e. iv

3. Tumor markers may be defined as
   a. Biologic substances synthesized and released by cancer cells or substances produced by the host in response to cancer cells
   b. Analytic tests (e.g., immunoassays) used to mark cancer cells
   c. Radioactive substances and chemicals used to help the physician identify cancer cells
   d. None of these

4. Which of the following is an oncofetal antigen?
   a. AFP
   b. CA-125
   c. β-hCG
   d. CEA

5. What are the major limitations of tumor markers?
   a. Sensitivity and specificity
   b. Cost
   c. Turnaround time
   d. Imprecision

6. The major clinical use for CA 15-3 is monitoring treatment response of
   a. Ovarian carcinoma
   b. Colorectal cancer
   c. Prostatic cancer
   d. Breast cancer

7. The most common immunoassays used to measure PSA detect which form of the enzyme?
   a. Total PSA
   b. Free PSA
   c. PSA complexed with α1-antichymotrypsin
   d. PSA complexed with α2-macroglobulin

8. Which of the following enzymes is commonly used as a tumor marker?
   a. LD
   b. Lipase
   c. PSA
   d. ALT

9. A tumor marker used in the assessment of choriocarcinoma or hydatidiform mole is
   a. β-hCG
   b. CEA
   c. AFP
   d. IgG

10. A serum PSA is used for all of the following except
   a. Diagnosis
   b. Screening
   c. Monitoring response
   d. Detecting recurrence

11. The following serum PSA measurements were obtained from two male patients who were being monitored over an 18-week period.

	Week 1	Week 6	Week 10	Week 15	Week 18
Patient A	21 ng/mL	26 ng/mL	46 ng/mL	79 ng/mL	78 ng/mL
Patient B	14 ng/mL	46 ng/mL	89 ng/mL	120 ng/mL	110 ng/mL

Which of the following statements most accurately describes these data?
   a. Patient A may have a more aggressive prostate cancer based on the velocity of these measurements.
   b. Patient A is most likely to have benign prostate cancer.
   c. Patient B is most likely to be experiencing an inflammatory reaction, and this is largely contributing to the elevated PSA above 100 ng/mL.
   d. Patient B may have a more aggressive prostate cancer based on the velocity of these measurements.
   e. Answers *a* and *c* most accurately describe these data.

12. When measuring tumor markers in the clinical laboratory, which of the following has been reported to contribute to 30% to 70% of the total amount of error?
   a. Preanalytical errors
   b. Analytical errors
   c. Hook effect
   d. Using different immunoassay methods
   e. Not comparing lot numbers between ELISA kits

13. Which of the following methods is commonly used to measure endocrine metabolites?
   a. Protein electrophoresis
   b. Immunoassays
   c. HPLC
   d. Electrochemistry
   e. Gas chromatography

suggested reading

Diamandis EP, Fritsche HA, Lilja H, et al. *Tumor Markers: Physiology, Pathobiology, Technology, and Clinical Applications.* Washington, DC: AACC Press; 2002.

Wu JT. *Circulating Tumor Markers of the New Millennium: Target Therapy, Early Detection, and Prognosis.* Washington, DC: AACC Press; 2002.

references

1. Howlader N, Noone AM, Krapcho M, et al., eds. *SEER Cancer Statistics Review*. Bethesda, MD: National Cancer Institute; 1975–2012. http://seer.cancer.gov/csr/1975_2012/
2. Abeloff MD, Armitage JO, Niederhuber JE, et al., eds. *Abeloff's Clinical Oncology*. 4th ed. Philadelphia, PA: Churchill Livingstone; 2008.
3. Hanahan D, Weinberg RA. The hallmarks of cancer. *Cell.* 2000;100:57–70.
4. Clinical and Laboratory Standards Institute. *Standards and Guidelines for Clinical Laboratories*. www.clsi.org. Accessed October 20, 2008.
5. Klee GG. Human anti-mouse antibodies. *Arch Pathol Lab Med.* 2000;124:921–923.
6. Harris L, Fritsche H, Mennel R, et al. American Society of Clinical Oncology 2007 update of recommendations for the use of tumor markers in breast cancer. *J Clin Oncol.* 2007;25:5287–5312.
7. Bader D, Riskin A, Vafsi O, et al. Alpha-fetoprotein in the early neonatal period—a large study and review of the literature. *Clin Chim Acta.* 2004;349:15–23.
8. Gupta S, Bent S, Kohlwes J. Test characteristics of alpha-fetoprotein for detecting hepatocellular carcinoma in patients with hepatitis C. A systematic review and critical analysis. *Ann Intern Med.* 2003;139:46–50.
9. Wu JT. Serum alpha-fetoprotein and its lectin reactivity in liver diseases: a review. *Ann Clin Lab Sci.* 1990;20:98–105.
10. Diamandis EP, Hoffman BR, Sturgeon CM. National Academy of Clinical Biochemistry laboratory medicine practical guidelines for the use of tumor markers. *Clin Chem.* 2008;54:1935–1939.
11. Raghavan D. *Germ Cell Tumors*. London and Ontario: BC Decker; 2003.
12. Yin BW, Lloyd KO. Molecular cloning of the CA125 ovarian cancer antigen: identification as a new mucin, MUC16. *J Biol Chem.* 2001;276:27371–27375.
13. Duffy MJ, Bonfrer JM, Kulpa J, et al. CA125 in ovarian cancer: European Group on Tumor Markers guidelines for clinical use. *Int J Gynecol Cancer.* 2005;15:679–691.
14. Bast RC Jr, Xu FJ, Yu YH, et al. CA 125: the past and the future. *Int J Biol Markers.* 1998;13:179–187.
15. Verheijen RH, von Mensdorff-Pouilly S, van Kamp GJ, et al. CA 125: fundamental and clinical aspects. *Semin Cancer Biol.* 1999;9:117–124.
16. Duffy MJ, van Dalen A, Haglund C, et al. Clinical utility of biochemical markers in colorectal cancer: European Group on Tumour Markers (EGTM) guidelines. *Eur J Cancer.* 2003;39:718–727.
17. Bower M, Rustin G. Serum tumor markers and their role in monitoring germ cell cancers of the testis. In: Vogelzang N, Scardino P, Shipley W, et al., eds. *Comprehensive Textbook of Genitourinary Oncology*. 2nd ed. Philadelphia, PA: Lippincott Williams & Wilkins; 2000:931.
18. Cole LA, Sutton JM, Higgins TN, Cembrowski GS. Between-method variation in human chorionic gonadotropin test results. *Clin Chem.* 2004;50:874–882.
19. Schröder FH, Hugosson J, Roobol MJ, et al. Screening and prostate-cancer mortality in a randomized European study. *N Engl J Med.* 2009;360(13):1320–1328.
20. Schröder FH, Hugosson J, Roobol MJ, et al. Prostate-cancer mortality at 11 years of follow-up. *N Engl J Med.* 2012;366(11):981–990.
21. Andriole GL, Crawford ED, Grubb RL, et al. Mortality results from a randomized prostate-cancer screening trial. *N Engl J Med.* 2009;360(13):1310–1319.
22. American Cancer Society Prostate Cancer Screening Decision Support. http://www.cancer.org/acs/groups/content/@editorial/documents/document/acspc-024618.pdf. Accessed March 21, 2016.
23. American Society for Clinical Oncology Prostate Cancer Screening Decision Support. https://www.asco.org/sites/www.asco.org/files/psa_pco_decision_aid:71612.pdf. Accessed March 21, 2016.
24. Centers for Disease Control Prostate Cancer Screening Decision Support. http://www.cdc.gov/cancer/prostate/basic_info/infographic.htm. Accessed March 21, 2016.
25. Smith RA, Cokkinides V, Eyre HJ. American Cancer Society guidelines for the early detection of cancer, 2006. *CA Cancer J Clin.* 2006;56:11–25; quiz 49–50.
26. Loeb S, Catalona WJ. Prostate-specific antigen in clinical practice. *Cancer Lett.* 2007;249:30–39.
27. Herschman JD, Smith DS, Catalona WJ. Effect of ejaculation on serum total and free prostate-specific antigen concentrations. *Urology.* 1997;50:239–243.
28. Crawford ED, Schutz MJ, Clejan S, et al. The effect of digital rectal examination on prostate-specific antigen levels. *JAMA.* 1992;267:2227–2228.
29. Chybowski FM, Bergstralh EJ, Oesterling JE. The effect of digital rectal examination on the serum prostate specific antigen concentration: results of a randomized study. *J Urol.* 1992;148:83–86.
30. Collins GN, Martin PJ, Wynn-Davies A, et al. The effect of digital rectal examination, flexible cystoscopy and prostatic biopsy on free and total prostate specific antigen, and the free-to-total prostate specific antigen ratio in clinical practice. *J Urol.* 1997;157:1744–1747.
31. Tarhan F, Orcun A, Kucukercan I, et al. Effect of prostatic massage on serum complexed prostate-specific antigen levels. *Urology.* 2005;66:1234–1238.
32. Thompson IM, Goodman PJ, Tangen CM, et al. The influence of finasteride on the development of prostate cancer. *N Engl J Med.* 2003;349:215–224.
33. Thompson IM, Pauler DK, Goodman PJ, et al. Prevalence of prostate cancer among men with a prostate-specific antigen level < or = 4.0 ng per milliliter. *N Engl J Med.* 2004;350:2239–2246.
34. Akamatsu S, Tsukazaki H, Inoue K, et al. Advanced prostate cancer with extremely low prostate-specific antigen value at diagnosis: an example of high dose hook effect. *Int J Urol.* 2006;13:1025–1027.
35. Park S, Wians FH Jr, Cadeddu JA. Spurious prostate-specific antigen (PSA) recurrence after radical prostatectomy: interference by human antimouse heterophile antibodies. *Int J Urol.* 2007;14:251–253.

36. Descotes JL, Legeais D, Gauchez AS, et al. PSA measurement following prostatectomy: an unexpected error. *Anticancer Res.* 2007;27:1149–1150.

37. Pound CR, Partin AW, Eisenberger MA, et al. Natural history of progression after PSA elevation following radical prostatectomy. *JAMA.* 1999;281:1591–1597.

38. Roach M III, Hanks G, Thames H Jr, et al. Defining biochemical failure following radiotherapy with or without hormonal therapy in men with clinically localized prostate cancer: recommendations of the RTOG-ASTRO Phoenix Consensus Conference. *Int J Radiat Oncol Biol Phys.* 2006;65:965–974.

33

Nutrition Assessment

LINDA S. GORMAN and MARIA G. BOOSALIS

key terms

Body Mass Index (BMI)
Celiac Disease
Dietary Reference Intake (DRI)
Essential Nutrients
Gluten
Hypervitaminosis
Hypovitaminosis
Kwashiorkor
Malnutrition
Marasmus
Nitrogen Balance
Nutrient
Parenteral Nutrition
Vitamin

chapter objectives

Upon completion of this chapter, the clinical laboratorian should be able to do the following:

- Discuss the contribution of individual nutrient classes to human metabolism.
- Discuss therapeutic nutrition support by enteral and parenteral routes.
- List biochemical parameters used to monitor nutritional status.
- Describe the biochemical roles of vitamins.
- Correlate alterations in vitamin status with circumstances of increased metabolic requirements, age-related physiologic changes, or pathologic conditions.
- Describe drug–nutrient interactions that influence vitamin status.
- Delineate laboratory procedures used in the assessment of vitamin status.
- Discuss the role of the laboratory in nutritional assessment and monitoring.
- List the populations at risk for malnutrition.
- Identify the plasma protein changes as a result of stress.
- Describe some of the electrolyte and mineral abnormalities associated with total parenteral nutrition.

For additional student resources, please visit thePoint®
at http://thepoint.lww.com

NUTRITION CARE PROCESS: OVERVIEW

The *nutrition care process (NCP)* is defined as "a systemic problem-solving method that dietetic professionals use to critically think and make decisions to address nutrition-related problems and provide safe and effective quality nutrition care."[1] In other words, this process is the systematic approach used by the registered dietitian (RD) to identify, diagnose, and treat any nutrition-related problems or disorders.

There are four components to the NCP: nutrition assessment, nutrition diagnosis, nutrition intervention, and nutrition monitoring and evaluation.[1]

The focus of this chapter is the first component of the NCP, specifically nutrition assessment. *Nutrition assessment* is defined as a "systematic process of obtaining, verifying, and interpreting data in order to make decisions about the nature and cause of nutrition-related problems."[1] Nutrition assessment includes the "A to Fs of assessment."[2]

A—anthropometric or body composition measurements
B—biochemical analyses, the prime focus of this chapter
C—clinical examination usually performed by the physician or other health care provider
D—dietary analysis and assessment to determine usual food intake generally performed by the RD
E—environmental assessment, which includes a consideration of all the other aspects of the individual's environment that may affect his/her ability to purchase, prepare, and consume food
F—focused nutrition physical examination or nutrition-focused physical examination, in which the RD essentially does a head-to-toe review, focusing on nutrition-related findings to supplement the A to E data collected

NUTRITION ASSESSMENT

A. Anthropometric measurements include, at a minimum, the measurement of height and weight and from those two measurements the calculation of the **body mass index (BMI)**. The BMI "describes relative weight for height, is significantly correlated with total body fat content," and should be "used to assess overweight and obesity and to monitor changes in body weight."[3]

Other measurements in this category that are helpful, especially when assessing an individual, include a weight history (amount or percentage of gain vs. loss; intentional vs. unintentional) and possibly a waist circumference measurement (to help identify additional comorbidity risk and the presence of metabolic syndrome).

Other anthropometric or body composition measurements that belong in this category include skinfold thickness, hydrostatic weighing, air-displacement plethysmography, dual-energy x-ray absorptiometry, and bioelectrical impedance analysis, all of which are beyond the scope of this chapter. All of these different types of measurements are used to determine the percentage of fat, lean body muscle, water, and/or bone mineral density in the human body.

Until this epidemic of overweight/obesity lessens, approximately two of every three adults measured may be either overweight (BMI 25 to 29.9 kg/m²) or obese (BMI ≥ 30 kg/m²) by the National Heart, Lung, and Blood Institute (NHLBI) standards. On the other side of the spectrum is the adult who may be malnourished/undernourished and possibly also underweight (BMI < 18.5 kg/m²).

B. Biochemical assessment/markers are divided into macronutrients and micronutrients. The macronutrients include markers of carbohydrate, protein, and fat metabolism and utilization. How these markers change during inflammation and disease can be important to know if treatment is to be effective. Health care providers appreciate the clinical laboratory assessment of these markers and expect to receive the results in a timely manner. Micronutrient measurements are often more difficult to obtain and yet may hold the key to why a patient straddles the fence between health and illness. Insufficient or excessive vitamins and/or minerals can have a serious impact on the enzymes and biochemistry of the human body. In particular, trace elements or minerals are especially important to many biologically significant metabolic reactions.

There is a close interrelationship between the function of certain organs in the body and **nutrient** balance/imbalance, both positive and negative. Liver function will be affected if there is insufficient protein and excess fats. Liver function within normal limits is critical to the adequate processing of ingested protein and fats and the packaging/storage of certain vitamins and minerals. An excessive intake of protein may also be harmful to kidney function due to the excess of nonprotein nitrogen compounds formed that must then be removed. On the other hand, normal renal function is critical to the amount of protein, sodium, and fluids that can be consumed. Other nutrient imbalances can affect the heart (fats, water imbalances, vitamin deficiencies or excesses, selenium, etc.), pancreas, and/or other glands. The thyroid in particular not only requires adequate iodine and tyrosine levels for hormone synthesis but also requires adequate iron levels as enzyme cofactors for the formation and degradation of T_4 and T_3.[4]

In addition, during hospitalization, biomarkers enable the health care team to monitor and detect acute stress and other systemic inflammatory conditions. The acute-phase reactant proteins and other circulating vitamins and/or minerals that are monitored can help pinpoint patients at risk and in need of nutritional intervention and aid in the identification of the systemic inflammatory response syndrome.[5–11] In addition, signs of a chronic inflammatory state can be ascertained with the aid of clinical laboratory tests.[12]

Assessing the biomarkers in a nutrition assessment is the responsibility of the clinical laboratory professional. These are discussed individually in a later section of this chapter.

C. The clinical component of the nutrition assessment consists of the history of present illness, the past medical history, and an inquiry into the family history. It also includes the physical examination and a careful review of systems looking for signs of disease/illness. It includes a measurement of blood pressure as well as presence of any physical limitations/restrictions regarding physical movement/activity.

For example, the *review of systems* is a head-to-toe examination looking for signs of **malnutrition** and/or disease. For instance, ease of pluckability of hair (>8 to 10 hairs at one time) may indicate a protein deficiency that requires biochemical verification via measurement of circulating proteins such as albumin and transthyretin. Changes in vision such as night blindness or Bitot's spots may indicate a deficiency of vitamin A.

Metabolic syndrome is defined by utilizing information derived from the first three components (A to C) of a nutrition assessment. Specifically, the presence of three or more of any of the following parameters defines the presence of the metabolic syndrome in adults according to the American Heart Association and the NHLBI.[13] These parameters include the following:

1. An elevated waist circumference. In women, ≥35 in. (88 cm); in men, ≥40 in. (102 cm)
2. Elevated triglyceride levels, that is, ≥150 mg/dL
3. Elevated fasting glucose, that is, ≥100 mg/dL
4. Reduced high-density lipoprotein (HDL) cholesterol. In women, <50 mg/dL; in men, <40 mg/dL
5. Elevated blood pressure, that is, ≥130/85 mm Hg

D. The dietary component of the nutritional assessment strives to determine the adequacy of the usual day's intake with respect to nutritional recommendations that are specific for an individual's age, gender, level of physical activity, and particular health conditions. In addition, if there are any specific dietary needs that must be met, an assessment to determine whether these needs are met must also be included. There are several ways to assess adequacy of intake—by general food groupings and respective servings using the USDA Food Guidance System ChooseMyPlate eating plans[14] or via specific nutrients compared with the **Dietary Reference Intake (DRI)** recommendations (recommended dietary allowance [RDA], adequate intake [AI], and/or tolerable upper limits [UL]).[15] Examples of tools used by the RD to determine dietary adequacy include the 24-hour recall, the 3-day food record or diary, and/or the food frequency questionnaire. Again, specific details of each methodology are beyond the scope of this chapter.

E. The environmental assessment takes into consideration all aspects of an individual's environment or living conditions that may affect his or her ability to purchase, prepare, and/or consume food.

For example, it includes financial status to determine if money is a limiting factor to obtaining one's nutritional needs/adequate nutrition.

An individual's physical living conditions (e.g., adequate cooking skills, preparation supplies, and running water), social support system, and religious beliefs (especially if it prevents the individual from consuming certain food groups) are other types of information included.

This assessment also evaluates the highest level of education attained to tailor educational materials and message. In essence, any aspect of the environment that may affect the ability to purchase, prepare, and/or consume food is included in this evaluation.

F. The focused nutrition physical examination or nutrition-focused physical examination is a process used to unify findings from the previous A to E assessment, culminating in findings that will help determine the nutrition diagnosis, the next step in the NCP. Specifically, it is a systematic review of the entire individual, looking for signs of malnutrition with respect to macronutrients as well as micronutrients, beginning at the head and working way down to the toes; it uses tools of inspection (observe), palpation (touch), percussion (tap), and auscultation (listen). As the RD performs this focused type of examination, she/he is integrating findings from the other components of the nutrition assessment, including any biochemical findings. Moreover, as a result of this focused nutrition physical examination, other biochemical tests may be ordered to verify some of the findings, in particular related to signs of protein–calorie malnutrition and/or or specific vitamin mineral deficiencies. Detailed description of this particular aspect of the assessment is beyond the scope of this chapter.[16,17]

The information obtained from all A to F aspects of a complete nutrition assessment is then summarized and reviewed by the RD or other health care professional to determine a nutrition diagnosis, the next step in the NCP. Once the nutrition diagnosis is made, a plan for the nutrition intervention is designed and implemented followed by monitoring and evaluation as the last component of the NCP.

BIOCHEMICAL MARKERS: MACRONUTRIENTS

Protein

The primary objective is to identify the patient who is malnourished and then, through nutritional therapy, to preserve or replenish the protein component of the body. Laboratory nutrition assessment is best accomplished by monitoring selected serum proteins that ideally have a short biologic half-life and reflect changes in protein status by measuring their concentration changes in the serum. These concentrations of protein markers are affected by protein malnutrition associated with end-stage liver and renal disease and severe infection and, most significantly, by stress injury. Because the effect of the inflammatory response is closely associated with the decline of essential transport proteins, a separation of the inflammatory state from protein malnutrition can be problematic, except by using an acute-phase reactant, such as C-reactive protein (CRP). The prognostic inflammatory nutritional index, using the ratio of the CRP–orosomucoid (α_1-acid glycoprotein) product to

Protein	Molecular Weight (kD)	Half-Life	Reference Range
Albumin	65,000	20 d	33–48 g/L
Fibronectin	250,000	15 h	220–400 mg/L
Prealbumin (transthyretin)	54,980	48 h	160–350 mg/L
Retinol-binding protein	21,000	12 h	30–60 mg/L
Insulin-like growth factor 1	7,650	2 h	0.10–0.40 mg/L
Transferrin	76,000	9 d	1.6–3.6 g/L

TABLE 33.1 **Characteristics of Plasma Proteins of Nutritional Interest**

the albumin–transthyretin product, is intended to resolve this issue.[18] Table 33.1 offers detailed information about these protein markers.

Albumin

Albumin has long been used in the assessment of hospitalized patients. The albumin concentration in the body is influenced by albumin synthesis, degradation, and distribution. Low levels of serum albumin may reflect low hepatic production or loss from transfer of albumin between the extravascular and the vascular compartment. The long biologic half-life of albumin (~20 days) allows changes in the serum concentration only after long periods of malnutrition. Low albumin levels have been identified as a predictor of mortality in patients in long-term care facilities. Hospitalized patients with low serum albumin levels experience a fourfold increase in morbidity and a sixfold increase in mortality.[19,20]

Serum albumin is not a good indicator of short-term protein and energy deprivation; however, albumin levels are good indicators of chronic deficiency. Traditionally, albumin has been used to help determine two important nutritional states. First, it helps identify chronic protein deficiency under conditions of adequate non–protein-calorie intake, which leads to marked hypoalbuminemia. This may result from the net loss of albumin from both the intravascular and extravascular pools, causing **kwashiorkor**. Second, albumin concentrations may help define **marasmus**, a deficiency of calories with adequate protein status. In this condition, the serum albumin level remains normal despite considerable loss of body weight. Studies have classified various levels of malnutrition by using albumin levels. Serum albumin levels of ≥35 g/L are considered normal. Albumin levels of 28–30 to 35 g/L indicate mild malnutrition, levels of 23–25 to 28–30 g/L indicate moderate malnutrition, and levels less than 23 to 25 g/L indicate severely depleted albumin. Serum albumin is an accurate marker of the catabolic stress of infection. A level of ≤32 g/L indicates that if a patient is in the hospital for up to 10 days, there is a 75% risk of developing decubitus ulcers. Serum albumin levels of less than 25 g/L can be used as an accurate measure of predicting survival prognosis in 90% of critically ill patients.

Transferrin

Transferrin is a glycoprotein with a biologic half-life of approximately 9 days (shorter than albumin). It is synthesized in the liver and binds and transports ferric iron.

Transferrin synthesis is regulated by iron stores. When hepatocyte iron is absent or low, transferrin levels rise in proportion to the deficiency. It is an early indicator of iron deficiency, and the elevated transferrin is the last analyte to return to normal when iron deficiency is corrected.

The half-life of transferrin is approximately one-half that of albumin, and the body pool is smaller than that of albumin; therefore, transferrin is more likely to indicate protein depletion before serum albumin concentration changes. The usefulness of transferrin in diagnosis of subclinical, marginal, or moderate malnutrition is questionable, however, because a wide range of values have been reported in various studies. Transferrin levels can be lowered by factors other than protein or energy deficiency, such as nephrotic syndrome, liver disorders, anemia, and neoplastic disease.

In hospital and nursing home settings, transferrin levels have been used as indices of morbidity and mortality.[21] Information shows, however, that serum transferrin concentrations are not sufficiently sensitive to detect a change in nutritional status that occurs after 2 weeks of total parenteral nutrition (PN).[22] In addition to being responsive to serum iron concentrations, transferrin is uniquely sensitive to some antibiotics and fungicides.

Transthyretin

Transthyretin is sometimes called thyroxine-binding prealbumin or prealbumin because it migrates ahead of albumin in the customary electrophoresis of serum or plasma proteins. In normal situations, each transthyretin subunit contains one binding site for retinol-binding protein (RBP). Transthyretin and RBP are considered the major transport proteins for thyroxine and vitamin A, respectively.

Because of its short half-life and small body pool, transthyretin is a better indicator of visceral protein status and positive nitrogen balance than albumin and transferrin.[22] Transthyretin is a superior indicator for monitoring short-term effects of nutritional therapy. The concentration of transthyretin and RBP complex, greatly decreased in protein-energy malnutrition,[23] returns toward normal values after nutritional replenishment. Transthyretin has a low pool concentration in the serum, a half-life of 2 days, and a rapid response to low energy intake, even when protein intake is inadequate for as few as 4 days.[24] Serum transthyretin concentrations are decreased postoperatively by 50 to 90 mg/L in the first week, with the ability to double in 1 week or at least increase from 40 to 50 mg/L in response to adequate nutritional support. If the transthyretin response increases less than 20 mg/L in 1 week as an outcome measure, this indicates either inadequate nutritional support or inadequate response.[22,25]

When transthyretin decreases to levels of less than 80 mg/L, severe protein–calorie malnutrition develops; however, nutritional support can cause a daily increase in transthyretin of up to 10 mg/L.[22] These concentrations do not appear to be significantly influenced by fluctuations in the hydration state. Although end-stage liver disease appears to affect all protein levels in the body, liver disease does not affect transthyretin as early or to the same extent as it affects other serum protein markers, particularly RBP. Although transthyretin levels may be elevated in patients with renal disease, if a trend in the direction of change is noted, the changes are likely to reflect alteration in nutritional status and nitrogen balance. Steroids can cause a slight elevation in transthyretin, but the nutritional trend can still be followed because transthyretin responds to both overfeeding and underfeeding.

Transthyretin is also used as an indicator of the adequacy of a nutritional feeding plan[22] because changes in plasma protein are correlated with nitrogen balance. Transthyretin concentrations increase in patients with positive nitrogen balance and decrease in patients with negative nitrogen balance. When the transthyretin level is ≥180 mg/L, this correlates with a positive nitrogen balance and indicates a return to adequate nutritional status. It has been shown in both the pediatric and neonate population to be a highly accurate and relatively inexpensive marker for nutritional status[7,26] and has been found to be the most sensitive and helpful indicator when looking at the nutritional status of very ill patients.[27]

In summary, transthyretin effectively demonstrates an anabolic response to feeding and is a good marker for visceral protein synthesis in patients receiving metabolic or nutritional support.[27–29]

Retinol-Binding Protein
RBP has been used in monitoring short-term changes in nutritional status.[30–32] Its usefulness as a metabolic marker is based on its biologic half-life of 12 hours and its small body pool size. As a single polypeptide chain, RBP interacts strongly with plasma transthyretin and circulates in the plasma as a 1:1 mol/L transthyretin–RBP complex.[33] A potential problem exists in using RBP as a nutritional marker, however. Although RBP has a shorter half-life than transthyretin (12 hours, compared with 2 days), it is excreted in the urine, and its concentration increases more significantly than transthyretin in patients with renal failure. In contrast to RBP, transthyretin concentration is only moderately elevated in advanced chronic renal insufficiency.

Insulin-Like Growth Factor 1
Insulin-like growth factor 1 (IGF-1) (formerly termed somatomedin C) is important for stimulation of growth. The molecular size and structure of IGF-1 are similar to proinsulin.[34] IGF-1 serum concentrations are regulated by growth hormone and nutritional intake. Growth hormone stimulates the liver to produce IGF-1, which circulates bound to IGF-BP3. IGF-BP3 modulates the biologic effect of IGF-1 in the stress response, causing both decreases and increases in biologic activity. IGF-1 has been used as a nutritional marker in adults and children,[35–37] although not routinely.

Fibronectin
Fibronectin is an opsonic glycoprotein with a half-life of about 15 hours in humans. This protein has repeating blocks of a homogeneous sequence of amino acids and is an α_2-glycoprotein that serves important roles in cell-to-cell adherence and tissue differentiation, wound healing, microvascular integrity, and opsonization of particulate matter. It is considered the major protein regulating phagocytosis. Synthesis sites include endothelial cells, peritoneal macrophages, fibroblasts, and the liver. Fibronectin concentrations may decrease after physiologic damage caused by severe shock, burns, or infection. Levels return to normal on recovery. Fibronectin is of interest because it is not exclusively synthesized in the liver,[38] and it is an indicator of sepsis in burn patients. Fibronectin levels have been shown to decrease during infection or severe stress, partly due to its opsonic property. The infection or trauma, however, does not significantly decrease fibronectin concentration.[39] Fibronectin only increases in severe infection, in which it remains flat and does not increase as soon as IGF-1. It is not routinely used as a nutritional marker.

Nitrogen Balance
Another nutritional evaluation tool, **nitrogen balance**, is the difference between nitrogen intake and nitrogen excretion. It is one of the most widely used indicators of protein change and/or adequacy of feeding in a controlled setting. In the healthy adult population, anabolic and catabolic rates are in equilibrium, and the nitrogen balance approaches zero. During stress, trauma, or burns, the nutritional intake decreases, and due to an increase in catabolism, nitrogen losses increase and may exceed intake, leading to a negative nitrogen balance. During recovery from illness, the nitrogen balance should become positive with either enteral or PN support. In humans, 90% to 95% of the daily nitrogen loss is accounted for by elimination through the kidneys. About 90% of this loss is in the form of urea. Therefore, the determination of 24-hour urinary urea nitrogen (UUN) is a method for estimating the amount of nitrogen excretion. The nitrogen balance is calculated as follows[40]:

$$\text{Nitrogen balance} = \frac{24 \text{ hour protein intake (g)}}{6.25} - (24 \text{ hour UUN (g)} + 4\text{g}) \quad \text{(Eq. 33-1)}$$

Protein intake includes grams of protein that are provided by intravenous amino acids or by enteral feeding. Protein intake (in grams) is converted into grams of nitrogen by dividing by 6.25. The factor of 4 in the equation represents an estimation of nonurinary losses of nitrogen (e.g., from skin, feces, hair, and nails).[40] Nitrogen balance, as calculated by this equation, is not valid in patients with severe stress or sepsis, as can be seen in critical care areas or in patients with renal disease. Determining the validity of this equation in other clinical conditions involving normally high nitrogen losses may be difficult or even incorrect.

C-Reactive Protein

CRP is an acute-phase protein that increases dramatically under conditions of sepsis, inflammation, and infection. CRP can increase dramatically up to 1,000 times after tissue injury, which are more than two or three orders of magnitude greater than any other acute-phase reactant. CRP rises in concentration 4 to 6 hours before other acute-phase reactants begin to rise.[5,10,12,41,42]

The flow phase of marked catabolism presents clinically with tachycardia, fever, increased respiratory rate, and increased cardiac output. During this time, synthesis rates of CRP and other acute-phase proteins increase and albumin and prealbumin decrease.[5] Even with this increase in acute-phase proteins, a significant negative nitrogen balance usually occurs secondary to the greater protein catabolism.[43] Whether this catabolic state produces a clinically defined malnutrition or a separate entity is unknown, but it certainly produces weight loss with decreased albumin and prealbumin levels.

High-sensitivity CRP is an additional marker for inflammation and has been applied as a predictor of cardiac disease and other cholesterol-related atherosclerotic disorders.

In summary, many of the biochemical markers mentioned in this section can also be used as biochemical markers of inflammation. For instance, coupled with decreases in circulating levels of the negative acute-phase reactants, albumin, transferrin, and prealbumin/transthyretin in the serum, an elevated circulating level of CRP as well as blood glucose may be observed. In addition, a change in white blood cell count (either decreased or increased) coupled with an increased percentage of neutrophils in the cell differential, decreased platelet count, and marked negative nitrogen balance as discussed previously, especially when more than one is present and/or taken in combination can suggest and/or identify the presence of inflammation in the individual.[44]

Cytokines

Nutrition research has recently focused on cytokines, in particular the interleukins, a complex group of proteins and glycoproteins that can exert pleiotropic effects on several different target cells. Most interleukins are produced by macrophages and T lymphocytes, in response to antigenic or mitogenic stimulation, and affect primary T-lymphocyte function. Most nutritional investigations regarding cytokines have been performed on interleukin-1 (IL-1), IL-6, and tumor necrosis factor-α (TNF-α). In addition to these cytokines released by the immune system, adipose cells (adipocytes) release similar compounds, including IL-6 and TNF-α as well as other adipokines such as leptin, resistin, visfatin, and adiponectin, to mention a few. These cytokines and adipokines are subsequently involved in many reactions and body systems that are beyond the scope and purpose of this chapter.

Gluten Sensitivity Antibodies

Antibodies to **gluten** have become the latest protein assay added to the arsenal used to assess nutritional disease. The upswing in **celiac disease** (CD) and the number of individuals with gluten sensitivities resulting in diarrhea, abdominal bloating, rashes and vitamin deficiencies necessitates that we assay for the antibodies that such patients express. These antibodies include antitissue transglutaminase antibodies (tTG-antibodies), endomysial antibodies (EMA), and deamidated gliadin peptide antibody (DGP). DGP has replaced testing for an antibody to unmodified gliadin protein, which has not proven to be that accurate. All of these antibodies may take the form of IgA or IgG isotypes.[45] Serological testing for the IgA forms of tTG-antibodies has been recommended for screening with EMA testing used to confirm.

Fat

Fat is a macronutrient that, in appropriate amounts, is needed for a balanced diet. Alterations in fat intake may also affect circulating lipid levels and lipid metabolism. Laboratory markers for total cholesterol as well as triglycerides enable us to assess some of these lipid changes. Excess fat and/or kilocalorie intake and the repercussions from such a diet can be assessed by looking at HDL and low-density lipoprotein cholesterol levels as well as various lipoproteins. These markers are further discussed in Chapter 15.

Carbohydrate

Nutrition assessment for type 1 and type 2 diabetes mellitus comes into play after diagnosis and requires periodic laboratory assessment for patient compliance/monitoring of treatment. Patients with diabetes have a chronic illness that can be regulated by medication and diet, if they are willing to change many of their habits and eating preferences. Dietitians and physicians rely on laboratory assessment of patient compliance by looking at glucose markers of blood glucose, glycosylated hemoglobin/proteins, and fructosamine. As the patient with diabetes has long-term health issues with their disease, additional laboratory tests for renal function such as microalbumin and estimated glomerular filtration rate will also be requested. The partnership between the laboratory and those treating the individual with diabetes is needed to assist the latter in attaining the highest quality of good health. These laboratory markers are further discussed in Chapter 14.

BIOCHEMICAL MARKERS: MISCELLANEOUS

Parenteral Nutrition

Parenteral nutrition is a means of intense nutritional support for patients who are malnourished or in danger of becoming malnourished because they are unable to take any nutrients when the gut (enteral route) does not work. PN therapy involves administering appropriate amounts of carbohydrate, amino acid, and lipid solutions, as well as electrolytes, vitamins, minerals, and trace elements, to meet the caloric, protein, and nutrient requirements while maintaining water and electrolyte balance.[46] PN can be provided peripherally or centrally, the latter being more frequently used. These central PN preparations are usually administered through a subclavian catheter. Preferably, an individual will eat by mouth or a feeding tube that is placed either in the stomach or ideally the upper duodenum. These aforementioned tube feedings deliver nutrients. Patients may also have gastrointestinal surgery to have a feeding gastrostomy or jejunostomy catheter put in place during the surgical procedure. Because PN administration bypasses normal absorption and circulation routes, careful laboratory monitoring of these patients is critical. The goal is to provide optimal nutritional status by whatever routes nutrients are administered. An unintended weight loss of more than 10% to 12% leads to suspicion of either disease or malnutrition. The patient's height, age, and activity level are also considered.[47]

It is important to monitor the PN patient to avoid possible complications. Such laboratory monitoring provides necessary information needed to properly administer PN therapy.

Electrolytes

Sodium regulation is a problem in children during PN. Daily sodium requirements may vary depending on renal maturity and the ability of the child's body to regulate sodium. Factors that increase the amount of sodium necessary to maintain normal serum sodium concentrations in both children and adults are glycosuria, diuretic use, diarrhea or other excessive gastrointestinal losses, and increased postoperative fluid losses.

Hyperkalemia is a common problem in children when blood is obtained by heel stick. The squeezing of the heel may cause red cell hemolysis, resulting in falsely high serum potassium levels. Although adequate nutrition may be supplied to promote anabolism, hypokalemia may develop as the extracellular supply is used for cell synthesis.

The primary function of chloride is osmotic regulation. Hyperchloremia metabolic acidosis is a problem when crystal amino acid solutions are used, but such acidosis can be prevented or treated by altering the amount of chloride salt in the PN solution. Supplying some of the sodium and potassium requirements as acetate or phosphate salts can reduce the required amount of chloride. The reformulation of synthetic amino acid solutions by commercial manufacturers has helped to avoid this serious complication. If hyperchloremia metabolic acidosis does occur, treatment with sodium and potassium acetate solutions is used because acetate is metabolized rapidly to bicarbonate. Acetate salts are compatible with all other common PN components and are ideal to use when acidosis is present. Sodium bicarbonate cannot be used in PN solutions containing calcium because calcium carbonate readily precipitates. The use of acetate not only increases serum bicarbonate but also decreases the amount of chloride delivered to the patient.

Urine Testing

In small premature infants, glycosuria during the early phase of PN is a signal that glucose infusion is too rapid. If glucose appears in the urine of small infants after glucose tolerance has been established, however, the clinician should question the presence of respiratory disease, sepsis, or cardiovascular changes.

Organ Function

In order to successfully feed an individual, whether by mouth or parenterally, the major organ systems need to function properly, including the liver that metabolizes nutrients and/or the kidneys that excrete nutrient waste products. For this reason, health/nutrition professionals measure various markers such as circulating enzymes and proteins to determine adequate organ function.

BIOCHEMICAL MARKERS: MICRONUTRIENTS

Vitamins

Vitamins have a wide range of functions in biologic tissue, serving as cofactors in many enzymatic reactions, so that these enzymes have low catalytic activity in cellular reactions if vitamins are not present. These compounds and their biologically inactive precursors must be partially obtained from food sources and, in some instances, from bacterial synthesis. When cellular vitamin and activity levels from diet or intestinal absorption are inadequate, it is termed vitamin deficiency. The term *vitamin* has a historical basis in deficiency states that were relieved by specific food intake. The most notable examples are scurvy (vitamin C, sailors and lime consumption, limeys), rickets (vitamin D in the early industrial age), beriberi (alcoholics and thiamine), pellagra (niacin) and night blindness (vitamin A), megaloblastic anemia (folic acid or vitamin B_{12}), spina bifida (folic acid), and pernicious anemia with neuropathy (vitamin B_{12}). Abnormal increases of metabolism requiring high supplies of one of these cofactors may be termed *vitamin insufficiency* or *vitamin dependency*, depending on the level of supply demanded for physiologic function.[48,49]

Variabilities in clinical expression of vitamin abnormalities result from differences in any of the following: in specific cause, degree, and duration of vitamin inadequacy; the simultaneous presence of nutritional insufficiencies; and/or the increased metabolic demands imposed by conditions such as pregnancy, infection, and cancer. The clinical symptoms of vitamin deficiencies are usually nonspecific in early stages and in mild, chronic deficiency states. A combination of clinical findings, dietary history, focused nutrition physical examination, and laboratory measurements is often required to diagnose a vitamin deficiency. Vitamin metabolism is complex, and vitamin supplementation of foods is common. It is not unusual to find vitamin toxicities from inappropriate use of vitamin supplementation.

For simplicity, vitamins of diverse chemical structure are classified as either water soluble or fat soluble. Fat-soluble vitamins include A, D, E, and K. Those vitamins soluble in water include the B complex of vitamins—thiamine, riboflavin, niacin, vitamins B_6 and B_{12}, biotin, folate, and vitamin C. Water-soluble vitamins are readily excreted in the urine and are less likely than fat-soluble vitamins to accumulate to toxic levels in the body. Vitamins, classified as fat or water soluble, and the symptoms usually seen in deficiency states are shown in Table 33.2.[50,51]

Investigating the dietary deficiency of vitamins (**hypovitaminosis**) is sustained primarily from knowledge of dietary sources and dietary practices that produce inadequate intake or absorption. In the early 1990s, the Food and Nutrition Board of the Institute of Medicine began the process of reviewing the previous nutritional recommendations known as RDAs to also include the prevention of chronic diseases. In addition, besides the RDA, there are additional categories such as estimated average requirement, AI, and tolerable upper intake level (UL).[51–53]

Chemical determination of human vitamin states has been approached in the following ways:

- Measurement of active cofactors or precursors in biologic fluids or blood cells
- Measurement of urinary metabolites of the vitamin
- Measurement of a biochemical function requiring the vitamin (e.g., enzymatic activity), with and without in vitro addition of the cofactor form

- Measurement of urinary excretion of vitamin or metabolites after a test load of the vitamin
- Measurement of urinary metabolites of a substance, the metabolism of which requires the vitamin after administration of a test load of the substance

Reduced serum concentrations of a vitamin do not always indicate a deficiency that interrupts cellular function. Conversely, values within the reference interval do not always reflect adequate function. Interpretation of laboratory values must be done with knowledge of the biochemistry and physiology of vitamins.[54–56]

Fat-Soluble Vitamins

Vitamin A

Retinol and retinoic acid are derived directly from dietary sources, primarily as retinyl esters, or from metabolism of dietary carotenoids (provitamin A), primarily beta carotene. Major dietary sources of these compounds include animal products and pigmented fruits and vegetables (carotenoids). Vitamin A is stored in the liver and transported in the circulation complexed to RBP and transthyretin. Vitamin A and related retinoic acids are a group of compounds essential for vision, cellular differentiation, growth, reproduction, and immune system function. A clearly defined physiologic role for retinol is in vision. Retinol is oxidized in the rods of the eye to retinal, which, when complexed with opsin, forms rhodopsin, allowing dim light vision. This vitamin and vitamin D act through specific nuclear receptors in the regulation of cell proliferation. Vitamin A deficiency leads to night blindness (nyctalopia) and, when prolonged, may cause total blindness. In vitamin A deficiency states, epithelial cells (cells in the outer skin layers and cells in the

TABLE 33.2 Vitamin and Deficiency States

Vitamin Name	Clinical Deficiency
Fat-Soluble Vitamins	
Vitamin A_1	Night blindness, growth retardation, abnormal taste response, dermatitis, recurrent infections
Vitamin E	Mild hemolytic anemia (newborn), red blood cell fragility, ataxia
Vitamin D	Rickets (young), osteomalacia (adult)
Vitamin K	Hemorrhage (ranging from easy bruising to massive bruising), especially posttraumatic bleeding
Water-Soluble Vitamins	
Vitamin B_1	Infants: dyspnea, cyanosis, diarrhea, vomiting Adults: beriberi (fatigue, peripheral neuritis), Wernicke–Korsakoff syndrome (apathy, ataxia, visual problems)
Vitamin B_2	Angular stomatitis (mouth lesions), dermatitis, photophobia, neurologic changes
Vitamin B_6	Infants: irritability, seizures, anemia, vomiting, weakness Adults: facial seborrhea
Niacin/niacinamide	Pellagra (dermatitis, mucous membrane inflammation, weight loss, disorientation)
Folic acid	Megaloblastic anemia
Vitamin B_{12}	Megaloblastic anemia, neurologic abnormalities
Vitamin C	First, vague aches and pains; if long term, scurvy (hemorrhages into skin, alimentary and urinary tract, anemia, wound healing delayed)

lining of the gastrointestinal, respiratory, and urogenital tracts) become dry and keratinized. Fruits and vegetables contain carotene, which is a precursor of retinol. Carotenes provide more than one-half of the retinol requirements in the American diet. Vitamin A deficiency is most common among children living in nonindustrialized countries and is usually a result of insufficient dietary intake. Deficiency may also occur because of chronic fat malabsorption or impaired liver function or may be associated with severe stress and protein malnutrition. Premature infants are born with lower serum retinol and RBP levels, as well as lower hepatic stores of retinol; therefore, these newborns are treated with vitamin A as a preventive measure.[56,57]

When ingested in high doses, either chronically or acutely, vitamin A causes many toxic manifestations and may ultimately lead to liver damage due to **hypervitaminosis**. High doses of vitamin A may be obtained from excessive ingestion of vitamin supplements or large amounts of liver or fish oils, which are rich in vitamin A. Carotenoids, however, are not known to be toxic because of a reduced efficiency of carotene absorption at high doses and limited conversion to vitamin A. The RDA of vitamin A is 900 μg retinol activity equivalent (RAE) per day for adult males and 700 μg RAE per day for adult females.[51] Measurement of retinol is the most common means of assessing vitamin A status in the clinical setting. Retinol is most commonly measured by high-performance liquid chromatography (HPLC). Toxicity is usually assessed by measuring retinyl ester levels in serum rather than retinol, which is accomplished by HPLC.[57]

Vitamin E
Vitamin E is a powerful antioxidant and the primary defense against potentially harmful oxidations that cause disease and aging, protecting unsaturated lipids from peroxidation (cleavage of fatty acids at unsaturated sites by oxygen addition across the double bond and formation of free radicals). The role of vitamin E in protecting the erythrocyte membrane from oxidant stress is presently its major documented role in human physiology. It has been shown to strengthen cell membranes and augment such functions as drug metabolism, heme biosynthesis, and neuromuscular function. The generic name for vitamin E is tocopherol, which includes several biologically active isomers.[58] Alpha-tocopherol is the predominant isomer in plasma and the most potent isomer by current biologic assays. About 40% of ingested tocopherol is absorbed, affected mainly by the amount and degree of unsaturated dietary fat, largely determining the physiologic requirement. Absorbed vitamin E is associated with circulating chylomicrons, very-low-density lipoprotein, and chylomicron remnants. Dietary sources of tocopherols include vegetable oil, fresh leafy vegetables, egg yolk, legumes, peanuts, and margarine. Diets suspect for vitamin E deficiency are those low in vegetable oils, fresh green vegetables, or unsaturated fats.

The major symptom of vitamin E deficiency is hemolytic anemia. Although the use is still controversial, premature newborns are commonly supplemented with vitamin E to stabilize red blood cells and prevent hemolytic anemia. There is evidence for preventive roles of vitamin E in retrolental fibroplasia, intraventricular hemorrhage, and mortality of small, premature infants. Premature infants receiving vitamin E in amounts that sustain serum levels above 30 mg/L have an increased incidence of sepsis and necrotizing enterocolitis.[58]

Patients with conditions that result in fat malabsorption, especially cystic fibrosis and abetalipoproteinemia, are also susceptible to vitamin E deficiency.[59] A relationship exists between vitamin E deficiency and progressive loss of neurologic function in infants and children with chronic cholestasis.[59] Absorption of dietary vitamin E is most efficient in the jejunum, where it combines with lipoproteins and is transported through the lymphatics. Vitamin E is stored in the liver and other tissues with high lipid content and excreted principally in the feces. Assessment of vitamin E status is, therefore, primarily indicated in newborns, patients with fat malabsorption states, and patients receiving synthetic diets. Synergistic with two other **essential nutrients**, selenium and ascorbic acid, vitamin E is also necessary for the maintenance of normal vitamin A levels.[59] This vitamin deficiency commonly occurs in two groups: premature, very-low-birth-weight infants and patients who do not absorb fat normally. Although megadoses of vitamin E do not produce toxic effects, high doses have no proven health benefit; the RDA is 15 mg/d for adult males and/or females.[51] The most widely distributed and most biologically active form of vitamin E is alpha-tocopherol, which is the form commonly measured in the laboratory using HPLC methods.[58]

Vitamin D
Vitamin D refers to a group of related metabolites used for proper skeleton formation and mineral homeostasis. Exposure of the skin to sunlight (ultraviolet light) catalyzes the formation of cholecalciferol from 7-dehydrocholesterol. The other major form of vitamin D is ergocalciferol (vitamin D_2). Vitamin D occurs in foods as cholecalciferol or ergocalciferol. The most active metabolite of vitamin D is $1,25(OH)_2D_3$. It stimulates intestinal absorption of calcium and phosphate for bone growth and metabolism and, together with parathyroid hormone, stimulates bone to increase the mobilization of calcium and phosphate. $1,25(OH)_2D_3$ has an important proapoptotic effect, acting through a vitamin D hormonal system, that depends on binding of the active ligand to a vitamin D receptor. This led to important drug discovery developments in which calcium and phosphate release is minimized, and proliferative and anti-inflammatory effects of D-analogues are modulated.[59]

In northern climates, it is difficult to receive enough ultraviolet exposure to fully meet minimum requirements (2 h/d). Major dietary sources of vitamin D include irradiated foods and commercially prepared milk. Small amounts are found in butter, egg yolks, liver, sardines, herring, tuna, and salmon. The RDA of vitamin D for adults is 15 to 20 µg/d, depending on age.[57] Absorbed in the small intestine, vitamin D requires bile salts for absorption. It is stored in the liver and excreted in the bile. Severe deficiency in children causes a failure to calcify cartilage at the growth plate in metaphysical bone formation, leading to the development of rickets. In adults, the deficiency leads to undermineralization of bone matrix in remodeling, resulting in osteomalacia. Low levels of vitamin D are reported with the use of anticonvulsant drugs and in small bowel disease, chronic renal failure, hepatobiliary disease, pancreatic insufficiency, and hypoparathyroidism. Vitamin D can be toxic, especially in children. Elevated levels of vitamin D are present in hyperparathyroidism and hypophosphatemia and during pregnancy. Excess vitamin D produces hypercalcemia and hypercalciuria, which can lead to calcium deposits in soft tissue and irreversible renal and cardiac damage.[59]

It is important to measure the metabolic form of vitamin D $[1,25(OH)_2D_3]$, parathyroid hormone, and calcium levels when diagnosing primary hyperparathyroidism and different types of rickets, when monitoring patients with chronic renal failure, and when assessing patients on $1,25(OH)_2D_3$ therapy. The most commonly measured form of vitamin D in the clinical laboratory is $25(OH)D_3$. $25(OH)D_3$ is the major circulating form of vitamin D; its measurement is a good indicator of vitamin D nutritional status, as well as vitamin D intoxication. The reference range is 22 to 42 ng/mL for $25(OH)D_3$. Quantitation of vitamin D has gone thru some major changes over the last decade. Immunoassays, especially on automated systems, have been preferred over the more laborious methods of liquid chromatography (LC) and RIA. Development of LC-MS/MS tandem methods for 25-OH vitamin D has been recognized as very accurate but expensive. Comparison of two LC-MS/MS tandem methods to four immunoassay methods and RIA has shown that immunoassay methods that use extraction prior to the assay compared favorably to LC-MS/MS and RIA.[12,60,61] The release from the National Standards Bureau of a 25-OH vitamin D reference material has been predicted to improve correlations between all methods for vitamin D in the future.[61]

Vitamin K

Vitamin K (from the German word "Koagulation") is the group of substances essential for the formation of prothrombin and at least five other coagulation proteins, including factors VII, IX, and X and proteins C and S. The quinone-containing compounds are a generic description for menadione and derivatives exhibiting this activity. Vitamin K helps convert precursor forms of these coagulation proteins to functional forms; this transformation occurs in the liver. Dietary vitamin K is absorbed primarily in the terminal ileum and, possibly, the colon. Vitamin K is synthesized by intestinal bacteria; this synthesis provides 50% of the vitamin K requirement. Major dietary sources are cabbage, cauliflower, spinach and other leafy vegetables, pork, liver, soybeans, and vegetable oils. Uncomplicated dietary vitamin K deficiency is considered rare in healthy children and adults.

CASE STUDY 33.1

A 4-year-old boy is brought to an Alaskan children's clinic by the Social Services System of Alaska. The child was living in a foster home. Infrequently outdoors, his diet consisted of few green vegetables, dairy products, or meats. He began walking at 14 months; his legs showed some bowing. There is tetany or convulsions. He is small for his age: 27 lb, 90.6 cm tall, third percentile. His laboratory test results are shown in Case Study Table 33.1.1.

CASE STUDY TABLE 33.1.1 Laboratory Results

Test	Result	Reference Range
Hgb	14.1 g/dL	12.0–18.0 g/dL
Hct	46%	34.0%–52.0%
WBC	$8.4 \times 10^3/\mu L$ normal differential	4.0–11.0 µL
Urinalysis		
Specific gravity	1.010	1.003–1.030
pH	6.8	5.0–9.0
Glucose	Negative	Negative
Protein	Negative	Negative
Microscopic	Negative	Negative
Amino acid screen	Negative	Negative
Serum		
Na	140 mmol/L	132–143 mmol/L
K	4.0 mmol/L	3.2–5.7 mmol/L
Cl	101 mmol/L	98–116 mmol/L
CO_2	24 mmol/L	23–29 mmol/L
Ca	7.0 mg/dL	8.9–10.3 mg/dL
Phosphate	1.1 mg/dL	3.4–5.9 mg/dL
Alkaline phosphatase	23 units	15–20 units
Total protein	6.6 g/dL	5.6–7.7 g/dL
Albumin	3.4 g/dL	3.1–4.8 g/dL

Questions

1. What are the most likely diagnosis and reason for this disorder?

2. What can be done to prevent this disorder/condition?

Vitamin K deficiency may be caused by antibiotic therapy, which results from decreased synthesis of the vitamin by intestinal bacteria. When vitamin K antagonists, such as warfarin sodium (Coumadin), are used for anticoagulant therapy, anticoagulant factors II, VII, IX, and X are synthesized but nonfunctional. An apparent vitamin K deficiency may lead to a hemorrhagic episode or may result when anticoagulants, such as warfarin sodium, are used.[62–64]

Prothrombin time (velocity of clotting after addition of thromboplastin and calcium to citrated plasma) determination is an excellent index of prothrombin adequacy. Prothrombin time is prolonged in vitamin K deficiency and in liver diseases characterized by decreased synthesis of prothrombin. Vitamin K deficiency also results in prolongation of the partial thromboplastin time, but the thrombin time is within the reference interval.

Toxicity from vitamin K is not commonly seen in adults. Large doses in infants may result in hyperbilirubinemia. The adult AI for vitamin K is 120 µg/d for males and 90 µg/d for females.[51] In most laboratories, vitamin K is not assayed; however, prothrombin time is used as a functional indicator of vitamin K status.[64] The normal prothrombin time is 11 to 15 seconds, which varies with the method. With a vitamin K deficiency, the prothrombin time is prolonged. Several herbal supplements (e.g., garlic, gingko, and ginseng) may enhance the effects of Coumadin or interact with platelets, increasing the risk of bleeding.

Water-Soluble Vitamins
Thiamine
Thiamine (vitamin B_1) or thiamin acts as a coenzyme in decarboxylation reactions in major carbohydrate pathways and in branched-chain amino acid metabolism. It is rapidly absorbed from food in the small intestine and excreted in the urine. The clinical condition associated with chronic thiamine deficiency is beriberi. Although usually occurring in underdeveloped countries of the world, beriberi may be found in the United States among persons with chronic alcoholism. Decreased intake, impaired absorption, and increased requirements all appear to play a role in the development of thiamine deficiency in persons with alcoholism. The RDA of thiamine is 1.2 mg/d for adult males and 1.1 mg/d for adult females.[51] Thiamine functional activity is best measured by erythrocyte transketolase activity, before and after the addition of thiamine pyrophosphate (TPP). Thiamine deficiency is present if the increase in activity after the addition of TPP is greater than 25%.[65]

Riboflavin
Riboflavin (vitamin B_2) functions primarily as a component of two coenzymes, flavin mononucleotide and flavin adenine dinucleotide. These two coenzymes catalyze various oxidation–reduction reactions. Dietary riboflavin is absorbed in the small intestine. The body stores of a well-nourished person are adequate to prevent riboflavin deficiency for 5 months. Excess riboflavin is excreted in the urine and has no known toxicity. Foods high in riboflavin include milk, liver, eggs, meat, and leafy vegetables. Riboflavin deficiency occurs with other nutritional deficiencies, alcoholism, and chronic diarrhea and malabsorption. Certain drugs antagonize the action or metabolism of riboflavin, including phenothiazine, oral contraceptives, and tricyclic antidepressants.[66] The RDA of riboflavin is 1.3 mg/d for adult males and 1.1 mg/d for adult females.[51] Reduced glutathione reductase activity greater than 40% is an indication of deficiency.

Pyridoxine
Pyridoxine (vitamin B_6) is ubiquitous. Vitamin B_6 is three related compounds: pyridoxine, occurring mainly in plants, and pyridoxal and pyridoxamine, which are present in animal products. The major dietary sources of vitamin B_6 are meat, poultry, fish, potatoes, and vegetables; dairy products and grains contribute lesser amounts. Readily absorbed from the intestinal tract, vitamin B_6 is excreted in the urine in the form of metabolites.[66] Vitamin B_6 deficiency rarely occurs alone; it is more commonly seen in patients deficient in several B vitamins. Those particularly at risk for deficiency are patients with uremia, liver disease, absorption syndromes, malignancies, or chronic alcoholism. High intake of proteins increases the requirements for vitamin B_6. Deficiency is associated with hyperhomocysteinemia. Vitamin B_6 has low toxicity because of its water-soluble nature; however, extremely high doses may cause peripheral neuropathy. The RDA of vitamin B_6 is 1.3 to 1.7 mg/d for adult males and 1.3 to 1.5 mg/d for adult females, depending on age.[51]

Niacin
The requirement for niacin in humans is met, to some extent, by the conversion of dietary tryptophan to niacin. Niacin is the generic term for both nicotinic acid and nicotinamide. Niacin functions as a component of the two coenzymes nicotinamide adenine dinucleotide and nicotinamide adenine dinucleotide phosphate, which are necessary for many metabolic processes, including tissue respiration, lipid metabolism, fatty acid metabolism, and glycolysis. Reduction of the coenzyme yields dihydronicotinamide (NADH or NADPH), which has a strong absorption at 340 nm, a feature widely used in assays of pyridine nucleotide-dependent enzymes.

Niacin is absorbed in the small intestine, and excess is excreted in the form of metabolites in the urine.[67] Pellagra, the clinical syndrome resulting from niacin deficiency, is associated with diarrhea, dementia, dermatitis, and death. Niacin deficiency may result from alcoholism. To decrease lipid levels, pharmacologic doses of nicotinic acid are given therapeutically. The toxicity of niacin is low. When large doses are ingested, however, as often occurs during lipid-lowering therapies, flushing of the skin and vasodilation may occur. The RDA of niacin is 16 mg/d for adult males and 14 mg/d for adult females.[51] Blood or urinary niacin levels are of value in assessing niacin nutritional status.

Folate

Folate is the generic term for components nutritionally and chemically similar to folic acid. Folate functions metabolically as coenzymes involved in various one-carbon transfer reactions. Folate and vitamin B_{12} are closely related metabolically. The hematologic changes that result from deficiency of either vitamin are indistinguishable. Folate in the diet is absorbed in the jejunum, and the excess is excreted in the urine and feces. Large quantities of folate are also synthesized by bacteria in the colon. Structural relatives of pteroylglutamic acid (folic acid) are metabolically active compounds usually referred to as folates. Food folates are primarily found in green and leafy vegetables, fruits, organ meats, and yeast. Boiling food and using large quantities of water result in folate destruction. The average American diet may be inadequate in folate for adolescents and for pregnant or lactating women.[68]

The major clinical symptom of folate deficiency is megaloblastic anemia. Laboratory indices of deficiency are, in order of occurrence, low serum folate, hypersegmentation of neutrophils, high urinary formiminoglutamic acid (a histidine metabolite accumulating in the absence of folate), low erythrocyte folate, macroovalocytosis, megaloblastic marrow, and anemia. Serum folate levels, although an early index of deficiency, can frequently be low despite normal tissue stores. Because most folate storage occurs after the vitamin B_{12}–dependent step, erythrocyte folate can also be reduced in deficiency of either vitamin B_{12} or folate. Despite this overlap, erythrocyte folate concentration is accepted as the best laboratory index of folate deficiency.[69] Most physicians order both serum and erythrocyte folate levels because serum levels indicate circulating folate, and erythrocyte levels better approximate stores. Homocysteine elevation in serum and urine occurs in folate deficiency.[70] Total homocysteine is generally measured, which is the sum of all homocysteine species, both free and protein-bound forms.[71]

Folate requirement is increased during pregnancy and especially during lactation. The increase during lactation results, in part, from the presence of high-affinity folate binders in milk. Dietary supplementation of folate in pregnant women reduces the incidence of fetal neural tube defects. Other instances of increased folate requirement include hemolytic anemia, iron deficiency, prematurity, and multiple myeloma. Patients receiving dialysis treatment rapidly lose folate. Clinical conditions[71,72] associated with folate deficiency include megaloblastic anemia, alcoholism, malabsorption syndrome, carcinoma, liver disease, chronic hemodialysis, and hemolytic and sideroblastic anemia. Certain anticonvulsants and other drugs that interfere

TABLE 33.3	Actions of Drugs and Oral Contraceptives on Vitamins

Drug or Nutrient
Pyridoxine—antagonized by isoniazid, steroids, penicillamine
Riboflavin—antagonized by phenothiazines, some antibiotics
Folate—antagonized by phenytoin, alcohol, methotrexate, trimethoprim
Ascorbate—antagonized by (increased excretion) aspirin, barbiturates, hydantoins
Ascorbate excess—interferes with actions of aminosalicylic acid, tricyclic antidepressants, anticoagulants; may cause "rebound scurvy" on withdrawal

Oral Contraceptive Agent Cause
Increased serum vitamin A, retinol-binding protein
Decreased requirement for vitamins K and C
Decreased vitamin B_6 status indices
Decreased riboflavin use
Increased niacin pathway of tryptophan
Decreased induction of thiamin deficiency
Decreased serum folate (cycle-day dependent)
Decreased induction of cervical folate deficiency

with folate metabolism include sulfasalazine, isoniazid, and cycloserine. Folate deficiency of dietary origin commonly occurs in older persons. Phenytoin (Dilantin) therapy accelerates folate excretion and interferes with folate absorption and metabolism. Alcohol interferes with folate's enterohepatic circulation, and methotrexate, a chemotherapeutic agent, inhibits the enzyme dihydrofolate reductase (Table 33.3). Low levels of serum folate can occur with use of oral contraceptives.

There are no known cases of folate toxicity; the RDA is 400 µg/d for adult males and females.[51] In women of childbearing age, 400 µg/d of folate is recommended to prevent or reduce the incidence of neural tube defects.[57]

Reference ranges are as follows:

Serum: 3 to 16 ng/mL (6.8 to 36.3 nmol/L)
Erythrocyte: 130 to 630 ng/mL (294.5 to 1,427.5 nmol/L)
Deficient stores: <140 ng/mL (<317.3 nmol/L)

Folate levels may be measured in serum using a microbiologic assay with *Lactobacillus casei* or a competitive protein-binding assay for levels in serum and erythrocytes. When folate deficiency develops, serum levels fall first, followed by a decrease in erythrocyte folate levels and ultimately hematologic manifestation.[71,72] Measuring both serum and erythrocyte levels is helpful because serum levels indicate circulating folate, and erythrocyte levels better approximate stores.[69]

Serum contains endogenous binding proteins that can bind folate and result in falsely low serum folate concentration measurements. Although measurement of red blood cell folate concentration has advantages over the serum assay for the diagnosis of megaloblastic anemia, analytic problems may result from the various forms of folate in erythrocytes. Folate in the serum is almost exclusively present in the monoglutamate form; however, in red blood cells, it is in the polyglutamate form and as high-molecular-weight complexes.[71,72]

Vitamin B₁₂

Vitamin B_{12} (cobalamin) refers to a large group of cobalt-containing compounds. Intestinal absorption of vitamin B_{12} takes place in the ileum and is mediated by a unique binding protein called intrinsic factor, which is secreted by the stomach. Vitamin B_{12} participates as a coenzyme in enzymatic reactions necessary for hematopoiesis and fatty acid metabolism. Excess vitamin B_{12} is excreted in the urine. Vitamin B_{12} bears a corrin ring (containing pyrroles similar to porphyrin) linked to a central cobalt atom. Different corrinoid compounds, or cobalamins, are distinguished by the substituent linked to the cobalt. The active cofactor forms of vitamin B_{12} are methylcobalamin and deoxyadenosylcobalamin. The primary dietary sources for vitamin B_{12} are from animal products (e.g., meat, eggs, and milk). Therefore, total vegetarian diets are likely to be deficient or low in vitamin B_{12}. Animals derive vitamin B_{12} from intestinal microbial synthesis. The average daily diet contains 3 to 30 µg of vitamin B_{12}, of which 1 to 5 µg is absorbed. The frequency of dietary deficiency increases with age, occurring in more than 0.5% of people older than 60,[72] although the symptoms resulting from dietary deficiency are rare.

Most vitamin B_{12} absorption occurs through a complex with intrinsic factor, a protein secreted by gastric parietal cells. This intrinsic factor–B_{12} complex binds with specific ileal receptors. "Blocking" intrinsic factor antibodies prevents binding of vitamin B_{12} to intrinsic factor, and "binding" antibodies can combine with either free intrinsic factor or the intrinsic factor–B_{12} complex, preventing attachment of the complex to ileal receptors and intestinal uptake of the vitamin. Parietal cell antibodies have also been identified as a cause of pernicious anemia. After release from the intrinsic factor complex within the mucosal cell, vitamin B_{12} circulates in plasma bound to specific transport proteins and is deposited in liver, bone marrow, and other tissues. There is a significant enterohepatic circulation of vitamin B_{12}. Plasma contains both types of transport proteins, transcobalamins, and the three forms of vitamin B_{12} (hydroxocobalamin, methylcobalamin, and deoxyadenosylcobalamin).

In the Schilling test, the patient receives a small, oral dose of radiolabeled vitamin B_{12}. Parenteral B_{12} is given simultaneously to saturate binding sites. Serum and urine are collected at intervals, and labeled B_{12} is measured in the specimens. Patients who cannot absorb vitamin B_{12} (usually a deficiency of intrinsic factor, as in pernicious anemia)[72] cannot absorb the labeled B_{12} and, therefore, have low levels in the blood and urine.

The term *pernicious anemia* is now most commonly applied to vitamin B_{12} deficiency resulting from lack of intrinsic factor. Antibodies to intrinsic factor and parietal cells are common in patients with pernicious anemia, their healthy relatives, and patients with other autoimmune disorders. Deficiency of B_{12} can occasionally occur in strict vegetarians because of dietary deficiency. A loss of vitamin B_{12} also occurs in individuals infected with fish tapeworm or because of malabsorption diseases, such as sprue or celiac disease. Low vitamin B_{12} levels occur with folate deficiency, and a vitamin B_{12} deficiency can be masked by large doses of folate. Toxicity of vitamin B_{12} has not been reported. The RDA of vitamin B_{12} for adults is 2.4 µg/d.[51] Assay methods for B_{12} are either microbiologic assay using *Lactobacillus leichmannii* competitive protein-binding RIA or an enzyme immunoassay.

Deficiency of vitamin B_{12} causes two major disorders—megaloblastic anemia (pernicious anemia) and a neurologic disorder called combined systems disorder.[71] The neurologic manifestations are variable and may be subtle. For this reason, vitamin B_{12} deficiency should be considered a cause of any unexplained macrocytic anemia or neurologic disorder, especially in an elderly person. Serum vitamin B_{12} may be used in the initial assessment.[71] Methylmalonic acid levels may be more definitive because the lower reference limit of B_{12} is unclear. Patients with pernicious anemia usually have atrophic gastritis and have an increased incidence of gastric carcinoma. The reference range for vitamin B_{12} is 110 to 800 pg/mL (81.2 to 590.4 pmol/L).[71,72] The most common methods for determination of vitamin B_{12} are the competitive protein-binding RIAs, which are based on the principle that vitamin B_{12} released from endogenous binding proteins can be measured by its competition with colabeled B_{12} for a limited amount of specific binding protein. The binding proteins typically used are animal intrinsic factors. Special measures must be taken to eliminate interference caused by other nonspecific protein binders of vitamin B_{12}. Several nonradioisotopic assays for vitamin B_{12} have been developed for routine laboratory use.

CASE STUDY 33.2

A 65-year-old woman was admitted to the hospital with mild congestive heart failure. She had been seen in the family practice clinic with complaints of numbness, tingling in the calves and feet, and weight loss. The physical examination revealed a slightly confused, depressed, pale woman. Her blood pressure was 110/70 mm Hg. Faint scleral icterus was present. There was 1+ pitting and ankle edema. The neurologic examination revealed loss of vibratory sensation in both legs, with exaggerated ankle and knee reflexes. Initial laboratory results are shown in Case Study Table 33.2.1.

CASE STUDY 33.2 (continued)

CASE STUDY TABLE 33.2.1 Laboratory Results

Test	Result	Reference Range
Hgb	9.3 g/dL	12–16 g/dL
Hct	28%	38%–47%
MCH	35 pg	27–31 pg
MCV	108 fL	80–96 fL
MCHC	32.4 g/dL	32–36 g/dL
Na	141 mmol/L	136–145 mmol/L
K	4.2 mmol/L	3.5–5.3 mmol/L
Cl	102 mmol/L	96–106 mmol/L
CO_2	26 mmol/L	22–29 mmol/L
Ca	9.7 mg/dL	8.4–10.3 mg/dL
Glucose	100 mg/dL	70–110 mg/dL
BUN	14 mg/dL	10–20 mg/dL
Creatinine	1.0 mg/dL	0.4–1.4 mg/dL
Serum B_{12}	130 pg/mL	180–900 pg/mL
Serum folate	6 ng/mL	5–12 ng/mL
RBC folate	105 ng/mL	200–700 ng/mL

Questions

1. What is the biologically active form of cobalamin in plasma?
2. Where is intrinsic factor made in the body?
3. What is the binding protein for vitamin B_{12}?
4. List food substances that contain vitamin B_{12}.
5. List food substances that contain folate.

Biotin

Biotin is a coenzyme for several enzymes that transport carboxyl units in tissue and plays an integral role in gluconeogenesis, lipogenesis, and fatty acid synthesis.[73] Dietary biotin is absorbed in the small intestine, but it is also synthesized in the gut by bacteria. Numerous foods contain biotin, although no food is especially rich (up to 20 µg/100 g). The dietary intake of biotin, while low in the neonatal period, increases as newborns switch from colostrum to mature breast milk. Biotin deficiency can be produced by ingestion of large amounts of avidin, found in raw egg whites that bind to biotin. Biotin deficiency has been noted in patients receiving long-term PN and in infants with genetic defects of carboxylase and biotinidase enzymes. The AI for biotin is 30 µg/d.[51]

Reference ranges of 200 to 500 pg/mL (0.82 to 2.05 nmol/L) have been established in whole blood and

serum.[73,74] Assays had been performed using microbiology functional assay and the *Lactobacillus* organism. Newer methods of isotopic dilution, chemiluminescent, and photometric assays are now available but rarely used in hospital laboratories. Specimens are usually sent to a reference laboratory for analysis.[74]

Pantothenic Acid

A growth factor occurring in all types of animal and plant tissue was first designated as vitamin B_3 and later named *pantothenic acid* (from Greek for "everywhere"). Dietary sources include liver and other organ meats, milk, eggs, peanuts, legumes, mushrooms, salmon, and whole grains. Approximately 50% of pantothenate in food is available for absorption. Pantothenate is metabolically converted to 4′-phosphopantetheine, which becomes covalently bound to either serum acyl carrier protein or coenzyme A. Coenzyme A is a highly important acyl-group transfer coenzyme involved in many reaction types. The AI for pantothenic acid in adults is 5 mg/d.[51] Whole blood pantothenate of less than 100 µg/dL and urinary excretion of less than 1 mg/d are regarded as indicative of deficiency.[75] Reference range for urine is 1 to 15 mg/d or 5 to 68 µmol/d. Assays using a load test look for excretion of the acetylated *p*-aminobenzoic acid that is formed.[75]

Ascorbic Acid

The most commonly discussed vitamin, ascorbic acid (vitamin C), is a strong reducing compound that has to be acquired via dietary ingestion. Major dietary sources include fruits (especially citrus) and vegetables (e.g., tomatoes, green peppers, cabbage, leafy greens, and potatoes). Ascorbic acid is important in formation and stabilization of collagen by hydroxylation of proline and lysine for cross-linking and conversion of tyrosine to catecholamines (by dopamine β-hydrolase). It increases the absorption of certain minerals, such as iron, and is absorbed in the upper small intestine and distributed throughout the water-soluble compartments of the body.[76] The deficiency state, known as scurvy, is characterized by hemorrhagic disorders, including swollen, bleeding gums and impaired wound healing and anemia.[76,77]

Although urine is the primary route of excretion, measurement of urinary ascorbate is not recommended for status assessment. Drugs known to increase urinary excretion of ascorbate include aspirin, aminopyrine, barbiturates, hydantoin, and paraldehyde. Ascorbic acid requirements are more increased with acute stress injury and chronic inflammatory states, but are also increased with pregnancy and oral contraceptive use. Excessive intake may interfere with vitamin B_{12} metabolism and drug actions (e.g., aminosalicylic acid, tricyclic antidepressants, and anticoagulants).[76,77]

The most widely used assay for ascorbic acid is the 2,4-dinitrophenylhydrazine method. In this procedure, ascorbic acid is first oxidized to dehydroascorbic acid and

2,3-diketogulonic acid with the formation of a colored product that absorbs at 520 nm. This method measures the total vitamin C content of the sample because ascorbic acid, dehydroascorbic acid, and diketogulonic acid are also measured, and it is subject to interference from amino acids and thiosulfates. HPLC has been developed to give increased sensitivity and specificity. The reference range for ascorbic acid is 0.4 to 0.6 mg/dL (23 to 34 μmol/L).[77] The RDA for vitamin C is 90 mg/d for adult males and 75 mg/d for adult females.[51]

Conditionally Essential Nutrients
Carnitine

Carnitine, which includes L-carnitine and its fatty acid esters (acylcarnitine), is described as a conditionally essential nutrient.[78] Meat, poultry, fish, and dairy products are the major dietary sources. Foods of plant origin generally contain little carnitine, except for peanut butter and asparagus.[78] Normal diets provide more than half the human requirement, but strict vegetarian diets provide only 10% of the total carnitine needed by humans.[78] Synthesis occurs in liver, brain, and kidney. L-Carnitine facilitates entry of long-chain fatty acids into mitochondria for oxidation and energy production.[78] The major signs of carnitine deficiency are muscle weakness and fatigue. Total carnitine is measured after hydrolysis of ester forms to free carnitine. Human deficiency can be either hereditary or acquired—by inadequate intake, increased requirement (pregnancy and breastfeeding), or increased urinary loss (valproic acid therapy). Infants and patients following a course of long-term PN and those on hemodialysis are most vulnerable to deficiency.[78]

CASE STUDY 33.3

A 27-year-old man was diagnosed with a carcinoid tumor in the lower portion of the small intestine. The tumor was debulked, with removal of a portion of the lower section of the small intestine. His recovery course was somewhat complicated by weight loss. Seven months after surgery, he underwent a laparotomy, which showed that the carcinoid tumor had not been entirely removed; more of the small bowel was removed because of the obstructing adhesions. He recovered from the second surgery, and tube feeding was discontinued. He came back to the clinic 18 months after the initial surgery slightly pale and stating that he was having trouble maintaining weight. His laboratory evaluation showed slight hypochromic, macrocytic anemia, normal renal function, and normal liver function. A stool specimen was negative for ova, parasites, and enteric pathogens. He was readmitted for intravenous fluid and electrolyte replacement.

CASE STUDY TABLE 33.3.1 Laboratory Results

Test	Result	Reference Range
Albumin	3.4 g/dL	3.5–5 g/dL
Prealbumin	15 mg/dL	18–40 mg/dL
Na	139 mmol/L	136–145 mmol/L
K	3.7 mmol/L	3.5–5 mmol/L
Cl	101 mmol/L	99–109 mmol/L
Bicarbonate	23 mmol/L	22–28 mmol/L
Ca	8.6 mg/dL	8.5–10.5 mg/dL
Mg	1.7 mg/dL	1.5–2.5 mg/dL
Phosphate	3 mg/dL	2.8–4 mg/dL
Prothrombin time	17 s	10–14 s
Ferritin	22 ng/mL	20–250 ng/mL
Vitamin A	207 μg/L	300–800 mg/L
Vitamin D	6 ng/mL	30–53 ng/mL
Vitamin E	2 mg/L	5–18 mg/L
Vitamin C	0.4 mg/dL	0.4–0.6 mg/dL
Vitamin B$_{12}$	100 pg/mL	110–800 pg/mL
Fecal fat	30 g/d	<6 g/d (72 h)

Questions

1. What biochemical evidence exists for fat malabsorption?
2. What nutritional parameters would be affected by fat malabsorption?
3. Identify the fat-soluble vitamins.
4. What condition results from vitamin B$_{12}$ deficiency?

Minerals
Calcium/Phosphorus

One of the most important aspects of PN monitoring is determining deficiencies and excesses of calcium, phosphorus, and magnesium. When regulated inadequately, these minerals not only affect bone mass but can also precipitate life-threatening situations. Calcium and phosphorus are related closely in the important role of bone mineralization. Calcium is present in serum in two forms—protein bound, or nondiffusible, and ionized diffusible calcium. Ionized calcium is the physiologically active form and constitutes only 25% of total serum calcium. Regardless of total serum calcium, a decrease in ionized calcium may result in tetany. Decreased ionized calcium is often caused by an increase in blood pH (alkalosis). It is important to monitor ionized serum calcium and blood pH, especially in a patient on PN who is receiving calcium supplementation along with ingredients in the PN solution that may alter blood pH. Although calcium imbalance is frequent in newborns undergoing PN, it is much less common in adolescents and adults. Hypercalciuria with nephrolithiasis has been reported, however, as a complication in patients on long-term PN.

A reciprocal relationship exists between calcium and phosphorus. Intracellular phosphate is necessary to promote protein synthesis and other cellular functions. Calcium and phosphorus must be monitored carefully to maintain the correct balance between these two minerals. Severe hypophosphatemia has been reported in patients undergoing prolonged PN.[79,80] Magnesium, as a PN solution additive, is closely related to calcium and phosphorus. A reciprocal relationship exists between magnesium and calcium and, in certain situations, between magnesium and phosphorus. Low levels of magnesium can cause tetany, whereas high levels can increase cardiac atrioventricular conduction time. Certain electrolyte and mineral abnormalities associated with PN are shown in Table 33.4.

Given the emergence of osteoporosis and osteopenia as women's health issues, new emphasis has been given to assessment of calcium and vitamin D. Postmenopausal women lack the estrogen levels that previously helped to maintain bone structure. In addition, they may also lack adequate vitamin D and calcium intakes that could maintain bone without estrogen assistance.

Iron

Iron plays a crucial role in respiration and transfer of oxygen to body tissues. The importance of iron in the nutritional sense has to do with its importance to several enzymes, as well as the fact that excess iron has been associated with increasing the amount of free radicals and infection in patients. Enzymes requiring iron cofactor include aconitase, succinate dehydrogenase, and isocitrate dehydrogenase from the tricarboxylic acid cycle. Catalase for the breakdown of both hydrogen peroxide and myeloperoxidase found in neutrophils requires iron as cofactor. The ribonucleotide reductase and xanthine oxidase involved in RNA and DNA metabolism both require iron as cofactor. Besides the enzyme part of the cytochrome P-450 mechanism, iron is also needed by tryptophan hydroxylase (production of serotonin), phenylalanine hydroxylase, homogentisic acid oxidase, and tyrosine hydroxylase (formation of L-DOPA catecholamine precursor).[81,82] There are many other enzymes that require iron, and without sufficient quantities, these enzymes are prevented from performing as they should in energy metabolism, growth and proliferation, biotransformations of drugs, myelinogenesis, cell differentiation, and nutrient absorption. Deficiencies of iron are associated with not only anemia but also akathisia or "restless leg syndrome." Increasing the iron supplies to these patients has led to improvement and a reduction in symptoms.[82,83]

Iron absorption by the gastrointestinal system will be affected by the level of iron present in the body and in ferritin storage form. Low levels of serum or body iron enhance absorption from the intestinal cells as the ferritin levels are low and the apotransferrin levels are high. Other absorption enhancers of iron include vitamin C, copper, cobalt, and manganese when present in the intestine. Inhibitors of absorption besides excess ferritin in mucosal cells include phytic acid, polyphenols of tea and wine, and calcium.[81,83]

Measurements of iron, transferrin, and ferritin have already been discussed elsewhere in this book. The nutritional assessment of iron uses these same methods and reference ranges.

The RDA for iron is 8 mg/d for adult males and adult females over 51 years of age and 18 mg/d for adult females 19 to 50 years of age.[51]

TABLE 33.4	Electrolyte and Mineral Abnormalities Associated with Parenteral Nutrition	
Abnormality	**Manifestations**	**Usual Causes**
Hypernatremia	Edema, hypertension, thirst, intracranial hemorrhage	Inappropriate sodium intake
	Weakness, hypotension, oliguria, tachycardia	Inadequate sodium intake relative to water
Hyperkalemia	Weakness, paresthesia, cardiac arrhythmias	Acidosis, renal failure, excessive potassium intake
	Weakness, alkalosis, cardiac abnormalities	Insufficient potassium intake associated with protein anabolism
Hyperchloremia	Metabolic acidosis	Excessive chloride intake, amino acid solutions with high chloride content
Hypocalcemia	Tetany, seizures, rickets, bone demineralization	Inadequate calcium, phosphorus, and/or vitamin D intake
Hypophosphatemia	Weakness, bone pain, bone demineralization	Insufficient phosphorus intake
Hypomagnesemia	Seizure, neuritis	Inadequate intake of magnesium

CASE STUDY 33.4

A 66-year-old postmenopausal woman complained of severe weakness and dyspnea during the past 6 months on exertion. She noted that her appetite had decreased, with resultant weight loss. Her past medical history revealed ulcers. On admission to the hospital, she had normal blood pressure and pulse. Skin, conjunctiva, and mucous membranes were pale. Lungs were clear at auscultation. A grade 3/6 systolic murmur was present, heard best at the lower left sternal border and radiating to the carotids and axilla. Stool guaiac examination was 2+. Nail beds were pale, with no pedal edema. Laboratory data on admission are shown in Case Study Table 33.4.1.

CASE STUDY TABLE 33.4.1 Laboratory Results

Test	Result	Reference Range
CBC		
Hct	15%	36%–48%
Hb	3.8 g/dL	12–16 g/dL
RBC	2.79×10^6/mL	$3.6–5.0 \times 10^6$/mL
MCV	53.8 fL	82–98 fL
MCHC	25.3 g/dL	31–37 g/dL
WBC	8.2×10^3/mL	$4.0–11.0 \times 10^3$/mL
Neutrophil	80%	40%–80%
Lymph	20%	15%–40%
Reticulocyte count	5.5%	0.5%–1.5%
Reticulocyte index	0.8%	>3%
Chemistry		
BUN	15 mg/dL	7–18 mg/dL
Glucose	150 mg/dL	Fasting 70–100 mg/dL Nonfasting 70–150 mg/dL
Electrolytes	Normal	
Bilirubin	1.0 mg/dL	0.2–1 mg/dL
Direct	0.4 mg/dL	0–0.2 mg/dL
T_3 and T_4	Normal	
Serum Fe	15 µg/dL	30–150 µg/dL
TIBC	439 µg/dL	241–421 µg/dL

Questions

1. This patient's anemia is probably best explained by
   a. Dietary habits
   b. Chronic blood loss
   c. Chronic intravascular hemolysis
   d. Chronic inflammatory disease
2. What are the clinical manifestations of her anemia?
3. The bone marrow iron stores are
   a. reduced
   b. normal
   c. absent
   d. increased but present only in reticuloendothelial cells
4. If the correct treatment for this anemia is with oral ferrous sulfate, the treatment should
   a. be stopped as soon as the hematocrit returns to normal
   b. be continued indefinitely, even if the cause of the deficiency has been corrected
   c. be continued for 3 to 6 months after the hematocrit returns to normal to replace body iron stores
   d. be continued only until there is a brisk response in the reticulocyte index and hematocrit

Trace Elements

Copper

This metal is essential for a number of biochemical reactions as it is an essential element to enzymes critical to these reactions. The enzyme cytochrome oxidase has a copper component and is involved in reactions in the electron transport system where ATP energy is generated. Copper is part of the enzyme dopamine monooxygenase, which is necessary for neuron activity and transmission of impulse. A lack of copper at this crucial juncture can lead to neurologic problems. The enzyme superoxide dismutase is involved in reaction to reduce the free radical superoxide. Copper is an essential part of this enzyme, so its function as a free radical scavenger is related to the superoxide dismutase activity. A deficiency of copper sizable enough to affect the superoxide dismutase activity leaves the patient's cells open to free radical damage and cellular destruction. Ceruloplasmin is the fourth enzyme listed here that requires copper for activity. Eight copper atoms, four covalently bound and four loosely bound, are needed for ceruloplasmin to convert iron from the 3 plus state to the absorbed 2 plus state. Ceruloplasmin is viewed as an acute-phase reactant protein,[84] but it has a biochemical action as an enzyme that converts iron atoms to an ingestible state.

Because copper has such a large impact on many biochemical reactions, it is understandable that the liver contains high levels of copper. The turnover of copper from the liver is closely regulated, with excesses excreted through the bile leaving the liver. Deficiencies of copper are rare due to the liver's close regulation of copper levels. However, preterm babies, Menkes disease, and deficiency due to high dietary intake of zinc, iron, or vitamin C can be potential causes of copper deficiencies. PN can also lead to deficiency of copper. The diets of most patients on PN must be supplemented to maintain optimal levels of several trace elements; these elements must also be monitored to prevent deficiency or toxicity. Copper and zinc are the most common trace elements added to PN solutions. Pallor, decreased pigmentation, vein enlargement, and rashes resembling seborrheic dermatitis are the major clinical signs of copper deficiency, which at times go unnoticed. Some other abnormalities include recurrent leukopenia (white blood cell count, less than 5×10^9/L) and neutropenia (neutrophils, less than 1.5×10^9/L).

The diagnosis of copper deficiency is confirmed when both serum copper and ceruloplasmin (the copper-binding glycoprotein) are low. It is difficult to make this diagnosis in premature infants, however, because their serum copper levels remain depressed until about 9 weeks of age. Low copper levels have also been reported in malabsorption syndrome, protein-wasting intestinal diseases, nephrotic syndrome, severe trauma, and burns. The anemia seen in copper deficiencies is related to the low ceruloplasmin activity and thus lack of iron absorption into the patient.

Menkes disease is an X-linked recessive disease in which copper transport is adversely affected. Lack of copper absorption leads to low liver and serum levels of copper. The symptoms for Menkes disease include kinky hair, mental retardation, seizures, arterial aneurysms, and bone demineralization.[84]

The opposite of copper deficiency is copper toxicity. RDs may be asked to help a patient with Wilson's disease reduce their intake of copper. Although Wilson's disease is a deficiency of ceruloplasmin protein, the copper that should be attached is in the serum and liver leading to a toxic copper state. Patients with Wilson's disease have blockages of copper excretion from the liver to bile or serum. This accumulation of copper in the liver can go into hepatitis, then a fibrosis, and then cirrhosis if not treated with chelation and diet restricted in copper content. Copper toxicity to brain leads to tremors, dysphasia, chorea, and drooling. Patients with Wilson's disease need lifelong monitoring and chelation treatment.

Indirect copper measurements are attained by measuring the ceruloplasmin levels. Ceruloplasmin serum levels are 123 to 230 mg/L.[80] The RDA for copper in adults is 900 µg/d.[51]

Zinc

Zinc is an essential metal for over 200 metalloenzymes in humans. Metalloenzymes using zinc include carbonic anhydrase, alkaline phosphatase, thymidine kinase, alcohol dehydrogenase, and RNA and DNA polymerases. The range of biochemical functions of zinc-containing metalloenzymes includes protein synthesis, gene expression, transport processes, immunologic reactions, and wound healing, to name a few. Carbonic anhydrase needs zinc to foster the reactions it catalyzes between carbon dioxide and water. When zinc is deficient, carbonic anhydrase activity is lower in the blood, stomach, and intestines of affected patients. Patients with sickle cell anemia are especially at risk for adverse effects due to the lack of zinc for the carbonic anhydrase reaction as well as insufficient zinc for their red cells.

The role of zinc in wound healing and immune function is the primary reason that this trace metal needs to be monitored when assessing nutritional adequacy in hospitalized patients. The biosynthesis of connective tissues and ability to fight off infections after surgery can be positively affected if the patient's nutritional status is monitored and zinc levels are kept within the therapeutic range.

Patients on PN may develop acute zinc deficiency.[85,86] They initially suffer from a massive urinary loss of zinc during phases of catabolism. When weight gain begins, the zinc-deficient patient may experience diarrhea, perioral dermatitis, and alopecia. Premature newborns are particularly predisposed to zinc deficiency because zinc normally is acquired at the rate of about 500 mg/d during the final month of gestation. To compensate for this deficiency, zinc supplements for the premature newborn should be 50% higher than those for the full-term newborn. This concentration is then gradually decreased until it is the same as for a full-term infant.

Zinc should be monitored even more frequently in patients with ongoing gastrointestinal losses, even if they are receiving zinc supplements in their parenteral solutions.[87] Normal zinc absorption is only 30% to 40% of dietary intake. This means that while the duodenum and proximal jejunum are sites of active transport of zinc absorption, this absorption area limits zinc intake. Given the competition between zinc and copper absorption, interference of other metals for the metalloprotein needed to transport zinc can further limit the level of zinc intake and absorption. Deficiency of zinc can thus be a problem in normal people, let alone one who has a compromised immune system and surgical trauma.

Zinc transport in serum uses albumin primarily and α_2-macroglobulin. Some zinc may be transported by transferrin and amino acids, but this is not significant in most patients. Excretion of zinc is via the feces, with 25% of the excreted zinc leaving with pancreatic secretions. Urinary loss of zinc is about 5% of dietary intake of zinc. Sweat and semen can also be routes of zinc loss from humans.

Zinc is required for vision, taste, and smell functions. It promotes tissue repair, connective tissue synthesis, bone growth, and insulin synthesis. Zinc is involved in carbohydrate, protein, and phosphorus metabolism. Its role in antibody production and white blood cell well-being fosters the finding that zinc is needed for immune functions.

Malnutrition, infertility, inflammation, and hair loss are often treated with zinc supplementation because it has such a wide array of body functions.

Deficiencies of zinc are usually due to lack of absorption. Whether dietary fiber prevents zinc absorption or a conflicting metal prevents zinc uptake, a deficiency of zinc can be seen in the array of its known functions. Wound healing is reduced or lacking, appetite is lost, skin lesions develop secondary infections, fertility declines, and RNA and DNA synthesis is hampered.

In addition to the direct methods for zinc assessment discussed in Chapter 18, the indirect methods look at the effects of zinc on proteins and metalloenzymes. Specimen collection without contamination has been hard to achieve, making zinc measurements higher than actual values. Red cells contain zinc, so hemolysis elevates zinc plasma values.[88] The RDA for zinc is 11 mg/d for adult males and 8 mg/d for adult females.[51]

Selenium

Selenium (Se) as a trace mineral is reported to have an influence on cancer, cardiovascular diseases (CVDs), diabetes, and arthritis. Trace amounts of selenium in humans necessitate a daily RDA for selenium in adults of 55 µg/d,[51] but most texts indicate a daily intake of over 100 mg. Selenium functions as an essential cofactor to the antioxidant enzyme glutathione peroxidase, which is involved in neutralizing hydrogen peroxide formed during lipid oxidation in cells. Free radicals like hydrogen peroxide need to be removed if cell membranes and DNA are to remain intact.[89,90] Selenium incorporation into proteins and enzymes occurs through the selenocysteine dietary form, but a secondary selenomethionine also comes from dietary sources. Selenomethionine is not advantageous as it may interfere with normal methionine incorporation into proteins. The selenocysteine form is desirable, and its positive effects are seen in the enzyme glutathione peroxidase as well as other selenium-containing enzymes.

CASE STUDY 33.5

A young woman 33 years old complains to her family physician that she is always tired and cannot get her weight to a normal level. Her father has type 2 diabetes, and her grandmother is being treated for cardiovascular disease (CVD) postmyocardial infarction. Her mother and brother are on medication for high blood pressure. Her physician performs a physical examination and determines that her waist circumference is increased at 90 cm. Her blood pressure is 135/90 mm Hg. Blood is drawn, and the results are listed in Case Study Table 33.5.1.

CASE STUDY TABLE 33.5.1 Laboratory Results

Test	Result	Reference Range
Albumin	3.4 g/dL	3.5–5 g/dL
Total protein	7.1 g/dL	6.0–8.0 g/dL
Na	141 mmol/L	136–145 mmol/L
K	3.7 mmol/L	3.5–5 mmol/L
Cl	103 mmol/L	99–109 mmol/L
Bicarbonate	23 mmol/L	22–28 mmol/L
Glucose	120 mg/dL	80–100 mg/dL
BUN	19 mg/dL	7–18 mg/dL
Creatinine	1.1 mg/dL	0.5–1.1 mg/dL
Total cholesterol	196 mg/dL	<200 mg/dL
LDL cholesterol (calc)	127 mg/dL	<100 mg/dL
HDL cholesterol	35 mg/dL	>50 mg/dL (women)
Triglycerides	167 mg/dL	<150 mg/dL
AST	40 U/L	5–30 U/L
ALT	45 U/L	6–37 U/L
ALP	41 U/L	30–90 U/L

Questions

1. Given the information in this case study, the suspected disease is
   a. Type 2 Diabetes
   b. Metabolic syndrome
   c. Cirrhosis
   d. Atherosclerosis leading to CVD

2. Of the indicators seen in this case, which ones indicate to you that your choice in question 1 is correct. Why?

3. What treatment modality is required for this patient? How will the laboratory contribute to that treatment plan?

Functions of selenium in humans include antiatherogenic effect, anticancer effect, antioxidant, improved fertility, and increasing the immune response.[91] Deficiency of selenium, obviously, will lead to decreased capabilities in these areas. Incidence of CVD and cancer seems to rise in populations lacking adequate selenium. Furthermore, cell damage and susceptibility to infections also increase when selenium is deficient. Cancer increases as well as cell damage and the susceptibility to infections when selenium is deficient. Fertility issues affected include low sperm motility and an increase in female miscarriages. Adequate levels of selenium promote white blood cell production, improved thyroid metabolism, and healthy eye lens, skin, and hair. Besides the heart, thyroid, and skin, selenium helps maintain normal liver function and aids in slowing down the aging process.[92]

Selenium deficiency decreases function of selenium-dependent enzymes like glutathione peroxidase. This compromises vitamin E actions in cell membranes and can lead to increased levels of free radicals like hydrogen peroxide. The damage that the free radicals cause to heart, liver, and other organ tissue can leave them susceptible to cancer, viral and bacterial infections, and even cell death and organ failure. The cardiovascular damage due to selenium deficiency has resulted in juvenile cardiomyopathy (Keshan's disease) and chondrodystrophy (Kashin–Beck disease).[92] Other effects of selenium deficiency associated with heart disease and stroke include cataracts, anemia, increased cancer risk, diabetes, arthritis, early aging, infertility, and decreased immune function.

The cardiomyopathy effects of selenium deficiency are seen in home PN (HPN). A case report describes a 46-year-old man who developed an enlarged heart and a myopathy.[93] The findings reported include that selenium-derived deficiency adversely affected the red blood cell selenium levels and the glutathione peroxidase levels. Red cells were then susceptible to the oxidative stress without a way to neutralize those compounds. Recognition of the problem resulted in the patient being started on selenium. In a month, he improved, once selenium was added to his HPN solutions. A second earlier study on selenium deficiency looked at patients with significant dilated cardiomyopathy.[89] The results indicated no significant difference in the patient group with the disease versus the age- and gender-matched control group without disease. While both groups had lower than normal selenium levels, the question as to why some developed disease while others did not remained an unresolved scientific question.

CASE STUDY 33.6

An 18-year-old female of small bone frame comes to her physician complaining about feeling tired and fatigued. She has had a recent severe cold and took various over-the-counter medications including zinc-containing cold lozenges to get some relief. She thinks her cold has made her weak, but after a month and half, she decides she needs a doctor to check her out for other infections. Her blood work is shown in Case Study Table 33.6.1.

CASE STUDY TABLE 33.6.1 Laboratory Results

Test	Result	Reference Range
CBC		
Hct	25%	36%–48%
Hb	7.8 g/dL	12–16 g/dL
RBC	3.1×10^6/mL	3.6–5.0×10^6/mL
MCV	67 fL	82–98 fL
MCHC	25.3 g/dL	31–37 g/dL
WBC	7.2×10^3/mL	4.0–11.0×10^3/mL
Neutrophil	56%	40%–80%
Lymph	20%	15%–40%
Reticulocyte count	2.5%	0.5%–1.5%
Reticulocyte index	1.7%	>3%
Chemistry		
BUN	15 mg/dL	7–18 mg/dL
Glucose	110 mg/dL	Fasting 70–100 mg/dL
		Nonfasting 70–150 mg/dL
Electrolytes	Normal	
Bilirubin	1.6 mg/dL	0.2–1 mg/dL
Direct	0.5 mg/dL	0–0.2 mg/dL
T_3 and T_4	Normal	
Serum zinc	125 µg/dL	60–120 µg/dL
Ceruloplasmin	15 mg/dL	17–54 mg/dL

Questions

1. What type of anemia does this patient exhibit?
2. Why do you think her ceruloplasmin value is decreased?
3. What do you think her physician will recommend for this patient?

Excessive selenium levels can occur with excessive supplementation. Effects of excess include fatigue, irritability, loss of hair and nails, vomiting, nerve damage, skin rashes, and brittle bones.[92,93] Specifically, a recent review found that indiscriminant use of selenium supplementation above RDA had adverse effects in individuals with diabetes.[94]

Celiac Disease Deficiencies

Celiac disease (CD) is a food intolerance to gluten that is being diagnosed more frequently as of late. The disease has a genetic basis in individuals that express HLA-DQ2 and HLA-DQ8 on chromosome 6.[45] The inflammatory gluten amino acid sequence is found in wheat, barley, and rye. Exposure in susceptible celiac patients leads to inflammatory damage to intestinal villi in the duodenum and jejunum and malabsorption. This damage occurs over time but can affect both fat-soluble and water-soluble vitamins. A study of untreated CD patients in the Netherlands[95] found that 87% of these CD patients were deficient in at least one nutrient. Deficiencies included vitamin A, vitamin B6, folic acid, and vitamin B_{12}, as well as zinc and ferritin.[95] While 17% of their study population were malnourished, 22% were underweight and 29% were overweight. The diagnosis of CD and the vitamin/nutrient deficiencies were present even in overweight patients.

Screening for the IgA tTG-antibodies followed by EMA IgA antibodies enables the clinical laboratory to assist in CD diagnosis. The gold standard continues to be an intestinal biopsy that confirms the villi atrophy although these immunoassays are less invasive for patients.

Vitamins and Cancer

Megadoses of vitamins and nutrients have been touted as a possible preventive measure to prevent cancer. The antioxidant nature of vitamin A, E, C, D, and selenium has been studied in an effort to find a natural way to curb cancer. Results have been varied, and the suspicion is that different cancers may be susceptible to different nutrients. The Third National Health and Nutrition Examination Survey or NHANES III data were examined for possible correlations of antioxidant vitamins and minerals on cancer.[96] A group of 16,008 adults from this study had 4,225 deaths over a 14-year follow-up. Blood samples were examined for the antioxidant vitamins and selenium. The findings showed that levels below 1.78 μmol/L of vitamin A were effective, but higher levels of vitamin A were not. B-carotene, a storage form of vitamin A, was also effective at levels below 0.20 μmol/L. Selenium was effective up to 1.71 nmol/L. Vitamin C showed effectiveness across a much wider range of values. It was recommended though that vitamin studies and cancer effectiveness would be better defined by prospective studies rather than retrospective ones.[96]

For additional student resources, please visit **thePoint** at http://thepoint.lww.com

questions

1. Which of the following describes the correct source, function, and deficient state of the vitamin listed?
a. Thiamine (B_1)—whole grains, carbohydrate metabolism, beriberi
b. Vitamin E—plant tissues, antioxidant, osteomalacia
c. Niacin—meat, oxidation–reduction reactions, scurvy
d. Folic acid—dairy products, myelin formation

2. Which vitamin would be affected if a patient was diagnosed with a disorder involving fat absorption?
a. Vitamin K
b. Vitamin B_{12}
c. Ascorbic acid
d. Thiamine

3. Which vitamin is a powerful antioxidant, protects the erythrocyte membrane from oxidative stress, and is found primarily in vegetable oils?
a. Vitamin E
b. Vitamin K
c. Vitamin C
d. Folic acid

4. A 70-year-old man presented to his physician with a broken arm. Laboratory work indicated an elevated prothrombin time, with all other laboratory results being normal. The man was also taking an antibiotic for an earlier respiratory infection. Which, if any, of the following vitamins might be involved?

a. Vitamin K
b. Vitamin D
c. Biotin
d. None of these

5. The most commonly used method for determination of vitamin B_{12} is
a. Competitive protein-binding RIA
b. Chemiluminescence assay
c. Magnetic separation immunoassay
d. HPLC

6. The term describing patients who are chronically calorie malnourished and lose both adipose and muscle tissue, but who do not demonstrate a protein deficiency, is
a. Marasmus
b. Kwashiorkor
c. Debilitated
d. None of these

7. Metabolic syndrome is a complex disorder with many parameters to measure. Which of the following is NOT needed to assess metabolic syndrome?
a. Elevated HDL cholesterol
b. Elevated triglyceride levels
c. Elevated fasting glucose
d. Elevated blood pressure

review questions (continued)

8. Which of the following nutritional markers has been found to be the most sensitive and helpful indicator of nutritional status in very ill patients?
a. Transthyretin
b. Transferrin
c. Albumin
d. Somatomedin C

9. Laboratory monitoring of the patient on TPN therapy is important to avoid possible complications. Which of the following trace elements should be monitored on a weekly basis?
a. Copper
b. Selenium
c. Molybdenum
d. Chromium

references

1. Lacey K, Pritchett E. Nutrition care process and model: ADA adopts road map to quality care and outcomes management. *J Am Diet Assoc.* 2003;103:1061–1072.
2. Sebastian JG, Boosalis MG. Nutritional aspects of home health care. In: Martinson IM, Widmer AG, Portillo CJ, eds. *Home Health Care Nursing.* 2nd ed. Philadelphia, PA: WB Saunders; 2002:140–179.
3. NHLBI. *Obesity Education Initiative Electronic Textbook: Treatment Guidelines.* http://www.nhlbi.nih.gov/guidelines/obesity/e_txtbk/txgd/40.htm. Accessed August 1, 2012.
4. Dillman E, Gala C, Green W, et al. Hypothermia in iron deficiency due to altered triiodo-thyroxine metabolism. *Am J Physiol.* 1980;239:377–381.
5. Boosalis MG, Ott L, Levine AS, et al. The relationship of visceral proteins to nutritional status in chronic and acute stress. *Crit Care Med.* 1989;17:741–747.
6. Boosalis MG, McCall JT, Solem LD, et al. Serum copper and ceruloplasmin and urinary copper levels in thermal injury. *Am J Clin Nutr.* 1986;44:899–906.
7. Boosalis MG, Solem LD, Ahrenholz DH. Serum and urinary selenium levels in thermal injury. *Burns Incl Therm Inj.* 1986;12:236–240.
8. Boosalis MG, McCall JT, Solem LD, et al. Serum and urinary silver levels in thermal injury. *Surgery.* 1987;101:40–43.
9. Boosalis MG, McCall JT, Solem LD, et al. Serum zinc response in thermal injury. *J Am Coll Nutr.* 1988;7:69–76.
10. Boosalis MG, Gray D, Walker S, et al. The acute phase response in autologous bone marrow transplantation. *J Med.* 1992;23:175–193.
11. Boosalis MG, Stiles NJ. Nutritional assessment in elders: biochemical analyses. *Clin Lab Sci.* 1995;8:31–33.
12. Boosalis MG, Snowdon DA, Tully CL, et al. The acute phase response and plasma carotenoid concentrations in older women: findings from the Nun Study. *Nutrition.* 1996;12:475–478.
13. National Heart, Lung, Blood Institute, NHLBI. http://www.nhlbi.nih.gov/health/health-topics/topics/ms/diagnosis.html. Accessed August 1, 2012.
14. USDA. *ChooseMyPlate.* http://www.choosemyplate.gov. Accessed August 1, 2012.
15. USDA Agricultural Research Service. http://www.ars.usda.gov/News/docs.htm?docid=9265. Accessed August 1, 2012.
16. Academy of Nutrition and Dietetics. *International Dietetics & Nutrition Terminology Reference Manual.* 4th ed. Chicago, IL: Academy of Nutrition and Dietetics; 2012:198–200, 269–271.
17. Academy Quality Management Committee and Scope of Practice Subcommittee of Quality Management Committee. Academy of Nutrition and Dietetics: revised 2012 standards of practice in nutrition care and standards of professional performance for dietetic technicians, Registered Dietitians *J Acad Nutr Diet.* 2013;113(6 Suppl 2):S56–S71.
18. Royle GT, Kettlewell MGW. Liver function tests in surgical infection and malnutrition. *Ann Surg.* 1980;192:459.
19. Apelgren KN, Rombeau JL, Twomey PL, et al. Comparison of nutritional indices and outcome in critically ill patients. *Crit Care Med.* 1982;10:305.
20. Ingenbleek Y, Van Den Schrieck H-G, De Nayer P, et al. Albumin, transferrin and thyroxine-binding prealbumin/retinol-binding protein (TBPA-RBP) complex in assessment of malnutrition. *Clin Chim Acta.* 1975;63:61.
21. Georgieff MK, Amarnath UM, Murphy EL, et al. Serum transferrin levels in the longitudinal assessment of protein-energy status in preterm infants. *J Pediatr Gastroenterol Nutr.* 1989;8:234.
22. Ingenbleek Y, De Visscher M, De Nayer P. Measurement of prealbumin as an index of protein-calorie malnutrition. *Lancet.* 1972;2:106.
23. Smith FR, Goodman DS, Zaklama MS, et al. Serum vitamin A, retinol-binding protein, and prealbumin concentrations in protein calorie malnutrition. I Functional defect in hepatic retinol release. *Am J Clin Nutr.* 1973;26:973.
24. Bernstein LH, Leukhardt-Fairfield CJ, Pleban W, et al. Usefulness of data on albumin and prealbumin concentrations in determining effectiveness of nutritional support. *Clin Chem.* 1989;35:271.
25. Large S, Neal G, Glover J, et al. The early changes in retinol-binding protein and prealbumin concentrations in plasma of protein-energy malnourished children after treatment with retinol and an improved diet. *Br J Nutr.* 1980;43:393.
26. Georgieff MK, Sasanow SR, Pereira GR. Serum transthyretin levels and protein intake as predictors of weight gain velocity in premature infants. *J Pediatr Gastroenterol Nutr.* 1987;6:775.
27. Moskowitz SR, Pereira G, Spitzer A, et al. Prealbumin as a biochemical marker of nutritional adequacy in premature infants. *J Pediatr.* 1983;102:749.
28. Church JM, Hill GL. Assessing the efficacy of intravenous nutrition in general surgical patients: dynamic nutritional assessment with plasma proteins. *J Parenter Enteral Nutr.* 1987;11:135.
29. Tuten MB, Wogt S, Dasse F, et al. Utilization of prealbumin as a nutritional parameter. *J Parenter Enteral Nutr.* 1985;9:709.

30. Cavarocchi NC, Au FC, Dalal FR, et al. Rapid turnover proteins as nutritional indicators. *World J Surg.* 1986;10:468.

31. Carlson DE, Cioffi WG Jr, Mason AD Jr, et al. Evaluation of serum visceral protein levels as indicators of nitrogen balance in thermally injured patients. *J Parenter Enteral Nutr.* 1991;15:440.

32. Ingenbleek Y, Van Den Schrieck HG, De Nayer P, et al. The role of retinol-binding protein in protein-calorie malnutrition. *Metabolism.* 1975;24:633.

33. Smith FR, Suskind R, Thanangkul O, et al. Plasma vitamin A, retinol-binding protein and prealbumin concentrations in protein-calorie malnutrition. III. Response to varying dietary treatments. *Am J Clin Nutr.* 1975;28:732.

34. Baxter RC. The somatomedins: insulin-like growth factors. *Adv Clin Chem.* 1986;25:49.

35. Isley WL, Lyman B, Pemberton B. Somatomedin-C as a nutritional marker in traumatized patients. *Crit Care Med.* 1990;18:795.

36. Clemmons DR, Underwood LE, Dickerson RN, et al. Use of plasma somatomedin-C/insulin-like growth factor I measurements to monitor the response to nutritional repletion in malnourished patients. *Am J Clin Nutr.* 1985;41:191.

37. Unterman TG, Vazquez RM, Slas AJ, et al. Nutrition and somatomedin. XIII Usefulness of somatomedin-C in nutritional assessment. *Am J Med.* 1985;78:228.

38. Mosher DF. Physiology of fibronectin. *Annu Rev Med.* 1984;35:561.

39. Saba TM, Blumenstock FA, Shah DM, et al. Reversal of opsonic deficiency in surgical, trauma, and burn patients by infusion of purified human plasma fibronectin. *Am J Med.* 1986;80:229.

40. Russell MK, McAdams MP. Laboratory monitoring of nutritional status. In: Matarese LE, Gottschlich MM, eds. *Contemporary Nutrition Support Practice: A Clinical Guideline.* Philadelphia, PA: WB Saunders; 1998:54.

41. Deodhar SD. C-reactive protein: the best laboratory indicator available for monitoring disease activity. *Cleve Clin J Med.* 1989;56:126.

42. Hokama Y, Nakamura RM. C-reactive protein: current status and future perspectives. *J Clin Lab Anal.* 1987;1:15.

43. Cerra FB. Hypermetabolism, organ failure, and metabolic support. *Surgery.* 1987;101:1.

44. White JV, Guenter P, Jensen GL, et al. Consensus statement: Academy of Nutrition and Dietetics and the American Society for Parenteral and Enteral Nutrition: Characteristics Recommended for the Identification and Documentation of Adult Malnutrition (Undernutrition). *JPEN J Parent Ent Nutr.* 2012;36:275–283;in *Nutr Clin Pract.* 2013;28:639–650.

45. Sapone A, et al. Spectrum of gluten-related disorders: consensus on new nomenclature and classification. *BMC Med.* 2012;10:13.

46. Dudrick SJ. A clinical review of nutritional support of the patient. *J Parenter Enteral Nutr.* 1979;3:444.

47. Howard L, Meguid MM. Nutritional assessment in total parenteral nutrition. *Clin Lab Med.* 1981;1:611.

48. Briggs MH, ed. *Vitamins in Human Biology and Medicine.* Boca Raton, FL: CRC Press; 1981.

49. Food and Nutrition Board. *Recommended Dietary Allowances.* 10th ed. Washington, DC: National Academy of Science; 1989.

50. Otten JJ, Hellwig JP, Meyers LD, eds. *Dietary Reference Intakes: The Essential Guide to Nutrient Requirements.* Washington, DC: Institute of Medicine, National Academies Press; 2006. http://www.nap.edu/catalog.php?record_id=11537. Accessed August 1, 2012.

51. Boosalis MG. Vitamins. In: Matarese LE, Gottschlich MM, eds. *Contemporary Nutrition Support Practice: A Clinical Guideline.* Philadelphia, PA: WB Saunders; 1998:145–162.

52. Boosalis MG. Micronutrients. In: Boosalis MG, ed. *The Science and Practice of Nutrition Support: A Case-Based Core Curriculum.* Dubuque, IA: Kendall/Hunt Publishing; 2001:85–106.

53. Otten JJ, Hellwig JP, Meyer LD, eds. *Dietary Reference Intakes: The Essential Guide to Nutrient Requirements.* Washington, DC: National Academies Press; 2006:5–19.

54. Ensminger AH, Ensminger ME, Konlande JE, et al. *Foods and Nutrition Encyclopedia.* 2nd ed. Boca Raton, FL: CRC Press; 1994:2257–2260.

55. Sauberlich HE. *Laboratory Tests for the Assessment of Nutritional Status.* 2nd ed. Boca Raton, FL: CRC Press; 1999:11–280.

56. Book LS. Fat soluble vitamins and essential fatty acids in total parenteral nutrition. In: Lebenthal E, ed. *Total Parenteral Nutrition: Indications, Utilization, Complications.* New York, NY: Raven Press; 1986:59–81.

57. Underwood BA. Methods for assessment of vitamin A status. *J Nutr.* 1990;120(Suppl 11):1459–1463.

58. Bieri JG, Evarts RP, Thorp S. Factors affecting the exchange of tocopherol between red cells and plasma. *Am J Clin Nutr.* 1977;30:686.

59. Institute of Medicine, Food and Nutrition Board. *Dietary Reference Intakes for Calcium and Vitamin D.* Washington, DC: National Academies Press; 2010. http://books.nap.edu/openbook.php?record_id=13050&page=1106. Accessed February 28, 2012.

60. Holick MF. The use and interpretation of assays for vitamin D and its metabolites. *J Nutr.* 1990;120(Suppl 11):1464–1469.

61. Farrell CJL, Martin S, McWhinney B, et al. State-of-the-art vitamin D assays: a comparison of automated immunoassays with liquid chromatography–tandem mass spectrometry methods. *Clin Chem.* 2012;58:3, 531–542.

62. Suttie JW. Vitamin K. In: Diplock AD, ed. *Fat-Soluble Vitamins: Their Biochemistry and Applications.* London: Heinemann; 1985:225–311.

63. Hazell K, Baloch KH. Vitamin K deficiency in the elderly. *Gerontol Clin.* 1970;12:10–17.

64. Sitren H. Vitamin K. In: Baumgartner TG, ed. *Clinical Guide to Parenteral Micronutrition.* New York, NY: Fujizawa USA, Inc.; 1991:411–430.

65. Sitren HS, Bailey LB, Cerda JJ, et al. Thiamin (vitamin B₁). In: Baumgartner TG, ed. *Clinical Guide to Parenteral Micronutrition.* New York, NY: Fujizawa USA, Inc.; 1991:431–449.

66. Bailey LB. Pyridoxine (vitamin B₆). In: Baumgartner TG, ed. *Clinical Guide to Parenteral Micronutrition.* New York, NY: Fujizawa USA, Inc.; 1991:521–539.

67. Sitren HS, Bailey LB, Cerda JJ, et al. Niacin (vitamin B₃). In: Baumgartner TG, ed. *Clinical Guide to Parenteral Micronutrition.* New York, NY: Fujizawa USA, Inc.; 1991:469–486.

68. Bailey LB. Folic acid. In: Baumgartner TG, ed. *Clinical Guide to Parenteral Micronutrition.* New York, NY: Fujizawa USA, Inc.; 1991:573–590.

69. Bailey LB. Folate status assessment. *J Nutr.* 1990;120(Suppl 11):1508–1511.

70. Ueland PM, Refsum H, Stabler SP, et al. Total homocysteine in plasma or serum: methods and clinical applications. *Clin Chem.* 1993;39:1764–1779.

71. Steinkamp RC. Vitamin B₁₂ and folic acid: clinical and pathophysiological considerations. In: Brewster MA, Naito IIK, eds. *Nutritional Elements and Clinical Biochemistry.* New York, NY: Plenum; 1980:169–240.

72. Bailey LB. Cobalamine (vitamin B$_{12}$). In: Baumgartner TG, ed. *Clinical Guide to Parenteral Micronutrition.* New York, NY: Fujizawa USA, Inc.; 1991:541–572.

73. Roth KS. Biotin in clinical medicine: a review. *Am J Clin Nutr.* 1981;34:1967.

74. Zempleni J, Mock DM. Advanced analysis of biotin metabolites in body fluids allows a more accurate measurement of biotin bioavailability and metabolism in humans. *J Nutr.* 1999;129:494S–497S.

75. McCormick DB, Greene HL. Vitamins. In: Burtis CA, Ashwood ER, eds. *Tietz Textbook of Clinical Chemistry.* 3rd ed. Philadelphia, PA: WB Saunders; 1999:999–1029.

76. England S, Seifter S. The biochemical functions of ascorbic acid. *Annu Rev Nutr.* 1986;6:265–304.

77. Jacob RA. Assessment of human vitamin C status. *J Nutr.* 1990;120(Suppl 11):1480–1485.

78. Tanphaichitr V, Leelahagul P. Carnitine metabolism and human carnitine deficiency. *Nutrition.* 1993;9:246–254.

79. Takala J, Neuvonen P, Klossner J. Hypophosphatemia in hypercatabolic patients. *Acta Anaesthesiol Scand.* 1985;29:65.

80. Tovey SJ, Benton KGF, Lee HA. Hypophosphatemia and phosphorus requirements during intravenous nutrition. *Postgrad Med.* 1977;53:289.

81. Ghosh K. Non-haematological effects of iron deficiency: a perspective. *Indian J Med Sci.* 2006;60:30–37.

82. Willis WT, Gohil K, Brooks GA, et al. Iron deficiency: improved exercise performance within 15 hours of iron treatment in rats. *J Nutr.* 1990;120:909–916.

83. Nuttall KL, Klee GG. Iron. In: Burtis CA, Ashwood ER, eds. *Tietz Fundamentals of Clinical Chemistry.* 5th ed. Philadelphia, PA: WB Saunders; 2001:596–601.

84. O'Dell BL. Copper. In: Ziegler EF, Filer EF Jr, eds. *Present Knowledge in Nutrition.* 7th ed. Washington, DC: ILSI Press; 1996:261–267.

85. Bogden JD, Klevay LM. *Clinical Nutrition of Essential Trace Elements and Minerals.* Totowa, NJ: Humana Press; 2000.

86. Gordon EF, Gordon RC, Passal DB. Zinc metabolism: basic clinical and behavioral aspects. *J Pediatr.* 1981;99:341.

87. Jeejeebhoy KN. Zinc and chromium in parenteral nutrition. *Bull N Y Acad Med.* 1984;60:118.

88. ARUP Lab. *Zinc, Serum.* http://www.aruplab.com/guides/ug/tests/0020097.jsp. Accessed August 1, 2012.

89. Fawzy ME, Yazigi AE, Stefadouros MA, et al. The role of selenium deficiency in dilated cardiomyopathy in Saudi Arabia. *Ann Saudi Med.* 1999;19:20–22.

90. Hussein O, Rosenblat M, Refael G, et al. Dietary selenium increases cellular glutathione peroxidase activity and reduces the enhanced susceptibility to lipid peroxidation of plasma and low density lipoprotein in kidney transplant recipients. *Transplantation.* 1997;63:679–685.

91. Girodon F, Galan P, Monget AL, et al. Impact of trace elements and vitamin supplementation on immunity and infections in institutionalised elderly patients. *Arch Intern Med.* 1999;159:748–754.

92. Fleet JC, Mayer J. Dietary selenium repletion may reduce cancer incidence in people at high risk who live in areas with low soil selenium. *Nutr Rev.* 1997;55:277–279.

93. Wamique YS. Cardiomyopathy in association with selenium deficiency: a case report. *J Parenter Enteral Nutr.* 2002;26:63–66.

94. Boosalis MG. The role of selenium in chronic disease. *Nutr Clin Pract.* 2008;23(2):152–160.

95. Wierdsma NJ, van Bokhorst-de van der Schueren MAE, Berkenpas M, et al. "Vitamin and mineral deficiencies are highly prevalent in newly diagnosed celiac disease patients." *Nutrients.* 2013;5(10):3975–3992.

96. Goyal A, Terry MB, Siegel AB. Serum antioxidant nutrients, vitamin A, and mortality in U.S. Adults. *Cancer Epidemiol Biomarkers Prev.* 2013;22(12):2202–2211.

34

Clinical Chemistry and the Geriatric Patient

LAURA M. HICKES and J. MARVIN MCBRIDE

chapter objectives

Upon completion of this chapter, the clinical laboratorian should be able to do the following:

- Define aging, atherosclerosis, geriatrics, gerontology, homeostasis, menopause, and osteoporosis.
- Discuss the impact of geriatric patients on the clinical laboratory.
- Appraise the physiologic changes that occur with the aging process.
- Identify the age-related changes in clinical chemistry analytes.
- Explain the problems associated with establishing reference intervals for the elderly.
- Describe the effects of medication on clinical chemistry results in the elderly.
- Discuss the effects of exercise and nutrition on chemistry results in the elderly.
- Correlate age-related physiologic changes and laboratory results with pathologic conditions.

For additional student resources, please visit **thePoint** at **http://thepoint.lww.com**

686

The number and proportion of older individuals in the total population is increasing rapidly in the United States and other developed nations. There are a number of physiological and metabolic changes unique to aging that may affect clinical laboratory values. In addition, aging is often accompanied by multiple medical conditions requiring diverse medications, which can also affect clinical laboratory values. This chapter will summarize the issues that should be given special consideration with regard to clinical chemistry in the geriatric patient.

THE AGING OF AMERICA

The age structure of the United States population is currently undergoing a change, and based on this change, there is increased focus and emphasis on the older subset of individuals. The population older than 65 is projected to nearly double by the year 2050 to over 83.7 million.[1] While in 2010, there were over 40 million individuals in the United States aged 65 years and older, which made up 13% of the population, the baby boomers began to turn 65 in 2011, which increased the percentage over the age of 65 to nearly 50 million in 2015. Not only is this the largest number of aged individuals and the largest percentage of the population ever reported in a US Census, this segment of the population is growing much more rapidly than the US population as a whole.

Aging of the "baby boomers," individuals born during the post–World War II surge from 1946 to 1964, coupled with increased life expectancy, has had a significant impact on the population breakdown in the United States. In 2010, the average female was expected to live to 80.8 years, while the average male was expected to live to 75.7 years.[2] Now it is estimated that one out of every three nursing home residents is an "Oldest Old Woman," that is, over the age of 85 years.[1] Further, approximately 10,000 boomers will turn 65 each day for the next two decades, more than doubling the number of Americans 65 years of age or older to 88.5 million by 2050.[2] Figure 34.1, taken from the U.S. Census Bureau 2010: "65+ In the United States," categorizes the age structure of the American population and the projected changes over the next 40 years. These changes are largely due to the aging of the baby boomers along with immigration trends.[3] Complementary data from the 2010 census document illustrate and characterize the increase in the population numbers over the past 110 years.[1] Depending on immigration, fertility, and longevity rates, these seniors are expected to constitute over 20% of the total US population by 2050 (Fig. 34.2).[3,4] The total population over the age of 65 (Fig. 34.3) is expected to reach 19 million in the United States by 2050, almost 4.5% of the total population.[3] With the burden of medical illness and medication use falling disproportionately on the elderly, a dramatic increase in the utilization of health care services, including clinical chemistry, is inevitable.

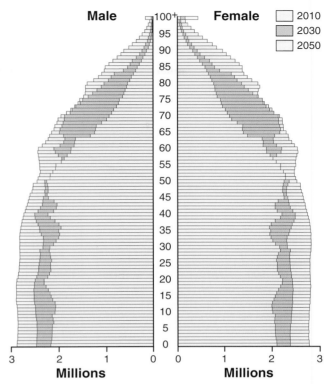

FIGURE 34.1 Data taken from the US Census Bureau 2008 display the age/gender structure of the population in this country and the projected changes that are expected to occur over the next 40 years. There is an anticipated shift in the age structure for the 13% of the population falling into the subclass of 65 or older. The distribution is expected to increase to nearly 20% by the year 2030.[3] (Source: Vincent GK, Velkoff VA. *The Next Four Decades: The Older Population in the United States: 2010 to 2050.* Washington, DC: US Census Bureau; 2008. http://www.census.gov/prod/2010pubs/p25-1138.pdf. Accessed August 26, 2012.)

AGING AND MEDICAL SCIENCE

Gerontology, the study of aging, and **geriatrics**, the subspecialty of clinical medicine that focuses on care of the aged, have much to tell us about normal aging, as well as the unique features of common illnesses in the elderly. The differentiation of "normal" or "healthy" aging versus the accumulation of multiple medical problems with age is an area of active research and debate. There are several analytical measurements that change when comparing a diseased individual to a healthy one, but because there are also a number of biochemical changes that occur as a consequence of normal aging, it can be difficult to differentiate between abnormal physiological changes and normal signs of aging in geriatric patients.

One important principle is that aging is extremely heterogeneous. The extent of differences between individuals of the same age is often quite significant. Indeed, an individual's overall health status and expected longevity are more closely related to their functional status than their chronologic age. Thus, an 86-year-old jet-setting international attorney may look very unlike a 60-year-old

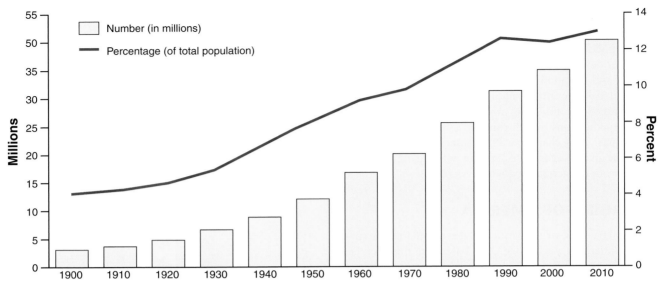

FIGURE 34.2 Population 65 years and older by size and percent of total population: 1900 to 2010. This figure shows the age growth over the past 110 years in the United States. Currently, over 40.3 million people are over age 65. This was an additional increase of 5.3 million over the numbers in the 2000 census. Additionally, the percentage of the population over age 65 has increased from 12.4% in 2000 to 13% in 2010. Further, the percentage of the US population greater than 85 years is expected to continue to increase, and in 2050, this age range is expected to make up over 20% of the US population. (Source: U.S. Census Bureau. Decennial census of population, 1900 to 2000. *2010 Census Summary File 1.*)

nursing home patient bedbound with dementia. Older adults may also mistake a health symptom for a normal part of aging, and may not seek medical attention as early as they should.[5]

An important consideration is the concept of diminished physiological reserve. While an aged person usually has the same adaptive mechanisms to stress as a younger person, those adaptations may not be as rapid

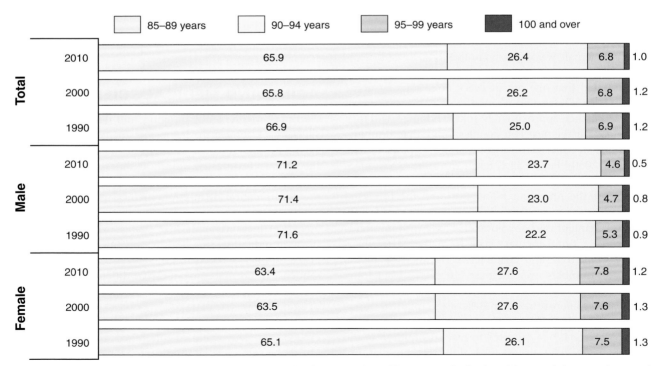

FIGURE 34.3 Projected population of Americans over the age of 65 by age and sex. The percent distribution of the population over the age of 85 is further broken down according to gender.[3] The largest percentage increase during the previous 20 years was in the 90 to 94 year age group, which saw an increase of 1.4% between the years 1990 and 2010. Females contribute a larger percentage to the oldest-old calculation compared with the male data. (Source: U.S. Census Bureau. *1990 Census Summary File 2C, Census 2000 Summary File 1, and 2010 Summary File 1.*)

TABLE 34.1	Changes in Selected Clinical Chemistry Analytes with Age[8-28]	
Increase	**Decrease**	**Unchanged**
ANP		ACTH
Alkaline phosphatase (females)	ADH	Calcium
Calcitonin	Albumin	Chloride
C-reactive protein		Cortisol
EPO	Aldosterone	Creatinine
Ferritin	Vitamin B_{12}	HDL-C
Fibrinogen	LDL-C	Insulin
Folic acid	Cholesterol	Sodium
FSH	DHEA-S	Total T4
Free T4	Estrogen	pH or slight decrease
Gamma globulins	Ferritin	
Homocysteine	Growth hormone	
Insulin	IGF-1	
Lactate	po_2	
Parathyroid hormone	Progesterone	
Potassium	Testosterone	
TBG	T3	
TSH (slight)	Total protein	
Transferrin	Uric acid	
Triglycerides	Vitamin D	
GGT		

ANP, atrial natriuretic peptide; ACTH, adrenocorticotropic hormone; ADH, antidiuretic hormone; EPO, erythropoietin; HDL-C, high-density lipoprotein cholesterol; LDL-C, low-density lipoprotein cholesterol; FSH, follicle-stimulating hormone; DHEA-S, sulfated dehydroepiandrosterone; IGF-1, insulin-like growth factor-1; TBG, thyroid binding globulin; TSH, thyroid-stimulating hormone; GGT, Gamma-glutamyl transferase; T3, triiodothyronine.

or as robust. Therefore, with diminished reserve, an aged individual may encounter adverse health effects much more quickly than a younger person. For example, an elderly person undergoing diuretic therapy for hypertension would not be able to withstand a long period of vomiting and diarrhea compared with a younger person. Age-associated decrease in total body water would favor dehydration and development of hypernatremia and delirium.[6]

While age-dependent changes in concentrations of analytes are shown to be important in a number of areas of chemistry, there are also several examples of chemistry values that are unchanged as a consequence of age.[7] Table 34.1 outlines some of the age-specific changes that occur in regard to certain chemistry analytes, and some of these changes will be specifically addressed in the coming section outlining physiologic changes with age. Ideally, the changes that impact laboratory results would be classified in age-specific reference ranges, but since these are not readily available; changes in analyte level over time can help to manage patient treatment.[7]

GENERAL PHYSIOLOGIC CHANGES WITH AGING

The aging process involves both biochemical and physiological changes and can be subdivided into various organ systems. The systems continue to function appropriately unless they are subjected to excess stress. With increasing

age, an individuals' ability to respond to stress decreases. This leads to an age-associated increase in the prevalence of pathological conditions. Table 34.2 outlines some of the more common factors impacting the interpretation of clinical laboratory results.

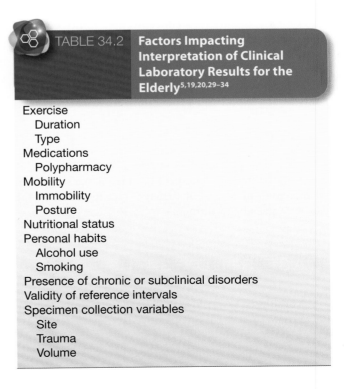

TABLE 34.2	Factors Impacting Interpretation of Clinical Laboratory Results for the Elderly[5,19,20,29-34]

Exercise
  Duration
  Type
Medications
  Polypharmacy
Mobility
  Immobility
  Posture
Nutritional status
Personal habits
  Alcohol use
  Smoking
Presence of chronic or subclinical disorders
Validity of reference intervals
Specimen collection variables
  Site
  Trauma
  Volume

Muscle

Total body muscle mass typically decreases with age, but the rate and extent of loss have a strong genetic component. This age-related decline (sarcopenia) results in a decrease in lean body mass and a decrease in total creatinine production, such that serum creatinine is no longer reliable for assessment of renal function in the aged.[8]

Bone

Total bone density and mass decreases with age in both men and women, though the changes are much more dramatic in women after **menopause**.[9] Serum calcitonin levels typically rise with age, but ionized calcium levels remain stable.[10] Parathyroid hormone (PTH) levels increase in postmenopausal women, and this increase is associated with changes in bone metabolism.[11]

Gastrointestinal System

The incidence of atrophic gastritis increases with age, with a consequent increase in vitamin B_{12} deficiency from poor absorption.[12] The incidence of achlorhydria (low or absent gastric acid production) also increases with age, which can result in decreased calcium and iron absorption, as well as an increased incidence of bacterial overgrowth in the small intestine.[13] Albumin levels decrease, and the incidence of malnutrition, leading to higher mortality rates, also increases.[35]

Kidney/Urinary System

The number of functional glomeruli decreases with age, resulting in a decrease in kidney size and weight. Glomerular filtration rate (GFR) declines, and renal blood flow is even more reduced, such that filtration fraction (GFR/renal plasma flow) actually increases.[15] Additionally, the kidney's concentrating ability declines. The result of all these changes is that acid/base, water, and electrolyte levels remain normal under optimal conditions, but physiologic reserve is diminished. The secretion of erythropoietin (EPO), the glycoprotein hormone that controls red blood cell production, increases with age, and the level of serum renin, an enzyme that regulates blood pressure, decreases. Renal responsiveness to atrial natriuretic peptide (ANP) decreases, and serum levels of ANP and brain natriuretic peptide increase with age.[16,36] Structural, neurological, and immune changes result in an increased incidence of urinary tract infection in the elderly, especially in women.[17]

CASE STUDY 34.1

A healthy 65-year-old man entered the hospital to have his appendix removed. Preoperative laboratory results are shown in Case Study Table 34.1.1.

CASE STUDY TABLE 34.1.1 Laboratory Results

Test	Result	Reference Range
Albumin	25 g/L	35–50 g/L
BUN	35 mg/dL	8–26 mg/dL
Creatinine	1.7 mg/dL	0.9–1.5 mg/dL
Serum osmolality	280 mOsm/kg	275–295 mOsm/kg
Sodium	140 mmol/L	135–145 mmol/L

Question

1. What is the BUN/Creatinine ratio for this patient?
2. What do these data suggest?
3. Which test results support this conclusion?

Immune System

The thymus shrinks with age, causing a decrease in thymosin levels and T-cell function. B-cell function slowly declines, as well, such that cellular and humoral immune responses are less vigorous and slower in the aged than in younger individuals.[18] Autoimmune antibody (antinuclear antibody [ANA]) levels increase,[37] and hematopoietic stem cell numbers decrease.[38] Examples of the consequences of declining cellular immunity in the elderly include reactivation of latent tuberculosis and herpes varicella zoster (HVZ) virus. HVZ is the virus responsible for the chicken pox, but in an adult, reactivation is termed shingles and presents as a painful, blistering skin rash. The prevalence of shingles in the United States is about a million cases per year, and susceptibility to shingles increases at the age of 50 years. This increase has led to the development of a live vaccine for elderly adults.[39]

Endocrine System

Serum adrenocorticotropic hormone and cortisol levels typically do not change with age, though response to stress may be delayed. Pulsatile secretion of growth hormone (GH) typically diminishes with age, resulting in a decrease in lean body mass/fat ratio, as well as loss of overall body mass. The peak but not the basal levels of melatonin secretion decrease with age, which may contribute to sleep cycle disorders as well as diminished protection from free radicals.[40] Norepinephrine secretion generally increases, which contributes to systemic vasoconstriction and decrease in myocardial relaxation; epinephrine levels remain stable. Aldosterone levels may decline, which can contribute to orthostatic hypotension, or a drop in blood pressure upon standing.[41] Thyroid hormone levels are typically well preserved or slightly increased into very old age.[42,43]

Sex Hormones

Although menopause in women typically occurs prior to the earliest ages considered "geriatric," the reduction in gonadal production of estrogen and progesterone and secondary increase in hypothalamic gonadotropin-releasing hormone persist through the remainder of a woman's life.[44] Testosterone levels in men typically exhibit a gradual decrease with increasing age—the term "andropause" has been used to describe this observation in analogy to menopause, but the decline in serum levels of sex hormone is not abrupt and not as significant in degree for men as it is for women. The distinction between a normal serum testosterone level for age and hypogonadism in an aged man is a point of some contention and includes consideration of sexual function, general perception of well-being by the individual, and other clinical factors in addition to the value of the serum testosterone level.[45] Dehydroepiandrosterone (DHEA), sulfated DHEA, and pregnenolone all decrease with age.

Glucose Metabolism

Insulin secretion is unchanged, though there are age-related changes at the cellular level in insulin signalling, receptors, and glucose transporters. An individual with the genetic predisposition to type II diabetes mellitus is more likely to manifest clinical illness with increasing age, body mass index, and lack of exercise. The combination of an aging population, increasing obesity, and an increasing number of individuals from racial/ethnic groups at increased risk of diabetes (African American, Hispanic American, American Indian) has resulted in a dramatic increase in the number of older adults with diabetes.[46] Many of these individuals will also suffer some of the consequences of diabetes, including damage to the eyes, kidneys, nerves, and blood vessels.

EFFECTS OF AGE ON LABORATORY TESTING

Basic biochemical and physiological changes accompany the aging process, and these changes can impact an individual's clinical laboratory test results. It is important that laboratorians understand how these changes can impact specific tests. It has been suggested that the presence of age-specific changes may warrant separate reference intervals for the elderly,[43,47] but these are not readily available. In addition, consideration of preanalytical variables must be factored into the interpretation of laboratory results. How does the aging process affect interpretations of drug levels in the elderly? What are the effects of exercise and nutrition on chemistry results? Table 34.3 describes some of the factors that laboratorians should consider when interpreting test results for the elderly and defines some of the laboratory values that are impacted by these changes.

Muscle

As muscles age, they begin to decrease in number and size. Creatinine levels correlate with both muscle mass and renal function. In the geriatric population, a decrease in muscle mass coupled with the decrease in renal function keeps the creatinine level nearly the same or slightly increased.

Bone

Adequate calcium intake and sufficient vitamin D are important in maintaining bone mass and density. **Osteoporosis** incidence is high in the elderly population, and this leads to increased risk of fracture. In addition, osteoporosis incidence coincides with increased risk of vitamin D deficiency. Vitamin D helps with absorption of dietary calcium from the intestine, thus decreased vitamin D levels can decrease the amount of dietary calcium that is absorbed. Inadequate calcium absorption may eventually lead to low serum calcium levels and increased PTH levels. This increased PTH then causes increased calcium loss from the bone, which increases alkaline phosphatase levels.[19]

Gastrointestinal System

The gastrointestinal system includes the digestive tract and accessory organs including the pancreas and the liver. There are a number of age-related changes with respect to the liver

TABLE 34.3	Effects of Age on Laboratory Testing[9,16,18,36,37,42–45,48–55]	
	Normal Physiological Changes With Age	**Laboratory Values that Correlate**
Muscle	↓ Muscle mass	↓ Creatinine
Bone	↓ Mineral content of bone, ↓ cartilage	↑ PTH (females), ↓ calcium, and calcitonin
GI	↓ Gastric motility, vitamin absorption, and drug absorption	↓ Vitamin B_{12}, calcium, and Fe absorption
Kidney	↓ Renal function	↑ Serum ANP, BNP, epo, and GFR, creatinine ↓ Renin
Immune	↑ Hematopoietic stem cells, bone marrow activity, thymosin, and T-cell function ↓ Autoimmune antibodies	↑ ANAs
Endocrine	↑ Cancer incidence	↓ Aldosterone ↑ Norepinephrine
Reproductive	↓ Sex hormones	↓ Testosterone, estrogen, progesterone, DHEA-S, and pregnenolone ↑ GnRH

PTH, parathyroid hormone; GI, gastrointestinal; ANP, atrial natriuretic peptide; BNP, brain natriuretic peptide; EPO, erythropoietin; GFR, glomerular filtration rate; ANA, antinuclear antibody; DHEA-S, sulfated dehydroepiandrosterone; GnRH, gonadotropin-releasing hormone.

PART four Specialty Areas of Clinical Chemistry

analytes. C-reactive protein, an acute phase reactant, has been shown to be elevated in the elderly.[56] This elevation is thought to be a nonspecific indicator of inflammation and typically is a poor prognostic indicator.[29] Gamma-glutamyl transferase (GGT) levels tend to increase with age in a gender-specific manner. Men do not show this age-related increase, but men tend to have higher levels of GGT than women. Fibrinogen, an acute phase reactant, is frequently elevated in geriatric patients, and this increase coincides with inflammatory disease, stroke, coronary dysfunction, and cancer.[20,30]

CASE STUDY 34.2

A healthy 70-year-old woman is seen by her primary care physician for an annual checkup. She complains of muscle weakness, drowsiness and confusion. Her laboratory results are shown in Case Study Table 34.2.1.

CASE STUDY TABLE 34.2.1 Laboratory Results

Test	Result (mg/dL)	Reference Range
Calcium	12.0	8.5–10.2 mg/dL
Parathyroid hormone	111	12–72 pg/mL

Questions

1. Based on the laboratory data, how might the PTH test be interpreted?

2. Should any additional testing be done?

Ferritin levels can be low in the elderly population, and when this is seen, it is usually due to iron deficiency anemia, similar to younger people. Transferrin levels can be reduced due to iron-deficient anemia or as a result of acute or chronic stress. Albumin levels are frequently decreased in the elderly population as a result of inflammation, malnutrition, and liver disease. Levels can be high in dehydration, but elevations above the upper limits of normal rarely occur in the elderly due to the prevalence of other health conditions that mask alterations.[21] Total protein levels are also frequently decreased in the elderly for the same reasons that albumin levels are low.

Urinary System

Serum creatinine levels are thought to be lower in the elderly due to decreased muscle mass. At the same time, a reduction in glomeruli filtration rate can offset this decrease.

Immune System

As age increases, infection-induced morbidity and mortality rise. This is in part due to a weakened immune system.

The innate immune system, commonly referred to as the "first line of defense," is the nonspecific antigen activation that confers short-term protection from a pathogen. Adaptive immune system, on the other hand, is activated by the innate system and refers to the protection from antigen that an individual develops throughout the life. Both the innate and adaptive immune systems become damaged and dysfunctional as individuals age, leading to increased prevalence of infection, and potentially also autoimmune disease and cancer.[57] Gastroenteritis is more frequently observed as individuals' age, but the increased frequency is thought to be a result of a weakened immune system.[22] Pathogenic bacteria can enter and infect the digestive tract and contribute to presentation. Additionally, there is an increase in ANA production, which correlates with incidence of arthritis and many other autoimmune disorders.[31]

Endocrine System

There are a variety of age-related changes to endocrine hormone regulation. These can be subclassified according to whether the hormone level increases or decreases.

Increased Hormone Level

Elevated levels of cortisol, though rarely present, have been reported to be associated with decreased cognitive function and memory loss.[48] A slight increase in thyroid-stimulating hormone (TSH) has been observed but is not profound.[42,43] Follicle-stimulating hormone (FSH) levels increase with aging, but with this increase, there is a down-regulation of FSH receptors, such that in menopause, there are no longer circulating cells with FSH receptors and thus no responsiveness to the high level of hormone. ANP levels increase with age, and the levels have been shown to be nearly four-fold higher in healthy elderly individuals than in younger people.[49] Anemia is common in the elderly population, and EPO, a marker for anemia, rises in elderly patients.[23] PTH levels are slightly higher in older individuals than gender-matched pairs.[50]

Decreased Hormone Level

In contrast to the finding with cortisol, DHEA levels have been shown to decrease by 40% to 60%.[24] Estrogen and progesterone levels decrease with age, and the reduction in estrogen further up-regulates FSH levels. Insulin-like growth factor (IGF-1) and GH levels decrease with age. Secretion rates and serum concentrations of aldosterone decrease with age as a consequence of a decreased level of renin.[51,58] Pituitary function declines with age, and hypothalamic antidiuretic hormone (ADH) levels are increased.

Sex Hormones

Levels of expression of all sex hormones diminish with age. Testosterone levels decrease with age, as do estrogen and progesterone levels.[45]

Glucose Metabolism

Insulin sensitivity decreases with age. As a result of this decreased sensitivity, there is an increase in the prevalence of type 2 diabetes, with the incidence reaching a peak between the ages of 60 and 74.[59]

ESTABLISHING REFERENCE INTERVALS FOR THE ELDERLY

Most laboratory tests have "gender-specific" reference ranges and/or "age-specific" reference ranges. The broad categories for the age ranges are very wide, and the adult reference range includes individuals between 18 and about 50 years. As people live longer, age-related criteria for the analysis and interpretation of test results become increasingly important. Because of the need to establish reference ranges in a healthy population, and the increased prevalence of at least one health condition in the aged, there are little data on more appropriate age-specific reference ranges for older adults. Based on this lack of data, there has been an increased interest in determining age-related reference ranges in order to more effectively identify individuals with early stage disease.[52,60,61] While the idea has a lot of merit, there are only a few publications establishing age-appropriate reference ranges for the elderly.[62] Laboratories should consult the current literature for latest age-related reference ranges.

Certain analyte fluctuations that are seen as individual's age are clearly the result of aging organs, but other analytes do not lend themselves to such apparent delineation.[63] In addition, coincident medical conditions can further complicate the issue. The requirement that reference values be obtained from healthy, normal individuals unfortunately limits a large number of geriatric patients from contributing to establishing these references. Recently, a strategy for reference interval data mining has been introduced to expand on age-appropriate reference intervals for all age groups.[64] Prior to this approach, the use of exclusion criteria caused the geriatric population to be vastly underrepresented in most randomized clinical trials, which further limited the validity of age-specific reference range generation.[65] In addition, there is a wide intraindividual variability among the various analytes, which has been seen as a major obstacle for determining age-appropriate reference ranges among the elderly. Instead, the current clinical approach that has been increasingly implemented is careful documentation of laboratory values and paying closer attention to changes over time instead of where the values fit in with the remainder of the population. This is not feasible among all elderly, as there is a small subset that resists treatment and thus does not see a medical professional on a regular basis.[66] A lack of baseline measurements coupled with the lack of age-specific reference ranges continues to make diagnosis challenging. Currently, most physicians who care for the geriatric patient population rely on established patient care, frequent routine examinations, and following changes in laboratory values over time as an early indicator of a problem.

PREANALYTICAL VARIABLES UNIQUE TO GERIATRIC PATIENTS

There are a number of factors that contribute to the accuracy and validity of test results in any population, but several of these factors have a greater impact in the geriatric patient. These include sample collection, sample handing, and physiological variables. Geriatric patients can present a challenge to phlebotomists due to disease, malnutrition, or dehydration.[67] With increased age, there is a reduction in healing rate and an increased risk of acquiring infection due in part to a gradual loss in the capacity of the immune system to fight off infections.[68] Further, the skin and veins are less elastic and can be injured more easily during venipuncture. The decrease in muscle mass and collagen leads to a decrease in vascular stability of veins and a subsequent decrease in blood flow. Physiological changes in the patient may impact laboratory results due to unavoidable issues that arise at the time of collection. Increased hemolysis or insufficient volume can ultimately impact the validity of the result. Other factors that may influence normal laboratory values in geriatric patients include diet, medications, exercise, smoking, alcohol consumption, physical activity, and body composition. While these factors influence results independent of age, geriatric patients are more likely to have one or several of these causing variations in test results. Caution should always be exercised when reporting results in a geriatric patient, but clearly an absurd result (one not compatible with life) should be investigated to identify potential causes of the discrepancy.

DISEASES PREVALENT IN THE ELDERLY

There are many diseases that are especially common in the elderly. Table 34.4 outlines the prevalence of some of these conditions in Americans 65 years and older as reported in the 2007 to 2008 National Health Interview Survey, a self-reported statistically valid sample of the US population.[69] The overall prevalence of these diseases is inadequately understood due to poor documentation and the presence of multiple conditions warranting many medications. There have been attempts to classify disease prevalence in the elderly population based upon pharmacy databases.[70]

TABLE 34.4	Diseases Prevalent in the Elderly: 2007–2008 National Health Interview Survey[67]
Hypertension	55.7%
Arthritis	49.5%
Heart disease	31.9%
Cancer	22.5%
Diabetes	18.6%
Asthma	10.4%
Chronic bronchitis/emphysema	9.0%
Stroke	8.8%

TABLE 34.5	Leading Causes of Death in the Elderly[71]
Heart disease	
Cancer	
Cerebrovascular disease	
Chronic obstructive pulmonary disease	
Pneumonia	
Diabetes	
Influenza	
Septicemia	
Nephritis	
Alzheimer's	

Classification in this population has been difficult due to inaccuracies related to misidentification of conditions or diseases, or incomplete medical records. Approaches to classify individuals at an earlier stage of disease have led clinicians and laboratorians to analyze drug combination therapies as markers of disease. A list of drugs that patients are prescribed is available in a pharmacy database, from which statistics can be generated calculating nationwide averages for disease prevalence.

The majority of the diseases noted in Table 34.5 are degenerative conditions, leading to concerns that increased life expectancy will increase the number of years with declining health. Health is defined as the state of being free from illness or injury, and deteriorating health is the number one reason that elderly leave their homes and enter retirement facilities.[72] Unfortunately, without baseline measurement, it can be difficult to identify noteworthy changes in analyte levels.

Menopause is defined as the time when the primary function of the human ovaries is permanently terminated. This time is variable for each individual, but typically, it begins between the ages of 35 and 58 years. This wide age range is based in part on the fact that functional disorders affecting the reproductive system can speed the transition to menopause. For instance, women with cancer of the reproductive tract, polycystic ovary syndrome, or endometriosis typically transition to menopause earlier than women without these conditions.[73–75] The precise definition of menopause is lack of menses for greater than 1 year. This transitional phase from reproductive to nonreproductive typically lasts about a year to a year and a half, and during this period of time, there is a gradual decline in ovarian function, thus a decrease in ovarian hormone production.[75] The changes that occur are caused by reduced estrogen levels that result from loss of the granulosa and interstitial cells lining the follicles.[76] The placenta normally produces hCG during pregnancy, but in addition to placental production, hCG can also arise from the pituitary. In perimenopausal women, hCG levels are often detected in the absence of pregnancy as a result of ovarian failure.[53] Pituitary hCG is more commonly detected in women ≥55 years, and marked elevations in this age group are most commonly associated with cancer.[77]

Osteoporosis, a bone disease that is prevalent in the elderly, leads to increased risk of bone fracture. Two types of tissue form bone, compact and spongy (trabecular). Compact bone accounts for 80% of the total bone mass of an adult, while trabecular bone accounts for the remaining 20%. Trabecular bone is highly porous (30% to 90%), while compact bone has a porosity of 5% to 30%. The risk of fracture is highest in bones with more compact tissue, which functions in whole body support. Bone mineral density (BMD) is reduced with age, and the World Health Organization has defined osteoporosis as BMD 2.5 standard deviations below peak bone mass.[78] This decreased density and an observed reduction in a number of bone-associated proteins both contribute to the weakened condition. Classifications of osteoporosis include primary type 1, primary type 2, and secondary (also known as type 3).[79] While primary type 1 is more frequently seen in elderly females, there is a growing precedence of osteoporosis in men. Secondary osteoporosis occurs in women or men who are older than 70 years of age and is typically associated with decreased bone formation and decreased renal production of dihydroxy vitamin D. Vitamin D deficiency causes decreased calcium absorption, which increases the PTH levels and promotes calcium mobilization from the bones, sacrificing skeletal calcium in order to maintain normal serum calcium levels. Type 3 osteoporosis is the only form of osteoporosis that affects individuals of any age. Most cases of type 3 osteoporosis are due to drug treatment or medication use, such as steroids,[80] and type 3 is not common in the elderly. Laboratory testing surrounding osteoporosis includes monitoring serum calcium, phosphate, creatinine, alkaline phosphatase, and 25-hydroxy vitamin D, and in men, testing also includes testosterone.[81]

Dementia is a syndrome defined as impairment of memory and at least one other cognitive domain (language, perceptual skills, attention, constructive abilities, orientation, and problem solving) that is severe enough to significantly impair day-to-day function.[82] Dementia is common in the elderly—approximately 10% of individuals over 65 years suffer from the syndrome; this rises to as high as 50% of those over 85 years.[83] Mild cognitive impairment (MCI) is a term used to describe similar cognitive problems that are not severe enough to significantly impair day-to-day function, but between 6% and 25% of individuals with MCI will go on to develop dementia in 1 year.

Dementia can be described in a number of ways, including the area of the brain that is most affected (cortical vs. subcortical), whether the etiology is known or unknown (secondary vs. primary), age of onset (presenile vs. senile), or by clinical syndrome. Many types of dementia can only be definitively diagnosed by pathological examination of brain tissue, which is obviously not helpful to the individual suffering from the illness, and correlation between the clinical syndromes and pathologic findings has historically been fairly poor. Recent advances in imaging and neurochemistry have improved this somewhat.[84] Conditions of cognitive impairment are largely clinical assessments and do not involve chemistry measurement in most cases. This is an opportunity for additional research as there are few proteins associated with these medical conditions (indicated below), and the data are not as terribly strong.

Alzheimer's disease (AD) is the most common form of dementia, responsible for approximately 70% of cases.[83] The pathologic findings of AD include amyloid plaques (made of beta amyloid) and neurofibrillary tangles (made of tau protein). Individuals with AD typically have a fairly slow but steady progression of impairment.

Vascular dementia is the second most common form of dementia and may be caused either by multiple clinically evident strokes (multi-infarct dementia) or by ischemic changes in the deep white matter of the brain. Individuals with vascular dementia typically have a "stuttering" or "stair-step" progression of impairment, but the speed of progression and specific manifestations may vary widely, depending on which areas of the brain are damaged.[71,84,85]

Dementia with Lewy bodies (DLB) is the third most common form of dementia and is characterized by prominent visual hallucinations, significant fluctuations in mental status, and parkinsonism (motor symptoms similar to those of Parkinson's disease). Lewy bodies are collections of alpha-synuclein protein inside neurons, but whether they are a cause or an effect of the illness is unclear, and Lewy bodies are also seen in Parkinson's disease, as well as in some cases of Alzheimer's. DLB typically progresses more quickly than AD.

There are also less common types of dementia including Pick's disease, frontotemporal dementia, Creutzfeldt-Jakob disease, normal pressure hydrocephalus, Huntington's disease, and Wernicke-Korsakoff syndrome. Typically, diagnosis of dementia is based on the patient's history and physical examination. Brain imaging and clinical laboratory testing may be performed to confirm or eliminate suspicion of specific clinical abnormalities.[86]

AGE-ASSOCIATED CHANGES IN DRUG METABOLISM

As adults age, changes occur that impact how the body metabolizes and utilizes drug compounds. Absorption, distribution, metabolism, and excretion of the drugs are impacted by the normal aging process. The prevalence of multiple health conditions in this subset of the population has highlighted the issue of polypharmacy[32] and the importance of therapeutic drug monitoring. Such testing in the laboratory helps prevent overdose and adverse drug reactions. Calculation of the actual in situ drug level is a key factor when looking at the result and metabolic rate, and elimination of these compounds needs to be considered for optimal dosing.[87]

Absorption

The rate of drug absorption from the small intestine slows with aging, leading to a lower peak serum concentration and a decrease in the time to reach peak. Typically, the total amount of drug absorbed (bioavailability) is the same in younger and older patients.[88] An exception arises due to an age-related decrease in hepatic function. Drugs that undergo extensive first-pass metabolism (such as nitrates) tend to have greater serum concentrations or greater bioavailability than drugs involved in conjugation or acetylation reactions.

Varying disease states or other drugs administered concurrently to the elderly may also cause changes in absorption. For example, calcium carbonate is frequently recommended for bone health in the elderly. This calcium salt requires gastric acid for absorption and should therefore be taken with food to stimulate gastric acid secretion. Patients with achlorhydria from natural causes or from acid-suppressing medications such as proton pump inhibitors or H_2 blockers should instead take calcium citrate, the absorption of which does not require gastric acid.[89]

Distribution

Volume of distribution (V_d) is the volume of plasma into which a fixed concentration of drug is dissolved. The larger the V_d, the greater the distribution of the compound. Older adults typically have less body water and lean body mass as a percent of total body mass—or in other words have more fat as a percent of total body mass. Drugs such as ethanol and lithium that are water soluble (*hydrophilic*) have a lower V_d in the elderly. Highly water-soluble drugs tend to be more concentrated in elderly individuals due to decreased body water. Additionally, drugs such as benzodiazepines and barbiturates that are fat soluble (*lipophilic*) have higher V_d in the elderly due to increased body fat and decreased lean body mass.[90] The extent to which a drug binds to plasma proteins also impacts its V_d. Many drugs bind to albumin, which is often decreased in the elderly. The unbound (free) portion of the drug is the pharmacologically active portion, and many drug assays measure total (bound and unbound) drug concentrations. Elderly patients with "normal" total drug levels may have excessive levels of free drug and exhibit signs of toxicity due in part to decreased albumin levels. Digoxin and phenytoin are examples of drugs that are significantly protein bound[91]—geriatricians will typically aim for the low end of the therapeutic range because of this issue.[92]

Metabolism

The liver is responsible for the majority of drug metabolism, and both hepatic blood flow and hepatic mass decrease with age. Phase I pathways of drug metabolism (hydroxylation, oxidation, dealkylation, and reduction) result in metabolites that may be of lesser, equal, or greater pharmacologic effect than the parent drug. In contrast, phase II pathways (glucuronidation, conjugation, or acetylation) result in inactive metabolites. Therefore, drugs metabolized by phase II pathways are generally preferred for the elderly because of decreased incidence of toxicity—for example, lorazepam is preferred over diazepam when benzodiazepine therapy is required in the elderly. The half-life of diazepam is

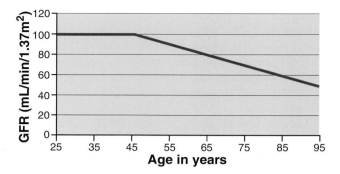

FIGURE 34.4 Rate of GFR decline in normal individuals with age. The course of GFR decline with normal aging was based on a cross-sectional study of iothalamate clearance in patients aged 17 to 70 years.[116] (Modified from Hebert L, Cody R, Slivka A, Sedmak D. Hypertension-induced kidney, heart, and central nervous system disease. In: Mandal AK, Jennette JC, eds. *Diagnosis and Management of Renal Disease and Hypertension.* 2nd ed. Durham NC: Carolina Medical Press; 1994.)

extremely long, and as a result of this prolonged half-life, its metabolites accumulate to unexpectedly high levels in the elderly with repeated dosing. Because of this, lorazepam is preferred in this patient population.[93]

Elimination

Kidney mass and blood flow decrease with age, which results in gradual decline in GFR. Figure 34.4 graphically represents this gradual, age-related decline over time. Further, the current estimates of the prevalence of chronic kidney disease in individuals over age 60 years are nearly 40%.[92,93] This decrease in GFR impairs elimination of therapeutic drugs and increases toxicity and adverse outcomes.[94,95] Therapeutic drug monitoring is an important consideration to ensure that compounds ingested are being metabolized and excreted appropriately. The gold standard for determining GFR is a measurement of iothalamate or iohexol measurement following intake. Another means of determining GFR is the measurement of creatinine in a 24-hour urine sample, though measurement of creatinine in a random serum sample is more commonly tested due to ease of collection. A number of formulas exist to calculate GFR, and no formula is ideal for all patient populations. The three equations used to estimate renal function are the Modification of Diet in Renal Disease (MDRD) equation, the Cockcroft-Gault equation (CG), and the Chronic Kidney Disease Epidemiology Collaboration equation (CKD EPI).[94–96] All three formulas use serum creatinine levels in combination with other factors to estimate GFR. The Food and Drug Administration traditionally uses the CG equation in its recommendations on appropriate dosing of therapies.[97] Most clinical laboratories estimate renal function using the MDRD equation because this equation requires serum creatinine, age, race, and gender, but not weight. There is growing movement based upon current recommendations to use the CKD-EPI equation, which uses serum creatinine, age, race, and gender. There is also interest in incorporating cystatin C as well as creatinine in

an estimating equation. There have been studies to assess the best equation for different demographics and patient populations. The findings of these studies have been contradictory, and based on the mixed results, there is no consensus equation used in the elderly patient population.[98,99] Different GFR results can change the dose of drug administered, and thus, there has been effort to find alternate methods to achieve the best estimation of GFR. There have been various methods proposed and tested, but eGFR measurement has been widely incorporated into clinical laboratory testing. Creatinine measurement alone should not be used to assess renal function.

Example 34.1 Diazepam

Diazepam is highly lipophilic—it is quickly and efficiently absorbed and accumulates with multiple doses. It is metabolized by phase I mechanisms to *N*-desmethyldiazepam and temazepam. Both of these metabolites are further metabolized to oxazepam—all three metabolites are pharmacologically active. Both temazepam and oxazepam are inactivated by glucuronidation (a phase II process) and eliminated via the kidney. Elimination half-life increases by approximately 1 hour for each year of age beginning with a half-life of 20 hours at 20 years of age.[100] This appears to be due to an increase in volume of distribution with age and a decrease in clearance. Consequently, the elderly may have lower peak concentrations, and on multiple dosing higher trough concentrations. It will also take longer to reach steady state.[12]

Example 34.2 Morphine Sulfate

Parenteral morphine has a smaller volume of distribution, higher plasma concentration, and slower clearance in elders compared with young adults. Older adults experience at least equivalent levels of pain relief with half the dose of intramuscular morphine sulfate as younger adults and the relief lasts longer. It is not clear if this is entirely due to age-related changes in pharmacokinetics or if there are age-related changes in pharmacodynamics at work here, as well. In any event, morphine should be administered at lower doses and longer intervals in the elderly, at least initially, to avoid toxicity.[88]

ATYPICAL PRESENTATIONS OF COMMON DISEASES

There are a number of medical problems that can occur in any age, but these conditions may present differently in the elderly. Differences in presentation or biological responsiveness to common conditions will typically be most evident to physicians or nursing staff who interact one-on-one with patients[5]; however, there are some unusual presentations that can be represented by the laboratory values. These are outlined below:

- Apathetic hyperthyroidism is hyperthyroidism with a paradoxical symptom of fatigue/apathy, instead of typical anxiety and hyperactivity. Thyroid disease in the elderly appears traditionally in the typical manner. Apathetic hyperthyroidism, a rare form of Graves' disease, presents in an unusual way in elderly patients. Unlike younger patients with Graves', older patients generally present with low to normal TSH. Before the advent of ultrasensitive TSH testing, the moderate variation in TSH made diagnosis difficult, but today laboratories routinely use ultrasensitive TSH tests, which make diagnosis of these patients more straightforward.[101,102]
- Acute myocardial infarction (AMI) is the leading cause of morbidity in the United States.[103] The incidence of myocardial infarction (MI) increases with age, and manifestations of MI can be unique. While the majority of younger patients (less than age 65) present with chest pain, the most common alternate AMI symptom in the elderly patient is shortness of breath.[104] The age-related respiratory changes, including shallow breathing and decreased respiratory rate, can complicate the diagnosis in some cases.

Geriatric Syndromes

There are a number of common constellations of symptoms in the elderly that are considered "geriatric syndromes." This concept emphasizes that certain issues commonly observed in the elderly population typically result from multiple coexisting and interacting problems. Since clinical training outside geriatrics tends to emphasize "Occam's razor"—looking for the simplest explanation for a patient's problems—the approach to geriatric syndromes requires a change in the diagnostic logical process.[105] Multiple parallel lines of investigation, rather than a single linear approach, are often required for adequate evaluation of these syndromes. The American Geriatric Society considers the conditions in Table 34.6 to be geriatric syndromes. The identification of a geriatric syndrome cannot be made with a specific laboratory test, but some tests can help explore the underlying cause of the symptoms that lead to patient presentation.

THE IMPACT OF EXERCISE AND NUTRITION ON CHEMISTRY RESULTS IN THE ELDERLY

Research indicates that regular exercise can increase the life span and improve the quality of life among geriatric patients. Maintaining physical activity improves physical strength and fitness, as well as balance. Exercise helps prevent depression, and manage and defend against diseases such as diabetes, heart disease, breast and colon cancer, and

TABLE 34.6	Geriatric Syndromes[104]

- Difficulty swallowing
- Malnutrition
- Sleep problems
- Bladder control problems
- Delirium
- Dementia
- Vision problems
- Hearing problems
- Dizziness
- Fainting
- Difficulty walking
- Falls
- Osteoporosis
- Pressure ulcers

osteoporosis.[33,106,107] Physical activities also improves endurance, flexibility sleep, mood, and self-esteem.[108] Increased physical activity may prevent more rapid deterioration. Fitness-related activities can reduce the risk of falling, and incorporation of exercise into lifestyle has been shown to be one of the best ways to improve bone mass throughout the life.[109] There have also been data linking the positive effects of exercise and long-term maintenance of cognitive function.[110] More importantly, lack of physical activity was shown to be a better predictor of all-cause mortality than being overweight or obese.[111]

The successful management of aging requires proper nutrition in addition to regular exercise. It is reported that 10% to 40% of hospitalized older adults suffer from malnutrition, which can be defined as any disorder of nutrition status resulting from a deficiency of nutrient intake, impaired metabolism, or overnutrition.[112] The difficulty recognizing the problem makes treatment a challenge.[35] Some of the laboratory values that can indicate undernutrition are low albumin and low prealbumin. There are a number of issues with the identification of malnutrition in the elderly. Based on this, there is increasing interest in establishing nutritional assessment tools for identification of undernourished individuals.[113]

Clearly, geriatric dietary intake is a concern in the area of undernourishment, but excessive calorie intake, resulting in obesity and increased prevalence of type 2 diabetes, is also a worry.[46] Based on increasing incidence of diabetes with aging, and the previously discussed benefits of physical activity, increasing numbers of elderly people are being encouraged to become active. Clinicians and laboratorians will need a better understanding of how exercise is likely to impact test results of older individuals. This will require closer attention to baseline measurements and observations of changes over time.

questions

1. High blood ammonia levels result in
   a. Respiratory acidosis
   b. Metabolic acidosis
   c. Metabolic alkalosis
   d. Respiratory alkalosis

2. Point-of-care testing is helpful when
   a. Results are needed quickly
   b. Only small sample sizes are available
   c. The device can be linked to the hospital LIS
   d. Quality control samples are not needed

3. The pituitary secretes which of the following hormones (more than one answer is possible)?
   a. Growth hormone
   b. Testosterone
   c. Insulin-like growth factor
   d. Thyroid-stimulating hormone

4. Aminoglycoside drug levels, such as gentamicin, should be measured
   a. 30 minutes after a dose
   b. 3 hours after a dose
   c. At steady state
   d. At any time

5. Which condition is least likely to be associated with increased alkaline phosphatase levels?
   a. Osteoporosis
   b. Paget's disease
   c. Hyperparathyroidism
   d. Osteomalacia

6. Which could account for drug toxicity following a normally prescribed dose?
   a. All of these
   b. Decreased renal clearance by the kidney
   c. Altered serum protein binding
   d. Liver impairment

7. Hearing loss is common among the elderly and may cause embarrassment. What should be done to facilitate the specimen collection process?
   a. Adjust your position to speak into the ear with the best hearing.
   b. Speak very loud and forcefully.
   c. Don't speak at all. Just give the patient printed instructions.
   d. Use a microphone.

8. Given the following information, calculate the creatinine clearance using the Cockcroft-Gault formula:
   Age = 85; weight = 70 kg; sex = male
   Serum creatinine = 1.0 mg/dL
   a. 53
   b. 72
   c. 47
   d. 35

9. Glucose intolerance, abnormal cholesterol level, high blood pressure, and upper body obesity are characteristics of
   a. Insulin resistance
   b. Chronic inflammatory disease
   c. Coronary heart disease
   d. Cerebrovascular disease

suggested readings

Busko M. Prevalence of CKD in the US Continues to Rise. *Medscape.com.* 2007. http://www.medscape.com/viewarticle/553492. Accessed August 26, 2012.

Cockcroft DW, Gault MH. Prediction of creatinine clearance from serum creatinine. *Nephron.* 1976;16: 31–41.

Hebert L, Cody R, Slivka A, et al. Hypertension-induced kidney, heart, and central nervous system disease. In: Mandal AK, Jennette JC, eds. *Diagnosis and Management of Renal Disease and Hypertension.* 2nd ed. Durham, NC: Carolina Medical Press; 1994.

Inouye SK, Studenski S, Tinetti ME, et al. Geriatric syndromes: clinical, research, and policy implications of a core geriatric concept. *J Am Geriatr Soc.* 2007;55:780–791.

Levey AS, Stevens LA, Schmid CH, et al. A new equation to estimate glomerular filtration rate. *Ann Intern Med.* 2009;150:604–612.

Passell JA, Cohn D. *U.S. Population Projections: 2005-2050.* Washington, DC: Pew Research Center; 2008. http://pewhispanic.org/files/reports/85.pdf. Accessed August 26, 2012.

Top 10 Causes of Death Among Adults Over Age 65. About.com Senior Health. 2010. http://seniorhealth.about.com/od/death-anddying/tp/cause_death.htm. Accessed August 26, 2012.

references

1. Colby SL, Ortman JM. Projections of the size and composition of the U.S. population: 2014 to 2060. *Current Population Reports, P25-1143.* Washington, DC: U.S. Census Bureau; 2014.

2. Ortman JM, Velkoff VA, Hogan H. An aging nation: the older population in the United States. *Current Population Reports, P25-1140.* Washington, DC: U.S. Census Bureau; 2014.

3. Vincent GK, Velkoff VA. *The Next Four Decades: The Older Population in the United States: 2010 to 2050.* Washington, DC: US Census Bureau; 2008. http://www.census.gov/prod/2010pubs/p25-1138.pdf. Accessed August 26, 2012.

4. Martin P, Midgley E. Immigration: shaping and reshaping America. *Popul Bull.* 2006;61:3–27.

5. Gray-Vickrey P. Gathering "pearls" of knowledge for assessing older adults. *Nursing.* 2010;40:34–42.

6. Gerber A. Navigating in evidence-poor waters—how much hydration is needed at the end of life? The recommendations of a Swiss expert group (Bigorio Group). *Ther Umsch.* 2012;69:91–92.

7. Faulkner WR. *Geriatric Clinical Chemistry Reference Values.* Washington, DC: American Association for Clinical Chemistry; 1993.

8. Burks TN, Cohn RD. One size may not fit all: anti-aging therapies and sarcopenia. *Aging (Albany, NY).* 2011;3:1142–1153.

9. Uusi-Rasi K, Sievänen H, Pasanen M, et al. Age-related decline in trabecular and cortical density: a 5-year peripheral quantitative computed tomography follow-up study of pre- and postmenopausal women. *Calcif Tissue Int.* 2007;81:249–253.

10. Phillips K, Aliprantis A, Coblyn J. Strategies for the prevention and treatment of osteoporosis in patients with rheumatoid arthritis. *Drugs Aging.* 2006;23:773–779.

11. Lombardi G, Di Somma C, Vuolo L, et al. Role of IGF-I on PTH effects on bone. *J Endocrinol Invest.* 2010;33:22–26.

12. Hausman DB, Johnson MA, Davey A, et al. The oldest old: red blood cell and plasma folate in African American and white octogenarians and centenarians in Georgia. *J Nutr Health Aging.* 2011;15:744–750.

13. Bhutto A, Morley JE. The clinical significance of gastrointestinal changes with aging. *Curr Opin Clin Nutr Metab Care.* 2008;11:651–660.

14. Tan JC, Workeneh B, Busque S, et al. Glomerular function, structure, and number in renal allografts from older deceased donors. *J Am Soc Nephrol.* 2009;20:181–188.

15. Tanner GA. Kidney function. In: Rhoades RA, Bell DR, eds. *Medical Physiology: Principles for Clinical Medicine.* 4th ed. Philadelphia, PA: Lippincott Williams & Wilkins; 2012:399–426. http://www.lww.com/webapp/wcs/stores/servlet/product_Medical-Physiology_11851_-1_12551_Prod-9781451110395

16. Baylis C, Schmidt R. The aging glomerulus. *Semin Nephrol.* 1996;16:265–276.

17. Matthews SJ, Lancaster JW. Urinary tract infections in the elderly population. *Am J Geriatr Pharmacother.* 2011;9:286–309.

18. Foster AD, Sivarapatna A, Gress RE. The aging immune system and its relationship with cancer. *Aging Health.* 2011;7(5):707–718.

19. Winzenberg T, van der Mei I, Mason RS, et al. Vitamin D and the musculoskeletal health of older adults. *Aust Fam Physician.* 2012;41:92–99.

20. Makarewicz-Wujec M, Kozlowska-Wojciechowska M. Nutrient intake and serum level of gamma-glutamyltransferase, MCP-1 and homocysteine in early stages of heart failure. *Clin Nutr.* 2011;30:73–78.

21. Llewellyn DJ, Langa KM, Friedland RP, et al. Serum albumin concentration and cognitive impairment. *Curr Alzheimer Res.* 2010;7:91–96.

22. del Val JH. Old-age inflammatory bowel disease onset: a different problem? *World J Gastroenterol.* 2011;17:2734–2739.

23. Vanasse GJ, Berliner N. Anemia in elderly patients: an emerging problem for the 21st century. *Hematology Am Soc Hematol Educ Program.* 2010;2010:271–275.

24. Laughlin GA, Barrett-Connor E. Sexual dimorphism in the influence of advanced aging on adrenal hormone levels: The Rancho Bernardo Study. *J Clin Endocrinol Metab.* 2000;85:3561–3568.

25. Carlsson L, Lind L, Larsson A. Reference values for 27 clinical chemistry tests in 70-year-old males and females. *Gerontology.* 2010;56:259–265.

26. Lapin A, Böhmer F. Laboratory findings in elderly patients: a forgotten aspect of laboratory medicine? *Z Gerontol Geriatr.* 1999;32:41–46.

27. Millán-Calenti JC, Sánchez A, Lorenzo-López L, et al. Laboratory values in a Spanish population of older adults: a comparison with reference values from younger adults. *Maturitas.* 2012;71(4):396–401. doi:10.1016/j.maturitas.2012.01.005.

28. Tietz NW, Shuey DF, Wekstein DR. Laboratory values in fit aging individuals—sexagenarians through centenarians. *Clin Chem.* 1992;38:1167–1185.

29. Kushner I. C-reactive protein elevation can be caused by conditions other than inflammation and may reflect biologic aging. *Cleve Clin J Med.* 2001;68:535–537.

30. Breitling LP, Claessen H, Drath C, et al. Gamma-glutamyltransferase, general and cause-specific mortality in 19,000 construction workers followed over 20 years. *J Hepatol.* 2011;55:594–601.

31. Rutger Persson G. Rheumatoid arthritis and periodontitis—inflammatory and infectious connections. Review of the literature. *J Oral Microbiol.* 2012;4:2066–2074.

32. Terrie YC. *Understanding and Managing Polypharmacy in the Elderly.* 2004. http://www.pharmacytimes.com/publications/issue/2004/2004-12/2004-12-9094. Accessed August 26, 2012.

33. Marks BL, Katz LM, Smith JK. Exercise and the aging mind: buffing the baby boomer's body and brain. *Phys Sportsmed.* 2009;37:119–125.

34. *High-Normal Uric Acid Linked with Mild Cognitive Impairment in the Elderly.* 2007. http://www.apa.org/news/press/releases/2007/01/uric-cognition.aspx. Accessed August 26, 2012.

35. Tsutsumi R, Tsutsumi YM, Horikawa YT, et al. Decline in anthropometric evaluation predicts a poor prognosis in geriatric patients. *Asia Pac J Clin Nutr.* 2012;21:44–51.

36. Sim V, Hampton D, Phillips C, et al. The use of brain natriuretic peptide as a screening test for left ventricular systolic dysfunction—cost-effectiveness in relation to open access echocardiography. *Fam Pract.* 2003;20:570–574.

37. Weksler ME, Goodhardt M. Do age-associated changes in "physiologic" autoantibodies contribute to infection, atherosclerosis, and Alzheimer's disease? *Exp Gerontol.* 2002;37:971–979.

38. Tuljapurkar SR, McGuire TR, Brusnahan SK, et al. Changes in human bone marrow fat content associated with changes in hematopoietic stem cell numbers and cytokine levels with aging. *J Anat.* 2011;219:574–581.

39. Zussman J, Young L. Zoster vaccine live for the prevention of shingles in the elderly patient. *Clin Interv Aging.* 2008;3:241–250.

40. Gooneratne NS, Edwards AY, Zhou C, et al. Melatonin pharmacokinetics following two different oral surge-sustained release doses in older adults. *J Pineal Res.* 2011;52(4):437–445. doi:10.1111/j.1600-079X.2011.00958.x.

41. Rockwood MRH, Howlett SE, Rockwood K. Orthostatic hypotension (OH) and mortality in relation to age, blood pressure and frailty. *Arch Gerontol Geriatr.* 2012;54(3):e255–e260. doi:10.1016/j.archger.2011.12.009.

42. Huber KR, Mostafaie N, Stangl G, et al. Clinical chemistry reference values for 75-year-old apparently healthy persons. *Clin Chem Lab Med.* 2006;44:1355–1360.

43. Bremner AP, Feddema P, Leedman PJ, et al. Age-related changes in thyroid function: a longitudinal study of a community-based cohort. *J Clin Endocrinol Metab.* 2012;97(5):1554–1562. doi:10.1210/jc.2011-3020.

44. Shaw ND, Srouji SS, Histed SN, et al. Differential effects of aging on estrogen negative and positive feedback. *Am J Physiol Endocrinol Metab.* 2011;301:E351–E355.

45. Barron AM, Pike CJ. Sex hormones, aging, and Alzheimer's disease. *Front Biosci (Elite Ed).* 2012;4:976–997.

46. Morley JE. Diabetes and aging: epidemiologic overview. *Clin Geriatr Med.* 2008;24:395–405.

47. Kokotas H, Grigoriadou M, Petersen MB. Age-related macular degeneration: genetic and clinical findings. *Clin Chem Lab Med.* 2011;49:601–616.

48. Lupien SJ, de Leon M, de Santi S, et al. Cortisol levels during human aging predict hippocampal atrophy and memory deficits. *Nat Neurosci.* 1998;1:69–73.

49. Davis KM, Fish LC, Minaker KL, et al. Atrial natriuretic peptide levels in the elderly: differentiating normal aging changes from disease. *J Gerontol A Biol Sci Med Sci.* 1996;51:M95–M101.

50. Sherman SS, Hollis BW, Tobin JD. Vitamin D status and related parameters in a healthy population: the effects of age, sex, and season. *J Clin Endocrinol Metab.* 1990;71:405–413.

51. Bauer JH. Age-related changes in the renin-aldosterone system. Physiological effects and clinical implications. *Drugs Aging.* 1993;3:238–245.

52. Ueda M, Araki T, Shiota T, et al. Age and sex-dependent alterations of serum amylase and isoamylase levels in normal human adults. *J Gastroenterol.* 1994;29:189–191.

53. Cole LA, Khanlian SA, Muller CY. Normal production of human chorionic gonadotropin in perimenopausal and menopausal women and after oophorectomy. *Int J Gynecol Cancer.* 2009;19:1556–1559.

54. Mulkerrin E, Epstein FH, Clark BA. Aldosterone responses to hyperkalemia in healthy elderly humans. *J Am Soc Nephrol.* 1995;6:1459–1462.

55. Glassock RJ, Winearls C. Ageing and the glomerular filtration rate: truths and consequences. *Trans Am Clin Climatol Assoc.* 2009;120:419–428.

56. Evrin PE, Nilsson SE, Oberg T, et al. Serum C-reactive protein in elderly men and women: association with mortality, morbidity and various biochemical values. *Scand J Clin Lab Invest.* 2005;65:23–31.

57. Castle SC. Clinical relevance of age-related immune dysfunction. *Clin Infect Dis.* 2000;31:578–585.

58. Flood C, Gherondache C, Pincus G, et al. The metabolism and secretion of aldosterone in elderly subjects. *J Clin Invest.* 1967;46:960–966.

59. Cowie CC, Rust KF, Ford ES, et al. Full accounting of diabetes and pre-diabetes in the U.S. population in 1988–1994 and 2005–2006. *Diabetes Care.* 2008;32:287–294.

60. Drion I, Joosten H, van Hateren KJ, et al. Employing age-related cut-off values results in fewer patients with renal impairment in secondary care. *Ned Tijdschr Geneeskd.* 2011;155:A3091.

61. Coin A, Giannini S, Minicuci N, et al. Limb fat-free mass and fat mass reference values by dual-energy X-ray absorptiometry (DEXA) in a 20-80 year-old Italian population. *Clin Nutr (Edinburgh, Scotland).* 2012;31(4):506–511. doi:10.1016/j.clnu.2012.01.012.

62. Faulkner WR, Meites S. *Geriatric Clincal Chemistry Reference Values.* Washington, DC: AACC Press; 1994.

63. Garry PJ. *Laboratory Medicine and the Aging Process.* Joseph A. Knight. Chicago, IL: ASCP Press; 1996:420, $45.00, ISBN 0–89189-397–0. *Clin Chem.* 1997;43:2444.

64. Jones G, Horowitz G, Katayev A, et al. Reference intervals data mining: getting the right paper. *Am J Clin Pathol.* 2015;144(3):527.

65. The New Old Age Blog. Clinical trials neglect the elderly. 2011. http://newoldage.blogs.nytimes.com/2011/08/19/clinical-trials-neglect-the-elderly/. Accessed August 26, 2012.

66. Mayo Clinic Staff. Caring for the elderly: dealing with resistance. *Mayo Foundation for Medical Education and Research (MFMER) MY01436.* 2010. http://www.mayoclinic.org/healthy-lifestyle/caregivers/in-depth/caring-for-the-elderly/art-20048403.

67. Isaac RM. Nutrition support makes more than sense/cents. *J Can Diet Assoc.* 1988;49:89–91.

68. Vukmanovic-Stejic M, Rustin MHA, Nikolich-Zugich J, et al. Immune responses in the skin in old age. *Curr Opin Immunol.* 2011;23:525–531.

69. Patricia M, Barnes MA, Barbara Bloom MPA, et al. *National Health Statistics Reports.* 2008;12.

70. Naughton C, Bennett K, Feely J. Prevalence of chronic disease in the elderly based on a national pharmacy claims database. *Age Ageing.* 2006;35(6):633–636.

71. Garcia A, Zanibbi K. Homocysteine and cognitive function in elderly people. *CMAJ.* 2004;171:897–904.

72. *Deteriorating Health Top Reason to Leave Home, Seniors Say. McKnight's.* 2008. http://www.mcknights.com/deteriorating-health-top-reason-to-leave-home-seniors-say/article/110638/. Accessed August 26, 2012.

73. Pamuk ON, Dónmez S, Cakir N. Increased frequencies of hysterectomy and early menopause in fibromyalgia patients: a comparative study. *Clin Rheumatol.* 2009;28:561–564.

74. Hermes GL, McClintock MK. Isolation and the timing of mammary gland development, gonadarche, and ovarian senescence: implications for mammary tumor burden. *Dev Psychobiol.* 2008;50:353–360.

75. Racho D, Teede H. Ovarian function and obesity—interrelationship, impact on women's reproductive lifespan and treatment options. *Mol Cell Endocrinol.* 2010;316:172–179.

76. McConnell DS, Stanczyk FZ, Sowers MR, et al. Menopausal transition stage-specific changes in circulating adrenal androgens. *Menopause (New York, NY).* 2012;19(6):658–663. doi:10.1097/gme.0b013e31823fe274.

77. Cole LA. HCG variants, the growth factors which drive human malignancies. *Am J Cancer Res.* 2012;2:22–35.

78. World Health Organization. Assessment of fracture risk and its application to screening for postmenopausal osteoporosis. Report of a WHO Study Group. *World Health Organ Tech Rep Ser.* 1994;843:1–129.

79. Koda-Kimble MA, Young LY, Alldredge BK. *Applied Therapeutics: The Clinical Use of Drugs.* Philadelphia, PA: Lippincott Williams & Wilkins; 2004.

80. Gourlay M, Franceschini N, Sheyn Y. Prevention and treatment strategies for glucocorticoid-induced osteoporotic fractures. *Clin Rheumatol.* 2007;26:144–153.

81. Lee J, Vasikaran S. Current recommendations for laboratory testing and use of bone turnover markers in management of osteoporosis. *Ann Lab Med.* 2012;32:105–112.

82. Buell JS, Dawson-Hughes B, Scott TM, et al. 25-Hydroxyvitamin D, dementia, and cerebrovascular pathology in elders receiving home services. *Neurology.* 2010;74:18–26.

83. *Alzheimer's Association—Latest Facts & Figures Report.* 2012. http://www.alz.org/alzheimers_disease_facts_and_figures.asp. Accessed August 26, 2012.

84. de la Torre JC. A turning point for Alzheimer's disease? *BioFactors (Oxford, England).* 2012;38(2):78–83. doi:10.1002/biof.200.

85. Engelborghs S, De Vreese K, Van de Casteele T, et al. Diagnostic performance of a CSF-biomarker panel in autopsy-confirmed dementia. *Neurobiol Aging.* 2008;29:1143–1159.

86. *Homocysteine: One of the Best Objective Markers of Your Health Status.* 2012. http://www.drbenkim.com/articles-homocysteine.html. Accessed August 26, 2012.

87. Ruiz JG, Array S, Lowenthal DT. Therapeutic drug monitoring in the elderly. *Am J Ther.* 1996;3:839–860.

88. Villesen HH, Banning AM, Petersen RH, et al. Pharmacokinetics of morphine and oxycodone following intravenous administration in elderly patients. *Ther Clin Risk Manage.* 2007;3:961–967.

89. Bo-Linn GW, Davis GR, Buddrus DJ, et al. An evaluation of the importance of gastric acid secretion in the absorption of dietary calcium. *J Clin Invest.* 1984;73:640–647.

90. Hughes SG. Prescribing for the elderly patient: why do we need to exercise caution? *Br J Clin Pharmacol.* 1998;46:531–533.

91. Dasgupta A. Clinical utility of free drug monitoring. *Clin Chem Lab Med.* 2002;40:986–993.

92. Tjia J, Field TS, Fischer SH, et al. Quality measurement of medication monitoring in the "meaningful use" era. *Am J Manage Care.* 2011;17:633–637.

93. Kraemer G. *Epilepsy in the Elderly: Clinical Aspects and Pharmacotherapy.* Stuttgart, Germany: Thieme; 1999.

94. Glassock RJ. The GFR decline with aging: a sign of normal senescence, not disease. *Nephrol Times.* 2009;2:6–8.

95. Euans DW. Renal function in the elderly. *Am Fam Physician.* 1988;38:147–150.

96. Levey AS, Bosch JP, Lewis JB, et al. A more accurate method to estimate glomerular filtration rate from serum creatinine: a new prediction equation. Modification of Diet in Renal Disease Study Group. *Ann Intern Med.* 1999;130:461–470.

97. Nacif MS, Arai AA, Lima JA, et al. Gadolinium-enhanced cardiovascular magnetic resonance: administered dose in relationship to United States Food and Drug Administration (FDA) guidelines. *J Cardiovasc Magn Reson.* 2012;14:18.

98. Carter JL, Stevens PE, Irving JE, et al. Estimating glomerular filtration rate: comparison of the CKD-EPI and MDRD equations in a large UK cohort with particular emphasis on the effect of age. *QJM.* 2011;104(10):839–847. doi:10.1093/qjmed/hcr077.

99. Gill J, Malyuk R, Djurdjev O, et al. Use of GFR equations to adjust drug doses in an elderly multi-ethnic group—a cautionary tale. *Nephrol Dial Transplant.* 2007;22:2894–2899.

100. *Drug Safety Labeling Changes—Valium (diazepam) Tablets 2009.* http://www.fda.gov/Safety/MedWatch/SafetyInformation/Safety-RelatedDrugLabelingChanges/ucm119276.htm. Accessed August 26, 2012.

101. *Hyperthyroidism: Thyroid Disorders: Merck Manual Professional.* 2012. http://www.merckmanuals.com/professional/endocrine_and_metabolic_disorders/thyroid_disorders/hyperthyroidism.html. Accessed August 26, 2012.

102. Reuben DB, Yoshikawa TT, Besdine RW, eds. *Geriatric Review Syllabus.* 3rd ed. Washington DC: American Geriatrics Society; 1996:296–297.

103. Smolina K, Wright FL, Rayner M, et al. Determinants of the decline in mortality from acute myocardial infarction in England between 2002 and 2010: linked national database study. *BMJ.* 2012;344:d8059.

104. Woon VC, Lim KH. Acute myocardial infarction in the elderly—the differences compared with the young. *Singapore Med J.* 2003;44:414–418.

105. Drachman DA. Occam's razor, geriatric syndromes, and the dizzy patient. *Ann Intern Med.* 2000;132:403–404.

106. American College of Sports Medicine Position Stand. Exercise and physical activity for older adults. *Med Sci Sports Exerc.* 1998;30:992–1008.

107. Rose DJ, Hernandez D. The role of exercise in fall prevention for older adults. *Clin Geriatr Med.* 2010;26:607–631.

108. Sarah Kovatch MFA, Melinda Smith MA, Segal J. *Senior Exercise and Fitness Tips.* 2012. Helpguide.org.

109. Gómez-Cabello A, Ara I, González-Agüero A, et al. Effects of training on bone mass in older adults: a systematic review. *Sports Med (Auckland, NZ).* 2012;42(4):301–325. doi:10.2165/11597670-000000000-00000.

110. Kraft E. Cognitive function, physical activity, and aging: possible biological links and implications for multimodal interventions. *Neuropsychol Dev Cogn B Aging Neuropsychol Cogn.* 2012;19:248–263.

111. van Dam RM, Li T, Spiegelman D, et al. Combined impact of lifestyle factors on mortality: prospective cohort study in US women. *BMJ.* 2008;337:a1440.

112. Milne AC, Potter J, Vivanti A, et al. Protein and energy supplementation in elderly people at risk from malnutrition. *Cochrane Database Syst Rev.* 2009;(2):CD0032882009. http://onlinelibrary.wiley.com/doi/10.1002/14651858.CD003288.pub3/abstract. Accessed August 26, 2012.

113. López-Contreras M-J, Torralba C, Zamora S, et al. Nutrition and prevalence of undernutrition assessed by different diagnostic criteria in nursing homes for elderly people. *J Hum Nutr Diet.* 2012;25(3):239–246. doi:10.1111/j.1365-277X.2012.01237.x.

35

Clinical Chemistry and the Pediatric Patient

TRACEY G. POLSKY and MICHAEL J. BENNETT

chapter outline

Developmental Changes from Neonate to Adult
Respiration and Circulation
Growth
Organ Development
Problems of Prematurity and Immaturity
Phlebotomy and Choice of Instrumentation for Pediatric Samples
Phlebotomy
Preanalytic Concerns
Choice of Analyzer
Point-of-Care Analysis in Pediatrics
Regulation of Blood Gases and pH in Neonates and Infants
Blood Gas and Acid–Base Measurement
Regulation of Electrolytes and Water: Renal Function
Disorders Affecting Electrolytes and Water Balance
Development of Liver Function
Physiologic Jaundice
Energy Metabolism
Diabetes
Nitrogen Metabolism
Nitrogenous End Products as Markers of Renal Function
Liver Function Tests

Calcium and Bone Metabolism in Pediatrics
Hypocalcemia and Hypercalcemia
Endocrine Function in Pediatrics
Hormone Secretion
Hypothalamic–Pituitary–Thyroid System
Hypothalamic–Pituitary–Adrenal Cortex System
Growth Factors
Endocrine Control of Sexual Maturation
Development of the Immune System
Basic Concepts of Immunity
Components of the Immune System
Neonatal and Infant Antibody Production
Immunity Disorders
Genetic Diseases
Cystic Fibrosis
Newborn Screening for Whole Populations
Diagnosis of Metabolic Disease in the Clinical Setting
Drug Metabolism and Pharmacokinetics
Therapeutic Drug Monitoring
Toxicologic Issues in Pediatric Clinical Chemistry
Questions
References

key terms

Drug metabolism
Endocrine system
Genetic disease
Growth
Immunity
Physiologic development
Point-of-care testing
Sexual maturation
Tandem mass spectrometry

For additional student resources, please visit thePoint® at http://thepoint.lww.com

chapter objectives

Upon completion of this chapter, the clinical laboratorian should be able to do the following:

- Define the adaptive changes that occur in the newborn.
- Describe the developmental changes that occur throughout childhood.
- Discuss the problems associated with collecting blood from small children.
- Understand the role of point-of-care testing in pediatric settings.
- Summarize the changes that occur in children with regard to electrolyte and water balance, endocrine function, liver function, and bone metabolism.
- Explain how drug treatment and pharmacokinetics differ between children and adults.
- Discuss the procedures used to diagnose inherited metabolic diseases.
- Describe the development and disorders of the immune system.

DEVELOPMENTAL CHANGES FROM NEONATE TO ADULT

Pediatric laboratory medicine provides many unique opportunities to study how the homeostatic and physiologic mechanisms that control normal human development evolve. With these opportunities to study development comes a completely new set of challenges, many based on failure of some component of the normal development process and resulting disease. With this scenario in mind, it becomes clear that the environment for the specialist pediatric laboratorian is different from the environment encountered in adult practice, in which **physiologic development** is not a major issue. The diseases encountered in pediatric practice, therefore, differ considerably from those in adult situations. Moreover, the nature of body size and, hence, available blood volume create additional problems for the analyst with regard to choice of instrumentation and testing menu.

The greatest pediatric challenge relates to the birth of an infant. There is a requirement at this time for rapid adaptation from intrauterine life, in which homeostasis is maintained by maternal and placental means, to the self-maintenance needed to adapt to extrauterine life. Issues related to this adaptation are further complicated by prematurity or intrauterine growth restriction (IUGR), when many organ systems have not reached sufficient maturity to enable the newborn to adapt to the necessary changes at the time of delivery.[1]

Respiration and Circulation

At birth, the normal infant rapidly adapts by initiating active respiration. The stimuli for this process include clamping of the umbilicus, cutting off maternal delivery of oxygen, and the baby's first breath. Initiation of breathing requires the normal expression of surfactant in the lungs. Surfactant is necessary for the normal expansion and contraction of alveoli and allows gaseous exchange to take place.

Initiation of respiration and expansion of lung volume causes increased pulmonary blood flow and reduced blood pressure. This, in turn, results in closure of the ductus arteriosus and a shift in blood flow through the heart that allows newly oxygenated blood from the lungs to be directed through the left side of the heart to the body. Blood flow now goes from the right side of the heart to the lungs for oxygenation. Closure of the ductus arteriosus is essential for this process to take place.

Growth

A normal baby delivered at term weighs about 3.2 kg. A baby whose birth weight is below the 10th percentile for gestational age is considered small for gestational age (SGA), a condition potentially caused by IUGR. Babies are regarded as premature when born at less than 37 weeks of gestational age. In the first days of life, weight loss is a result of insensible water loss through the skin. This is generally offset by weight gain of 6 g/kg/d as feeding is initiated. An infant's body weight will double in 4 to 6 months. Premature babies tend to grow at a slower rate and often still weigh less than does a term baby at the equivalent of term.

Organ Development

Most organs are not fully developed at birth. Glomerular filtration rate (GFR) of the kidney and renal tubular function mature during the first year of life at which point laboratory markers of renal function approximate adult values. Liver function can take 2 to 3 months to fully mature. Motor function and visual acuity develop during the first year of life. This development is accompanied by changes in the electroencephalogram until the normal "adult" picture is seen. There are dramatic changes in hematopoiesis as the switch from fetal hemoglobin to adult hemoglobin takes place. This coincides with significant hyperbilirubinemia as fetal hemoglobin is broken down, coincident with immature hepatic pathways of bilirubin metabolism. Bone growth in the rapid growth phases in the first few years of life and at puberty results in cyclical changes in bone growth markers. **Sexual maturation** results in significant endocrine changes, particularly of the hypothalamic–pituitary–gonadal hormone pathway, which eventually lead to the constitutive development of adult secondary sexual characteristics and eventually to the adult.

Problems of Prematurity and Immaturity

Intrauterine development is programmed for a normal 38 to 40 weeks of gestation.[1] Many organs are not fully ready to deal with extrauterine life before this time. This organ immaturity results in many of the clinical problems that we see associated with prematurity, which include respiratory distress (lung immaturity), electrolyte and water imbalance (kidney immaturity), and excessive jaundice (liver immaturity). Infants born before their due date constitute a major burden on the laboratory. They not only have abnormal biochemical parameters that require frequent blood drawing, they also have small blood volumes from which to draw on.

PHLEBOTOMY AND CHOICE OF INSTRUMENTATION FOR PEDIATRIC SAMPLES

Phlebotomy

Blood collection from infants and young children is complicated by the patient's size and frequently by the ability of the patient to communicate with the phlebotomist. The small blood volume of small patients dictates both the number of tests that can be performed safely on the patient and the number of times that blood can be drawn safely for repeat analysis.[2] Table 35.1 shows the percentage of total body blood volume that is drawn from an individual with a 10-mL blood draw. This volume is standard in adult laboratory medicine, but the table clearly shows that this amount of blood represents about 5% of total blood volume in a premature neonate. Clearly, frequent blood draws of this nature quickly will lead to anemia and the need for blood transfusion. Table 35.2 shows the guidelines for blood volume collection developed at Children's Hospital of Philadelphia. Infants and children have smaller veins than adults; to ensure that small veins do not collapse, narrow-gauge needles are generally used for venipuncture. Smaller needles increase the risk of hemolysis and hyperkalemia.

Frequently, good access to veins is impossible in a pediatric patient with intravenous and central lines in place. Capillary samples often are collected when suitable veins

TABLE 35.1	Implications of a 10-mL Blood Draw in an Infant Population	
Age	Weight (kg)	Total Blood Volume (%)
26 weeks of gestation	0.9	9.0
32 weeks of gestation	1.6	5.5
34 weeks of gestation	2.1	4.0
Term	3.4	2.5
3 mo	5.7	2.0
6 mo	7.6	1.6
12 mo	10.1	1.4
24 mo	12.6	1.0

TABLE 35.2	Recommended Blood Draw Volumes for Pediatric Patients		
Weight (kg)	Maximum Volume for a Single Blood Draw (mL)	Weight (kg)	Maximum Volume for a Single Blood Draw (mL)
2	4	30	60
4	8	32.5	65
6	12	35	70
8	16	37.5	75
10	20	40	80
12.5	25	42.5	85
15	30	45	90
17.5	35	47.5	95
20	40	50	100
22.5	45	52.5	105
25	50	55	110
27.5	55		

Courtesy of Dr. David Friedman, Children's Hospital of Philadelphia, Philadelphia, Pennsylvania.

are not available. However, capillary blood obtained by skin puncture has the potential to be contaminated, at least to some extent, by interstitial fluid and tissue debris. The concentration of protein (and protein-bound constituents) is approximately three times lower in interstitial fluid than in plasma. Table 35.3 highlights the major differences in analyte composition between venous serum and capillary serum. The lower concentrations of protein, bilirubin, and calcium in capillary specimens likely reflect mixing (and dilution) with interstitial fluid. Capillary samples, by either heel or finger stick, should be collected by phlebotomists with pediatric expertise. The heel should be warmed and well perfused to "arterialize" the capillaries, and the lancet puncture should be in an area of the heel away from bone. Excessive squeezing or milking of the lancet site can result in both hemolysis and factitious hyperkalemia from tissue fluid leakage.

Preanalytic Concerns

There is a growing trend toward complete front-end automation in clinical chemistry laboratories. The clear advantage with automation of sample handling is that traditional bottlenecks at sites of data entry and centrifugation are removed and turnaround times are reduced. Several issues have prevented the introduction of full-scale automation in pediatrics. A typical pediatric chemistry laboratory receives samples in tubes of many different sizes, varying from standard adult tubes to small pediatric tubes or Microtainers. While several of the large chemistry analyzers can directly sample from small pediatric tubes, as of this time, no manufacturer of laboratory equipment has developed a fully automated system that can handle this range of tubes. Although there have been reports in the literature from individual laboratories that have modified existing robotic instrumentation to allow complete automation

TABLE 35.3 Differences in Composition of Capillary and Venous Serum

Capillary Value Greater Than Venous Value (%)		No Difference Between Capillary and Venous Values	Capillary Value Less Than Venous Value (%)	
Glucose	1.4	Phosphorous	Bilirubin	5.0
Potassium	0.9	Urea	Calcium	4.6
			Chloride	1.8
			Sodium	2.3
			Total Protein	3.3

Source: Burtis CA, Ashwood ER, eds. *Tietz Fundamentals of Clinical Chemistry*. 5th ed. St. Louis, MO: WB Saunders; 2012.

of the testing process using pediatric tubes,[3,4] this is not routine practice.

A second important issue relates to evaporation of sample from open tubes. Most automated sample handling systems require open-topped tubes for processing. With large sample volumes, the effect of evaporation is minimal. With small volumes that have relatively large surface areas to total volume, evaporation can be significant and may affect results by as much as 10%.

Choice of Analyzer

Careful inspection and choice of analytic systems remain crucial for handling pediatric samples. Until recently, only a few analyzers were capable of performing multiple analytic procedures on small sample volumes (5 to 50 μL). Today, most analyzers can perform this function. Choice of analyzer becomes dependent on issues such as the following:

1. How much dead volume is there in the system? The smaller the dead volume, the greater is the number of tests that can be run.
2. Does clot or bubble detection allow for salvage of sample? All analyzers can detect a clot, but not all will allow retrieval of sample.
3. Is the system truly random access? This allows selectivity of menu for a given sample.

Typically, sample throughput time is less of an issue, as pediatric facilities tend to run fewer samples than busy adult services.

POINT-OF-CARE ANALYSIS IN PEDIATRICS

Point-of-care testing (POCT), or near-patient testing, plays an important and expanding role in pediatric practice.[5] Testing devices that are portable and easy to use, require small specimen volume, do not require sample preparation, and provide rapid results at the bedside are providing the momentum for increased POCT. To provide cost-effective and appropriate quality assurance for POCT, several factors need to be addressed.[5]

1. Does the analyte really require immediate turnaround for optimal patient management? Analyzers are becoming available that measure increasing numbers of different

analytes at the patient's bedside. Typically, the cost of POCT measurement is higher than the traditional laboratory measurement. The idea of instant results is so seductive that nonlaboratorian users often discount economic factors. In the author's institution, the clinical laboratory has played a leading role in determining which POCT assays will be available and in which clinical settings they have real value (Table 35.4).

2. Who chooses the POCT device? As the field of POCT expands, the number of devices on the market is also increasing. The clinical laboratory should be the setting in which POCT devices for institutional use should be first evaluated. The laboratory should make choices for instrumentation. Important features of a good POCT device should include the following:

- The ability to lock out untrained users. Only individuals accredited to use the device should be allowed access via a personal code.
- The device should not be allowed to proceed to patient sample analysis without running and validating appropriate quality assurance procedures.

TABLE 35.4 Important Pediatric Point-of-Care Tests and Testing Sites

Test
Blood gas
Electrolyte
Glucose
Activated clotting time
Hemoglobin
Glycated hemoglobin
Pregnancy
Urinalysis
Prothrombin time
Rapid *Streptococcus*

Testing Sites
Coronary care unit/intensive care unit
Trauma unit/emergency department
Diabetes clinic
Transport
Surgery
Extracorporeal membrane oxygenation sites

- The data should be downloadable to the hospital laboratory information system (LIS) for evaluation by the hospital quality assurance officer. Downloading the data also allows for billing and data entry into patient charts, features readily lost when analyzers are used that cannot be linked to the LIS.

The data generated by POCT devices have limitations. Typically, analytic performance is not as good as that with the main laboratory analyzer. POCT data are less precise and not suited to monitoring therapy in instances where small changes are important. The linear range for most POCT devices is not as broad as that of the main chemistry analyzer, and users need to be aware of these limitations. A prime example in the authors' institution is the use of POCT glucose analyzers. The instrument used for acute diabetic management in the outpatient setting loses linearity above 400 mg/dL, while the main chemistry analyzer measures up to 600 mg/dL (and the range can be extended even higher with sample dilution). Hypoglycemia is also particularly common in pediatrics and characteristically difficult to accurately quantitate using POCT devices. Low glucose levels should be confirmed using a more sensitive main laboratory analyzer.

REGULATION OF BLOOD GASES AND PH IN NEONATES AND INFANTS

Primary maintenance of blood gas and pH homeostasis following birth requires that the lungs and kidneys are sufficiently mature to regulate acid and base metabolism. At about 24 weeks of gestation, the lung expresses two distinct types of cells: type 1 and type 2 pneumocytes. Type 2 pneumocytes are responsible for the secretion of surfactant, which contains the phospholipids lecithin and sphingomyelin. Surfactant is required for the lungs to expand and the transfer of blood gases following delivery. Oxygen crosses into the circulation, and carbon dioxide is removed and expired. Immaturity of the surfactant system as a result of prematurity or IUGR results in respiratory distress syndrome (RDS). In RDS, there is failure to excrete carbon dioxide and, as a result, carbon dioxide levels rise, causing respiratory acidosis; oxygen levels are low and result in additional oxygen requirements for the baby.

The relative amounts of lecithin and sphingomyelin are critical for normal surfactant function. The measurement of amniotic fluid lecithin/sphingomyelin (L/S ratio) has been used for many years to predict fetal lung maturity. A ratio of less than 1.5 is considered indicative of surfactant deficiency.

The fetal fibronectin (fFN) test is a newer test used to determine the likelihood of premature delivery and risk for fetal maturity in women at high risk for preterm delivery.[6,7] fFN is a protein secreted uniquely by the fetus; toward term, or when preterm labor is potentially imminent, it is found in maternal cervical fluid. A POCT device is available that has been designed for use in the obstetrician's office. A negative test has a high predictive value that preterm delivery of the baby (within 7 to 14 days following testing) is unlikely.[6] A positive test is moderately predictive of preterm delivery,

TABLE 35.5	Causes of Acidosis and Alkalosis in Neonates and Infants
Respiratory Acidosis	**Hypoventilation/CO$_2$ Retention**
Metabolic acidosis	Renal tubular bicarbonate wasting
	Anoxia
	Poor tissue perfusion
	Metabolic disease
Respiratory alkalosis	Hyperventilation
	High blood ammonia/metabolic disease
Metabolic alkalosis	Pyloric stenosis/loss of gastric acid
	Excessive bicarbonate administration
	Low blood potassium

warrants close follow-up, and can be used to alert the pediatrician to the potential for RDS.

The trauma and relative anoxia during delivery can also induce acidosis in the newborn. This is typically a metabolic acidosis associated with increased lactic acid production. Serum bicarbonate levels are reduced in this situation compared with the respiratory acidosis in RDS. Persistent metabolic acidosis in the newborn that is difficult to correct with bicarbonate replacement is an indication for further intensive evaluation for possible inborn error of metabolism or other etiologies that require differentiation (Table 35.5).

Alkalosis is an unusual finding in pediatric medicine. One important cause of alkalosis is hyperammonemia, which may be secondary to a number of etiologies, including liver disease and inborn errors of metabolism (Table 35.5).

Blood Gas and Acid–Base Measurement

Oxygen status can readily be measured using noninvasive transcutaneous monitoring. Good correlation has been demonstrated between the arterial pressure of oxygen and transcutaneous measurement. Transcutaneous carbon dioxide monitors are also in widespread use. The measurement of acid–base status requires blood sampling. Most blood gas/acid–base analyzers can be adapted to take the small capillary samples routinely collected in pediatric settings. It is important for the person drawing the capillary blood to do so anaerobically, which requires thorough warming of the capillary site and collection of a freely flowing blood sample from a lancet stick. The sample needs to be sealed to ensure minimal gas exchange. Analysis should be performed immediately to not compromise the sample integrity. The author's laboratory maintains a goal of a 10-minute turnaround time from the sample receipt.

Most blood gas analyzers measure pO_2, pCO_2, and pH by ion-specific electrodes and calculate bicarbonate concentration by the Henderson-Hasselbalch equation. The Henderson-Hasselbalch equation is less valid when pH is far outside the normal physiologic range (extreme acidosis or alkalosis). On these occasions, it may become important to measure the bicarbonate concentration using a direct measurement.

Many blood gas analyzers have been upgraded in recent years to measure additional analytes, including blood sodium, potassium, and chloride, using ion-specific electrodes and lactate and urea and several instruments measure bilirubin and creatinine. The major advantage of this type of analyzer in pediatrics is that whole blood can be used. The volumes are typically smaller than those required for the main chemistry analyzer, and the lack of need for centrifugation shortens the turnaround time. One disadvantage of using whole blood is that the analyst cannot detect whether a sample is hemolyzed.

REGULATION OF ELECTROLYTES AND WATER: RENAL FUNCTION

From the 35th week of gestation, the fetal kidneys develop rapidly in preparation for extrauterine life.[1] The kidneys, critical organs for the maintenance of electrolyte and water homeostasis, control the rate of salt and water loss and retention. At term, neither the glomeruli nor the renal tubules function at the normal rate. The GFR is about 25% of the rate seen in older children and does not reach full potential until age 2 years (Table 35.6). Tubular function also develops at a similar rate. The maximal concentrating power of the kidney is only about 78% of that of the adult kidney at this time, although the tubular response to antidiuretic hormone appears to be normal. This gradual process of renal development in the newborn results in diminished filtration and impaired reabsorption of salt and water; therefore, in the newborn period and early infancy, large shifts in serum electrolyte levels can be observed. These problems are exacerbated in the preterm infant with renal function that is even less mature.

The kidneys also primarily maintain water loss and retention. However, in the newborn period, insensible water loss through the skin is also an important cause of water and electrolyte imbalance. Water loss and consequent hemoconcentration frequently result from the use of radiant heaters that are used to maintain body temperature. Increased water loss also occurs via respiration in children with RDS. Up to one third of insensible water loss may occur through this route. The total body water content of a newborn is about 80%; 55% is intracellular fluid, and 45% is extracellular fluid. The extracellular water is 20% plasma

TABLE 35.7	**Causes of Hypernatremia and Hyponatremia**

Hypernatremia
Excessive loss of water through overhead heater
Gastrointestinal fluid loss
Fluid deprivation
Renal loss of water/nephrogenic diabetes insipidus
Administration of hypertonic fluids containing sodium

Hyponatremia
Inappropriate ADH secretion due to trauma or infection
Administration of hypotonic fluids
Renal tubular acidosis
Salt-losing congenital adrenal hyperplasia
  (21-hydroxylase deficiency)
Cystic fibrosis
Diuretics
Renal failure

water and 80% interstitial. During the first month of extrauterine life, the total body water content decreases to about 60%, mostly a result of loss of the interstitial component.[1]

Disorders Affecting Electrolytes and Water Balance

The causes of hypernatremia (sodium, >145 mEq/L) and hyponatremia (sodium, <130 mEq/L) are listed in Table 35.7. Both disturbances can have dire outcomes, with a high risk of seizures. This is a result of the shift of water out of or into brain cells, with concurrent shrinkage or expansion of these cells. Hypernatremia results from hypotonic fluid loss, and hyponatremia results from hypertonic fluid loss. Hyponatremia may also be a result of excessive body water content and needs to be distinguished from hypertonic loss. Clinical evaluation and measurement of other components, including hematocrit, serum albumin, creatinine, and blood urea nitrogen, can be used to differentiate these etiologies. All of these compounds will be elevated with hemoconcentration. Clinically, it is usually possible to distinguish dehydration from excessive hydration.

Treatment of electrolyte and water loss is directed at replacing the loss to regain normal physiologic levels. Care must be taken to avoid too rapid a replacement, particularly with hypertonic dehydration. If water replacement is done too quickly, a rapid expansion of neuronal cell volume can occur, which results in seizures.

The causes of hyperkalemia and hypokalemia are listed in Table 35.8. The symptoms of hyperkalemia (serum potassium, >6.5 mEq/L) include muscle weakness and cardiac conduction defects that may lead to heart failure. In pediatrics, it is particularly important to recognize factitious hyperkalemia as a result of hemolysis and bad capillary blood collection, without hemolysis but with high potassium tissue leakage.

Because the situation regarding electrolyte and water homeostasis can change rapidly in small infants, it is important

TABLE 35.6	**Development of Glomerular Filtration in the Newborn**	

Age	Glomerular Filtration Rate (mL/min per 1.73 m² Mean)	Range
1 d	24	3–38
2–8 d	38	17–60
10–22 d	50	32–68
37–95 d	58	30–86
1–2 y	115	95–135[a]

[a]Adult values.

TABLE 35.8 Causes of Hyperkalemia and Hypokalemia

Hyperkalemia
Fluid deprivation/dehydration causing tissue leakage
Intravascular hemorrhage causing release from
  red cells
Trauma/tissue damage
Acute renal failure
Salt-losing adrenal hyperplasia (see *hyponatremia*)
Exchange transfusion using stored blood

Hypokalemia
Inappropriate ADH secretion
Diuretics, particularly frusemide
Alkalosis
Pyloric stenosis
Renal tubular acidosis secondary to bicarbonate loss

to monitor therapeutic intervention on a frequent basis.[1,2] The availability of POCT devices that use small volumes of whole blood helps with management of these imbalances, with the only caution being that it is impossible to detect hemolysis and factitious hyperkalemia on a whole blood sample.

DEVELOPMENT OF LIVER FUNCTION

Physiologic Jaundice

The liver is an essential organ for many metabolic processes. The processing of many normal metabolic pathways and the metabolism of exogenous compounds, in particular, pharmacologic agents, proceed slower in neonates. The most striking effect of an immature liver, even in a normal-term baby, is the failure to adequately metabolize bilirubin. Bilirubin is an intermediate of the breakdown of the heme molecules, which accumulate as fetal hemoglobin is rapidly destroyed and replaced by adult hemoglobin. Normally, the liver conjugates bilirubin to glucuronic acid using the enzyme bilirubin UDP-glucuronosyltransferase. Conjugated bilirubin can be readily excreted in the bile or through the kidneys. At birth, this enzyme is too immature to complete the process, and increased levels of unconjugated bilirubin and "physiologic" jaundice result. At this time, a normal baby may have a serum bilirubin level of up to 15 mg/dL, most of which is unconjugated. This level, which would be alarming in adult practice, should fall back to baseline by about 10 days of age. Because excessive jaundice can lead to kernicterus and result in severe brain damage, the measurement of blood conjugated and unconjugated bilirubin has an important role in pediatrics. An alternative means of reducing high unconjugated circulating bilirubin levels is phototherapy with ultraviolet light, which causes bilirubin to be converted to a potentially less toxic and more readily excreted metabolite. Severe cases may require an exchange transfusion. Complete absence of the bilirubin-conjugating enzyme results in severe persistent jaundice and Crigler-Najjar disease, a rare genetic disease. It is important to differentiate Crigler-Najjar from physiologic immaturity because treatment options vary considerably.

CASE STUDY 35.1

A newborn infant was born with a bilirubin level of 7 mg/dL (mostly unconjugated) that rose to 10 mg/dL by the 3rd day of life. The infant was breast-fed normally, and the bilirubin levels returned to normal values within 2 weeks without treatment.

Questions

1. What is the most likely diagnosis? Are there likely to be any long-term adverse health effects?
2. What is the most likely biochemical cause of the elevated bilirubin level?
3. What other disorders can cause unconjugated hyperbilirubinemia in neonates?

Energy Metabolism

The liver plays an essential role in energy metabolism for the whole body (Table 35.9). Carbohydrates derived from the diet as disaccharides or polysaccharides form the bulk of our energy sources. They are broken down into simpler monosaccharides, which reach the liver via the portal blood system. The primary sugars in newborns and infants come from the breakdown of disaccharide lactose in milk. Lactose is broken down to glucose and galactose. When it reaches the hepatocytes, galactose is converted to glucose by a series of enzymic reactions that have unique pediatric significance. Genetic deficiency of any of the reactions results in failure to convert galactose to glucose and essentially reduce the energy content of milk by 50%. The most common cause of failure to convert galactose to glucose results in galactosemia or deficiency of galactose-1-phosphate uridyltransferase, a serious genetic disease of the newborn. In this

TABLE 35.9 Important Biochemical Pathways in the Liver

Catabolic
Transamination
Amino acid oxidation to make ketones and acetyl-CoA
Fatty acid oxidation to make ketones
Urea cycle to remove ammonia
Bilirubin metabolism (hemoglobin breakdown)
Drug and exogenous xenobiotic compounds
  metabolized

Anabolic
Albumin synthesis
Clotting factor synthesis
Lipoprotein synthesis, very-low-density lipoprotein
Gluconeogenesis (synthesis of glucose)
Bile acid synthesis

disease, galactose-1-phosphate accumulates inside liver cells and causes hepatocellular damage and rapid liver failure. Other organs are also involved with this disease, including the renal tubules and the eyes. Galactose-1-phosphate accumulation causes acute renal tubular failure and tubular loss of glucose, phosphate, and amino acids. The loss of glucose in cooperation with the liver damage results in severe hypoglycemia. Accumulation of galactose in the eye results in cataract formation. A simple test that directs us to the diagnosis of galactosemia is the urine-reducing substance test. This detects the presence of non–glucose-reducing sugars (galactose) in urine when a child is symptomatic. The clinical significance of establishing a diagnosis is clear; galactosemia is often fatal if undiscovered but completely treatable by dietary lactose restriction when diagnosis is made.

Another critical pathway of carbohydrate energy metabolism in the newborn involves the pathway of gluconeogenesis. At birth, a term baby has sufficient liver glycogen stores to provide glucose as an energy source and maintain euglycemia. If the delivery is particularly stressful, these reserves of energy may become depleted prematurely. At this time, the normal physiologic role of gluconeogenesis, which essentially converts the amino acid alanine into glucose, becomes critical in maintaining glucose homeostasis. This pathway is not always mature at birth, and suboptimal operation results in what is termed *physiologic hypoglycemia*. Newborns can survive blood glucose levels below 30 mg/dL, although adults would fall into rapid hypoglycemic coma and risk sudden death at these levels. Physiologic hypoglycemia usually corrects quickly as the enzyme systems mature or by simple intravenous glucose infusion. Persistent and severe hypoglycemia should alert the physician to a possible inborn error of metabolism, such as galactosemia, gluconeogenesis, or disorders of fatty acid oxidative metabolism.

Diabetes

Blood glucose homeostasis and hepatic metabolism of glucose are maintained by the concerted actions of several hormones.[8] Following a meal, the level of glucose in the circulation rises, which triggers increased synthesis and release of insulin by the pancreatic β cells of the islets of Langerhans. Increased levels of insulin in the circulation cause glucose to be taken up by certain cells, such as hepatocytes and muscle cells, and to be converted into glycogen as a future source of energy. As a result of the insulin action, blood glucose levels begin to fall to the preprandial level. Glucagon, a hormone secreted by the α cells of the islets of Langerhans, has an opposing effect to that of insulin. It is generally believed that the insulin–glucagon ratio, rather than absolute amounts of either, is the primary endocrine modulator of circulating glucose levels. Other hormones, including cortisol, epinephrine, and insulin-like growth factor (IGF), can also affect glucose levels. These hormones are secreted in response to stress and can affect glucose measurement when samples are collected under stressful situations.

Diabetes mellitus, a condition in which the endocrine control of glucose metabolism is abnormal, is usually related to failure of the insulin regulatory pathway. Type 1 diabetes (insulin dependent) is the most common in pediatrics.

This may be caused by failure of the pancreas to secrete insulin or by the presence of circulating insulin antibodies that reduce the ability for endocrine action. This type of diabetes can be further classified as immune mediated or idiopathic. In the immune-mediated form (the most common form), the insulin-secreting beta cells are destroyed by a T-cell–mediated autoimmune response. This form of diabetes was previously termed "juvenile diabetes" because it is the predominant form in children. A patient typically presents with diabetic ketoacidosis, with profound hyperglycemia and metabolic acidosis that result from the liver increasing fatty acid metabolism and producing excess ketone bodies.

Type 2 diabetes (non–insulin dependent) is normally associated with increased resistance to normally secreted insulin in obese individuals. Obesity, particularly of the central (abdominal) region, is the most important risk factor for developing type 2 diabetes as it is strongly associated with insulin resistance, which, when coupled with relative insulin deficiency, leads to the overt development of type 2 diabetes. During the past 30 years, the number of children diagnosed as being overweight has increased by >100%, and this epidemic of childhood obesity is causing children to suffer from chronic complications that were previously only seen in adults.[9] Type 2 diabetes now accounts for a considerable proportion of newly diagnosed cases of diabetes in the pediatric population.

To be diagnosed with diabetes mellitus, an individual must demonstrate one of the following diagnostic criteria: fasting plasma glucose level ≥126 mg/dL (7.0 mmol/L), plasma glucose ≥ 200 mg/dL (11.1 mmol/L) 2 hours after a 75-g oral glucose load, symptoms of hyperglycemia and random plasma glucose ≥200 mg/dL (11.1 mmol/L), or glycated hemoglobin (Hb A1$_C$) ≥ 6.5%.[10] A positive result on any of the above should be repeated on a different day prior to the diagnosis of diabetes.

Urbanization, unhealthy diets, and increasingly sedentary lifestyles have contributed to increase the prevalence of childhood obesity, particularly in developed countries.[11] The metabolic syndrome is a combination of medical disorders that when occurring together, greatly increase the chance of cardiovascular disease and diabetes. Several definitions of the metabolic syndrome exist but generally include diabetes or impaired glucose resistance, hypertension, dyslipidemia (increased triglycerides and decreased HDL), and central obesity. The link between obesity, metabolic syndrome, and type 2 diabetes has been well characterized in adult populations but has been increasingly observed in pediatric populations. In children and adolescents, a number of studies have demonstrated a link between childhood metabolic syndrome and elevated cardiovascular risk in later life.[11]

It is important to recognize diabetes as a cause of hyperglycemia in children and to distinguish it from other medical causes of high blood sugar, including acute pancreatic disease or hypersecretion of counterregulatory hormones such as growth hormone (GH), cortisol, or catecholamines. Chronic hyperglycemia can be readily distinguished from acute causes by simply measuring the blood concentration of glycated hemoglobin or hemoglobin A1$_C$, a well-established marker for long-term hyperglycemia. In addition to being included as a diagnostic criteria of diabetes, this assay also plays a major role in monitoring compliance in diabetic patients on treatment.[10]

Nitrogen Metabolism

The liver plays a central role in nitrogen metabolism. It is involved with the metabolic interconversions of amino acids and the synthesis of nonessential amino acids. The liver synthesizes many body proteins, including most proteins found in the circulation, such as albumin, transferrin, and the complement clotting factors. The liver does not synthesize immunoglobulins. The liver is also responsible for complete metabolism of the breakdown products of nitrogen turnover, such as ammonia and urea through the urea cycle and creatinine and uric acid from energy stores and nucleic acids, respectively. Blood ammonia levels are higher in the newborn period than in later life, presumably due to immaturity of urea cycle enzymes and the portal circulation. A blood ammonia level of 100 µmol/L in a newborn would be regarded as less significant than the same level in a 1-year-old. Persistently elevated ammonia levels should alert the investigator to possible liver damage and secondary failure of the urea cycle. High ammonia levels suggest a possible primary defect in the urea cycle, and patients should be evaluated for such a defect.

Nitrogenous End Products as Markers of Renal Function

In contrast to the high neonatal ammonia levels, creatinine and uric acid levels are lower in newborns. Both metabolites rise eventually to normal adult ranges. Creatinine concentrations in blood increase with muscle mass and may vary with diet (i.e., meat ingestion). It is filtered at the glomerulus and not extensively reabsorbed by the renal tubules. Its measurement as a clearance ratio in blood and in a 24-hour urine sample has been used as a marker for the GFR for many years. Creatinine clearance is calculated from the creatinine concentration in the collected urine sample, the urine flow rate, and the plasma creatinine concentration. Creatine clearance calculations are not commonly performed anymore due to the difficulties in collecting a complete 24-hour urine specimen and the fact that newer, more convenient methods to estimate the glomerular filtration rate (eGFR) using a single plasma creatinine value are commonly used.

While several different equations exist to estimate GFR from plasma creatinine values in adults, the most widely used is the Modification of Diet in Renal Disease (MDRD) formula.[12] The equation estimates GFR from the patient's serum creatinine (mg/dL), age, sex, and ethnicity as follows:

$$GFR\left(mL/min/1.73\,m^2\right)=175\times S_{cr}^{-1.154}$$
$$\times\left(age\right)^{-0.203}\times\left(0.742\text{ if female}\right)$$
$$\times\left(1.212\text{ if African American}\right)$$

This equation has only been validated on patients greater than 18 years old, and since this equation does not adjust for body mass, it may underestimate eGFR for heavy people and overestimate it for underweight people. In children, the most widely used and extensively validated equation

is the updated or "bedside" Schwartz equation,[13] which estimates GFR from serum creatinine (mg/dL), the child's height (cm) and a constant as follows:

$$GFR\left(mL/min/1.73\,m^2\right)=\frac{\left(0.41\times\text{height in cm}\right)}{\text{Serum creatinine in mg/dL}}$$

The use of both of the above equations requires the use of a creatinine assay that has been standardized and its calibration traceable to the gold standard measurement technique, isotope dilution mass spectrometry (IDMS).

The worldwide standardization of creatinine to a single gold standard methodology was a major undertaking by several of the world's leading clinical chemistry organizations, medical societies, and instrument manufacturers with a goal of reducing the interlaboratory variation in creatinine assay calibration. This has allowed for more accurate estimations of GFR, which has allowed health care providers to better identify and treat chronic kidney disease and improve patient outcomes. As of 2012, virtually all manufacturers of creatinine assays have standardized their assays to the IDMS gold standard.

Serum cystatin C, a newer and possibly more sensitive marker of GFR, is considered a potential replacement for creatinine[14] as its concentration is independent of muscle mass and recent meat ingestion. Cystatin C (an inhibitor of cysteine protease) is a ubiquitous protein secreted by most cells in the body. Cystatin C is freely filtered at the glomerulus and reabsorbed by the tubular epithelial cells with only a very small amount being excreted in the urine. Several recent studies have proposed equations to relate cystatin C concentrations to GFR, and some of the proposed equations actually incorporate both creatinine and cystatin C values. A recent study proposed a modification of the Schwartz equation for use in children with chronic kidney disease; one that utilizes both serum creatinine and cystatin C.[15] This marker could potentially replace the creatinine clearance assay and remove the need for difficult 24-hour urine collections from children. Incomplete collections form the basis of most errors in this assay.

Liver Function Tests

As discussed, the liver is responsible for performing a large number of synthetic and catabolic processes, and normal liver function is central to maintaining body homeostasis. Several laboratory tests have emerged that are generally classified as liver function tests.

The measurements of serum albumin and total and conjugated bilirubin are true tests of liver function because they measure the synthetic and metabolic pathways for these compounds. In protein–calorie malnutrition, the reduced of availability of amino acids for synthesis of new proteins results in diminished functional synthetic rate and low levels of newly synthesized proteins, such as albumin. Very low levels of albumin indicate a long exposure to protein restriction, and its measurement in blood is often used as a guide to nutritional status and chronic liver disease of other causes.

Impaired hepatocellular function also results in reduced ability to conjugate bilirubin, with subsequent increase in the unconjugated form, which is normally barely detectable.

Other tests, such as measurement of liver enzymes, more truly reflect tests of liver cell integrity and are not strictly functional assays. Large elevations in serum AST and ALT indicate hepatocellular damage and subsequent leakage of cellular contents into the serum, and elevated ALP suggests hepatic biliary damage but gives little functional information.

CALCIUM AND BONE METABOLISM IN PEDIATRICS

Normal bone growth, which parallels body growth, requires integration of calcium, phosphate, and magnesium metabolism with endocrine regulation from vitamin D, parathyroid hormone (PTH), and calcitonin.[8] The active metabolite of vitamin D is 1,25-dihydroxy vitamin D. Hydroxylation of vitamin D from the diet takes place in the liver and in the kidneys and requires normal functioning of these organs. Absorption of vitamin D from the gastrointestinal tract, conversion to its active form in the kidney, and incorporation of calcium and phosphate into growing bone require normally active PTH. Secretion of PTH is, in turn, modulated by serum calcium and magnesium levels. Low levels of both divalent cations inhibit PTH secretion. Calcitonin has an antagonistic effect on PTH action.

Much recent attention has been given to the study of vitamin D deficiency and the role of vitamin D in maintaining optimal health. Vitamin D deficiency can result from inadequate nutritional intake of vitamin D coupled with inadequate sunlight exposure or use of sunscreens, disorders that limit vitamin D absorption, and conditions that impair the conversion of vitamin D into active metabolites including certain liver and kidney diseases. Deficiency results in impaired bone mineralization and leads to bone softening diseases including rickets in children and osteoporosis and osteomalacia in adults. According to numerous recent studies, vitamin D may be helpful in preventing other diseases, including several types of cancer, diabetes, multiple sclerosis, obesity, and hypertension.[16]

Vitamin D deficiency is common in children. The American Academy of Pediatrics recommends that all infants (beginning in the first few days of life) receive 400 IU/d of vitamin D supplementation.[16] This dose is required to prevent rickets and osteomalacia and possibly help prevent other chronic diseases. The serum concentration of 25-hydroxyvitamin D is typically used to determine vitamin D status. It reflects vitamin D produced in the skin as well as that acquired from the diet and has a fairly long circulating half-life.

Several assay manufacturers produce immunoassays that are convenient for hospital-based clinical laboratories; however, the gold standard reference method is liquid chromatography coupled with **tandem mass spectrometry**. There have been ongoing issues with variability in results of 25-hydroxyvitamin D levels measured by different methods and immunoassays

TABLE 35.10	**Causes of Hypocalcemia**
Prematurity	
Metabolic acidosis	
Vitamin D deficiency	
Liver disease (failure to activate vitamin D)	
Renal disease (failure to activate vitamin D)	
Hypoparathyroidism	
Low calcium intake	
High phosphorus intake	
Diuretic use	
Hypomagnesemia	
Exchange transfusion (anticoagulants in transfused blood)	

produced by different manufacturers. A standard reference material is commercially available, which should allow assay manufacturers and laboratories to better standardize their assays. In addition, several new proficiency schemes have been developed to help ensure consistency between laboratories.

The rapid bone growth that occurs during infancy, and later during puberty, requires optimal coordination of mineral absorption, transport, and endocrine-controlled incorporation of the minerals into growing bone. Approximately 98% of total body calcium content is present in bone and less than 1% is measurable in the blood. Serum calcium is present as the unbound ionized fraction (about 50% of total in blood), with the rest bound to protein (40%) or chelated to anions in the circulation, such as phosphate and citrate. Serum ionized and bound calcium levels are highly regulated and maintained within strict homeostatic limits. Abnormalities in any of the regulatory components have profound clinical effects on children.

Hypocalcemia and Hypercalcemia

Hypocalcemia is defined as total serum calcium below 7.0 mg/dL or ionized calcium below 3.0 mg/dL. In the newborn and particularly the immature newborn, these levels may be commonly encountered with few symptoms. However, hypocalcemia can result in irritability, twitching, and seizures. Serum calcium is usually measured in infants with seizures of unknown etiology. Prolonged hypocalcemia can result in reduced bone growth and rickets. The causes of hypocalcemia are listed in Table 35.10. Hypomagnesemia frequently occurs with hypocalcemia. Because low levels of serum magnesium also inhibit PTH secretion, it is important to consider the possibility of concurrent hypomagnesemia in a child with hypocalcemic seizures and to correct any abnormalities that may be identified in the magnesium status as calcium is also corrected.

Hypercalcemia is defined as total serum calcium of greater than 11.0 mg/dL. This is an unusual finding in pediatrics (Table 35.11) but has potentially severe clinical implications. Patients with hypercalcemia have poor muscle tone, constipation, and failure to thrive and may develop kidney stones leading to renal failure.

TABLE 35.11	**Causes of Hypercalcemia**

Hyperparathyroidism
Acute renal failure
Excessive intake of vitamin D
Idiopathic hypercalcemia of infancy

Hypercalcemia is less common than hypocalcemia in infants.

ENDOCRINE FUNCTION IN PEDIATRICS

The field of endocrinology provides numerous examples of the "differences" that occur in clinical chemistry between children and adults.[2] The process of maturation from a prepubertal child into a sexually fertile adult, for example, requires a complex, endocrine-mediated, developmental process switching on during childhood. As addressed in the previous section, the bone growth that accompanies systemic **growth** also requires a complex process, which is also under endocrine control.

Hormone Secretion

The **endocrine system** relates to a group of hormones that are typically produced and secreted by one specialized cell type into the circulation, where the hormonal effect is exerted in other target cells through the binding of the hormones to specialized receptors. Some of these hormones are polypeptides; others are amino acid derivatives or steroids.

Four major endocrine systems have been described, all of which play critical roles in normal human development. These systems all involve the hypothalamus as a major higher brain control center, the pituitary gland as a major secretor of hormones, and then various end organs, which have responsive elements for the pituitary hormone and affect many metabolic and developmental functions. These end organs include the thyroid gland, adrenal cortex, liver, and gonads. Each system involves regulated secretion of a trophic hormone by the hypothalamus, which in turn is transported to and controls endocrine secretion by the pituitary and, occasionally, secondary hormonal secretion by the end organ, which then produces the appropriate cellular endocrine effect. There is feedback on the hypothalamus by the final product of the pathway (long loop feedback) and also by the endocrine product of the pituitary (short loop feedback). The feedback regulates hypothalamic control of the pathway. Clearly, there are many areas that can go wrong in each of these pathways, all of which result in disease. Certain disease conditions are uniquely pediatric, and they are discussed further.

Hypothalamic–Pituitary–Thyroid System

The hypothalamus secretes thyrotropin-releasing hormone (TRH), a 3-amino acid peptide into the portal blood system between the hypothalamus and anterior pituitary.[8] TRH binds to a receptor on specialized cells in the anterior pituitary, which stimulates the secretion of thyroid-stimulating hormone (TSH), a polypeptide made up of two chains (α and β). The α chain is common to human chorionic

gonadotropin (hCG), follicle-stimulating hormone (FSH), and luteinizing hormone (LH), and the β chain confers specificity to all of these hormones. TSH is released into the circulation and targets its end organ, the thyroid gland. Unique TSH receptors on the thyroid gland, when occupied by a TSH molecule, cause the follicular cells of the thyroid gland to synthesize and release thyroid hormones into the circulation. The synthesis of thyroid hormone involves several complex steps in which iodine is trapped within the thyroid tissue and used to iodinate tyrosine residues on a prohormone thyroglobulin, which is then cleaved to release the iodinated amino acid triiodothyronine (T_3) and tetraiodothyronine (T_4). Thyroid hormones in the circulation are greater than 99% bound to specific transporter proteins called *thyroid-binding globulins*. Free thyroid hormone, in particular free T_3, is the active form of the hormone and reacts with receptors on many peripheral tissues to cause increased metabolism and simulate normal growth and development. T_4, T_3 (long loop), and TSH (short loop) levels feedback on the hypothalamus to regulate TRH production.

Two major areas of dysfunction in this endocrine pathway need consideration in pediatrics: primary hypothyroidism and secondary hypothyroidism. Primary hypothyroidism results from any defect that causes failure of the thyroid gland to synthesize and secrete thyroid hormone. This results in a common disease known as *congenital hypothyroidism* (CH), which is present in 1 of 4,000 births and is screened for in all newborns in the developed world. Untreated patients with this disease have severe mental retardation with unusual facial appearances. Treatment by thyroid replacement therapy is usually successful when diagnosis is established. The best diagnostic test is to measure TSH levels in blood spots from newborns or serum if CH is suspected in later childhood. TSH levels are high as a result of failure of the long feedback loop. Thyroid hormone levels, typically total T_4 but also free T_4, in untreated patients are very low.

Secondary hypothyroidism is a result of the failure of the pituitary gland to secrete TSH, which results in lack of thyroid gland stimulation and subsequent low production of thyroid hormone. The differential diagnosis is established by measuring low circulating TSH levels. Because the pituitary is involved with all major endocrine systems, it is important to study the other pituitary pathways to determine if hypothyroidism is the result of an isolated TSH defect or due to panhypopituitarism involving all other pathways. Panhypopituitarism is clinically complex and may include features of hypoglycemia, salt loss, poor somatic and bone growth, failure to thrive, and, in later childhood, failure to develop secondary sexual characteristics.

Hypothalamic–Pituitary–Adrenal Cortex System

This system is essential for regulating mineral and carbohydrate metabolism.[4] The hypothalamus secretes corticotrophin-releasing hormone (CRH), a 41-amino acid polypeptide, into the portal blood system, which binds to receptors on specialized anterior pituitary cells, resulting in the release of corticotrophin or adrenocorticotropic hormone (ACTH) into the circulation. ACTH binds to receptors on cells in the adrenal cortex, which are stimulated to secrete the steroid hormones, cortisol and aldosterone. This pathway is also stimulated by stress at the higher cerebral center. ACTH acts as a short loop feedback control on the hypothalamus, while cortisol and aldosterone are long loop regulators. Aldosterone functions in the kidneys to regulate salt and water homeostasis. Cortisol interacts in many peripheral tissues and has many metabolic functions, involving the regulation of carbohydrate, protein, lipid, and overall energy metabolism. Cortisol also plays a poorly understood role in the provision of resistance to infection and inflammation that accounts for the therapeutic use of steroids in many clinical situations. As with all endocrine systems, diseases occur that result from hyperfunction or hypofunction of the hypothalamic–pituitary–adrenal pathway. Diseases may be primary, resulting from end-organ dysfunction, or secondary, resulting from pituitary or hypothalamic disease. Pediatric diseases associated with primary disorders of the adrenal cortex are shown in Table 35.12. Many of the disorders listed are rare genetic diseases. However, steroid 21-hydroxylase deficiency is sufficiently common (about 1 of 5,000 births) to merit whole population screening in most developed countries in the world by measurement of blood spot 17-hydroxyprogesterone levels. This disorder results in failure to adequately synthesize both aldosterone and cortisol. Aldosterone deficiency results in renal salt-losing crises, and patients in the newborn period can be profoundly hyponatremic and hyperkalemic. Failure to synthesize cortisol results in stress-induced hypoglycemia. Furthermore, intermediates of steroid metabolism, which build up as a result of the metabolic block, cause androgenization. Girls born with this disorder frequently have ambiguous genitalia and may be first classed as boys. Boys may not have such pronounced abnormalities at birth but may still develop electrolyte crises.[17] Defects of the other enzymes in the steroid pathway result in a variety of clinical signs and symptoms including salt loss, androgenization, hypertension, and hypoglycemia, and diagnosis frequently requires steroid profiling.

TABLE 35.12	Congenital Diseases of the Adrenal Cortex
	Metabolic Profile
21-Hydroxylase[a]	↑ 17-Hydroxyprogesterone, ↓ cortisol
3β-Hydroxy dehydrogenase	↑ Dehydroepiandrosterone (DHEA)
11β-Hydroxylase	↑ 11-Deoxycortisol, ↓ cortisol
17α-Hydroxylase	↑ 17-Ketosteroids, ↓ testosterone
18-Hydroxylase	↓ Aldosterone, ↑ renin

[a]Common disorder screened for in all newborns.

Growth Factors

The hypothalamus secretes two regulatory hormones that affect growth. GH-releasing hormone is a 40-amino acid polypeptide that stimulates release of GH from the anterior pituitary. GH-inhibiting factor, also known as *somatostatin*, inhibits GH secretion. Additional factors from higher cerebral centers (cerebral cortex), including catecholamines, serotonin, ghrelin, and endorphins, have a positive effect on GH secretion. Inhibition of GH secretion also occurs when infants are socially deprived. The mechanism for this reversible inhibition is not known, but neglect and potential child abuse are major differentials in infants with retarded growth.

CASE STUDY 35.2

A 5-year-old boy presents to his pediatrician with a 2-week history of lethargy, anorexia, and weight loss. Upon further questioning, his parents admit that he seems more thirsty during the day, and he recently started wetting the bed at night (which was never an issue previously). A random venous plasma glucose drawn later that day is 250 mg/dL.

Questions

1. What is the most likely diagnosis?

2. What are the diagnostic criteria for this disease?

3. What is the pathophysiology of the two forms of this disease?

GH is a 191-amino acid polypeptide, with the liver as its primary site of action. GH receptors on the liver that are occupied by a GH molecule cause the liver to secrete a group of related polypeptide hormones, called *insulin-like growth factors (IGFs)*, and their binding proteins, called *IGF-binding proteins*. IGF-1 and IGF-BP3 are the most significant products of GH activity on the liver. IGF-1 has a molecular structure similar to insulin; however, it is a much more potent stimulator of linear growth and increased metabolism in infants.

This pathway probably represents the most important endocrine pathway responsible for normal childhood growth. Deficiencies of any component of the pathway are known to result in poor growth, resulting in short-statured adults.

There are difficulties in measuring GH in serum, which result from diurnal variation of secretion and stress-related effectors including catecholamines. A single, low level of GH is not sufficient to confirm GH deficiency. It is important to determine true organic deficiency, caused by hypothalamic or pituitary disease, from emotional deficiency because only organic deficiency responds to expensive GH replacement therapy, while nonorganic GH deficiency will respond to emotional lifestyle changes. Trauma to the head may also cause failure of GH secretion by the pituitary through direct anoxic damage to the very sensitive specialized GH-secreting cells. This type of growth failure will respond to GH therapy. Several stimulation tests have been devised to test the absolute capacity of the pituitary to secrete GH. These stimulation tests include inducement of hypoglycemia with insulin, arginine, or clonidine or direct stimulation with glucagon. These tests require that up to five blood samples be collected in the 2 hours poststimulation and the peak level of GH secretion determined. If this is less than 7 ng/mL, the patient has organic GH deficiency and is likely to respond to GH therapy.[18]

Downstream testing for serum IGF-1 and IGF-BP3 levels is available and shows great promise in the identification of GH deficiency because these compounds are not secreted by the liver in GH deficiency and their basal levels do not seem to have the large variation that occurs for GH. In addition, defects of both IGF and IGF-BP synthesis and secretion have been recognized as a cause of growth failure in certain infants. Individuals with these defects are unlikely to respond to GH replacement.

Endocrine Control of Sexual Maturation

The hypothalamus secretes a 10-amino acid peptide called *gonadotropin-releasing hormone (GnRH)* into the portal blood system. GnRH bind to a specific receptor and causes the release of two larger polypeptide hormones, called *follicle-stimulating hormone (FSH)* and *luteinizing hormone (LH)*, from the anterior pituitary in both males and females.

Baseline levels of the gonadotropins FSH and LH are very low in infants and young children as a result of GnRH suppression.

FSH and LH have different effects in males and females, both before and during puberty. In males, the target hormonal activity is directed to the testis and causes the release of androgens, primarily the steroid hormones testosterone and androstenedione that are released into the circulation. In females, the primary site of action is the ovary and results in the secretion of a different family of steroid hormones—estrogens, primarily estradiol into the circulation. Prior to puberty, the circulating levels of androgens and estrogens are very low. The measurement of pediatric gonadotropin levels and sex steroid hormones provide excellent examples of the need for unique pediatric reference ranges for these biomarkers as the pediatric clinical laboratory is often requested to measure these hormones when a child appears to be going into premature puberty. Testosterone is particularly difficult to measure in prepubertal children as many commercial immunoassays detect an interfering compound, which results in false elevation of the hormone level. Measurement by mass spectrometry appears to overcome these interferences.

During puberty, the GnRH suppression is removed and there is a gradual increase in FSH and LH secretion, with concomitant increase in androgen levels in males and estrogen and progesterone levels in females. These changes result in the development of secondary sexual characteristics and

onset of menarche in females. This period of childhood is also associated with a major surge in linear and bone growth until adult proportions are achieved.

Disorders of this endocrine pathway are associated with either premature or precocious puberty or delayed onset of puberty. The measurement of serum FSH, LH, testosterone, and estradiol levels is useful in evaluating disordered puberty. Often, disorders of other endocrine systems affect puberty. Congenital adrenal hyperplasia results in excess secretion of androgen-like steroids that can affect puberty. Disorders of the hypothalamus and pituitary can affect secretion of FSH and LH, which if reduced will result in delayed puberty.

DEVELOPMENT OF THE IMMUNE SYSTEM

In pediatric clinical facilities, the vast majority of hospital visits and admissions are related to complications arising from infectious diseases. At the same time, although the parents or caregivers may be exposed to the same infectious etiologies, they do not become so ill as to require medical attention. This is because the child does not have the same degree of **immunity** to disease at birth or during infancy.[1]

Basic Concepts of Immunity

The immune system is divided into two functional divisions: the innate immune system and the adaptive immune system. The innate immune system is the first line of defense, particularly in the newborn and infant not exposed to infection. The adaptive immune system generates a specific reaction following exposure to an infectious agent and provides greater immunity with subsequent exposure to that agent. Initially, however, the first response to exposure may be suboptimal and result in illness related to that exposure.

Components of the Immune System
Skin

The skin is normally an effective barrier to most microorganisms, although in premature babies this barrier is less well developed and can easily become a source of infection. Many newborns with congenital infections manifest profound skin lesions. Most infectious agents enter the body by the nasopharynx, gastrointestinal tract, lungs, or genitourinary tract. Normally, various physical and biochemical defenses protect the nonsurgical sites of entry. Lysozyme, an enzyme widely distributed in different secretions, for example, is capable of partially digesting a chemical bond in the membrane of many bacterial cell walls thus reducing the infectivity. In premature babies, this pathway of defense is less effective. Surgical incisions and intravenous or central lines are also potential sites of entry for infectious agents.

Phagocytes

Phagocytes are present in many cell types. When a foreign organism such as a bacterium penetrates an epithelial surface, it encounters phagocytic cells, which are derived from bone marrow and recruited into tissue in response to the organism. These cells engulf and digest particles. Phagocytic cells include polymorphonuclear cells, which are short-lived in the circulation, and monocytes that, when exposed to a foreign particle, develop into macrophages that subsequently recognize the organism when the individual is re-exposed and mount a concerted defense, which is typically more potent than that of the first exposure.

B Cells
B cells are lymphocytes that are characterized by the presence of surface immunoglobulins. These cells can differentiate into plasma cells that are able to respond to foreign antigens in the circulation by producing neutralizing antibodies. Activation, proliferation, and differentiation of B cells are assisted by cytokine secretion from T-cell lymphocytes, which do not produce antibodies. On binding antigen, antibodies can activate a cascade involving the complement pathway, which ultimately produces lysis and cellular death of foreign organisms.

Natural Killer Cells
Natural killer (NK) cells are leukocytes capable of recognizing cell surface changes on host cells infected by viral particles. The NK cells bind to these target cells and can kill them and the virus. The NK cells respond to interferons, which are cytokine molecules produced by the host cells when infected by virus. Interferons are also part of the innate immune system capable of providing resistance to infection in host cells not virally infected.

Acute-Phase Proteins
Acute-phase proteins are defense proteins produced by the liver in response to infection, particularly bacterial infection. Certain proteins can increase in the serum by 2-fold to 100-fold. The most significant acute-phase protein is called *C-reactive protein (CRP)* because of its ability to bind to the C protein of *pneumococci*. CRP bound to bacteria promotes the binding of complement that, in turn, aids phagocytosis. Serum CRP levels are routinely measured to determine degree of infection in pediatric patients. The required sensitivity of the CRP assay for this clinical purpose is less than that used for the high-sensitivity CRP assay used clinically as an independent risk factor for cardiac disease. In the pediatric application of this assay, rapid turnaround of results

is most important. The complement system consists of at least 20 proteins, most of which are acute-phase proteins. They interact sequentially with each other, with antigen–antibody complexes and with cell membranes in a coordinate manner to ultimately destroy bacteria and viruses. Clinically, the complement proteins that are measured most often are C3 and C4. Low levels of either of these proteins indicate poor ability to destroy foreign particles. A more detailed description of acute-phase proteins can be found in the chapter in this volume on amino acids and proteins.

Antibody Production
Immunoglobulins are classified into five major groups, based on structure and function: IgG, IgM, IgA, IgD, and IgE. Secreted by plasma cells derived from B lymphocytes, their properties are listed in Table 35.13. IgG is the major immunoglobulin subclass providing antibody response in adults and represents 70% to 75% of total immunoglobulin content. IgG is further broken down into four additional subclasses: IgG.[1–3,5] Each immunoglobulin is built from similar structural units, based on two heavy polypeptide chains (A, G, M, D, and E) and two light chains (k and λ). The ability to recognize large numbers of foreign antigens is a result of the infinite ability of the genes for the so-called variable region of the immunoglobulin molecule to rearrange. This area recognizes foreign antigens, and a gene rearrangement with production of a unique antibody covers each new foreign antigen exposed to the body. Because of the large number of different immunoglobulin species within each subgroup, electrophoretic separation of these serum proteins on an isoelectric focusing gel during serum protein electrophoresis (SPEP) analysis generates a region that is diffuse, unlike the albumin or transferrin bands, which are distinct bands.

Neonatal and Infant Antibody Production
The human fetus is able to synthesize a small amount of IgM and, to a lesser degree, IgA. IgG has a lower molecular weight than IgM and readily crosses the placenta. IgG is also transferred from mother to baby in breast milk. Transplacental and breast milk–derived IgG offer the baby a passive immunologic protection until endogenous IgG production becomes a significant protective factor. The half-life of IgG is about 30 days and, with prolonged breast-feeding, the infant can derive additional protection. The process of antibody

TABLE 35.13 Properties of Immunoglobulin (Ig) Classes

	IgG[a]	IgA	IgM	IgD	IgE
Mass (kD)	160	160	970	184	188
Percent of total Ig	70–75	10–15	5–10	<1	Trace
Crosses placenta	Yes	No	No	No	No
In breast milk	Yes	Yes	No	Unknown	Unknown
Activates complement	Yes	Yes	Yes	No	No
In secretions	No	Yes	No	No	No
Binds to mast cells	No	No	No	No	Yes

[a]Present as four subclasses (IgG1–4).

production in infants takes several years to complete when based on total serum levels of the immunoglobulin subclasses, which take up to 4 years to be attained and provide another example of how age-related reference ranges are particularly important in pediatric laboratory medicine. Premature babies have an even greater immunoglobulin deficit than term babies because of diminished transplacental delivery of antibodies.

Immunity Disorders

Given the complexity of the immune system, there are many stages at which acquired or genetically inherited defects can result in inappropriate infectious disease in the pediatric population.[19] Transient hypogammaglobulinemia of infancy may occur because of prematurity or, in certain infants, may be a result of delayed onset of immunoglobulin production of unknown etiology. These infants eventually develop a normal immune system but will be prone to repeated bouts of severe infection until this time. At the opposite end of the spectrum, complete absence of γ-globulins occurs in boys in an X-linked disorder known as *agammaglobulinemia*, or Bruton's disease. This disorder presents early in life with recurrent febrile infections. Patients do not have B cells and have low levels of all endogenous immunoglobulin subclasses. The disease process probably begins the moment that any maternally derived immunoglobulins have been lost. The most common infections are of the upper and lower respiratory tracts, causing otitis, pneumonia, sinusitis, meningitis, sepsis, and osteomyelitis. Without early γ-globulin therapy, these children die from respiratory complications. Other immune pathways are normal in these children.

Severe Combined Immune Deficiency

One of the most graphic examples of unique pediatric disease comes from infants who lack both humoral and cellular pathways for killing bacteria and viruses. These children are at risk of severe infection each time they are exposed to an infectious agent. The vivid image is of the "boy in the bubble," existing in a completely sterile environment to avoid contact with any bacteria or virus particles. Severe combined immune deficiency (SCID) may be inherited as an X-linked disorder only seen in boys, or it may be autosomal recessive and girls may also inherit the disease. There are several causes of SCID, including genetic diseases of purine metabolism and disorders of lymphocyte development and maturation, in which both T cells and B cells, if present, are nonfunctional. The most common purine disorder, adenosine deaminase deficiency, is responsible for 15% of SCID cases. It is diagnosed by measuring elevated levels of adenosine in body fluids. Establishing this diagnosis is important because enzyme replacement therapy using recombinant enzyme has been successfully used to treat the disorder.

GENETIC DISEASES

Analytic methods for the identification of **genetic disease** play an important part in the pediatric clinical chemistry laboratory.[1,20–22] The presentations of many genetic diseases are unique to the pediatric population and require

physicians and clinical laboratorians who provide services to have specialized knowledge and training. Most diseases that present with clinical signs in infants and children are inherited in an autosomal recessive mode, which means that the patient has two disease-causing mutations in the gene for that disorder, one inherited maternally and one inherited paternally. Parents are almost always without any symptoms. Several examples of diseases with this inheritance pattern have already been introduced in this chapter, including galactosemia, due to inability to metabolize the milk sugar galactose, which results in severe hepatic and renal failure in the newborn, associated with congenital cataracts and congenital adrenal hyperplasia as a result of steroid 21-hydroxylase deficiency. Treatments for these two conditions are readily available. Galactosemia responds very well to dietary restriction of milk and milk products, and hormone replacement is available for congenital adrenal hyperplasia. Certain other diseases are recessive but are inherited on the X chromosome. Typically, boys inherit a mutated X chromosome from their mothers; because they do not inherit a paternal X chromosome, they show signs of disease with only one mutation. Girls carrying an X chromosome mutation may also demonstrate disease signs due to the fact that one of their X chromosomes becomes inactivated and if the active X chromosome carries the mutation they will have the disease or a spectrum of the disease depending upon the relative amount of X-chromosome inactivation. Dominantly inherited diseases, which can be inherited as a single mutation through either parental line, frequently tend not to present as unique childhood diseases. Examples include familial hypercholesterolemia, Huntington's disease, and factor V Leiden thrombophilia, all of which are generally regarded as diseases of the adult population, although the mutation is inherited at birth. All of the disease examples described above are diseases of DNA that replicates in the cell nucleus. Mitochondria, the organelles responsible for generating cellular energy and other important metabolic pathways, also contain DNA (mtDNA), which encodes proteins involved in energy generation. mtDNA has a high rate of spontaneous mutation and results in a large number of energy-wasting diseases many of which present with high blood lactate levels. Mitochondria are only inherited from the mother, so that mtDNA mutations that are not spontaneous can only come from the maternal lineage.

Cystic Fibrosis

Cystic fibrosis (CF) is one of the most commonly inherited genetic diseases encountered by pediatric clinical chemistry laboratories. The rate of this debilitating disease in Western populations is one of 2,400 live births, which results from recessively inherited mutations in the cystic fibrosis transmembrane regulator (*CFTR*) gene. Patients may present in the newborn period with severe pancreatic insufficiency caused by accumulated thick mucous secretions in the pancreatic ducts, which inhibit the secretion of pancreatic digestive enzymes. These babies have steatorrhea and fail to thrive. Patients with CF do not always develop pancreatic symptoms; however, in most patients, the thick mucus that accumulates in the lungs causes respiratory disease and makes them particularly susceptible to rare infectious diseases, such as *Pseudomonas*. Although palliative therapies have improved over the past few generations because of the availability of better antibiotics, CF is still regarded as untreatable.

The gold standard diagnostic test for CF has been available for many years. It involves measurement of chloride content in sweat collected after pilocarpine iontophoresis. The dynamic range for sweat chloride concentration differs from that of blood, and therefore, sweat cannot be run on a major chemistry analyzer. Analysis has to be made with a specialist chloride meter. This type of testing is time consuming and requires specialist experience from the operator. The genetic basis for CF has been established. Although there are some mutations that are frequently encountered in the population, such as the ΔF508, there are hundreds of other mutations. The American College of Medical Genetics and the American College of Obstetrics and Gynecology recommended heterozygote screening in selected couples.[23] This recommendation poses an analytic challenge because of the large number of mutations and is dependent upon the availability of clinically and cost acceptable mutation detection technology such as next-generation sequencing (see Chapter 28).

Newborn Screening for Whole Populations

Certain inherited diseases are sufficiently common in the population to be considered candidates for whole population screening.[20,21] Phenylketonuria (PKU) was the first genetic metabolic disorder to be screened in every baby born in the developed world and increasingly in emerging counties. Other diseases that are readily treatable were added to the list in following years, including steroid 21-hydroxylase deficiency, sickle cell disease, and CH and, in some states and countries, galactosemia. These genetic diseases mostly respond well to simple therapy, which is often dietary. In most states in the United States, this process takes place in the state-screening laboratory, a facility that has the ability to easily follow up abnormal test results. The nature of the testing procedure requires a sensitive screening test that has few false-negative results and an acceptable level of false positives. There should then be confirmation using a test that is more specific to rule out false-positive results. Confirmatory testing may take place in a specialist laboratory.

Tandem mass spectrometric analysis allows many different biochemical genetic diseases to be screened on a single sample at the same time, and the technology was introduced about 15 years ago into many programs. This technique allows whole groups of similar compounds, in particular amino acids for the diagnosis of amino acid disorders and acylcarnitines for the diagnosis of fatty acid oxidation and some organic acid disorders, to be analyzed

on small sample volumes without complex sample preparation (Table 35.14). The analytic time is about 2 minutes per sample, which means that it is possible to readily perform analysis for an entire state. The birth rate in the United States is approximately 4.4 million births per year. Tandem mass spectrometry has been shown to be capable of handling this workload, and all states currently offer this program. This approach is increasingly being utilized for global screening of metabolic diseases.

The present status of newborn screening for metabolic diseases comprises a panel of 29 recommended conditions, referred to as the uniform panel, of which 20 can presently be diagnosed using tandem mass spectrometry. The most common of these additional disorders is medium-chain acyl-CoA dehydrogenase (MCAD) deficiency, which is a defect of the pathway in which we derive energy from fatty acids during periods of fasting or high energy demand such as fever. Prior to including this defect in newborn screening

TABLE 35.14	Metabolic Diseases Detectable by Newborn Screening Using Tandem Mass Spectrometry

Amino Acids
Phenylketonuria (PKU)
Maple syrup urine disease (MSUD)
Tyrosinemia, types 1 and 2
Homocystinuria
Hypermethioninemia

Urea Cycle
Argininemia
Citrullinemia
Argininosuccinic aciduria (ASA)

Organic Acids
Propionic acidemia (PA)
Methylmalonic acidemia (MMA)
Isovaleric acidemia (IVA)
Glutaric acidemia, types 1 and 2 (GA1, GA2)
β-Ketothiolase deficiency
3-Hydroxy-3-methylglutaryl-CoA lyase (HMG-CoA lyase) deficiency
3-Methylcrotonyl-CoA carboxylase (MCC) deficiency
Malonyl-CoA decarboxylase deficiency
2-Methyl-3-hydroxybutyryl-CoA dehydrogenase*

Fatty Acids
MCAD deficiency
Short-chain acyl-CoA dehydrogenase deficiency (SCAD)*possibly a benign biochemical condition
Very-long-chain acyl-CoA dehydrogenase (VLCAD) deficiency
Carnitine palmitoyltransferase, types 1A and 2 (CPT1A, CPT2)
Carnitine-acylcarnitine translocase (CAT) deficiency
Long-chain 3-hydroxyacyl-CoA dehydrogenase deficiency (LCHAD)
Mitochondrial trifunctional protein (MTP) deficiency

*Clinical significance not established.

programs, infants would develop fasting-induced hypoglycemia and liver failure often leading to death or neurological damage. Subsequent to screening by measurement of blood spot octanoylcarnitine (C8) and presymptomatic diagnosis with early management, the outcomes for children with MCAD deficiency have improved greatly. In addition to the core screening diseases, a number of secondary diseases can also be identified using tandem mass spectrometry some of which are very rare and have less data to confirm sensitivity and specificity. Many additional metabolic diseases can be diagnosed by tandem mass spectrometry; however, the current evidence to support a substantial benefit at the population level by uniform screening is less strong. Methods to diagnose additional diseases by tandem mass spectrometry are constantly being developed, and it is likely that routine population-based screening will be expanded in the near future. The next group of conditions that will be included in all screening programs will be lysosomal storage diseases, which were long considered to be untreatable and therefore unsuitable. However, treatment modalities are currently being investigated for many lysosomal storage diseases, and it is likely that the most success in treatment will come from early diagnosis in the newborn period. A number of states in the United States have already included some lysosomal disorders in their programs, and others are considering doing so.

TABLE 35.15 Examples of Large Molecule Storage Disorders

Mucopolysaccharide (MPS) or Glycosaminoglycan Storage Diseases
Hurler's disease (MPS, type I)
Hunter's disease (type II)
Morquio's disease (type IV)

Complex Lipid Storage
Gaucher's disease
Tay-Sachs disease
Niemann-Pick disease (types A, B, C)

Glycogen Storage Diseases
von Gierke (type 1)
Pompe (type 2)
McArdle (type 5)

Peptide Storage
Neuronal ceroid lipofuscinoses, types 1–10 (Batten's disease)

Posttranslational Protein Modification
Carbohydrate-deficient glycoprotein syndromes

CASE STUDY 35.3

An infant presented to the pediatrician with failure to thrive, steatorrhea (foul-smelling, fatty stool), and persistent respiratory infections. An older sibling with the same clinical presentation has a confirmed genetic disease.

Questions

1. What is the likely diagnosis?
2. How is the disease inherited?
3. What is the molecular mechanism of this disease?
4. What is the gold standard diagnostic test?

Diagnosis of Metabolic Disease in the Clinical Setting

At the present time, the clinical laboratory is needed to confirm the diagnosis of newborns screened positive for the disorders listed in Table 35.14[24] and also for the rest of the approximately 500 single gene defects that result in biochemical genetic disease not presently detectable by tandem mass spectrometry. These inborn errors of metabolism can be broken down generally into two main types.

Large Molecule Diseases

Large molecule diseases have an accumulating intermediate of metabolism composed of large complex molecules; examples are listed in Table 35.15. Many of these diseases involve intracellular accumulation of the abnormal chemical with relatively small excretion in body fluids. In glycogen storage diseases, the glycogen accumulates in the liver and muscle but cannot be seen in blood or urine samples. The histopathologist, using microscopic examination of tissue, often makes these diagnoses. A few, mostly urine, tests are available for gathering clues to large molecule diseases, including glycosaminoglycan (mucopolysaccharide [MPS]) analysis using high-voltage electrophoresis to identify unusual metabolites associated with the MPS storage diseases. These tests are relatively insensitive, and improvements made by using mass spectrometry are currently being investigated. Confirmation of the diagnosis requires measurement of deficient enzyme activity or identification of defined disease-causing mutations. Fortunately, many enzymes that result in large molecule storage diseases can be found in white blood cells, enabling confirmation to be made on a blood sample. Enzymic confirmation can be difficult to establish in small babies because large blood samples may be required for diagnostic testing.

Small Molecule Diseases

Small molecule diseases result from defects in metabolic pathways of intermediary metabolism. Usually, the abnormal compounds that are present in these diseases are low molecular weight compounds that are readily excreted in body fluids; the types of pathways involved are listed in Table 35.16. Initially, the clinical chemistry laboratory had few diagnostic tools capable of identifying the large number of metabolic intermediates that may accumulate in these diseases, and a number of simple, colorimetric urine tests, such as the dinitrophenylhydrazine (DNPH) test for ketoacids, were developed to establish diagnosis. These methods lack both sensitivity and specificity and have no role to play in the modern clinical chemistry laboratory. They have been

TABLE 35.16	**Pathways Involved with Small Molecule Metabolic Disease and Examples**

Amino acids—phenylketonuria
Fatty acids—medium-chain acyl-coA dehydrogenase deficiency
Organic acids—propionic acidemia
Urea cycle—citrullinemia
Oxidative phosphorylation—mitochondrial DNA diseases
Vitamin metabolism—pyridoxine responsive seizures
Steroid biosynthesis and breakdown—21-hydroxylase–deficient congenital adrenal hyperplasia
Cholesterol synthesis—Smith-Lemli-Opitz syndrome
Purine and pyrimidine metabolism—adenosine deaminase form of severe combined immunodeficiency
Neurotransmitter metabolism—4-hydroxybutyric aciduria
Plasmalogen synthesis—Zellweger's syndrome
Glutathione metabolism—pyroglutamic aciduria
Oxalate metabolism—hyperoxaluria types 1 and 2
Creatine metabolism—guanidinoacetic acidemia

multiple different metabolites, many of which were not easily measurable prior to the introduction of this technology.

CASE STUDY 35.4

A newborn infant was identified with a newborn screen that was positive for elevated galactose levels. Mother had been breast-feeding the baby who presented with acute and rapid onset of liver failure. Ophthalmological examination also identified that the baby had congenital cataracts.

Questions

1. What is the most likely diagnosis?
2. Why did the baby develop liver failure when being breast-fed?
3. What is the treatment for this condition?
4. What group of genetic diseases is currently being incorporated into whole population screens?

superseded by assays with greater sensitivity and specificity, often based on separation technology and mass spectrometry.

Small molecule diseases have a variable clinical presentation and could present to almost any medical subspecialty with any organ system involved. (Table 35.16 lists certain pathways that may be involved.) Biochemical testing for these diseases is usually described in two phases. First, it is important to recognize the degree of tissue compromisation at presentation. This requires routine chemistry evaluation for blood gas status, if acidotic; anion gap measurement; liver function testing; analysis of skeletal and cardiac muscle markers, such as creatine kinase or troponin levels; lactic acid; and ammonia measurement. All of these analyses should be available stat and used to monitor management once a diagnosis is established. The second phase of analysis should be to look for metabolic markers that pinpoint the site of a defect. These tests involve a form of separation technology, such as ion-exchange chromatography or ultra-performance liquid chromatography for amino acids. The preferred material for amino acid analysis is serum because the renal tubules have efficient transport systems for reabsorbing filtered amino acids. It is possible to miss an amino acid abnormality if only urine is analyzed. Urine amino acid analysis is of value if a tubular defect such as cystinuria is suspected. The most useful test for detecting abnormal metabolic intermediates is organic acid analysis. This test is performed on urine and should only be performed using the technique of gas chromatography–mass spectrometry. It is a method that is capable of identifying metabolic markers for up to 100 genetic diseases and is a form of metabolomics. As mentioned earlier, tandem mass spectrometry is another technique seeing rapid growth in the metabolic disease diagnosis field. This technique is being applied to newborn screening and is playing an increasing role in analysis of

DRUG METABOLISM AND PHARMACOKINETICS

There are several important differences in the way that infants and children handle pharmacologic agents compared with adults.[1] This area of pediatric laboratory medicine provides many good examples of why children should not be regarded as "small adults." It is not clinically appropriate to prorate the amount of drug prescribed to a child based on relative body weight compared with an adult dose.

Drug metabolism depends on the following factors: absorption, circulation, and volume of distribution, and metabolism and clearance. Often, the medium in which a drug is provided to a child differs from the adult version of the same drug. Syrups, for instance, provide a more rapid release of a drug and greater availability for gastrointestinal absorption than tablets, which have the drug trapped in a solid matrix that requires digestion. Children are more likely to be given medication in a palatable form, such as syrup, and to require lower doses. The pH of gastric secretions differs in infants. At birth, the gastric pH is nearly neutral, not reaching the adult level of acidity for several years. This pH difference can affect the absorption of certain drugs, including some frequently prescribed penicillins. The distribution of drugs often differs between adults and children. Lipid-soluble drugs are taken up into lipid reserves and only slowly released into the circulation. Because infants have relatively little adipose tissue, these drugs are not stored as efficiently. The overall effect is that lipid-soluble drugs reach a higher level more quickly than in individuals with sizable fat stores; however, the drug is also cleared more rapidly. It becomes appropriate for drugs to be provided in smaller, more frequent doses to optimize the effect. Hepatic metabolism of many drugs is immature in young infants. This may delay the metabolic conversion to an active drug

TABLE 35.17	Drugs with Well-Defined Therapeutic Indices	
Drug	**Therapeutic Range**	**Toxicity**
Phenytoin	10–20 mg/L	>20 does not enhance seizure control, may cause ataxia and involuntary eye movement, >35 causes seizure
Phenobarbital	15–40 mg/L	>35 causes CNS depression; >65 coma
Carbamazepine	4–12 mg/L	>15 causes drowsiness
Theophylline[a]	6–13 mg/L	>20 can cause cardiac arrhythmia
Caffeine[a]	8–20 mg/L	Less toxic than theophylline
Methotrexate	Depends on therapy	High levels cause myelosuppression
Gentamicin	5–10 mg/L (peak)[b]	>10 ototoxicity, nephrotoxicity

[a]Theophylline is metabolized to caffeine in neonates but not in adults. Used to treat apnea.
[b]Peak level should be drawn 30 minutes after last dose for aminoglycoside drugs. Children are particularly prone to hearing loss at toxic levels.
Source: Wu AHB, ed. *Tietz Clinical Guide to Laboratory Tests.* 4th ed. St. Loius, MO: WB Saunders; 2006.

or increase the time in which an active drug is circulating. Good hepatic function is important for clearing those drugs metabolized by the liver, as good renal function is important for clearing drugs that have water-soluble end products.

Therapeutic Drug Monitoring

The principles of therapeutic drug monitoring remain the same in adult and pediatric clinical chemistry. It is important to measure the blood levels of various drugs if that information can provide important guidance to the physician with regard to optimal dosing. This is most important if a drug has a well-defined therapeutic index. This means that the drug is known to be ineffective if the blood level is below a certain value, that there is a well-defined therapeutic range over which the drug is effective, and that there is a higher level at which the drug becomes toxic. It is important to monitor levels of drugs with these characteristics. Table 35.17 lists drugs for which the importance of therapeutic monitoring is established.

Toxicologic Issues in Pediatric Clinical Chemistry

Issues related to the provision of a toxicologic service can be divided into two distinct groups in pediatrics. The first group involves infants and young children who

unknowingly consume pharmacologic and other chemical agents. This usually involves the child finding access to medication belonging to another individual in the household and consuming the medication as if it were candy. It is relatively easy for the investigator to ascertain the nature of the medication by identifying what is available in the household. Toxicologic investigation can usually be restricted to a few specific tests.

A rare, but potentially dangerous condition, is that of Munchausen's syndrome by proxy. In this condition, mental illness in a caregiver causes them to give unnecessary and illness-causing drugs to an otherwise well child. This can go unrecognized and result in multiple hospitalizations and even death of the child. Clinical suspicion of this form of child abuse should involve performing a comprehensive drug screen to identify causative agents. Because of the intermittent nature of clinical presentation of Munchausen's syndrome by proxy, it can often be confused with metabolic disease. Metabolic studies, in addition to comprehensive toxicologic studies, may be necessary.

Because the likelihood of self-ingestion of street drugs of abuse is present in older children, pediatric clinical chemistry laboratories should make assays available for street drugs similar to those in adult practice.

For additional student resources, please visit the**Point** at http://thepoint.lww.com

questions

1. All of the following represent normal physiology of the newborn except
a. Weight of 2.4 kg
b. Immature liver function and inability to eliminate excess bilirubin
c. Closure of the ductus arteriosus and a shift of blood flow through the heart
d. 4 to 6 months for the infant's body weight to double

2. Which of the following choices is false concerning blood obtained by heel stick (capillary) and venipuncture (venous)?
a. The chemical composition of the sera derived from each is identical.
b. The capillary specimen is likely contaminated with interstitial fluid and tissue debris.
c. Venous blood contains higher bilirubin and calcium concentrations.
d. Capillary blood contains less concentrated proteins due to mixing with interstitial fluid.

review questions (continued)

3. Under normal conditions, what is the maximum amount of blood that should be drawn from a 30-kg child during a single blood draw?
   a. 60 mL
   b. 80 mL
   c. 40 mL
   d. 20 mL

4. When choosing a chemistry analyzer for a pediatric laboratory, it is necessary to
   a. Incorporate total laboratory automation
   b. Be able to analyze from small volumes
   c. Have a rapid turnaround time
   d. Ensure a minimum specimen dead volume

5. Which of the following is true regarding POCT?
   a. Results are generally available more rapidly than with traditional laboratory tests.
   b. POCT is usually less expensive than traditional laboratory measurements.
   c. The device cannot be linked to the hospital information system.
   d. Quality control samples are not needed.

6. Which of the following conditions are related to acidosis in the newborn?
   a. Anoxia and trauma during delivery
   b. Respiratory distress syndrome
   c. Hyperammonemia caused by liver disease
   d. Hyperventilation

7. Which of the following are characteristics of renal development and function during the neonatal period?
   a. Control the rate of salt and water loss and retention
   b. GFR about 50% of the rate seen in older children
   c. Completely developed by 24 weeks of gestation
   d. Have a maximum solute concentrating power of approximately 30% of an adult kidney

8. Which of the following statements about the neonatal thyroid system is true?
   a. Secondary hypothyroidism is usually diagnosed by measuring a low TSH level.
   b. Thyroid hormones (T_4 and T_3) are less than 50% bound to thyroid-binding globulins.
   c. CH is a very rare and untreatable disorder.
   d. A low measured TSH level may be due to a global pituitary gland dysfunction (panhypopituitarism).

9. Cystic fibrosis
   a. Is diagnosed by the measurement of elevated chloride concentration in sweat following iontophoresis
   b. Is a very uncommon genetic disease
   c. Is caused by only a single type of mutation in the CF transmembrane regulator (CFTR) gene
   d. Is characterized by thin, watery mucous secretions in the lungs and pancreatic ducts

references

1. Green A, Morgan I, Gray J. *Neonatology and Laboratory Medicine*. London: ACB Venture Publications; 2003.
2. Soldin SJ, Rifai N, Hicks JMB, eds. *Biochemical Basis of Pediatric Disease*. Washington, DC: American Association for Clinical Chemistry; 1992.
3. Rautenberg MW, van Solinge WW, Heunks JJ, et al. Pediatric tube direct sampling by the Abbott Architect Integrated ci8200 Chemistry/Immunochemistry Analyzer. *Clin Chem.* 2006;52:768–770.
4. Demir AY, van Solinge WW, Kemperman H. Handling of and direct sampling from primary barcode-labeled pediatric tubes on Vitros Clinical Chemistry Analyzers integrated into an enGen Work Cell. *Clin Chem.* 2005;51:920–921.
5. Gill FN, Bennett MJ. The pediatrics unit. In: Price CP, Hicks JM, eds. *Point of Care Testing*. Washington, DC: American Association for Clinical Chemistry; 1999.
6. Andersen FH. Use of fetal fibronectin in women at risk for preterm delivery. *Clin Obstet Gynecol.* 2000;43:746–758.
7. Goldenberg RL, Mercer BM, Iams JD. The preterm prediction study: patterns of cervicovaginal fetal fibronectin as predictors of spontaneous preterm delivery. *Am J Obstet Gynecol.* 1997;177:8–12.
8. Polak M, Van Vliet G. Disorders of the thyroid gland. In: Sargoglou K, Hoffman G, Roth K, eds. *Pediatric Endocrinology and Inborn Errors of Metabolism*. New York, NY: McGraw-Hill; 2009:353–382.
9. Hannon TS, Rao G, Arslanian SA. Childhood obesity and type 2 diabetes mellitus. *Pediatrics.* 2005;116(2):299–306.
10. American Diabetes Association. Summary of the Revisions for the 2010 Clinical Practice Recommendations. *Diabetes Care.* 2010;33(suppl 1):S3.
11. Zimmet P, Alberti K, George MM, et al.; IDF Consensus Group. The metabolic syndrome in children and adolescents—an IDF consensus report. *Pediatr Diabetes.* 2007;8:299–306.
12. Levey AS, Coresh J, Greene T, et al. Chronic Kidney Disease Epidemiology Collaboration. Using standardized serum creatinine values in the modification of diet in renal disease study equation for estimating glomerular filtration rate. *Ann Intern Med.* 2006;145(4):247–254.
13. Schwartz GJ, Work DF. Measurement and estimation of GFR in children and adolescents. *J Am Soc Nephrol.* 2009;4(11):1832–1643.

14. Newman DJ. Cystatin C. *Ann Clin Biochem.* 2002;39: 89–104.

15. Schwartz GJ, Munoz A, Schneider MF, et al. New Equations to Estimate GFR in Children with CKD. *J Am Soc Nephrol.* 2009;20:629–637.

16. Wagner C, Greer FR. Prevention of rickets and vitamin D deficiency in infants, children, and adolescents . *Pediatrics.* 2008;122:1142.

17. Austin A, Finkielstain GP. Adrenal disorders. In: Dietzen DJ, Bennett MJ, Wong ECC, eds. *Biochemical and Molecular Basis of Pediatric Disease.* 4th ed. Washington, DC: AACC Press; 2010:135–153.

18. Winter WE, Rosenbloom AL. Disorders of growth. In: Dietzen DJ, Bennett MJ, Wong ECC, eds. *Biochemical and Molecular Basis of Pediatric Disease.* 4th ed. Washington, DC: AACC Press; 2010:171–194.

19. Loechelt BJ. Primary immunodeficiency diseases. In: Dietzen DJ, Bennett MJ, Wong ECC, eds. *Biochemical and Molecular Basis of Pediatric Disease.* 4th ed. Washington, DC: AACC Press; 2010:409–427.

20. Valle D, Beaudet AL, Vogelstein B, et al., eds. In: *Online Metabolic and Molecular Bases of Inherited Disease (OMMBID).* http://ommbid.com. Accessed July 30, 2012.

21. Sargoglou K, Hoffman G, Roth K, eds. *Pediatric Endocrinology and Inborn Errors of Metabolism.* New York, NY: McGraw-Hill; 2009.

22. Hommes FA, ed. *Techniques in Diagnostic Human Biochemical Genetics.* New York, NY: Wiley-Liss; 1991.

23. American College of Obstetricians & Gynecologists, American College of Medical Genetics. *Preconception and Prenatal Carrier Screening for Cystic Fibrosis: Clinical and Laboratory Guidelines.* Washington, DC: American College of Obstetricians & Gynecologists; 2001.

24. Dietzen, DJ, Rinaldo P, Whitley RJ, et al. National Academy of Clinical Biochemistry Laboratory Medicine Practice Guidelines: Follow-up testing for metabolic diseases identified by expanded newborn screening using tandem mass spectrometry; Executive summary. *Clin Chem.* 2009;55:1615–1626. http://www.aacc.org/members/nacb/LMPG/OnlineGuide/DraftGuidelines/EN_Metabolic_Disease/Pages/default.aspx

Index

CCS0419